Compliments of

THE MANUAL OF INTERVENTIONAL CARDIOLOGY

THIRD EDITION

Robert D. Safian, M.D.
Mark S. Freed, M.D.

Division of Cardiology

William Beaumont Hospital

Royal Oak, Michigan

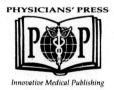

PHYSICIANS' PRESS

Innovative Medical Publishing

www.physicianspress.com

ABOUT PHYSICIANS' PRESS

Physicians' Press was established in 1990 to provide innovative and user-friendly references to the Interventional Cardiology, General Cardiology, and Internal Medicine communities. Physicians' Press stands apart from all other medical publishers in being able to produce completely current publications, with literature references *less than 2 weeks old* at the time of book release, compared to 9-18 months old for most other textbooks. We frequently receive comments such as, "I am astounded at how current your information is. The only books I read are yours; the rest are outdated." Physicians' Press is committed to providing its readers with the most current, practical, and user-friendly information available, as we continue to distinguish ourselves as the gold-standard in medical publishing.

Mark S. Freed, M.D.
President and Editor-in-Chief

Be sure to visit our bookstore at www.physicianspress.com for a complete listing of our medical titles. If you would like to place an order, or have comments, questions, or suggestions, please contact us at:

Physicians' Press
620 Cherry Street
Royal Oak, Michigan 48073
Tel: (248) 616-3023
Fax: (248) 616-3003
www.physicianspress.com

Printed in the United States of America   ISBN 1-890114-29-4

DEDICATION

To my beautiful wife, Maureen, who has given me the most
precious gift in the world: A loving family with four wonderful children,
Ryan, Luke, Noah, and Sierra

— Rob Safian

To Mom, Dad, Ralph, Susie, Bradley, Paulie, Boomer, Wrigley, and Dallas,
The Joys of My Life

— Mark Freed

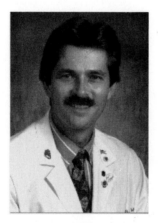

Robert D. Safian, M.D.

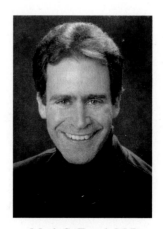

Mark S. Freed, M.D.

NOTICE

The explosive growth of new equipment, techniques, and drug therapy has led to the rapid evolution and acceptance of practice patterns that are often based on observational studies and personal experience. Their ultimate role will require close inspection of prospective randomized trials. The clinical recommendations set forth in this book are those of the authors; they are offered as *general guidelines and are not to be construed as specific instructions for individual patients.* In addition, not all medications have been accepted by the U.S. Food and Drug Administration (USFDA) for usages described in this manual. The use of any drug should be preceded by a careful review of the package insert, which provides indications and dosages approved by the USFDA. The reader is advised to consult the package insert before using any therapeutic agent or interventional device. The authors and publisher disclaim all responsibility for any liability, loss, injury, or damage incurred as a direct or indirect consequence of the use and application of any material contained herein, including omissions or undetected errors.

TABLE OF CONTENTS

EXPANDED TABLE OF CONTENTS

PREFACE

Since its debut in 1990, *The Manual of Interventional Cardiology* has been the most practical and popular reference in the field. Now, the Cardiology Division of William Beaumont Hospital and leading interventionalists from around the world proudly present the much awaited Third Edition. In addition to complete and extensive revision of 38 previous chapters on patient triage, device selection and technique, adjunctive imaging and pharmacotherapy, hemodynamic support, intraprocedural complications, and clinical follow-up, the Third Edition features:

- **Special Emphasis on Stents, Acute Coronary Syndromes, Adjunctive Pharmacotherapy, and Peripheral Vascular Intervention**

- **New Chapters** on Cardiovascular Risk Reduction, Atherogenesis and Thrombosis, Radiation Principles and Safety, and Percutaneous Intervention for Adult Congenital Heart Disease

- **Up-to-the-Minute Data,** including literature references less than 2 weeks old at the time of book release

- **User-friendly Information** presented in easy-to-read outline format, including more than 750 tables, figures, and management algorithms

- **The Mini-Manual,** a portable pocket companion with concise summaries and key management algorithms from the Unabridged Edition — a perfect review for the busy clinician!

We hope you enjoy reading *The Manual of Interventional Cardiology*, and find it a practical resource for patient care.

Robert D. Safian, M.D.
Mark S. Freed, M.D.

ACKNOWLEDGMENTS

To accomplish the tremendous task of presenting the data contained in the *Manual*, a small, dedicated team of professionals was assembled. This team focused their energy and discipline for many months into typing, designing, illustrating, and formatting the many chapters that make up this text. We wish to publicly recognize the abilities of this talented team. We sincerely thank them, and would like to acknowledge:

Monica Crowder-Kaufman: As project manager, Monica Crowder-Kaufman supervised, coordinated, and participated in every aspect of production, from library research to design and formatting. Her commitment, enthusiasm, work ethic, and expertise over the last 18 months has been unsurpassed.

Rebecca Smith: As assistant project manager, Ms. Smith spent many hours formatting the revisions that went into creating the *Manual*. Her skillful work, commitment, and indefatigable work ethic were essential to successful completion of this project.

We would also like to thank the many authors who graciously contributed their time and energy amidst busy professional lives, Alan Winick for proofreading, Steven Kronenberg for figure design, Norman Lyle for cover design, Cindy Gillespie, Dianna Frye, and Darcy Brunette for typing and literature searches, the staff at Dickinson Press for their printing expertise, and the many companies who provided information on their products, including Guidant, Boston Scientific Scimed, Medtronic AVE, Cordis/Johnson & Johnson, JOMED, InterVentional Technologies, and others.

We are indebted to these individuals, and hope their efforts are well received.

Robert D. Safian, M.D.
Mark S. Freed, M.D.

CONTRIBUTORS

STEVEN L. ALMANY, M.D.
Division of Cardiology
William Beaumont Hospital
Royal Oak, MI

CHRISTIE M. BALLANTYNE, M.D.
Clinical Director, Section of Atherosclerosis
Professor of Medicine
Baylor College of Medicine
Houston, TX

THOMAS M. BASHORE, M.D.
Division of Cardiology
Professor of Medicine
Duke University Medical Center
Durham, NC

PHILLIP J. BENDICK, PH.D.
Director, Peripheral Vascular Diagnostic Center
William Beaumont Hospital
Royal Oak, MI

ALAN BENNETT, R.C.I.S.
Carnegie Institute
Troy, MI

TERRY T. BOWERS, M.D.
Division of Cardiology
William Beaumont Hospital
Royal Oak, MI

JANICE CAMPBELL, M.S.
Division Radiation Safety Officer
William Beaumont Hospital
Troy, MI

GEORGE DANGAS, M.D., PH.D.
Director of Clinical Cardiology and
Interventional Pharmacology
Cardiovascular Research Foundation
Lenox Hill Hospital
New York, NY

ANTHONY C. DE FRANCO, M.D.
Director, Heart and Vascular Institute
McLaren Regional Medical Center
Flint, MI

DANIEL J. DIVER, M.D.
Chief, Section of Cardiology
Director, Cardiac Catheterization Laboratory
St. Francis Hospital
Hartford, CT

SIMON DIXON, M.D.
Division of Cardiology
William Beaumont Hospital
Royal Oak, MI

MARK DOORIS, M.B.B.S.
Division of Cardiology
Royal Brisbane Hospital
Queensland, Australia

LISA W. FORBESS, M.D.
Division of Cardiology
Mount Auburn Hospital
Cambridge, MA

MARK S. FREED, M.D.
Division of Cardiology
William Beaumont Hospital
Royal Oak, MI

HAROLD Z. FRIEDMAN, M.D.
Division of Cardiology
William Beaumont Hospital
Royal Oak, MI

JAMES J. FERGUSON, III, M.D.
Associate Director, Cardiology Research
Texas Heart Institute/St. Luke Episcopal Hospital
Houston, TX

CONTRIBUTORS

VALENTIN FUSTER, M.D., PH.D.
Director, The Zena and Michael A. Wiener
Cardiovascular Institute
Professor of Cardiology
Mount Sinai School of Medicine
New York, NY

BARRY S. GEORGE, M.D.
Midwest Cardiology Research Foundation
Grant/Riverside Methodist Hospitals
Columbus, OH

SHELDON GOLDBERG, M.D.
Director of Interventional Cardiology
Cooper Hospital University Medical Center
Camden, NJ

JAMES A. GOLDSTEIN, M.D.
Director of Cardiovascular Research and
Education
William Beaumont Hospital
Royal Oak, MI

ADAM B. GREENBAUM, M.D.
Co-Director, Cardiac Catheterization Lab
Henry Ford Hospital
Detroit, MI

JAMES HERMILLER, M.D.
Director, Cardiac Catheterization Lab
The Care Group
St. Vincent Hospital
Indianapolis, IN

NORMAN M. KAPLAN, M.D.
Professor of Medicine
University of Texas Southwestern Medical Center
Dallas, Texas

KEVIN L. KELCO, M.A., R.C.I.S.
Division of Cardiology
William Beaumont Hospital
Royal Oak, MI

ALEXANDRA J. LANSKY, M.D.
Director, Angiographic Core Laboratory
Cardiovascular Research Foundation
Lenox Hill Hospital
New York, NY

DANIEL LEE, M.D.
Division of Cardiology
William Beaumont Hospital
Royal Oak, MI

VINCENT MCCORMICK, M.S.
Medical Physiologist for Cardiology
William Beaumont Hosptial
Royal Oak, MI

RAYMOND G. MCKAY, M.D.
Division of Cardiology
Hartford Hospital
Hartford, CT

STEVEN E. NISSEN, M.D.
Vice Chairman, Department of Cardiology
Cleveland Clinic Foundation
Cleveland, OH

JAMES H. O'KEEFE, JR., M.D.
Director, Preventive Cardiology
Mid-America Heart Institute
Kansas City, MO

WILLIAM W. O'NEILL, M.D.
Director, Division of Cardiology
William Beaumont Hospital
Royal Oak, MI

MICHAEL A. PETERSON, M.D.
Division of Cardiology
Washington Hospital Center
Washington, D.C.

STEPHEN R. RAMEE, M.D.
Director, Cardiac Catheterization Laboratory
Ochsner Hospital
New Orleans, LA

CONTRIBUTORS

MARK REISMAN, M.D.
Director, Cardiac Catheterization Laboratory
Swedish Medical Center
Seattle, WA

KENNETH ROSENFIELD, M.D.
Assistant Professor of Medicine
Tufts University School of Medicine
Director, Interventional Laboratory
St. Elizabeth Medical Center
Boston, MA

ROBERT D. SAFIAN, M.D.
Director of Interventional Cardiology
William Beaumont Hospital
Royal Oak, MI

MARC P. SAKWA, M.D.
Division of Cardiovascular Surgery
William Beaumont Hospital
Royal Oak, MI

CHERYL CULVER SCHULTZ, M.S.
Corporate Radiation Safety Office
William Beaumont Hospital
Royal Oak, MI

FRANCIS L. SHANNON, M.D.
Division of Cardiovascular Surgery
William Beaumont Hospital
Royal Oak, MI

GREGG W. STONE, M.D.
Director of Cardiovascular Research and
Education
Cardiovascular Research Foundation
Lenox Hill Heart and Vascular Institute
New York, NY

JAMES E. TCHENG, M.D.
Associate Professor of Medicine
Duke University Medical Center
Durham, NC

ON TOPAZ, M.D.
Director, Interventional Cardiovascular
Laboratory
McGuire VA Medical Center
Richmond, VA

E. MURAT TUZCU, M.D.
Director, Intravascular Ultrasound Core
Laboratory
Cleveland Clinic Foundation
Cleveland, OH

CHRISTOPHER J. WHITE, M.D.
Chairman, Department of Cardiology
Ochsner Clinic
New Orleans, LA

STEVEN J. YAKUBOV, M.D.
Midwest Cardiology Research Foundation
Grant/Riverside Methodist Hospitals
Columbus, OH

KHALED M. ZIADA, M.D.
Department of Cardiology
Cleveland Clinic Foundation
Cleveland, OH

JAMES ZIDAR, M.D.
Associate Professor of Medicine
Duke University Medical Center
Durham, NC

I

Simple and Complex Intervention

1

CORONARY INTERVENTION:
PREPARATION, EQUIPMENT & TECHNIQUE

Robert D. Safian, M.D.
Mark S. Freed, M.D.

PREPROCEDURAL PREPARATION

Percutaneous transluminal coronary angioplasty (PTCA) has enjoyed explosive growth and popularity since first introduced by Andreas Gruentzig in 1977. Although initially restricted to patients with single, discrete, concentric, noncalcified stenoses, percutaneous revascularization is now routinely applied to patients with acute coronary syndromes, multivessel disease, and left ventricular (LV) dysfunction. Improvements in PTCA hardware, adjunctive pharmacotherapy, and other mechanical techniques have turned yesterday's "complex" procedure is today's "simple" case. Meticulous attention to patient selection, procedural technique, and early recognition of complications are mandatory.

A. **EVALUATION OF THE PATIENT PRIOR TO PERCUTANEOUS INTERVENTION.** The medical history, physical examination, and laboratory data are essential considerations prior to intervention (Table 1.1).

1. **History.** Cardiac history should be ascertained, including previous myocardial infarction, coronary artery bypass grafting (CABG), heart failure, arrhythmias, valvular heart disease, and complications during previous cardiac catheterization or percutaneous intervention. Additional history should identify active infection, peripheral or cerebrovascular disease, renal insufficiency, chronic obstructive pulmonary disease (COPD), hypertension, diabetes, pregnancy, hepatic dysfunction, bleeding tendencies, and relative or absolute contraindications to thrombolytic therapy or platelet glycoprotein IIb/IIIa receptor antagonists (such as gastrointestinal or urinary tract bleeding, recent major surgery, or stroke). It is important to obtain a history of allergic reactions to radiographic contrast, iodine, latex, aspirin, or other routine medications. A history of eczema, asthma, or hay fever should be documented, as these conditions are associated with increased risk of contrast reactions. Finally, a variety of noncardiac medications have important interactions with cardiac medications and radiographic contrast; adequate patient preparation is essential (Table 1.2).

2. **Physical Examination.** The physical examination is directed toward estimating the patient's volume status (peripheral edema, jugular venous distension, pulmonary rales), the presence and severity of valvular heart disease and LV dysfunction, and the degree of compensation. Focal neurologic deficits, vascular bruits, peripheral pulses, and evidence of COPD should also be recorded.

3.   **Laboratory Studies.** A complete blood count, platelet count, electrolyte panel, BUN, creatinine, and PT/PTT are standard laboratory evaluations prior to PTCA. A 12-lead electrocardiogram (ECG) should be obtained before and after intervention. A chest x-ray is recommended if there is an abnormality on examination of the lungs. Thyroid function tests and drug levels (e.g., digoxin, theophylline, antiarrhythmics) are ordered as appropriate. A blood type and screen for antibodies should be obtained in case urgent transfusion or CABG is needed. For patients with peripheral vascular disease, noninvasive studies will help determine the site and severity of obstructive disease to plan the safe use of large-bore introducing sheaths, an intra-aortic balloon pump (IABP), or percutaneous cardiopulmonary bypass (CPS) as required. Review of previous angiograms, cardiac catheterization records, and operative reports is essential to help determine procedural risk, vascular approach (femoral, brachial, or radial), dilatation strategy, equipment selection, and the likelihood of adverse reactions to contrast agents and other medications.

Table 1.1. Medical Conditions Requiring Postponement of Elective Intervention

Allergy
- Contrast
- Aspirin

Cardiovascular
- Heart failure, decompensated
- Severe hypertension
- Uncontrolled arrhythmias
- AV block (Type II 2° or 3°)

Pulmonary disease, decompensated

Diabetes
- Poorly-controlled
- Glucophage treatment (Table 1.2)

Electrolyte abnormalities
- $K^+ < 3.3$ or > 6.0 mEq/L
- $Na^+ < 125$ or > 155 mEq/L

Gastrointestinal
- Acute hepatitis
- Active GI bleeding

Hematologic
- Platelet count $< 50,000/mm^3$
- Leukocytosis, unexplained
- Hemoglobin < 10 gm/dL, acute
- Prothrombin time > 16 seconds

Neurologic
- Neurologic deficit, unexplained or progressive
- Cerebral hemorrhage, recent

Renal insufficiency, unexplained or progressive

Systemic
- Bacterial infection
- Unexplained fever

Table 1.2. Important Noncardiac Medications in Patients Undergoing Angiography

Drug	Drug Class	Cath Lab Significance	Recommendations
Metformin (Glucophage)	Oral hypoglycemic agent	Associated with a small risk of lactic acidosis, which carries a mortality rate of 50%. Risk is increased with contrast-induced renal dysfunction, especially in patients with pre-existing hypovolemia or renal insufficiency. Presents as abdominal pain, obtundation, hypotension, tachypnea; diagnosed by high serum lactic acid levels; treated with hemodialysis	• Normal renal function (serum creatinine < 1.5 mg/dL): Discontinue metformin 48 hrs before contrast exposure if possible (do not cancel procedure); ensure adequate hydration before and after procedure; resume metformin when renal function is shown to be normal • Abnormal renal function (baseline serum creatinine ³ 1.5 mg/dL): Postpone study until metformin has been discontinued for 48 hrs; correct hypovolemia; use low-osmolar contrast; closely monitor urine output and renal function. In emergency situations, weigh risk of lactic acidosis against benefit of procedure • If metformin is taken within 48 hrs of contrast exposure, avoid periprocedural cimetidine, nifedipine, furosemide, and alcohol, which increase metformin concentration or potentiate the effects of metformin on lactic acidosis
Warfarin (Coumadin)	Oral anticoagulant	Increases the risk of bleeding and vascular complications	• Elective cath: Defer cath until INR < 1.5 (PT < 16 seconds). Stop warfarin for 2-4 days prior to procedure; if necessary, heparinize the patient while warfarin is held • Urgent cath: Use fresh frozen plasma to reverse INR; avoid parenteral vitamin K (may induce hypercoagulable state); use vascular closure device if available
Sildenafil (Viagra)	Phosphodiesterase inhibitor used for impotence	Potentiates the hypotensive effects of nitrates; unknown significance of antiplatelet effects	• Elective cath: Stop sildenafil for at least 24 hrs. • Urgent cath: Do not postpone procedure; stop sildenafil; use nitroglycerin only if necessary; treat hypotension (fluids, pressors, IABP)
Meperidine (Demerol)	Narcotic analgesic	Associated with unpredictable reactions with MAO inhibitors, including a narcotic overdose-like syndrome (respiratory depression, hypotension, coma), or a hyperexcitatory syndrome (paradoxical agitation, seizures, hypertension, hyperpyrexia). Can also induce seizures in patients with renal failure	• Stop MAO inhibitors at least 2 weeks prior to procedure, if possible; otherwise, use a different narcotic and/or a benzodiazepine for conscious sedation • Treat severe reactions with hydrocortisone (100-250 mg IV); consider chlorpromazine (2 mg q 2-5 min; max. 25 mg) for hypertension or hyperpyrexia

B. THERAPEUTIC MEASURES

    1. Routine Pre-PTCA Medications (Table 1.3)

    2. Aspirin Allergy. Aspirin reduces the incidence of acute occlusion following PTCA by 50-75% and is considered essential therapy prior to non-emergent interventions. At our institution, aspirin (325 mg PO) is administered at least 1 day prior to elective PTCA. Select patients with aspirin allergy may be considered for aspirin desensitization, although most physicians use other antiplatelet agents such as clopidogrel (75 mg QD). The likelihood of effective desensitization depends on the nature of the previous allergic reaction (bronchospasm, rhinosinusitis, urticaria, angioedema, anaphylaxis).

      a. Aspirin-Induced Asthma and Rhinosinusitis

        1. Features. Over 10% of adults with asthma and 30% of those with asthma and rhinosinusitis develop aspirin sensitivity. Reactions range from exacerbations of nasal congestion, chest tightness, and sneezing to life-threatening bronchospasm and anaphylaxis. Aspirin sensitivity can develop at any time in susceptible individuals; the absence of a prior adverse reaction does not predict continued tolerance. Most aspirin-allergic patients have nasal polyps (80%), eosinophils (90%) and mast cells (50%) on nasal smear, and abnormal sinus radiographs (90%) ranging from mild mucoperiosteal thickening to complete opacification.

Table 1.3. Preprocedural Medication Orders

Routine orders	• NPO after midnight except medications (may have clear liquid breakfast if PTCA is late in the day) • Aspirin 325 mg PO started at least 1 day prior to the procedure • Clopidogrel 300-475 mg PO (load) and 75 mg QD for planned stent • Void on call to the cath lab • Sedative/narcotic on call to the cath lab
Diabetics	• Give ½ usual A.M. insulin dose on the day of the procedure. IV fluids should contain dextrose. If possible, PTCA should be performed early in the day • See Table 1.2 for metformin recommendations
Renal insufficiency	• The patient must be well-hydrated prior to the procedure. IV crystalloids are usually administered for 6-12 hours (100-150 ml/hr) in hospitalized patients • Supplemental diuretics may be necessary when ventricular dysfunction is present • See Chapter 25
Dye allergy	• Premedication regimens vary and none are completely protective • One approach is to give prednisone 60 mg, diphenhydramine 50 mg, and cimetidine 300 mg the afternoon and evening before the procedure, and the morning of the procedure • See Chapter 25
Aspirin allergy	• Elective PTCA is deferred • For a history of aspirin-induced anaphylaxis, we empirically administer clopidogrel (300-475 mg PO load prior to PTCA; 75 mg QD thereafter)

Table 1.4. Aspirin Desensitization Protocol at Scripps Clinic

1. Inclusion criteria: Asthma in remission, baseline $FEV_{1.0}$ >1.5 L and >70% of predicted value

2. Preprocedural medication: Patient may continue steroids and methylxanthines but must stop antihistamines, cromolyn, and inhaled bronchodilators

3. Oral aspirin challenge:*+ Progressively larger doses are administered until a positive reaction occurs (fall in $FEV_{1.0}$ >20% from baseline or marked nasal congestion and rhinorrhea) or 650 mg is tolerated. If a positive reaction develops, the same dose is readministered once the $FEV_{1.0}$ has returned to baseline and symptoms have completely resolved

	Day 1	Day 2	Day 3
8 AM	Placebo	30 mg*	150 mg
11 AM	Placebo	45-69 mg	325 mg
2 PM	Placebo	60-100 mg	650 mg

4. Monitoring: $FEV_{1.0}$ and symptoms hourly

5. Treatment of a positive reaction: For bronchospasm, administer aerosolized bronchodilator (albuterol 2.5 mg in 3cc normal saline) every 10 minutes until asthma is controlled. Treat nasal congestion with Afrin (2 sprays intranasally) and Vasacon A (2 drops each eye), repeated every 30 minutes as necessary

* Regimens vary (e.g., may give aspirin every 2 hours to complete sequence in one day, although 2-day sequence provides a greater safety margin)
+ For patients suspected of being highly sensitive, the initial dose should be 3 mg
Courtesy of Donald Stevenson, MD, Scripps Clinic, La Jolla, CA.

2. **Desensitization.** Scripps Clinic and Research Foundation developed an aspirin desensitization protocol that has proven to be very safe and effective. Desensitization involves the oral administration of progressively larger doses of aspirin at specified time intervals (Table 1.4), and results in a refractory period during which aspirin can be safely administered. This desensitization period can be maintained indefinitely as long as aspirin therapy is not interrupted (325 mg every 48 hours or 80 mg QD). If aspirin has not been given for two or more days, repeat desensitization may be necessary. Patients who require desensitization should be referred to a center experienced in this technique.

b. **Aspirin-Induced Cutaneous Reactions.** Despite the success of desensitizing aspirin-sensitive patients with asthma and rhinosinusitis, desensitization of individuals with aspirin-induced urticaria is not recommended. Fortunately, a previous cutaneous reaction to aspirin does not place the individual at increased risk of anaphylaxis upon readministration of drug. If PTCA is required, aspirin is dosed in routine fashion; H1 and H2 antagonists can usually control cutaneous symptoms during the periprocedural period.

c. **Anaphylaxis.** Desensitization has not been attempted in individuals who have had an anaphylactic reaction to aspirin; readministration of aspirin is not recommended. If PTCA is required, we empirically administer other agents (see below).

    d.   **Alternative Antiplatelet Agents (Chapter 34).** There are isolated case reports of the use of other antiplatelet agents in aspirin-allergic patients, such as low-molecular-weight dextran, sulfinpyrazone, and dipyridamole. There are insufficient data with these drugs to recommend their use in such patients. Other more potent platelet inhibitors, such as ticlopidine and clopidogrel, have demonstrated value in unstable angina and cerebral ischemia, and may have value in patients with aspirin-allergy; pretreatment for 2-4 days prior to intervention is recommended to achieve optimal platelet inhibition. Platelet glycoprotein IIb/IIIa receptor antagonists have been shown to reduce ischemic complications following high-risk and elective coronary interventions (Chapter 34); their role in aspirin-allergic patients has not been defined but is theoretically appealing. Oral IIb/IIIa receptor antagonists are currently investigational.

C.   **INFORMED CONSENT.** It is the obligation of the interventionalist to discuss the risks and benefits of intervention, bypass surgery, and medical therapy with the patient, family, and referring physician. The likelihood of immediate success and complications (including emergency bypass surgery and restenosis) should be explained. In general, the risks of percutaneous intervention include death (< 1%), nonfatal myocardial infarction (4%), and emergency bypass surgery (1%). Certain clinical and angiographic characteristics increase the risk of adverse outcomes after PTCA (Table 1.5), but many of these characteristics may be less important if stent implantation is feasible. Additional complications include stroke (< 0.5%), vascular injury (2-5%), infection, blood transfusion (2-8%), contrast nephropathy, allergic reactions, and systemic atheroembolization. Restenosis occurs in approximately 30% of patients after PTCA and repeat revascularization is necessary in 20%; these outcomes are reduced by 30-50% with stenting.

EQUIPMENT AND TECHNIQUE

A. **PROCEDURAL OVERVIEW**

    1.   **Intraprocedural Medication (Chapter 34).** At the time of intervention, a narcotic and benzodiazepine are usually employed for analgesia and conscious sedation. A continuous infusion of nitroglycerin (30-100 mcg/min) may be used to attenuate ischemia and vasospasm. Heparin is universally employed during all interventional procedures (IV bolus 100 units/kg); an activated clotting time (ACT) > 300 seconds is recommended before advancing PTCA hardware into the coronary artery. If adjunctive glycoprotein IIb/IIIa receptor antagonists are utilized, weight-adjusted heparin (70 units/kg) is recommended to achieve an ACT of 250 seconds (Chapter 34). Patients receiving continuous heparin prior to the procedure may manifest drug resistance and require a higher dose to achieve a therapeutic ACT. Supplemental heparin is administered as necessary to maintain the target ACT. Low-molecular-weight heparin (e.g., enoxaparin 1 mg/kg IV bolus) may be used as an alternative to unfractionated heparin.

2. **Vascular Access**

   a. **Femoral Approach.** To obtain vascular access, the femoral artery with the strongest pulse is identified, followed by administration of a local anesthetic (10-20 cc of 2% lidocaine). If pulses in both groins are equal, the femoral artery with the stronger peripheral pulse is chosen. If the femoral artery has been punctured within the last week, the contralateral artery is used for access. Synthetic grafts older than one month may be used for vascular access; sequential dilatation with progressively larger introducers may be necessary before the sheath can be inserted. Access is obtained by percutaneous puncture of the anterior wall of the common femoral artery using a beveled hollow needle and a modified Seldinger technique (Figure 1.1). It is important to access the *common* femoral artery, as sheath placement in the superficial or profunda femoral artery increases the risk of vascular complications. Anatomic and radiographic landmarks can be used to identify the site for arterial access and are especially useful in obese patients. The most reliable landmark is the junction between the middle and lower third of the femoral head; arterial access at this location will almost always be in the common femoral artery (Figure 1.2). Femoral venous access is recommended as a port for medications, a pacemaker, or a pulmonary artery catheter, especially in high-risk patients. In "simple" cases, many operators do not obtain central venous access.

Table 1.5. Factors Associated with Increased Complications or Decreased Success During PTCA

Clinical	Angiographic
Advanced age	Multivessel/multilesional disease
Aortic stenosis	Left main or equivalent
Pulmonary hypertension	Single patent vessel
Ejection fraction < 40%, particularly with CHF	Lesion characteristics:
Diabetes mellitus	Long
Female gender	Bend-point (^{3}45°)
Hypotension	Bifurcation
Severe hypertension	Thrombus
Previous MI	Eccentric
Previous CABG	Irregular contour
Peripheral vascular disease	Proximal vessel tortuosity
Unstable angina	Calcification
Acute MI	Chronic total occlusion
Multiple PVCs	Ostial location
	Diffuse disease
	Degenerated vein graft

Abbreviations: CHF = congestive heart failure; MI = myocardial infarction; PVCs = premature ventricular contractions

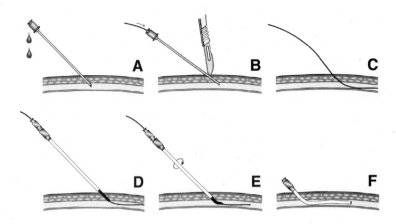

Figure 1.1. Arterial Access: Single-Wall Technique

Once pulsatile blood flow is obtained through the needle (A), a 0.035-0.038" guidewire is advanced into the vessel (B), followed by needle removal (C). An arterial sheath and dilator are then advanced over the wire (D, E) into the femoral artery, followed by removal of both guidewire and dilator (F). The sheath is then aspirated and flushed.

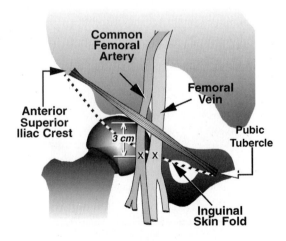

Figure 1.2. Landmarks for Vascular Access

Arterial access should be obtained at the junction between the middle and lower third of the femoral head, which corresponds to a site 2-3 cm below the inguinal ligament. The inguinal ligament runs between the anterior superior iliac spine and the pubic tubercle. The inguinal skinfold is a misleading landmark and should not be used to determine the site of access.

b. **Brachial and Radial Approaches.** Successful mastery of these alternative approaches to femoral vascular access greatly increases the range of options available to the interventionalist, and in selected cases, may increase the comfort, safety, and efficacy of catheter-based intervention (Chapter 2).

3. **Pacemaker Insertion.** Most operators reserve prophylactic pacing for patients with pre-existing high-grade conduction abnormalities, and for those at increased risk for severe bradycardia or heart block. These cases include degenerated vein grafts or thrombus-associated lesions in large RCA or left circumflex arteries, and Rotablator atherectomy of the RCA.

4. **Equipment Setup.** A guiding catheter of appropriate size and configuration is advanced over a 0.035- or 0.038-inch guidewire. Once in the ascending aorta, the wire is removed and the guiding catheter is connected to a manifold assembly and Y-adapter, then flushed. The manifold is connected to a pressure transducer, which continuously records central arterial pressure (Figure 1.3). The guiding catheter is maneuvered until it engages the coronary ostium; baseline angiograms are taken in orthogonal views to visualize the lesion and serve as a roadmap. Common angiographic views are listed in Figure 1.4.

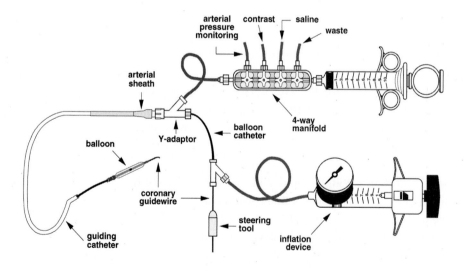

Figure 1.3. Basic Angioplasty Equipment and Setup

5. **Balloon Sizing.** The diameter of the final balloon is chosen to match the diameter of the reference segment (balloon-to-artery ratio of 1.0). The reference diameter is frequently estimated by comparing the target vessel to the guiding catheter (7F guide = 2.3mm, 8F = 2.7mm, 9F = 3.0mm, 10F = 3.3mm, 11F = 3.6mm). Visual estimates of reference diameter are the simplest and most popular method, but reference vessel diameter may also be estimated by on-line digital quantitative angiography or intravascular ultrasound (IVUS) (Chapter 31). Balloon sizing should be performed carefully, as undersizing (balloon-to-artery ratio < 0.9) frequently results in significant residual stenosis, and oversizing (balloon-to-artery ratio ≥ 1.2) increases the risk of complications. Accurate sizing is also important for optimal stent implantation.

6. **Guidewire Shaping.** Selection of the guidewire is based on coronary anatomy, lesion morphology, and operator preference. The guidewire is shaped to accommodate the morphology of the target vessel; this is easily accomplished by gentle manipulation of the wire between thumb and index finger, or by rolling the guidewire tip over the guidewire introducer. In general, the length of the distal bend should approximate the diameter of the vessel, since a small distal bend limits steerability and a large distal bend increases the risk of wire prolapse. A double-bend is very useful for steering into steeply angled vessels (Figure 1.5).

7. **Advancing the Guidewire and Balloon.** The guidewire and balloon are inserted through the O-ring of the Y-adapter into the guiding catheter, and air must be purged from the system. The balloon catheter and guidewire are then advanced to the guiding catheter tip. Standard angioplasty equipment and set-up are demonstrated in Figure 1.3.

8. **Crossing the Lesion with the Guidewire.** To reduce the risk of vasospasm, intracoronary nitroglycerin (100-200 mcg) is recommended prior to guidewire advancement. The guidewire should pass smoothly through the stenosis; if buckling occurs, the wire should be retracted and readvanced rather than forcefully prolapsed beyond the lesion to avoid vessel injury.

9. **Balloon Dilatation.** With the guidewire fixed in place, the balloon is advanced into the target lesion. After confirming proper balloon position using contrast injections, the balloon is gradually inflated using an inflation device filled with a 50:50 mixture of contrast and saline. The inflation pressure is increased until the lesion no longer indents the balloon or the rated burst pressure has been reached. Inflation times usually last 1-2 minutes, but range from 15 seconds to several minutes depending on patient tolerance, response of the lesion, and operator preference. With the balloon inflated, the patient is questioned regarding chest pain and a 12-lead ECG is obtained; these may prove useful in diagnosing abrupt closure after the patient leaves the angioplasty suite.

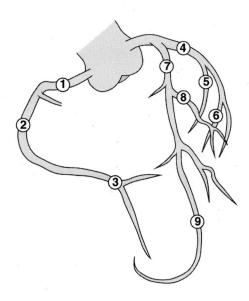

Figure 1.4. Frequently Used Angiographic Views

RCA	LCX	LAD
(1) Proximal RCA • 30° LAO, 30° caudal • 20° RAO, 20° caudal • 90° LAO, 20° caudal	**(4)** Proximal LCX • 30° RAO, 30° caudal • 30° LAO, 30° caudal	**(7)** Proximal LAD • 20° LAO, 20° cranial • 30° RAO, 30° caudal • 50° LAO, 30° caudal
(2) Mid-RCA • 30° LAO • 20° RAO • 90° LAO	**(5)** Obtuse Marginal • 20° RAO, 20° caudal • 50° LAO, 30° caudal	**(8)** Mid-LAD • 50° LAO, 30° cranial • 60° RAO, 20° cranial • 90° LAO • 50° LAO, 30° caudal
(3) Distal RCA • 30° LAO, 30° cranial • 90° LAO	**(6)** Distal LCX • 30° RAO, 30° caudal • 30° LAO, 30° cranial	**(9)** Distal LAD • 20° RAO, 20° caudal • 40° LAO • 20° LAO, 20° cranial

Abbreviations: RCA = right coronary artery; LCX = left circumflex artery; LAD = left anterior descending coronary artery; LAO = left anterior oblique; RAO = right anterior oblique

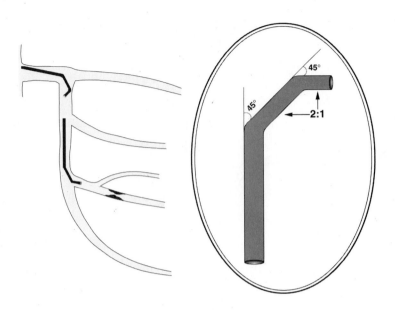

Figure 1.5. Double-Bend Guidewire

The proximal bend allows the operator to steer the wire from the left main into the left circumflex artery. Once in the circumflex, the smaller distal bend allows entry into the marginal branch.

10. **Evaluation of Acute Angiographic Outcome.** Following PTCA, the balloon is retracted into the guiding catheter, leaving the guidewire across the lesion. Angiograms are obtained in orthogonal views to assess vessel patency and residual stenosis. The angiogram should be carefully evaluated for residual stenosis, thrombus, dissection, sidebranch occlusion, distal embolization, spasm, perforation, and no-reflow. If the patient is clinically stable and a good angiographic outcome has been obtained, all hardware is removed and final angiograms are taken. If a suboptimal angiographic result is obtained, various technical approaches may be employed (Figure 1.6); most operators rely on stents to manage suboptimal PTCA.

B. **EQUIPMENT SELECTION**
1. **Vascular Sheaths.** Arterial sheaths commonly used for interventional procedures are 6-8F in diameter; larger sheaths are required for atherectomy (9-11F), valvuloplasty (12F), and percutaneous cardiopulmonary bypass (18-22F). Long sheaths (23cm) may be useful for straightening tortuous femoral and iliac arteries, facilitating guiding catheter support, and improving torque-control.

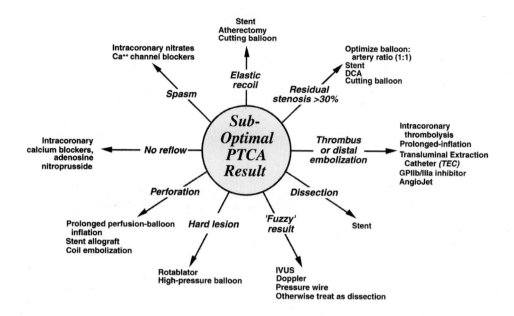

Figure 1.6. Suboptimal Angiographic Outcome Following PTCA: Causes and Management

2. **Guiding Catheter Selection (Table 1.8, Figure 1.7).** The enormous variety of guiding catheters has improved the technique of coronary intervention. Many companies now manufacture guiding catheters from 6-10F, and each guide has its own unique design and construction. For a given size guiding catheter, the internal diameter is either a standard lumen, large lumen, or giant lumen better opacification, support, and pressure monitoring; disadvantages include an increased risk of ostial trauma, vascular complications, and kinking of the catheter shaft. Compared to diagnostic catheters used for coronary arteriography, guiding catheters have a stiffer shaft, larger internal diameter, a shorter and more angulated tip (110° vs. 90°), and re-enforced construction (3 vs. 2-layers) (Figure 1.8). Guiding catheter selection is based on aortic root width, coronary ostial origin (high, anterior), and ostial orientation (superior, horizontal, inferior) (Tables 1.8, 1.9, Figure 1.9).

Table 1.6. Internal Diameters of Standard, Large, and Giant-Lumen Guiding Catheters

French	Standard (in.)	Large (in.)	Giant (in.)
6	≤ 0.061	0.062 - 0.065	≥ 0.066
7	≤ 0.071	0.072 - 0.075	≥ 0.076
8	≤ 0.079	0.080 - 0.085	≥ 0.086
9	≤ 0.089	0.090 - 0.095	≥ 0.096
10	≤ 0.099	0.100 - 0.107	≥ 0.108

Table 1.7. Minimum Recommended Guiding Catheter Internal Diameters

Technique	Device	Internal Diameter (inch)
PTCA	Simple	0.056
	Kissing balloon*	0.076
Stents	Various	0.062-0.076
Rotablator Burr	1.25 mm	0.053
	1.50 mm	0.063
	1.75 mm	0.073
	2.0 mm	0.083
	2.15 mm	0.089
	2.25 mm	0.093
	2.38 mm	0.098
	2.50 mm	0.102
ELCA Probe	1.4 mm	0.076
	1.7 mm	0.076
	2.0 mm	0.084
DCA Atherocath	5F	0.104
	6F	0.104
	7F,7FG	0.104
	Flexi-Cut	0.087
TEC Catheter	5.5F, 6F	0.088
	6.5F	0.090
	7F	0.096
	7.5F	0.103
IVUS		0.062

Abbreviations: ELCA = excimer laser coronary angioplasty; DCA = directional coronary atherectomy (AtheroCath);
TEC = transluminal extraction catheter; IVUS = intravascular ultrasound; F = French size
* Virtually all low-profile 0.014-inch compatible systems and fixed-wire devices can be used. To determine kissing
  balloon and guiding catheter combinations, add balloon profiles for each balloon plus 0.010" for clearance; the total
  must be less than the guide ID.

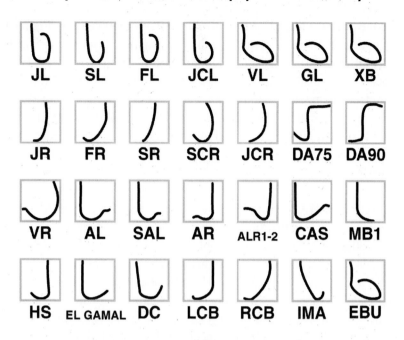

Figure 1.7. Selected Guiding Catheter Configurations

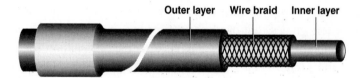

Figure 1.8. Guiding Catheter Construction

The outer layer consists of either polyurethane or polyethylene for overall stiffness. The middle layer is composed of a wire matrix for torque generation. The inner layer is composed of a Teflon coating for smooth passage of the balloon dilatation catheter.

a. **Left Anterior Descending (LAD) Coronary Artery Intervention (Figure 1.9, Table 1.9).**
A JL4 guide is the catheter of choice in the vast majority of cases involving the LAD, which normally arises in an anterior and superior position. If the ostium of the left main is high or the aortic root is small, a JL3.5 catheter may be preferred. Once in the left main, gentle counter-clockwise rotation of the guiding catheter will frequently direct it anteriorly. An out-of plane femoral guiding catheter (30° anterior orientation) is available, though rarely needed. If the left main is short, a short-tip guide may provide better coaxial alignment, which is best confirmed in the LAO (50°)-Caudal (30°) view or in the shallow RAO (5°)-Caudal (20°) view.

b. **Left Circumflex (LCX) Intervention (Figure 1.9, Table 1.9).** LCX angioplasty is sometimes associated with difficulties in guidewire passage and balloon tracking due to the inherent tortuosity of this vessel. Stable coaxial alignment may be facilitated by gentle clockwise rotation of a JL4 guiding catheter once engaged in the left main. A JL5 may be of benefit in a dilated aortic root or when the tip of a JL4 points anteriorly. An Amplatz left guiding catheter should be considered for a sharply angulated or inferiorly-positioned circumflex ostium. Amplatz catheters can also be extremely useful in providing additional back-up support for balloon advancement when proximal vessel tortuosity, chronic total occlusion, or a distal target lesion is present. If an Amplatz guide becomes deeply engaged, it should be partially withdrawn over an extended balloon to prevent vessel injury. Amplatz catheters must be carefully disengaged from the coronary artery; simple withdrawal from the vessel in a manner similar to Judkins guides can cause the tip to advance farther into the vessel. To disengage an Amplatz catheter, it is first advanced slightly to prolapse the tip out of the artery, and then rotated away from the ostium prior to withdrawal. In addition to JL5 and Amplatz left guides, out-of-plane (30° posterior orientation) guiding catheters are available. Geometric catheter configurations offer the best support for interventions in the left coronary artery (e.g., Voda-left guide); unlike Amplatz and Judkins curves, which derive their support from the left Sinus of Valsalva, geometric guides derive their support from the opposite wall of the aorta.

c. **Right Coronary Artery (RCA) Intervention (Figures 1.9, 1.10, Table 1.9).** The right coronary artery is more difficult to engage than the left coronary artery. For horizontally-oriented RCAs and most proximal lesions in gently superior or inferior orientations, a JR4 guiding catheter will usually suffice. However, when additional back-up support is needed, a left Amplatz guide or Hockey-stick may be required. For marked superior orientations ("Shepherd's Crook"), a left Amplatz, Hockey-stick, internal mammary, El Gamal, Voda-right, or double-loop Arani catheter (75°) provide better coaxial alignment than a standard Judkin's catheter (Figure 1.10). Although double-loop Arani catheters provide excellent back-up, they are often very difficult to engage; a Voda-right guide provides similar back-up and is much easier to engage the ostium. Like the left Voda, the right Voda and double-loop Arani derive support from the opposite wall of the aorta rather than the Sinus of Valsalva.

For marked inferior orientations, a Multipurpose or Amplatz catheter (left or right) is preferred for better coaxial alignment and backup.

d. **Saphenous Vein Graft Intervention (Table 1.9) (Chapter 17).** Saphenous vein bypass grafts to the RCA usually arise from the anterior wall of the aorta several centimeters above the aortic root, and are best approached with a Multipurpose or Amplatz (left or right) guiding catheter. Grafts to the LAD and left circumflex are usually positioned above and lateral to RCA grafts, and may require an El Gamal, left coronary bypass, Hockey-stick, right Judkins, or Amplatz guiding catheter.

e. **Internal Mammary Artery Intervention (Chapter 17).** Internal mammary guiding catheters are used most frequently for internal mammary artery intervention.

f. **"Dampening" of the Arterial Pressure Tracing (Figure 1.11).** Occasionally, guiding catheter engagement obstructs coronary flow, causing an immediate fall in diastolic pressure ("ventricularization"), or a fall in both systolic and diastolic pressures ("dampened" pressure). Ventricularization and dampening are most commonly due to the presence of a diseased ostium, but may be caused by coronary spasm, non-coaxial alignment between the guide and vessel wall, or mismatch between the vessel diameter and the diameter of the guide. In these instances, forceful contrast injections increase the risk of coronary dissection and must be avoided. When dampening is caused by a small coronary artery or an ostial obstruction, the guiding catheter should be replaced with a sidehole catheter to allow passive entry of aortic blood into the guiding catheter and coronary artery. If a sidehole catheter is not available, sideholes can be created with a sidehole cutter or the beveled end of the vascular access needle. Potential problems with sidehole catheters include suboptimal opacification (contrast escapes through the sideholes), decreased back-up support due to weakness of the catheter shaft, and kinking at the sideholes, particularly with giant lumen guides. When sidehole guides are used for ostial lesions, the presence of sideholes will permit passive perfusion but does not reduce the risk of guiding catheter injury to the vessel ostium.

3. **Guidewires (Table 1.10)**
   a. **Composition.** Guidewires consist of 3 basic components, including a central core or shaft (usually stainless steel or nitinol), a distal flexible spring coil (usually platinum or tungsten), and a lubricious coating (silicone, PTFE, or other hydrophilic coating) (Figure 1.12). Virtually all guidewires can be used for most coronary interventions, although guidewire construction does influence performance, particularly in difficult anatomy such as severe tortuosity or angulation (Chapter 11). In general, wires with single-core construction provide a smoother transition, enhanced torque response, and less prolapse compared to wires with a shaping ribbon construction. Guidewires with nitinol cores are virtually kink-resistant, while those with stainless steel cores may be more susceptible to kinking.

Table 1.8. Guiding Catheter Configurations

Catheter	Description	Recommended Use
JL	Judkins left	Most left coronary artery interventions
FL	Femoral left	Most left coronary artery interventions
JCL	Judkins "C" left	Same relationship of tip to shaft as JL, but more gentle transition; useful for DCA of left coronary artery, biliary stents, Rotablator
VL	Voda left	Back-up support from opposite wall of aorta; excellent for difficult anatomy (tortuous, angulated, calcified, total occlusion) in left coronary artery
VLHT	Voda left, high takeoff	Back-up support from opposite wall of aorta; excellent for difficult anatomy (tortuous, angulated, calcified, total occlusion) in left coronary artery with high takeoff
XB	Extra-backup	Back-up support from opposite wall of aorta; excellent for difficult anatomy (tortuous, angulated, calcified, total occlusion) in left coronary artery
GL	Geometric left	Back-up support from opposite wall of aorta; excellent for difficult anatomy (tortuous, angulated, calcified, total occlusion) in left coronary artery
EBU	Extra Back Up	Back-up support from opposite wall of aorta; excellent for difficult anatomy (tortuous, angulated, calcified, total occlusion) in left coronary artery
LS	Left Support	Back-up support from opposite wall of aorta; excellent for difficult anatomy (tortuous, angulated, calcified, total occlusion) in left coronary artery
AL	Amplatz left	Versatile configuration; particularly useful for Shepherd Crook RCA, high-anterior RCA, tough anatomy in left coronary artery (especially left circumflex), virtually all vein grafts
JR	Judkins right	Most RCA interventions; also useful for many interventions on vein grafts to the left coronary artery; may not provide coaxial alignment for vein grafts to the RCA
FR	Femoral right	Most RCA interventions; also useful for many interventions on vein grafts to the left coronary artery; may not provide coaxial alignment for vein grafts to the RCA
NTR	No-torque right	Most RCA interventions; minimal catheter manipulation required
SCR	Shepherd Crook right	Shepherd Crook RCA; may be useful for vein grafts to the left coronary artery with vertical upward origin
S/R	Shani right	Shepherd Crook RCA; excellent support for difficult anatomy in RCA; minimal catheter manipulation required
JCR	Judkin's "C" right	DCA of RCA and vein grafts to the left coronary artery with horizontal or slightly inferior origin; also used for biliary stents
DA 75,90	Double-loop Arani (75°, 90°)	Excellent back-up support for difficult anatomy in RCA or Shepherd Crook; difficult catheters to manipulate
VR	Voda right	Excellent back-up support for difficult anatomy in RCA, Shepherd Crook RCA, or vein grafts to the left coronary artery with vertical upward origin

Table 1.8. Guiding Catheter Configurations

Catheter	Description	Recommended Use
VRSC	Voda right, Shepherd Crook	Excellent back-up support for difficult anatomy in RCA, Shepherd Crook RCA, or vein grafts to the left coronary artery with vertical upward origin
AR	Amplatz right	Useful for interventions in RCA or vein grafts to RCA with inferior origin
ALR 1-2	Amplatz left-right (modified Amplatz)	Similar to AL and AR; slightly longer reach than AR and shorter reach than AL
MP	Multipurpose	Useful for RCA or vein grafts to RCA with inferior origin; also useful for many vein grafts to the left coronary artery with gentle inferior or horizontal origin
SON	Sones	Useful for RCA or vein grafts to RCA with inferior origin; also useful for many vein grafts to the left coronary artery with gentle inferior or horizontal origin
HS	Hockey-Stick	Good guiding catheter for horizontal or gentle superior origin of RCA or vein grafts to left coronary artery
Champ	Champ	Good guiding catheter for horizontal or gentle superior origin of RCA or vein grafts to left coronary artery
ELG	El Gamal bypass	Good guiding catheter for horizontal or gentle superior origin of RCA or vein grafts to left coronary artery
LCB	Left coronary bypass	Similar to JR and HS; useful for vein grafts to left coronary artery with horizontal or slightly superior origin
RCB	Right coronary bypass	Useful for vein grafts to the left coronary artery with horizontal origin; may not provide coaxial alignment with vein grafts to the RCA with inferior origin
IMA	Internal mammary	Target lesions in LIMA, RIMA, or native vessel beyond anastomosis; sometimes useful for upward vertical origin of vein graft to left coronary artery or native RCA
CAS	Castillo	Left Amplatz type of confirguration; intended use from brachial approach (similar to Simmons)
DC	Doctor's choice	Multipurpose catheter for RCA or left coronary artery; extra backup from opposite wall of aorta
RAD	Radial	Multipurpose catheter for RCA or left coronary artery; intended use from radial artery access
HBD	Hybrid	Multipurpose catheter for RCA or left coronary artery; intended use from radial artery or femoral artery access

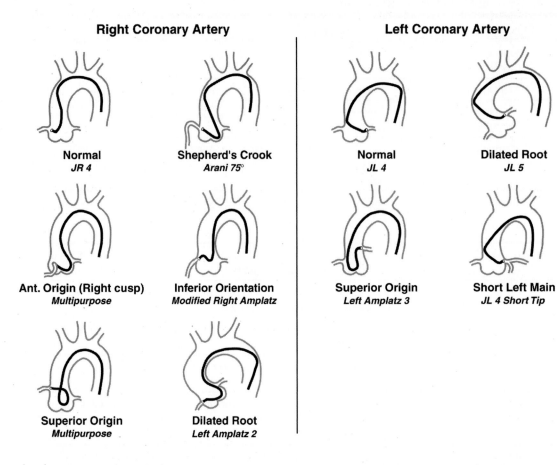

Right Coronary Artery

Normal
JR 4

Shepherd's Crook
Arani 75°

Ant. Origin (Right cusp)
Multipurpose

Inferior Orientation
Modified Right Amplatz

Superior Origin
Multipurpose

Dilated Root
Left Amplatz 2

Left Coronary Artery

Normal
JL 4

Dilated Root
JL 5

Superior Origin
Left Amplatz 3

Short Left Main
JL 4 Short Tip

Figure 1.9. Guide Selection Based on Aortic Root Width and Coronary Artery Orientation

Table 1.9. Guiding Catheter Selection

Target Vessel	Configuration	Guiding Catheters
Right Coronary Artery (RCA)	Aortic root	
	Normal	JR4, AL1, AR1
	Dilated	JR $\geq$ 5, AL $\geq$ 2, AR $\geq$ 2
	Narrow	JR 3, AL $\leq$ 0.75
	Orientation*	
	Normal	JR, AL, AR
	Anterior, Superior	AL, HS, MP
	Inferior	MP, AR, JR
	Shepherd Crook	AL, SCR, VR, VRSC, DA, ELG, SHR, Champ, IMA
	Horizontal	JR, HS
Left Coronary Artery (LCA)	Aortic root	
	Normal	JL4, AL2, VL4, GL4, XB3.5, XBU4
	Dilated	JL $\geq$ 5, AL $\geq$ 2, VL $\geq$ 4, GL $\geq$ 4, XB $\geq$ 4, XBU $\geq$ 4
	Narrow	JL3.5, VL3.5, GL3.5, XB3.0, XBU3.5
	Orientation*	
	Normal, Anterior	JL, AL, VL, GL, XB, XBU
	Posterior	AL, VL, GL, XB, XBU
	Superior	JL, VL, GL, XB, XBU
	Supraselect	
	LAD	JL3.5, JL (anterior)
	LCX	JL4.5, AL, JL (posterior)
SVG to RCA	Orientation*	
	Inferior	MP, AL, AR, JR
	Horizontal	JR, AL, MP
SVG to LCA	Orientation*	
	Horizontal	JR, HS, MP, AL, RCB, AR
	Superior	HS, ELG, LCB, MP, SCR, Champ, SHR

Abbreviations: SVG = saphenous vein graft; see Table 1.8 and Figure 1.7 for guiding catheter descriptions
* Size of curve depends on the diameter of the aortic root

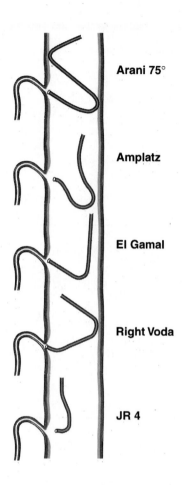

Arani 75°

Amplatz

El Gamal

Right Voda

JR 4

Figure 1.10. Guide Catheter Selection for Shepherd's Crook RCA

Note suboptimal alignment with JR4 catheter compared to Arani 75°, Amplatz, El Gamal, and right Voda guides.

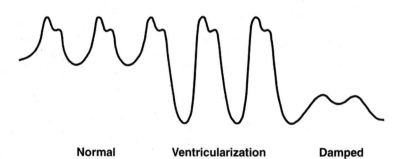

Normal   Ventricularization   Damped

Figure 1.11. Arterial Pressure Tracings Recorded from Guiding Catheter

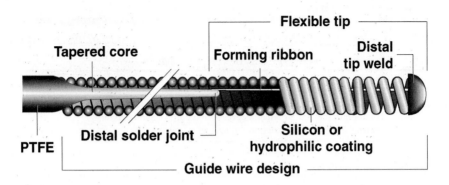

Figure 1.12. Guidewire Construction

---

b. **Characteristics.** Features to consider when choosing a guidewire include its torque-control, steerability, visibility, flexibility, and support for device advancement. Unfortunately, the perfect angioplasty guidewire does not exist: Wires with increased flexibility have decreased steerability, and wires with increased torque-control have decreased flexibility. Although larger wires (0.016-0.018-inch) have increased steerability, result in greater straightening of tortuous coronary segments, and provide more support for catheter advancement, they have been largely replaced by an exceptional variety of 0.014-inch guidewires. Guidewire tips are manufactured with either a preformed "J" or are straight and require shaping. Most guidewires have radiopaque tips (usually platinum) in short (2-3 cm) and long (25-40 cm) lengths. Although there are no differences in performance per se, each has its own advantages and disadvantages: Long radiopaque tips are readily visible in the guiding catheter and target vessel, making the wire path and kinks or loops in the wire apparent at all times. However, the radiopacity of the guidewire frequently interferes with assessment of fine details of lumen morphology, such as intraluminal filling defects, haziness, or dissection, particularly in small vessels. In addition, most on-line digital QCA programs are unable to quantitate lumen diameter if such radiopaque wires are in place. Because of these limitations, guidewires with long radiopaque tips are not routinely recommended.

c. **Exchange-Length and Extension Wires.** Exchange-length wires are available in 270, 300, and 400 cm lengths. Many conventional length guidewires can be extended using special extension wires (e.g., DOC, DOC-Tite, Cinch-QR, Linx-EZ, Trooper/Patriot).

d. **Specialty Wires**
   1. **Magnum Wire.** The Magnum wire, which is available in 0.014, 0.018, 0.021-inch

Table 1.10. Coronary Guidewires

Name	Description	Intended Use
— BOSTON SCIENTIFIC SCIMED —		
ChoICE® Floppy	Hydrophilic-coated, polymer sleeve, spring coil tip front-line guidewire	Simple-to-complex PTCA
Luge™	Hydrophilic-coated, polymer sleeve, spring coil tip front-line moderate support guidewire	Stent delivery
ChoICE® Extra Support	Hydrophilic-coated, polymer sleeve, spring coil tip guidewire with extra rail support	Extra support stent delivery
ChoICE® Intermediate	Hydrophilic-coated, polymer sleeve, spring coil tip guidewire with slightly stiffer tip	Added pushability; stiffer tip
ChoICE® Standard	Hydrophilic-coated, polymer sleeve, spring coil tip guidewire with stiff tip	Total occlusions
ChoICE® PT	High performance polymer tip crossing wire with hydrophilic-coated polymer sleeve for distal trackability	Simple-to-complex PTCA; crossing severe tortuosity and tight lesions
PT Graphix™	High performance polymer tip crossing wire with hydrophilic-coated polymer sleeve for distal trackability and enhanced rail support	Stent delivery; crossing severe tortuosity and tight lesions
ChoICE® PT Extra Support	High performance polymer tip crossing wire with hydrophilic-coated polymer sleeve for distal trackability and extra rail support	Extra support stent delivery
Trooper™ Floppy	Silicone-coated, full spring coil floppy guide wire with unibody corewire for enhanced torque and steerability	Simple-to-complex PTCA
Patriot™	Silicone-coated, full spring coil moderate support guide wire with unibody core wire for enhanced torque and steerability	Stent delivery
Trooper™ Extra Support	Silicone-coated, full spring coil guidewire with extra rail support	Extra support stent delivery
Trooper™ Intermediate	Silicone-coated, full spring coil guidewire with slightly stiffer tip	Added pushability; stiffer tip
Trooper™ Standard	Silicone-coated, full spring coil guidewire with stiff tip	Chronic total occlusions
Mailman™	Hydrophilic-coated, polymer sleeve, spring coil tip highly supportive guidewire	Super support; vessel straightening
Platinum Plus™	Silicone-coated, full spring coil highly supportive guidewire	Super support; vessel straightening
Crosswire™	High performance polymer tip crossing wire with hydrophilic-coated polymer sleeve	Chronic total occlusions
Glidewire® Gold*	High performance polymer tip crossing wire with hydrophilic-coated polymer sleeve	Chronic total occlusions

Table 1.10. Coronary Guidewires

Name	Description	Intended Use
— CORDIS / J & J —		
ATW™ All Track Wire	Highly steerable 1 piece corewire, moderate support, flexible broad distal transition, floppy tip, lubricious PTFE sleeve	Simple and complex PTCA; stent delivery
ATW™ Marker Wire	ATW wire with 4 radiopaque markers spaced 10 mm apart. Distal marker is 4.5 cm from wire tip	Useful for measuring lesion length
STABILIZER® Balanced Performance SuperSoft	Very steerable 1 piece corewire, flexible distal broad transition, moderate support, lubricious PTFE sleeve	Simple and complex PTCA; stent delivery
STABILIZER® Balanced Performance Soft	Very steerable 1 piece corewire, flexible distal broad transition, moderate support, lubricious PTFE sleeve, slightly stiffer tip	Added pushability with stiffer tip
STABILIZER® Marker Wire	STABILIZER Balanced Performance with 6 radiopaque markers spaced 15 mm apart. Distal marker is 4.5 cm from wire tip	Useful for measuring lesion length; simple and complex PTCA; stent delivery
STABILIZER® Plus	Extra support and excellent steerability, lubricious PTFE sleeve	Extra support stent delivery; some vessel straightening
STABILIZER® XS	Highest level of extra-support, steerable 1 piece corewire, lubricious PTFE sleeve	Highest level extra support stent delivery; vessel straightening
WIZDOM® SuperSoft	Light support, very steerable and flexible 1 piece corewire, lubricious PTFE sleeve	Highest level extra support stent delivery, vessel straightening
WIZDOM® Soft	Light support, very steerable and flexible 1 piece corewire, lubricious PTFE sleeve, slightly stiffer tip	Added pushability with stiffer tip
WIZDOM® ST	Light support, short distal transition corewire that can be prolapsed, 1 piece corewire for enhanced torque control, lubricious PTFE sleeve	Simple PTCA; stent delivery
REFLEX® .012"/.014"	Hybrid wire with very flexible .012" distal diameter, silicone-coated, radiopaque wire	PTCA, tight lesions
REFLEX® .014" SuperSoft	Very steerable, flexible radiopaque wire, silicone coated	Simple and complex PTCA
REFLEX® Soft	Very steerable, flexible radiopaque wire, silicone coated, slightly stiffer tip	Added pushability with stiffer tip
SHINOBI®	Highly steerable 1 piece corewire, PTFE sleeve extends over firm tip for crossing	Uncrossable lesions
SHINOBI® Plus	Extra support, highly steerable 1 piece corewire, PTFE sleeve extends over firm tip for crosssing	Uncrossable lesions; extra support
CINCH® QR	.014", 145 cm length extension wire	Extension wire for Cordis coronary steerable guidewires

Table 1.10. Coronary Guidewires

Name	Description	Intended Use
— GUIDANT —		
Hi-Torque Balance MiddleWeight™	Soft, floppy tip, medium support. Nitinol core for steering and durability. Hydrocoat hydrophilic coating	Workhorse wire, medium support
Hi-Torque Balance Trek™	Soft floppy tip. Nitinol core for steering and durability. Hydrocoat hydrophilic coating.	Workhorse wire, medium support. Low profile for tight catheter inner lumens
High-Torque Floppy II Extra Support™	Soft floppy tip; more supportive stainless steel core	Workhorse wire, medium support
High-Torque Floppy II™	Soft floppy tip; flexible stainless steel core	Workhorse wire, light support
Hi-Torque Balance HeavyWeight™	Soft floppy tip. Nitinol core for steering and durability. Hydrocoat hydrophilic coating	Rail support when some vessel straightening is needed
Hi-Torque Extra S'Port™	High-support stainless steel core. Core-to-tip design for precise steering	Rail support when some vessel straightening is needed
Hi-Torque All Star™	High-support stainless steel core. Core-to-tip design for precise steering. Teflon jacket for smooth movement	Rail support when some vessel straightening is needed
Hi-Torque Iron Man™	Super-support stainless steel core; soft tip	Super rail support when vessel straightening is needed
Hi-Torque Balance™	Soft floppy tip; light support. Nitinol core for steering and durability. Hydrocoat hydrophilic coating	Tortuousity or acute take-offs
Hi-Torque Traverse™	Soft core-to-tip design, with broad transitions for tracking. Hydrocoat hydrophilic coating	Tortuousity or acute take-offs
Hi-Torque Cross-It XT™ series (100, 200, 300)	Unique tapered tip, increasing tip support levels for tight lesions. Hydrocoat hydrophilic coating	Severe stenoses
Hi-Torque Wiggle Wire™	Wiggles built into wire near distal tip	Helps 'wiggle' catheter tip around obsturction
— MEDTRONIC AVE —		
Fusion	0.014" Nitinol PTCA guidewire	Workhorse wire for PTCA and device delivery
Floppy	0.014" Stainless steel PTCA guidewire	PTCA; minimal support devices
Direct	0.014" Stainless steel PTCA guidewire	PTCA; medium support devices
Light Support	0.014" Stainless steel PTCA guidewire	Workhorse wire for PTCA and device delivery
Support	0.014" Stainless steel PTCA guidewire	Extra support for device delivery
Silk	0.012" Stainless steel PTCA guidewire	Tracking through tortuosity
Standard	0.014" Stainless steel PTCA guidewire	Crossing subtotal occlusions
Hi-per Flex	0.014" Stainless steel PTCA guidewire	PTCA; medium support devices
Lumisilk	0.012" Stainless steel PTCA guidewire	Tracking through tortuosity

* Crosswire and Glidewire Gold wires manufactured by Terumo Corp; available through Boston Scientific Scimed in USA.

diameters, consists of a stainless steel core, a flexible gold-plated tungsten spring, and a 1-mm olive-shaped tip. Its principal use has been in recanalizing chronic total occlusions (Chapter 16).

   2. Hydrophilic Guidewires. There are numerous 0.014- and 0.018-inch hydrophilic wires with kink-resistant nitinol cores and low-friction hydrophilic polymer coatings to facilitate smooth passage through high-grade obstructions and total occlusions (Table 1.10).

4. Balloon Dilatation Catheters. Angioplasty balloon catheters are arbitrarily classified into three different categories: over-the-wire (OTW) systems; single-operator-exchange (SOE) or monorail systems; and fixed-wire systems (formerly called "balloon-on-a-wire"). In addition, several specialty balloons have unique "niche" applications (Figure 1.13).

a. Classification of Balloon Catheters

   1. Over-the-Wire (OTW) Systems. In the United States, the majority of operators use OTW systems that accommodate 0.014-inch guidewires. The availability of many ultra-low profile balloons have led most manufacturers to eliminate or markedly curtail the production of balloons that accommodate other guidewires. Although the standard usable length of most balloons is 135 cm, longer shaft balloons (145,150 cm) are available and may be useful for dilating target lesions in distal vessels, particularly beyond bypass graft anastomoses.

   The two techniques of guidewire manipulation with OTW balloons are the "thru-wire" and "bare-wire" techniques — both are equally acceptable. In the *thru-wire technique*, the operator advances the guidewire-loaded balloon into the O-ring and through the guiding catheter just proximal to the vessel ostium. The guidewire is then advanced beyond the stenosis, and the balloon is tracked over the wire and into the lesion. If the operator has difficulty with guidewire crossing, the balloon catheter can be advanced into the target vessel for additional support and torque control. If the lesion still cannot be crossed, the balloon catheter can be left in place to function as a transfer catheter, and the operator can fashion a different curve on the guidewire or use a new guidewire as necessary. The *bare-wire technique* involves advancing the guidewire across the lesion *without* the balloon. This technique may allow better visualization during contrast injections, but does not permit use of the balloon to enhance support or facilitate exchanges.

   2. Single-Operator Exchange (SOE) Systems. Outside the United States, SOE systems, also commonly referred to as "monorail" or "rapid-exchange" balloons, comprise the overwhelming majority of balloon catheter sales. SOE balloons are modified over-the-wire balloons in which only the distal portion of the balloon catheter tracks coaxially over the guidewire; the remaining portion of the catheter shaft does not have a guidewire thru-lumen. Compared to over-the-wire balloons, SOE balloons have a lower profile and are better suited for single operator use. Standard-length (175 cm) guidewires are recommended using a bare-wire technique; exchange-length guidewires are not necessary. Disadvantages of SOE balloons include less pushability and trackability, inability to reshape or exchange the guidewire without a transfer catheter, and difficulty using the balloon catheter for additional guidewire back-up support while crossing a difficult lesion.

3. **Fixed-Wire Systems.** Formerly referred to as "balloon-on-a-wire" systems, these devices do not permit independent movement of the guidewire and balloon. Although fixed-wire devices have always had the lowest profile of all balloon catheters, a significant limitation is the inability to exchange balloons or guidewires without having to recross the lesion. The important role of PTCA as an adjunct to virtually all laser, atherectomy, and stent devices—which themselves require a movable guidewire—and the availability of ultra-low-profile systems have substantially reduced the need for fixed-wire devices. Nevertheless, fixed-wire balloons are occasionally useful when other balloons have failed in tortuous vessels, highly angulated lesions, and for gaining access to sidebranches "jailed" by stents (Chapter 11).

4. **Specialty Balloons.** There are a variety of "specialty" balloons that can be used for specific niche indications (as well as for routine PTCA). The most common specialty balloon is the perfusion balloon catheter, which is available as an over-the-wire or single-operator-exchange balloon. Multiple sideholes in the catheter shaft proximal and distal to the balloon permit passive flow of arterial blood to the distal myocardial bed during balloon inflation (perfusion rates are 30-60 cc/min). Although perfusion balloons were useful in patients unable to tolerate conventional balloon inflations (due to severe angina or hemodynamic dysfunction) and to manage suboptimal PTCA, the availability of numerous stent designs has virtually eliminated the need for perfusion balloons in contemporary practice. Because of their perfusion capabilities, these catheters may be used as bailout devices during triage of patients to emergency CABG. Other specialty balloons are also available: The tapered balloon, which tapers by 0.5 mm from distal-to-proximal ends of a 25-mm balloon, had been used successfully for tapering vessels, but is no longer available. The Focus balloon (Cardiovascular Dynamics, Santa Clara, CA) is an interesting and potentially useful balloon for adjunctive PTCA before and after stenting. The balloon is 20-mm long, and consists of a central PE segment (10 mm) and two PET segments on each end (5 mm each); during high-pressure inflations (>12 ATM), the central PE segment is 0.2-0.5 mm larger than the PET segments on either end. The "cutting balloon" (InterVentional Technologies, San Diego, CA) contains several longitudinal microtomes that incise plaque and create controlled, localized dissection during balloon inflation.

b. **Characteristics of Balloon Catheters**
    1. **Balloon Material, Compliance, and Creep.** Balloon compliance, defined as the change in balloon diameter per atmosphere of inflation pressure, is an index of the stretchability

of a balloon. Balloon materials can be classified as highly-compliant, moderately-compliant, and minimally-compliant; more compliant balloons are generally associated with more "creep," which refers to the tendency of a balloon to enlarge after serial inflations at the same pressure. Balloon compliance ranges from 0.095mm/ATM (POC balloons) to 0.010 mm/ATM (PET balloons). Although in-vitro testing suggests that PET balloons are less compliant than POC or PE balloons, most studies have found that these differences are not clinically relevant (Chapter 20). In fact, high compliance is marketed by some manufacturers as an advantage (sizing "flexibility") and by others as a disadvantage ("less predictable" balloon sizing). Concerns about balloon compliance and creep have been heightened by clinical studies suggesting that accurate balloon sizing (ideal balloon-to-artery ratio = 0.9-1.1) is needed to minimize the risk of dissection, abrupt closure, and ischemic complications. Despite the recognized importance of proper balloon sizing, there are no data to suggest clear superiority of certain balloon materials. Only two retrospective studies reported different results for compliant and noncompliant balloons; one reported better results for noncompliant balloons, and the other reported better results for compliant balloons. In contrast, several nonrandomized and randomized studies failed to show any difference in angiographic results or ischemic complications (Chapter 20). Although early studies suggested that angulated lesions may respond better to noncompliant balloons, more recent data from a prospective randomized study suggested no difference in outcome for angulated lesions, lesions > 20 mm, ostial lesions, calcified lesions, or eccentric lesions. Nevertheless, noncompliant balloons are associated with higher burst pressures (see below), and are clearly useful as adjuncts to stenting and for rigid lesions that cannot be dilated at inflation pressures < 10 ATM.

2. **Burst Pressure.** Nominal pressure refers to the inflation pressure required to achieve the inflated balloon diameter on the package label, and usually ranges from 3-10 ATM. Burst pressure (usually reported as rated burst pressure [RBP]) is defined as the pressure below which 99.9% of balloons will not rupture. RBP is an important component of product labeling (and is monitored by the FDA), providing the operator with a good idea about the safe range of inflation pressures. RBP commonly ranges from 6-16 ATM. Mean burst pressure (MBP), defined as the pressure at which 50% of balloons will rupture, is higher than RBP and ranges from 10-27 ATM. Many manufacturers do not publish data about MBP.

3. **Profile.** There are considerable data about deflated profile (measured diameter of the deflated balloon and distal catheter shaft). Although measured profile was relevant 10 years ago, contemporary PTCA products from virtually all manufacturers are extremely low-profile. Although measured differences in profile do exist, their clinical relevance is probably less important than differences in trackability and pushability (see below). While

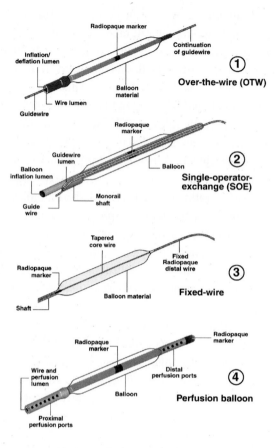

Figure 1.13. Balloon Dilatation Catheter Designs

deflated profiles after one or more initial balloon inflations are extremely important, virtually no companies report these data. Clinical experience suggests that inadequate refolding of the balloon ("winging") is worse for PET balloons, which may explain the recognized difficulty recrossing lesions after a series of initial balloon inflations.

4. **Pushability and Trackability.** Unlike compliance, creep, nominal pressure, burst pressure, and profile (all of which can be measured in-vitro), there are no reliable in-vitro methods for measuring "trackability" (the ease of tracking a balloon over the guidewire up to the target lesion) or "pushability" (the ability to advance the balloon across the lesion). However, trackability and pushability are more important to the practice of interventional cardiology than any other in-vitro measurement. The guiding catheter, guidewire, and operator experience also influence the operator's perception of trackability and pushability.

5. **Balloon Diameter and Length.** Most PTCA balloons are available in 0.5 mm increments from 2.0-4.0 mm in diameter; 1.5-mm balloons, 4.5-6.0 mm balloons, and quarter-sizes are also available from many manufacturers. Although the "standard" PTCA balloon is 20 mm in length, long balloons (30 and 40-mm) and short balloons (8, 9, 10, 13, 15-mm) are also available. Long balloons are particularly useful for long segments of diffuse disease, ostial lesions, and angulated lesions, whereas short balloons are useful for very focal lesions and for adjunctive PTCA after stenting.

6. **Accessories.** Y-adapters attach to the guiding catheter and provide a means of maintaining hemostatic control while advancing interventional hardware and injecting contrast. Standard adapters consist of two channels (one for PTCA hardware, the other for contrast); a three-channel adapter is useful for bifurcation angioplasty. It is important to verify that accessories such as Y-adapters, guidewire introducers, and torque devices can accommodate planned devices and guidewires.

7. **Transfer and Infusion Catheters.** A variety of end-hole transfer catheters can be used for guidewire exchanges; sideholes are usually absent. Infusion catheters and wires are designed for selective drug infusion, and can be used as transfer catheters; most contain multiple sideholes and variable infusion lengths.

8. **Coating.** There are a variety of lubricious coatings for guidewires, guiding catheters, and balloon catheters which reduce friction, facilitate advancement of hardware, and enhance lesion crossing. Examples include hydrophilic polymer, silicone, and PTFE.

POSTPROCEDURAL CONSIDERATIONS

A. **TRIAGE AND MONITORING.** After an uncomplicated procedure, patients are observed for 12-24 hours in a skilled nursing telemetry unit. If the intervention was complicated by persistent dissection, prolonged hypotension, hemodynamic compromise, serious bleeding, or vascular complications, a longer period of observation may be prudent. A 12-lead ECG is obtained immediately after the case and the following morning to identify silent ischemia and new conduction disturbances, and to serve as a new baseline if chest pain recurs. We routinely obtain a complete blood count, CPK, and creatinine 12-24 hours post-procedure to identify potential complications.

B. **COMPLICATIONS.** Recurrent chest pain is not uncommon after intervention. The decision to return to the catheterization laboratory is based on the character of the chest pain and the presence of ECG changes (particularly when compared to pre-PTCA) (Chapter 20). Mild hypotension may be caused by medications (sedatives, nitrates, calcium antagonists, beta blockers) and volume depletion

(NPO status, contrast-induced diuresis); hypotension from these causes should respond promptly to saline administration. Postprocedural hypotension may also be caused by more serious conditions such as acute vessel closure, retroperitoneal bleeding, coronary perforation and tamponade, or sepsis. It is important to systematically exclude concomitant non-cardiac causes of hypotension even if acute closure is present. The recognition, diagnosis, and management of acute closure are reviewed in Chapter 20.

C. **POST-PTCA PHARMACOTHERAPY.** If a good final result has been obtained (< 30% stenosis, normal flow, absence of significant dissection or thrombus), additional heparin is not recommended. However, if a suboptimal angiographic result is obtained, the ideal regimen is unknown. We empirically administer intravenous nitroglycerin (30-100 mcg/min) until the vascular sheaths have been discontinued, followed by oral or transdermal nitrates for 1-6 months and aspirin (325 mg PO QD) indefinitely. Platelet receptor antagonists and other adjunctive medications are discussed in Chapter 34. Risk factor modification including the use of antihypertensive and antidyslipidemic agents is discussed in Chapter 41. Antiplatelet therapy for stent patients is discussed in Chapter 26.

D. **SHEATH REMOVAL, AMBULATION, AND PATIENT DISCHARGE.** Femoral sheaths are removed 4-6 hours after discontinuing heparin; if thrombolytics have been given, the fibrinogen level should be > 150 mg/dL prior to sheath removal. When the ACT is 140-160 seconds, the sheaths are pulled and the site meticulously compressed until bleeding stops (usually 30-45 minutes). In patients receiving warfarin, administration of fresh frozen plasma or use of an arterial closure device is recommended prior to sheath removal if the INR > 2.0; parenteral vitamin K is not recommended, due to the risk of inducing a hypercoagulable state and difficulty in achieving subsequent therapeutic anticoagulation. The use of special femoral compression and arterial closure devices is described in Chapter 25. Patients are kept recumbent in bed for a minimum of one hour for each French size of the arterial sheath (e.g., 6F = 6 hrs, 10F = 10 hrs). The evaluation and management of a new bruit, pulsatile mass, or loss of distal pulses is discussed in Chapter 25. The majority of uncomplicated patients are discharged within 24 hours after the procedure; the patient is instructed to immediately report any new or recurrent symptoms.

* * * * *

BRACHIAL AND RADIAL APPROACH
TO CORONARY INTERVENTION

2

Steven L. Almany, M.D.
Steven J. Yakubov, M.D.
Barry S. George, M.D.

Percutaneous revascularization via the brachial or radial approach is useful as an alternative to the femoral approach or when the femoral approach is undesirable or impossible.[1-3] Brachial cutdown requires considerable expertise not routinely obtained in most training programs. More recently, radial artery cannulation has been introduced for diagnostic and interventional catheterization, and does not require cutdown techniques. Successful mastery of these alternative approaches greatly increases the range of options available to the interventionalist, and in selected cases, may increase the comfort, safety, and efficacy of catheter-based intervention.

A. **PROCEDURAL OVERVIEW**. The selection of access site (femoral, brachial, radial) is mostly determined by operator preference, although there are advantages and disadvantages to each technique (Tables 2.1, 2.2).[4] Overall, less than 3% of angioplasty procedures are performed via the brachial or radial route. However, given the important role of potent new antithrombin and antiplatelet agents, which increase the risk of bleeding complications, it is possible that brachial and radial techniques may become more widely used.

Table 2.1. Comparison of Femoral, Brachial, and Radial Catheterization Techniques

	Femoral	Brachial	Radial
Physician Factors			
Training	Common	Uncommon	Uncommon
Experience	Extensive	Minimal	Minimal
Catheter manipulation	Easy	More difficult	More difficult
Radiation exposure	Less	More	More
Superselective intubation	Difficult	Easy	Difficult
Complications			
Bleeding	More common	Less common	Less common
Loss of pulse	Less common	More common	More common
Transfusion	More common	Less common	Uncommon
Surgical repair	Uncommon	Uncommon	Uncommon
Technical Factors			
Percutaneous	Yes	Yes	Yes
Cutdown/repair	No	Yes	No
Repeated access	Yes	Limited	Limited
Bedrest > 8 hours	Common	Not necessary	Not necessary

Table 2.2. Advantages and Disadvantages of the Femoral and Radial Approach

Approach	Advantages	Disadvantages
Femoral approach	• Long history of use • Technically easy access • Availability of equipment • Larger caliber vessel • Facilitates larger devices	• Strict bed rest required (1 hr per French size) • Closure devices are costly • More vascular complications, transfusions, neuropathy, urinary retention
Radial approach	• Dual blood supply • Applicable to patients with severe aorto-iliac disease, back pain, obesity • Earlier ambulation • No closure device needed • Lower equipment costs • Vascular complications less frequent • Patient preference	• Operator unfamiliarity with anatomy and equipment • Small vessel size • Fewer equipment options • Learning curve • Radial artery spasm is common

1. **Cutdown Approach to Brachial Artery Access (Figure 2.1)**

    a. **Cutdown Technique.** A variety of techniques have been used for brachial artery access.[3,5,6] Regardless of the approach, strict sterile technique (cap, gown, mask) is essential to limit infection. We have found the following technique to be simple and reliable:

    • Sterilize the antecubital fossa with a povidone-iodine solution

    • Anesthetize the area just above the elbow crease over the brachial pulse with a subdermal injection of 2% lidocaine

    • Make a horizontal incision (0.75 to 1.5 inches) over the brachial artery

    • Use a Wheatlander retractor and curved hemostat to carefully perform blunt dissection and isolate the brachial artery

    • Identify the artery just below the bicipital aponeurosis and carefully separate other soft tissue from the artery. Extreme care should be taken to avoid injury to the median nerve

    • Retract a 1-inch segment of brachial artery to the skin surface using curved or right-angle hemostats

    • Place cotton umbilical tapes under the artery proximally and distally for hemostatic control

- With traction on the proximal tape, inject 3000-5000 units of dilute heparin into the distal brachial artery using a 22-gauge needle (or a 22-gauge angiocath after the arteriotomy is created)

- Create a vertical arteriotomy (3-4 mm) using a No. 11 blade. Use of a 6-8F arterial sheath and a 0.035" guidewire permits easy exchange of guiding catheters for PTCA, stent implantation, and other interventional devices

b. Brachial Artery Repair (Figure 2.1)
- Maintain traction on the proximal and distal umbilical tapes while removing the sheath; traction may be released slightly to ensure flow in antegrade and retrograde directions

- Repair the brachial artery arteriotomy with 6-0 or 7-0 prolene using interrupted sutures placed 1 mm apart. Meticulous attention to suture technique is necessary to achieve complete hemostasis; subdermal oozing may be managed with gentle pressure, electrocautery, topical thrombin or Gelfoam

- Close the skin with interrupted silk sutures or an absorbable subcuticular repair. Gentle pressure over the arteriotomy may be necessary if oozing persists despite adequate arterial repair

- If an adequate radial artery pulse is not obtained, consider revision of the arteriotomy and Fogarty catheter embolectomy; liquid hematoma is manually "milked" from the antecubital fossa at this time to decrease the risk of brachial artery or median nerve compression

Table 2.3. Contraindications to Radial Artery Access

Absolute Contraindications
    Abnormal Allen test*
    Known upper extremity arterial occlusive disease
    Need for large sheaths ($\geq$ 8F)
    Raynaud's phenomenon
    Buerger's disease
    Need for radial artery as a conduit for bypass or dialysis

Relative Contraindications
    Contralateral IMA graft

* We prefer the modified Allen test using plethysmography and oximetry (see text)

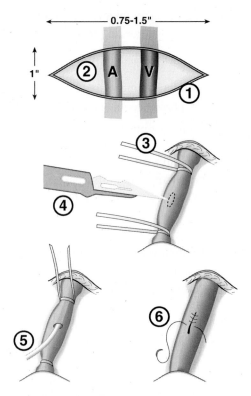

Figure 2.1. Brachial Artery Access: Cutdown Technique

1. Horizontal incision 1 cm above antecubital crease
2. Blunt dissection to expose brachial artery (A) and vein (V)
3. Tag the artery with umbilical tape and the vein with 3-0 silk
4. With traction on proximal tape, create arteriotomy
5. Insert vascular sheath and catheter
6. Repair brachial artery with 6-0 prolene (interrupted sutures)

2. **Percutaneous Approach to Brachial Artery Access (Figure 2.2).** Local sterilization and anesthesia are identical to the cutdown technique. After careful palpation of the brachial pulse, a modified Seldinger or micropuncture technique is used to cannulate the brachial artery. Usually, a 6-8F sheath can be inserted without difficulty.

3. **Radial Artery Approach (Figure 2.2).** Contraindications to radial access are listed in Table 2.3. Although either radial artery may be used, access via the left radial artery is preferred because of better engagement of the coronary ostia. Modifications in technique continue to evolve, but the following technique is commonly employed:
   a. **Perform the Allen Test.** The Allen test is used to assess the presence and adequacy of a dual arterial circulation to the hand prior to radial artery cannulation. It is performed by

simultaneously compressing both the radial and ulnar artery of the same hand for 30-60 seconds, followed by release of the ulnar artery (Figure 2.3). The test is considered normal (i.e., good dual blood supply present) when hand color returns to normal within 10 seconds after release of the ulnar artery. A more objective assessment of the arterial circulation can be obtained by using a *modified* Allen test. Instead of relying on hand color, this test uses a pulse oximeter on the index finger or thumb for continuous assessment of the vascular integrity of the radial/ulnar system. A persistent fall in oxygen saturation during ulnar artery release indicates an abnormal response; radial access should not be used. In patients who require a second procedure through the same radial site, it may be helpful to perform a *reverse* Allen test. In this situation, the physician releases pressure over the radial artery to detect asymptomatic proximal radial artery occlusion. Patients with an abnormal reverse Allen test should not undergo a repeat transradial procedure from that site.

b. Radial Artery Cannulation Technique
- Abduct the arm to 70° and hyperextend the wrist. The wrist should be adequately "cocked" to facilitate arterial access; this can be accomplished with either a small towel, rolled gauze, or a splint-like device (Accumed Systems, Inc.). The armboard should allow access at a 45-degree angle from the patient, and then allow the arm and wrist to be placed next to the hip. Specialized radial drapes are now available.

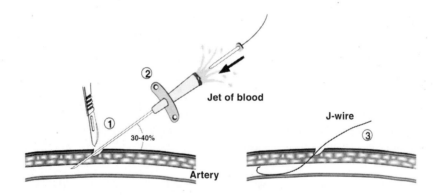

Figure 2.2. Arterial Access: Percutaneous Technique

1. Create a skin-nick inferior to the arterial pulsation
2. Use single-wall puncture technique to enter the vessel lumen
3. After brisk blood return is achieved, insert wire and sheath

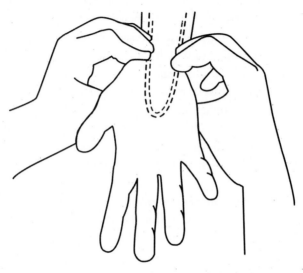

Figure 2.3. The Allen Test

See text for description

- Sterilize and anesthetize the area locally with povidone-iodine solution and a subdermal injection of 2% lidocaine. It is important to cannulate the radial artery 2-3 cm proximal to the flexion crease of the wrist to avoid reticulum and smaller superficial branches, which will be encountered more distally.

- Puncture the radial artery with a 2-cm, 21-gauge needle (micropuncture kit) at a 45° angle, 1 cm from the styloid process. Longer needles may cause the operator to miss the flash of blood as the needle enters the artery.

- Once there is pulsatile blood return, advance a 30-50 cm floppy-tip 0.025" straight or angled guidewire (not J) into the brachial artery.

- Predilate the radial artery with a 4-5F dilator, followed by insertion of a 6-7F introducing sheath over a 0.035" J-guidewire. A 23-cm hydrophilic sheath is preferable to a 10-cm sheath to prevent radial artery spasm and facilitate movement of guiding catheters; intra-arterial nitroglycerin (100-200 mcg) or verapamil (250-500 mcg) delivered through the sheath will minimize spasm. Dilute heparin (5,000-10,000 units) should also be given. Special attention should be directed toward selection of guiding catheters to ensure coaxial alignment and adequate backup (Table 2.4).

Table 2.4. Guiding Catheter Selection for Radial Intervention

Catheter	Comments
Judkins	From the right radial artery, select a curve 0.5 cm smaller than normally used from the femoral approach or use a short-tip guide to engage the LCA. Use a curve 1 cm larger for the RCA. From the left radial artery, standard sizes usually work well
Hockey stick	Can be used to engage the LCA and RCA
Geometric guides	Well-suited for the LCA from the left radial approach
Multipurpose	Well-suited for the LCA, RCA, and vein grafts from either radial artery; MP-A is better suited for RCAs with inferior takeoff, whereas MP-B is better suited for horizontal or superior takeoffs
Kimny	Specifically designed for radial intervention; well-suited for LCA and RCA from either radial artery
Long-tip	New, modified long-tip guiding catheters have been designed for the LCA and RCA from the right radial approach.[33] Similar to geometric guides designed for the femoral approach, these guides derive support from the opposite wall of the aorta
Barbeau	Modified MP-A catheter; best suited for the RCA and vein grafts from the right radial artery

Abbreviations: LCA = left coronary artery; RCA = right coronary artery; MP = multipurpose catheter

c. **Radial Artery Sheath Removal and Hemostasis.** The arterial sheath can removed immediately after completion of most cases. Thereafter, apply a specially-made tourniquet (Hemoband, Radial clamp, Radistop) at the radial puncture site for at least 30 minutes, then gradually release pressure until hemostasis is achieved. If a special tourniquet is not available, manual compression is adequate. Following hemostasis, apply a pressure bandage and instruct the patient to restrict wrist movement for 6 hours. The patient may ambulate when sedation wears off.

d. **Important Anatomic Tips.** It is important to review the pertinent anatomy and anatomic variants. In one study of transradial intervention, routine ultrasound demonstrated radial artery anomalies is 9.5%, but transradial intervention failed or was not attempted in only 2.6% of patients[34] (Table 2.5). In most patients the brachial artery divides into the radial and ulnar arteries just below the elbow, which pass along the outer and inner aspects of the forearm, respectively. In some cases the radial artery originates from the upper brachial or axillary artery. At the wrist, the ulnar artery divides into two branches that join the radial artery to form the deep and superficial palmar arches. It is not uncommon for a patient to display adequate ulnar and radial pulses, yet have abnormal plethysmography (or Allen test). Whether this represents true radial or ulnar dominance or incomplete palmar circulation (reported in up to 10-23% of patients) is difficult to ascertain; in any case, patients who display radial or ulnar dominance should not have radial intervention.

Table 2.5. Anatomic Variants of the Radial Artery[34]

Variant	Incidence (%)	Implications for Transradial Intervention (TRI)
Severe tortuosity	5.2	TRI feasible, but guidewire advancement may be difficult
Stenosis	1.7	TRI feasible
Hypoplasia (ulnar dominance)	1.7	Use alternative approach
Radioulnar loop	0.9	Use alternative approach

Table 2.6. Technical Problems During Radial Intervention

Problem	Solution
Difficult access	Obtain access on the first try. The radial artery is prone to spasm and it is common to find a diminished pulse after multiple failed attempts. If this occurs, options include: • Wait before trying again • Cannulate artery more proximally • Give nitroglycerin IV or SL • Have the patient clench and open hand • Use another site
Difficult guidewire movement	After successful access is achieved, it may be difficult to advance the guidewire. Causes include tortuosity, spasm, radial artery occlusion or stenosis, guidewire lodged in a side branch (usually too distal in the artery), abnormal take-off of the radial artery from the brachial artery, or subintimal position. If this occurs, the following options should be tried: • Rotate the needle to change the angle of the bevel • Perform a radial angiogram • Use a hydrophilic guidewire • Try a 0.018-inch PTCA wire • Give vasodilators through the needle and then try to readvance the wire
Difficulty removing sheath	This is an uncommon problem (especially with a hydrophilic sheath) but may be seen in smaller patients with intense radial spasm. Options include: • Give vasodilators and pain medications • Gently rotate the sheath upon removal • Hold the skin distal to the incision to avoid "buckling"
Difficult guide placement	Guiding catheter technique differs between radial and femoral approaches. Several maneuvers facilitate guide placement: • Advance the guide below the ostium (especially when approaching the left coronary artery) and push down on the catheter so the tip bends up toward the left main. Pull the catheter back to allow the tip to cannulate the ostium • Always use an exchange-length wire when changing catheters to avoid the need to recross the great vessels • Have the patient take a deep breath to facilitate catheter movement

　　e.　Troubleshooting. Common technical problems during radial intervention and their solutions are described in Table 2.6.

　　f.　Post-Procedural Management. Our policy is to pull radial lines immediately after intervention; hemostasis is rarely a problem. In general, the hemostasis band is left on for 30 minutes after a diagnostic procedure and 60 minutes after an interventional procedure (even with platelet IIb/IIIa receptor antagonists). If bleeding persists, the band is left in place for another 30 minutes. Persistent bleeding may be due to a lacerated artery; an inflatable blood pressure cuff can be used to control bleeding while a surgical consult is obtained. Patients who undergo diagnostic angiography can be discharged within two hours, but should be instructed to avoid wrist flexion and extension for the remainder of the day. Local swelling is treated with ice and analgesics. Rebleeding is treated with hand elevation and local pressure.

B.　SPECIAL INDICATIONS FOR BRACHIAL AND RADIAL TECHNIQUES

　1.　Peripheral Vascular Disease. Femoral artery access may be difficult (morbid obesity, extensive post-operative scarring, severe peripheral vascular disease), impossible (aortic occlusion), or relatively contraindicated (coagulopathy). For these patients, the brachial and radial techniques allow alternative approaches for coronary angiography, peripheral angiography, and percutaneous intervention. Many operators routinely perform diagnostic lower extremity angiography through the brachial approach; renal angiography is easier and requires less contrast.

　2.　Patient Preference. Brachial and radial artery angioplasty allow immediate ambulation, which may be important in patients with severe back pain aggravated by prolonged bed rest. A single-center randomized trial reported a strong patient preference for the radial approach compared to the femoral approach.[30]

　3.　Need for Uninterrupted Anticoagulation. Brachial artery repair and radial catheterization allow continuous anticoagulation (with heparin or warfarin) and infusions of glycoprotein platelet receptor antagonists, and have been used successfully in select patients undergoing primary stenting for acute MI.[31]

　4.　Difficult Internal Mammary Artery Cannulation. In some cases, selective angiography of the internal mammary artery cannot be accomplished via the femoral route because of severe tortuosity of the subclavian or brachiocephalic artery. In these cases, selective angiography (and intervention, if necessary) can usually be performed via the ipsilateral brachial or radial artery (right Judkins or internal mammary artery catheter) or contralateral brachial artery (Simmons catheter).

　5.　Severe Coronary Artery Tortuosity. The left brachial approach facilitates deep intubation with the guiding catheter, which is particularly useful when severe tortuosity of the target vessel precludes advancement of interventional hardware from the femoral approach.

Table 2.7. Preferred Guiding Catheters from the Brachial Approach

Target Vessel	Preferred Guide(s)
Right Coronary Artery	
Right or left brachial approach	Right Judkins (especially good fit from the left brachial approach); Amplatz (may have greater difficulty navigating the subclavian artery and aortic arch); Multipurpose
Left Coronary Artery*	
Right brachial approach	Amplatz (excellent support and maneuverability)
Left brachial approach	Left Judkins (first choice), Amplatz, Voda
Saphenous Vein Grafts	
Right or left brachial approach	Amplatz, Multipurpose
Internal Mammary Grafts	
Ipsilateral	Internal mammary (first choice), right Judkins
Contralateral	Simmons, Castillo

* Due to the orientation of the left subclavian artery and aortic arch, the left guide catheter should be 0.5F smaller than the typical corresponding femoral guide

C. INTERVENTIONAL CONSIDERATIONS

1. **Guide Catheter Selection (Tables 2.4, 2.7)**

2. **Non-Balloon Devices.** Rotational atherectomy and stents can be safely and easily performed via the brachial technique as long as the appropriate sheath can be placed in the brachial artery.[7] Elective PTCA or stenting via the brachial or radial approach is particularly appealing because it can decrease length of stay, allow uninterrupted full-dose anticoagulation, minimize bed rest and immobility, and decrease the incidence of bleeding and vascular complications.[8,9,27-29] Insertion of an IABP via the brachial artery is feasible, but may predispose to infection and vascular injury if the IABP is needed for several days.

D. COMPLICATIONS

1. **Brachial Approach.** In general, the incidence of peripheral vascular complications associated with brachial cutdown and percutaneous femoral techniques are similar, including significant hematoma (1.3%), retroperitoneal hemorrhage (0.4%), false aneurysm (0.4%), vessel occlusion (0.1%), infection (0.1%), and cholesterol embolization (0.1%).[10] However, femoral vascular complications are usually associated with greater patient morbidity.[8] Compiled data from the TAMI trials show comparable success rates using brachial and femoral access sites, but complication rates were slightly lower from the brachial site.[11-14]

2. **Radial Approach (Table 2.8).** In a study of 1300 coronary interventions from the radial approach, vascular access complications occurred in 1.1% (mainly hematomas); only 0.15% of patients required surgery and no blood transfusions were needed.[20] In a study of 100 patients treated with

elective PTCA from the radial artery, there were no major cardiac complications, blood transfusions, or vascular surgical repairs,[15] although the incidence of stroke was 2% in one report.[16] Other studies have reported asymptomatic radial artery occlusion in 6-10%,[15-17,25] although 40-60% spontaneously recanalize after 1 month.[17,35] In centers with extensive experience in radial and femoral arterial access, bleeding and vascular complications were virtually eliminated, length of stay was shorter, and hospital costs were lower after transradial stenting, despite use of femoral closure devices.[32] Risk factors for radial artery occlusion after intervention include radial artery diameter < 2 mm by ultrasound, mismatch between the sheath size and radial artery diameter, and diabetes.[36] The ACCESS study was a prospective randomized study of PTCA with 6F catheters using the transradial, transbrachial, and transfemoral approaches (Table 2.9). Analysis of 900 patients revealed more access-site failures and fewer bleeding complications after transradial PTCA, although PTCA success and cardiac events were similar among all three approaches.[18] Another prospective randomized study of transradial and transfemoral PTCA with 6F catheters revealed fewer vascular complications, shorter length of stay, and lower hospital charges using the radial approach (Table 2.10).[19]

Table 2.8. Results of Transradial Intervention

Study	Technique	N	Success (%)	In-hospital Outcome (%) MACE	Bleeding
ESPRIT[37] (2001)	TRI-stent	144	-	11.1*	0.7
	TFI-stent	1886	-	9.4*	6.6
Mann[32] (2000)	TRI-stent	109	100	1.9	0
	TFI-stent	109	99	1.9	3.7
Byers[35] (1999)	TRI-stent	100	100	0	0
Saito[21] (1998)	TRI	1360	97.7	1.0	0.2
	TFI	793	98.1	2.0	3.3
Mann[23] (1998)	TRI-stent	68	96	0	0
	TFI-stent	77	96	0	4
Benit[22] (1997)	TBI-stent	36	-	0	0
	TFI-stent	55	-	8	6
	TRI-stent	50	-	2	2
Wu[24] (1997)	TRI	75	91	7	-
El-Shiekh[25] (1997)	TRI-stent	38	97	3.3	0
Lotan[26] (1997)	TRI	250	94.8	2.4	0.4

Abbreviations: ESPRIT = Enhanced Suppression of the Platelet IIb/IIIa Receptor with Integrilin Therapy; MACE = major adverse cardiac events (death, Q-wave MI, CABG, rePTCA); TBI = transbrachial intervention; TFI = transfemoral intervention; TRI = transradial intervention; - = not reported
* Includes non-Q-wave MI

Table 2.9. Results of ACCESS: A Randomized Comparison of PTCA Approaches [18]

	Transradial	Transbrachial	Transfemoral
No. patients	300	300	300
PTCA success (%)	91.7	90.7	90.7
Failed access (%)	7.0	4.3	0.3*
Major bleeding (%)	0	2.3	2.0**
Cardiac events (%)	6.7	8.3	5.3

ACCESS = A Randomized Comparison of Transradial, Brachial, and Femoral Coronary Angioplasty with 6F Guide Catheters
* $p \leq 0.001$
** $p = 0.03$

Table 2.10. Randomized Study of Transradial and Transfemoral PTCA [19]

	Transradial	Transfemoral
No. patients	73	95
PTCA success (%)	95	97
Emergency CABG (%)	1	0
Vascular complications (%)	0	4*
Length of stay (days)	2.1	2.6*
Hospital charge ($)	14,374	15,796*

Abbreviations: CABG = coronary artery bypass surgery
* $p < 0.05$

* * * * *

REFERENCES

1. Sones FM, Shirey EK. Cine coronary arteriography. Mod Conc Cardiovasc Dis 1962;31:735.

2. Judkins MP. Selective coronary arteriography: A percutaneous transfemoral technique. Radiology 1967;89:815-824.

3. Stertzer SH. Brachial approach to transluminal coronary angioplasty. In *Angioplasty* (New York, McGraw-Hill), 1986, pp 260-294.

4. Yakubov SJ, George, BS. Coronary Intervention: Brachial Technique. In *Interventional Cardiovascular Medicine: Principles and Practice* (New York, Churchill-Livingston), 1994, pp 451-64.

5. Huepler F. Coronary arteriography and left ventriculography: Sones technique. In *Coronary Arteriography and Angioplasty* (New York, McGraw-Hill), 1985, pp 137-181.

6. Kamada RO, Fergusson DJ, Itagaki RK. Percutaneous entry of the brachial artery for transluminal coronary angioplasty. Cathet Cardiovasc Diagn 1988;15:132-133.

7. George BS. Brachial technique to intervention. In *Textbook of Interventional Cardiology*, Vol. 2 (Philadelphia, W.B. Saunders Company), 1994, pp 549-564.

8. Kiemeneij F, Laarman, GJ. Percutaneous transradial artery approach for coronary stent implantation. Cath Cardiovasc Diagn 1993;30:173-178.

9. Keimeneij F, Laarman GJ, Slagboom T, Stella P. Transradial Palmaz-Schatz coronary stenting on an outpatient basis: Results of a prospective pilot study. J Invas Cardiol 1995;7:5A-11A.

10. Johnson LW, Esenta P, Giambartolomei A, et al. Peripheral vascular complications of coronary angioplasty by the femoral and brachial techniques. Cath Cardiovasc Diagn 1994;31:165-172.

11. George BS, Candela RJ, Topol EJ, et al. The brachial approach to emergency cardiac catheterization during thrombolytic therapy for acute myocardial infarction. Cathet Cardiovasc Diagn 1990;20:221-226.

12. Topol EJ, Califf RM, George BS, et al. A randomized trial of immediate vs. delayed elective angioplasty after intravenous tissue plasminogen activator in acute myocardial infarction. N Engl J Med 1987;317:581-588.

13. Topol EJ, Califf RM, George BS, et al. Coronary arterial thrombolysis with combined infusion of recombinant tissue-type plasminogen activator and urokinase in patients with acute myocardial infarction. Circulation 1988;77:1100-1107.

14. Topol EJ, George BS, Kereiakes DJ, et al. A randomized controlled trial of intravenous tissue plasminogen activator and early intravenous heparin in acute myocardial infarction. Circulation 1989;79:281-286.

15. Kiemeneij, F, Laarman GJ, de Melker E. Transradial artery coronary angioplasty. Am Heart J 1995;129:1-7.

16. Lotan C, Hasin Y, Mosseri M, Rozenman Y, et al. Transradial approach to coronary angiography and angioplasty. Am J Cardiol 1995;76:164-167.

17. Stella P, Kiemeneij F, Laarman G, et al. Incidence and outcome of radial artery occlusion following transradial artery coronary angioplasty. Circulation 1995;92:I-225.

18. Kiemeneij F, Laarman GJ, et al. A randomized comparison of percutaneous transluminal coronary angioplasty by the radial, brachial and femoral approaches: The ACCESS study. J Am Coll Cardiol 1997;29:1269-75.

19. Cubeddu MG, Arrowood ME, Mann JT. Right radial access for PTCA: a prospective study demonstrates reduced complications and hospital charges. Circulation 1995;92:I-662.

20. Fajadet J, Brunel P, Cassagneau B, et al. Transradial approach for interventional coronary procedures: analysis of complications. J Am Coll Cardiol 1996; 27:392A.

21. Saito S. Update on coronary intervention through the radial approach. J Interven Cardiol 1998;11(suppl.):S80-82.

22. Benit E, Missault L, Eeman T, et al. Brachial, radial, or femoral approach for elective Palmaz-Schatz stent implantation: A randomized comparison. Cathet Cardiovasc Diagn 1997;41:124-130.

23. Mann T, Cubeddu G, Bowen J, Schneider JE, et al. Stenting in acute coronary syndromes: A comparison of radial versus femoral access sites. J Am Coll Cardiol 1998;32:572-576.

24. Wu CJ, Lo PH, Chang KC, et al. Transradial coronary angiography and angioplasty in Chinese patients. Cathet Cardiovasc Diagn 1997;40:159-163.

25. El-Shiekh RA, Burket MW, Mouhaffel A, et al. U.S. experience of transradial coronary stenting utilizing Palmaz-Schatz stents. Cathet Cardiovasc Diagn 1997; 40:166-169.

26. Lotan C, Hasin Y, Salmoirago E, et al. The radial artery: an applicable approach to complex coronary angioplasty. J Invas Cardiol 1997;9:518-522.

27. Barbeau GR, Carrier G, Ferland S, Larriviere MM. Transradial approach for coronary angiography, angioplasty and stent delivery: Procedural results. Circulation 1995;92:I-196.

28. Kiemeneij F, Laarman GJ, Slagboom T, van der Wieken R. Transradial coronary stenting in outpatients. Circulation 1995;92:I-535.

29. Vallabhan RC, Anwar A, Bret JR, et al. Radial artery access for cardiac catheterization and coronary angioplasty. Circulation 1995;92:I-602.

30. Cooper CJ, El-Shiekh RA, Cohen DJ, et al. Effect of transradial access on quality of life and cost of cardiac catheterization: A randomized comparison. Am Heart J 1999;138:429-436.

31. Ochiai M, Isshiki T, Toyaizumi H, et al. Efficacy of transradial primary stenting in patients with acute myocardial infarction. Am J Cardiol 1999;83:966-968.

32. Mann T, Cowper PA, Peterson ED, et al. Transradial coronary stenting: comparison with femoral access closed with an arterial suture device. Cathet Cardiovasc Interven 2000;49:150-156.

33. Ochial M, Ikari Y, Yamaguchi T, et al. New long-tip guiding catheters designed for right transradial coronary intervention. Cathet Cardiovasc Inter 2000;49:218-224.

34. Yokoyama N, Takeshita S, Ochiai M. Anatomic variations of the radial artery in patients undergoing transradial coronary intervention. Cathet Cardiovasc Interven

2000;49:357-362.

35. Byers J, Brown S, Robertson R, Smucker M. Procedural outcome and clinical results after stent deployment from the radial approach. Am J Cardiol 1999;84:1088-1090.

36. Nagai S, Abe S, Sato T, et al. Ultrasonic assessment of vascular complications in coronary angiography and angioplasty after transradial approach. Am J Cardiol 1999:83:180-186.

37. O'Shea JC, Mann T, Hellkamp A, et al. Fewer bleeding complications with comparable efficacy with the transradial approach in coronary artery stenting: An analysis of the ESPRIT trial. J Am Coll Cardiol 2001;1123(29):33A.

SINGLE-VESSEL AND MULTIVESSEL INTERVENTION

3

Daniel J. Diver, M.D.
Mark S. Freed, M.D.
Robert D. Safian, M.D.

SINGLE-VESSEL DISEASE

A. **BALLOON ANGIOPLASTY.** Patients with single-vessel coronary artery disease (CAD) have excellent long-term survival (annual mortality < 1%), but may have persistent angina, decreased functional capacity and employment status, and need for long-term medical therapy. Observational and randomized studies (Table 3.1) provide insight into the benefits of medical therapy, percutaneous revascularization, and bypass surgery (Table 3.2). Revascularization guidelines for patients with single-vessel disease and stable angina depend on symptom status and the amount of jeopardized myocardium (Figure 3.1). Two older randomized trials (ACME, MASS) compared medical therapy to percutaneous or surgical revascularization in patients with single vessel disease, good LV function, and stable angina (Table 3.3). Compared to medical therapy, PTCA resulted in less angina and better exercise performance, but did not reduce death or MI.[5,69] For patients with severe stenosis of the proximal LAD, LIMA-CABG resulted in better event-free survival than PTCA or medical therapy.[69] More recently, the AVERT (Atorvastatin vs. Revascularization Treatments) trial demonstrated a 36% reduction in ischemic events at 18 months in patients treated with aggressive lipid-lowering therapy vs. PTCA (mainly due to less target lesion revascularization),[65] and RITA-2 reported better infarct-free survival at 2.7 years in medically-treated patients with 1- or 2-vessel disease vs. PTCA.[97] Anginal status was better in PTCA patients in both AVERT and RITA-2. Taken collectively, these data suggest that compared to medical therapy, PTCA results in better anginal status and exercise performance, but results in more late revascularization and possibly more ischemic events. In patients with severe stenosis of the proximal LAD, CABG results in better survival than PTCA or medical therapy. Single-vessel disease associated with acute coronary syndromes is discussed in Chapter 5.

B. **STENTS.** In a randomized study comparing stenting vs. PTCA in 120 patients with isolated proximal LAD disease, stenting resulted in less angiographic restenosis (10% vs. 40%) and better event-free survival (87% vs. 70%) at 1-year.[53] The New York State PTCA Registry evaluated early and late outcomes after PTCA and stenting in nearly 20,000 patients with single-vessel intervention,[56] and observed better outcomes in stent patients with regard to in-hospital CABG and 2-year event-free survival (death, CABG, or repeat PTCA). Compared to PTCA, 2-year mortality after stenting was better in diabetics, target vessels in the RCA or left circumflex, and intervention within 24 hours of acute MI. Although randomized trials of PTCA vs. CABG for single-vessel disease (ACME, RITA) did not routinely incorporate stents, the randomized SIMA (Stenting vs. Internal Mammary Artery) trial

Table 3.1. Medical Treatment and Revascularization for Single-Vessel Disease: Acute and Long-term Outcomes

Series	Modality	N	Success (%)	In-hospital (%) D / QMI / CABG	Follow-up (%) Yrs	D / MI / TLR	Other
Bossi[111] (2001)	PCI (Stents 79%)	224	-	0 / 1.8 / 1.3	1.6	2.6 / 1.3 / 16.5	Stents had better long-term outcome
Thiele[112] (2001)	Stent (Prox. LAD)	110	-	-		-	In-stent restenosis (27%); stenosis > 50% at distal anastomosis (16%); relief of angina better with MIDCAB
	MIDCAB (Prox. LAD)	110	-	-	0.5	-	
SIMA[94]* (2000)	Stent (prox. LAD)	62	98	1.6 / 0 / 0	2.4	2 / 5 / 24	Composite primary endpoint (D, MI, or TLR) at 2.4 yrs lower in CABG-IMA group (7% vs. 31%, p < 0.004)
	CABG-IMA (prox. LAD)	59	98	0 / 0 / -		4 / 4 / 0	
Espinol-Klein[70] (2000)	Medicine (CASS)	107	-	-	10	18 / 10 / -	PTCA cohort from 1983-86 compared to medical and CABG patients reported in CASS
	CABG (CASS)	107	-	-		15 / 16 / -	
	PTCA	509	78	-		14 / 9 / -	
O'Keefe[61] (1999)	PTCA (LAD)	469	-	1.1 / 0.6 / 0.4	2.3	3.9 / - / 30	Results of PCI worse in proximal LAD vs. mid-LAD
	Stent (LAD)	137		0 / 0.7 / 0		2.6 / - / 24	
	CABG-IMA (LAD)	98		0 / 1.0 / 0		1.1 / - / 5	
AVERT[65]† (1999)	Medicine	164	-	-	1.5	0.6 / 2.4 / 12	Any ischemic event (medicine 13% vs. PTCA 21%, p = 0.048). Anginal status better with PTCA. Atorvastatin with 46% reduction in LDL (mean = 77 mg/dL)
	PTCA	177	-	-		0.6 / 2.4 / 17	
MASS[69] (1999)	PTCA	72	96	-	5	5.6 / 5.6 / 30.3	Asymptomatic at follow-up (PTCA 65% vs. CABG 73% vs. medicine 26%)
	CABG-IMA	70		-		2.8 / 4.3 / 0	
	Medicine	72		-		2.8 / 4.2 / 16.7	
RITA[1,62]* (1999)	PTCA + devices	68	94	0 / 0 / 3	50	1.5++ / 15 / 38	Class 0-1 angina (PTCA 74% vs. CABG 71%); exercise duration similar; ≥ 2 antianginals (PTCA 35% vs. CABG 26%)
	CABG-IMA	66**		1 / 0 / -		1.5++ / 4 / 9	
	PTCA	456	-	-	4.7	3.8 / 5.1 / 40.5	Angina at 3 years (PTCA 17.5% vs CABG 16.1%)
	CABG			-		3.8 / 10.8 / 9.5	

Table 3.1. Medical Treatment and Revascularization for Single-Vessel Disease: Acute and Long-term Outcomes

Series	Modality	N	Success (%)	In-hospital (%) D / QMI / CABG	Follow-up (%) Yrs	Follow-up (%) D / MI / TLR	Other
Mark[3] (1994)	Medicine	2919	-	-	5	6 / - / -	Class 0-1 angina (PTCA 81% vs. CABG 90%); hospital stay (PTCA 3 days vs. CABG 8.7 days)
	PTCA	1693		-		5 / - / -	
	CABG	339		-		7 / - / -	
Cameron[4] (1994)	PTCA	254	93	- / 3 / 3	5.5	3 / 8 / 33	
	CABG	104		1 / - / -		7 / 2 / 1	
ACME[5,6]* (1992)	Medicine	107	82	-	0.5	1 / 3 / 1	Asymptomatic (medicine 46% vs. PTCA 63%); increase in exercise duration (medicine 0.5 min. vs. PTCA 2.1 min)
	PTCA	105		0 / 1 / 2		0 / 5 / 23	
	Medicine				4+++	11 / 7 / 38	Unstable angina (medicine 27% vs. PTCA 7%)
	PTCA					10 / 8 / 14	
Frierson[7] (1992)	PTCA	537	96	0.4 / 0.9 / 3	4.6	5.2 / 2.5 / 19	Asymptomatic 76%

Abbreviations: D = death; QMI = Q-wave myocardial infarction; CABG = coronary artery bypass grafting; TLR = target lesion revascularization; IMA = internal mammary artery; MIDCAB = minimally invasive bypass surgery; PCI = percutaneous coronary intervention

Acronyms: ACME = Angioplasty Compared to Medicine Trial; AVERT = Atorvastatin Versus Revascularization Treatment Trial; MASS = Medicine, Angioplasty or Surgery Study; RITA = Randomized Intervention Treatment of Angina; SIMA = Stenting vs. Internal Mammary Artery Trial

*   Randomized trial

**   6 patients assigned to CABG group actually treated by PTCA

+   Class 0 = asymptomatic, Class 1 = angina during strenuous exercise

++   Cardiac death

+++ Follow-up events occurring between 6 months to 4 years after randomization

†   AVERT trial: Patients with 1- or 2-vessel disease, normal LV function, no/mild/moderate symptoms randomized to atorvastatin (80 mg) or PCI + usual medications; stents in 30%.

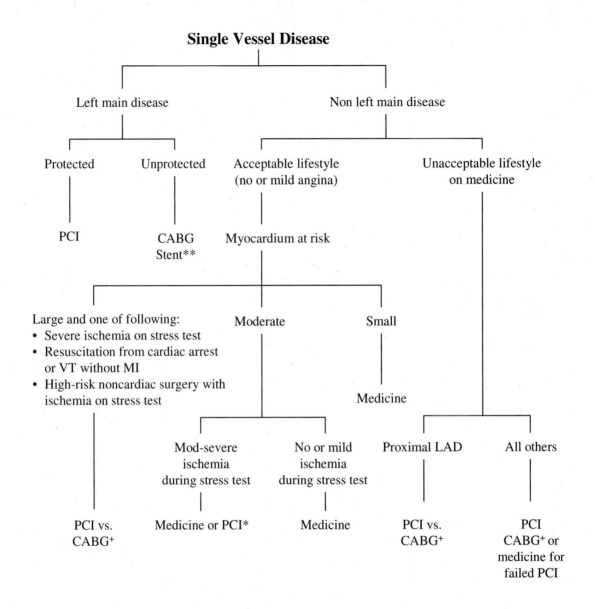

Figure 3.1. Revascularization Guidelines for Single-Vessel Disease and Chronic Angina

PCI = percutaneous coronary intervention; medicine = risk factor modification plus antianginal therapy
*   High-risk occupation (pilot, bus driver) favors PCI; consider CABG for proximal LAD stenosis
**   Non-surgical candidates
+   *Factors tending to favor PCI* = younger age, cerebrovascular disease, severe COPD, illness limiting survival, Type A
      lesion, patient desires to avoid CABG and accepts 20-30% risk of repeat procedures
      Factors tending to favor CABG = severe LV dysfunction, older age, severe mitral regurgitation, diabetes, renal dialysis,
      complex lesion morphology, patient desires to minimize number of procedures

recently reported their results in 123 patients (Table 3.1).[94] Using a composite primary endpoint of death, MI, or TLR, IMA-CABG resulted in better event-free survival at 2.4 years (93% vs. 69%, p < 0.004) due to less TLR (0% vs. 24%); there were no differences in death, MI, functional class, need for antianginal therapy, or quality of life.

Table 3.2. Treatment Strategies for Single-Vessel Disease

Modality	Advantages
Medical therapy	**Advantages over percutaneous revascularization:** • No procedural risk **Advantages over CABG:** • No procedural risk, protracted convalescence, or concern about SVG disease • Severe progression of underlying CAD can be treated with first CABG (as opposed to repeat CABG, which is associated with lower angina-free survival)
Percutaneous revascularization	**Advantages over medical therapy:** • Less angina • Fewer antianginal medications • Better functional capacity • Better quality of life • Fewer late revascularizations **Advantages over CABG:** • Shorter and less expensive hospitalization • Shorter convalescence • Earlier functional recovery and return to work • No concern about SVG disease • Severe progression of underlying CAD can be treated with first CABG (as opposed to repeat CABG, which is associated with lower angina-free survival)
CABG	**Advantages over medical therapy:** • Less angina • Fewer antianginal medications • Better functional capacity • Better quality of life **Advantages over percutaneous revascularization:** • IMA used more often when CABG is elective rather than emergent (for failed PTCA) • Less angina • Fewer antianginal medications • Fewer late revascularizations

Abbreviations: CAD = coronary artery disease; SVG = saphenous vein graft; IMA = internal mammary artery; CABG = coronary artery bypass grafting

MULTIVESSEL DISEASE

A. MULTIVESSEL ANGIOPLASTY IN PATIENTS WITH PRESERVED LV FUNCTION

1. **Randomized Trials of Medical Therapy vs. Revascularization (Table 3.3).** Four randomized trials compared medical therapy to percutaneous or surgical revascularization in patients with multivessel disease, good LV function, and stable angina. These studies are characterized by small sample size, low overall cardiac event rates, and completion before routine availability of stents, GP IIb/IIIa receptor antagonists, and statins. Despite these limitations, revascularization consistently improved anginal status and exercise capacity. In contrast, the impact of revascularization on infarct-free survival varied: two trials showed no difference (AVERT, ACME-2), one showed better survival after revascularization (ACIP), and one showed better survival in medically-treated patients (RITA-2). A recent metanalysis of randomized trials of medical therapy vs. PTCA for patients with stable angina and single- or multivessel disease suggested significant improvement in anginal status in PTCA patients (relative risk 0.70, p < 0.001), but a strong trend towards less death, fatal and non-fatal MI, and need for revascularization in medically-treated patients.[103]

2. **Randomized Trials of PTCA vs. CABG.** To determine the optimal revascularization technique for patients with multivessel disease, more than 4000 patients were randomized in six PTCA vs. CABG trials (Table 3.4). Most of these trials were completed prior to widespread availability of stents and GP IIb/IIIa inhibitors, thus limiting their application to current practice.

   a. **Inclusion and Exclusion Criteria (Table 3.4).** Specific entry criteria differ between each trial; most excluded patients with previous PTCA or CABG, evolving MI, left main disease, or severe non-cardiac illness. *Less than 10% of patients with symptomatic multivessel coronary disease were actually enrolled into these trials*, suggesting that the results of these trials may not be applicable to all patients with multivessel disease.

   b. **Study Design and Baseline Characteristics (Tables 3.5, 3.6).** PTCA was generally confined to diameter stenoses > 50% in vessels > 1.5 mm in diameter supplying viable myocardium and causing ischemia (complete "functional" revascularization). Lesions in small vessels and those supplying nonviable myocardium were generally not dilated. New device intervention was permitted only in CABRI (atherectomy and stents) and BARI (bailout stents). Internal mammary arteries were used in > 75% of CABG patients but in only 37% of patients in GABI. *Most patients enrolled into these trials had 2-vessel disease and preserved LV function.*

c. **In-hospital Outcome (Table 3.7).** In these randomized studies, PTCA success was achieved in 87-92%, with death in 0.7-1.5%, MI in 2.1-6.3%, and emergency CABG in 1.5-10.1%. Mortality rates were similar between PTCA and CABG groups, but PTCA patients had less in-hospital MI and a shorter length of stay. The incidence of these ischemic complications would be considered unacceptably high by contemporary standards utilizing stent techniques.

d. **Late Outcome (Table 3.8)**

   1. **Overall.** Clinical follow-up at 1-5 years revealed no difference in death, MI, or exercise capacity between groups. However, compared to CABG, PTCA patients had more recurrent angina (30-40% vs. 20-25%), greater need for antianginal therapy (66-88% vs. 51-75%), and a 3-10 fold increase in repeat target vessel revascularization (32-54% vs. 2-13%). At least 20% of PTCA patients with multivessel disease required CABG during follow-up. A recent report from BARI suggested better survival at 7 years for CABG patients, and the expected late attrition due to vein graft degeneration was not observed.[67]

   2. **Diabetics.** Results from BARI, the largest of the randomized trials, prompted the NIH to issue a clinical alert in September 1995 regarding excess mortality in diabetics treated by multivessel PTCA; at 5 years, mortality was 35% for PTCA vs. 19% for CABG ($p < 0.01$). The lower mortality after CABG was unrelated to periprocedural mortality (CABG 1.2% vs. PTCA 0.6%), but was explained by a striking reduction in late cardiac mortality (CABG 5.8% vs. PTCA 20.6%, $p = 0.0003$) in diabetics receiving at least one internal mammary graft.[49] Although CABG is often the preferred mode of revascularization for diabetics with multivessel coronary disease who meet the BARI inclusion criteria, BARI data do not reflect the improving results of multivessel angioplasty or stenting.[54] Interestingly, there was no survival difference in diabetic patients with multivessel disease treated with PTCA or CABG in the nonrandomized BARI Registry or Duke University database,[50,51,74] suggesting that it may be possible to select patients for PTCA or CABG without jeopardizing late outcome, even in diabetics. Nevertheless, these results may have profound implications for coronary revascularization, since 20-30% of all multivessel angioplasties are performed on diabetics.

Table 3.3.   **Randomized Trials of Medicine vs. Revascularization for Single and Multivessel Coronary Artery Disease**[100,103]

Study	N	Extent of CAD	Results
COURAGE[99] (1999)	3260	1, 2, 3-VD	In progress
AVERT[65] (1999)	341*	1, 2-VD	Less MACE at 18 months in patients treated with aggressive lipid-lowering therapy (13% vs. 21%, p < 0.05). Anginal status better with PTCA
RITA-2[97] (1997)	1018+	1, 2-VD	Medicine group had better infarct-free survival at 2.7 years (96.7% vs. 93.7, p = 0.02)
ACME-2[95] (1997)	101+	2-VD	Similar clinical outcomes
ACIP[96] (1995)	558+	1, 2, 3-VD	Revascularization (PTCA or CABG) was associated with better infarct-free survival at 2 years than medical therapy
MASS[69] (1995)	214+	1-VD (proximal LAD)	CABG (LIMA) had better EFS at 3 years compared to PTCA or medical therapy (97% vs. 76% vs. 83%, p < 0.01); CABG and PTCA resulted in less angina and better exercise performance than medicine
ACME[5] (1992)	212**+	1-VD	Similar infarct-free survival (5% vs. 4%) at 6 months; PTCA resulted in better exercise tolerance and fewer medications, but more CABG (7% vs. 0%, p < 0.01)

Abbreviations: CABG = coronary artery bypass grafting; CAD = coronary artery disease; LAD = left anterior descending coronary artery; MACE = major adverse cardiac events; VD = vessel disease
Acronyms: ACIP = Asymptomatic Cardiac Ischemia Pilot trial; ACME = Angioplasty Compared to Medicine trial; ACME-2 = Angioplasty Compared to Medical Therapy in Two-Vessel Disease trial; AVERT = Atorvastatin Versus Revascularization Treatment trial; COURAGE = Clinical Outcomes Utilizing Revascularization and Aggressive Drug Evaluation trial; MASS = Medicine, Angioplasty or Surgery Study trial; RITA-2 = Second Randomized Intervention Treatment of Angina trial
+   Studies were performed prior to availability of stents, platelet IIb/IIIa receptor antagonists, and routine use of statins
*   Significant selection bias, as thousands of patients at participating centers underwent elective PTCA and were not enrolled in the study; most of the difference in MACE was due to recurrent angina, not endpoints such as death or MI
** 9500 patients were screened, but only 4% were enrolled

     e.   **Conclusions From the Randomized PTCA vs. CABG Trials (Table 3.9).** A metanalysis of randomized trials concluded that PTCA and CABG resulted in a similar risk of death and nonfatal MI at 1-3 years, but CABG resulted in less angina and repeat revascularization procedures.[43] In BARI, 5-year cardiac mortality after PTCA was 2.6-fold higher in insulin-dependent diabetics, and 5-year cardiac mortality after CABG was 4.1-fold higher in patients with ST-elevation (compared to other PTCA and CABG patients). Overall mortality after percutaneous or surgical revascularization was highest in insulin-dependent diabetics, the elderly, and patients with baseline heart failure or renal failure.[73] Although initial procedural costs were higher for CABG than PTCA, the cost-advantage for PTCA was lost over 5-7 years because of the frequent need for additional procedures.[101]

Table 3.4. Randomized Trials of PTCA vs. CABG: Inclusion and Exclusion Criteria

Trial	N	Randomized (%)	Criteria
RITA[10]	1011	6	**Inclusion:** 1, 2, or 3-vessel disease ($\geq$ 70% stenosis); lesion supplying $\geq$ 20% of myocardium; angina or objective evidence of ischemia; equivalent revascularization by PTCA or CABG. **Exclusion:** Previous PTCA or CABG; left main disease, hemodynamically-severe valve disease; noncardiac illness threatening survival.
ERACI[11]	127	9	**Inclusion:** Multivessel disease ($\geq$ 2 vessels with $\geq$ 70% stenosis) and either significant angina despite medical therapy or a large area of myocardium at risk by exercise testing. **Exclusion:** Dilated ischemic cardiomyopathy; severe 3-vessel disease with EF $\leq$ 35%; significant left main stenosis; severe valvular or hypertrophic heart disease; evolving acute MI; noncardiac illness threatening survival.
GABI[12]	359	4	**Inclusion:** Age < 75 years; angina $\geq$ Class 2; multivessel disease ($\geq$ 2 vessels with $\geq$ 70% stenosis). **Exclusion:** Previous PTCA or CABG; total occlusion; left main stenosis $\geq$30%; > 50% of LV at risk during abrupt closure; lesion length > 2 cm; diffuse disease; coronary aneurysm; MI within 4 weeks.
CABRI[13]	1054	4.6	**Inclusion:** Age $\leq$ 76 years with multivessel disease ($\geq$ 2 vessels with $\geq$ 50% stenosis); clinical ischemia; equivalent degrees of revascularization not required. **Exclusion:** Previous PTCA or CABG; left main stenosis $\geq$ 50%; last remaining vessel; acute MI within previous 10 days; EF $\leq$ 35%; overt heart failure; recent stroke; severe concomitant illness.
EAST[14]	392	7.6	**Inclusion:** Patients of any age with 2 or 3-vessel disease with angina or objective evidence of ischemia. **Exclusion:** Previous PTCA or CABG; chronic total occlusion > 8 weeks; left main stenosis $\geq$ 30%; $\geq$ 2 total occlusions; EF < 25%; MI within 5 days; noncardiac illness threatening survival.
BARI[15]	1829	7	**Inclusion:** Age > 17 and < 80; multivessel disease ($\geq$ 2 vessels with $\geq$ 50% stenosis); and clinically severe angina (class III-IV or unstable angina; recent non-Q-MI; or class I-II angina either with severe ischemia on exercise testing, recent Q-MI, or EF < 50%), or no angina if severe ischemia was present on noninvasive testing and either a prior Q-MI or history of angina. **Exclusion:** Emergency revascularization; left main stenosis $\geq$ 50%; noncardiac illness that was a contraindication to PTCA or CABG or might limit survival; primary coronary spasm; severe ascending aortic calcification; need for other major surgery at same time as revascularization; known or suspected pregnancy.

CONCLUSIONS: Only a small percentage (< 25%) of patients with multivessel disease met inclusion criteria, and even fewer (< 10%) were actually randomized.

Abbreviations: MVD = multivessel disease; LV = left ventricle; EF = ejection fraction; MI = myocardial infarction; QMI = Q-wave myocardial infarction; CABG = coronary artery bypass grafting
Acronyms: BARI = Bypass Angioplasty Revascularization Investigation; CABRI = Coronary Angioplasty vs. Bypass Revascularization Intervention; EAST = Emory Angioplasty vs. Surgery Trial; ERACI = Argentine Randomized Trial Coronary Angioplasty vs. Bypass Surgery in Multivessel Disease; GABI = German Angioplasty Bypass Surgery Investigation; RITA = Randomized Intervention Treatment of Angina Trial

Table 3.5. Randomized Trials of PTCA vs. CABG: Study Design and Baseline Characteristics

	RITA[10]	ERACI[11]	GABI[12]	CABRI[13]	EAST[14]	BARI[15]
No. Patients	1011	127	359	1054	392	1829
Study Design						
Planned follow-up (yrs)	10	3	1	5-10	5	10
Complete revascularization required**	Yes	No	Yes	No	No	No
Total occlusion eligible	Yes	Yes	No	Yes	No	Yes
New devices	No	No	No	Yes+	No	Yes*
CABG-IMA (%)	74	77	37	81	90	82
Baseline Characteristics						
Age (yrs)	57	57	-	60	61	61
Male (%)	81	54	80	78	73	74
Previous MI (%)	43	31	47	43	41	55
Unstable angina (%)	59	53	14	15	62	65
LVEF (%)	-	61	56	63	62	57
No. diseased vessels (%)						
1	45	0	0	0	0	0
2	43	55	82	58	60	59
3	12	45	18	40	40	41

CONCLUSIONS:
- **Complete revascularization goal varied between trials**
- **Patients with total occlusions were excluded from some trials but not others**
- **Use of new devices and IMA grafting varied between trials**
- **Most patients had 2-vessel disease and normal LV function**

Abbreviations: IMA = internal mammary artery; LVEF = left ventricular ejection fraction; CABG = emergency coronary artery bypass grafting; - = not reported
Acronyms: See Table 3.4
+ Atherectomy or stenting
* Bailout stenting
** Complete anatomical revascularization whenever possible

Table 3.6. Randomized Trials of PTCA vs. CABG: PTCA Success and Revascularization Goals

Trial	PTCA Success* (%)	Staged PTCA (%)	PTCA Revascularization Goal
RITA[10]	87	7	Complete functional revascularization. Among patients with 2- or 3-vessel disease, attempted PTCA of all lesions occurred in 81% and 63%, respectively
ERACI[11]	92	-	Complete functional revascularization in 89%
GABI[12]	92	30	Complete anatomic revascularization in 86%
CABRI[13]	91	-	Complete functional revascularization
EAST[14]	88	40	Complete functional revascularization; dilate lesions thought to be contributing to ischemia
BARI[15]	88	17	Complete functional revascularization

CONCLUSIONS:
- **PTCA success rates were high**
- **Usual goal of PTCA was to dilate significant stenoses supplying viable myocardium; obstructions supplying nonviable myocardium or small territories were generally left untreated**

Definitions: Complete anatomical revascularization = PTCA of all lesions regardless of viability of myocardial territory; *Complete functional revascularization* = PTCA of only those lesions thought to be causing ischemia; lesions with small territories or nonviable myocardium were rarely dilated
Acronyms: See Table 3.4
* At least one lesion successfully dilated
- Not reported

3. **Nonrandomized Studies of Multivessel Angioplasty (Table 3.10)**
   a. **Ischemic Endpoints.** The Multivessel Angioplasty Prognosis Study (MAPS)[16] compared the results of multivessel PTCA in 1991 vs. 1986-87 (when many of the randomized trials enrolled patients). Despite older age and lower ejection fraction, the 1991 cohort had *higher* procedural success, *more complete* revascularization, and *better* clinical outcome than the earlier cohort (Table 3.10).[16] Other studies reported continued improvement in hospital outcomes for multivessel angioplasty in 1994 compared to 1990-1991 (in-hospital MACE 2% vs. 5%, $p < 0.05$),[17,102] and a 40% reduction in ischemic complications in 1995 compared to 1993-1994 due to elective stenting (1.7% vs. 3.0%, $p = 0.004$).[41] Studies of multivessel stenting report high procedural success, good long-term event-free survival, and low rates of repeat revascularization.[52,54] These findings have important implications for proper interpretation of the randomized PTCA vs. CABG trials, which enrolled patients 10 years ago.

Table 3.7. Randomized Trials of PTCA vs. CABG: In-Hospital Results

Trial	Group	Complications (%)			Other
		D	MI	CABG	
RITA[10]	PTCA	0.7	3.5	4.5	Length of stay (4 days vs. 12 days)
	CABG	1.2	2.4	-	
ERACI[11]	PTCA	1.5	6.3	1.5	Stroke (1.5% vs. 3.1%)
	CABG	4.6	6.2	-	
GABI[12]	PTCA	1.1	2.3	2.8	Stroke (0% vs. 1.2%); post-procedure pneumonia (1.1% vs.
	CABG	2.5	8.1*	-	10.6%, < 0.001); length of stay (5 days vs. 19 days); angina (18% vs. 7%, p < 0.005)
CABRI[13]	PTCA	1.3	-	3.3	-
	CABG	1.3	-	-	
EAST[14]	PTCA	1	3	10.1	Stroke (0.5% vs. 1.5%)
	CABG	1	10.3*	-	
BARI[15]	PTCA	1.1	2.1	6.3	Stroke (0.2% vs. 0.8%); respiratory failure (1% vs. 2.2%,
	CABG	1.3	4.6*	-	p < 0.05)

CONCLUSIONS:
- **In-hospital mortality was similar between PTCA and CABG groups**
- **In-hospital MI was higher in CABG group**
- **Emergency CABG for failed PTCA was required in 1.5-10%**
- **Length of hospital stay was 2-3 fold higher in CABG group**

Abbreviations: D = death; Q-MI = Q-wave myocardial infarction; CABG = emergency coronary artery bypass grafting; - = not reported. *Acronyms:* See Table 3.4
* p < 0.01

    b. **Restenosis**. Symptomatic status is not a reliable indicator of restenosis after multivessel PTCA.[13] Patients with asymptomatic restenosis managed medically had 6-year outcomes similar to patients *without* restenosis. These data support functional assessment of borderline lesions rather than routine repeat intervention based on angiographic findings alone ("oculostenotic reflex").

B. MULTIVESSEL STENTING. Large, contemporary multicenter registries from the Society of Coronary Angiography and Intervention (SCAI),[59] the Northern New England Cardiovascular Disease Study Group,[60] and others [64] demonstrate that despite application of percutaneous techniques to increasingly complex patients, the rate of ischemic complications has decreased, a trend which parallels the increasing utilization of stents (Tables 3.11, 3.12). Although most of the multicenter randomized stent trials enrolled patients with normal LV function requiring single-vessel intervention, several observational studies reported excellent results in multivessel stenting with and without LV dysfunction (Table 3.13).[54,55,57,58] These data are remarkable for procedural success rates > 95%, in-hospital ischemic complications < 5%, and the need for urgent CABG in < 2%. Furthermore, event-free survival rates are 75-80% at 2-3 years, and late target lesion revascularization was required in only 10-20% of patients. There are limited data from randomized trials of stents vs. CABG for multivessel disease. The ARTS trial randomized 1200 patients to stents or CABG, and reported no difference in 1-year infarct-free survival (90.5% vs. 91.2%). However, there was greater need for late revascularization in stent patients (16.8% vs. 3.4%, p < 0.001).[107] In the smaller Argentine ERACI-II trial, stenting of high-risk patients (90% had unstable angina) resulted in less death or MI at 30 days and 1 year, but more late revascularization (Table 3.13).[110]

C. **MULTIVESSEL ANGIOPLASTY IN PATIENTS WITH LV DYSFUNCTION**. Data from the Coronary Artery Surgery Study (CASS) Registry established the powerful adverse impact of LV dysfunction on the natural history of coronary artery disease by demonstrating that medically-treated patients with single-vessel disease and poor LV function had *higher* mortality than patients with 3-vessel disease and normal LV function (Table 3.14). Randomized trials of medicine vs. CABG clearly demonstrate the benefit of revascularization on total- and event-free survival. Likewise, nonrandomized studies of PTCA vs. CABG suggest that CABG results in better 2-5-year event-free survival and less angina (Table 3.15).[18,91] However, late outcome after PTCA vs. CABG was influenced most by the *completeness, not the mode*, of revascularization; patients with complete revascularization demonstrated similar event-free survival regardless of treatment mode. These data suggest that CABG may be preferred if PTCA cannot achieve complete revascularization, particularly in patients with diabetes, LV dysfunction, or proximal LAD disease.[19,20] Other nonrandomized studies of PTCA and CABG in patients with multivessel disease and LV dysfunction are shown in Tables 3.16 and 3.17.

D. **REVASCULARIZATION STRATEGY (Figure 3.2)**
   1. **Complete vs. Incomplete Revascularization.** The concept of complete revascularization evolved from the early surgical experience, which demonstrated improved anginal status, exercise capacity, and 5-7 year event-free survival when all stenoses > 50% were bypassed.[21-25] The early PTCA experience seemed to corroborate the benefits of this approach.[26-28] However, patients with incomplete revascularization are generally older and have more LV dysfunction and comorbidities than patients with complete revascularization. After adjusting for these differences, completeness of revascularization had no impact on infarct-free survival.[29,30,93] Revascularization can be categorized as complete "anatomical" revascularization or complete "functional" revascularization (Table 3.18). Data from EAST suggest that when equivalent "functional" revascularization can be achieved with PTCA and CABG, similar long-term outcomes might be expected.[47] Complete anatomic revascularization may be more important in patients with LV dysfunction (possibly explaining the survival advantage of CABG), whereas complete functional revascularization may be sufficient in most patients with good LV function.

Table 3.8. Randomized Trials of PTCA vs. CABG: Late Outcome

Trial	Follow-up (yrs)	Modality	Late Outcome (%) D / MI / TLR / ASX	Other Results
BARI[67] (2000)	7.8	PTCA CABG	19.1 / 7.4 / 72.8 / 84.9 15.6[+] / 9.1 / 13.8[+++] / 89.6	Better survival at 7 years for CABG
		Diabetic[++] PTCA CABG	44.3[+++] / 5.7 / 70 / - 25.6 / 9.2 / 11.1 / -	Survival advantage for CABG at 5 years (19% vs. 35%)[15,44,48] continued to increase between 5-7 years of follow-up
EAST[66] (2000)	8	PTCA CABG	21.7 / - / 65.3 / - 17.3 / - / 26.5 / -	No survival difference. Late revascularization in first 3 years was more frequent after PTCA; between 3-8 years, late TLR was similar. Survival in diabetics was similar for CABG and PTCA
GABI[12,88] (2000) (1994)	3	PTCA (1986-91) CABG (1986-91)	- / - / 37 / 60 - / - / 3.2[+] / 80[+]	Compared to PTCA patients in GABI-I (1986-91), PCI patients in GABI-II (1996-97) had more stents (63% vs. 0%), IIb/IIIa antagonists (7% vs. 0%), and statins (93% vs. 48%), but less TLR (28% vs. 44%), CABG (7% vs. 21%), and class III-IV angina (1% vs. 9%) at 1 year
	1	PTCA(1986-91) CABG (1986-91) PCI (1996-97)	2.6 / 4.5 / 44 / 71 6.5 / 9.4 / 6 / 74 - / - / 28 / -	
ERACI[42] (1996)	5	PTCA CABG	12.7 / 11.1 / 38 / 54 9.4 / 9.4 / 6.3 / 73	PTCA was less expensive than CABG
CABRI[13] (1995)	1	PTCA CABG	3.9 / 4.9 / 35.6 / 67 2.7 / 3.5 / 2.1 / 75[+]	Need for antianginals was greater after PTCA (84% vs. 65%)
EAST[14,46] (1994)	3	PTCA CABG	7.1 / 14.6 / 54 / 80[+] 6.2 / 19.6 / 13[+] / 88[+]	Abnormal thallium stress (9.6% vs. 5.7%) and use of antianginals (66% vs. 51%, p < 0.05) was greater after PTCA, but PTCA was less expensive. No difference in LVEF
RITA[10] (1993)	2.5	PTCA CABG	3.1 / 6.7 / 35 / 69 3.6 / 5.2 / 3.8[+] / 79[+]	Death, MI, or reintervention was greater after PTCA (38% vs. 11%, p < 0.05); severe angina 6% in both groups; 40% of those not working at baseline had returned to work at 6 months. Revascularization had no effect on LVEF. PTCA was less expensive

CONCLUSIONS:
- **Infarct-free survival at 1-year was similar; diabetics treated with PTCA had higher late mortality***
- **PTCA resulted in more angina, antianginal therapy, and repeat revascularization (3-10 fold) compared to CABG; 20% of PTCA patients required CABG at 1-3 years, and 40% of PTCA patients required CABG at 5-7 years**

Abbreviations: ASX = asymptomatic; D = death; Q-MI = Q-wave myocardial infarction; CABG = coronary artery bypass grafting; EF = ejection fraction; TLR = target lesion revascularization; PCI = percutaneous coronary intervention; - = not reported.
Acronyms: See Table 3.4

*   In BARI, the survival advantage for diabetics treated with CABG increased during 5-7 years of follow-up; in EAST, diabetics had better survival 8 years after CABG compared to PTCA, but the difference was not statistically significant.

\+   p < 0.05

++   Patients receiving oral hypoglycemics or insulin at study entry

+++ p < 0.001

Table 3.9. Randomized PTCA vs. CABG Trials: Summary of Conclusions

Trial	In-hospital (%)		Late (%)				Other (PTCA vs. CABG)
	D	MI	D	MI	TLR	Angina	
RITA[10]	ND	ND	ND	ND	↑	↑	Severe angina (ND); cost (↓); exercise capacity (ND)
ERACI[11]	ND	ND	ND	ND	↑	↑	Cost (↓)
GABI[12]	ND	↓	ND	ND	↑	ND	Death or MI (↓); need for antianginals (↑)
CABRI[13]	-	-	ND	ND	↑	ND	Need for antianginals (↑)
EAST[14]	ND	↓	ND	ND	↑	↑	Abnormal thallium (ND); need for antianginals (ND); cost (ND); exercise capacity (ND)
BARI[15,67]	ND	↓	↑*	ND	↑	ND	

CONCLUSIONS:

- **For patients with multivessel disease and significant ischemia who are candidates for either PTCA or CABG and meet entry criteria for the randomized trials (no previous PTCA or CABG; preserved LV function; and no left main stenosis, evolving or very recent MI, or severe noncardiac illness):**
  - **PTCA and CABG result in similar acute and long-term (1-5 yr) infarct-free survival. However, there is a trend toward better survival at 5-7 years after CABG. The survival advantage increases further at 5-7 years after CABG**
  - **Diabetic patients treated by PTCA have higher mortality than CABG patients**
  - **Patients treated by PTCA have more angina, require more antianginal therapy, and need more revascularization procedures in the first 1-5 years, including CABG in 20% at 5 years and 40% at 7 years Beyond 5 years after initial revascularization, the need for later revascularization is similar for PTCA and CABG patients**
  - **Patients initially treated with CABG have a longer convalescence**
- **For patients with multivessel disease and either left main stenosis, single stenosis supplying > 50% of viable myocardium, severe LV dysfunction, diffusely diseased vessels, or undilatable occlusions supplying viable myocardium, CABG may be preferred over PTCA**

Abbreviations: D = death; MI = Q-wave myocardial infarction; CABG = coronary artery bypass grafting: TLR = target lesion revascularization; - = not reported. *Acronyms:* See Table 3.4
ND = no difference between PTCA and CABG groups
↑ Incidence higher in PTCA group
↓ Incidence lower in PTCA group
* Nondiabetics and diabetics had higher 7-year mortality after PTCA

Table 3.10. Nonrandomized Series of Multivessel PTCA

Series	Subset	N	Success (%)	In-hospital (%) D / Q-MI / CABG	Follow-up Years	Follow-up Event (%)	
						Death	CABG
Weintraub[32]	1-VD	7604	-	0.2 / 0.4 / 1.2	1,5,10	1 / 7 / 14	8 / 13 / 23
(1995)	2-VD	2587	-	0.8 / 0.9 / 0.2		3 / 11 / 24	11 / 21 / 42
	3-VD	592	-	1.7 / 3.0 / 3.2		5 / 10 / 30*	14 / 27 / 41+
Ellis[16]	1991	200	90	1 / 1.5 / 1	1	1991 vs. 1986-87:	
(1995)	1986-87	400	84	1 / 2 / 5.5		EFS (74% vs. 64%);	
						CABG (8.1% vs. 13.4%);	
						complete revascularization	
						(35% vs. 21%); use of new	
						devices (26% vs. 0%)	
Cowley[31]		370	92	-	3	EFS (77%);	
(1993)						asymptomatic (74%)	
LeFeuvre[33]		703	91	0 / 2.5 / 1.5	6	Death (7.1%); MI (9.2%);	
(1993)						class 0-1 angina (84%)	

Abbreviations: VD = vessel disease; D = death; Q-MI = Q-wave myocardial infarction; CABG = coronary artery bypass grafting; EFS = event-free survival; - = not reported
* 9-year
+ 8-year

a. **Nondiabetics with 2- or 3-Vessel Disease and Good LV Function.** The goal of revascularization in patients with 2- or 3-vessel disease and normal LV function is to improve symptomatic status and functional capacity, which can be achieved by revascularizing all severe stenoses in vessels with moderate or large myocardial distributions. Revascularization of vessels which supply nonviable myocardium or small vascular distributions is not necessary to achieve good long-term outcomes.[31] In ERACI , there was no difference in 1-year outcome between CABG patients who had complete "anatomic" revascularization and patients who had PTCA only of lesions causing ischemia (complete "functional" revascularization). In CABRI, incomplete revascularization was predictive of the need for reintervention, but not death or MI at 1 year.[10] An intended strategy of incomplete percutaneous revascularization was associated with a greater risk of late CABG in BARI, but had no apparent influence on death or MI at 5 years.[72,75] It may be important to distinguish complete revascularization at the time of intervention from complete revascularization which persists at the time of follow-up, particularly since bypass grafts may become occluded. To help address this issue, a BARI angiographic substudy performed routine angiography 1 year after revascularization in 270 patients. Despite the fact that 21% of CABG patients developed total occlusion of at least one graft, myocardial jeopardy scores were lower after CABG than after PTCA, suggesting more complete revascularization. In addition, lower jeopardy scores were associated with less angina at follow-up.[71] More complete revascularization at follow-up may help explain the emerging trend toward enhanced survival at 7 years after CABG in BARI patients with and without diabetes.[67]

b.   **Nondiabetics with 3-Vessel Disease and Poor LV Function.** The goal of revascularization in patients with multivessel disease and LV dysfunction is to improve symptomatic status, functional capacity, and prolong survival. Patients at high-risk for acute complications or restenosis should be referred for CABG. Select patients with low-risk lesions may be considered for percutaneous intervention if complete revascularization can be achieved. When PTCA and other devices are used, we attempt to revascularize all stenoses in vessels ≥ 2.0 mm, including chronic total occlusions supplying nonviable myocardium, since they can serve as a source of collaterals.

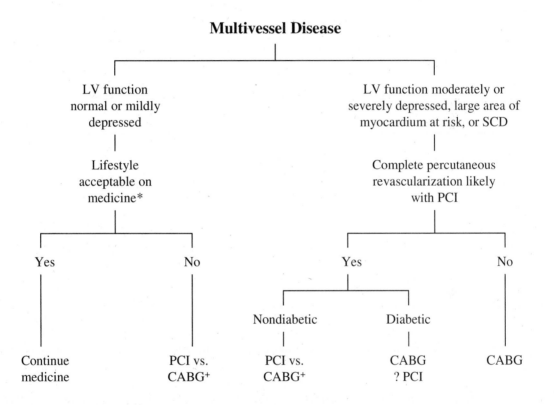

Figure 3.2. Revascularization Guidelines for Multivessel Disease and Chronic Stable Angina

Abbreviations: PCI = percutaneous coronary intervention; SCD = resuscitated sudden cardiac death
*   Medicine = risk factor modification + antianginal therapy
+   *Factors tending to favor PCI* = younger age, cerebrovascular disease, severe COPD, illness limiting survival, lesion suitable for stenting, no proximal LAD disease, patient desires to avoid CABG and accepts 20-30% risk of repeat procedures. *Factors tending to favor CABG* = older age, severe mitral regurgitation, diabetes, renal dialysis, lesion unsuitable for stenting, severe proximal LAD disease, patient desires to minimize number of procedures

Table 3.11. Percutaneous Revascularization: SCAI Experience in 19,510 Procedures[59]

Description	1996	1997	1998	Composite
Clinical Characteristics (%)				
Age > 65	43	42	45	44
Prior CABG	16	15	17	16
Diabetes	20	20	23	22
Renal failure	2	2	2	2
Multivessel disease	45	43	47	46
Unstable angina	58	60	66	63
MI < 24 hr	10	8	8	9
Procedural Factors (%)				
Emergent or urgent PCI	22	19	28	25
SVG	7	6	6	6
ACC/AHA type B lesion	75	63	67	66
ACC/AHA type C lesion	15	17	17	17
Device Selection (%)				
PTCA	51	37	26	33
DCA	0.7	0.6	0.3	0.5
Rotablator	4	6	6	6
Any stent	44	58	71	63
Planned stent	25	43	63	51
In-hospital Outcome (%)				
Death	0.3	0.6	0.4	0.5
CABG	0.4	0.4	0.6	0.5

Abbreviations: ACC/AHA = American College of Cardiology/American Heart Association lesion classification; CABG = coronary artery bypass grafting; DCA = directional coronary atherectomy; MI = myocardial infarction; PTCA = percutaneous transluminal coronary angioplasty; SCAI = Society for Cardiac Angiography and Interventions; SVG = saphenous vein graft

c.　**Diabetics with 2- or 3-Vessel Disease.** BARI suggests that diabetics undergoing CABG (with a LIMA graft to the LAD) have better long-term survival than after multivessel PTCA, particularly in patients with LV dysfunction. However, these data do not reflect the results of multivessel stenting and use of GP IIb/IIIa receptor antagonists, which improve late outcomes after percutaneous intervention (Chapter 7). Furthermore, there was no difference in survival among diabetics treated with CABG vs. PTCA in 2 nonrandomized trials,[104,105] including 5-year survival in the nonrandomized BARI registry.[104] These data suggest that carefully selected diabetics can be successfully managed by percutaneous revascularization. Regardless of whether CABG or PTCA is performed, long-term mortality rates are high, emphasizing the need for aggressive risk factor modification, tight glycemic control, and close follow-up. The relative role of CABG, PTCA, and other devices in diabetics is detailed in Chapter 7.

Table 3.12. Changing Outcomes After PCI: Northern New England Experience[60]

Description	1990-1993	1994-1995	1995-1997	p-Value
No. Procedures	13,014	7248	14,490	
Clinical Characteristics (%)				
Age > 80	4.0	5.6	6.3	< 0.001
Diabetes	21.2	21.4	22.3	0.021
Prior MI	29.8	26.5	23.5	< 0.001
Prior CABG	10.5	13.3	15.4	< 0.001
Heart failure	-	4.5	7.2	< 0.001
3-vessel disease	11.1	11.4	11.5	NS
EF < 40%	5.2	3.9	5.5	NS
Unstable angina	71.4	70.4	70.7	NS
Acute MI	2.5	4.1	5.2	< 0.001
Procedural Factors (%)				
Emergent or urgent PCI	64.7	64.5	65.3	< 0.01
Multiple lesions treated	29.1	27.0	29.8	< 0.001
SVG	3.5	5.4	6.0	< 0.001
ACC/AHA lesion type B_2/C	10.1	20.1	31.7	< 0.001
GP IIb/IIIa antagonist	-	-	6.8	-
Devices (%)				
Atherectomy	5.2	13.0	9.2	< 0.001
Stent	-	3.9	48.5	< 0.001
In-hospital Outcome (%)				
Success*	88.2	89.1	91.9	< 0.001
MI	2.4	2.1	1.9	0.001
CABG	3.1	3.3	1.8	< 0.001
Death	1.2	1.1	1.1	0.007

Abbreviations: ACC/AHA = American College of Cardiology/American Heart Association lesion classification; PCI = percutaneous coronary intervention; MI = myocardial infarction; CABG = coronary artery bypass graft; EF = ejection fraction; SVG = saphenous vein graft

* Success = final stenoses < 50% and no death, MI, or CABG

Table 3.13. Results of Stents for Multivessel Disease

Study	Modality	N	Success (%)	In-hospital (%) D / MI / CABG	Follow-up (%) D / MI / TVR	Comments
ERACI-II[110+] (2001)	Stent CABG	225 225	- -	- -	3.1* / 2.3* / 16.8* 7.5 / 6.6 / 4.8	Follow-up at 19 months
Abizaid[106] (2001)	Stent Diabetic Stent Nondiabetic	195 560	97 98	1.5 / 0.5 / 1 1.6 / 0.2 / 0.2	12.5 / 8.6 / 17.7 4.1* / 5.1 / 9.1*	1-yr MACE lower in nondiabetics (19.2% vs. 34.8%, p < 0.001)
Patel[113] (2001)	Stent PTCA CABG	260 308 260	- - -	1.6 2.6 1.2	- - -	In-hospital stroke (0% vs. 0.3% vs. 3.5%). No difference in survival between stent and CABG at 5 years; both better than PTCA
Kim[58] (2000)	Stent CABG	100 100	- -	1 / 3 / 2 2 / 3 / 0	0 / 1 / 19 1 / 2 / 2*	CR was higher for CABG (95% vs. 69%, p < 0.05); more recurrent angina in stent patients (19% vs. 8%, p = 0.03)
Moussa[108] (2000)	Stent	100	97	1 / 2 / 2	3 / 2 / 30	Restenosis (37%)
ARTS[107+] (1999)	Stent CABG	600 600	- -	- -	1-yr MACE (2.3% vs. 9.5%*)	No difference in combined endpoint of death, stroke, or MI at 1 year
Hernandez-Antolin[55] (1999)	Stent	136	95	0.7 / 4.4 / 0	2.2 / 0.7 / 11.0	EFS at 3 years (75%); freedom from restenosis (65%)
Kornowski[54] (1999)	Stent-MVD Stent-SVD	398 1941	96 97	0.5 / 0.9 / 0.5 0.6 / 0.7 / 1.6	0.7 / 0 / 15 1.4 / 1.2 / 16	EFS 78% in both groups at 2 years
Mathew[57] (1999)	Stent	175	98	1.7 / 0 / 0	- / - / 18.3	EFS at 1 year (80%); CR in 57%

Abbreviations: D = death; MI = myocardial infarction; CABG = coronary artery bypass graft; TVR = target vessel revascularization; EFS = event-free survival; CR = complete revascularization; SVD = single vessel disease; MVD = multivessel disease; MACE = death, MI, stroke, TLR

Acronyms: ARTS = Arterial Revascularization Therapy Study; ERACI = Argentine Randomized Study: Coronary Angioplasty (with stents) vs. Coronary Bypass Surgery in Multivessel Disease

* Statistically significant result (at least p < 0.05)

+ Randomized trial

Table 3.14. The Impact of LV Function and Extent of Coronary Disease on 4-Year Survival in Medically-Treated Patients[38]

LV Function*	No. Diseased Vessels		
	1	2	3
Good	94	91	79
Poor	67	61	42

* Systolic contraction was assessed in 5 selected LV segments and assigned a value of 1 (normal wall motion) to 6 (dyskinetic). Systolic contraction score was the sum of all segmental values; scores of 5-11 and 17-30 represented good and poor LV function, respectively.

2. **Approach to "Moderate" Stenoses.** Moderate (50-70%) stenoses may not be clinically significant. Factors favoring revascularization include ischemic ECG changes, a corresponding regional wall motion abnormality, reversible perfusion defect, an unstable plaque, intracoronary thrombus, or coronary flow reserve < 2.0 (Chapter 33).

3. **Order of Revascularization (Figure 3.3).** The order in which stenoses are treated can directly impact the safety of multivessel intervention. Total occlusions which supply large jeopardized areas or furnish collaterals are dilated first, followed by lesion(s) that supply moderate-to-large myocardial regions. If the culprit lesion cannot be identified, the most severe stenosis supplying the largest area of jeopardized myocardium should be revascularized first. When proximal and distal stenoses are present, the distal lesion should be treated first, unless the device impedes flow or cannot be advanced across the proximal stenosis.

4. **Staging**
    a. **Elective Intervention.** For most patients with multivessel disease, complete functional revascularization is attempted during the initial procedure. If further intervention compromises patient comfort or safety, other stenoses are "staged" at a later time (Table 3.19). A "next-day" staging strategy is useful, allowing most patients to be completely revascularized during their initial hospital stay (Figure 3.4). Alternatively, the operator may defer further percutaneous intervention for 2-4 weeks.

    b. **Urgent Intervention.** When PTCA is performed for acute coronary syndromes, the culprit lesion should be treated during the initial procedure. Timing of revascularization of other high-grade stenoses depends on symptom status and LV function (Figure 3.5).

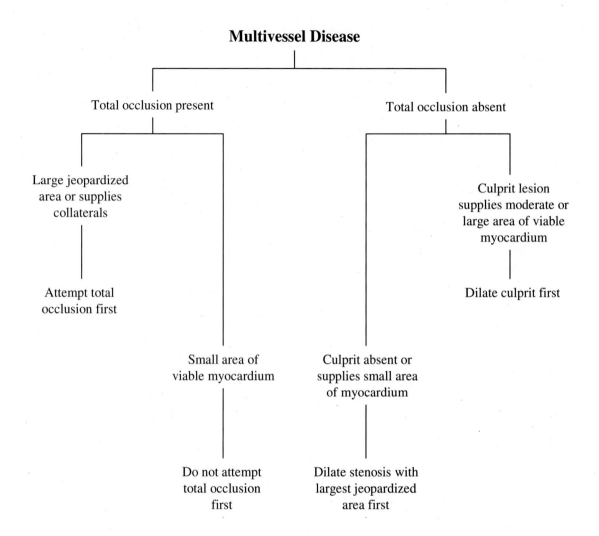

Figure 3.3. Dilatation Order for Patients Requiring Elective Multivessel Intervention

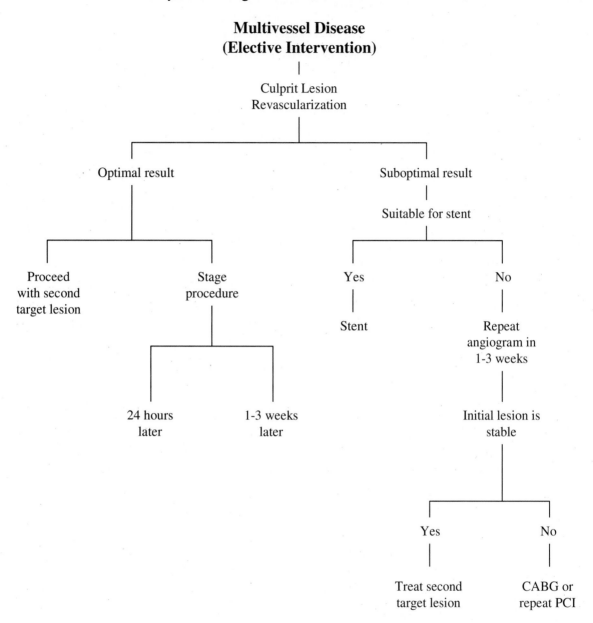

Figure 3.4. Staging of Multivessel Disease During Elective Intervention

CABG = coronary artery bypass surgery; PCI = percutaneous coronary intervention

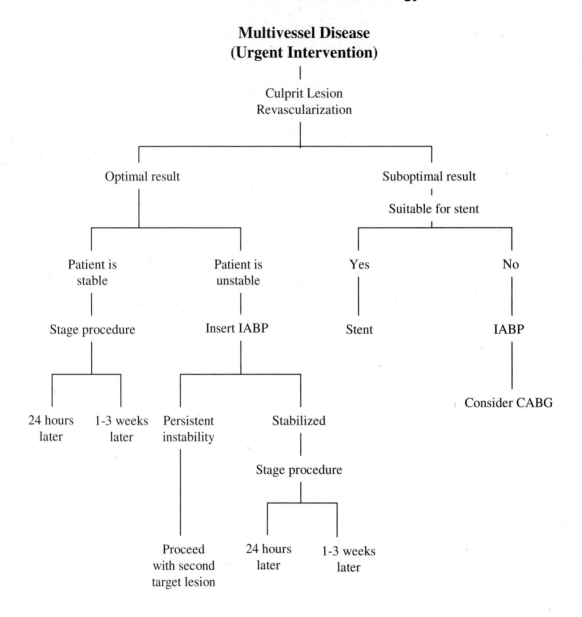

Figure 3.5. Staging of Multivessel Disease During Urgent Percutaneous Intervention

CABG = coronary artery bypass surgery; IABP = intra-aortic balloon pump

Table 3.15. PTCA vs. CABG for Patients with Multivessel Disease and LV Dysfunction*

Event (%)	O'Keefe[18] (1993)		Malenka[91]** (2000)	
	PTCA (n = 100)	CABG (n = 100)	PTCA (n = 534)	CABG (n = 1817)
In-hospital Outcome (%)				
Complete revascularization	37	82	-	-
Death	3	5	-	-
Q-MI	2	2	-	-
Stroke	0	7	-	-
Length of stay	4.3	12.8	-	-
Follow-up (%)	**5 years**	**5 years**	**4 years**	**4 years**
Death	33	24	22	16
Death or MI	54	24	-	-
Repeat revascularization	50	0	-	-
Class III-IV angina	11	1	-	-

*   EF < 40%

**   Various devices; no difference in survival between percutaneous revascularization vs. CABG for EF $\geq$ 40%

D. SPECIAL SUBSET OF MULTIVESSEL DISEASE: PTCA OF ONE MAJOR ARTERY WHEN THE OTHER IS OCCLUDED. Several studies have evaluated the results of PTCA in a major artery when the other vessel is occluded and is not amenable to percutaneous intervention.[34-36] As shown in Table 3.20, success and complications rates are acceptable. Nevertheless, many interventionalists refer such patients for bypass surgery, particularly when the occluded vessel supplies a large myocardial territory, LV function is poor, or the target lesion has high-risk morphology for acute complications or restenosis (e.g., thrombus, angulation, long). These patients should understand that although PTCA or stenting may be viable alternatives to CABG, repeat revascularization (including CABG) may be required.

Table 3.16. Results of PTCA in Patients with Left Ventricular Dysfunction

Series	EF (%)	N	Success (%)	Complications (%) D / MI / CABG	Follow-up
Malenka[91] (2000)	< 40	534	-	-	Death at 4 years (CABG 16% vs. PTCA 22%)
Siegal[92] (2000)	< 30	317	93	0.3 / - / 0.9	Outcomes at 1 year: death (6.7%); TLR (7.6%); EFS (8.5%). Mean EF increased from 28% to 38% at 1 year
Eltchaninoff[79] (1994)	< 40	343	95	2.6 / 2.6 / 3.2	Outcomes at 3 years: death (18%); repeat PTCA (13%); CABG (9.4%)
Holmes[81] (1993)	< 45	1802	-	0.8 / 4.9 / 4.5	Survival (87%); EFS (77%)
O'Keefe[80] (1993)	< 40	100	-	3 / - / -	Survival at 1 year (84%) and 5 years (66%); EFS at 1 year (75%) and 5 years (40%)
Terrien[82] (1993)	< 31	72	-	11 / - / -	Survival at 29 months (70%)
Serota[77] (1991)	< 40	73	85	5 / - / -	Survival at 1 year (79%) and 5 years (57%)
Stevens[76] (1991)	< 40	845	93	4 / - / 2	Outcomes at 33 months: CABG (15%); repeat PTCA (27%). Survival at 1 year (87%) and 4 years (69%)
Kohli[78] (1990)	< 35	61	90	3.2 / 5 / 5	Outcomes at 21 months: death (23%); EFS (51%)

Abbreviations: CABG = coronary artery bypass grafting; EF = ejection fraction; EFS = event-free survival; MI = myocardial infarction;- = not reported

Table 3.17. Results of CABG in Patients with Left Ventricular Dysfunction

Series	EF (%)	N	Complications (%) Death / MI	Follow-up
Whang[109] (2000)	< 36	342 (diabetics) 558 (nondiabetics)	-	CABG Patch trial (ICD). Diabetics had more post-op sternal wound infection and renal failure, more rehospitalization at 4 years (85% vs. 69%), but similar all-cause mortality (26% vs. 24%)
Mickleborough[63] (2000)	< 20	125	4 / 4	In-hospital stroke (4%); 4-yr survival (78%)
Malenka[91] (2000)	< 40	1817	-	Long-term survival better for CABG than PTCA; survival similar if EF > 40%
BARI[35] (1996)	< 50	-	-	No difference in survival for CABG vs. PTCA at 5 years
Veterans[86] (1995)	< 50	150	-	Survival at 7 years (74%) and 11 years (53%)
Elefteriades[87] (1993)	< 30	83	8.4 / -	Survival at 1 year (87%) and 3 years (80%)
O'Keefe[80] (1993)	< 40	100	5 / -	Survival at 1 year (91%) and 5 years (77%)
Alderman[83] (1983)	< 36	231	6.9 / 10.8	Survival at 5 years (63%)
Hochberg[84] (1983)	< 40	466	-	Survival at 3 years: EF < 20% (15%); EF 20-39% (60%)
Rahimtoola[85] (1983)	-	520	2 / -	Survival at 1 year (91%) and 5 years (79%)

Abbreviations: BARI = Bypass Angioplasty Revascularization Investigation; CABG = coronary artery bypass grafting; CASS = Coronary Artery Surgery Study; EF = ejection fraction; EFS = event-free survival; MI = myocardial infarction; - = not reported

Table 3.18. Percutaneous Revascularization Strategies and Expected Clinical Outcome

Strategy	Definition	Expected Clinical Outcome
Complete anatomic revascularization	Dilatation of all stenoses > 50% in vessels ≥ 2.0 mm in diameter	Similar to complete functional revascularization in patients with preserved LV function; may be preferred in patients with LV dysfunction or diabetes
Complete functional revascularization	Dilatation of only those lesions causing ischemia	Similar to complete anatomic revascularization in patients with preserved LV function; anatomic revascularization may be preferred in patients with LV dysfunction or diabetes
Incomplete functional revascularization	Inability to dilate ≥ 1 lesion thought to be causing ischemia	Worse than either of the other two groups

Table 3.19. Indications for Staging

Thrombus immediately after PTCA

Severe dissection or impaired flow after intervention

Procedure duration > 3 hours

Contrast media volume > 400 cc

Borderline lesions (50-70% stenosis) without objective evidence for ischemia

Table 3.20. PTCA of One Major Artery When the Other Is Occluded

Series	Group	N	In-hospital (%) D/Q-MI/CABG	Mos.	Follow-Up (%) D/Q-MI/PTCA/CABG/ASX
Lafont[34+] (1993)	PTCA of LAD or RCA when other is occluded	193	0.5 / 0.5 / 5.7	33	4.7 / 3.7 / 23.6 / 13.1 / 76
	PTCA of LAD + RCA	214	0.5 / 0.5 / 3.3 1.5		5.3 / 4.3 / 11.6 / 8.2 / 80
	CABG of LAD + RCA	194	/ 1.0 / 0		8.5 / 3.7 / 1.6 / 2.1 / 74
DeBruyne[35] (1991)	PTCA of LAD or LCX when RCA is occluded	61	0 / 0 / 4.9	5	- / - / 25 / 5 / 65
Teirstein[36] (1990)	PTCA of left coronary:				
	RCA occluded	65	1.5 / - / 0	17	8 / 3 / - / 18 / 61
	RCA not occluded	105	0 / - / 1.5		7 / 1 / - / 9 / 84

Abbreviations: ASX = asymptomatic; CABG = coronary artery bypass grafting; D = death; LAD = left anterior descending coronary artery; LCX = left circumflex artery; Q-MI = Q-wave myocardial infarction; RCA = right coronary artery;
+ Groups matched for number and location of stenoses, ejection fraction, age, gender, and study period
- Not reported

Chapter 3. Single & Multivessel Intervention

REFERENCES

1. Henderon RA, Pocock SJ, Hampton JR. Revascularization for patients with single vessel disease: Results from the randomized interventional treatment of angina (RITA) trial at 4.7 years. Circulation 1995;92:1-476.

2. Goy JJ, Eckhout E, Burnand B, et al. Coronary angioplasty versus left internal mammary artery grafting for isolated proximal left anterior descending artery stenosis. Lancet 1994;343:1149-1453.

3. Mark DB, Nelson CL, Califf RM, et al. Continuing evolution of therapy for coronary artery disease. Initial results from the era of coronary angioplasty. Circulation 1994;89:2015-2025.

4. Cameron J, Mahanonda N, Aroney C, et al. Outcome five years after percutaneous transluminal coronary angioplasty or coronary artery bypass grafting for significant narrowing limited to the left anterior descending coronary artery. Am J Cardiol 1994;74:544-549.

5. Parisi A, Folland E, Hartigan P. A comparison of angioplasty with medical therapy in the treatment of single-vessel coronary artery disease. N Engl J Med 1992;326:10-16.

6. Morris KG, Folland ED, Hartigan PM, et al. Unstable angina in late follow-up of the ACME trial. Circulation 1995;92:I-725.

7. Frierson JH, Dimas AP, Whitlow PL, Hollman JL. Angioplasty of the proximal left anterior descending coronary artery: Initial success and long-term follow-up. J Am Coll Cardiol 1992;19:745-751.

8. Henderson RA, Karani S, Dritsas A, et al. Long-term results of coronary angioplasty for single vessel, proximal left anterior descending disease. Eur Heart J 1991;12:642-47.

9. Kramer JR, Proudfit W, Loop FD, et al. Late follow-up of 781 patients undergoing PTCA or bypass surgery for an isolated obstruction in the left anterior descending coronary artery. Am Heart J 1989;118:1144-53.

10. Coronary angioplasty versus coronary artery bypass surgery: The randomized intervention treatment of angina (RITA) trial. RITA Trial Participants. Lancet 1993;341:573-80.

11. Rodriguez A, Boullon F, Perez-Balino N. Argentine randomized trial of percutaneous transluminal coronary angioplasty versus coronary artery bypass surgery in multivessel disease (ERACI): In-hospital results and 1-year follow-up. J Am Coll Cardiol 1993;22:1060-1067.

12. Hamm C, Reimers J, Ischinger T, Rupprecht H. A randomized study of coronary angioplasty compared with bypass surgery in patients with symptomatic multivessel coronary disease. N Engl J Med 1994;331:1037-1043.

13. First-year results of CABRI Coronary Angioplasty versus Bypass Revascularization Investigation). CABRI Trial Participants. Lancet 1995;346:1179-84.

14. King S, Lembo N, Weintraub W, Kosinski A. A randomized trial comparing coronary angioplasty with coronary bypass surgery. N Engl J Med 1994;331:1044-1150.

15. The Bypass Angioplasty Revascularization Investigation (BARI) Investigators. Comparison of Coronary Bypass Surgery with Angioplasty in Patients with multivessel disease. N Engl J Med 1996;335:217.

16. Ellis S, Cowley M, Whitlow P, et al. Prospective case-control comparison of percutaneous transluminal coronary revascularization in patients with multivessel disease treated in 1986-1987 versus 1991: Improved in-hospital and 12-month results. J Am Coll Cardiol 1995;25:1137-42.

17. Danchin N, Cador R, Dibon O, et al. Changes in immediate outcome of PTCA in multivessel coronary artery disease: Implications for the interpretation of randomized trials of PTCA versus CABG. Circulation 1995;92:I-475.

18. O'Keefe JH, Allan JJ, McCallister BD, McConahay DR. Angioplasty versus bypass surgery for multivessel coronary artery disease with left ventricular ejection fraction <40%. Am J Cardiol 1993;71:897-901.

19. Ellis SG, Vandormael MG, Cowley MJ, et al. Coronary morphologic and clinical determinants of procedural outcome with angioplasty for multivessel coronary disease: Implications for patient selection. Circulation 1990;82:1193-1202.

20. Ellis SG, Cowley MK, DiSciascio G, et al. Determinants of 2-year outcome after coronary angioplasty in patients with multivessel disease on the basis of comprehensive preprocedural evaluation: Implications for patient selection. Circulation 1991;82:1905-1914.

21. LaVee J, Rath S, Hoa, et al. Does complete revascularization by the conventional method truly provide the best possible results? Analysis of results and comparison with revascularization of infarct-prone segments (systematic segmental myocardial revascularization): The Sheba Study. J Thorac Cardiovasc Surg 1986;92:279-290.

22. Schaff HV, Gersh BJ, Pluth JR, et al. Survival and functional status after coronary artery bypass grafting: Results 10 to 12 years after surgery in 500 patients. Circulation 1983;68:II-200-204.

23. Lawrie GM, Morris GC, Silvers A, et al. The influence of residual disease after coronary bypass on the 5-year survival rate of 1274 men with coronary artery disease. Circulation 1982;66:717-723.

24. Jones EL, Craver JM, Guyton RA, et al. Importance of complete revascularization in performance of the coronary bypass operation. Am J Cardiol 1983;51:7-12.

25. Cukingham RA, Carey JS, Wittig JH, et al. Influence of complete coronary revascularization on relief of angina. J Thorac Cardiovasc Surg 1980;79:188-193.

26. Mabin TQA, Holmes DR, Smith HC, et al. Follow-up clinical results in patients undergoing percutaneous transluminal coronary angioplasty. Circulation 1985;71:754-760.

27. Vandormael MG, Chaitman BR, Ischinger T, Aker UT. Immediate and short-term benefit of multilesion coronary angioplasty: Influence of degree of revascularization. J Am Coll Cardiol 1985;6:983-991.

28. Bourassa MG, Yeh W, Detre K, for the NHLBI PTCA Investigators. Five-year event rates after multivessel PTCA when complete revascularization is not possible or not intended. J Am Coll Cardiol 1994;February:223A.

29. Bell M, Bailey K, Reeder G, Lapeyre A, Holmes D.

Percutaneous transluminal angioplasty in patients with multivessel coronary disease: How important is complete revascularization for cardiac event-free survival? J Am Coll Cardiol 1990;16:553-562.

30. Reeder GS, Holmes DR, Detre K, et al. Degree of revascularization in patients with multivessel coronary disease: A report from the National Heart, Lung and Blood Institute Percutaneous Transluminal Coronary Angioplasty Registry. Circulation 1988;3:638-644.

31. Cowley M, Vandermael M, Topol E, et al. Is traditionally defined complete revascularization needed for patients with multivessel disease treated by elective coronary angioplasty? J Am Coll Cardiol 1993;22:1289-1297.

32. Weintraub W, King S, Douglas J, Kosinski A. Percutaneous transluminal coronary angioplasty as a first revascularization procedure in single-, double-, and triple-vessel coronary artery disease. J Am Coll Cardiol 1995;26:142-151.

33. Le Feuvre C, Bonan R, Cote Gilles, et al. Five-to-10 year outcome after multivessel percutaneous transluminal coronary angioplasty. Am J Cardiol 1993;71:1153-1158.

34. Lafont A, Dimas AP, Grigera F, Pearce G. Percutaneous transluminal coronary angioplasty of one major coronary artery when the contralateral vessel is occluded. J Am Coll Cardiol 1993;22:1298-1303.

35. De Bruyne B, Renkin J, Col J, Wijns W. Percutaneous transluminal coronary angioplasty of the left coronary artery in patients with chronic occlusion of the right coronary artery: Clinical and functional results. Am Heart J 1991;122:415.

36. Teirstein P, Giorgi L, Johnson W, et al. PTCA of the left coronary artery when the right coronary artery is chronically occluded. Am Heart J 1990;119:479.

37. Le Feuvre C, Bonan R, Lesperance J, et al. Predictive factors of restenosis after multivessel percutaneous transluminal coronary angioplasty. Am J Cardiol 1994;73:840-844.

38. Mock M, Ringqvist I, Fisher L, et al. Survival of medically treated patients in the Coronary Artery Surgery Study (CASS) Registry. Circulation 1982;66:562-8.

39. Hueb WA, Bellotti G, de Oliveira A, et al. The Medicine, Angioplasty or Surgery Study (MASS): A prospective, randomized trial of medical therapy, balloon angioplasty or bypass surgery for single proximal left anterior descending artery stenoses. J Am Coll Cardiol 1995;26:1600-5.

40. Breeman A, Boersma E, Deckers JW, et al. The impact of the completeness of revascularization on adverse cardiac events at 1 year follow-up in 1021 CABRI patients. J Am Coll Cardiol 1996;27:55A.

41. Ellis SG, Whitlow PL, Guetta V, et al. A highly significant 40% reduction in ischemic complications of percutaneous coronary intervention in 1995: Beginning of a new era? J Am Coll Cardiol 1996;27:253A.

42. Mele E, Rodriguez, A, et al. Final follow up of Argentine randomized trial coronary angioplasty vs. bypass surgery in multivessel disease (ERACI): Clinical outcome and cost analysis. Circulation 1996;94:I-435.

43. Sim I, Gupta M, McDonald K, Bourassa MG, Hlatky MA. A meta-analysis of randomized trials comparing CABG with PTCA in multivessel coronary artery disease. Am J Cardiol 1995;76:1025-9.

44. Hlatky MA, Rogers WJ, Johnstone I, et al. Medical care costs and quality of life after randomization to coronary angioplasty or coronary bypass surgery. N Engl J Med 1997;336:92-99.

45. Jones RH, Kesler K, Phillips HR, et al. Long-term survival benefits of coronary artery bypass grafting and percutaneous transluminal angioplasty in patients with coronary artery disease. J Thorac Cardiovasc Surg 1996;111:1013-1025.

46. Weintraub WS, Mouldin PD, Becker E, Kosinski A, et al. A comparison of the cost of and quality of life after coronary angioplasty or coronary surgery for multivessel CAD. Result from the Emory Angioplasty versus Surgery Trial (EAST). Circulation 1995;92:2831-2840.

47. Zhao X-D, Brown BG, Stewart DK, et al. Effectiveness of revascularization in the Emory Angioplasty versus Surgery Trial. Circulation 1996;93:1954-1962.

48. Jacobs AK, Kelsey SF, Brooks MM, et al. Better outcome for women compared with men undergoing coronary revascularization. A report from the BARI investigation. Circulation 1998;98:1279-1285.

49. The BARI Investigators. Influence of diabetes on 5-year mortality and morbidity in a randomized trial comparision CABG and PTCA in patients with multivessel disease. Circulation. 1997;96:1761-1769.

50. Detre KM, Guo P, Holubkov R, et al. Coronary revascularization in diabetic patients. A comparison of the randomized and observational components of the BARI investigation. Circulation 1999;99:633-640.

51. Barsness GW, Peterson ED, Ohman EM, et al. Relationship between diabetes mellitus and long-term survival after coronary bypass and angioplasty. Circulation 1997;96:2551-6.

52. Moussa I, Reimers B, Moses J, et al. Long-term angiographic and clinical outcome of patients undergoing multivessel coronary stenting. Circulation 1997;96:3873-9.

53. Versaci F, Gaspardone A, Tomai F, et al. A comparison of coronary artery stenting with angioplasty for isolated stenosis of the proximal left anterior descending coronary artery. N Engl J Med 1997;336:817-822.

54. Kornowski R, Mehran R, Satler L, et al. Procedural results and late clinical outcomes following multivessel coronary stenting. J Am Coll Cardiol 1999;33:420-6.

55. Hernandez-Antolin R, Alfonso F, Goicole, J, et al. Results (> 6 months) of stenting > 1 major coronary artery in multivessel coronary artery disease. Am J Cardiol 1999;84:147-151.

56. Hannan E, Racz M, Arani D, et al. A comparison of short- and long-term outcomes for balloon angioplasty and coronary stent placement. J Am Coll Cardiol 2000;36:395-403.

57. Mathew V, Garratt K, Holmes D, Jr,. Clinical outcome after multivessel coronary stent implantation. Am Heart J 1999;138:1105-10.

58. Kim SW, Hong MK, Lee CW, et al. Multivessel coronary stenting versus bypass surgery in patients with multivessel coronary artery disease and normal left ventricular function: Immediate and 2-year long-term follow-up. Am Heart J 2000;139:638-42.

59. Laskey, W, Kimmel S, Krone, R. Contemporary trends in coronary intervention: A report from the registry of the Society for Cardiac Angiography and Interventions. Cathet. Cardiovasc. Intervent. 2000;49:19-22.

60. McGrath P, Malenka D, Wennberg D, et al. Changing

outcomes in percutaneous coronary interventions. A study of 34,752 procedures in northern New England, 1990 to 1997. J Am Coll Cardiol 1999;34:674-80.

61. O'Keefe J, Kreamer T, Jones P, et al. Isolated left anterior descending coronary artery disease: percutaneous transluminal coronary angioplasty versus stenting versus left internal mammary artery bypass grafting. Circulation 1999:100 (suppl II):II-114.

62. Goy JJ, Eeckhout E, Moret C, et al. Five-year outcome in patients with isolated proximal left anterior descending coronary artery stenosis treated by angioplasty or left internal mammary artery grafting: a prospective trial. Circulation. 1999;99:3255-3259.

63. Mickleborough MD, Carson S, Tamariz M, et al. Results of revascularization in patients with severe left ventricular dysfunction. J Thorac Cardiovasc Surg 2000;119:550-7.

64. Holubkov R, Detre K, Sopko G, et al. Trends in coronary revasculatization 1989 to 1997: The Bypass Angioplasty Revascularization Investigation (BARI) survey of procedures. Am J Cardiol 1999;84:157-161.

65. Pitt B, Waters D, Virgil W, et al. Aggressive lipid-lowering therapy compared with angioplasty in stable coronary artery disease. N Engl J Med 1999;341:70-6.

66. King S, Kosinski A, Guyton R, et al. Eight-year mortality in the Emory Angioplasty versus Surgery Trial (EAST). J Am Coll Cardiol 2000;35:1116-21.

67. The BARI Investigators. Seven-year outcome in the Bypass Angioplasty Revascularization Investigation (BARI) by treatment and diabetic status. J Am Coll Cardiol 2000;35:1122-9.

68. Pocock SJ, Henderson R, Clayton T, et al. Quality of life after coronary angioplasty or continued medical treatment for angina: three-year follow-up in the RITA-2 trial. J Am Coll Cardiol 2000;35:907-14.

69. Hueb W, Soares P, de Oliveira S, et al. Five-year follow-up of the medicine, angioplasty, or surgery study (MASS): A prospective, randomized trial of medical therapy, balloon angioplasty, or bypass surgery for single proximal left anterior descending coronary artery stenosis. Circulation. 1999;100[suppl II]:II-107-II-113.

70. Espinola-Klein C, Rupprecht HJ, Ergel R, et al. Ten-year outcome after coronary angioplasty in patients with single-vessel coronary artery disease and comparison with the results of the coronary artery surgery study (CASS). Am J Cardiol 2000;85:321-326.

71. Whitlow P, Dimas A, Bashore T, et al. Relationship of extent of revascularization with angina at one year in the Bypass Angioplasty Revascularization Investigation (BARI). J Am Coll Cardiol 1999;34:1750-9.

72. Bourassa M, Kip K, Jacobs A, et al. Is a strategy of intended incomplete percutaneous transluminal coronary angioplasty revascularization acceptable in nondiabetic patients who are candidates for coronary artery bypass graft surgery? The Bypass Angioplasty Revascularization Investigation. J Am Coll Cardiol 1999;33:1627-36.

73. Brooks M, Jones R, Bach R, et al. Predictors of mortality from cardiac causes in the Bypass Angioplasty Revascularization Investigation (BARI) randomized trial and registry. Circulation 2000;101:2682-9.

74. Feit F, Brooks M, Sopko G, et al. Long-term clinical outcome in the Bypass Angioplasty Revascularization Investigation registry: Comparison with the randomized trial. Circulation 2000;101:2795-2802.

75. Kip K, Bourassa M, Jacobs A, et al. Influence of pre-PTCA strategy and initial PTCA result in patients with multivessel disease: The Bypass Angioplasty Revascularization Investigation (BARI). Circulation 1999;100:910-917.

76. Stevens T, Kahn JK, McCallister BD, et al. Safety and efficacy of percutaneous transluminal coronary angioplasty in patients with left ventricular dysfunction. Am J Cardio 1991;68:313-319.

77. Serota H, Deligonul U, Lee WH, et al. Predictors of cardiac survival after percutaneous transluminal coronary angioplasty in patients with severe left ventricular dysfunction. Am J Cardiol 1991;67:367-372.

78. Kohli RS, DiSciascio G, Cowley MJ, et al. Coronary angioplasty in patients with severe left ventricular dysfunction. J Am Coll Cardiol 1990;16:807-811.

79. Eltchaninoff H, Franco I, Whitlow PK, et al. Late results of coronary angioplasty in patients with left ventricular ejection fractions $\leq 40\%$. Am J Cardiol 1994;73:1047-52.

80. O'Keefe JH, Allan JJ, McCallister, et al. Angioplasty versus bypass surgery for multivessel coronary artery disease with left ventricular ejection fraction < 40%. Am J Cardiol 1993;71:897-901.

81. Holmes DR, Detre KM, Williams DO, et al. Long term outcome of patients with depressed left ventricular function undergoing percutaneous transluminal coronary angioplasty. The NHLBI PTCA Registry. Circulation 1993;87:21-9.

82. Terrien EF, Siegel N, O'Neill WW, et al. Angioplasty in patients with severe left ventricular dysfunction: an analysis of immediate and long term survival. J Am Coll Cardiol 1993;21:272A.

83. Alderman EL, Fisher LD, Litwin P, et al. Results of coronary artery surgery in patients with poor left ventricular function (CASS). Circulation 1983;68:785-795.

84. Hochberg MS, Parsonnet V, et al. Coronary artery bypass grafting in patients with ejection fractions below forty percent. J Thorac Cardiovasc Surg 1983;86:519-527.

85. Rahimtoola SH, Nunley D, Grunkemeier G, et al. Ten year survival after coronary artery bypass surgery for unstable angina. N Engl J Med 1983;308:676-681.

86. The Veterans Administration Coronary Artery Bypass Surgery Cooperative Group. Eleven year survival in the Veterans Administration trial of coronary bypass surgery for stable angina. N Engl J Med 1995;311:1333-1339.

87. Elefteriades JA, Tolis G, Levi E, et al. Coronary artery bypass grafting in severe left ventricular dysfunction: excellent survival with improved ejection fraction and functional state. J Am Coll Cardiol 1993;22:1411-7.

88. Baldus S, Kerckhoff H, Nauheim B, et al. Cost effectiveness of current interventional technique for the treatment of multivessel coronary disease. Circulation 2000;102:II-549.

89. Rodriguez A. Bernardi V, Navia J, et al. Argentine randomized study of coronary angioplasty with stents versus coronary bypass surgery in multiple vessel disease (ERACI II). One year follow-up results. J Am Coll Cardiol 2000;35:8A

90. Rodriguez A, Saavedra S, Fernandez C, et al. Percutaneous transluminal coronary revascularization versus coronary bypass surgery in patients with multiple vessel disease and proximal

left anterior descending artery stenosis: Results from the ERACI II study. J Am Coll Cardiol 2000;35:9A.

91. Malenka D, O'Connor G, Quinton H, et al. Longterm survival following surgical versus percutaneous coronary revascularization in patients with low and preserved ejection fractions. J Am Coll Cardiol 2000;35:31A.

92. Siegel R, Vermillion J, Bhaskaran A, et al. Long-term clinical outcomes of percutaneous coronary intervention in patients with severe left ventricular dysfunction. J Am Coll Cardiol 2000;35:11A.

93. Muhlestein JB, Frommater DN, Bair TL, et al. Incomplete revascularization, long-term outcome and functional status in patients undergoing percutaneous coronary interventions. J Am Coll Cardiol 2000;35:79A.

94. Goy JJ, Kaufmann U, Goy-Eggenberger D, et al. A prospective randomized trial comparing stenting to internal mammary artery grafting for proximal, isolated de novo left anterior coronary artery stenosis: The SIMA trial. Mayo Clin Proc 2000;75:1116-1123.

95. Folland ED, Hartigan PM, Parisi AF, et al. Percutaneous transluminal coronary angioplasty vs. medical therapy for stable angina pectoris. J Am Coll Cardiol 1997;29:1501-11.

96. Davies RF, Goldberg AD, Forman S, et al. Asymptomatic cardiac ischemia pilot (ACIP) study two-year follow-up. Circulation 1997;95:2037-43.

97. RITA-2 Investigators. Coronary angioplasty vs. medical therapy for angina: The Second Randomized Intervention Treatment of Angina (RITA-2) trial. Lancet 1997;350:461-8.

98. Pitt B, Waters D, Virgil W, et al. Aggressive lipid-lowering therapy compared with angioplasty in stable coronary artery disease. N Engl J Med 1999;341:70-6.

99. O'Rourke RA, Boden WE, Weintraub WS, Hartigan P. Medical therapy vs. percutaneous coronary interventions: Implications of the AVERT study and the COURAGE trial. Curr Pract Med 1999;2:225-7.

100. Blumenthal RS, Cohn G, Schulman SP. Medical therapy versus coronary angioplasty in stable coronary artery disease: A critical review of the literature. J Am Coll Cardiol 2000;36:668-73.

101. Weintraub WS, Becker ER, Mauldin PD, et al. Costs of revascularization over eight years in the randomized and eligible patients in the Emory Angioplasty versus Surgery Trial (EAST). Am J Cardiol 2000;86:747-752.

102. Singh M, Rihal CS, Berger PB, et al. Improving outcome over time of percutaneous coronary interventions in unstable angina. J Am Coll Cardiol 2000;36:674-8.

103. Buchner HC, Hengstler P, Schindler C, Guyatt GH. Percutaneous transluminal coronary angioplasty versus medical treatment for non-acute coronary heart disease: Meta-analysis of randomized controlled trials. BMJ 2000;321:73-7.

104. Detre KM, Guo P, Holubkov R, et al. Coronary revascularization in diabetic patients: A comparison of the randomized and observational components of the Bypass Angioplasty Revascularization Investigation (BARI). Circulation 1999;99:633-640.

105. Barsness GW, Peterson ED, Ohman EM, Nelson CL, DeLong ER, Reves JG, Smith PK, Anderson D, Jones RH, Mark DB, Califf RM. Relationship between diabetes mellitus and long-term survival after coronary bypass and angioplasty. Circulation 1997;96:2551-2556.

106. Abizaid A, Dangas G, Mehran R, et al. One-year results after multivessel stenting in diabetic vs. non diabetic patients. J Am Coll Cardiol 2001;37(2):68A.

107. Serruys PW, Erasmus Univ the Netherlands, et al. Arterial revascularisation therapy study: The ARTS study, a randomised trial of bypass-surgery versus stenting in multivessel coronary disease. Circulation 2000; I498: 2620.

108. Moussa I, Di Mario C, Reimers B, et al. Long-term outcome of multivessel coronary stenting. Cardiology Review 2000;17:8.

109. Whang W, Bigger J. Diabetes and outcomes of coronary artery bypass graft surgery in patients with severe left ventricular dysfunction: Results from the CABG patch trial database. J Am Coll Cardiol 2001;36:1166-72.

110. Rodriguez A, Bernardi V, Navia J, et al. Argentine randomized study: Coronary angioplasty with stenting versus coronary bypass surgery in patients with multiple-vessel disease (ERACI II): 30-day and one-year follow-up results. J Am Coll Cardiol 2001;37:51-8.

111. Bossi I, Klersy C, Jordan C, et al. Isolated proximal left anterior descending coronary artery stenosis: Long-term clinical outcome after percutaneous interventions. J Am Coll Cardiol 2001;37(2):15A.

112. Thiele H, Diegelen A, Lauer B, et al. Minimal invasive bypass surgery versus stent implantation in isolated proximal high lesions of the LAD in more than 200 patients. J Am Coll Cardiol 2001;37(2):370A.

113. Patel V, Marso S, Jones P, et al. Multivessel stenting: Is it time to reconsider recommendations for coronary artery bypass surgery? J Am Coll Cardiol 2001;37(2):51A.

4 HIGH-RISK INTERVENTION

James E. Tcheng, M.D.
Robert D. Safian, M.D.

RISK STRATIFICATION

The risk of major ischemic complications (death, myocardial infarction, emergency repeat intervention or coronary bypass surgery) during and after percutaneous coronary intervention (PCI) varies considerably, depending on baseline clinical and angiographic characteristics and procedural factors. The risk can be minimized by careful case selection, risk factor modification, optimal technique, adjunctive pharmacotherapy, supplemental imaging modalities, circulatory support, and early recognition and management of complications.

One large multicenter study by the Registry Committee of the Society for Cardiac Angiography and Interventions (SCAI)[1] identified risk factors for major in-hospital complications among 10,622 patients undergoing angioplasty. After developing an integrated, simplified, predictive index based on the number of "high-risk" variables, the index was validated in a separate cohort of 5250 PTCA patients (Table 4.1). A number of older studies developed models to predict the risk of coronary intervention.[2-8] Factors which consistently increased the risk of abrupt closure after PTCA included unstable angina, lesion thrombus, multivessel disease, multilesion angioplasty, lesion angulation > 45°, branch point or ostial stenosis, long lesion length, suboptimal ACT, lack of aspirin therapy, residual stenosis > 30%, complex dissection (NHLBI class C-F), depressed ejection fraction, increasing age, and acute or recent MI. However, most of these studies antedated the routine availability of stents and platelet glycoprotein IIb/IIIa receptor blockers, which have markedly decreased the incidence of ischemic complications.

Table 4.1. Risk of Major Complications After PTCA[1]

Risk Class	Risk Factors (N)†	Patients (N)	Complications (%)*
Low	0	37,333	1.3
Moderate	1-2	5400	2.6
High	3	326	8.6
Very high	> 3	79	23

† Risk factors = aortic valve disease, left main PTCA, shock, acute MI < 24 hours, Type C lesion, multivessel disease, and unstable angina

* In-hospital death, MI (within 24 hours of the procedure), and emergency CABG

More recent studies indicate that clinical factors (e.g., LVEF < 35%, left main or multivessel disease, recent are MI) are more important than angiographic factors for predicting risk.[30] In contemporary practice (including stents, atherectomy), the incidence of in-hospital major ischemic complications has decreased from 3.6% to 1.6%.[29] Independent predictors of adverse outcome include cardiogenic shock (odds ratio 8.6), renal failure (odds ratio 3.3), evolving myocardial infarction (odds ratio 2.8), and congestive heart failure (odds ratio 2.2); unfavorable lesion morphology is an important determinant of procedural success, but is not a strong predictor of ischemic complications. A multivariable risk factor equation for hospital death after PTCA has been used to estimate risk in New York State (Table 4.2),[33] New England,[34] and the Cleveland Clinic.[35] These clinical characteristics can also be used to estimate risk in patients treated with stents and other devices. Lesion morphology (except for Type C lesions) adds little to risk assessment.[30,34]

Table 4.2. Multivariable Risk Factors for In-Hospital Death After PTCA[33]

Risk Factor	Odds Ratio
Demographic Factors	
Age	1.06
Female gender	1.31
Ventricular Function	
EF < 20%	3.68
EF 20-39%	1.49
Symptomatic heart failure	2.38
Prior MI	
< 6 hours	5.22
6-23 hours	3.67
1-7 days	2.10
Comorbidities	
Hemodynamic instability	4.15
Shock	18.31
Renal failure	3.51
Femoral popliteal disease	1.78
Diabetes mellitus	1.41
Procedural Factors	
IABP	2.39
Prior PTCA	0.59
Multivessel PTCA	1.82
Prior CABG	1.43

Abbreviations: CABG = coronary artery bypass surgery; EF = left ventricular ejection fraction; IABP = intra-aortic balloon pump; MI = myocardial infarction; PTCA = percutaneous transluminal coronary angioplasty

---

RISK REDUCTION

Figure 4.1 summarizes important prophylactic and therapeutic measures aimed at reducing the risk of high-risk PCI. Many of these issues are detailed elsewhere, however, a few deserve special emphasis.

A. **PRE-PROCEDURAL CONSIDERATIONS**

1. **Patient Referral.** Procedures involving high-risk lesions and/or high-risk patients should be performed at high-volume interventional centers with experienced operators and support staff. Expertise with stents, thrombectomy devices, IABP and CPS is essential.[9]

2. **Timing of Intervention.** Diabetics receiving metformin with baseline creatinine levels > 1.5 mg/dL should have their medication discontinued for at least 24 hours before and 48 hours after intervention, if possible, to reduce the risk of lactic acidosis, which carries a 50% mortality rate. Elective intervention should be deferred until the PT is < 16 seconds for patients taking warfarin, and for at least 24 hours after sildenafil (Viagra) has been discontinued (Chapter 1).

3. **Optimizing Volume Status and Electrolytes.** Careful assessment of intravascular volume is mandatory during high-risk intervention; intravascular volume depletion exaggerates the hypotensive effects of contrast agents, nitrates and ischemia, while aggressive administration of IV fluids can induce heart failure in patients with marginal LV reserve. A pulmonary artery catheter should be inserted in patients with labile hemodynamic performance or overt heart failure, and electrolyte disturbances should be corrected before intervention to reduce arrhythmia.

4. **Surgical Standby.** In high-risk intervention, consultation with cardiothoracic surgery *before* the procedure is advised to review options and plan strategies. An operating room should be on standby during the procedure to minimize the time to emergency CABG, particularly if a high-risk intervention is performed on a patient who is not a candidate for stenting.

5. **Prophylaxis Against Renal Failure.** Patients with pre-existing renal insufficiency or a history of renal dysfunction following contrast exposure must be well hydrated before intervention. The only pre-procedural measure documented to reduce renal dysfunction is saline hydration, although preliminary data with N-acetylcysteine and fenoldopam (dopamine-1 receptor agonist) are encouraging (Chapter 25).[10,11] In hospitalized patients, initiation of IV crystalloid infusion (75-150 cc/hr of normal saline starting ≥ 8 hours before the case) is advisable. Supplemental diuretics may be necessary to prevent pulmonary congestion if concomitant LV dysfunction is present. Upon completion of the case, crystalloid infusion is usually continued for an additional 8-24 hours to facilitate excretion of the contrast agent. In patients without heart failure, one or more bolus infusions of normal saline (200 cc) may be given if urine output falls below 40 cc/hr. If urine output remains low in patients with LV dysfunction, supplemental diuretics (e.g., furosemide 20-80 mg IV bolus) may improve urine flow.

6. **Choice of Contrast and Prophylaxis Against Reactions (Chapter 25).** A recent prospective multicenter randomized trial reported a 45% reduction in in-hospital ischemic complications with low-osmolar nonionic iodixanol (Visipaque) compared to low-osmolar ionic ioxaglate (Hexabrix).[31]

7. **Hemodynamic and Pacemaker Support.** A pulmonary artery catheter should be considered to ensure optimal volume status and continuously monitor pulmonary artery pressure in patients with severe LV dysfunction, a large area of jeopardized myocardium, or unstable hemodynamic performance. A prophylactic transvenous pacemaker should be considered when a pre-existing high-grade conduction disturbance is present or when no-reflow is anticipated in the distribution of a dominant RCA or left circumflex artery. No-reflow should be anticipated in the presence of a large thrombus, vein graft intervention, or when using the Rotablator. Contralateral femoral arterial access with a 4 or 5 French sheath is reasonable to assure central arterial access when an IABP or CPS might be needed. For selected high-risk cases, prophylactic insertion of a balloon pump or CPS may be indicated (Chapter 6).

8. **Other Considerations.** The support staff of the cardiac catheterization suite must be alerted to the high-risk nature of the procedure. Both groins should be prepped to minimize the delay in initiating emergency IABP or CPS. Placement of R-2 pads on the patient before placing the sterile drape will expedite defibrillation.

B. INTRAPROCEDURAL CONSIDERATIONS

1. **Limiting Ischemia.** Strict attention to procedural technique is necessary to avoid inadvertent or prolonged ischemia during high-risk intervention.

   1. **Limiting Ischemia During Guide Catheter Engagement.** Poor guide catheter technique can induce ischemia by ostial trauma, obstruction of flow from deep intubation (Figure 4.2), or size mismatch between the guide and ostium. Dampening of the arterial pressure or delayed clearance of contrast from the vessel should prompt immediate repositioning of the guide or selection of an alternate guide catheter (e.g., short-tip guide, sideholes, or a different configuration).

   b. **Limiting Ischemia During Intervention.** Even before balloon inflation, ischemia may be induced by the guidewire or the shaft of the deflated balloon catheter, particularly if the baseline stenosis is severe. Measures to reduce ischemic time include short duration (15-30 sec) inflations, pre-treatment with a beta-blocker,[12] and rarely IABP support (or even CPS). If stenting is indicated, inflation duration > 15 seconds is rarely necessary. To ensure maximal perfusion of non-target vessels, the guide catheter should be disengaged from the ostium during balloon inflation. Finally, when dilating a stenosis near a branch-point, the balloon should be positioned to minimize obstruction of uninvolved side branches (Figure 4.2). During balloon inflation, a small injection of contrast through the guide can detect impaired flow in the sidebranch; if present, prompt repositioning of the balloon is required.

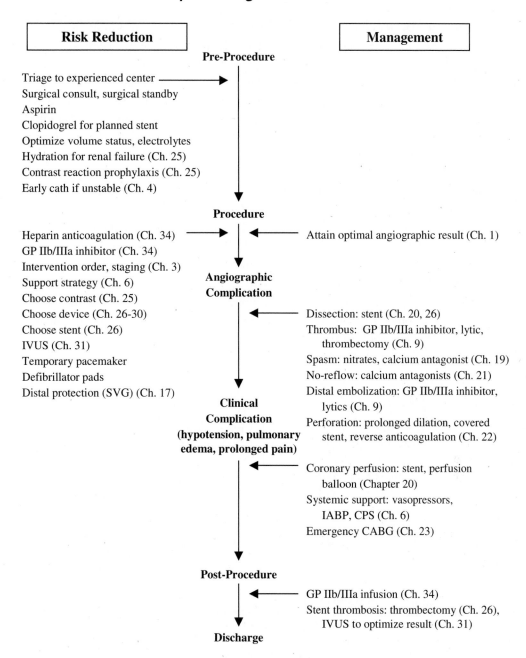

Figure 4.1. Overview of High-Risk Intervention: Risk Reduction and Management

CABG = coronary artery bypass surgery; CPS = percutaneous cardiopulmonary bypass support; IVUS = intravascular ultrasound; SVG = saphenous vein graft

2. **Interventional Devices.** The immediate goal of coronary intervention is to attain an optimal result without complications. Planned stent implantation is the most straightforward approach to reduce the potential for abrupt closure and subsequent restenosis[13] (Chapter 26). Rotablator is an important adjunct to stenting, particularly when balloon angioplasty is expected to fail (e.g., heavily calcified lesions) (Chapter 27). Other useful measures include distal protection to reduce ischemic complications during vein graft intervention (Chapter 17), intravascular ultrasound to optimize the result after high-risk stenting (Chapter 31), and coronary blood flow measurements to help guide further intervention (Chapter 33).

3. **Adjunctive Pharmacotherapy (Chapter 34).** Adjunctive pharmacotherapy remains a keystone of management. Aspirin and clopidogrel should be administered before the procedure to reduce complications if stent implantation is anticipated.[14] In the absence of contraindications, all high-risk patients should be considered for GP IIb/IIIa treatment, regardless of the device.[15-17,32] Treatment should be started before intervention to *prevent* complications, rather than reserved for salvage. Heparin should be administered to maintain a target ACT of 200-250 seconds when GP IIb/IIIa inhibitors are used since higher degrees of anticoagulation lead to excessive bleeding and adverse outcomes, particularly in high-risk patients.[18,19] When a GP IIb/IIIa inhibitor is used, additional heparin should not be given following the procedure.

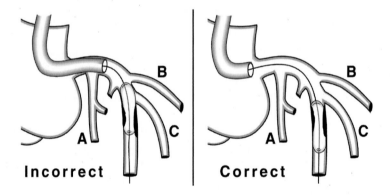

Figure 4.2. Guide Catheter and Balloon Positioning

Left panel: *Incorrect technique.* Deep intubation of the guide catheter obstructs flow down circumflex artery (A); mismatch between guide and proximal LAD obstructs flow down 1st diagonal (B); and poor balloon positioning obstructs flow down 2nd diagonal (C). Right panel: *Correct technique.* Guide is retracted 1-2 cm into the aorta after inflation of a properly positioned balloon. Coronary flow is maintained to branches A, B and C.

4. **Assessing Results.** Multiple views of the target lesion are required to accurately assess procedural outcome and exclude dissection, filling defect, residual stenosis, side branch occlusion, or flow impairment (Figure 1.6). Since abrupt closure in high-risk patients is associated with in-hospital mortality rates as high as 50%, stents and prophylactic GP IIb/IIIa inhibitors should be used in high-risk cases to reduce the risk of ischemic complications.[20,21] Intravascular ultrasound (IVUS) is particularly useful for optimizing procedural results,[22] especially in high-risk stent implantation, to ensure optimal stent expansion, apposition, and symmetry. Angioscopy can differentiate intimal flaps from intraluminal thrombus (Chapter 32),[23] but is not available in most centers.

5. **Use of Regional and Systemic Support Systems (Chapter 6).** A perfusion balloon catheter may be used when prolonged balloon inflations are required to treat perforations or reverse abrupt closure, particularly if stenting is not an option. Intra-aortic balloon pumping, which can increase coronary blood flow, improve ventricular function, and support the systemic circulation, is useful for patients who develop procedural hypotension or heart failure. CPS is recommended for hypotension refractory to IABP and vasopressors, and for abrupt circulatory collapse.

C. POSTPROCEDURAL CONSIDERATIONS

1. **Triage and Monitoring.** Patients should be transferred to a telemetry unit after high-risk intervention. Overnight observation in a cardiac intensive care unit is preferred if the procedure is complicated by a suboptimal angiographic result or the continued need for a pacemaker, IABP, or CPS. Invasive hemodynamic monitoring and support should remain in place until the patient is stable, usually for 24 hours or less.

2. **Complications.** Recurrent chest pain associated with ECG changes or hemodynamic instability mandates immediate return to the cath lab to exclude abrupt closure or stent thrombosis. Asymptomatic hypotension may be caused by medications (sedatives, nitrates, calcium antagonists, beta-blockers) or mild hypovolemia (NPO status, contrast-induced diuresis). More serious conditions such as tamponade, retroperitoneal hemorrhage, perforation, and sepsis should be considered and promptly excluded.

LEFT MAIN DISEASE

Left main coronary disease is present in 7% and 15% of patients with stable and unstable angina, respectively. Among 1484 patients enrolled in the CASS Registry with > 50% obstruction of the left main, median survival was 13.3 years for the surgical group, but only 6.6 years for the medical group.[24] The survival benefit was confined mainly to patients with > 60% stenosis, particularly if LV dysfunction was present. Balloon angioplasty of unprotected left main disease is technically feasible, but procedural and 3-year mortality rates are high: 9% and 64% for elective cases, and 50% and 70% for acute MI.[25,37,38] More favorable results with stents have recently been reported by a number of groups[26-28,36,37,39] (Chapter 26), although death or CABG at 12 months has been reported in up to 20% of patients.[36,39] Despite improving outcomes with stents and potent antiplatelet regimens, unprotected left main stenosis should still be considered a surgical disease; further studies of percutaneous intervention are required, particularly in patients who refuse surgery or who are poor surgical candidates. In contrast, when the left main is protected, catheter-based interventions can be performed with acceptable early and late outcomes.[25]

CARDIOGENIC SHOCK

The incidence of cardiogenic shock complicating acute MI varies from 6-20%,[40] depending on the definitions of MI and shock, whether shock is present on admission or develops during hospitalization, and on the use of early reperfusion therapy. A reasonable estimate of the incidence of cardiogenic shock is 0.8-1.8% at the time of admission and 7% during the hospitalization.[40-43] Although the incidence of cardiogenic shock has not declined over the last 25 years, there was a trend toward higher survival in the mid-to-late 1990s, which seems to parallel increasing trends in the use of coronary reperfusion strategies.[44]
Nevertheless, the risk of in-hospital death is nearly 6-fold higher in patients with cardiogenic shock than in those without it (72% vs. 12%). Virtually all patients with cardiogenic shock should receive an IABP to improve clinical and hemodynamic status, although an IABP alone is insufficient treatment to improve survival. Two multicenter randomized trials compared emergency revascularization to initial medical stabilization for cardiogenic shock complicating acute MI.[44,45] Although neither demonstrated differences in 30-day survival, the SMASH trial (Swiss Multicenter Trial of Angioplasty for Shock) was prematurely terminated because of selection bias.[46] Importantly, the SHOCK trial demonstrated significantly better 6-month survival (50% vs. 37%, p = 0.027) and 1-year survival (46.7% vs. 33.6%, p < 0.03)[48] in the early revascularization group, even though 30-day mortality was similar. Among patients with non-ST-elevation acute coronary syndromes who developed cardiogenic shock in the PURSUIT trial, eptifibatide reduced the risk of death at 30 days (odds ratio = 0.51, p = 0.03),[47] suggesting a potential role for antiplatelet therapy.

* * * * * *

REFERENCES

1. Kimmel SE, Berlin JA, Strom BL, Laskey WK. Development and validation of a simplified predictive index for major complications in contemporary percutaneous transluminal coronary angioplasty practice. J Am Coll Cardiol 1995;26:931-938.

2. Thel MC, Califf RM, Tcheng JE, et al. Clinical risk factors for ischemic complications after percutaneous coronary interventions: results from the EPIC trial. Am Heart J 1999;137:264-73.

3. Hong MK, Popma JJ, Baim DS, et al. Frequency and predictors of major in-hospital ischemic complications after planned and unplanned new-device angioplasty from the New Approaches to Coronary Intervention (NACI) registry. Am J Cardiol 1997; 80(10A):40K-49K.

4. King SB, Yeh W, Holubkov R, et al. Balloon angioplasty versus new device intervention: clinical outcomes. A comparison of the NHLBI PTCA and NACI registries. J Am Coll Cardiol, 1998;31:558-66.

5. Garot P, Himbert D, Juliard JM, et al. Incidence, consequences, and risk factors of early reocclusion after primary and/or rescue percutaneous transluminal coronary angioplasty for acute myocardial infarction. Am J Cardiol 1998;82:554-8.

6. Maynard C, Chapko MK, Every NR, et al. Coronary angioplasty outcomes in the Healthcare Cost and Utilization Project, 1993-1994. Am J Cardiol 1998;81:848-52.

7. Malenka DJ, O'Connor GT, Quinton H, et al. Differences in outcomes between women and men associated with percutaneous transluminal coronary angioplasty. A regional prospective study of 13,061 procedures. Circulation 1996; 94(9 Suppl):II 99-104.

8. Waksman R, Ghazzal ZM, Baim DS, et al. Myocardial infarction as a complication of new interventional devices. Am J Cardiol 1996; 78:751-6.

9. Hirshfeld JW Jr, Ellis SG, Faxon DP. Recommendations for the assessment and maintenance of proficiency in coronary interventional procedures: Statement of the American College of Cardiology. J Am Coll Cardiol 1998;31:722-43.

10. Solomon R, Werner C, Mann D, J DE, Silva P. Effects of saline, mannitol, and furosemide to prevent acute decreases in renal function induced by radiocontrast agents. N Engl J Med 1994;331:1416-1420.

11. Stevens MA, McCullough PA, Tobin KJ, et al. A prospective randomized trial of prevention measures in patients at high risk for contrast nephropathy: results of the P.R.I.N.C.E. Study. Prevention of Radiocontrast Induced Nephropathy Clinical Evaluation. J Am Coll Cardiol 1999;3:403-11.

12. Zalewski A, Goldberg A, Dervan JP, et al. Myocardial protection during transient coronary artery occlusion in man: beneficial effects of regional ß-adrenergic blockade. Circulation 1986;73:734-9.

13. Versaci F, Gaspardone A, Tomai F, et al. A comparison of coronary artery stenting with angioplasty for isolated stenosis of the proximal left anterior descending coronary artery. N Engl J Med 1997;336:817-22.

14. Moussa I, Oetgen M, Roubin G, et al. Effectiveness of clopidogrel and aspirin versus ticlopidine and aspirin in preventing stent thrombosis after coronary stent implantation. Circulation 1999;99:2364-2366.

15. Lincoff AM, Califf RM, Anderson KM, et al. Evidence for prevention of death and myocardial infarction with platelet membrane glycoprotein IIb/IIIa receptor blockade by abciximab (c7E3 Fab) among patients with unstable angina undergoing percutaneous coronary revascularization. J Am Coll Cardiol 1997;30:149-56.

16. The EPISTENT Investigators. Randomized placebo-controlled and balloon-angioplasty-controlled trial to assess safety of coronary stenting with use of platelet glycoprotein IIb/IIIa blockade. Lancet 1998;352:87-92.

17. Bhatt DL, Topol EJ. The benefit of abciximab in interventional cardiology is not device-specific. Circulation 1998;98:I-17 (abstract).

18. Mandak JS, Blankenship JC, Gardner LH, et al. Modifiable risk factors for vascular access site complications in the IMPACT II Trial. J Am Coll Cardiol 1998;31:1518-24.

19. Blankenship JC, Hellkamp AS, Aguirre FV, et al. Vascular access site complications after percutaneous coronary intervention with abciximab in the Evaluation of c7E3 for the Prevention of Ischemic Complications (EPIC) trial. Am J Cardiol 1998;81:36-40.

20. Belli G, Ellis SG, Topol EJ. Stenting for ischemic heart disease. [Review] Prog Cardiovasc Dis 1997;40:159-82.

21. Madan M, Berkowitz SD, Tcheng JE. Glycoprotein IIb/IIIa integrin blockade. [Review] Circulation 1998;98:2629-35.

22. Oesterle SN, Whitbourn R, Fitzgerald PJ, et al. The stent decade: 1987 to 1997. Stanford Stent Summit faculty. [Review] Am Heart J 1998;136(4 Pt 1):578-99.

23. Annex BH. Coronary angioscopy. Clinical applications. [Review] Cardiol Clin 1997;15:131-7.

24. Caracciolo EA, Davis KB, Sopko G, et al. Comparison of surgical and medical group survival in patients with left main coronary artery disease. Long-term CASS experience. Circulation 1995;91:2325-2334.

25. Ellis SG, Tamai H, Nobuyoshi M, et al. Contemporary percutaneous treatment of unprotected left main coronary stenoses: initial results from a multicenter registry analysis 1994-1996. Circulation 1997;96:3867-72.

26. Kornowski R, Klutstein M, Satler LF, et al. Impact of stents on clinical outcomes in percutaneous left main coronary artery revascularization. Am J Cardiol 1998;82:32-7.

27. Laruelle CJ, Brueren GB, Ernst SM, et al. Stenting of "unprotected" left main coronary artery stenoses: early and late results. Heart 1998;79:148-52.

28. Park SJ, Park SW, Hong MK, et al. Stenting of unprotected left main coronary artery stenoses: immediate and late outcomes. J Am Coll Cardiol 1998;31:37-42.

29. Harrell L, Schunkert H, Palacios I, Risk predictors in patients scheduled for percutaneous coronary revascularization. Catheterization and Cardiovascular Interventions 1999;48:253-260.

30. Rihal CS, Grill DE, Bell MR, et al. Prediction of death after percutaneous coronary interventional procedures. Am Heart J 2000;1031-1038.

31. Davidson CJ, Laskey WK, Jermiller JB, et al. Randomized trial of contrast media utilization in high-risk PTCA.

Circulation 2000; 2172-2177.

32. Weintraub WS, Culler S, Boccuzzi, SJ et al. Economic impact of GPIIB/IIIA blockade after high-risk angioplasty. J Am Coll Cardiol 1999;34:1061-1066.

33. Hannan EL, Racz M, Ryan TJ, et al. Coronary angioplasty volume-outcome relationships for hospitals and cardiologists. JAMA 1997; 277:892-8.

34. O'Connor GT, Malenda DJ, Quinton H, et al. Multivariate predication of in-hospital mortality after percutaneous coronary interventions in 1994-1996. J Am Coll Cardiol 1999;34:681-690.

35. Moscucci M, O'Conner GT, Ellis SG, et al. Validation of risk adjustment models for in-hospital percutaneous transluminal coronary angioplasty mortality on an independent data sheet. J Am Coll Cardiol 1999;35:692-6.

36. Silvestri M, Barragan P, Sainsous J, et al. Unprotected left main coronary artery stenting: immediate and medium-term outcomes of 140 elective procedures. J Am Coll Cardiol 2000;35:1543-52.

37. Marso SP, Steg G, Plokker T, et al. Catheter-based reperfusion of unprotected left main stenosis during acute myocardial infarction (the ULTIMA experience). Am J Cardiol 1999;83:1513-16.

38. Kosuga K, Tamai H, Ueda K, et al. Inital and long-term results of angioplasty in unprotected left main coronary artery disease. Am J Cardiol 1999;83:32-7.

39. Wong P, Wong V, Tse K, et al. A prospective study of elective stenting in unprotected left main coronary disease. Catheterization and Cardiovascular Interventions 1999;46:153-159.

40. Califf RM, Bengston JR. Cardiogenic shock. N Engl J Med 1994;330:1724-30.

41. Edep ME, Brown DL. Effect of early revascularization on mortality from cardiogenic shock complicating acute myocardial infarction in california. Am J Cardiol 2000;85:1185-88.

42. Holmes DR, Bates ER, Kleiman NS, et al. Contemporary reperfusion therapy for cardiogenic shock. The GUSTO-1 trial experience. J Am Coll Cardiol 1995;26:668-74.

43. Goldberg RJ, Samad NA, Yarzebski J, et al. Temporal trends in cardiogenic shock complicating acute myocardial infarction. N Engl J Med 1999;340:1162-68.

44. Brodie BR, Stuckey TD, Hansen C, et al. Intra-aortic balloon counterpulsation before primary percutaneous transluminal coronary angioplasty reduces catheterization laboratory events in high-risk patients with acute myocardial infarction. Am J Cardiol 1999;84:18-23.

45. Hochman JS, Sleeper LA, Webb JG, et al. Early revascularization in acute myocardial infarction complicated by cardiogenic shock. N Engl J Med 1999;341:625-634.

46. Urban P, Stauffer JC, Bleed D et al. A randomized evaluation of early revascularization to treat shock complicating acute myocardial infarction. Eur Heart J 1999;20:1030-1038.

47. Hasdai D, Harrington RA, Hochman JS, et al. Platelet glycoprotein IIb/IIIa blockade and outcome of cardiogenic shock complication acute coronary syndromes without persistent ST-segment elevation. J Am Coll Cardiol 2000;36:685-92.

48. Hochman JS, Sleeper LA, White HD, et al. One-year survival following early revascularization for cardiogenic shock. JAMA 2001;285:190-192.

PERCUTANEOUS INTERVENTION FOR ACUTE CORONARY SYNDROMES

Alexandra J. Lansky, M.D.
Gregg W. Stone, M.D.

ACUTE MYOCARDIAL INFARCTION

The widespread availability of intravenous thrombolytic therapy has revolutionized the medical management of patients with acute MI, by prolonging survival and preserving left ventricular function. Despite these important beneficial effects, there are many deficiencies of thrombolysis:

- Only 33% of acute MI patients receive thrombolytic therapy

- 20% of vessels remain occluded and 45% have TIMI flow ≤ 2

- The median time to reperfusion is 45 minutes

- No bedside clinical markers reliably predict reperfusion

- Recurrent ischemia occurs in 15-30% of patients

- Life-threatening intracranial bleeding develops in 0.5-1.5% of patients

To overcome these deficiencies, several PTCA strategies for acute MI have emerged, including primary PTCA (no prior thrombolytics); salvage or rescue PTCA (for failed thrombolysis); immediate PTCA (after successful thrombolysis); and delayed PTCA (before hospital discharge) (Table 5.1). Other techniques such as mechanical thrombectomy, stents, and potent platelet receptor antagonists have been developed as adjuncts to PTCA.

Table 5.1. Angioplasty Approaches for Acute MI

Approach	Description
Primary (Direct)	PTCA without antecedent thrombolytic therapy
Rescue (Salvage)	PTCA after failed thrombolysis (TIMI 0-1 in the infarct vessel)
Immediate	PTCA for significant residual stenosis immediately after successful thrombolysis
Delayed (Deferred)	PTCA for significant residual stenosis 1-7 days after thrombolysis, prior to discharge

Table 5.2. Primary (Direct) PTCA

Advantages Compared to Thrombolysis

 Applicable to thrombolytic-ineligible patients

 Immediate definition of coronary anatomy and left ventricular function

 Early risk stratification

 Superior restoration of acute vessel patency and TIMI 3 flow

 Less recurrent ischemia, reinfarction and reocclusion

 Better survival in high-risk patients

 Less reperfusion injury and myocardial rupture

 Lower risk of life-threatening intracranial hemorrhage

 Shorter length of hospital stay

 Reduced cost

Disadvantages Compared to Thrombolysis

 Skilled interventional cardiologist and cath lab facilities must be available

 Logistic delays in mobilizing lab and support staff

PRIMARY (DIRECT) PTCA

Primary PTCA refers to the use of balloon angioplasty without prior thrombolytic therapy, and is associated with several potential advantages and disadvantages compared to thrombolysis (Table 5.2). Importantly, compared to lytics, PTCA results in better acute arterial patency (TIMI 2 or 3 flow in 95-99% vs. 70-80%), less recurrent ischemia, and improved survival, especially in high-risk patients (elderly, women, anterior infarction, cardiogenic shock). Many studies have also demonstrated serial improvement in left ventricular function after primary PTCA, as well as less reperfusion injury, cardiogenic shock, and myocardial rupture. Even in centers that do not regularly perform elective PTCA, low rates of recurrent ischemia, reinfarction and need for emergency CABG have been described, raising the issue of whether on-site surgical backup is necessary for primary PTCA.[1-4] Although early series reported early and late reocclusion rates in 8% and 20% of patients, contemporary in-hospital and 6-month reocclusion rates are 2-3% and 9-13%, respectively, due to more frequent use of antiplatelet agents, optimal heparin dosing, and improved PTCA and stent techniques.[5-9]

Over the last 10 years, pooled data from single-center observational studies of primary PTCA reported acute patency in 93%, in-hospital mortality in 7.4%, and predischarge reocclusion in 10% of patients (Table 5.3).[8,10-21] Independent predictors of in-hospital mortality included cardiogenic shock, triple vessel disease, reduced ejection fraction, advanced age, anterior infarction, and failed PTCA.[22] Mortality at 1 month, 1 year, and 3 years was 5%, 9%, and 13%, respectively.[23] The Myocardial Infarction Triage and Intervention (MITI) investigators tracked the outcomes of 3750 consecutive patients with acute MI in metropolitan Seattle over a three-year period,[24] including 653 (17%) patients treated with thrombolytic therapy and 441 (12%) patients treated with primary PTCA. Compared to thrombolytics, primary PTCA patients had fewer strokes (0.6% vs. 2.1%, p = 0.12), shorter hospital stay (7.0 vs. 8.1 days, p < 0.001), and less recurrent ischemia (20% vs. 30%, p = 0.009). Primary PTCA also had superior long-term outcomes compared to intracoronary tPA.[26]

A. **PRIMARY PTCA FOR LYTIC-INELIGIBLE PATIENTS.** About 75% of acute MI patients have absolute or relative contraindications to thrombolytic therapy based on TIMI 2B criteria. Compared to lytic-eligible patients, these patients are more likely to be older, female, and have prior MI, multivessel disease, low ejection fraction, and high in-hospital mortality (18.7% vs. 3.9%, p < 0.001).[25,27] As shown in Table 5.4, primary PTCA can be applied to most MI patients irrespective of lytic eligibility.[10,11,23,28] However, procedure-related mortality is higher in lytic-ineligible patients due to underlying comorbid disease.[10,11] Certain patient groups are better suited for primary PTCA than thrombolytic therapy, including the elderly (less intracranial hemorrhage), patients who present late after symptom onset (higher patency rates with PTCA), and patients with vein graft occlusions (low patency rates with intravenous thrombolytics due to large thrombus burden and reduced run-off).[10,11,21,29] The randomized SMART trial of PTCA vs. medical therapy for lytic-ineligible patients reported less ischemia and reinfarction after PTCA.[30] At our institution, all lytic-ineligible patients who present within 12 hours of acute MI (or later if symptoms persist) undergo emergency catheterization followed by primary PTCA or stenting if appropriate. When a skilled interventionalist and cath lab are not immediately available for lytic-ineligible patients, transfer to a tertiary center for emergency PTCA is recommended, especially if high-risk features are present (Figure 5.2).

B. **PRIMARY PTCA FOR LYTIC-ELIGIBLE PATIENTS**
  1. **Registry Experience.** The PAR (Primary Angioplasty Revascularization)[50] registry and others[10,11] reported high procedural success (92-97%) and a relatively low incidence of in-hospital ischemic complications after primary PTCA (mortality 2-4%, recurrent MI 2-3%, recurrent ischemia 2-12%) (Table 5.5). These results compared favorably to the 60-80% patency rates, 4-11% mortality rates, and 30% reocclusion rates reported after thrombolytic therapy.[51-63]

  2. **Randomized Trials.** A total of 10 trials have been performed in 2606 patients randomized to primary PTCA vs. streptokinase (4 studies), a 3- or 4-hour t-PA regimen (3 studies), or accelerated t-PA (3 studies).[5,64,65-70] Most of these trials demonstrated superiority of primary PTCA with regard to acute patency, TIMI-3 flow, recurrent ischemia, reinfarction, infarct artery reocclusion, stroke, intracranial bleeding, mortality, and length of hospital stay. The largest trial, the GUSTO-2B

angioplasty substudy, demonstrated that PTCA was superior to accelerated tPA in reducing recurrent ischemia, intracranial bleeding (0% vs. 1.4%, p = 0.008), and the 30-day primary composite endpoint of death, reinfarction, or disabling stroke (9.6% vs. 13.6%, p = 0.03).[71] At 6 months, the early advantage of primary angioplasty was less dramatic,[72] in contrast to the PAMI trial (benefits of PTCA were maintained) and the Zwolle study (benefits of primary PTCA improved during follow-up). These studies were too small to demonstrate mortality differences, but several metanalyses[70,73] demonstrated better short-term mortality and less nonfatal MI and stroke after PTCA. High-risk patients (age > 70, anterior MI, heart rate > 100, or Killip class > 1) had the most striking reduction in death and stroke, whereas low-risk patients had less recurrent ischemia, reinfarction, and shorter hospital stay. The definitive metanalysis of all 10 randomized trials (Tables 5.6, 5.7)[291] demonstrated marked benefits for PTCA, including lower mortality at 30 days (4.4% vs. 6.6%, p = 0.02) and 6 months (5.1% vs. 7.5%, p = 0.039); less nonfatal reinfarction at 30 days (2.9% vs. 5.3%, p = 0.002) and 6 months (4.2% vs. 8.4%, p = 0.0001); fewer strokes at 30 days (0.66% vs. 1.88%, p = 0.01); and virtual elimination of intracranial hemorrhage (0.07% vs. 1.09%). The relative reduction in death or non-fatal reinfarction after primary PTCA was striking: 40% at at 30 days (7.2% vs. 11.9%, p = 0.001) and 37% at 6 months (9.6% vs. 15.2%, p = 0.0001). These results strongly support the superiority of primary PTCA for reducing death, reinfarction, stroke, and intracranial hemorrhage. The mechanism of improved outcome after primary PTCA (vs. thrombolysis) is multifactorial:

- **Improved Vessel Patency and Coronary Flow:** TIMI-3 flow is an important determinant of left ventricular functional recovery and patient survival.[74] A metanalysis of angiographic trials after thrombolysis[60] and the GUSTO angiographic substudy[74] reported acute patency rates (TIMI 2 or 3 flow) of 50% (with streptokinase) and 80% (with accelerated tPA); TIMI-3 flow was restored in only 40-52% of patients after thrombolysis. In contrast, primary PTCA achieved acute patency in 98-99% of patients, TIMI-3 flow in 93-94%, and a residual stenosis < 50% in 93-97%.[5,7,8,64,65,73]

- **Less Reocclusion (Table 5.8):** Late angiographic follow-up demonstrated less reocclusion after primary PTCA compared to successful thrombolysis (5-13% vs. 30-40%).[5,7,8,75-79] (Restenosis after primary PTCA occurs in 35-45% of patients, necessitating repeat revascularization in 25% of patients within 5 months.)

- **Early Triage:** Emergency angiography allows early definition of coronary anatomy, assessment of left ventricular function and filling pressures, and facilitates risk stratification and appropriate therapy. Based on clinical and angiographic findings, patients may be referred for PTCA or stents, immediate or delayed cardiac surgery, or medical therapy.[1,64,80,81] In PAMI, there was an 18-fold difference in mortality between high-and low-risk patients based on clinical and angiographic variables.[81]

- **Less Intracranial Bleeding.** As more elderly patients are treated with thrombolytic therapy, intracranial hemorrhage rates have risen to ~1%. In the GUSTO trial, 85% of intracranial bleeds resulted in death or severe disability. Primary PTCA virtually eliminates this risk.

3. **Cost.** Because of fewer complications, less recurrent ischemia, and shorter hospital stay, the cost of primary PTCA is less than the cost of thrombolysis. In PAMI-2, low-risk patients (age ≤ 70, 1-2 vessel disease, ejection fraction > 45%, successful PTCA of a native coronary, no serious arrhythmia)[80] were safely discharged on day 3 (in-hospital mortality 0.4%, similar to elective PTCA), resulting in a cost-savings of $4000 per patient compared to traditional care.[82,83]

4. **Time to Reperfusion.** The time from patient arrival in the emergency room to completion of angiography was 75 minutes in GUSTO-2B and 120 minutes in the PAMI trials. However, high rates of TIMI-3 flow (>90%) are restored even when primary PTCA is performed up to 12 hours after symptom onset. The multicenter AIR-PAMI trial is randomizing 430 high-risk MI patients (at sites without PTCA facilities) to emergency transfer for PTCA at a tertiary center or accelerated t-PA without routine transfer.

C. **PRIMARY PTCA FOR CARDIOGENIC SHOCK.** Patients in cardiogenic shock are typically taken to the catheterization laboratory for hemodynamic stabilization with an intra-aortic balloon pump, angiography, and emergency revascularization. Nonrandomized studies suggested a 50% reduction in mortality if TIMI-3 flow was restored (Table 5.9);[31-48] survival rates of 40-86% after PTCA were reported in this extremely high-risk patient population, compared to 30% after lytic therapy and 10% after medical therapy. In GUSTO-1, an aggressive revascularization strategy of PTCA or CABG was independently associated with improved 30-day survival[45] despite infrequent use of early intervention and balloon pumps.[49] Most recently, the multicenter randomized trial SHOCK compared the 30-day mortality of 302 patients treated by emergency catheterization followed by revascularization when appropriate (PTCA or CABG) vs. initial medical stabilization and later revascularization, if indicated. Intra-aortic balloon pumps were placed in 86%, right heart catheterization was performed in 95%, systemic thrombolytic therapy was administered in 49% of the invasive group and 64% of the conservative group, and revascularization was performed in 87% of the invasive group and 34% of the conservative group (p < 0.001). Among PTCA patients, TIMI-3 flow was restored in 61%, which was associated with a 1-month mortality of 35% compared to 65% if TIMI-3 flow was not restored (p < 0.001). At 30 days, mortality was significantly reduced in several important subgroups with the invasive approach, including patients < 75 years old (41% vs. 57%, p < 0.05), patients randomized within 6 hours of MI onset (37% vs. 63%, p < 0.01), and patients with prior MI (40% vs. 68%, p < 0.01). Survival benefit persisted at 1 year for patients in the emergency revascularization group (47.6% vs. 33.6%, p < 0.03); 83% of 1-year survivors were in NYHA heart failure class I or II.[308] These compelling data suggest that patients in cardiogenic shock should be considered for immediate angiography, IABP placement, and revascularization, particularly those < 75 years old.

D. **RECOMMENDATIONS.** Primary PTCA should be strongly considered for patients who are ineligible for thrombolytic therapy or have high-risk features (anterior MI, advanced age, tachycardia, hypotension, or heart failure). Even in low-risk, thrombolytic-eligible patients, primary PTCA will reduce recurrent ischemia, reinfarction, length of hospital stay and cost, and minimize the risk of life-threatening intracranial hemorrhage. As discussed below, IIb/IIIa receptor inhibitors and stents have improved the outcome of primary PTCA. Our approach to the interventional management of acute MI is summarized in Figure 5.1.

Table 5.3. Observational Studies of Primary PTCA: In-hospital Outcome

Study	N	Patency (%)	Mortality (%)	Reocclusion (%)
Stone[21] (1995)	47	86	6.3	13
O'Keefe[10] (1993)	1000	94	7.7	13
Nakagawa[13] (1993)	190	90	4	-
O'Neill[8] (1992)	63	92	6.3	-
Brodie[11] (1991)	383	91	9	-
Beauchamp[12] (1990)	214	92	7.9	-
Rothbaum[14] (1987)	151	87	9	9
Miller[15] (1987)	127	92	8.6	8
Dageford[16] (1987)	65	97	1.5	9
Marco[18] (1987)	43	95	9.3	-
O'Neill[19] (1986)	29	83	6.8	8
Pooled Results	**2370**	**93**	**7.4**	**10**

Table 5.4. Primary PTCA: Results in Thrombolytic Eligible vs. Ineligible Patients

Study	N	Success (%)		In-hospital Mortality (%)	
		TE	TI	TE	TI
Stone[28] (1995)	395	-	-	2.4	2.9
O'Keefe[10] (1993)	1000	96	92	3	14
Brodie[11] (1991)	383	92	88	4	24

Abbreviations: TE = thrombolytic-eligible; TI = thrombolytic-ineligible

Table 5.5. Primary PTCA in Lytic-Eligible Patients: In-hospital Outcomes

	N	Success	In-hospital Outcome (%)		
			Death	Reinfarction	Recurrent Ischemia
Danchin[320] (1999)	152	-	7.0	-	-
Tiefenbrunn[321] (1998)	4052	-	5.6	2.5	-
Stone[28] (1995)	127	-	2.4	3.1	11.8
O'Neill[50] (1994)	245	97	3.7	3	10
O'Keefe[10] (1993)	568	96	3	-	-
Brodie[11] (1991)	282	92	4	-	1.8

- not reported; reinfarction = recurrent myocardial infarction; Recurrent Ischemia = recurrent ischemia

Table 5.6. Metanalysis of Randomized Trials of Primary PTCA vs. Thrombolytic Therapy[*291]

	Primary PTCA (n = 1348)	Lytic Therapy (n = 1377)	p-Value
30-day Outcomes (%)			
Mortality	4.4	6.6	0.02
Reinfarction	2.9	5.3	0.002
Stroke	0.7	1.9	0.02
Hemorrhagic stroke	0.7	1.1	0.01
6-month Outcomes (%)			
Mortality	5.1	7.5	0.039
Reinfarction	4.2	8.4	0.0001
Death or MI	9.6	15.2	0.0001

* Pooled analysis of 10 prospective randomized trials of primary PTCA versus thrombolytic therapy from the Primary Coronary Angioplasty Trialists (PCAT) Collaboration

Table 5.7. Primary PTCA vs. Thrombolytic Therapy: Subgroup Analysis[291*]

Subgroup	30-day Death or Reinfarction (%)		Odds Ratio	Events prevented per 1000 pts
	Primary PTCA (n = 1348)	Lytic Therapy (n = 1377)		
Age < 60	4.3	8.2	0.48	41
60-70	6.3	12.8	0.51	64
> 70	13.3	23.6	0.43	118
Male	5.7	12.2	0.53	61
Female	11.7	16.4	0.29	82
No Diabetes	6.5	11.8	0.45	59
Diabetes	9.2	19.3	0.52	97
No Prior MI	6.6	11.5	0.43	58
Prior MI	9.7	22.7	0.57	114
Non-Anterior MI	6.2	12.0	0.48	60
Anterior MI	8.2	14.5	0.43	73

* Pooled analysis of 10 prospective randomized trials of primary PTCA versus thrombolytic therapy from the Primary Coronary Angioplasty Trialists (PCAT) Collaboration

Table 5.8. Primary PTCA: Angiographic Follow-up

	Follow-up (N) Angio/Clinical	Time (months)	Occluded (%)	Restenosis* (%)	TVR (%) PTCA	CABG
Brodie[7] (1994)	154 / 271	6	13	45	15.5	3.3
Zijlstra[5] (1993)	130 / 152	3 / 12	5	20	13.8	6.6
Grines[64] (1993)	199 / 175	6	-	34	13.7	7.4
Gibbons[71] (1993)	- / 47	5	-	-	4.3	4.3
O'Neill[8] (1992)	90	6	13	38	-	-

Abbreviations: TVR = target vessel revascularization

Table 5.9. Results of PTCA for Cardiogenic Shock

Study	N	Success (%)	Survival Overall	(+) Reperfusion	(-) Reperfusion
SHOCK[303] (2000)	302	-	40	65	35
Brown[38] (1995)	28	61	43	58	18
O'Neill[39] (1995)	27	88	70	75	33
Hochman[47] (1995)	55	69	40	-	-
Holmes[48] (1995)	406	-	62	-	39*
O'Keefe[10] (1993)	79	82	56	63	21
Gacioch[33] (1992)	48	73	46	61	7
Bengtson[34] (1992)	46	85	54	-	-
Lee[32] (1991)	69	71	55	69	20

* Reperfusion status unknown since angiography not performed; - = not reported; (+) = successful reperfusion; (-) = unsuccessful reperfusion

RESCUE (SALVAGE) PTCA FOR FAILED THROMBOLYSIS

A. **NONRANDOMIZED STUDIES.** Compared to patients with normal flow after thrombolytic therapy, patients with impaired (TIMI $\leq$ 2) flow have worse left ventricular function, more mechanical complications (ventricular septal defect, papillary muscle rupture), and greater mortality.[74] Rescue PTCA is often attempted in patients with failed thrombolysis to re-establish antegrade flow, salvage myocardium, and improve survival. Although rescue PTCA (Table 5.10)[84-93] restored acute patency in 71-100% of occluded vessels after failed thrombolysis, reocclusion occurred in 18% (range 3-29%; 2-3-fold higher than after primary PTCA), in-hospital mortality in 10.6% (range 0-17%), and improvement in ejection fraction was unusual. Although in-hospital and late mortality were similar after successful thrombolysis and successful rescue PTCA after failed thrombolysis,[94] failed rescue PTCA was associated with a mortality of 28-39%[95,96] (or higher in patients with cardiogenic shock or multivessel disease). Although the initial success of rescue PTCA was independent of the type of lytic agent, reocclusion rates were higher (20-30%) after t-PA. Better understanding of the importance of aspirin, high-dose heparin, and angioplasty technique have resulted in lower reocclusion rates. In the GUSTO angiographic substudy, there was no difference in immediate patency or in-hospital reocclusion among various thrombolytic regimens.[97] Likewise, reocclusion at 24 hours occurred in only 4% of patients in TIMI-4.[98]

B. **RANDOMIZED TRIALS.** There are few randomized trials of rescue PTCA compared to medical therapy (Table 5.11).[58,99,100,102,305] In TAMI-5,[66] rescue PTCA resulted in greater pre-discharge vessel patency, better wall motion in the infarct zone, and less recurrent ischemia than medical therapy. In RESCUE, patients with first anterior MI undergoing rescue PTCA of an occluded LAD had better left ventricular function, less heart failure, and a trend toward lower mortality at 1 month and 1 year than medically-treated patients.[99] The utility of abciximab during rescue angioplasty was evaluated in the GUSTO III substudy and was associated with a lower 30-day mortality (3.6% vs. 9.7%, p = 0.076),[102] although the risk of hemorrhagic complications was slightly higher. Rescue PTCA improves regional wall motion and left ventricular function, and may reduce the risk of heart failure, shock, and death in high-risk patients. The prognosis of patients after successful rescue PTCA is similar to that after successful thrombolysis, but patients requiring rescue PTCA are at increased risk for reocclusion compared to patients treated with primary PTCA or successful thrombolytic therapy. Early mortality is high if rescue PTCA is unsuccessful.

C. **RECOMMENDATIONS.** Since clinical signs of reperfusion are not reliable, we recommend emergency angiography in any acute MI patient with ongoing chest pain, hemodynamic compromise, or persistent ST-elevation 90 minutes after thrombolytic therapy for anterior MI. PTCA or stenting with adjunctive IIb/IIIa inhibitors should be performed on high-grade lesions with impaired (TIMI $\leq$ 2) flow. Small observational series suggest higher procedural success and fewer ischemic complications at 1 year with rescue stenting vs. rescue PTCA. Rescue PTCA for TIMI-3 flow has not been studied.

Table 5.10. Observational Studies of Rescue PTCA for Failed Thrombolysis: In-hospital Outcome

Study	N	Success (%)	Reocclusion (%)	Mortality (%)
GUSTO III[102]	83	-	-	3.6*
(1999)	309	-	-	9.7**
TIMI 9B[322]	218	87	4	0.5
(1997)				
CORAMI[101]	72	90	7	4
(1994)				
Ellis[99]	78	92	8	5
(1994)				
Ross[97]	214	90	12	-
(1993)				
Ellis[84]	24	78	20	13
(1992)				
Belenkie[100]	28	89	-	14
(1992)				
Grines[88]	36	-	11	-
(1991)				
Whitlow[93]	44	85	27	-
(1990)				
Abbottsmith[94]	192	88	21	9.9
(1990)				
Grines[90]	10	90	12	10
(1989)				
Holmes[89]	34	71	-	11
(1989)				
O'Connor[91]	90	89	14	17
(1989)				
Califf[85]	52	85	10	-
(1988)				
Baim[92]	37	92	26	5.4
(1988)				
Topol[104]	22	86	3	0
(1987)				
Fung[86]	13	92	16	7.6
(1986)				

Abbreviations: - = not reported
* Abciximab
** No abciximab

Table 5.11. Randomized Trials of Rescue PTCA vs. Medicine for Failed Thrombolysis

Study	TIMI Flow*	MI (%)		Death (%)		Relative Benefit of PTCA vs. Medicine
		PTCA	Medicine	PTCA	Medicine	
PRAGUE[351] (2000)	0-1	0	9	18.1	20	Trend for reduction in 30-day death, MI, revascularization, or heart failure (20% vs. 45%, p = 0.09)
Vermeer[352] (1999)	0-1	5.4	12	9.4	6.7	Trend for reduction in 30-day death or MI (5% vs. 12%, p = 0.15)
RESCUE II	2	-	-	7.1	6.7	No demonstrable benefit
RESCUE I (1994)	0-1	-	-	5.1	9.6	No difference in LVEF or death at 30 days, but significant reduction in death or heart failure (16.6% vs. 6.4%, p = 0.05)
Belenkie[353] (1992)	0-1	-	-	6.3	33.3	Non-significant reduction in in-hospital death
TAMI I (1986)	2	-	-	6.1	1.7	Slight improvement in LVEF at 14 days (p = 0.02)

Abbreviations: LVEF = left ventricular ejection fraction; PRAGUE = Primary Angioplasty in Patients Transferred from General Community Hospitals to Specialized Units with or without Emergency Thrombolysis; RESCUE = Randomized Evaluation of Salvage Angioplasty with Combined Utilization of Endpoints; TAMI = Thrombolysis and Angioplasty in Myocardial Infarction

* TIMI 0-1 = totally occluded vessels; TIMI-2 = partially occluded vessels

IMMEDIATE PTCA IN ASYMPTOMATIC PATIENTS FOLLOWING SUCCESSFUL THROMBOLYSIS

After successful thrombolysis, immediate PTCA of a high-grade stenosis may be performed in the hope of improving left ventricular function and preventing recurrent ischemia, reinfarction, and reocclusion.

A. **Randomized Trials.** Several randomized trials demonstrated that early routine PTCA after successful thrombolysis was associated with *more* transfusions and emergency CABG, a trend toward *higher* mortality, and *no* improvement in pre-discharge ejection fraction compared to deferred PTCA or medical therapy.[55,70,100,103-105] Limitations in some of these studies included failure to prescribe preprocedural aspirin (which is known to increase the risk of acute vessel closure), inadequate doses of heparin, and failure to monitor ACTs. In some cases, PTCA was performed on modest (> 60%) stenoses,[78,106] subjecting the patient to the risk of PTCA without anticipated benefit. Use of IIb/IIIa receptor antagonists and stents may improve outcomes after immediate PTCA, though this has not yet been tested in a randomized trial.

B. **RECOMMENDATIONS**. Based on the available data, routine PTCA cannot be recommended after successful thrombolysis. We do, however, recommend emergency angiography for ongoing signs or symptoms of ischemia or hemodynamic instability. PTCA should be performed when a critical stenosis (> 75%) and impaired (TIMI $\leq$ 2) coronary flow are evident. Preprocedural aspirin is necessary in all patients, and heparin should be given to maintain the ACT > 300 seconds.

DELAYED PTCA

A. **DELAYED PTCA IN ASYMPTOMATIC PATIENTS AFTER <u>SUCCESSFUL</u> THROMBOLYSIS.** PTCA of a high-grade stenosis may be performed 1-7 days after successful thrombolysis in the hope of preventing recurrent ischemia, reinfarction, and reocclusion, and improving ventricular function.

1. **Randomized Trials.** Several trials [107-111] compared an "invasive" (routine PTCA before discharge) vs. "conservative" approach (PTCA only for spontaneous or inducible ischemia) after successful thrombolysis (Table 5.12). These studies showed no differences in mortality, reinfarction, or ejection fraction. However, patients treated conservatively had more residual ischemia on pre-discharge exercise testing, and patients with prior MI treated conservatively had higher in-hospital mortality (12% vs. 4%, p < 0.001).[112] In contrast, in-hospital mortality in diabetic patients without prior MI was lower with the conservative approach (4% vs. 15%, p < 0.001).

2. **Limitations of Studies**. In TIMI-2B,[107] the intention-to-treat analysis may have attenuated the beneficial effect of PTCA, since PTCA was performed in only 54% of patients in the invasive arm and 13% in the conservative arm. Furthermore, 40% of deaths occurred *before* PTCA was performed, and 69% of all deaths in the invasive arm occurred in patients who never received PTCA or CABG. In fact, in-hospital mortality was lower if patients underwent mechanical revascularization, irrespective of assignment to invasive or conservative approaches (2.6% vs. 6.7%, p = 0.0001) (Table 5.13). Furthermore, PTCA patients may have received inadequate doses of heparin (ACT was not monitored) and aspirin (not given until the time of PTCA). Finally, total occlusions (identified in 12% of infarct vessels) were not dilated, omitting an important subgroup likely to benefit from revascularization.

3. **Recommendations.** Available data do not support routine delayed PTCA in the asymptomatic patient after thrombolysis without objective evidence of ischemia. However, limitations of available studies and the high (25-30%) incidence of late reocclusion after thrombolysis suggest that revascularization may be warranted in patients with:

- History of prior MI
- Reduced left ventricular function
- Multivessel disease
- Stenosis ≥ 90% supplying a moderate or large amount of myocardium
- Physiologic significance documented by intravascular Doppler or pressure gradient assessment

B. DELAYED PTCA IN ASYMPTOMATIC PATIENTS AFTER <u>FAILED</u> THROMBOLYSIS

1. **Nonrandomized Studies.** After failed thrombolysis, successful delayed PTCA of the occluded infarct artery may improve left ventricular function[113] and survival.[114-116] Potential mechanisms include improved remodeling (less left ventricular dilatation, aneurysm formation, and intracavitary thrombus formation), better recovery of viable but hibernating myocardium (if collaterals are present), and fewer arrhythmias.

2. **Randomized Trials.** In TAMI-6, left ventricular function at 6 weeks was improved in patients treated with PTCA at 48 hours compared to those treated medically. However, this difference was not sustained, and the reocclusion rate was 40% at 6 months.[117]

3. **Recommendations.** Due to limited data, absolute recommendations cannot be given. We recommend late PTCA of an occluded vessel in an asymptomatic patient if there is a large amount of myocardium supplied by the infarct vessel and/or evidence of viability (collaterals, preserved wall motion, retained R-waves, PET viability). Since reocclusion is common, stents are favored to maintain vessel patency.

C. PTCA FOR POST-MI ISCHEMIA

1. **Randomized Trials.** PTCA is commonly used for post-MI ischemia after thrombolytic therapy. Until recently, there was no proof that this practice improved clinical outcomes. In the DANAMI study,[118] 1008 patients with spontaneous or inducible post-infarction ischemia after thrombolysis were randomized to catheterization and revascularization (PTCA or CABG) vs. medical therapy (PTCA or CABG for refractory symptoms). The routine invasive approach resulted in less reinfarction (5.8% vs. 10.5%, p = 0.0038) and unstable angina (17.9% vs. 29.5%, p < 0.001) at 24 months, but no difference in mortality (Table 5.14).

2. **Recommendations.** Patients with post-infarction ischemia (either spontaneous angina or provocable ischemia on a pre-discharge exercise test) should undergo catheterization and revascularization if anatomically feasible.

Table 5.12. Delayed PTCA After Thrombolysis: In-hospital Results

Study	N	Drug	LVEF (%)		Reinfarction (%)		Death (%)	
			Inv	Cons	Inv	Cons	Inv	Cons
Van den Brand[110] (1992)	3262	tPA	50	50	5.9	5.4	5.2	4.6
SWIFT[108] (1991)	800	APSAC	52	51	12.1	8.2	2.7	3.3
Barbash[109] (1990)	194	tPA	50	49	-	-	8.2	3.8
Ozbek[111] (1990)	218	tPA	51	50	2.7	1	1.8	2.9
TIMI-2B[107] (1989)	324	SK	55	55	11.3	16.8	8.8	6

Abbreviations: Inv = invasive strategy (routine predischarge PTCA if appropriate); Cons = conservative strategy (PTCA only for spontaneous or inducible ischemia); LVEF = left ventricular ejection fraction; SK = streptokinase; tPA = tissue plasminogen activator; APSAC = anistreplase (Eminase)

Table 5.13. In-hospital Mortality After Delayed PTCA: TIMI 2B Results[107]

	Invasive*		Conservative*		
	N	Mortality (%)	N	Mortality (%)	p-Value
Intention to treat	1636	5.2	1626	4.6	NS
Received assigned therapy	1084	2.4	1319	5	0.0009
Did not receive assigned therapy	522	10.7	307	3.3	0.0001

* Invasive strategy = routine predischarge PTCA (if appropriate); conservative strategy = PTCA only for spontaneous or inducible ischemia

Table 5.14. Post-MI Ischemia: Outcome After Revascularization vs. Conservative Care[295]

	Revascularization*	Conservative+	p-Value
Anti-ischemic drugs (%)			
3 months	56	81	0.001
6 months	49	79	0.001
12 months	43	75	0.001
Unstable angina (%)			
3 months	22	52	0.001
6 months	23	58	0.001
12 months	22	43	0.001
Cardiac events at 24 months (%)			
MI	5.6	10.5	0.004
Death	3.6	4.6	NS

* CABG or PTCA
+ Medical therapy; CABG or PTCA for refractory symptoms

STENTS AND OTHER DEVICES FOR ACUTE MI (Table 5.15)

A. **STENTS.** The use of stents during acute MI is discussed in detail in Chapter 26.

   1. **Observational Studies.** The early experience with stents supported the feasibility and safety of stenting in the setting of recent or acute MI. Procedural success exceeded 90%, but stent thrombosis occurred in 0-9.6%.[171-186,298] The Stent-PAMI Pilot demonstrated the feasibility and safety of Palmaz-Schatz stenting in acute MI, with success in 98%, low early mortality (0.8%) and reinfarction (2%), angiographic restenosis in 27.5%, and infarct artery reocclusion in 6.4%.[187,292]

   2. **Randomized Trials (Table 5.16).** The safety and efficacy of primary stenting has been evaluated in numerous prospective randomized trials. The Stent-PAMI Trial enrolled 1458 patients presenting within 12 hours of acute MI, including 900 patients randomized to the Palmaz-Schatz heparin-coated stent (n = 452) or PTCA (n = 448).[188] Bail-out stenting was performed in 15% of PTCA patients for suboptimal results. Primary stenting was associated with higher procedural success (97.6% vs. 85%, p < 0.001); less death, MI, stroke, or TVR (12.6% vs. 20.1%, p < 0.01); and less angiographic restenosis at 6 months (20.3% vs. 33.5%, p < 0.001). Subacute thrombosis occurred infrequently in both groups (1.1% vs. 1.8%, p = 0.39). However, an unexpected finding was that final TIMI-3 flow was more frequent after PTCA than after stenting (93% vs. 89%, p = 0.006), and 6-month mortality was higher in the stent group (4.3% vs. 2.8%, p = 0.06). In contrast,

Table 5.15. Devices for Acute Coronary Syndromes

Device	Results
IABP	• Decrease in recurrent ischemia, but not death, reinfarction or reocclusion after primary PTCA; no late improvement in left ventricular function (PAMI-2) • Decrease in congestive heart failure in high-risk patients • Clear utility in acute MI complicated by shock
Stents	• High success rates and few complications in acute MI, with less restenosis and TVR at 6 months. Less TIMI-3 flow compared to PTCA alone and higher mortality in Stent-PAMI were not observed in CADILLAC • Stents in unstable angina are safe (with proper technique and antiplatelet therapy)
DCA	• Increase in peri-procedural MI and distal embolization compared to PTCA in unstable angina; slight reduction in angiographic restenosis compared to PTCA with optimal DCA. Limited role in acute MI.
TEC	• Extracts thrombus and atheroma; may decrease distal embolization in thrombotic lesions and vein grafts; high rates of restenosis • TOPIT trial demonstrated fewer non-Q-MI in acute ischemic syndromes in native coronary arteries
AngioJet	• Extracts fresh thrombus • VeGAS-II showed better acute outcomes in thrombotic vein grafts compared to urokinase • Acute MI Registry is complete; effective thrombus removal; additive benefits to primary PTCA are unproven
X-Sizer	• Extracts thrombus and soft atheroma • Randomized trial in progress
Rotablator	• Not recommended in thrombotic lesions or saphenous vein grafts
Laser	• Excimer registry in progress. Randomized trial of the holmium laser showed no benefits in acute ischemic syndromes compared to stand alone PTCA (LAVA trial)
Ultrasound Thrombolysis	• Limited registry data (ACUTE) is favorable for acute MI • Randomized trial (ATLAS) underway
Local Drug Delivery	• Local heparin delivery in LOCAL-PAMI was safe; no additive benefits to primary PTCA alone

Abbreviations: IABP = intraaortic balloon pump, DCA = directional coronary atherectomy; TEC = transluminal extraction catheter; TVR = target vessel revascularization
Acronyms: ACUTE = Analysis of Coronary Ultrasound Thrombolysis Endpoints; ATLAS = Acolysis During Treatment of Lesions Affecting SVGs; LAVA = Laser Facilitated Balloon Angioplasty Versus Angioplasty; PAMI-2 = Second Primary Angioplasty in Myocardial Infarction; VEGAS II = Vein Graft AngioJet Study - Phase II

Table 5.16. Randomized Trials of PTCA vs. Stenting for Acute MI

Trial	N	Stent	Summary (Stent vs. PTCA)	Comment
CADILLAC[329] (2000)	2082	MultiLink MultiLink-Duet	See Tables 26.37, 26.38	See Table 26.39
STENTIM-2[338] (2000)	211	Wiktor	Less ARS (23.3% vs. 39.6%, p < 0.05); no difference in procedural success, EFS, or TLR at 6 and 12 months	Stents associated with less angiographic restenosis
STOPAMI[339] (2000)	140	-	Stent + abciximab vs. t-PA; smaller infarct size (p < 0.05), better myocardial salvage (p < 0.001) and lower MACE at 6 months (8.5% vs. 23.2%, p < 0.05)	Stents plus abciximab resulted in better myocardial salvage and event-free survival than t-PA
FRESCO[340] (2000)	150	GR	Less MACE (9% vs. 28%, p < 0.01) and ARS (17% vs. 43%, p < 0.001) at 6 months	Stents associated with less MACE and restenosis
STENT-PAMI[341] (1999)	900	HCPSS	Less TIMI-3 flow (89% vs. 93%, p < 0.05); less ischemic TVR at 6 months (7.7% vs. 17%, p < 0.001) and 1 year (10.6% vs 21%, p < 0.0001); less ARS at 6 months (23% vs. 35%, p < 0.001); less MACE (17% vs. 24.8%, p < 0.01) but higher mortality at 1 year (5.8% vs. 3.0%, p = 0.054)	Stents associated with less ischemic complications but worse TIMI-3 flow and a trend toward higher mortality at 1 year
PASTA[342] (1999)	136	PSS	Similar success (99% vs. 97%); less in-hospital MACE(6% vs. 19%, p < 0.05) and 1-year MACE (22% vs. 49%, p < 0.001); less ARS at 6 months (17% vs. 37.5%, p < 0.05)	Stents associated with better in-hospital and late outcome
STAT (1999)	123	-	Stent vs. t-PA: Less recurrent MI (6.5% vs. 16.4%, p = 0.09), TVR (14.5% vs. 50.8%, p < 0.001), and MACE (24.2% vs. 57.4%, p < 0.001) at 6 months	Stents associated with less recurrent ischemia and better outcomes at 6 months
GRAMI[344] (1998)	104	GR-II	Similar procedural success; less in-hospital MACE (3.8% vs. 19.2%, p = 0.05) and better TIMI-3 flow (98% vs. 83%, p < 0.01); better EFS (82.7% vs. 65.4%, p < 0.01) but similar TLR at 1 year	Stents superior to PTCA for in-hospital complications, TIMI-flow, and late MACE
Jacksch[345] (1998)	462	Various	Less in-hospital MACE (9.9% vs. 15.6%, p < 0.001); less ARS (23% vs. 42%, p < 0.001) at 6 months	Stents associated with less in-hospital MACE and restenosis
ESCOBAR[346] (1998)	225	PSS	Less recurrent MI (1% vs. 7%, p < 0.05), TLR (4% vs. 17%, p < 0.01), and MACE (5% vs. 20%, p < 0.01) at 6 months; no mortality difference	Stents associated with better outcome at 6 months
PRISAM (1997)	300	Wiktor	Better lumen dimensions and less TLR (11% vs. 36%, p < 0.01) at 3 months	Stents associated with less TLR at 3 months

Abbreviations: ARS = angiographic restenosis; EFS = event-free survival; TLR = target lesion revascularization; MACE = major adverse cardiac events; - not reported

Table 5.17. The CADILLAC Trial: 6-Month Clinical Outcome[289]

	PTCA (n = 516)	PTCA + abciximab (n = 529)	Stent (n = 512)	Stent + abciximab (n = 525)	p-Value
MACE (%)	19.3	15.2	10.9	10.8	< 0.001
Death (%)	4.3	2.3	2.8	3.8	NS
Stroke (%)	0.8	0.8	1.2	1.7	NS
Reinfarction (%)	1.6	2.1	1.2	2.3	NS
TVR (%)	14.2	12.1	7.4	5.0	< 0.000001

Abbreviations: CADILLAC = Controlled Abciximab and Device Investigation to Lower Late Angioplasty Complications; MACE = major adverse cardiac events; TVR = target vessel revascularization

the CADILLAC trial randomized 2665 patients with acute MI to MultiLink stent or PTCA, and abciximab or placebo (Table 5.17).[289] There was a marked improvement in 6-month event-free survival with MultiLink stents, and no increase in mortality as observed in Stent-PAMI. Interestingly, abciximab had a favorable impact in primary PTCA patients but no impact in stent patients.

3. **Recommendations.** Based on the recently completed CADILLAC trial, it is reasonable to use primary stenting as the default (routine) reperfusion strategy for patients with acute MI, and for patients with failed PTCA or suboptimal results. The role of IIb/IIIa inhibitors is discussed below.

Table 5.18. Acute MI: Indications for Emergency or Urgent CABG

Left main stenosis > 50%; LAD or circumflex infarct vessel

Left main stenosis > 75%; right coronary infarct vessel

Severe proximal multivessel disease not suitable for PTCA, particularly if the infarct vessel is patent

Severe multivessel disease with cardiogenic shock

Failed mechanical reperfusion with infarct duration < 6 (and occasionally < 12) hours, a large amount of jeopardized myocardium at risk, and ongoing ischemic pain, especially in the presence of well-formed collaterals

B. **OTHER PERCUTANEOUS DEVICES.** A variety of percutaneous techniques have been used as adjuncts to PTCA and stents for primary revascularization of acute MI (Table 5.15). In general, these devices rely on thrombus extraction (DCA, TEC, AngioJet), thrombus ablation (ELCA, Acolysis), or thrombus dissolution (local drug delivery). At this time, none have shown superiority to conventional PTCA, although most operators recommend thrombus extraction (using TEC or the AngioJet) in thrombotic vein grafts. Distal embolic protection with the GuardWire reduced ischemic complications by 50-60% following elective vein graft intervention in the SAFER trial (Chapter 17); studies of distal embolic protection devices are planned in patients with acute coronary syndromes.

C. **INTRA-AORTIC BALLOON PUMP.** The routine use of IABP in the setting of PTCA for acute MI is somewhat controversial. Early studies of routine IABP after successful primary PTCA improved left ventricular function and reduced reocclusion.[167,168] In PAMI-2, prophylactic IABP for 36-48 hours after primary PTCA resulted in less recurrent ischemia and repeat PTCA, but failed to improve left ventricular function or reduce death, recurrent MI, heart failure, stroke, or reocclusion.[6,169,170] The value of IABP in patients with evolving acute MI complicated by hypotension, shock, or refractory heart failure develops is uncontested.

D. **EMERGENCY BYPASS SURGERY**. CABG is not widely utilized during acute MI because of logistical considerations and concerns about the adverse effects of general anesthesia and cardiopulmonary bypass. However, CABG should be considered part of an integrated revascularization strategy, especially for patients with cardiogenic shock. Indications for emergency CABG in the setting of acute MI are described in Table 5.18.

ADJUNCTIVE PHARMACOTHERAPY IN
PERCUTANEOUS INTERVENTION FOR ACUTE MI

Despite the benefits of primary PTCA compared to thrombolytic therapy, complete tissue perfusion is only achieved in one-third of patients; two-thirds of patients manifest delayed ST-segment resolution[309] and reduced myocardial blush scores.[310] Potential mechanisms for decreased myocardial perfusion despite normal epicardial coronary flow include microvascular spasm, endothelial swelling, or small vessel plugging by microembolic debris or in-site thrombosis. One potential means to improve myocardial perfusion is through adjunctive pharmacology aimed at earlier and more complete reperfusion.

A. **GLYCOPROTEIN IIb/IIIa INHIBITORS (Table 5.19)**
    1. **Abciximab (ReoPro)**
        a. **Primary PTCA.** In EPIC, patients with acute MI treated by primary or rescue PTCA had fewer Q-wave reinfarctions (0% vs. 17.4%, p = 0.05) and repeat PTCA (0% vs. 34.8%, p =

0.003) at 6 months if they received abciximab rather than placebo.[235] In contrast, although abciximab reduced the 30-day incidence of death, MI, or urgent revascularization by 62% (5.8% vs. 11.1%, p = 0.04) in RAPPORT,[236] there was no difference in death, reinfarction, or TVR at 6 months (28.1% vs. 28.2%, p = NS). Furthermore, as an adjunct to PTCA, abciximab did not improve TIMI flow, residual stenosis, dissection, distal embolization, no-reflow, or sidebranch closure. For PTCA patients in CADILLAC, abciximab was associated with a trend toward better event-free survival, but had no impact in stent patients.

b. **Primary Stenting.** The utility of abciximab as an adjunct to primary stenting has been studied in several randomized trials. In the Munich trial, 200 patients with acute MI were randomized to abciximab or placebo.[288] Patients treated with abciximab had less in-hospital death, reinfarction, or urgent TVR (2.0% vs. 9.2%, p < 0.05), and better regional wall motion, global left ventricular function, and peak coronary blood flow, consistent with better microcirculatory function and less distal embolization. In ADMIRAL, TIMI-3 flow at 24 hours was more common in abciximab patients (85.6% vs. 78.4%, p < 0.05). The primary endpoint (death, reinfarction, and urgent TVR at 30 days) was lower in the abciximab group (10.7% vs. 20.0%, p < 0.03), and left ventricular ejection fraction was better at 24 hours and 30 days (55% vs 51%, p < 0.05). Event-free survival did not improve with abciximab in ISAR-2, but 14-day left ventricular ejection fraction was higher with abciximab (62% vs. 56%, p < 0.05). In CADILLAC, primary stenting was superior to primary PTCA, but there was no incremental benefit for abciximab during primary stenting (Table 5.17).[289] The impact of abciximab on left ventricular function is under evaluation.

2. **Tirofiban (Aggrastat).** In RESTORE, 134 patients underwent primary PTCA. Tirofiban was associated with a 56% reduction in adverse events at 1 week (p = 0.022) and a nonsignificant 22% reduction at 1 month.

3. **Recommendations for IIb/IIIa Inhibitors in Acute MI**. Results from available trials are somewhat discordant, which precludes definitive recommendations about their use. Nevertheless, CADILLAC suggests a role for abciximab as an adjunct to primary PTCA for acute MI. Although the value of IIb/IIIa inhibitors during primary stenting has not been demonstrated, future recommendations may change if left ventricular function improves after abciximab.

B. **HEPARIN.** Several randomized trials have clearly shown the benefit of IV heparin in patients with acute MI, and its use is considered mandatory.

1. **Pre-PTCA.** In acute MI patients, a heparin bolus of 10,000 units does not improve the 20% patency rate due to spontaneous recanalization.[64,237] Although the HEAP (Heparin in Early Patency) Pilot study suggested that high-dose heparin (300 units/kg)[238] achieved infarct artery patency in 56% within 90 minutes, the randomized HEAP trial failed to show an early patency benefit.

2. **During PTCA.** An ACT >300 seconds during elective PTCA is recommended to reduce the risk of abrupt closure.[240] However, higher ACT levels may be necessary in patients with unstable angina or acute MI due to heparin resistance, to achieve better inhibition of platelet activation and aggregation.[241] In PTCA for unstable angina, higher levels of heparin anticoagulation reduced ischemic events—acute closure was reduced by 1.3% for each 10 second increase in ACT[242]— and there was an inverse linear relationship between acute closure and ACT.[243] Although higher ACT levels increased the risk of bleeding, one risk/benefit analysis suggested an optimal ACT of 425-525 seconds,[244] a level which is virtually never achieved or recommended during percutaneous intervention. Bleeding complications are markedly increased by high ACT levels when abciximab and high-dose heparin are combined, without additional clinical benefit;[230] standard practice consists of weight-adjusted heparin (70 U/kg) and a target ACT of 200-250 seconds when abciximab is used (Chapter 34).

3. **Post-PTCA.** The optimal dose and duration of heparin infusion after PTCA for acute MI or unstable angina is unknown. In a nonrandomized study examining the outcomes following short (24 hours) versus prolonged heparin (72 hours) after primary PTCA,[246] prolonged heparin was associated with more bleeding complications and no difference in reocclusion. The randomized HAPI trial (Heparin After Percutaneous Intervention) showed no benefit for post-procedural heparin after successful PTCA in patients with unstable or post-infarct angina.[247] In patients who receive heparin for ≥ 2 days, heparin should be discontinued *slowly* over 12 hours to decrease the risk of rebound thrombosis.[246,248-251] If adjunctive IIb/IIIa inhibitors are used, heparin should be discontinued immediately after the procedure to minimize bleeding complications.

4. **Recommendations**. For PTCA or stenting in acute MI, we recommend an ACT of 350-400 seconds. When IIb/IIIa inhibitors are used, we recommend weight-adjusted heparin (70 U/kg) and an ACT of 200-250 seconds. Since ACT measurements may vary by 40-60 seconds, it may be prudent to obtain multiple ACTs to confirm the desired level. ACTs should be checked every 30 minutes and additional heparin given if necessary to maintain the ACT at the desired level for the duration of the procedure.

C. **DIRECT THROMBIN INHIBITORS**. Direct thrombin inhibitors bind more effectively to fibrin-bound thrombin than heparin, and are not affected by anti-thrombin III, platelet factor 4, or heparinase. Since thrombin is the most potent endogenous platelet activator, there was hope that potent thrombin inhibition would improve PTCA outcomes in patients with acute coronary syndromes. Hirudin, a peptide derived from the medicinal leech, reduces platelet deposition and restenosis in animal models. The GUSTO 2B substudy randomized 1138 acute MI patients undergoing primary PTCA to heparin or hirudin; a nonsignificant 24% reduction in death, reinfarction or disabling stroke was demonstrated with recombinant hirudin (lepirudin) (8.2% vs. 10.6%, p = 0.037).[71] Hirulog (bivalirudin), a synthetic peptide analog of hirudin, has not been evaluated in the setting of primary intervention for acute MI.

D. THROMBOLYTIC THERAPY (Table 5.20). In the setting of unstable angina, multiple randomized trials have consistently demonstrated *worse* clinical outcomes for PTCA patients treated with intravenous or intracoronary thrombolytic therapy (Table 5.31),[1,125,256-260] even when angiographic features most likely to benefit from lytics (e.g. complex lesions, filling defects) are present.[260] In acute MI, the ability of thrombolytic therapy to restore early patency prior to primary PTCA was evaluated in 606 patients in the Plasminogen Activator Angioplasty Comparability Trial (PACT).[349] The administration of a 50 mg t-PA bolus immediately prior to angiography resulted in better TIMI-3 flow prior to PTCA (33% vs. 15%, p < 0.001), and less need for immediate intervention. Furthermore, patients with TIMI-3 flow prior to PTCA had greater recovery of left ventricular function than patients in whom TIMI-3 flow was restored by PTCA without t-PA. Finally, low dose t-PA did not cause additional bleeding complications or recurrent ischemic events compared to primary angioplasty alone. Combined therapy may therefore be the preferred strategy especially in patients intended for primary intervention when relatively long time delays are anticipated. Further studies are in progress.

E. COMBINATION THERAPY WITH THROMBOLYTICS AND GLYCOPROTEIN IIb/IIIa INHIBITORS. Since thrombolytic therapy is a potent platelet activator (by exposing clot-bound thrombin), adjunctive antiplatelet therapy with IIb/IIIa inhibitors has been evaluated in the hope of improving the speed and frequency of reperfusion, which correlates closely with prognosis.

1. **Trials.** In acute MI, TIMI-3 flow is established in only 50-60% after lytic therapy and 15-32% after abciximab.[268,269] In contrast, reperfusion rates exceed 90% after primary PTCA or stenting, but the availability of percutaneous revascularization is limited and often delayed, and good epicardial blood flow does not ensure good microvascular perfusion. A number of recent trials have therefore evaluated combined therapy with thrombolytics and IIb/IIIa inhibitors (Table 5.21). TAMI 8 evaluated the safety of t-PA (100 mg), aspirin, and graded-doses of abciximab in patients with acute MI, and demonstrated a dose-dependent reduction in platelet aggregation with increasing doses of abciximab.[270] IMPACT AMI demonstrated that the speed and frequency of reperfusion was enhanced by eptifibatide plus t-PA without an increase in bleeding.[271] In PARADIGM,[272] there was no improvement in clinical outcome and more bleeding complications with lamifiban, but ST-segment monitoring indicated that lamifiban was associated with more rapid reperfusion. The TIMI 14a Pilot study found that half dose t-PA bolus (15mg) + infusion (35mg over 60 min) combined with standard dose abciximab (bolus + 12 hour infusion) resulted in TIMI-3 flow at 90 minutes in 79%.[273] The SPEED (GUSTO IV Pilot) study evaluated abciximab with or without reteplase (5U vs. 7.5U vs. 10U vs. two 5U doses 30 minutes apart) in patients presenting within 6 hours of acute MI. Double-bolus reteplase (5U) plus standard-dose abciximab resulted in the highest TIMI-3 flow rate (73%) at 90 minutes.[274] GUSTO IV AMI is comparing standard intravenous reteplase vs. half-dose reteplase plus full-dose abciximab in 17,000 patients with acute MI.[275] CADILLAC II will determine whether combination therapy with TNK tPA and tirofiban immediately prior to PTCA/stenting will offer any additional clinical benefit over current mechanical reperfusion approaches.

2. **Recommendations.** Results from the current dose ranging trials suggest that combination therapy with low-dose fibrinolytics, IIb/IIIa inhibitors, aspirin, and low-dose heparin is a promising and safe strategy for patients with acute MI, enhancing reperfusion without excess bleeding complications. Whether this approach also improves clinical outcomes (with or without percutaneous intervention) is currently under evaluation in several randomized trials.

DEFICIENCIES OF PTCA FOR ACUTE MI

A. **REPERFUSION ARRHYTHMIA**
    1. **Incidence.** Profound hypotension and bradycardia (the Bezold-Jarisch reflex from stimulation of vagal afferents) or sudden ventricular fibrillation may occur after PTCA of an occluded coronary artery, especially the RCA.[119] One study[122] found that minor events were more common after primary PTCA of the RCA; major adverse events (death, CPR, defibrillation, cardioversion, IABP, or urgent surgery) however, were uncommon, except in patients with cardiogenic shock. In PAMI-I,[64] ventricular fibrillation occurred in 6.7% of PTCA patients, and was more common in patients with inferior MI than anterior MI (9.7% vs. 1.4%, p = 0.03).

    2. **Recommendations.** To reduce reperfusion arrhythmia during primary intervention for acute MI, we recommend IV beta-blockers prior to intervention, low-osmolar ionic contrast (ioxaglate), and optimization of oxygen saturation, filling pressures, and electrolyte status (especially potassium and magnesium levels).

B. **BLEEDING COMPLICATIONS**
    1. **Incidence.** In older primary PTCA literature, blood transfusion was required in 14% of cases [64,80,50,5] and was associated with use of thrombolytic agents, prolonged anticoagulation, and indwelling sheaths. Contemporary data indicate marked reductions in bleeding complications due to optimal antiplatelet and anticoagulation dosing, and fastidious attention to vascular access (Chapter 25).

    2. **Recommendations.** Bleeding and vascular complications can be minimized by meticulous attention to vascular access technique, careful monitoring of ACT levels, and avoidance of post-procedural heparin. Weight-adjusted heparin and early sheath removal are recommended when IIb/IIIa inhibitors are used (Chapter 34).

C. **ISCHEMIC COMPLICATIONS.** In-hospital reinfarction after lytic therapy is a common cause of death after MI. Early reocclusion increases in-hospital mortality from 4.0% to 12.8% and results in more heart failure, life-threatening arrhythmia, repeat revascularization, and cost.[123,124] The incidence of in-hospital recurrent ischemia is 30% after thrombolytic therapy, 15% after primary PTCA, and 3% after stenting. The incidence of early reinfarction is 8% after thrombolytic therapy, 1-2% after primary PTCA, and < 1% after stenting.[50,64,125] PTCA for acute MI is associated with a 5% risk of reocclusion prior to discharge,[6] and reocclusion after successful rescue PTCA after failed thrombolytic therapy is as high as 29%.[94] Most of these ischemic complications are now avoided by stenting. In addition, the risk of late reocclusion (10-15%) and restenosis (40%) are significantly improved by stents.[5,7,8,126]

Table 5.19. Major Trials of IIb/IIIa Antagonists for Coronary Intervention in Acute MI

Study	Antagonist	1° Endpoint	Result	Comments
CADILLAC[329] (n = 2082)	Abciximab (PTCA vs. stent)	Death, MI, or ischemia-driven TVR at 6 months	PTCA: 19.3% PTCA/abcix: 15.2% Stent: 10.9% Stent/abcix: 10.8% (p < 0.0001)	Stenting superior to PTCA; adverse effects of stents on TIMI flow and late mortality in PAMI-STENT not observed in CADILLAC. Abciximab was associated with a trend toward better event-free survival in PTCA patients, but no benefit in stent patients
RAPPORT[330] (n = 483)	Abciximab (primary PTCA)	Death, MI, or revascularization at 6 months	Placebo: 16.1% Abciximab: 13.3% (p = 0.32)	No benefit for abciximab in primary PTCA patients
ADMIRAL[331] (n = 299)	Abciximab (stent 85%, PTCA 15%)	Death, MI, or ischemia-driven TVR at 30 days	Placebo: 20% Abciximab: 10.7% (p < 0.03)	Substantial benefit for abciximab in primary stent patients
Munich Trial[332] (n = 200)	Abciximab (primary stenting)	Hospital death, MI, revascularization	Placebo: 9.2% Abciximab: 2.0% (p < 0.05)	Abciximab group also had better regional wall motion, global LV function, and peak coronary blood flow. Short-term benefits on primary endpoint were no longer significant at 30 days (p = 0.16)
ISAR-2[333] (n = 401)	Abciximab (primary stenting)	Angiographic restenosis	No effect on restenosis	Abciximab led to reduction in 30-day MACE (5.0% vs. 10.5%). No additional benefit over time
EPIC[334] (n = 64)	Abciximab (direct or rescue PTCA)	Death, MI, or urgent revascularization at 30 days	*30-day*: Placebo 26.1% vs. abciximab[+] 4.8% (p = 0.06) *6-month*: Placebo 47.8% vs. abciximab[+] 4.5% (p = 0.002)	Study group represented 64 of 2099 patients in EPIC with acute MI; 42 direct PTCA, 22 rescue PTCA
GRAPE[335] (n = 60)	Abciximab (PTCA)	Infarct artery patency	TIMI-3: 18%	Abciximab before primary PTCA is safe
RESTORE[336,337] (n = 134)	Tirofiban (primary PTCA)	Death, MI, or any revascularization	56% reduction at 7 days and 22% reduction at 30 days (p = NS)	Study group represented 134 of 2141 patients in RESTORE with acute MI

Abbreviations: IVUS = intravascular ultrasound; MI = myocardial infarction; TVR = target vessel revascularization
+   Bolus plus infusion
Acronyms: See Table 34.31

Table 5.20. PTCA Outcome For Unstable Angina or Acute MI: Impact of Lytic Therapy

Series	N	Lytic	Dose (units)	Results
Mehran[260] (1995)	469	UK	250-500,00 IC	More acute closure in complex lesions (15% vs. 5.9%, p = 0.03) after UK
Grines[125] (1995)	172	UK	Variable doses	More ischemia (18.4% vs. 10.6%, p = 0.10) after UK
Ambrose[259] (1994)	469	UK	250-500,000 IC	More acute closure (10.2% vs. 4.3%, p = 0.02) and major cardiac events (12.9% vs. 6.3%, p = 0.02) after UK
Buller[258] (1994)	471	tPA	80 mg IV	More major cardiac events (11% vs. 4%, p = 0.06) after tPA
O'Neill[8] (1992)	122	SK	1.5 MU IV	More emergency CABG (10.3% vs. 1.6%, p = 0.03), transfusion (39% vs. 8%, p = 0.0001), hospital stay, and cost after SK
Ambrose[257] (1991)	66	UK	150,000 IC	No difference in abrupt closure
Spielberg[256] (1990)	660	UK	1670-6670 IC	More abrupt closure after UK

Abbreviations: CABG = coronary artery bypass surgery; IC = intracoronary; IV = intravenous; MU = million units; SK = streptokinase; tPA = tissue plasminogen activator; UK = urokinase

Table 5.21. Combined IIb/IIIa Inhibitors and Thrombolytic Therapy in Acute MI

Study	N	Agent	Design	Results
— FULL-DOSE THROMBOLYSIS AND GP IIb/IIIa INHIBITION —				
TAMI 8[270]		Abciximab	Full dose tPA + graded doses of abciximab	Dose-dependent reduction in platelet aggregation with increasing doses of abciximab (TIMI 3 flow rates 80-90% without excess bleeding)
IMPACT AMI[271]	132	Eptifibatide	Eptifibatide (180 mcg/kg bolus, 0.75 mcg/kg/min infusion) + full dose tPA vs. tPA alone	Combined therapy improved 90 minute TIMI 3 flow rates (66% vs. 39%, p = 0.006) without excess bleeding
PARADIGM[272]	353	Lamifiban	Full dose tPA or SK + dose ranging lamifiban	No obvious clinical benefit for lamifiban when added to lytics; increased rate of major bleeding
— REDUCED-DOSE THROMBOLYSIS AND GP IIb/IIIa INHIBITION —				
TIMI 14	888	Abciximab	tPA alone vs. abciximab alone vs. abciximab + reduced SK	Abciximab + half-dose tPA improved reperfusion (77% TIMI 3 at 90 min vs. 62% for tPA alone, p = 0.01) without excess major bleeding complications. TIMI 3 flow with abciximab alone (32%)
GUSTO IV Pilot (SPEED)		Abciximab	Abciximab alone vs. abciximab + rPA (5U vs. 7.5U vs. 10U) vs. abciximab + rPA (5U x 2 30 min apart)	Combined abciximab + double bolus rPA resulted in highest TIMI 3 flow rates at 90 min (73%)
GUSTO IV AMI	17	Abciximab	Abciximab + half-dose rPA vs. rPA alone	Ongoing
INTRO AMI	394	Eptifibatide	Eptifibatide (180/90 bolus; 1.33 mcg/kg/min infusion) + half-dose tPA vs. eptifibatide (180/90 bolus; 2.0 mcg/kg/min infusion) + half-dose tPA vs. full-dose tPA	Ongoing

UNSTABLE ANGINA

Prior to the availability of potent platelet receptor antagonists and contemporary interventional techniques, medical therapy for unstable angina was associated with in-hospital mortality in 1% and myocardial infarction in 7-9%. At one year, cardiac death occurred in 8-18% and myocardial infarction in 14-22% of patients.[127] With novel antithrombotic and antiplatelet agents, the outcome of medical therapy has improved, though patients still remain at high risk for adverse cardiac events.[128]

A. **PATHOPHYSIOLOGY.** Coronary thrombus, plaque rupture, and mural hemorrhage are common findings in patients who die after unstable angina.[129,130,121] Angiography early in the course of unstable angina typically demonstrates complex lesions with ulceration, intraluminal haziness, and thrombus. Patients with a history of antecedent angina are more likely to have significant multivessel disease and collaterals, whereas patients with new onset unstable angina often have a fissured, ulcerated plaque without collaterals. The pathophysiology of unstable angina is described in Chapter 40.

B. **SUCCESS AND COMPLICATIONS OF PTCA IN UNSTABLE ANGINA.** Although the technical success rate of PTCA in unstable angina is similar to stable angina, the incidence of peri-procedural complications is higher, especially when thrombus is present.[132-137] Patients with rest angina and ECG changes or CPK-MB or troponin elevation (non-Q-wave MI) have more complications after PTCA and other devices.[137-149] However, PTCA complication rates are decreasing, particularly with increasing use of stents and potent platelet receptor antagonists.[150,151]

C. **RISK STRATIFICATION AND TARGETED THERAPY FOR UNSTABLE ANGINA.** The spectrum of unstable angina is broad, and risk stratification based on clinical, electrocardiographic, enzymatic, and functional parameters can identify patients who will benefit from early cardiac catheterization and revascularization (Table 5.22).[152,153] Patients with high-risk characteristics and those at intermediate risk who fail medical stabilization are most appropriately managed with early cardiac catheterization and revascularization, including patients with inducible ischemia,[118] left ventricular impairment,[154] or left main or left main equivalent disease. The optimal timing of revascularization in patients with acute coronary syndromes is discussed below.

Table 5.22. Risk Stratification of Unstable Angina Patients*

High Risk	Prolonged rest pain (> 20 min)
	Angina at rest with ST segment changes = 1mm
	Angina complicated by heart failure, mitral regurgitation, or hypotension
	Elevated CPK-MB or troponins (non-Q-wave MI)
Intermediate Risk	Angina with dynamic T wave changes
	Recent onset angina (<2 weeks)
	Q waves or ST depression in multiple lead groups
	Nocturnal angina
Low Risk	Angina pattern is more frequent, longer duration, and more severe
	Lower threshold of inducible angina
	Normal electrocardiogram

* See Figure 5.3

D. COMPARISONS OF MEDICAL THERAPY, PTCA AND CABG IN UNSTABLE ANGINA

1. **Medical Therapy vs. CABG.** Two randomized trials have compared medical and surgical therapy in unstable angina associated with reversible ECG changes: The National Cooperative Group Study and the Veterans Administration Cooperative Study. Both reported better symptom-relief and functional capacity after CABG. Though no difference in overall survival was present at 2-3 years, post-hoc analysis showed a significant survival advantage after CABG for patients with left ventricular dysfunction. The Duke registry also reported better 5-year survival after CABG in patients with 2 or 3 vessel disease, but no difference in outcome for single vessel disease.

2. **Medical Therapy vs. PTCA (Table 5.23).** Whether to manage patients with acute coronary syndromes invasively (routine catheterization followed by PTCA or CABG when appropriate) vs. conservatively (reserving angiography and revascularization for refractory symptoms) has been the subject of 5 randomized trials. In **TIMI-3B**, there was no difference in death or MI, but PTCA resulted in earlier discharge, fewer readmissions, and less need for medication. Furthermore, angiography was ultimately performed in 57% and revascularization in 40% of the "conservatively treated" patients before hospital discharge, which increased to 73% and 58% respectively at 1 year.[159] Thus, most patients ultimately required catheterization and angioplasty. In contrast, the invasive arm in **VANQWISH** was associated with higher in-hospital mortality and MI, largely due to the 11.6% surgical mortality in the invasive group.[160] Other important limitations of VANQWISH included marked delays in angiography (2 days) and revascularization (8 days) in the invasive group, and the fact that PTCA or CABG was only performed in 21% of patients in the invasive strategy. Furthermore, use of PTCA was more frequent in the conservative group (33% vs. 22%), and patients at "very high risk" (those who may benefit the most from intervention) were excluded from the trial. Both TIMI-3B and VANQWISH were performed prior to the availability

of stents and IIb/IIIa inhibitors, and may have limited relevance to current practice. In FRISC 2, 2457 patients with unstable angina or non-Q-wave MI were randomized to an early invasive versus conservative strategy. If possible, patients were also treated with low-molecular-weight heparin (dalteparin) for 4-5 days prior to angiography. At 1 year, patients randomized to the early invasive strategy (including stents in 61%) had less death (2.2% vs. 3.9%, p = 0.016), MI (8.6% vs. 11.6%, p = 0.015), and revascularization (7.5% vs. 31%, p < 0.001).[350] In TACTICS-TIMI 18, 2220 patients with unstable angina or non-ST-elevation MI were treated with aspirin, heparin, beta-blockers, and tirofiban on admission to the hospital, with subsequent randomization to an early invasive strategy (cardiac catheterization and revascularization within 48 hours) or a conservative strategy (cardiac catheterization only for recurrent ischemia). The primary endpoint of death, MI, or rehospitalization for acute coronary syndromes at 6 months was reduced by 18% in the invasive group (15.9% vs 19.4%, p = 0.025), with the greatest benefit among patients with positive troponins. In light of GUSTO-4 ACS, which failed to demonstrate benefit in the 30-day endpoint of death and MI among 7800 patients with ACS randomized to medical therapy with abciximab or placebo, the current weight of evidence favors an early invasive approach for patients presenting with unstable angina or non-Q-wave MI.

3. **PTCA vs. CABG.** Unstable angina was present in 14-83% of the patients enrolled in the randomized trials of PTCA vs. CABG. [161-166] In BARI, death or Q-wave MI at 5 years was similar in unstable angina patients treated with PTCA or surgery; outcome was unrelated to lesion morphology, extent of multivessel disease, or left ventricular function. Mortality was significantly greater in PTCA patients with diabetes mellitus, with and without unstable angina. Stents and IIb/IIIa inhibitors were not available during patient recruitment, limiting the applicability of these studies to contemporary practice (Chapter 3).

E. **RECOMMENDATIONS FOR TIMING OF CORONARY INTERVENTION IN UNSTABLE ANGINA AND NON-Q-WAVE MI.** Among high- to intermediate-risk patients with acute coronary syndromes, including troponin-positive patients, current evidence favors a strategy of intensive medical therapy (aspirin, heparin, GPIIb/IIIa inhibitors) with cardiac catheterization and revascularization within 48 hours of presentation (Figure 5.3). Adjunctive antiplatelet and antithrombin therapy is discussed below.

Table 5.23. Aggressive Versus Conservative Therapy in Patients with Acute Coronary Syndromes

Study	N	In-hospital Outcome Invasive vs. Conservative	Late Outcome Invasive vs. Conservative	Comments
FRISC II (2001)	2457	-	1-year death (2.2 vs. 3.9%, p = 0.016), MI (8.6% vs. 11.6%, p = 0.015), death or MI (10.4% vs. 14.1%, p = 0.005), TVR (7.5% vs. 31%, p < 0.01)	Invasive approach with clear benefit at 6 months and 1 year
TACTICS-TIMI 18[325] (2000)	2220	-	6-month endpoint of death, MI, or readmission for ACS (15.9% vs 19.4%, p = 0.025)	In ACS patients treated with tirofiban, early invasive approach is superior to conservative approach
VANQWISH[160] (1998)	920	Death (4.5% vs 1.3%, p = 0.007), death/MI (7.8% vs 3.3%, p = 0.004)	1-year death (12.6% vs 7.9%, p = 0.025), death/MI (24% vs 18.6%, p = 0.05)	High mortality in the invasive group was due to high mortality after CABG rather than PTCA (10.4% vs 0%) at 30 days
TIMI-3B[158] (1994)	1473	Death (2.4% vs 2.5%, p = NS), MI (5.1 vs 5.7%, p = NS), LOS (10.2 days vs 10.9 days, p = 0.01)	6-week death (2.5% vs 2.4%, p = NS), MI (5.7% vs 5.1%, p = NS)	At 6 weeks, invasive strategy had less readmission (7.8% vs 14.1%, p = 0.001) and less need for > 2 antianginals (44% vs 52%, p = 0.02). Invasive group had shorter LOS

Abbreviations: ACS = acute coronary syndromes; LOS = length of stay; MI = myocardial infarction; TVR = target vessel revascularization

DEVICES FOR THROMBOTIC LESIONS IN UNSTABLE ANGINA

A. **STENTS (Chapter 26).** Immediate and long-term results of stent implantation for stable and unstable angina are similar,[312-317] although the presence of Braunwald class II or III unstable angina was associated with more MI and target vessel revascularization at 1-2 years in one report.[306] In more than 7000 patients with unstable angina treated with stents or PTCA, stents resulted in fewer in-hospital ischemic complications, including death (1.5% vs. 2.6%, p = 0.003), recurrent angina (23.5% vs. 47.4%, p < 0.00001), Q-wave MI (0.4% vs. 1.9%, p < 0.00001), repeat PTCA (13.8% vs. 30.6%, p < 0.00001), and CABG (6.5% vs. 19.6%, p < 0.00001),[318] but no difference in mortality at 1 year. In the presence of thrombotic lesions, thrombectomy devices and adjunctive pharmacology are typically utilized prior to stent implantation (Chapter 9).

B. **DIRECTIONAL CORONARY ATHERECTOMY (Chapter 28).** DCA in patients with recent MI and thrombotic lesions resulted in lower success and higher rates of complications, despite anecdotal favorable results.[189-191] In CAVEAT, 65% of the patients randomized to DCA had unstable angina, and DCA was associated with more non-Q-wave MI in-hospital and at 6 months (8.2% vs. 3.8%, p = 0.0031).[192] In BOAT, optimal DCA resulted in slightly lower angiographic restenosis rates than PTCA, but no difference in TVR. CK elevation was more common after DCA, but there was no independent effect on late outcome.[307] DCA is not recommended in acute or post-MI patients, or in patients with acute coronary syndromes and thrombus, unless the lesion is unsuitable for PTCA or stenting; abciximab is recommended to decrease CPK elevation in these patients.[186]

C. **TEC ATHERECTOMY (Chapter 29).** TEC may be useful in thrombotic lesions in native vessels and degenerated saphenous vein grafts.[193-198] The multicenter randomized TOPIT trial (TEC Or PTCA In Thrombus) demonstrated less CPK elevation after TEC in patients with acute coronary syndromes (Chapter 9, Table 9.4).[280] TEC may be considered in degenerated vein grafts, in patients with acute coronary syndromes and large thrombus burden, or thrombus refractory to other treatment modalities.

D. **ANGIOJET.** The Possis AngioJet Rheolytic Thrombectomy System is FDA-approved for treatment of thrombus-containing lesions. The randomized VeGAS II trial showed better acute outcomes in vein grafts and thrombotic lesions compared to urokinase infusion (Chapter 9, Table 9.6). The VeGAS II AMI Registry evaluated the AngioJet in native arteries and saphenous vein grafts in 107 patients presenting with acute MI; there was no definite benefit compared to PTCA alone. Nonetheless, the AngioJet is a therapeutic alternative for lesions with a large thrombus burden; it is most effective in removing fresh thrombus, but lacks efficacy for organized clot and grumous in saphenous vein grafts.

E. ROTABLATOR ATHERECTOMY. The Rotablator is not recommended in thrombotic lesions due to the risk of distal thromboembolization and no-reflow, but may be considered in patients with acute coronary syndromes and heavily calcified or non-dilatable lesions without clot.

F. LASER (Chapter 30). Although the excimer and holmium infrared lasers have been utilized in patients with thrombus, data are limited in acute MI.[199-202] The LAVA trial (Laser Angioplasty vs. Angioplasty) found no benefit for the holmium laser in patients with acute coronary syndromes.[281] The holmium laser has been used in selected patients with AMI, though incremental benefit compared to PTCA alone has not been established.[282] The Excimer Laser in Thrombotic Ischemic Syndromes (ELTIS) Trial is an ongoing registry evaluating the outcomes of excimer laser in thrombotic lesions in 100 patients with acute coronary syndromes. "Blind" lasing has been utilized for chronic total occlusions resistant to guidewire crossing, but complication rates are high. Further studies are required to establish a role for laser thrombolysis as an adjunct to PTCA. Lasers are rarely utilized in most interventional programs.

G. THERMAL BALLOON ANGIOPLASTY. Laser balloon angioplasty was effective in desiccating thrombus and reversing PTCA induced abrupt closure,[203-206] but was withdrawn due to high restenosis rates. Other thermal angioplasty systems have been studied, with similar results.[207-208]

H. LOCAL DRUG DELIVERY (Chapter 35). Heparin infused locally into the vessel wall adheres to and permeates the intima, resulting in high local concentrations that persist for hours to days. Local heparin also inhibits platelet deposition at the site of intervention,[209-214] potentially reducing recurrent ischemia, reocclusion, restenosis, and bleeding complications.[215] Local delivery of urokinase using the hydrogel-coated balloon was evaluated in 108 patients with acute MI (CORAMI II trial); patients treated with urokinase had less no-reflow (3.7% vs. 24.6%, p = 0.03), but no difference in reocclusion.[216] Intramural heparin using the LocalMed infusasleeve in acute MI (Local PAMI Trial) was associated with a clinical restenosis rate of only 7.5%, but the role of locally delivered heparin during acute MI remains unclear.[283,284]

I. ULTRASOUND (Chapter 9). Therapeutic ultrasound may ablate fresh thrombus. The Analysis of Coronary Ultrasound Thrombolysis Endpoints in Acute Myocardial Infarction (ACUTE) Trial evaluated ultrasound thrombolysis in 15 patients; procedure success was 87%. The ATLAS (Acolysis during Treatment of Lesions Affecting SVGs) MI trial is a multicenter registry evaluating acolysis in patients with acute MI and saphenous vein graft occlusion; results are pending.

J. DISTAL PROTECTION DEVICES. The PercuSurge GuardWire was recently shown to reduce ischemic complications by 50-60% after elective vein graft intervention in the SAFER trial. A number of novel distal protection devices are currently under evaluation in the setting of unstable angina and acute myocardial infarction (Chapters 17, 36).

ADJUNCTIVE PHARMACOTHERAPY FOR UNSTABLE ANGINA (Chapter 34)

A. ANTIPLATELET AGENTS

1. **Aspirin** reduces the incidence of acute closure by 30-50% after balloon angioplasty, and is considered routine pharmacotherapy prior to and after intervention. The importance of aspirin is well established in acute MI[56] and acute coronary syndromes.[285] However, despite its ability to inhibit cyclooxygenase and the arachidonic acid pathway, up to 10% of patients with CAD are aspirin-resistant,[354] and platelet aggregation still occurs in response to thrombin, catecholamines, ADP, serotonin, and shear-stress.[217] In one report, patients with unstable angina or MI were shown to have heightened platelet activity and thrombus formation despite aspirin therapy.[218] High dose oral,[219] chewable, and intravenous aspirin[220] may reduce platelet aggregation and thrombus formation more effectively than standard doses of oral aspirin.

2. **Ticlopidine** is a thienopyridine derivative which is a more potent platelet antagonist than aspirin, and works by antagonizing ADP-induced platelet aggregation. Although ticlopidine exerts its maximal effect on in-vitro platelet aggregation at 3-5 days, antiplatelet effects can be detected within hours of ingestion. In one report, loading with 500 mg BID for the first 2-3 days resulted in greater platelet inhibition than the 250 mg dose.[221] In randomized trials, the combination of aspirin and ticlopidine has been shown to reduce stent thrombosis compared to aspirin alone or aspirin and warfarin.[222] Aspirin and ticlopidine have shown a synergistic effect in reducing platelet deposition[223] and thrombin generation after PTCA[224] and stenting. Use of ticlopidine in the interventional setting has been replaced by clopidogrel, which is equally effective, better tolerated, and associated with fewer hematologic side effects (neutropenia, TTP).

3. **Clopidogrel** is another thienopyridine derivative, similar to ticlopidine, that inhibits ADP-dependent platelet aggregation. The CAPRIE trial established the safety and efficacy of clopidogrel (75mg daily) compared to aspirin in 19,185 patients with atherosclerotic vascular disease.[225] Recent results from the CURE trial establish the benefit of aspirin plus clopidogrel vs. aspirin alone in acute coronary syndromes (Table 34.32, p. 779). Compared to ticlopidine, clopidogrel has equally low rates of stent thrombosis (0.2% vs. 0.7%, p = 0.20), fewer side effects, and lower cost.[226] When clopidogrel is used for intracoronary stenting, we recommend a loading dose of 300-450 mg at least 4 hours before the procedure, if possible, followed by 75 mg daily for 2-4 weeks.

4. **Glycoprotein IIb/IIIa Receptor Antagonists (Chapter 34).** The most potent antiplatelet agents block the GP IIb/IIIa receptor, the final common pathway of platelet aggregation. These agents have improved the safety of coronary intervention in patients with acute coronary syndromes. There is now compelling evidence from large-scale randomized clinical trials for benefit of IIb/IIIa receptor blockers as adjuncts to coronary intervention and as primary therapy for acute ischemic syndromes, to passivate the unstable plaque and reduce adverse event rates before and after revascularization.

a. **IIb/IIIa Inhibitors in the Medical Management Unstable Angina and Non-Q-Wave MI.** Multiple randomized studies have demonstrated the utility of IIb/IIIa inhibitors for patients with acute coronary syndromes (Chapter 34, Tables 34.15, 34.16). Benefits are established for tirofiban and eptifibatide in patients not undergoing percutaneous intervention, but GUSTO-IV ACS failed to show benefit for abciximab.

b. **IIb/IIIa Inhibitors n the Interventional Management of Unstable Angina and Non-Q-Wave MI (Table 5.24).**

1. **Abciximab (ReoPro).** The EPIC trial randomized 2099 high-risk patients (unstable angina, non-Q-wave MI, complex angiographic morphology, large thrombus) undergoing PTCA or DCA to abciximab bolus,[230] abciximab bolus and infusion, or placebo. Abciximab bolus plus infusion reduced the primary endpoint (death, MI, and urgent reintervention at 30 days) by 35% (8.3% vs. 12.8%, p = 0.008). Among 489 patients with unstable or post-MI angina, recurrent MI was significantly reduced by abciximab (1.8% vs. 9.0%, p = 0.01).[231] At 3 years, bolus plus infusion abciximab patients with acute coronary syndromes had a 60% reduction in mortality (5.1% vs. 12.7%, p = 0.01); no long-term benefits were observed in patients treated with bolus abciximab alone.[232] Bleeding complications were markedly increased in EPIC, but in the subsequent EPILOG trial, low-dose weight-adjusted heparin, procedural ACT of 200-250 seconds, and early sheath removal reduced the risk of hemorrhagic complications.[287] The EPISTENT trial was a randomized trial of abciximab versus placebo in 2399 patients undergoing PTCA or stenting.[233] The event rate (death, MI or urgent TVR at 30 days) was lowest for stent plus abciximab compared to PTCA plus abciximab or stent alone (5.3% vs. 6.9% vs. 10.8%; p < 0.01). Among 487 patients with unstable angina, abciximab was associated with a 70% reduction in the 30-day primary endpoint (4.7% vs. 11.8%, p = 0.002).[234] At 1 year, mortality was significantly lower for stent plus abciximab compared to PTCA plus abciximab or stent alone (1.0% vs. 2.1% vs. 2.4%, p = 0.037). The CAPTURE trial randomized 1265 patients with refractory unstable angina and planned percutaneous intervention to aspirin and intravenous heparin with or without abciximab (bolus 0.25mg/kg plus infusion 10mcg/hour initiated 18-24 hours before and continued for one hour after intervention).[227] The primary endpoint (death, MI, or ischemia-driven TVR at 30 days) was reduced with abciximab (11.3% vs. 15.9%, p = 0.012), primarily due to a reduction in MI before (0.6% vs. 2.1%, p = 0.029) and after (2.6% vs. 5.5%, p = 0.009) PTCA. Benefits were most pronounced in patients with elevated troponin prior to intervention.[286] Major bleeding was more frequent with abciximab (3.8% vs. 1.9%, p = 0.043), but this was due to non-weight adjusted heparin, multiple femoral instrumentations, and prolonged in-dwelling sheath times. At 6 months there was no difference in the composite endpoint.[227] Nonetheless, this study showed that abciximab can passivate the unstable plaque and prevent ischemic complications prior to PTCA.

2. **Tirofiban (Aggrastat).** In the RESTORE trial, 2141 patients with unstable angina, recent MI or acute MI undergoing PTCA or DCA were randomized to IV tirofiban (10 mcg/kg bolus + 0.15 mcg/kg/min infusion for 36 hours) or placebo. Tirofiban patients had lower primary endpoints (death, MI, reinfarction, TVR, or bail-out stent) at 2 days, (5.4% vs. 8.7%, p = 0.005), and 7 days (7.6% vs. 10.4%, p = 0.02), but not at 30 days (10.3% vs. 12.2%, p = 0.16). In TACTICS TIMI 18, 2220 patients with unstable angina or non-ST-elevation MI were treated with aspirin, heparin, beta-blockers, and tirofiban on admission to the hospital, with subsequent randomization to an early invasive strategy (cardiac catheterization and revascularization within 48 hours) or a conservative approach (cardiac catheterization only for recurrent ischemia). The primary endpoint of death, MI, or rehospitalization for ACS at 6 months was reduced by 18% in the invasive group (15.9% vs 19.4%, p = 0.025), with the greatest benefit among patients with positive troponins. The TARGET trial was a "head-to-head" comparison of tirofiban and abciximab in 4812 patients undergoing stent implantation, and demonstrated a 26% relative benefit for abciximab in the primary composite endpoint of death, MI, or revascularization at 30 days (6.0% vs 7.5%, p = 0.037); abciximab benefits were greatest among patients with acute coronary syndromes (6.3% vs. 9.3%).

3. **Eptifibatide (Integrelin).** The use of eptifibatide as an adjunct to coronary intervention was evaluated in the elective setting in IMPACT I and ESPRIT (Chapter 34), and in patients with acute coronary syndromes in IMPACT II and a subgroup of PURSUIT. IMPACT II randomized patients with stable or unstable angina to eptifibatide 135 mcg/kg bolus and 0.5 mcg/kg/min versus 0.75 mcg/kg/min infusion for 20-24 hours compared to placebo. There was a non-significant 19% reduction in the primary endpoint (30-day death, MI, or revascularization) in the low-dose group (9.2% vs 11.4%, p = 0.063) and in the high-dose group (9.9% vs 11.4%, p = 0.22). There was no difference in bleeding complications with eptifibatide. In the PURSUIT trial subgroup of 1250 patients with unstable angina who underwent coronary interventions within 72 hours of randomization, eptifibatide dosed at 180 mcg/kg bolus and 2.0 mcg/kg/min infusion reduced the 30-day primary endpoint of death or MI by 31% (11.6% vs 16.7%, p = 0.01).

4. **Recommendations for Platelet IIb/IIIa Inhibitors in Unstable Angina and Non-Q-Wave MI (Figures 5.3, 5.4).** The present data support the routine use of abciximab, eptifibatide, and possibly tirofiban in patients with non-Q-wave MI or high-risk unstable angina (elevated troponin, fluctuating ST segments, or recurrent chest pain despite aspirin and heparin). Based on FRISC-II and TACTICS TIMI-18, most patients with acute coronary syndromes should undergo cardiac catheterization followed by percutaneous or surgical revascularization when appropriate. If percutaneous intervention is performed on a patient receiving eptifibatide or tirofiban, the drug should be continued for 18-24 hours after intervention. If a patient has not been receiving a IIb/IIIa inhibitor and PTCA or stenting is planned, abciximab should be administered in the cath lab prior to the first balloon inflation, with weight-adjusted heparin (70 U/kg) to maintain an ACT of 200-250

seconds. After intervention, the infusion should be continued for 12 hours, no additional heparin should be given, and sheaths should be removed when the ACT falls below 170 seconds.

B. HEPARIN. Several randomized trials have clearly shown benefits of IV heparin (with and without aspirin) in patients with unstable angina. Although retrospective studies suggested that prolonged heparinization (3-7 days) improved the safety of PTCA for unstable angina, other studies reported no benefit for prolonged heparin.[239] In many centers, delayed PTCA is not practical because of increased length of hospital stay and cost; we recommend PTCA as soon as possible to reduce recurrent ischemia, MI, and death. For PTCA or stenting in unstable angina, non-Q-wave MI, or acute MI, we recommend an ACT of 350-400 seconds. If adjunctive IIb/IIIa inhibitors are used, weight-adjusted heparin (70 U/kg) and an ACT of 200-250 seconds is recommended, especially for abciximab (Chapter 34). Since ACT measurements may vary by 40-60 seconds, it may be prudent to obtain multiple ACTs to confirm the desired level. ACTs should be checked every 30 minutes and additional heparin given as necessary to maintain the ACT at the desired level for the duration of the procedure. It is very important to recognize that patients with ongoing heparin infusions often require as much intraprocedural heparin as those not on heparin.[252] Bivalirudin (Angiomax) has been approved for procedural anticoagulation in patients with unstable angina (dose: 1mg/kg IV bolus just prior to PTCA followed by a 4-hour IV infusion of 2.5 mg/kg/hr; may give an additional 0.2 mg/kg/hr up to 20 hours, if needed).

C. LOW-MOLECULAR-WEIGHT HEPARIN (LMWH) (Chapter 34, Tables 34.8, 34.9). Numerous trials of LMWH have been completed or are in progress, including randomized placebo-controlled trials in patients with acute coronary syndromes (FRISC,[176,178] FRISC-II[181]), randomized comparative trials to unfractionated heparin in patients with acute coronary syndromes treated conservatively (FRIC,[177] ESSENCE,[179] TIMI-11-B), randomized trials during percutaneous intervention (ENTICES, ATLAST), and observational studies evaluating combination therapies during percutaneous intervention (NICE-1, NICE-3, NICE-4) (Chapter 34, Tables 34.8, 34.9). These trials are difficult to compare to each other because of different inclusion criteria, primary endpoints, duration of therapy and follow-up, and use of different LMWH preparations. Despite these differences, the results of these trials can be summarized as follows: First, in patients presenting with acute coronary syndromes, LMWH is superior to placebo with respect to reduction in early (< 45 days) ischemic events (FRISC, FRISC-II), but the benefit may not be sustained at 3 months (FRISC-II). Combination therapy with IIb/IIIa inhibitors appears to be safe (NICE-3), but superior efficacy has not yet been demonstrated. Second, when patients with acute coronary syndromes undergo percutaneous revascularization, there is no incremental benefit for prolonged therapy with LMWH compared to placebo (FRISC-II). In these patients, the addition of IIb/IIIa inhibitors is safe (NICE-1, NICE-3, NICE-4, ENTICES, ATLAST), and although reduction in early ischemic events was reported in ENTICES, this benefit was not observed in ATLAST. Third, reliable anticoagulation is achieved with LMWH, and the risk of bleeding complications is similar to or less than that of unfractionated heparin. Finally, there does not appear to be any significant incremental value for one month of LMWH therapy after high-risk or suboptimal stenting compared to conventional antiplatelet therapy (ATLAST trial). The ongoing CRUISE

(Coronary Revascularization Utilizing Integrelin and Single Bolus Enoxaparin) trial will determine the relative benefit of enoxaparin vs. unfractionated heparin in eptifibatide patients undergoing coronary intervention.

D. DIRECT THROMBIN INHIBITORS (Chapter 34, Table 34.13). Direct thrombin inhibitors more effectively bind to fibrin-bound thrombin than heparin, and are not influenced by anti-thrombin III, platelet factor 4, or heparinase. Since thrombin is the most potent endogenous platelet activator, the hope was that potent thrombin inhibition would improve PTCA outcomes in patients with acute coronary syndromes.

1. **Hirudin.** Hirudin is a peptide derived from the medicinal leech shown to reduce platelet deposition and restenosis in animal models. The HELVETICA multicenter trial randomized 1141 patients with unstable angina to one of three arms: (1) 10,000 U heparin bolus plus 24-hour infusion; (2) hirudin 40 mg bolus plus 24-hour infusion; or (3) hirudin 40 mg bolus plus subcutaneous hirudin twice daily for 3 days after coronary intervention. Hirudin was associated with a significant reduction in adverse events at 30 days (11.0% vs. 7.9% vs. 5.6%, p = 0.023), but not at 6 months.[254] These studies suggest an initial but non-sustained benefit for hirudin in patients with acute coronary syndromes undergoing PTCA.

2. **Hirulog (Bivalirudin).** Hirulog is a synthetic peptide analog of hirudin. In 4088 patients undergoing PTCA for unstable or post-MI angina,[145] hirulog did not reduce ischemic events compared to heparin (11.4% vs. 12.2%), but did result in less bleeding. In the subgroup of patients with post-MI angina, hirulog was associated with fewer early ischemic events, but no benefit at 6 months. The Comparison of Abciximab Complications with Hirulog Events Trial (CACHET) trial will evaluate adjunctive anticoagulation with hirulog, clopidogrel, and abciximab in patients undergoing coronary intervention.[255] Bivalirudin is approved for procedural anticoagulation in patients with unstable angina.

E. THROMBOLYTIC AGENTS. Although a few early studies of unstable angina found immediate angiographic improvement after thrombolytic therapy, multiple recent randomized trials have consistently demonstrated *worse* clinical outcomes for PTCA patients treated with intravenous or intracoronary thrombolytic therapy,[1,125,256-260] even when angiographic features most likely to benefit from lytics were present (e.g., complex lesions, filling defects).[260] Potential mechanisms by which thrombolytic agents potentiate vessel occlusion after PTCA include enhanced platelet aggregation[261-263] and intramural hemorrhage.[264-267] Furthermore, coronary dissections that occur during PTCA may be more difficult to "tack-up" when thrombolytics have been given. Thus, routine use of thrombolytic agents should be avoided in patients undergoing PTCA for unstable angina.

F. CONTRAST AGENTS (Chapter 25). Ionic contrast agents are preferred by many operators for PTCA in acute coronary syndromes, since they prolong PTT and clotting time, inhibit platelet aggregation and degranulation, and shorten the time to thrombolysis. The GUSTO IIb contrast media substudy of 454 patients demonstrated fewer ischemic events at 30 days among patients receiving ionic vs. nonionic contrast (5.5% vs. 11.0%, p = 0.04).[319] However, although several observational and randomized trials demonstrated less acute closure, no-reflow, recurrent ischemia and MI with ionic contrast compared to low-osmolar nonionic contrast, other studies showed no difference (Chapter 25).[276-278] The ionic, low-osmolar contrast agent ioxaglate (Hexabrix) was compared to the non-ionic isosmolar agent Visipaque in the randomized COURT trial (Contrast Media Utilization in High Risk PTCA), which included 787 high-risk patients with unstable angina, acute MI, or post-MI angina. Visipaque resulted in a lower composite primary endpoint (in-hospital emergent revascularization, abrupt closure, stroke, thromboembolic events, cardiac death, or MI) (5.2% vs. 9.5%, p = 0.018). The secondary endpoint of angiographic success by independent angiographic core laboratory analysis (≤ 50% residual stenosis, TIMI 3 flow, > 20% reduction in diameter stenosis) was higher with Visipaque (90.1% vs. 84.6%, p = 0.016). These data suggest that osmolarity and ionicity are both important determinants of safety; Hexabrix and Visipaque are safe during coronary intervention for acute coronary syndromes.

Table 5.24. Results of IIb/IIIa Inhibitors for PCI in Acute Coronary Syndromes

Study	Antagonist	1° Endpoint	Result	Comments
CAPTURE[323] (n = 1265)	Abciximab (PCI for refractory unstable angina)	Death, MI, or urgent TVR at 30 days	Placebo: 15.9% Abciximab:0 11.3% (p = 0.012)	More major bleeding with abciximab; no difference in outcome at 6-months, suggesting the need for 12-hour drug infusion post-intervention
IMPACT-II[324] (n = 4010)	Eptifibatide (elective and urgent PCI for ACS)	Death, MI, or urgent TVR at 30 days	Placebo: 11.4% LD eptifib: 9.2% (p = 0.062) HD eptifib: 9.9% (p = 0.22)	No difference in bleeding; insignificant trend toward benefit with low-dose eptifibatide may have been due to inadequate drug dose
TARGET[354] (n = 4082)	Tirofiban vs. abciximab (stent for ACS and non-ACS)	Death, MI, or ischemia-driven TVR at 30 days	Tirofiban: 7.6% Abciximab: 6.0% (p = 0.037)	Greatest benefit for abciximab in ACS patients (6.3% vs. 9.3%); no difference in bleeding complications or outcome in non-ACS patients
TACTICS[325] (n = 2220)	Tirofiban (conservative vs. invasive strategy for ACS)	Death, MI, or rehospitalization at 30 days	Invasive: 7.4% Conservative: 10.5% (p < 0.001)	Benefits for early invasive strategy persisted at 6 months (15.9% vs. 19.4%, p = 0.025)
RESTORE[326,327] (n = 2141)	Tirofiban (PCI for ACS or MI)	Death, MI, or TVR at 48 hours	Placebo: 8.7 % Tirofiban: 5.4% (p = 0.005)	No difference in bleeding; used different endpoints that abciximab trials; tirofiban with persistent (but not significant) benefit at 30 days and 6 months
EXCITE[328]	Xemilofiban (PCI for ACS)	Death, MI, or urgent TVR at 30 days	Placebo: 8.1% 10 mg: 8.1% 20 mg: 7.3% (p = NS)	Oral xemilofiban had no benefit; diabetics had slight benefit with xemilofiban

Abbreviations: ACS = acute coronary syndromes; HD = high-dose; IVUS = intravascular ultrasound; LD = low-dose; MI = myocardial infarction; RRR = relative risk reduction; SD = standard dose; TVR = target vessel revascularization
Acronyms: See Table 34.31

SUMMARY: CLINICAL APPROACH TO ACUTE CORONARY SYNDROMES

A. UNSTABLE ANGINA AND NON-Q-WAVE MI. Figure 5.3 depicts our approach to the patient with unstable angina or non-Q-wave MI. When PTCA is performed, technical details are identical to acute MI (see below).

B. ACUTE MI. All MI patients with ST-segment elevation presenting within 12 hours of symptom onset are candidates for emergency reperfusion therapy. As shown in Figure 5.1, if a skilled interventionalist is available, the optimal reperfusion strategy is emergency PTCA with or without stenting. If a skilled interventionalist is not available and the patient is eligible for thrombolysis, intravenous thrombolytic therapy should be administered (Figure 5.2). For a large infarction with continued or recurrent ischemia, hemodynamic instability, or shock, catheterization should be performed as soon as possible, even if inter-hospital transfer is required. Our general recommendations include:

- Chewable aspirin 325mg, clopidogrel 300-450 mg PO, IV heparin (ACT 350-400 seconds, or 200-250 seconds if abciximab or other IIb/IIIa inhibitors are used), and IV beta-blockers prior to reperfusion
- Ionic contrast (or low osmolar Hexabrix or Visipaque)
- PTCA or stenting of culprit vessel only (goal is residual stenosis < 30% and TIMI-3 flow); multivessel intervention may be required and life-saving for patients in cardiogenic shock
- Stent for residual stenosis > 30% or significant dissection after PTCA
- Consider TEC, AngioJet, or abciximab for large intracoronary thrombus
- Treat no-reflow with intracoronary calcium antagonists, sodium nitroprusside, or adenosine
- IABP for continued ischemia, hypotension, pulmonary edema, left ventricular dysfunction and multivessel disease
- Consider bypass surgery for high-risk anatomy not amenable to PTCA or stenting
- Low-risk patients with successful PTCA may be managed in the step-down unit rather than the CCU, and discharged on the third hospital day if stable.

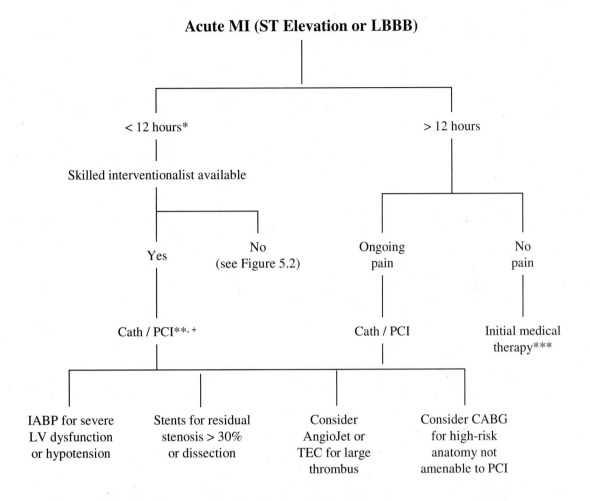

Figure 5.1. Interventional Management of Acute MI

Abbreviations: CABG = coronary artery bypass grafting; IABP = intra-aortic balloon pump; LV = left ventricular; PCI = percutaneous coronary intervention

*   Aspirin 325 mg chewed, IV heparin, IV beta-blocker

**   During PCI: Clopidogrel 300 mg (stent), ACT $\geq$ 350 sec, Hexabrix for heart failure or unstable hemodynamics
      After PCI: *Medical Therapy*: Aspirin, clopidogrel 75 mg QD x 1 month (stent), beta-blocker long-term, ACE
      inhibitor. *Stress test*: Not routinely recommended. *Discharge*: Day 3 if low-risk (age < 70, EF > 45%, 1 or 2-vessel
      disease, successful PCI). *Follow-up*: Manage lipid disorder, smoking cessation

*** Aspirin indefinitely, beta-blocker, ACE inhibitor

+   Abciximab is recommended for PTCA, optional for stents (use weight-adjusted heparin and ACT 250-300
      seconds). No data to support use of eptifibatide or tirofiban

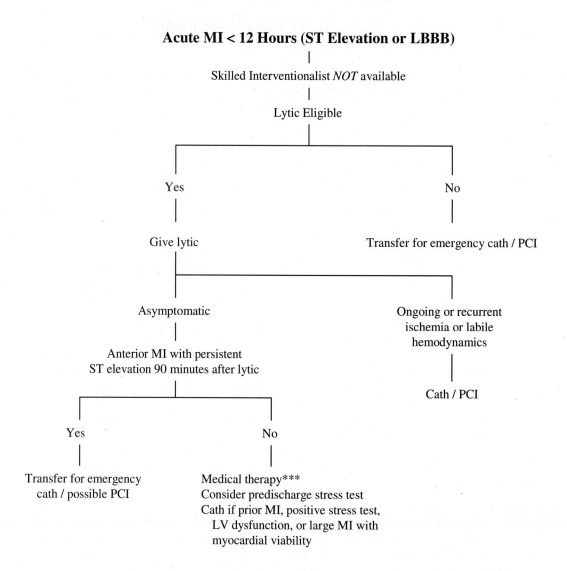

Figure 5.2.   Management of Acute MI: Cath Lab & Skilled Interventionalist *NOT* available

Abbreviations: LV = left ventricular; PCI = percutaneous coronary intervention
*** Aspirin indefinitely, beta-blocker, ACE inhibitor

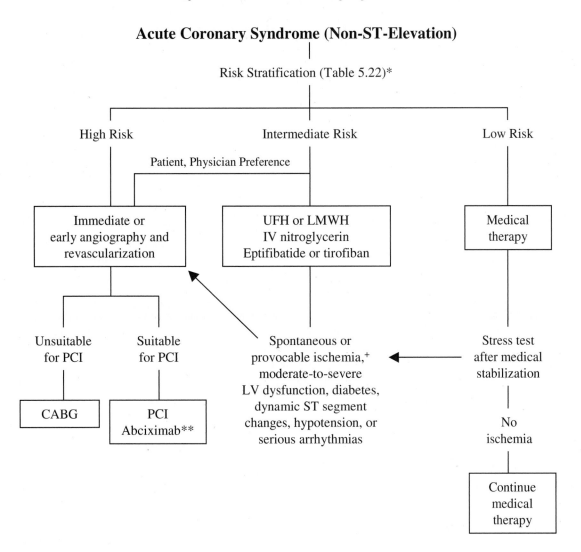

Figure 5.3. Interventional Management of Unstable Angina or Non-Q-Wave MI

Abbreviations: CABG = coronary artery bypass grafting; LMWH = low-molecular-weight heparin; LV = left ventricular; PCI = percutaneous coronary intervention; UFH = unfractionated heparin

* All patients should receive aspirin, beta-blockers (unless contraindicated), and possibly clopidogrel

** Patients who receive eptifibatide or tirofiban prior to angiography should continue to receive that agent during and after PCI (see Figure 5.4)

\+ Stress test after medical stabilization

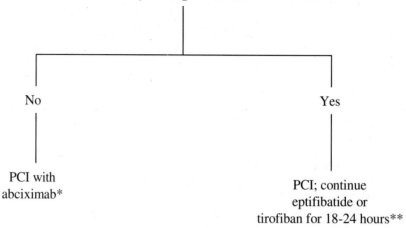

Patient is Already on Eptifibatide or Tirofiban

No

PCI with
abciximab*

Yes

PCI; continue
eptifibatide or
tirofiban for 18-24 hours**

Figure 5.4. Approach to Patients with Acute Coronary Syndromes Who Require PCI

Abbreviations: PCI = percutaneous coronary intervention
*   Bolus 0.25 mg/kg IV, then 0.125 mcg/kg/min IV x 12 hrs; heparin (70 U/kg to achieve ACT ~ 250 seconds),
      clopidogrel (300 mg bolus, then 75 mg QD for 30 days); no post-procedural heparin
** Target ACT ~ 250 seconds; no post-procedural heparin

REFERENCES

1. Weaver WD, Parsons L, Every N. Primary coronary angioplasty in hospitals with and without surgery backup. J Invas Cardiol 1995;7:34F-39F.
2. Ayers M. Coronary angioplasty for acute myocardial infarction in hospitals without cardiac surgery. J Invas Cardiol 1995;7:40F-46F.
3. Weaver W, Parsons L, Martin JS, Every N. Direct PTCA for treatment of acute myocardial infarction: A community experience in hospitals with and without surgical back-up. Circulation 1995;92:I-138.
4. Wharton TP, Schmitz JM, Fedele FA, McNamara NS, Gladstone AR, Jacobs MI. Primary angioplasty in acute myocardial infarction at community hospitals without cardiac surgery: Experience in 195 cases. Circulation 1995;92:I-138.
5. Zijlstra F, Jan de Boaer M, Hoorntje JCA, Reiffer S, Reiber JHC, Suryapranata H. A comparison of immediate coronary angioplasty with intravenous streptokinase in acute myocardial infarction. N Engl J Med 1993;328:680-684.
6. Griffin J, Grines CL, Marsales D, et al. A prospective, randomized trial evaluating the prophylactic use of balloon pumping in high-risk myocardial infarction patients: PAMI-2. J Am Coll Cardiol 1995;25:86A.
7. Brodie BR, Grines CL, Ivanhoe R, Knopf W, Taylor G, O'Keefe J, Weintraub RA, Berdan LG, Tcheng JE, Woodlief LH, Califf RM, O'Neill WW. Six -month clinical and angiographic follow-up after direct angioplasty for acute myocardial infarction. Circulation 1994;90:156-162.
8. O'Neill WW, Weintraub R, Grines CL, Meany TB, Brodie BR, Friedman HZ, Ramos RG, Gangadharan V, Levin RN, Choksi N, Westveer DC, Strzelecki RN, Timmis GC. A prospective placebo-controlled randomized trial of intravenous streptokinase and angioplasty therapy of acute myocardial infarction. Circulation 1992;86:1710-1717.
9. Zahn R, Koch A, et al. (1997), Primary angioplasty versus thrombolysis in the treatment of acute myocardial infarction. Am J Cardiol 79:264-259.
10. O'Keefe JO, Bailey WL, Rutherford BD, Hartzler GO. Primary angioplasty for acute myocardial infarction in 1000 consecutive patients. Am J Cardiol 1993;72:107G-115G.
11. Brodie BR, Weintraub RA, Stuckey TD, et al. Outcomes of direct coronary angioplasty for acute myocardial infarction in candidates and non-candidates for thrombolytic therapy. Am J Cardiol 1991;67:7-12.
12. Beauchamp GD, Vacek JL Robuck W. Management comparison for acute myocardial infarction: direct angioplasty versus sequential thrombolysis-angioplasty. Am Heart J 1990;120:237-242.
13. Nakagawa Y, Iwasaki Y, Takeshi, Nobuyoshi M. Serial angiographic follow-up after successful direct angioplasty for acute myocardial infarction; single center experience. Circulation 1993;88(Suppl I):I-106 (abstr.).
14. Rothbaum DA, Linnemeier TJ, Landin RJ, et al. Emergency percutaneous transluminal coronary angioplasty in acute myocardial infarction: a 3 year experience. J Am Coll Cardiol l987;10:264-272.
15. Miller PF, Brodie BR, Weintraub RA, et al. Emergency coronary angioplasty for acute myocardial infarction. Arch Intern Med 1987;147:1565-1570.
16. Dageford DA, Genovely HC, Goodin RR, Allen RD. Emergency percutaneous transluminal coronary angioplasty in acute myocardial infarction. J Kentucky Med Assn 1987;85:368-372.
17. Kimura T, Nosaka H, Ueno K, Nobuyoshi M. Role of coronary angioplasty in acute myocardial infarction. Circulation 1986;74(Suppl II):II-22(abstr).
18. Marco J, Caster L, Szatmary LF, Fajadet J. Emergency percutaneous transluminal coronary angioplasty without thrombolysis as initial therapy in acute myocardial infarction. Int J Cardiol 1987;15:55-63.
19. O'Neill W, Timmis GC, Bourdillon PD, et al. A prospective randomized clinical trial of intracoronary streptokinase versus coronary angioplasty for acute myocardial infarction. N Engl J Med 1986;314:812-818.
20. Stone GW, Rutherford BD, McConahay DR, et al. Direct coronary angioplasty in acute myocardial infarction: outcome in patients with single vessel disease. J Am Coll Cardiol 1990;15:534-43.
21. Stone GW, Grines CL, Topol EJ. Update on percutaneous transluminal coronary angioplasty for acute myocardial infarction. Book chapter. Current Review of Interventional Cardiology. Ed. .E. Topol, M.D., P. Serruys, M.D., Current Medicine, Philadelphia, PA, 1995.1-56.
22. Stone CW, Grines CL, Browne KF, Marco J, Rothbaum D, O'Keefe J, Hartzler GO, Overlie P, Donohue B, Chelliah N, Timmis GC, Vlietstra R, Strzelecki M, Puchrowicz-Ochocki S, O'Neill WW. Predictors of in-hospital and 6 month outcome after acute myocardial infarction in the reperfusion era: The Primary Angioplasty in Myocardial Infarction (PAMI) Trial J Am Coll Cardiol 1995:25:370-377.
23. Waldecker B, Waas W, Haberbosch W, Voss R, Kistler P, Tillmanns H. Long-term follow-up (2.5 years) of 300 consecutive patients with primary angioplasty for acute myocardial infarction. Circulation 1995;92:I-461.
24. Maynard C, Weaver D, Litwin PE, et al. Hospital mortality in acute myocardial infarction in the era of reperfusion therapy (the Myocardial Infarction Triage and Intervention Project). Am J Cardiol 1993;72:877-82.
25. Rogers WJ, Chandra NC, Gore JM, for the NMRI Investigators. National registry of myocardial infarction (NMRI): What have we learned from the first 100,000 patients? J Am Coll Cardiol 1993;21:349A.
26. Aoki H, Suzuki T, et al. A prospective randomized trial of intracoronary t-PA versus coronary angioplasty in acute myocardial infarction: Japanese intervention trial in myocardial infarction (JIMI). Circulation 1997;96:1-536.
27. Cragg DR, Friedman HZ, Bonema JD, et al. Out come of patients with acute myocardial infarction who are ineligible for thrombolytic therapy. Ann Int Med 1991;115:173-177.
28. Stone GW, Grines CL, Brown KF, Marco J, Rothbaum D, O'Keefe J, Overlie P, Donohue B, Puchrowicz S, O'Neill WW. Outcome of different reperfusion strategies in thrombolytic "eligible" versus "ineligible" patients with acute myocardial infarction . J Am Coll Cardiol February 1995;401A.
29. Grines CL, Booth D, Nissen S, Gurley J, Bennett K, O'Connor

WN, DeMaria A. Mechanism of acute myocardial infarction in patients with prior coronary artery bypass grafting and therapeutic implications. Am J Cardiol 1990;65:1292-96.

30. McKendall GR, Drew TM, Kelsey SF, et al. What is the optimal treatment for thrombolytic ineligible AMI Preliminary results of the Study of Medicine vs. Angioplasty Reperfusion Trial (SMART). J Am Coll Cardiol 1994;1A-484A:225A.

31. Kaplan AJ, Bengtson JR, Aronson LG, et al. Reperfusion improves survival in patients with cardiogenic shock after acute myocardial infarction. J Am Coll Cardiol 1990;15:155 (abstr).

32. Lee L, Erbel R, Brown TM, et al. Multi-center registry of angioplasty therapy of cardiogenic shock: initial and long-term survival. J Am Coll Cardiol 1991;17:599-603.

33. Gacioch GM, Ellis SG, Lee L, et al. Cardiogenic shock complicating acute myocardial infarction: the use of coronary angioplasty and the integration of the new support devices into patient management. J Am Coll Cardiol 1992;19:647-653.

34. Bengtson JR, Kaplan AJ, Pieper KS, et al. Prognosis in cardiogenic shock after acute myocardial infarction in the interventional era. J Am Coll Cardiol 1992;20:1482-1489.

35. Hibbard MD, Holmes Dr, Gersh BJ, Reeder GS. Coronary angioplasty for acute myocardial infarction complicated by cardiogenic shock. Circulation 1990;82:III-511.

36. Moosvi AR, Villanueva L, Gheorghiade M, et al. Early revascularization improves survival in cardiogenic shock. Circulation 1990;82:III-308.

37. Eltchaninoff H, Simpendorfer C, Whitlow PL. Coronary angioplasty improves both early and 1 year survival in acute myocardial infarction complicated by cardiogenic shock. J Am Coll Cardiol 1991;17:167.

38. Brown TM, Lannone LA, Gordon DF, et al. Percutaneous myocardial reperfusion reduces mortality in acute myocardial infarction complicated by cardiogenic shock. Circulation 1995;72:III-309.

39. O'Neill WW, Erbel R, Laufer N, et al. Coronary angioplasty therapy of cardiogenic shock complication g acute myocardial infarction. Circulation 1995;72:III-309.

40. Meyer P, Blanc P, Badouy M, Morand P. Treatment de choc cardiogenique primaire par angioplastie transluminale coronarienne a la phase aigue de l'Infarctus. Arch Mal Cœur 1990;83:329-334.

41. Lee L, Bates ER, Pitt B, Walton JA, et al. Percutaneous transluminal coronary angioplasty improves survival in acute myocardial infarction complicated by cardiogenic shock. Circulation 1998;78:145-151.

42. Seydoux C, Goy J-J, Beuret P, et al. Effectiveness of percutaneous transluminal coronary angioplasty in cardiogenic shock during acute myocardial infarction. Am J Cardiol 1992;68:968-969.

43. Heuser RR, Maddoux GL, Goss JE, et al. Coronary angioplasty in the treatment of cardiogenic shock: the therapy of choice. J Am Coll Cardiol 1986;7:219.

44. Shani J, Rivera M, Geengart A, et al. Percutaneous transluminal coronary angioplasty in cardiogenic shock. J Am Coll Cardiol 1986;7:149.

45. Disler L, Haitas B, Benjamin J, et al. Cardiogenic shock in evolving myocardial infarction: treatment by angioplasty and streptokinase. Heart Lung 1987;16:649.

46. Verna E, Repetto S, Boscarina m, et al. Emergency coronary angioplasty in patients with severe left ventriculardysfunction of cardiogenic shock after acute myocardial infarction. Eur Heart J 1989;10:958-966.

47. Hochman JS, Boland J, Sleeper LA, Porway M, Brinker J, Col J, Jacobs A, Slater J, Miller D, Wasserman H, Menegus MA, Talley D, McKinlay S, Sanborn T, LeJemtel T, and the SHOCK Registry Investigators. Current spectrum of cardiogenic shock and effect of early revascularization on mortality. Circulation 1995;91:372-881

48. Holmes DR, Bates EF, Kleiman NS Sadowski z, Horan JHS, Morris DC, Califf RM, Berger PB, Topol EJ. Contemporary reperfusion therapy for cardiogenic shock: the GUSTO-I trial experience. J Am Coll Cardiol 1995;26:668-674.

49. Anderson RD, Stebbins AL, Bates E, Stomel R, Granger CB, Ohman EM. Underutilization of aortic counter pulsation in patients with cardiogenic shock: Observations from the GUSTO-1 study. Circulation1995;92:I-139.

50. O'Neill WW, Brodie BR, Ivanhoe R, Knopf W, Taylor G, O'Keefe J, Grines CL, Weintraub R, Sickinger B, Berdan LG, Tcheng JE, Woodlief LG, Strzelecki M, Hartzler G, Califf RM. Primary coronary Angioplasty for Acute Myocardial Infarctin (the Primary Angioplasty Registry). Am J Cardio 1994;73:627-634.

51. Gruppo Italiano per lo Studio della Streptochinasi nell'Infarto Miocardico (GISSI): Effectiveness of intravenous thrombolytic treatment in acute myocardial infarction. Lancet 1986;1:397-402.

52. ISIS-2 (Second International Study Group of Infarct Survival) collaborative group: Randomized trial of intravenous streptokinase, oral aspirin, both or neither among 17,187 case of suspected acute myocardial infarction. Lancet 1988;2:349-360.

53. Wilcox RG, Olsson CG, Skene AM, Von Deer Lippe G, Jensen G, Hampton JR. Trial of tissue plasminogen activator for mortality reduction in acute myocardial infarction. Anglo Scandinavian Study of Early Thrombolysis (ASSET). Lancet 1988;2:525-530.

54. AIMS Trial Study Group: Effect of intravenous APSAC on mortality after acute myocardial infarction: Preliminary report of placebo-controlled clinical trial. Lancet 1998;1:515-549.

55. Chesebro JH, Knatterud G, Roberts R, et al. Thrombolysis in Myocardial Infarction (TIMI) Trial, phase I: a comparison between intravenous tissue plasminogen activator and intravenous streptokinase. Circulation 1987;76:142-154.

56. Topol EJ, Califf RM, George BS, Kereiakes DJ, Lee KL. Insights derived from the Thrombolysis and Angioplasty in Myocardial Infarction (TAMI) trials. J Am Coll Cardiol 1988;12:24A-31A.

57. Grines CL, Nissen SE, Booth DC, et al. A prospective, randomized trial comparing half-dose tissue-type plasminogen activator with streptokinase to full-dose tissue-type plasminogen activator. Circulation 1991;84:540-549.

58. Califf RM, Topol EJ, Stack RS, et al. Evaluation of combination thrombolytic therapy and timing of cardiac catheterization in acute myocardial infarction: results of Thrombolysis and Angioplasty in Myocardial Infarction-

Phase 5 randomized trial. Circulation 1991;83;1543-1556.

59. Carney RJ, Murphy GA, Brandt TR, et al. Randomized angiographic trial of recombinant tissue-type plasminogen activator (alteplase) in myocardial infarction. J Am Coll Cardiol 1992;20:17-23.

60. Granger CB, Ohman EM, Bates E. Pooled analysis of angiographic patency rates from thrombolytic therapy trials. Circulation 1992;86(suppl I):I-269 (abstr).

61. Kennedy JW, Martin GV, Davis KB, et al. The Western Washington Intravenous Streptokinase in Acute Myocardial Infarction randomized trial. Circulation 1988;77:345-352.

62. Schroder R, Neuhaus K-L, Leizorovicz A, Linderer T, Tebbe U. A prospective placebo-controlled double-blind multi-center trial of intravenous streptokinase in acute myocardial infarction (ISAM) long term mortality and morbidity. J Am Coll Cardiol 1987;9:197-203.

63. Meinertz T, Kasper W, Schumacher M, Just H. The German multi-center trial of anisoylated plasminogen streptokinase activator complex versus heparin for acute myocardial infarction. Am J Cardiol 1988;62:347-351.

64. Grines CL, Browne KF, Marco J, Rothbaum D, Stone GW, O'Keefe J, Overlie P, Donohue B, Chelliah N, Timmis GC, Vlietstra RE, Strzelecki M, Puchrowicz-Ochocki S, O'Neill W. A comparison of immediate angioplasty with thrombolytic therapy for acute myocardial infarction. N Engl J Med 1993;328:673-679.

65. Gibbons RJ, Holmes DR, Reeder GS, Bailey KR, Hopenspirger MR, Gersh BJ. Immediate angioplasty compared with the administration of a thrombolytic agent followed by conservative treatment for myocardial infarction. N Engl J Med 1993;328:685-691.

66. O'Neill W, Timmis GC, Bourdillon PD Lai P, Ganghadarhan V, Walton J, Ramos R, Laufer N, Gordon S. Schork MA, Pitt B. A prospective randomized clinical trial of intracoronary streptokinase versus coronary angioplasty for acute myocardial infarction. N Engl J Med 1986;341:812-818.

7. DeWood MA, Fisher MJ, for the Spokane Heart Research Group. Direct PTCA versus intravenous rtPA in acute myocardial infarction: Preliminary results from a prospective randomized trial. Circulation 1989;80:II-418.

68. Ribeiro EE, Silva LA, Carneiro R, D'Oliveria LG, Gasquez A, Jose GA, Tavares JR, Petrizzo A, Torossian s. Duprat R, Buffolo E, Ellis SG. Randomized trial of direct coronary angioplasty versus intravenous streptokinase in acute myocardial infarction. J Am Coll Cardiol 1993;22:376-380.

69. Elizaga J, Garcia EJ, Delcan JL, Garcia-Robles JA, Bueno H, Soriano J, Abeytua M, Lopez-Bescos L. Primary coronary angioplasty versus systemic thrombolysis in acute anterior myocardial infarction: in -hospital results from a prospective randomized trial. Circulation 1993;88:I-411.

70. Michels KB, Yusif S. Does PTCA in acute myocardial infarction affect mortality and reinfarction rates? A quantitative overview (meta-analysis) of the randomized clinical trials. Circulation 1995;91:476-485.

71. Investigators, G.I. A Clinical trail comparing primary coronary angioplasty with tissue plasminogen activator for acute myocardial infarction. N Engl J Med. 1997;336:1621-1628.

72. Granger C, Betriu A, et al. Nearly half of early benefit of direct angioplasty lost in longer-term follow-up: 6 month results from the gusto lib direct angioplasty substudy. Circualtion 1998;96:1-205.

73. O'Neill WW, de Boaer MJ, Gibbons RJ, Holmes Dr, Timmis GC, Sachs D, Grines CL, Zijlstra F. Data from three prospective randomized clinical trials of thrombolytic versus angioplasty therapy of acute myocardial infarction. Preliminary results from a pooled analysis. Book chapter in Primary Coronary Angioplasty in Acute Myocardial Infarction. Ed. Menko Jan de boer, Proefschrift Rotterdam: Erasmus University, 1994, 99. 165-171.

74. The GUSTO Angiographic Investigators. The effects of tissue plasminogen activator, streptokinase, or both on coronary-artery patency, ventricular function, and survival after acute myocardial infarction. N Engl J Med 1993;329:1615-1622.

75. Topol EJ, Califf RM, Vandormael M, et al. The Thrombolysis and Angioplasty in Myocardial Infarction (TAMI-6) Study Group. A randomized trial of late reperfusion therapy for acute myocardial infarction. Circulation 1992;85:2090-2099.

76. Meijer A, Verhjeugt FWA, Werter CJPJ, Lie KI, vander Pol JMJ, van Eenige MJ. Aspirin versus coumadin in the prevention of reocclusion and recurrent ischemia after successful thrombolysis: A prospective placebo-controlled angiographic study. Results of the APRICOT study. Circulation 1993;87:1524-1530.

77. Meijer A, Verheugt F, Eenigem M, Werter C. Left ventricular function at 3 months after successful thrombolysis. Impact of reocclusion without reinfarction on ejection fraction, regional function and remodeling. Circulation 1994;90:1706-1714.

78. Veen G, Meyer A, Verheugt F, et al. Culprit lesion morphology and stenosis severity in the prediction of reocclusion after coronary thrombolysis: Angiographic results of the APRICOT study. J Am Coll Cardiol 1993;22:1755-62.

79. White H, French J, Hamer A, et al. Frequent reocclusion of patent infarct-related arteries between 4 weeks and 1 year: Effects of antiplatelet therapy. J Am Coll Cardiol 1995;25:218-23.

80. Grines Cl, Griffin JJ, Brodie BR, Stone GW, Donohue BC, Balestrini CE, Wharton TP, Spain MG, Shimshak T, Jones D, Mason D, Sachs D, O'Neill WW. The second Primary Angioplasty for Myocardial Infarction study (PAMI-II): Preliminary Report. Circulation 1994;90:I-433.

81. Grines C, Marsalese D, Brodie B, Griffin J, Donohue BC, Sampaolesi A, Costantini C, Stone G, Spain M, Jones D, Sachs D, Mason D, O'Neill W. Acute cath provides the best method of risk stratifying MI patients. Circulation, 1995;92:I-531.

82. Brodie B, Grines CL, Spain M, et al. A prospective, randomized trial evaluating early discharge (day 3) without non-invasive risk stratification in low risk patients with acute myocardial infarction: PAMI-2. J Am Coll Cardiol 1995;25:5A.

83. Donohue BC, O'Neill WW, Jackson EJ, Brodie B, Griffin J, Balestrini C, Stone G, Wharton T, Jones DE, Grines CL. Cost analysis of different management strategies for myocardial infarction. J Am Coll Cardiol 1996;27:221A.

84. Ellis SG, Vande Weft F, Da Silva ER, et al. Present status of

rescue coronary angioplasty: Current polarization of opinion and randomized trials. J Am Coll Cardiol 1992;19:681-686.

85. Califf RM, Topol EJ, George BS, et al. Characteristics and outcomes of patients in whom reperfusion with tissue-type plasminogen activator fails: results of the thrombolysis and Angioplasty in Myocardial Infarction (TAMI) Trial. Circulation 1988;77:1090-1099

86. Fung AY, Lai P, Topol EJ, et al. Value of percutaneous transluminal coronary angioplasty after unsuccessful intravenous streptokinase therapy in acute myocardial infarction. Am J Cardiol 1986;58:686-691.

87. Topol EJ, Califf RM, George BS, et al and the TAMI Study Group. Coronary arterial thrombolysis with combined infusion of recombinant tissue-type plasminogen activator and urokinase in patients with acute myocardial infarction. Circulation 1988;77:1100-1107.

88. Grines CL, Nissen SE, Booth DC, et al and the KAMIT study group. A new thrombolytic regimen for acute myocardial infarction using combination half dose tissue-type plasminogen activator with full dose streptokinase: a pilot study. J Am Coll Cardiol 1989;14:573-580.

89. Holmes DR, Gersh BJ, Baily KR, et al. "Rescue" percutaneous transluminal coronary angioplasty after failed thrombolytic therapy: 4-year follow-up. J Am Coll Cardiol 1989;13:193(abstr).

90. Grines CL, Nissen Booth DC, et al and the Kentucky Acute Myocardial Infarction Trial (KAMIT) Group. A prospective, randomized trial comparing combination half-dose tissue-type plasminogen activator and streptokinase with full-dose tissue-type plasminogen activator. Circulation 1991;84:540-549.

91. O'Connor CM, Mark DB, Honohara T, et al. Rescue coronary angioplasty after failure of intravenous streptokinase in acute myocardial infarction: in-hospital and long-term outcomes. J Invasive Cardiol 1989;1:85-95.

92. Baim DS, diver DJ, Knatterud GL and the TIMI II-A Investigators. PTCA "salvage" for thrombolytic failures: implications from TIMI II-A. Circulation 1988;78(Suppl II):II-112(abstr).

93. Whitlow PL. Catheterization/rescue angioplasty following thrombolysis (Craft) study: :Results of rescue angioplasty. Circulation 1990;82(Suppl III):III-308 (abstr).

94. Abbottsmith CW, Topol EJ, George BS, et al. Fate of patients with acute myocardial infarction with patency of the infarct-related vessel achieved with successful thrombolysis versus rescue angioplasty. J Am Coll Cardiol 1990;16:770-778.

95. Gibson CM, Cannon CP, Piana RN, et al. Rescue PTCA in the TIMI 4 trial. J Am Coll Cardiol 1994;1A-48A:225A.

96. Wnqk A, Krupa H, Gasior M, Kalarus Z, Borkowski B, Wqs T, Lekston A, Wester A, Chodor P, Pasyk S. Results of rescue-angioplasty after unsuccessful intracoronary streptokinase therapy in patients with acute myocardial infarction. European Congress of Cardiology, abstract, 1995.

97. Ross AM, Reiner JS, Thompson MA, et al. Immediate and follow-up procedural outcome of 214 patients undergoing rescue PTCA in the GUSTO trial: no effect of the lytic agent. Circulation 1993;88(Suppl I):I-410(abstr).

98. Gibson M, Cannon C, et al. Rescue angioplasty in the thrombolysis in myocardial infarction (TIMI) 4 trial. Am J Cardiol 1997;80:21-26.

99. Ellis SG, Ribeiro da Silva E, Heyndrickx G, Talley D, Cernigliaro C, Steg G, Spaulding C, Nobuyoshi M, Erbel R, Vassanelli C, Topol EJ. Randomized comparison of rescue angioplasty with conservative management of patients with early failure of thrombolysis for acute anterior myocardial infarction. Circulation 1994;90:2280-2284.

100. Belenkie I, Traboulsi M, Hall CA, Hansen JL, Roth DL, Manyari D, Filipchuck NG, Schnurr LR, Rosenal TW, Smith ER, Knudtson M. Rescue angioplasty during myocardial infarction has a beneficial effect on mortality: A tenable hypothesis. Can J Cardiol 1992;8:357-362.

101. The CORAMI Study Group. Outcome of attempted rescue coronary angioplasty after failed thrombolysis for acute myocardial infarction. Am J Cardiol 1994;74:172-174.

102. Miller J, Ohman E, et al. Survival benefit of aboiximab administration during early rescue angioplasty: Analysis of 387 patients from the GUSTO-III trial. J Am Coll Cardiol 1998;31:191A.

103. Rogers WJ, Baim DS, Fore JM, et al for the TIMI-IIA investigators. Comparison of immediate invasive, delayed invasive, and conservative strategies after tissue-type plasminogen activator. Circulation 1990;81:1457-1476.

104. Topol EJ, Califf RM, George BS, et al and the Thrombolysis and Angioplasty in Myocardial Infarction Study Group. A randomized trial of immediate versus delayed elective angioplasty after intravenous tissue plasminogen activator in acute myocardial infarction. N Engl J Med 1987;317:581-588.

105. Simoons ML, Arnold AET, Bertriu A, et al. Thrombolysis with tissue plasminogen activator in acute myocardial infarction: No additional benefit from immediate percutaneous coronary angioplasty. Lancet 1988;1:197-202.

106. Gibson C, Cannon C, Piana R. Angiographic predictors of reocclusion after thrombolysis: Results from the thrombolysis in myocardial infarction (TIMI-4) trial. J Am Coll Cardiol 1995;25:589-9.

107. The TIMI Study Group. Comparison of invasive and conservative strategies after treatment with intravenous tissue plasminogen activator in acute myocardial infarction. Results of the Thrombolysis in Myocardial Infarction (TIMI) Phase II Trial. N Engl J Med 1989;320:

108. SWIFT (Should We Intervene Following Thrombolysis?) Trial Study Group. SWIFT trial of delayed elective intervention vs. conservative treatment after thrombolysis with anistreplase in acute myocardial infarction. Br Med J 1991;302:555-560.

109. Barbash GI, Roth A, Hod H, et al. Randomized controlled trial of late in-hospital angiography and angioplasty versus conservative management after treatment with recombinant tissue-type plasminogen activator in acute myocardial infarction. Am J Cardiol 1990;66:538-545.

110. Van den Brand MJ, Betrui A, Bescos LL, et al. Randomized trial of deferred angioplasty after thrombolysis for acute myocardial infarction. Coronary Artery Disease 1992;3:393-401.

111. Ozbek C, Dyckmans, J, Sen S, et al. Comparison of invasive and conservative strategies after treatment with streptokinase in acute myocardial infarction: results of a randomized trial (SIAM). J Am Coll Cardiol 1990;15:63A (abstr).

112. Mueller HS, Cohen LS, Braunwald E, et al, for the TIMI

Investigators. Predictors of early morbidity and mortality after thrombolytic therapy of acute myocardial infarction. Analysis of patient subgroups in the Thrombolysis in Myocardial Infarction (TIMI) Trial, Phase II. Circulation 1992;85:1254-1264.

113. Guerci AD, Gerstenblith G, Brinker JA, et al. A randomized trial of intravenous tissue plasmingogen activator for acute myocardial infarction with subsequent randomization to elective coronary angioplasty. N Engl J Med 1987;317:1613-1618.

114. Van de Werf F. Discrepancies between the effects of coronary reperfusion on survival and left ventricular function. Lancet 1989;I:1367-1369.

115. Galvani M, Ottani F, Ferrini D, Sorbello F, Rusticali F. Patency of the infarct-related artery and left ventricular function as the major determinants of survival after Q-wave acute myocardial infarction. Am J cardiol 1993;71:I-7.

116. Anderson JL. Overview of patency as an endpoint of thrombolytic therapy. Am J Cardiol 1991;67:11-16E.

117. Topol EJ, Califf RM, Vandormael M, Grines CL, George BS, Sanz ML, Wall T, O'Brien M, Schwaiger M, Aguirre FV, Young S, Popma JJ, Lee KL, Ellis SG and the Thrombolysis and Angioplasty in Myocardial Infarction-6 Study Group. A randomized trial of late reperfusion therapy for acute myocardial infarction. Circulation 1992;85:2090-2099.

118. Madsen J, Grande P, et al. Danish multi-center randomized study of invasive versus conservative treatment in patients with inducible ischemia after thrombolysis in acute myocardial infarction (DANAMI). Circulation 1997;96:748-755.

119. Kaplan B, Safian R, Grines C, et al. Differences in outcome after angioplasty for AMI: The left anterior descending artery vs. the right coronary. J Am Coll Cardiol 1996;27:166A.

120. Bates ER. Reperfusion therapy in inferior myocardial infarction. J Am Coll Cardiol 1988;12:44A-51A.

121. Gacioch GM, Topol EJ. Sudden paradoxic clinical deterioration during angioplasty of the occluded right coronary artery in acute myocardial infarction. J Am Coll Cardiol 1989;14:1202-9.

122. Kahn JK, Rutherford BD, McConahay DR, et al. Catheterization laboratory events and hospital outcome with direct angioplasty for acute myocardial infarction. Circulation 1990;82:1910-1915.

123. Ohman EM, Califf RM, Topol EJ, et al. Consequences of reocclusion after successful reperfusion therapy in acute myocardial infarction. Circulation 1990;82:781-91.

124. Stone GW, Grines CL, Browne KF, Marco J, Rothbaum D, O'Keefe J, Hartzler GO, Overlie P, Donohue B, Chelliah N, Vlietstra R, Puchrowicz-Ochocki S, O'Neill WW. Implications of recurrent ischemia after reperfusion therapy in acute myocardial infarction: A comparison of thromboytic therapy and primary angioplasty. J Am Coll Cardiol 1995;26:66-72.

125. Grines C, Brodie B, Griffin J, Donohue B, Sampaoiesi A, Costantini C, Sachs D, Wharton T, Esente P, Spain M, Stone G. Which primary PTCA Patients may benefit from new technologies? Circulation 1995;92:I-146.

126. Nunn C, O'Neill W, Rothbaum D, O'Keefe J, Overlie P, Donohue B, Mason D, Catlin T, Grines C. Primary

angioplasty for myocardial infarction improves long-term survival: PAMI-I follow-up. J Am Coll Cardiol 1996;27:153A.

127. Braunwald E, Mark DB, Jones RH, Cheitlin MD, Fuster V, McCauley K, Edwards C, Green LA, Mushlin AL, Swain JA, Smith EE, Cowan M, Rose GC, Concannon CA, Grines CL, Brown L, Lytle BW, Goldman LA, Topol EJ, Willerson JT, Brown J, Archibald N. Unstable Angina: Diagnosis and Management-Clinical Practice Guidelines. U.S. Department of Health and Human Services AHCPR Publication No> 94-0682, March 15, 1994.

128. Liebson P, Klein L, et al. The non Q-wave myocardial infarction revisited: 10 years later. Prog Cardiovasc Dis 1997;39:399-444.

129. Cohen M, Fuster V. Insights into the pathogenic mechanisms of unstable angina. Circulation 1990;98:734-741.

130. Falk E, Shah P, et al. Coronary plaque disruption. Circulation 1995;92:657-671.

131. Roberts W, Kragel A, Gertz S, Roberts S. Coronary arteries in unstable angina, acute myocardial infarction and sudden coronary death. Am J Cardiol 1994;127:1588-1593.

132. DeFeyter P, Serruys P. Percutaneous transluminal coronary angioplasty for unstable angina. In: Textbook of Interventional Cardiology. Ed. EJ Topol, M.D., W. B Saunder Co., 1994, p. 274.

133. Steffenino G, Meier B, Finci L, et al. Follow-up results of treatment of unstable angina by coronary angioplasty. Br Heart J 1987;57:416.

134. Myler RK, Shaw RE, Stertzer SH, et al. Unstable angina and coronary angioplasty. Circulation 1990;82:II-88-95.

135. Stammen F, De Scheerder I, Glazier JJ, et al. Immediate and follow-up results of the conservative coronary angioplasty strategy of unstable angina pectoris. Am J Cardiol 1992;69:1533.

136. de Feyter PJ, Suryapranata H, Serruys PW, et al. Coronary angioplasty for unstable angina: Immediate and late results in 200 consecutive patients with identification of risk factors for unfavorable early and late outcome. J Am Coll Cardiol 1988;12:324.

137. Plokker HWT, Ernst SMPG, Bal ET, et al. Percutaneous transluminal coronary angioplasty in patients with unstable angina pectoris refractory to medical therapy. Cathet Cardiovasc Diagn 1988;14:15.

138. Perry RA, Seth A, Hunt A, et al. Coronary angioplasty in unstable angina and stable angina: A comparison of success and complications. Br Heart J 1988;60:367.

139. Bentivoglio LG, Holubkov R, Kelsey SF, et al. Short and long term outcome of percutaneous transluminal coronary angioplasty in unstable versus stable angina pectoris: a report of the 1985-1986 NHLBI PTCA Registry. Cathet Cardiovasc Diagn 1991;23:227.

140. Rupprecht HJ, Brennecke R, Kottmeyer M, Bernhard G, Erbel R, Pop T, Meyer R. Short and long-term outcome after PTCA in patients with stable and unstable angina. Eur Heart j 1990;11:964.

141. Morrison DA. Coronary angioplasty for medically refractory unstable angina within 30 days of acute myocardial infarction. Am Heart J 1990;120:256.

142. Ambrose J, Almeida O, Sharma S, et al. Adjunctive

thrombolytic therapy during angioplasty for ischemic rest angina. Results of the TAUSA trial. Circulation 1994;90:69-77.

143. Lincoff A, Califf R, Anderson K, et al. Striking clinical benefit with platelet GPIIb/IIIa inhibition by C7E3 among patients with unstable angina: Outcome of the EPIC trial. Circulation 1994;90:I-21.

144. Williams D, Sharaf B, Braunwald E, et al. Percutaneous transluminal coronary angioplasty (PTCA) for acute myocardial ischemia: the TIMI-3 experience. Circulation 1994;90:I-433.

145. Bittl J, Strong J, Brinker J, et al. Treatment with Bivalirudin (Hirulog) as compared with heparin during coronary angioplasty for unstable or post infarction angina. N Engl J Med 1995;333:764-9.

146. Serruys P, Herrman J, Simon R, et al. A comparison of Hirudin with heparin in the prevention of restenosis after coronary angioplasty. N Engl J Med 1995;333:757-63.

147. Bengtson J, Wilson J, Interventions in unstable angina. In: Interventional Cardiovascular Medicine-Principals and Practice. Eds. Roubin, Califf, O'Neill, Phillips, Stack. Churchill Livingstone,Inc. New York, New York, 1996

148. huang Y, Popma J, Satler LF, et al. Increasing angina predicts an unfavorable outcome after new device angioplasty. J Am Coll Cardiol 1994:289A.

149. Hong M, Popma J, Wong S, et al. Incidence of and factors associated with abrupt closure in patients undergoing elective, new device angioplasty in native coronary arteries. J Am Coll Cardiol 1995;122A.

150. Marzocci, A, Piovaccari G, et al. Results of coronary stenting for unstable angina pectoris. Am J Cardiol 1997;79:1314-1318.

151. Singh M, Holnmes D, et al. Changing outcome of percutaneous intervention in patients with unstable angina. Circulation 1999;33:31A.

152. White H. Targeting therapy in unstable angina. J Invas Cardiol 1998;10:12D-21D.

153. Kuntz K, Fleishmann K, et al. Cost effectiveness of diagnostic strategies for patients with chest pain. An Intern Med 1999;130:709-718.

154. Luchi R, Scott S, et al. Comparison of medical and surgical treatment of unstable angina pectoris: Results from the veterans administration cooperative study. N Eng J Med 1987;316:977-984.

155. Antoniucci D, Santoro G, et al. Early coronary angioplasty as compared with delayed coronary angioplasty in patients with high-risk unstable angina pectoris. Coron Artery Dis 1996;7:75-80.

156. Moreyra A, Palmeri s, et al. Coronary angioplasty in unstable angina: Contemporary experience. Can J Cardiol 1995;11:385-390.

157. Schartz G, Oliver M, et al. Rationale and design of the myocardial ischemia reduction with aggressive cholesterol lowering study that evaluates atorvastatin in unstable angina pectoris and in non Q-Wave myocardial infarction. Am J Cardiol 1995;81:578-581.

158. TIMI-3B Investigators. Effects of tissue plasminogen activator and a comparison of early invasive and conservative strategies in unstable angina and non Q-wave myocardial infarction.. Circulation 1994;89:1545-1556.

159. Anderson H, Cannon C, Stone P, et al. One year results of the thrombolysis in myocardial infarction (TIMI) 3B clinical trial J Am Coll Cardiol 1995;26:1643-1650.

160. Boden W, O'Rourke R, et al. Outcomes in patients with acute non-Q-Wave myocardial infarction randomly assigned to an invasive as compared with a conservative management strategy. N Engl J Med 1998;338:1785-92.

161. CABRI Trial Participants. First-year results of CABRI (Coronary Angioplasty vs. Bypass Revascularization Investigation). Lancet 1995;346:1179-84.

162. RITA Trial Participants. Coronary angioplasty versus coronary artery bypass surgery: The Randomized Intervention Treatment of Angina (RITA) trial. Lancet 1993;343:573-80.

163. King SB, Lembo NJ, Kosinski AS, et al. A randomized trial comparing coronary angioplasty with coronary bypass surgery. N Engl J Med 1994;331:1044-50.

164. Hamm CW, Riemers J, Ischinger T, et al. A randomized study of coronary angioplasty compared with bypass surgery in patients with symptomatic multi-vessel coronary disease. N Engl J Med 1994;331:1037-1043.

165. Rodriguez A, Boullon F, Prez-Balino N, et al. Argentine randomized trial of percutaneous transluminal coronary angioplasty versus coronary artery bypass surgery in multi-vessel disease (ERACI): in-hospital results and 1-year follow-up. J Am Coll Cardiol 1993;22:1060-67.

166. Bypass Angioplasty Revascularization Investigation (BARI). N Engl J Med 1996, in press.

167. Ohman GM, George B, White C, et al. Use of aortic counterpulsation to improve sustained coronary patency during acute MI. Results of a randomized trial. Circulation 1994;90:792-799.

168. Ishihara M, Sato H, Tateishi H, et al. Intraaortic balloon pumping as the post-angioplasty strategy in acute myocardial infarction. Am Heart J 1991;122:385-389.

169. Grines CL, Brodie BR, Griffin JJ, Donohue BC, Costantini C, Balestrini C, Stone G, Jones DE, Sachs D, O'Neill WW. Prophylactic intraaortic balloon pumping for acute myocardial infarction does not improve left ventricular function. J Am Coll Cardiol 1996;27:167A.

170. Stone G, Marsalese D, et al. A prospective randomized evaluation of prophylactic intraaortic balloon counterpulsation in high-risk patients with acute myocardial infarction treated with primary angioplasty. J Am Coll Cardiol 1997;29:1459-67.

171. Malosky S, Hirschfeld J, Herman H. Comparison of results of intracoronary stenting in patients with unstable vs. stable angina. Cath and CV Diagn 1994;31:95-101.

172. Levy G, deBoisgelin, Volpiliere R, Bouvagnet P. Intracoronary stenting in direct infarct angioplasty: Is it dangerous? Circulation 1995;92:I-139.

173. Neumann F, Walter H, Schmitt C, Alt E, Schomig. Coronary stenting as an adjunct to direct balloon angioplasty in acute myocardial infarction. Circulation 1995;92:I-609.

174. Monassier JP, Elias J, Meyer P, et al. STENTIMI I: The French Registry of stenting at acute myocardial infarction. J Am Coll Cardiol 1996;27:68A.

175. Verna E, Castiglioni B, Onofri M, et al. Intracoronary stenting of the infarct-related artery without anticoagulation

in acute myocardial infarction. Euro Heart j 1995;16:12.

176. Benzuly KH, Goldstein JA, Almany SL, et al. Feasibility of stenting in acute myocardial infarction. Circulation 1995;92:I-616.

177. Romero M, Medina A, Suarez J, et al. Elective Palmaz-Schatz stent implantation in acute coronary syndromes induced by thrombus-containing lesions. Euro Heart J 1995;16:179.

178. Verna E, Castiglioni B, Onofri M, et al. Intracoronary stenting of the infarct-related artery without anticoagulation in acute myocardial infarction. Euro Heart J 1995;16:12.

179. Levy G, deBoisgelin, Volpiliere R, Bouvagnet P. Intracoronary stenting in direction infarct angioplasy: Is it dangerous? Circulation 1995;92:I-139.

180. Romero M, Medina A, Suarex J, et al. Elective Palmaz-Schatz stent implantation in acute coronary syndromes induced by thrombus-containing lesions. Euro Heart J 1995;16:179.

181. Repetto S, Onofri M, Castiglioni B, et al. Stenting of the infarct related artery during complicated angioplasty in acute myocardial infarction. J Invas Cardiol 1996;8:177-183.

182. Rodriquez A, Fernandez M, Santaera O, et al. Coronary stenting in patients undergoing PTCA during acute myocardial infarction. Am J Cardiol 1996;77:685-689.

183. Steinhubl S, Moliterno O, Teirstein P, et al. Stenting for acute myocardial infarction: the early United States multicenter experience. J Am Coll Cardiol 1996;22:279A.

184. Benzuly K, Allen D, Mason D, et al. A prospective pilot study of primary stenting for acute myocardial infarction (STAMI). J Invas Cardiol 1996;8:38.

185. Stone G, Marice M, Brodie B, et al. Primary stenting in acute MI: Interim report from the PAMI-3 stent pilot study. European Congress of Cardiology. August, 1996

186. Lefkovits J, Anderson K, Weisman H, Topol E. Increased risk of non-Q-MI following DCA: Evidence for a platelet dependant mechanism from the EPIC Trial. Circulation 1994;90:I-214.

187. Stone G, Brodie B, et al. Prospective multi-center study of the safety and feasibility of primary stenting in acute myocardial infarction: In-hospital and 30 day results of the PAMI stent pilot trial. J Am Coll Cardiol 1998;31:23-30.

188. Grines C, Cox D, et al. A randomized trial of primary angioplasty compared to heparin-coasted stent implantation for acute myocardial infarction. NFJM 1999 (in press).

189. Ghazzal ZMB, Hinohara T, Scott NA, et al. Directional coronary atherectomy in patients with recent myocardial infarction: a NACI Registry report. J Am Coll Cardiol 1993;21:32A.

190. Robertson G, Hinohara T, Vetters J, et al. Directional coronary atherectomy for patients with recent myocardial infarction. J Am Coll Cardiol 1994;219A.

191. Abdelmeguid A, Sapp S, Lynch D, et al. Immediate and follow-up results of directional coronary atherectomy for the treatment of unstable angina. Circulation 1993;88:I-496.

192. Topol EJ, Leya F, Pinkerton CA, et al. A comparison of directional atherectomy with coronary angioplasty in patients with coronary artery disease. N Engl J Med 1993;329:221-7.

193. Smucker ML, Sarnat WS, Kil D, Scherb DE, Howard PF. Salvage from cardiogenic shock by atherectomy after failed emergency coronary artery angioplasty. Cath Cardiovasc Diagn 1990;21:23-5.

194. Lasorda DM, Incorvati DL, Randal RR. Extraction atherectomy during myocardial infarction in a patient with prior coronary artery bypass surgery. Cath Cardiovasc Diag 1992;26:117-121.

195. Larkin TJ, Niemyski PR, Parker MA, Kramer BL. Primary and rescue extraction atherectomy in patients with acute myocardial infarction. Circulation 1991;84:II-537.

196. Larkin TJ, O'Neill WW, Safian RD, Schreiber TL, May MA, Kazziha S, Niemyski PR, Parker MA, Kramer BL, Grines CL. A prospective study of transluminal extraction atherectomy in high-risk patients with acute myocardial infarction. J Am Coll Cardiol 1994;226A.

197. Kaplan BM, O'Neill WW, Safian RD, Schreiber TL, Larkin TJ, Dooris M, May M, Grines CL. Clinical and angiographic follow-up to a prospective study of transluminal extraction atherectomy in high-risk patients with acute myocardial infarction. J Am Coll Cardiol 1995;331A

198. Dooris M, Hoffman M, Flazier S, et al. Comparative results of transluminal extraction coronary atherectomy in saphenous vein graft lesions with and without thrombus. J Am Coll Cardiol 1995;25:1700-1705.

199. Topaz O. Holmium laser coronary thrombolysis-a new treatment modality for revascularization in acute myocardial infarction: Review . J Clin Laser Med & Surg 1992;10:427-31.

200. De Marchena E, Mallon S, Posada JD, et al. Direct holmium laser-assisted balloon angioplasty in acute myocardial infarction. Am J Cardiol 1993;71:1223-5.

201. Topaz O, Rozenbaum EA, Battista S, Peterson C, Wysham DG. Laser facilitated angioplasty and thrombolysis in acute myocardial infarction complicated by prolonged or recurrent chest pain. Cath Cardiovasc Diag 1993;28:7-16.

202. Topaz O, Minisi A, Luxenberg M, et al. Laser angioplasty for lesions unsuitable for PTCA in acute myocardial infarction: Quantitative coronary angiography and clinical results. Circulation 1994;90:I-434.

203. Spears JR, Jundu SK, McMath LP. Laser balloon angioplasty: Potential for the reduction of the thrombogenicity of the injured arterial wall and for local application of bioprotective materials. J Am Coll Cardiol 1991;17:179B-188B.

204. Spear JR, Dsgisn TF, Douglas JS, et al. Multi-center acute and chronic results of laser balloon angioplasty for refractory abrupt closure after PTCA. Circulation 1991;84:II-517.

205. Reis GJ, Pomerantz RM, Jenkins RD, et al. Laser balloon angioplasty: clinical , angiographic and histologic results. J Am Coll Cardiol 1991;18:193-202.

206. Schwartz L, Andrus S, Sinclair IN, et al. Restenosis following laser balloon angioplasty - a randomized pilot multi-center trial. Circulation 1991;84:II-361.

207. Makowski S, O'Neill B, Sarkis A, et al. Physiological low stress angioplasty at 60°C. Initial results and 6 month follow-up. J Am Coll Cardiol 1993;21:440A.

208. Saito S, Arai H, Kin K, et al. Initial experience of unipolar radio-frequency hot balloon angioplasty for bail-out from abrupt coronary closure after conventional balloon angioplasty. J Am Coll Cardiol 1993;21:338A.

209. Moura A, Lam JYT, Hebert D, Letchacovski G, Robitaille D, Grant G, Kaplan A. Local heparin delivery decrease the thrombogenicity of the balloon-injured artery. Circulation 1994;90:I-449.

210. Thomas CN, Barry JJ, King SB, Scott NA. Local delivery with heparin with a PTCA infusion balloon inhibits platelet-dependent thrombosis. J Am Coll Cardiol 1994;23:4A.

211. Azrin MA, Mitchel JF, Fram DB, Pedersen CA, Cartun RW, Barry JJ, Bow LM, Waters D, McKay RG. Decreased platelet deposition and smooth muscle cell proliferation following intramural heparin delivery with hydrogel-coated balloons. Circulation 1994;90:433-441.

212. Fram DB, Mitchel JF, Azrin MA, Schwedick, MW, Waters DD, McKay RG. Local heparin delivery in porcine coronary arteries with the Dispatch catheter delivery, washout and effect on platelet deposition following balloon angioplasty. Circulation 1994;90:I-493.

213. Mitchel JF, Azrin MA, Schwedwick MW, Bow LM, Waters DD, McKay RG. Local delivery of heparin with a novel iontophoretic catheter – quantitative heparin delivery and effect on platelet deposition following balloon angioplasty. Circulation 1994;90:I-492.

214. Lopez-Sendon J, Sobrino N, Gamallo C, Lorenzo A, Jimenez J, Calvo L, Sobrino JA, Rico J, de Miguel E. Locally delivered heparin reduces intimal hyperplasian and lumen stenosis following arterial balloon injury in swine. Euro Heart J 1993;14:191.

215. Camenzind E, van der Giesen W, Ligthart J, Ruygrok P, de Jaegere P, de Feyter P, Serruys PW. Local, low-pressure heparin delivery following angioplasty in man: the solution to restenosis? J Am Coll Cardiol 1995:376A

216. Stag G. CORAMI II. Cohort of rescue angioplasty in myocardial infarction II. Circulation 1997 96:1-532.

217. Coller BS. Platelets and thrombolytic therapy. N Engl J Med 1990;322:33-42.

218. Lacoste L, Lam JYT. Enhanced platelet thrombus formation in unstable angina. Circulation 1994;90:1374.

219. Lacoste L, Lam JYT, Letchacovski G. Comparative antithrombotic efficacy of aspirin: 80mg vs. 325mg daily. Circulation 1994;90:I-552.

220. Dabaghi SF, Damat S, Hendricks O, Payne J, Kleiman NS. Low dose aspirin inhibits in vitro platelet aggregation within minutes after ingestion. Circulation 1992;86:I-261.

221. Khurana S, Westley S, Mattson J, Safian R. Is it possible to expedite the antiplatelet effect of ticlopidine? Presented at the TCT, February 1996.

222. Leon M, Baim D, et al. A clinical trial comparing three antithrombotic drug regimens after coronary artery stenting. N Engl J Med 1998;339:1665-71.

223. Jeong M, Owen W, Staabon, et al. Does ticlopidine effect platelet deposition and acute stent thrombosis? Circulation 1995;92:I-489.

224. Gregorini L, Marco J, Fajadet J, et al. Ticlopidine alternates post angioplasty thrombin generation. Circulation 1995;92:I-608.

225. Committee, C.S. A randomized, blinded, trial of clopidofrel versus aspirin in patients at risk of ischemic events (CAPRIE). Lancet 1996;348:1329-39.

226. Berger P, Bellot V, et al. Clopidogrel versus Ticlopidine for

coronary stents. Circulation 1999;33:34A.

227. Investigators, T.C. Randomized placebo-controlled trial of aboiximab before and during coronary intervention in refractory unstable angina. Lancet 1997;349:1429-35

228. Investigarors, P.P. Inhibition of the platelet glycoprotien IIb/IIIa receptor with tirofiban in unstable angina and non-Q-wave myocardial infarction. N Engl J Med 1998;338:1488-97.

229. Investigators, P.T. Inhibition of platelet glycoprotein IIb/IIIa with eptifibatide in patients with acute coronary syndromes. N Engl J Med 1998 339:436-43.

230. Investigators, T.E. Use of a monoclonal antibody directed against the platelet glycoprotein IIb/IIIa receptor in high-risk coronary angioplasty. N Engl J Med 1994;330:956-961.

231. Lincoff A, Callif, R, et al. Evidence for prevention of death and myocardial infarction with platelet membrane glycoprotein IIb/IIIa receptor blockade by aboiximab (c7E3 Fab) among patients with unstable angina undergoing percutaneous coronary revascularization. J Am Coll Cardiol 1997;30:149-56.

232. Topol E, Ferguson J, et al. Long-term protection from myocardial ischemic stents in a randomized trial of brief integrin blockade with percutaneous coronary intervention. J Am Med Assoc 1997;278:479-484.

233. Investigators, T. E. Randomized placebo controlled and balloon angioplasty controlled trial to assess safety of coronary stenting with use of platelet glycoprotein IIb/IIIa blockade. Lancet 1998;352:87-92.

234. Kereiakes D, Lincoff A, et al GpIIb/IIIa blockade during coronary intervention for unstable angina: longer is not better. Am J Cardiol 1998;7:Suppl:95S.

235. Lefkovitss J, Ivanhoe R, et al. Effects of platelet glycoprotein IIb/IIIa receptor blockade by a chimeric monoclonal antibody (aboiximab) on acute and six month outcomes after percutaneous transluminal coronary angioplasty for acute myocardial infarction. Am J Cardiol 1996;77:1045-1051.

236. Brener S, Barr L, et al. Randomized placebo-controlled trial of platelet glycoprotein IIb/IIIa blockade with primary angioplasty for acute myocardial infarction. Circulation 1998;98:734-741.

237. Wharton TP, Marsalese D, Brodie BR, Griffin JJ, Donohue BC, Costantini CRF, Balestrini CE, Stone GW, Esente P, Moses J, McNamara NS, Jones D, Sachs D, Grines CL. How often do infarct-related arteries show early perfusion without prior thrombolytic therapy, and should these vessels be dilated acutely? Results from PAMI-2. Circulation 1995;92:I-530.

238. Verheugt R, Liem A, et al. High does bolus heparin as initial therapy before primary angioplasty for acute myocardial infarction: Results of the heparin in early patency (HEAP) pilot study. J Am Coll Cardiol 1998;31:289-93.

239. Ambrose J, Almeida D, Ratner D, et al. Heparin administered prior to angioplasty does not decrease angioplasty complications. TAUSA trial results. Circulation 1994;90:I-374.

240. Ferguson J, Dougherty K, Gaos C, et al. Relation between procedural activated coagulation time and outcome after percutaneous transluminal coronary angioplasty. J Am Coll Cardiol 1994;23:1061-1065.

241. Naqvi T, Ivy P, Linn P, et al. Low dose heparin enhances and high dose heparin suppresses platelet P-selection expression and platelet aggregation. Circulation 1995;92:I-673.

242. Ahmed W, Meckel C, Grines C, et al. Relation between ischemic complications and activated clotting times during coronary angioplasty: Different profiles for heparin and Hirulog. Circulation 1995;92:I-608.

243. Nairns CR, Hillegass WG, Nelson CL, et al. Activated clotting time predicts abrupt closure risk during angioplasty. J Am Coll Cardiol 1994;23:470A.

244. Hillegass W, Narins C, Brott B, et al. Activated clotting time predicts bleeding complications from angioplasty. J Am Coll Cardiol 1994;184A.

245. Investigators T. E. Platelet glycoprotein IIb/IIIa receptor blockade and low dose heparin during percutaneous coronary revascularization. N Engl J Med 1997;336:1689-1696.

246. Granger C, Armstong P. For the GUSTO IIa investigators. Reinfarction following discontinuation of intravenous heparin or hirudin for unstable angina and acute myocardial infarction. Circulation 1995;92:I-460.

247. Rabah M, Mason D, Muller DWM, Hundley R, Kugelmass AD, Weiner B, Cannon L, O'Neill WW, Safian RD. Heparin after percutaneous intervention (HAPI): A prospective multicenter randomized trial of three heparin regimens after successful coronary intervention. J am Coll Cardiol 1999;34:461-467.

248. Granger C, Miller J, Bovill E, et al. Rebound increase in thrombin generation and activity after cessation of intravenous heparin in patients with acute coronary syndromes. Circulation 1995;921:1929-35.

249. Flather M, Weitz J, Campeau J, et al. Evidence for rebound activation of the coagulation system after cessation of intravenous anticoagulant therapy for acute MI. Circulation 1995;92:I-485.

250. Strony J, Ahmed W, Meckel C, et al. Clinical evidence for thrombin rebound after stopping heparin but not hirulog. Circulation 1995;92:I-609.

251. Khan M, Sepulveda J, Jeroudi M, et al. Rebound increase in thrombin activity with associated decrease in antithrombin III levels after PTCA. Circulation 1995;92:I-785.

252. Blumenthatl R, Wolff M, Resar J, et al. Preprocedural anticoagulation does not reduce angioplasty heparin requirements. Am Heart J 1993;125:1221.

253. Zidar J. New Insights in the prevention of thrombosis in coronary stents. The ENTCES Trial Ann Hematology 1997;Suppl II:A152.

254. Serruys P, Herrmann J, et al. A comparison of Hirudin with heparin in the prevention of restenosis after coronary angioplasty. HELVETICA Investigators. N Engl J Med 1995;333:757-63.

255. Topol E. Towards a new frontier in myocardial reperfusion therapy: emerging platelet preeminence. Circulation 1988;97:211-218.

256. Spielberg C, Schnitzer L, Linderer T, et al. Influence of catheter technology and adjuvant medication on acute complications in percutaneous coronary angioplasty. Cathet Cardiovasc Diagn 1990;21:72.

257. Ambrose JA, Torre SR, Sharma SK, et al. Adjuvant urokinase for PTCA in unstable angina: final angiographic results of TAUSA pilot study. Circulation 1991;84:II-590.

258. Buller CE, Fung AY, Thompson CR, Ricci DR, Thompson B, Schractman M, Williams DO. Does pre-treatment with tPA improve safety of coronary angioplasty in acute coronary syndrome? Results from TIMI II-B. Circulation 1994;90:I-22.

259. Ambrose JA, Almeida OD, Sharma SK, Torre SR, Marmur JD, Israel DH, Ratner DE, Weiss MB, Hjemdahl-Monsen CE, Myler TK, Moses J, Unterecker WJ, Grunwald AM, Garrett JS, Cowley MJ, Anwar A, Sobolski J for the TAUSA Investigators. Adjunctive thrombolytic therapy during angioplasty for ischemic rest angina. Results of the TAUSA Trial. Circulation 1994;90:69-77.

260. Mehran R, Ambrose JA, Bongu RM, Almeida OD, Israel DH, Torre S, Sharma SK, Ratner ED for the TAUSA study group. Angioplasty of complex lesions in ischemic rest angina: Results of the Thrombolysis and Angioplasty in UnStable Angina (TAUSA) trial. J Am Coll Cardiol 1995;26:961-966.

261. Kerins DM, Roy L, FitzGerald GA, Pitzgerald DJ. Platelet and vascular function during coronary thrombolysis with tissue-type plasminogen activator. Circulation 1989;80:1718.

262. Bennett WR, Yawn DH, Migliore PJ, et al. Activation of the complement system by recombinant tissue plasminogen activator. J Am Coll cardiol 1987;10:1718.

263. Fitzgerald DJ, Roy L, Wright F, Fitzgerald GA. Functional significance of platelet activation following coronary thrombolyisis. Circulation 1987;76:IV-153.

264. Castaneda-Zuniga WR, Sibley R, Amplatz K. The pathologic basis of angioplasty. Angiology 1984;35:195.

265. Kohchi K, Taebayashi S, Block PC. Arterial changes after percutaneous transluminal coronary angioplasty: results at autopsy. J Am Coll Cardiol 1987;10:592.

266. Waller BF, Rothbaum DA, Pinkeron CA, et al. Status of the myocardium and infarct-related coronary artery in 19 necropsy patients with acute recanalization using pharmacologic (streptokinase, r-tissue plasminogen activator), mechanical (percutaneous transluminal coronary angioplasty) or combined types of reperfusion therapy. J Am Coll Cardiol 1987;9:785.

267. Colavita PG, Ideker RE, Reimer KA, et al. The spectrum of pathology associated with percutaneous transluminal coronary angioplasty during acute myocardial infarction. J Am Coll Cardiol 1986;8:855.

268. Merkhof van den L, Aijlstra F, et al. Aboiximab in the treatment of acute myocardial infarction eligible for primary percutaneous transluminal coronary angioplasty. Results of the Glycoprotein Receptor Antagonist Patency Evaluation (GRAPE) Pilot Study. J Am Coll Cardiol 1999;33:1528-32.

269. Verheught F, Ohman E, et al. Emergency room infusion of aboiximab speeds up reperfusion in acute myocardial infarction eligible for primary PTCA. J Am Coll Cardiol 1999;33:354A.

270. Kleiman N, Ohman E, et al. Profound inhibition of platelet aggregation with monoclonal antibody 7E3Fab after thrombolytic therapy: Results from the Thrombolysis and Angioplasty in myocardial infarction (TAMI)8 pilot study. J Am Coll Cardiol 1993;22:381-389

271. Ohman E, Kleiman N, et al. Combined accelerated tissue plasminogen activator and platelet glycoprotein IIb/IIIa

integrin receptor blockade with integrin in acute myocardial infarction: Results of a randomized placebo controlled dose ranging trial. Circulation 1997;95:846-854.

272. Investigators, T.P. Combined thrombolysis with the platelet glycoprotein IIb/IIIa inhibitor lamifiban: Results of the platelet aggregation receptor antagonist dose investigation and reperfusion gain in myocardial infarction (PARADIGM) trial. J Am Coll Cardiol 1998;32:2003-2010.

273. Antman E. Results of the TIMI 14 A Trial. J Am Coll Cardiol 1998:abstract.

274. Ohman E. Results of the SPEED (Strategy for patency enhancement in the emergency department) study. J Am Coll Cardiol 1998:abstract.

275. Topol E. Evolution of improved antithrombotic and antiplatelet agents genesis of the Comparison of Aboiximab complications with Horologe Events Trial (CACHET). Am J Cardiol 1998;82(8B):63P-68P.

276. Grines C, Schreiber T, Savas V, et al. A randomized trial of low osmolar ionic versus non-ionic contrast media in patients with acute myocardial infarction or unstable angina undergoing PTCA. J Am Coll Cardiol 1996;27:1381-6.

277. Piessens JH, Stammen F, Brolix MC, et al. Effects of ionic versus a non-ionic low osmolar contrast agent on the thrombotic complications of coronary angioplasty. Catheterization and Cardiovascular Diagnosis. 1993;28:99-105.

278. Aguirre F, Topol EJ, Donohue T. Impact of ionic and non ionic contrast media on post PTCA ischemic complications: Results from the EPIC trial. J Am Coll Cardiol 1995;25:8A.

279. FRISC Study Group. Low-molecular-weight heparin during instability in coronary artery disease: Fragmin during Instability in coronary Artery Disease (FRISC) Study Group. Lancet. 1996;347:561-568.

280. Schreiber T, Kaplan B, Gregory M, et al. Transluminal extraction atherectomy vs. balloon angioplasty in acute ischemic syndromes (TOPIT): hospital outcome and six-month status. J Am Coll Cardiol 1999;34:461-467.

281. Stone GW, de Marchena E, Dageforde D, et al. A prospective, randomized multicenter comparison of laser facilitated balloon angioplasty versus stand alone balloon angioplasty in patients with obstructive coronary artery disease. J Am Coll Cardiol 1997;30:1714-1721.

282. Topaz O, McIvor M, Stone GW, et al. Acute results, complications and effect of lesion characteristics on outcome with the solid-state, mid-infrared laser angioplasty system: final multicenter registry report. Lasers in surgery and Medicine 1998;22:228-239.

283. Kaplan AV, Vandormael M, Hofmann M, et al. Heparin delivery at the site of angioplasty with a novel drug delivery sleeve. Am J Cardiol 1996;77:307-310.

284. Esente P, Kaplan AV, Ford JK, et al. Local intramural heparin delivery during primary angioplasty for acute myocardial infarction: results of the Local PAMI pilot study. Catheter Cardiovasc Interv 1999;47:237-42.

285. Theroux P, Ouimet H, McCans J, et al. Aspirin, heparin or both to treat acute unstable angina. N Engl J Med 1988;319:1105-1111.

286. Hamm C et al. N Engl J Med 1999.

287. The EPILOG Investigators. Platelet glycoprotein IIb/IIIa receptor blockade and low-dose heparin during percutaneous coronary revascularization. N Engl J Med 1997;336:1689-1696.

288. Neumann FJ, Blasini R, Schmitt C, et al. Effect of glycoprotein IIb/IIIA receptor blockade on recovery of coronary flow and left ventricular function in and after the placement of coronary-artery stents in acute myocardial infarction. Circulation 1998;98:2695-2701.

289. Stone GW. Stenting and Glycoprotien IIb/IIIA Receptor Blockade in Acute Myocardial Infarction: An Introduction to the CADILLAC Trial. J Inv Cardiol 1998;10:36B-47B.

290. Wallentin L. Presented at the 48th annual scientific sessions of the American College of Cardiology, March 1999.

291. Weaver WD, Simes RJ, Ellis SG, et al. Comparison of primary coronary angioplasty and intravenous thrombolytic therapy for acute myocardial infarction. A quantitative review JAMA 1997;278:2093-2098.

292. Stone GW, Brodie BR, Griffin JJ, et al. Clinical and Angiographic follow-up after primary stenting in acute myocardial infarction: The PAMI Stent Pilot Trial. Circulation 1999;99:1548-1554.

293. Ellis S, Gusto IIB Angioplasty Substudy. Presented at the ACC Scientific Sessions, March 1996.

294. Erbel R, Pop T, Diefenbach C, Meyer J. Long-term results of thrombolytic therapy with and without percutaneous transluminal coronary angioplasty. J Am Coll Cardiol 1989;14:276-285.

295. DANAMI Study. Results presented at the American Heart Association, 1995 Plenary Session.

296. Kamp O, Beatt KJ, de Feyter PJ, et al. Short-, medium-, and long-term follow-up after percutaneous transluminal coronary angioplasty for stable and unstable angina pectoris. Am Heart j 1989;117:991.

297. Faxon DP, Detre KM, McCabe CH, et al. Role of percutaneous transluminal coronary angioplasty in the treatment of unstable angina. Report from the national Heart, Lung, and Blood Institute Percutaneous Transluminal Coronary Angioplasty and Coronary Artery Surgery Study Registries. Am J Cardiol 1994;53:131C.

298. Saito S, Hosokawa G, Kin K, et al. Primary stent implantation without coumadin in acute myocardial infarction. J Am Coll Cardiol 1996;8:74-81.

299. Suryapranta H, Hoorntje JC, de Boer MJ, et al. Randomized comparison of primary stenting with primary balloon angioplasty in acute myocardial infarction. Circulation 1997;96:I-327.

300. Antoniucci D, Santoro G, et al. A clinical trial comparing primary stenting of the infarct related artery with optimal primary angioplasty for acute myocardial infarction. Results from the FRESCO Trial. J Am Coll Cardiol 1996;31:1234-9.

301. Rodriguez A, Bernardi V, et al. Coronary stents improve outcome in acute myocardial infarction: immediate and long term results of the GRAMI Trial. J Am Coll Cardiol 1998;31:64A.

302. Nishida Y, Nonaka H, et al. In-Hospital outcome of primary stenting for acute myocardial infarction using wiktor coil stent: Results from multicenter randomized (PRISAM) Trial. Circulation 1997;96:1-531.

303. Investigators, T. R. Effects of platelet glycoprotein IIb/IIIa

receptor blockade with tirofiban on adverse cardiac events in patients with unstable angina or acute myocardial infarction undergoing coronary angioplasty. Circulation 1997;96:1453-1455.

304. Investigators, T.P. International randomized controlled trial of lamifiban, heparin or both in unstable angina. Circulation 1998;97:2386-2395.

305. (Montelescot G. The ADMIRAL trial. Presented at the 48th annual scientific sessions of the American College of Cardiology, March 1999.

306. (Angioi M et al. AJC 2000;85:1065-70)

307. [Baim DS, Cutlip DE, Sharma SK, et al. Final results of the balloon vs. optimal atherectomy trial (BOAT). Circulation 1998;97:322-331].

308. Hochman JS, Sleeper LA, White HW, et al. One-year survival following early revascularization for cardiogenic shock. JAMA 2001;282:190-192.

309. Van't Hof AW et al. Lancet 1997;350:615-9

310. Van't Hof AW et al. Circulation 1999

311. Ross AM, Coyne KS, Reiner JS et al A Randomized trial comparing primary angioplasty with a strategy of short acting thrombolysis and immediate planned rescue angioplasty in acute myocardial infarction: the PACT trial. JACC 1999;34:1954-1962

312. Malosky S, Hirshfeld J, Herrmann H. Comparison of results of intracoronary stenting in patients with unstable vs. stable angina. Cathet Cardiovasc Diagn 1994;31:95-101.

313. Robinson NMK, Thomas MR, Wainwright RJ, Jewitt DE. Is unstable angina a contraindication to intracoronary stent insertion? J Invas Cardiol 1996;8:351-356.

314. Marzocchi A, Piovaccari G, Marrozzini C, et al. Results of coronary stenting for unstable versus stable angina pectoris. Am J Cardiol 1997;79:1314-1318.

315. Shimada K, Kawarabyashi T, Ryuushi K, et al. Efficacy and safety of early coronary stenting for unstable angina. Cath Cardiovasc Diagn 1998;43:381-385.

316. Chauhan A, Ricci DR, Buller C, et al. Multiple coronary stenting in unstable angina: Early and late clinical outcomes. Cath Cardiovasc Diagn 1998;43:11-16.

317. Chauhan A, Vu E, Ricci DR, Bullr CE, et al. Multiple coronary stenting in unstable angina: Early and late clinical outcomes. Cathet Cardiovasc Diagn 1998;43:11-16.

318. Singh M, Holmes DR, Garratt KN, et al. Stents versus conventional PTCA in unstable angina. J Am Coll Cardiol 1999;33:29A.

319. Bachelor WB, et al. Am J Cardiol 2000;85:692-97.

320. Danchin et al. Circulation 1999;99:2639-44.

321. Tiefenbrunn et al. J Am Coll Cardiol 1998;31:1260-65.

322. McKendall et al. J Am Coll Cardiol 1997;29:389A

323. The CAPTURE Investigators. Randomised placebo-controlled trial of abciximab before and during coronary intervention in refractory unstable angina: the CAPTURE study. Lancet 1997; 349:2429-35.

324. The IMPACT-II Investigators. Randomized placebo-controlled trial of effect of eptifibatide on complications of percutaneous coronary intervention: IMPACT-II. Lancet 1997; 349:1422-28.

325. Cannon CP. TACTICS/TIMI 18 - Oral presentation. TCT 2000

326. The RESTORE Investigators. Effects of platelet glycoprotein IIb/IIIa blockade with tirofiban on adverse cardiac event in-patients with unstable angina or acute myocardial infarction undergoing coronary angioplasty. Circulation 1997; 96:1445-53.

327. Gibson CM, Goel M, Cohen DJ, et al. Six-month angiographic and clinical follow-up of patients prospectively randomized to receive either tirofiban or placebo during angioplasty in the RESTORE trial. J Am Coll Cardiol 1998; 32:28-34.

328. O'Neill WW, Serruys P, Knudtson M, van Es GA, Timmis GC, van der Zwaan C, Kleiman J, Gong J, Roecker EB, Dreiling R, Alexander J, Anders R. Long-term treatment with a platelet glycoprotein-receptor antagonist after percutaneous coronary revascularization. EXCITE Trial Investigators.

329. Stone GW. CADILLAC - Oral presentation. TCT 2000.

330. Brener SL, Barr LA, Burchenal JE, et al. Randomized, placebo-controlled trial of platelet glycoprotein IIb/IIIa blockade with primary angioplasty for acute myocardial infarction. ReoPro and Primary PTCA Organization and Randomized Trial (RAPPORT) Investigators. Circulation 1998; 98:734-741.

331. Barragan P, Beauregard C. Montalescot G, Wittenberg O, Ecollan P, Elhadad S, Villain P, Boulenc JM, Maillard L, Pinton P. Abciximab associated with primary angioplasty and stenting in acute myocardial infarction: The Admiral Study, 6-month results. Circulation 2000; 102(18):II-663 (Abstract).

332. Neumann FJ, Blasini R, Schmitt C, et al. Effect of glycoprotein IIb/IIIa receptor blockade on recovery of coronary flow and left ventricular function after the placement of coronary-artery stents in acute myocardial infarction. Circulation 1998;98:2695-701.

333. Neumann F-J, Kastrati A, Schmitt C, Blasini R, Hadamitzky M, Mehilli J, Gawaz M, Schleef M, Seyfarth M, Dirschinger J, Schömig A. Effect of glycoprotein IIb/IIIa receptor blockade with abciximab on clinical and angiographic restenosis rate after the placement of coronary stents following acute myocardial infarction. J Am Coll Cardiol 2000; 35:915-21.

334. Lefkovits J, Ivanhoe RJ, Califf RM, Bergelson BA, Anderson KM, Stoner GL, et al for the EPIC Investigators. Effects of platelet glycoprotein IIb/IIIa receptor blockade by a chimeric monoclonal antibody (abciximab) on acute and 6-month outcomes after percutaneous transluminal coronary angioplasty for acute myocardial infarction. Am J Cardiol 1996; 77:1045-51.

335. Theroux P, Kouz S, Roy L, et al. Platelet membrane receptor glycoprotein IIb/IIIa antagonism in unstable angina: The Canadian lamifiban study. Circulation 1996;94:899-905.

336. The RESTORE Investigators. Effects of platelet glycoprotein IIb/IIIa blockade with tirofiban on adverse cardiac event in-patients with unstable angina or acute myocardial infarction undergoing coronary angioplasty. Circulation 1997; 96:1445-53.

337. Gibson CM, Goel M, Cohen DJ, et al. Six-month angiographic and clinical follow-up of patients prospectively randomized to receive either tirofiban or placebo during angioplasty in the RESTORE trial. J Am Coll Cardiol 1998; 32:28-34.

338. Maillard L, Hamon M, Khalife K, et al. A comparison of systematic stenting and conventional balloon angioplasty during primary percutaneous transluminal coronary angioplasty for acute myocardial infarction. J Am Coll Cardiol 2000;35:1729 –36.

339. Schoming A, Kastrati A, Dirschinger J, et al. Coronary stenting plus platelet glycoprotein IIb/IIIa blockade compared with tissue plasminogen activator in acute myocardial infarction. Stent versus thrombolysis occluded coronary arteries in patients with acute myocardial infarction study investigators. N Engl J Med. 2000;43:385-91.

340. Antoniucci D, Santoro G M, Bolognese L, et al. A clinical trial comparing primary stenting of the infarct-related artery with optimal primary angioplasty of acute myocardial infarction. Results from the Florence Randomized Elective Stenting in Acute Coronary Occlusions (FRESCO) trial. J Am Coll Cardiol 1998;31: 1234 – 9.

341. Grines C L, Cox D A, Stone G W, et al. Coronary angioplasty with or without stent implantation for acute myocardial infarction. N Engl J Med 1999;341:1949-56.

342. implantation is superior to balloon angioplasty in acute myocardial infarction: Final results the primary angioplasty versus stent implantation in acute myocardial infarction (PASTA) Trial. Cathet Cardiovasc Intervent. 1999;48: 262-8.

343. Investigators, T.P. International randomized controlled trial of lamifiban, heparin or both in unstable angina. Circulation 1998;97:2386-2395.

344. Rodriquez A, Bernardi V, Fernandez M, et al. Hospital and late results of coronary stents versus conventional balloon angioplasty in acute myocardial infarction (GRAMI Trial). Am J Cardiol 1998;81: 1286-91.

345. Jacksch R, Niehues R, Knobloch W, Schiele T. PTCA vs. stenting in acute myocardial infarction (AMI). Circulation 1998;98 (Suppl I): I-307.

346. Suryapranata H, Van't Hof AW, Hoorntje J, et al. Randomized comparison of coronary stenting with balloon angioplasty in selected patients with acute myocardial infarction. Circulation 1998;97:2502-05.

347. Ahmed W, Meckel C, Grines C, et al. Relation between ischemic complications and activated clotting times during coronary angioplasty: Different profiles for heparin and Hirulog. Circulation 1995;92:I-608.

348. Gibson CM, Goel M, Cohen DJ, et al. Six-month angiographic and clinical follow-up of patients prospectively randomized to receive either tirofiban or placebo during angioplasty in the RESTORE trial. J Am Coll Cardiol 1998; 32:28-34.

349. Ross AM, Coyne KS, Reiner JS, et al. A randomized trial comparing primary angioplasty with a strategy of short acting thrombolysis and immediate planned rescue angioplasty in acute myocardial infarction: the PACT trial. JACC 1999;34:1954-1962.

350. Wallentin L, Lagerqvist B, Konty F, et al. Outcome at 1 year after an invasive compared with a non-invasive strategy in unstable coronary-artery disease: the FRISC II invasive randomised trial. Lancet 2000;356:9

351. Widminsky P, Groch L, Zelizke, M et al. Multicentre randomized trial comparing transport to primary angioplasty vs. immediate thrombolysis vs. combined strategy for patients with acute myocardial infarction presenting to community hospital without a catheterization laboratory. The PRAGUE study. Eur Heart J 2000;21 (10):832:31.

352. Vermeer F, Oude Ophuis AJ, vd-Berg EJ, et al. Prospective randomized comparison between thrombolysis, rescue PTCA, and primary PTCA in patients with extensive myocardial infarction admitted to a hospital without PTCA facilities: a safety and feasibility study. Heart 1999:82 (4):426-31.

353. Belenkie I, Traboulsi M, Hall CA, et al. Rescue angioplasty during myocardial infarction has a beneficial effect on mortality: a tenable hypothesis. Can J Cardiol 1992;8 (4);357-62.

354. Gum PA, Kottke-Marchant K, Poggio ED, et al. Profile and prevalence of aspirin resistance among patients with heart disease: A prospective, comprehensive assessment. Circulation 2000;18:II-418.

INTERVENTIONAL STRATEGIES IN PATIENTS WITH LEFT VENTRICULAR DYSFUNCTION

6

Steven L. Almany, M.D.
Robert D. Safian, M.D.

When angioplasty was originally introduced in the late 1970's, it was estimated that only 5% of patients with coronary artery disease would be acceptable candidates.[1] Absolute contraindications to angioplasty included the presence of multivessel disease and severe left ventricular (LV) dysfunction. Since then, the development of circulatory support systems, advances in catheter technology, and increased operator experience have extended the application of percutaneous techniques. The single most important advance in the application of percutaneous methods to high-risk patients is the coronary stent (Chapter 26).

A. **HISTORICAL RESULTS.** There are limited published data regarding PTCA in patients with LV dysfunction (Table 3.15). In general these patients were older, more symptomatic, and had more previous myocardial infarction, coronary artery bypass grafting, and multivessel disease than patients with normal LV function. Patients with coronary artery disease and LV dysfunction treated medically have 4-year survival rates of 35-60%.[9] The nonrandomized Coronary Artery Surgery Study Registry (CASS) reported a 4-year survival of 72% after CABG compared to 61% after medical therapy in patients with LV ejection fraction < 35%.[10] Patients with LV dysfunction and 1- or 2-vessel disease had better total survival after PTCA or CABG compared to medical therapy, but there was no difference in event-free survival.[11]

B. **DETERMINATION OF NEED FOR SUPPORTED ANGIOPLASTY.** In the past, the hemodynamic significance of target lesions and the viability of the myocardial perfusion bed was assessed by the "jeopardy score," which correlated with the risk of death after acute closure. In this scoring system the coronary tree was divided into 6 segments of equal myocardial perfusion (Figure 6.1).[17] "Closure score" was the sum of all segments likely to become akinetic if the target vessel developed acute closure during PTCA.[18] Although stents have markedly decreased the risk of acute closure, the impact of vessel occlusion after PTCA or stenting may still by accurately estimated by the jeopardy and closure scores. Clinical and angiographic descriptors were previously used to select patients for supported angioplasty (Table 6.1), but in contemporary practice, most of the decision-making about supported angioplasty depends on whether or not stent implantation is feasible (Figures 6.2, 6.3). Mechanical circulatory support systems (Table 6.2) and pharmacologic methods for attenuating myocardial ischemia are rarely needed if elective stent implantation is feasible. However, if stenting is not feasible or is expected to be difficult, hemodynamic support is recommended in patients with severe LV dysfunction.

Table 6.1. Potential Candidates for Supported Angioplasty

Target vessel supplies the majority of viable myocardium*

Ejection fraction < 20-30%*

Jeopardy score > 3*

Cardiogenic shock and multivessel disease

* Supported angioplasty may not be necessary if stenting is readily performed. Patients in cardiogenic shock require hemodynamic support.

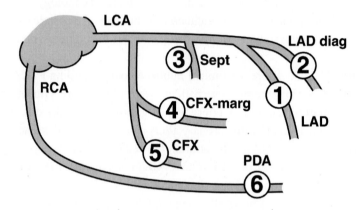

Figure 6.1. Jeopardy Score

Six arterial segments are used to calculate the jeopardy score, which considers the total region of jeopardized myocardium (supplied by the target vessel and providing collaterals to other regions) and the degree of baseline LV dysfunction. Scoring system:
- 1 point for each myocardial region supplied by the target lesion
- 1 point for each myocardial region supplied by a vessel with diameter stenosis $\geq$ 70%
- 0.5 point for each myocardial region that is hypokinetic at baseline and not supplied by a vessel with significant stenosis.

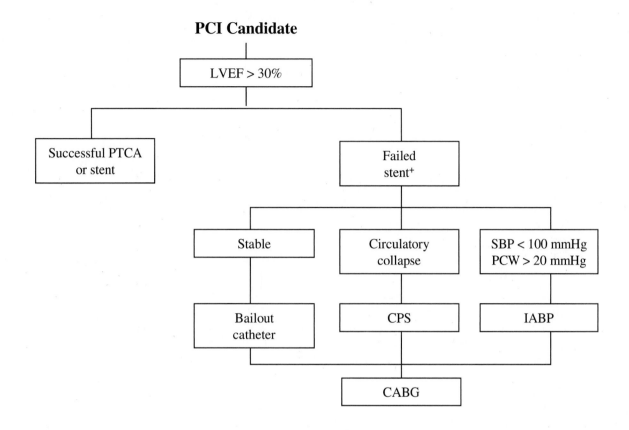

Figure 6.2. Selection of Patients for Supported Angioplasty: LV Ejection Fraction > 30%

Abbreviations: CABG = emergency coronary bypass grafting; CPS = percutaneous cardiopulmonary bypass support; IABP = intra-aortic balloon pump; LVEF = left ventricular ejection fraction; PCI = percutaneous coronary intervention; PCW = pulmonary capillary wedge pressure; SBP = systolic blood pressure;
+ Bailout catheters are recommended if emergency CABG is needed

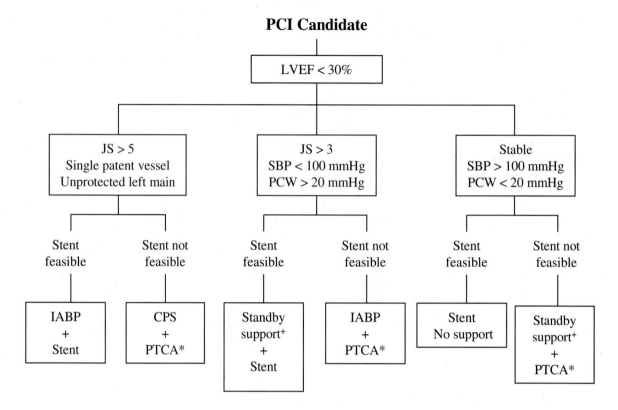

Figure 6.3. Selection of Patients for Supported Angioplasty: LV Ejection Fraction < 30%

Abbreviations: CABG = emergency coronary bypass grafting; CPS = percutaneous cardiopulmonary bypass support; IABP = intra-aortic balloon pump; JS = jeopardy score (see Figure 6.1); LVEF = left ventricular ejection fraction; PCW = pulmonary capillary wedge pressure; SBP = systolic blood pressure

*   Autoperfusion balloons may be useful

\+   Contralateral femoral vascular access; IABP or CPS ready if needed

Table 6.2. Overview of Supported Angioplasty

SYSTEMIC SUPPORT	
Intra-aortic balloon pump (IABP)	**Advantages**: Extensive clinical experience. Provides afterload reduction. May result in improved outcome for selected high-risk PTCA patients and for those unable to be weaned from CPS. **Disadvantages**: Requires stable cardiac rhythm for optimal function. Probable slight increase in vascular complications.
Percutaneous cardiopulmonary bypass support (CPS)	**Advantages**: Provides systemic support independent of ventricular function or cardiac rhythm. **Disadvantages**: Does not prevent myocardial ischemia during balloon inflation (or during acute closure). Not intended for long-term support. Does not unload ventricle.
Ventricular assist devices	**Advantages**: Systemic support independent of ventricular function or cardiac rhythm. Long-term support possible. **Disadvantages**: Surgical placement required. Limited clinical experience.
Left atrial-femoral artery bypass	**Advantages**: Systemic support independent of ventricular function or cardiac rhythm. Able to provide support for longer periods than CPS. **Disadvantages**: Requires transseptal puncture. Limited clinical experience. New systems can achieve flow rates of 4 liters/min.
REGIONAL MYOCARDIAL SUPPORT	
Autoperfusion catheters	**Advantages**: Allows better tolerance of prolonged balloon inflations. Better outcome for patients with abrupt closure. **Disadvantages**: Large profile limits access to distal lesions or tortuous vessels. Requires mean arterial pressure > 65 mmHg for effective passive perfusion. Mostly replaced by stents.
Active hemoperfusion	**Advantages**: Less ischemia during balloon inflations. **Disadvantages**: Limited clinical experience. Potential for hemolysis at high flow rates.
Coronary sinus retroperfusion	**Advantages**: Improves myocardial oxygenation during inflations. Retrograde delivery of drugs possible. Does not require crossing lesion. **Disadvantages**: Requires separate venipuncture (usually internal jugular). Not consistently effective for right coronary and circumflex arteries. Coronary sinus rupture may occur. Placement may be difficult. Not widely available.
Perfluorochemicals	**Advantages**: High oxygen carrying capacity. Low viscosity. Hemolysis absent at high flow rates. **Disadvantages**: Removed from commercial market in 1995. Expensive. Time required for thawing. Increased incidence of pulmonary edema.
Adjunctive pharmacotherapy	**Advantages**: Ease of administration. **Disadvantages**: Least effective of all regional approaches.

SYSTEMIC SUPPORT

A. INTRA-AORTIC BALLOON COUNTERPULSATION

1. **Description.** Intra-aortic balloon counterpulsation (IABP) is the most commonly used method of cardiac support, and consists of an inflatable 40 cc balloon attached to an external control console (32 cc balloons are recommended in patients < 62 inches tall). Once properly positioned (just distal to the origin of the left subclavian artery), the balloon is triggered to inflate with helium immediately after aortic valve closure. This results in an increase in aortic diastolic pressure and coronary blood flow. The balloon is deflated as the aortic valve opens in early systole, markedly decreasing resistance to ventricular ejection (afterload) and improving stroke work.

   a. **Preparation of the IABP.** A one-way valve is connected to the helium port of the IABP. All air is aspirated from the balloon by applying negative pressure to the one-way valve. A 0.025-0.030-inch J-tipped IABP wire is inserted through the central lumen after removing the stylet and flushing the catheter.

   b. **Access Site Evaluation.** In a non-emergent setting, the aorto-iliac system should be assessed by noninvasive assessment or contrast injection for severe tortuosity or high-grade obstruction.

   c. **Arterial Access.** The femoral artery is predilated with an 8F sheath to facilitate insertion of the larger 8.0-10.5F sheath, using a 0.035-inch wire for support.

   d. **Balloon Pump Insertion.** After removing the sheath dilator, the guidewire is advanced beyond the distal end of the IABP, and the IABP is positioned so the marker is at the level of the tracheal carina (this is a good anatomic landmark for the aorta distal to the left subclavian artery). If resistance is met during balloon advancement, the wire is removed and the location of the balloon is checked by a hand injection of contrast through the distal lumen. In patients with small or diseased iliofemoral systems, or those who are hemodynamically stable but require prophylactic IABP, an 8F IABP may be used.

   e. **Balloon Pump Positioning.** The guidewire is advanced into the ascending aortic arch as the balloon is positioned approximately 2 cm distal to the left subclavian artery (at the tracheal carina). Proper position is confirmed by the presence of an adequate arterial wave form, augmentation of diastolic pressure, and afterload reduction. Adequate balloon positioning and full inflation should be confirmed under fluoroscopy. If incomplete filling is detected, refilling of the balloon should be performed by depressing the "autofill" button. If the balloon remains unwrapped, a brief hand injection and aspiration of 30 cc of helium may be attempted.

2. **Advantages**. Intra-aortic balloon counterpulsation decreases myocardial oxygen demand, increases coronary perfusion pressure (by augmenting diastolic blood pressure and decreasing left ventricular filling pressure), and increases cardiac output by 20-39%.[19] It is easily placed in 90% of patients, and prolonged treatment is possible.

3. **Disadvantages.** IABPs were previously associated with a high incidence of vascular complications (9-43%), including AV fistulae, pseudoaneurysms, iliofemoral thrombosis, and local bleeding. In contrast, the PAMI-2 study found no increase in vascular complications in patients randomized to IABP after PTCA for acute MI. Complications are more common in patients with pre-existing vascular disease, diabetics, and females (4 times more common than men); however, complication rates are not affected by age, adequacy of anticoagulation, or body surface area.[20] The 8F IABP may reduce the incidence of vascular and bleeding complications. Unlike percutaneous cardiopulmonary support (CPS), which can maintain circulatory support independent of cardiac rhythm, IABP requires a stable cardiac rhythm for effective diastolic augmentation.[21] Moderate hemolysis and thrombocytopenia are common, although platelet counts < 50,000/mm^3 are quite unusual.

4. **Outcome.** Several small studies suggest that prophylactic placement of an IABP may allow successful revascularization in over 95% of high-risk patients.[22,23] In the setting of abrupt closure, IABPs were associated with hemodynamic stabilization and resolution of ST segment changes.[24] However, stents have nearly eliminated abrupt closure and its hemodynamic consequences, thereby reducing the need for prophylactic or emergent use of IABP. Although some studies suggest that an IABP during primary angioplasty for acute MI results in fewer reocclusions and improved ventricular function,[25-27] the PAMI-2 trial showed no difference in reocclusion, reinfarction, death, or LV function at 1 and 6 months in high-risk patients with or without IABP. Less established roles for IABP include mitigation of myocardial necrosis during acute myocardial infarction,[28] and treatment of intractable ventricular arrhythmias due to ischemia.[29]

5. **Applications.** Prophylactic IABP should be considered in selected high-risk PTCA patients who are not ideal candidate for stents,[22] and those with refractory angina,[30] cardiogenic shock,[31] and failure to wean from CPS (Figures 6.2, 6.3).[32]

B. PERCUTANEOUS CARDIOPULMONARY SUPPORT (CPS)

1. **Description.** Femoral vein-to-femoral artery bypass has been employed by surgeons for over thirty years. Advances in technology and design have led to the development of a portable system, allowing extended application to patients undergoing high-risk percutaneous revascularization procedures.[33] The cardiopulmonary support system collects venous blood from a cannula within the right atrium, pumps it through a semipermeable membrane oxygenator and heat exchanger, and then returns oxygenated blood to the arterial system via a cannula in the femoral artery (Figure 6.4).

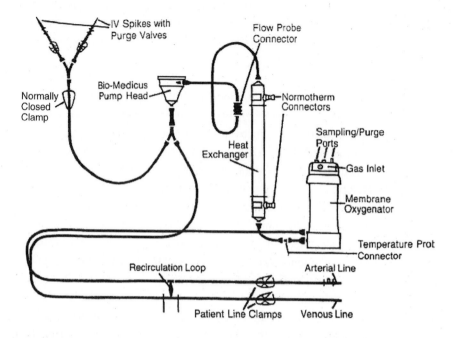

Figure 6.4. CPS Circuitry

2. **Technique of Cardiopulmonary Support**
    a. **Obtain Vascular Access** in the right femoral artery and vein.

    b. **Optimize Volume Status.** Prior to initiating CPS, a pulmonary artery catheter is inserted to optimize filling pressures and cardiac output. Systemic and pulmonary artery pressures are recorded continuously during the procedure.

    c. **Evaluate Suitability of Peripheral Vasculature.** Because of the large caliber of the CPS sheaths, patency, size, and tortuosity of the aorto-iliac system should be assessed by angiography before placement of the cannulas. The arterial cannula must be inserted into the common femoral artery; insertion into the superficial femoral or profunda femoral artery greatly increases the risk of vascular complications.

    d. **Venous Cannula Insertion.** An 0.038-inch Amplatz or other stiff wire is inserted through the venous sheath and positioned under fluoroscopy at the junction between the right atrium and inferior vena cava. The femoral vein is progressively dilated with 8F, 12F and 14F dilators. The CPS venous cannula (18F or 20F depending on body size and desired flow) is inserted under fluoroscopy and positioned in the right atrium. The guidewire and internal dilator are removed as the patient performs the Valsalva maneuver, ensuring that external air is not introduced into the system. The thumb-clamp is applied, and the cannula is immediately sutured to the skin to prevent migration.

e. **Arterial Cannula Insertion.** As with venous cannula placement, 8F, 12F and 14F dilators are inserted into the common femoral artery over a stiff guidewire. The arterial cannula is advanced under fluoroscopy into position between the renal arteries and aortic bifurcation. The guidewire and internal dilator are removed and the thumb-clamp applied. This must be performed quickly to minimize blood loss. The cannula is immediately sutured to the skin.

f. **Anticoagulation.** Intravenous heparin is given as a bolus of 300 U/kg (average 20,000-25,000 units) and supplemented as needed to ensure the ACT remains > 400 seconds during CPS. Prophylactic blood transfusion should be considered in patients undergoing CPS with baseline hemoglobin levels < 10 gm/dL.

g. **Connect Cannulae to the CPS Console.** Hold the polyvinyl chloride (PVC) venous cannula tubing vertically in the left hand and the PVC tubing from the venous port of the CPS console vertically in the right hand, side-by-side. An assistant fills both ends of the tubing with saline and the two ends are quickly connected, minimizing air trapping. The thumb-clamp is released and the perfusionist vents any air trapped in the venous line through the console. The same steps are followed for the arterial cannula; it is absolutely critical that no air is trapped in the arterial line before releasing the thumb-clamp.

h. **Initiate CPS Flow and Perform PTCA.** Monitored continuously by a perfusionist, CPS flow is rapidly increased to an average rate of 3-5 L/min. Maximum flow rates are dependent on volume status and the size of the CPS cannulae (18F = 3-5L/min, 22F = 4-7L/min). Pulmonary capillary wedge pressure should be maintained above 5mmHg and mean arterial pressure between 60-80 mmHg.

i. **After CPS Has Been Discontinued,** thumb-clamps are reapplied to both arterial and venous cannulas, PVC tubing is cut just proximal to the clamps, and plungers from 5-cc syringes are inserted into the cut ends of the PVC tubing connected to the cannulas. The cannulas are sutured in place to prevent migration, and the patient is transferred to the cardiac care unit for observation.

3. **Special Considerations**
   a. **Hypotension.** Hypotension is very common within the first few minutes of CPS and usually responds to a bolus of normal saline (100-300 cc) rather than increasing the flow rate. Hypotension is due to a decrease in systemic vascular resistance from CPS-induced volume shifts or vasodilation. On occasion, decreasing CPS flow may improve systemic vascular resistance and restore blood pressure. When vasopressors are required, neosynephrine (1 mg) can be given directly through the CPS unit. Vibration in the venous line

is frequently caused by volume depletion or excessive flow.

b. **Weaning.** Following conclusion of the case, CPS is gradually weaned by decreasing flow rates. On occasion, placement of an IABP is required for hemodynamic support during the weaning process. The IABP can usually be discontinued 4-12 hours later, depending on hemodynamic performance.

c. **Cannulae Removal.** Arterial and venous cannulas are removed 4-6 hours after the last heparin dose; protamine is not used. Initially, manual pressure is applied for 5-20 minutes, followed by placement of a compression device. Surgical removal is recommended when manual compression is not possible (e.g., poor patient cooperation) or continued anticoagulation is required. Pressure should be sufficient to maintain hemostasis without loss of pedal Doppler signals; pressure is gradually released over several hours once the ACT falls below 150 seconds. Total compression time up to 18 hours is sometimes required. Once hemostasis is achieved, heparin may be restarted and continued until prothrombin times are therapeutic. Warfarin is recommended for 1-6 months following CPS to reduce the risk of iliofemoral venous thrombosis. In some cases, antecedent use of the Perclose arterial closure device prior to insertion of the arterial cannula will permit successful vascular repair without groin compression or surgical intervention.

4. **Advantages.** CPS provides excellent systemic perfusion independent of ventricular function or intrinsic cardiac rhythm. Although patient perception of chest pain was less common in CPS-supported patients treated with prolonged balloon inflations,[34] stents have virtually eliminated the need for inflations > 1 minute.

5. **Disadvantages.** The most significant deficiency of CPS-supported angioplasty is that although systemic support is maintained, myocardial ischemia (regional wall motion abnormalities and anaerobic metabolism) still occurs during balloon inflations.[35] In addition, CPS cannot be continued beyond 6 hours due to the increased risk of disseminated intravascular coagulation, hemolysis, third-spacing of fluids, hypokalemia, and hypomagnesemia. Other disadvantages include vascular injury, large heparin requirements, the need for a perfusionist, and the need for surgical removal of lines or prolonged compression. Other effects of CPS include an immediate fall in hemoglobin $\geq$ 3 gm/dL (due to the dilutional effect of pump priming), suppression of respiratory drive, inadequate CNS perfusion, and varying degrees of aortic insufficiency. Peripheral vascular complications include bleeding, pseudoaneurysm, AV fistula, and arterial occlusion. Transfusion rates in the 1989 CPS registry varied from 31% after percutaneous CPS to 69% after cut-down techniques.[36] Because of these problems and others, CPS-supported angioplasty has essentially been replaced by stenting, with or without adjunctive IABP (Figures 6.2, 6.3).

Table 6.3. High-Risk PTCA: Indications for CPS

Probably Indicated
 Cath lab circulatory collapse

Possible Indications (in poor stent candidates)
 Poor LV function (EF < 20%)
 Large area of myocardium at risk
 PTCA of unprotected left main

Contraindications
 Peripheral vascular disease
 Moderate or severe aortic insufficiency

6. **Outcome**. The National Registry of Supported Angioplasty has collected data on patients undergoing elective supported angioplasty. Patients with poor LV function (EF < 20%), single patient coronary vessel, and inoperable disease underwent CPS-supported angioplasty with an in-hospital mortality rate of 6%; more than 90% of these patients improved by at least one anginal class.[37] Thus, CPS-supported angioplasty can be performed with a high degree of success and low mortality in selected patients. Patients who experienced cardiac arrest or cardiogenic shock and were immediately placed on CPS (within 15 minutes) and then revascularized (PTCA or CABG) had a survival rate of 48%; CPS in these cases was superior to other hemodynamic support systems.[38]

7. **Indications (Table 6.3).** Because of the many drawbacks associated with prophylactic CPS, standby CPS has emerged as an accepted support strategy when stent implantation is not possible (Figure 6.2). When this approach is employed, 5-6F sheaths are usually placed in the left femoral artery and vein after angiographic views demonstrate their suitability for CPS cannulae placement. Experienced operators can usually prime the support system and insert cannulas in less than 5 minutes.[39] Registry data indicate that only 5-10% of patients with standby CPS will actually require initiation of circulatory support. Mortality rates in patients who underwent standby CPS (6%) were similar to those in whom prophylactic placement was performed. Several reports suggest that patient outcomes improve when CPS is initiated within 10 minutes of cardiac arrest unresponsive to conventional ACLS measures.

C. VENTRICULAR ASSIST DEVICES

1. **Description.** There are limited data on the use of adjunctive assist devices during high-risk angioplasty.[40] The Hemopump (Nimbus left ventricular assist device) utilizes the Archimedes screw principle to create antegrade aortic flow while decompressing the left ventricle. The screw is encased in a flexible tube that is inserted and removed surgically through the femoral artery. The Hemopump lies across the aortic valve and generates flow up to 3.5 L/minute. The system is highly dependent upon adequate pulmonary venous return.

2. **Advantages.** The system is light (less than 25 lbs), does not require a membrane oxygenator, may be run on rechargeable batteries, and results in marked left ventricular unloading. It also appears to lack the fluid and coagulation abnormalities of prolonged CPS, and systemic support is achieved independent of ventricular function or cardiac rhythm. The cable drive shaft is 11F and has been well-tolerated during periods of prolonged support without limb ischemia. Long-term support is possible and the system requires only low-dose heparin.

3. **Disadvantages.** Surgical placement is required. Complications include cannulae migration, coagulopathy, emboli, arrhythmias, and sepsis. Contraindications to the Hemopump include the presence of aortic dissection, significant peripheral vascular disease, moderate or severe aortic insufficiency, significant aortic stenosis, and the presence of left ventricular thrombus.

4. **Outcome.** Animal studies suggest that the Hemopump can be used for several weeks without significant clinical or biochemical sequelae.[41] When compared to intra-aortic balloon counterpulsation in dogs, the Hemopump was better able to maintain aortic pressure, unload the left ventricle, and reduce dyskinesis of the ischemic region during balloon inflation.[42] Hemodynamic measurements obtained during Hemopump supported angioplasty demonstrated a 23% improvement in cardiac index and a 17% reduction in pulmonary capillary wedge pressure. Hematological complications were limited to mild hemolysis and moderate thrombocytopenia, although a 14F device has been associated with severe hemolysis.

5. **Applications.** Current indications for this investigational device include inability to wean from CPS, intractable cardiogenic shock, and as a bridge to cardiac transplantation.

D. LEFT ATRIAL-FEMORAL ARTERY BYPASS (PERCUTANEOUS LVAD)

1. **Description.** Involves placement of a 21F catheter into the left atrium (by transseptal technique), which returns blood to a femoral artery catheter.[43] The system is highly dependent upon adequate pulmonary venous return, and is functionally a percutaneous left ventricular assist device.

2. **Advantages.** LA-FA bypass results in significant unloading of the left ventricle, does not require use of a membrane oxygenator, and can provide longer support than CPS.

3. **Disadvantages.** This device requires transseptal puncture; left-to-right heart shunting has been recognized. It is also less effective in the setting of pulmonary edema or severe right heart failure, and has limited flow rates (< 4.5 L/min).

REGIONAL MYOCARDIAL SUPPORT

A. **AUTOPERFUSION CATHETERS.** Many patients who were unable to tolerate prolonged balloon inflations due to severe angina, arrhythmias, or hemodynamic instability were safely and effectively treated with autoperfusion catheters. However, these have been nearly completely replaced by stents.

1. **Description.** There are several types of perfusion balloon catheters (Chapters 1, 35). All except the Dispatch catheter have sideholes permitting passive blood flow during balloon inflation. The Dispatch catheter consists of an over-the-wire catheter with a spiral inflation coil wrapped around a non-porous polyurethane sheath. When the spiral inflation coil is inflated, it forms an internal lumen that allows antegrade blood flow (60-100 cc/min); it can also be used for local drug delivery (Chapter 35).

2. **Technique.** These catheters are inserted over 0.014-0.018-inch guidewires. Because of their large profile and limited trackability, they may be difficult to place in tortuous vessels or distal coronary segments. Once properly positioned, the balloon is inflated to 6 atmospheres; higher inflation pressures may impair blood flow. The guidewire is withdrawn proximal to the sideholes and the central lumen intermittently flushed with heparinized saline to prevent thrombosis. The guiding catheter is retracted to allow blood to enter the proximal side holes. Distal flow is directly related to the perfusion pressure; rates as high as 40-60 ml/min have been reported.[44] Hypotension must be corrected as flow rates are dependent on arterial pressure; fluids, IABP or vasopressors may be necessary. "Bailout" catheters have a similar design to autoperfusion catheters except they lack a balloon at their distal end. Use of this catheter is confined to failed stenting while preparing for emergency surgical revascularization. Flow rates are similar to those achieved with autoperfusion balloon catheters.

3. **Advantages.** Subjective and objective evidence of ischemia, ST segment shifts, and segmental wall motion abnormalities improve with autoperfusion catheters.[45] Among patients in whom a bailout catheter could be properly positioned during acute closure, there was a lower incidence of Q-wave infarction (9% vs. 75%), less ST segment elevation, and greater subsequent use of internal mammary grafts.[46]

4. **Disadvantages.** The large profile often limits catheter placement to proximal and mid-coronary vessel segments, and the relatively inflexible shaft contributes to the difficulty navigating tortuous vessels.

5. **Applications.** Perfusion balloons were indicated when PTCA resulted in severe symptoms or hemodynamic instability, or when prolonged balloon inflations were required (e.g., in treating suboptimal angiographic outcomes, including coronary dissection and acute closure). However, perfusion balloons are rarely used today because of the superior efficacy of coronary stents (Chapter 26).

B. ACTIVE CORONARY HEMOPERFUSION. These systems actively deliver oxygenated blood obtained from the side arm of an arterial sheath via hand injection, roller pump or power injector. Use of active hemoperfusion during balloon inflation has resulted in fewer subjective and objective manifestations of ischemia.

C. PERFLUOROCHEMICALS. Fluosol was taken off the commercial market in 1995. Randomized trials demonstrated that fluorocarbons have the potential to relieve or prevent regional ischemia,[42-48] although other studies have shown that autologous blood infusion may be just as effective.[49]

D. CORONARY SINUS RETROPERFUSION. The concept of coronary vein perfusion was advanced in the early 1940's when Beck and colleagues surgically interposed a vein graft between the aorta and coronary sinus. This technique allowed blood to travel through the coronary sinus retrograde into ischemic myocardium, resulting in improved patient symptomatology. However, myocardial edema and hemorrhage led to a marked decline in enthusiasm. Percutaneous coronary sinus retroperfusion was later developed as a method for delivering oxygenated blood to the myocardial bed during balloon inflation.

1. **Description.** The retroperfusion catheter consists of a triple lumen 8.5F radiopaque catheter with a balloon 10 mm from its distal end. Arterial blood is pumped from the femoral artery to the coronary sinus. The 7 or 8F arterial cannula is connected to the console, which can deliver flow rates up to 250 ml/minute.[50] The coronary sinus balloon is synchronized with the R wave of the electrocardiogram, preventing regurgitation of arterial blood into the right atrium during systole.

2. **Technique.** Cannulation of the coronary sinus is usually performed via the right internal jugular or subclavian vein under fluoroscopic guidance. For optimal retroperfusion of the LAD territory, the catheter should be advanced into the distal segment of the great cardiac vein.

3. **Advantages.** Coronary sinus retroperfusion allows for retrograde delivery of pharmacologic agents and does not require crossing of diseased coronary arterial segments.[51] When used in the setting of high-risk angioplasty, it has been shown to reduce wall motion abnormalities, ST segment changes, and allow longer inflations; there was no difference in hemodynamic performance.[52-53]

4. **Disadvantages.** Inability to cannulate the coronary sinus precludes its use in 10-15% of patients.[54] It also does not provide systemic support, and is not consistently effective for the circumflex and right coronary arteries. Infrequent complications include transient atrial fibrillation, hematoma, and coronary sinus staining.[55]

5. **Outcome.** In 28 patients who underwent LAD angioplasty, retroperfusion was successfully performed in 87%.[49] The incidence of balloon-induced angina was reduced by 50%.[55]

6. **Applications.** Coronary sinus retroperfusion allows regional support and subselective administration of pharmacologic agents during complex PTCA of the LAD.

E. PHARMACOTHERAPY. Although definitive data are lacking, nitroglycerin, beta blockers, and calcium antagonists reduce myocardial oxygen consumption; however, none augment collateral flow. These strategies are rarely employed in the stent era.

1. **Beta Blockers.** These agents delay the onset of ischemia and may allow for longer balloon inflations.[56] In patients demonstrating evidence of high adrenergic tone (i.e., hypertension, tachycardia), supplemental use of intravenous beta blockers (e.g., metoprolol 5 mg q 5 min x 3, propranolol 1-2 mg, or esmolol 0.15 mg/kg) may allow for longer inflation times; however PTCA-induced bradycardia may be accentuated.

2. **Calcium Antagonists and Nitrates.** Pre- and intra-procedural calcium antagonists and nitrates are routinely administered during angioplasty. These agents have been shown to delay the onset of angina, ECG evidence of ischemia, and increases in left ventricular end-diastolic pressure during balloon inflation.[57]

* * * * *

REFERENCES

1. Gruentzig AR, Senning A, Siegenthaler WE. Nonoperative dilation of coronary artery stenosis: percutaneous transluminal coronary angioplasty. N Engl J Med 1979;301:61-68.
2. Stevens T, Kahn JK, McCallister BD, et al. Safety and efficacy of percutaneous transluminal coronary angioplasty in patients with left ventricular dysfunction. Am J Cardio 1991;68:313-319.
3. Serota H, Deligonul U, Lee WH, et al. Predictors of cardiac survival after percutaneous transluminal coronary angioplasty in patients with severe left ventricular dysfunction. Am J Cardiol 1991;67:367-372.
4. Kohli RS, DiSciascio G, Cowley MJ, et al. Coronary angioplasty in patients with severe left ventricular dysfunction. J Am Coll Cardiol 1990;16:807-811.
5. Eltchaninoff H, Franco I, Whitlow PK, et al. Late results of coronary angioplasty in patients with left ventricular ejection fractions ≤ 40%. Am J Cardiol 1994;73:1047-52.
6. O'Keefe JH, Allan JJ, McCallister, et al. Angioplasty versus bypass surgery for multivessel coronary artery disease with left ventricular ejection fraction < 40%. Am J Cardiol 1993;71:897-901.
7. Holmes DR, Detre KM, Williams DO, et al. Long term outcome of patients with depressed left ventricular function undergoing percutaneous transluminal coronary angioplasty. The NHLBI PTCA Registry. Circulation 1993;87:21-9.
8. Terrien EF, Siegel N, O'Neill WW, et al. Angioplasty in patients with severe left ventricular dysfunction an analysis of immediate and long term survival. J Am Coll Cardiol 1993;21:272A.
9. Pigott JD, Kouchoukos NT, Oberman A, et al. Late results of surgical and medical therapy for patients with coronary artery disease and depressed left ventricular function. J Am Coll Cardiol 1985;5:1036-1045.
10. Alderman EL, Fisher LD, Litwin P, et al. Results of coronary artery surgery in patients with poor left ventricular function (CASS). Circulation 1983;68:785-795.
11. Miller TD, Christian TF, Taliercio CP, et al. Impaired left ventricular function, one- or two-vessel coronary artery disease, and severe ischemia: outcome with medical therapy versus revascularization. Mayo Clin Proc 1994;69:626-31.
12. Hochberg MS, Parsonnet V, et al. Coronary artery bypass grafting in patients with ejection fractions below forty percent. J Thorac Cardiovasc Surg 1983;86:519-527.
13. Rahimtoola SH, Nunley D, Grunkemeier G, et al. Ten year survival after coronary artery bypass surgery for unstable angina. N Engl J Med 1983;308:676-681.
14. The Veterans Administration Coronary Artery Bypass Surgery Cooperative Group. Eleven year survival in the Veterans Administration trial of coronary artery bypass surgery for stable angina. N Engl J Med 1995;311:1333-1339.
15. Elefteriades JA, Tolis G, Levi E, et al. Coronary artery bypass grafting in severe left ventricular dysfunction: excellent survival with improved ejection fraction and functional state. J Am Coll Cardiol 1993;22:1411-7.
16. BARI Investigators. The bypass angioplasty revascularization investigation (BARI): five year mortality and morbidity in a randomized study comparing CABG and PTCA in patients with multivessel coronary artery disease. N Engl J Med 1996;335:217.
17. Califf R, Phillips H, Hindman M, et al. Prognostic value of a coronary artery jeopardy score. J Am Coll Cardiol 1985;5:1055-63.
18. Ellis SG, Roubin GS, King SB III, et al. In-hospital cardiac mortality after acute closure after coronary angioplasty: analysis of risk factors from 8207 procedures. J Am Coll Cardiol 1988;11:211-216.
19. Kaltenbach M, Gruentzig A, Rentrop P, et al. In: Transluminal Coronary Angioplasty and Intracoronary Thrombolysis, 1982;145-150.
20. Alderman JD, Gabliani GI, McCabe CH, et al. Incidence and management of limb ischemia with percutaneous wire-guided intraaortic balloon catheters. J Am Coll Cardiol 1987;9:524-530.
21. Fuchs RM, Brin KP, Brinker JA, et al. Augmentation of regional coronary blood flow by intra-aortic balloon counterpulsation in patients with unstable angina. Circulation

1983;68:117-123.

22. Kahn JK, Rutherford BD, McConahay DR, et al. Supported "high risk" coronary angioplasty using intraaortic balloon pump counterpulsation. J Am Coll Cardiol 1990;15:1151-1155.

23. Meany TB, Pavlides G, Cragg D, et al. Prophylactic percutaneous cardiopulmonary bypass versus intraaortic balloon pump support for high risk angioplasty. J Am Coll Cardiol 1992;19:349A.

24. Murphy DA, Craver JM, Jones EL, et al. Surgical management of acute myocardial ischemia following percutaneous transluminal coronary angioplasty. J Thorac Cardiovasc Surg 1984;87:332-339.

25. Ishihara M, Sato H, Tateishi H, et al. Intraaortic balloon pumping as the postangioplasty strategy in acute myocardial infarction. Am Heart J 1991;122:385-388.

26. Ohman EM, George BS, White CJ, et al. Use of aortic counterpulsation to improve sustained coronary artery patency during acute myocardial infarction. Results of a randomized trial. Circulation 1994;90:792-9.

27. Ohman EM, Califf RM, George BS, et al. The use of intraaortic balloon pumping as an adjunct to reperfusion therapy in acute myocardial infarction. Am Heart J 1991;895-901.

28. Leinbach RC, et al. Early intraaortic balloon pumping for anterior myocardial infarction without shock. Circulation 1978;58:204.

29. Hanson EC, et al. Control of post infarction ventricular irritability with intraaortic balloon pump. Circulation 1978;62:30.

30. Aroesty J, Weintraub R, Paulin S, et al. Medically refractory unstable angina pectoris. Ii. Hemodynamic and angiographic effects of intraaortic balloon counterpulsation. Am J Cardiol 1979;43:887.

31. DeWood MA, Notske RN, Hensley GR, et al. Intraaortic balloon counterpulsation with and without reperfusion for myocardial infarction shock. Circulation 1980;61:1105-1112.

32. Tomasso CL. Use of percutaneously inserted cardiopulmonary bypass in the cardiac catheterization laboratory. Cathet Cardiovasc Diagn 1990;20:32-38.

33. Sturm JT, McGee MG, Fuhrman TM, et al. Treatment of postoperative low output syndrome with intraaortic balloon pumping: experience with 419 patients. Am J Cardiol 1980;45:1033-1036.

34. Vogel RA, Shawl F, Tommaso C, et al. Initial report of the national registry of elective cardiopulmonary bypass supported coronary angioplasty. J Am Coll Cardiol 1990;15:23-29.

35. Stack RK, Pavlides GS, Miller R, et al. Hemodynamic and metabolic effects of venoarterial cardiopulmonary support in coronary artery disease. Am J Cardiol 1991;67:1344-1348.

36. Vogel RA et al. Chapter 26 in Textbook of Interventional Cardiology 1994. Editor Topol (W.B. Saunders).

37. Shawl FA, et al. Cardiopulmonary bypass supported PTCA: long term follow-up of 85 consecutive patients. Circulation 1990;82:III-653A.

38. Overlie PA, Walter PD, Hurd HP, et al. Emergency cardiopulmonary support with circulatory support devices. Cardiology 1994;84(3):231-7.

39. Overlie PA. Emergency use of portable cardiopulmonary bypass. Cathet Cardiovasc Diagn 1990;20:27-31.

40. Loisance D, Dubois-Rande JL, et al. Prophylactic use of Hemopump in high risk coronary angiography. J Am Coll Cardiol 1990;15:249A.

41. Wampler RK, Moise JC, Frazier OH, et al. In vivo evaluation of a peripheral vascular access axial flow blood pump. Trns Am Soc Artif Intern Organs Trans 1988;34:450-454.

42. Smalling RW, Cassidy DB, Merhige M, et al. Improved hemodynamic and left ventricular unloading during acute ischemia using the Hemopump left ventricular assist device compared to intra aortic balloon counterpulsation. J Am Coll Cardiol 1989;13:160A.

43. Babic UU, Grujicic S, Djurisic Z, et al. Percutaneous left atrial aortic bypass with a roller pump. Circulation 1989;80:II-272.

44. Stack RS, Quigley PJ, Collins G, et al. Perfusion balloon catheter. Am J Cardiol 1988;61:77G-80G.

45. Turi ZG, Campbell CA, Gottimukkala MV, et al. Preservation of distal coronary perfusion during prolonged balloon inflation with an autoperfusion angioplasty catheter. Circulation 1987;75:1273-1280.

46. Banka VS, Trivedi A, Patel R, et al. Prevention of myocardial ischemia during coronary angioplasty: a simple new method for distal antegrade arterial blood perfusion. Am Heart J 1989;118:830-836.

47. Bell MR, Nishimura RA, Holmes DR, et al. Does intracoronary infusion of Fluosol prevent left ventricular diastolic dysfunction during coronary balloon angioplasty? J Am Coll Cardiol 1990;16;4:959-966.

48. Robalino BD, Marwick T, Lafont A, et al. Protection against ischemia during prolonged balloon inflation by distal coronary perfusion with use of an autoperfusion catheter or Fluosol. J Am Coll Cardiol 1992;20:1378-84.

49. Christensen CW, Reeves WC, Lassar TA, et al. Inadequate subendocardial oxygen delivery during perfluorocarbon perfusion in a canine model of ischemia. Am Heart J 1988;115:30-37.

50. Hajduczki I, Kar S, Areeda J, et al. Reversal of chronic regional myocardial dysfunction (hibernating myocardium) by synchronized diastolic coronary venous retroperfusion during coronary angioplasty. J Am Coll Cardiol 1990;15:238-242.

51. Drury JK, Yamazaki S, Fishbein MC, et al. Synchronized diastolic coronary venous retroperfusion: results of a preclinical safety and efficacy study. J Am Coll Cardiol 1985;6:328-335.

52. Incorvati RL, Tauberg SG, Pecora MJ, et al. Clinical applications of coronary sinus retroperfusion during high risk percutaneous transluminal coronary angioplasty. J Am Coll Cardiol 1993;22:127-34.

53. Nanto S, Nishida K, Hirayama A, et al. Supported angioplasty with synchronized retroperfusion in high risk patients with left main trunk or near left main trunk obstruction. Am Heart J 1993;125:301-9.

54. Carday E, Kar S, Drury JK, et al. Coronary venous retroperfusion for support of ischemic myocardium. Cardiovascular Rev Rep 1988:9:50-53.

55. Kar S, et al. Reduction of PTCA induced ischemia by Synchronized Coronary Venous Retroperfusion: Results of a Multicenter Clinical Trial. J Am Coll Cardiol 1990;15:250A.

56. Zalewski A, Goldberg S, Dervan JP, et al. Myocardial protection during coronary occlusion in man: beneficial effects of regional beta blockade. J Am Coll Cardiol 1985;5:445.

57. Zalewski A, Savage M, Goldberg S. Protection of the ischemic myocardium during percutaneous transluminal coronary angioplasty. Am J Cardiol 1988;61:54-60G.

REVASCULARIZATION BASED ON PATIENT CHARACTERISTICS

7

Mark S. Freed, M.D.
Robert D. Safian, M.D.

YOUNG PATIENTS (AGE < 40 YEARS)

A. BACKGROUND. Although coronary artery disease typically occurs with advancing age, 5% of patients are less than 40 years old. Compared to older patients, young patients typically have more cardiac risk factors and less extensive disease. Coronary artery bypass grafting (CABG) can be performed with high success and low mortality (0-2%). However, since young patients may require reoperation due to vein graft failure, catheter-based intervention may offer an alternative to CABG.

B. BALLOON ANGIOPLASTY. Patients as young as 15 years old have been treated by PTCA;[1] larger series indicate that PTCA can be performed with success rates of 86-96% and major complication rates < 5% (Table 7.1).

C. FOLLOW-UP. Among successfully treated patients followed over 3-5 years, repeat PTCA was required in 30%, survival was 87-100%, and more than 80% were asymptomatic and employed.[3,5]

Table 7.1. PTCA in Young Patients: Acute Outcome

Series	Age	N	Success (%)	Complications (%) D / Q-MI / CABG	Other
Ellis[106] (1998)	< 40	86	90	0 / 3.5 / 2.3	5-yr survival (95%); 10-yr survival (91%); 5-yr EFS (89%); 10-yr EFS (68%)
Mehan[2] (1994)	≤ 40 > 40	89 1916	90 86	0 / 0 / 0 5 / 1 / 1	5-yr survival (100%). Follow-up at 30 mos: CABG (5%); re-PTCA (34%)
Buffett[3] (1994)	< 40	140	86	5.7 / 6.4 / 0	10-yr survival (96%); return to work (93%); restenosis (28%)
Kofflard[4] (1994)	<35	57	92	3.4 / 1.7 / 1.7	5-yr survival (87%). Follow-up at 4 yrs: MI (14%); CABG (11%); re-PTCA (32%)
Stone[5] (1989)	≤ 35	71	96	0 / 1 / 0	3-yr survival (98%)

Abbreviations: D = in-hospital death; MI = in-hospital Q-wave myocardial infarction; CABG = emergency coronary artery bypass grafting; EFS = event-free survival

D. CONCLUSIONS. Balloon angioplasty has a high success rate, low complication rate, and excellent long-term survival, and may be preferred over surgical revascularization for young patients with coronary disease. The need for repeat PTCA (for restenosis or new disease) is similar to other PTCA patients.

ELDERLY PATIENTS (AGE 65-75 YEARS)

A. BACKGROUND. In 1990, the United States Census estimated that 25% of the 31 million people over age 65 had symptomatic coronary artery disease. By 2020, this number is expected to increase by 65%. From 1987 to 1990, the rates of PTCA and CABG among the elderly increased by 55% and 18%, respectively.

B. PERCUTANEOUS REVASCULARIZATION. Compared to younger patients, elderly patients undergoing coronary revascularization are more often female, and are more likely to have diffuse disease, calcified lesions, unstable angina, prior MI, comorbid conditions, and low ejection fractions. Nevertheless, elective CABG (Table 7.2), PTCA (Tables 7.2, 7.3) and other devices (Table 7.4) can be performed with success rates > 90% and major complication rates of 3-13%. Although the elderly are at increased risk for death after acute closure, the risk of acute closure and the need for emergency CABG have been dramatically reduced by stents. However, there is still a 2-3-fold higher risk of peripheral vascular complications (pseudoaneurysm, AV fistula, large hematoma) and blood transfusions, and there is a strong correlation between advancing age and in-hospital mortality and late death.[188,189]

C. ACUTE MI. In general, advanced age is a risk factor for adverse outcome following acute MI. Primary PTCA is associated with better 30-day survival than either conservative therapy without reperfusion or intravenous thrombolytic therapy,[184] although outcomes following primary PTCA and lytic therapy are similar at 1-year.[184,185] A prospective multicenter randomized trial (PAMI-Elderly) is in progress, which is comparing intravenous thrombolytic therapy to primary percutaneous intervention (PTCA, stents) in elderly patients with acute MI.

D. FOLLOW-UP. More than 75% of successfully revascularized elderly patients have symptomatic improvement. Survival rates at 1 year and 3 years are 95% and 90%, respectively, with late MI in 5%, CABG in 15%, and PTCA in 20%—similar to other PTCA patients.

Table 7.2. Effect of Age on Coronary Revascularization

Series	Modality	Age	N	Complications (%)[++] D / Q-MI / CABG	Other Results
Kobayashi[208] (2001)	Stent	< 70 70-79 ≥80	476 251 94	0.2 / 0.5 / 0.2 0.4 / 0.4 / 0 0 / 0 / 0	No difference in 30-day CABG (~ 0.1%), mortality (~1.5%), or MACE (~1.5%). Vascular complications were highest in patients ≥ 80 years (1.0% vs. 1.6% vs. 4.3%, p = 0.05)
Batchelor[214] (2000)	PCI	≥ 80 < 80	7472 102,236	3.8 / 1.9 / 4.4 1.1 / 1.3 / 4.5	Patients ≥ 80 years had lower procedural success (84% vs. 89%) and more stroke (0.58% vs. 0.23%), renal failure (3.2% vs. 1.0%), and vascular complications (6.7% vs. 3.3%). Procedural success and complications improved during the 4 year study period
ARTS[192‡] (2000)	CABG Stent CABG Stent	< 54 < 54 > 68 > 68	139 162 156 145	- - - -	1-yr MACE (%): 5.4 23.5 15.4 24.1
Lucas[205] (2000)	CABG PTCA	≥ 75 ≥ 75	4993 (total)	- -	Overall 1-yr survival (90%); 4-yr survival (78%). CABG with 25% reduction in death vs. PTCA
Wennberg[188] (1999)	PTCA	< 60 60-69 70-79 ≥ 80	5217 3752 2696 507	- - - -	Angiographic success was independent of age, but in-hospital death was strongly associated with advancing age
Pliam[187] (1999)	CABG	> 80* > 80**	202 202	12.9 / 1.0 / - 5.4 / 0 / -	Strongest predictors of in-hospital death were emergency CABG (OR 10.5) and need for IABP (OR 8.6)
Mullany[90] (1997)	CABG PTCA CABG PTCA	< 65 < 65 ≥ 65 ≥ 65	1120 709	1.1 / - / - 0.7 / - / - 1.7 / - / - 1.7 / - / -	5-yr outcomes (%): Survival TLR 91.5 10 89.5 56 85.7 5 81.4 53
Thompson[87] (1996)	PTCA	> 65+ > 65++	982 768	3.3 / 3.9 / 5.5 1.4 / 2.2 / 0.7	No difference in survival
Hannan[6] (1994)	CABG	40-49 50-59 60-64 65-69 70-74 75-79 ≥ 80	2448 6118 5352 6268 5563 3561 1372	1.1 / - / - 1.7 / - / - 2.2 / - / - 2.8 / - / - 3.4 / - / - 5.3 / - / - 8.3 / - / -	Older cohorts include more females, emergency surgery, unstable angina, previous CABG, heart failure, renal failure, EF < 20%, previous stroke, peripheral vascular disease
O'Keefe[7] (1994)	CABG PTCA	> 70 > 70	195 195	9 / 6 / 5 2 / 1 / 0	5-yr survival (%): 65 63

Abbreviations: ARTS = Arterial Revascularization Therapy Study; CABG = emergency coronary artery bypass grafting; D = in-hospital death; EF = ejection fraction; MI = in-hospital Q-wave myocardial infarction; OR = odds ratio; TLR = target lesion revascularization; - = not reported

+   Elderly patients undergoing PTCA between 1980-1989; ++ Elderly patients undergoing PTCA between 1990-1992

*   1986-1993

**   1994-1996

‡   Randomized trial of multivessel stenting vs. CABG

++ In-hospital complications

Table 7.3. PTCA for Patients Over Age 65: Acute Outcome

Series	Age	N	Success (%)	Complications (%) D / Q-MI / CABG	Comments
BARI[90] (1997)	65-80	709*	-	1.7 / - / -	5-yr survival (81.4%); 5-yr TLR (53%)
Laster[88] (1996)	> 80	55	96	16 / - / 0	Primary PTCA for acute MI
Jollis[12]† (1995)	65-69 > 80	- 20,006	- -	1.8 / - / - 7 / - / -	1-yr survival (94.8% vs. 83%); 3-yr survival (89.6% vs. 70.4%)
Lindsay[10] (1994)	55-64 65-74 ≥ 75	914 996 474	93 92 94	0.5 / 0.3 / 3.7 1.1 / 0.5 / 2.2 2.1 / 1.3 / 3.6	Vascular repair (1% vs. 1.9% vs. 3.6%); non-balloon devices used in 35%
Burstein[11] (1994)	< 50 50-69 ≥ 70	172 938 622	- - -	0.7 / - / 4.7 1.3 / - / 3.5 3.6 / - / 2.1	
Thompson[13] (1994) 1980-89 1990-92	> 65 > 65	982 768	88 94	3.3 / 3.9 / - 1.4 / 2.2 / -	Death/MI at 6 months (10.3% vs. 9.9%)
Little[14] (1993)	< 80 > 80	500 118	88 89	0.2 / 1.4 / 2.6 2.1 / 0.8 / 0.8	Octogenarians: 1-yr survival (76%); 3-yr survival (61%)
Foreman[15] (1992)	60-69 70-79 ≥ 80	570 270 67	88 88 84	2 / 6 / 5 2 / 5 / 4 6 / 5 / 2	3-yr survival (96% vs. 80% vs. 72%)
Thompson[17] (1991)	65-69 70-74 ≥ 75	326 233 193	82 82 93	1.2 / 2.7 / 10.7 2.2 / 4.3 / 9 6.2 / 6.7 / 3	EFS (%): 1-yr / 3-yr / 5-yr 74 / 60 / 51 72 / 55 / 48 58 / 36 / 24

Abbreviations: BARI = Bypass Angioplasty Revascularization Investigation; CABG = emergency coronary artery bypass grafting; D = in-hospital death; EFS = event-free survival (no death, MI, CABG, PTCA, angina); MI = in-hospital Q-wave myocardial infarction; TLR = target lesion revascularization; - = not reported
*   PTCA + CABG
†   From the Medicare Provider Analysis and Review (MEDPAR) file

Table 7.4. Results of Interventional Devices in the Elderly

Series	Modality	Age	N	Success[*†] (%)	Complications (%)[+] D / Q-MI / CABG	Comments
Kobayashi[208] (2001)	Stent	< 70 70-79 ≥ 80	476 251 94	- 	0.2 / 0.5 / 0.2 0.4 / 0.4 / 0 0 / 0 / 0	No difference in 30-day CABG (~0.1%), mortality (~ 0.5%), or MACE (~1.5%). Vascular complications higher in patients ≥ 80 years (1.0% vs. 1.6% vs. 4.3%, p = 0.05)
Trabattoni[221] (2001)	Stent	> 75 51-75 31-50	130 200 150	91 95 96	3.8 / - / 0.7 1.0 / - / 0 0 / - / 0	No difference in late MACE or restenosis between groups
Baklanov[222] (2001)	Stent	> 80	197	93	2 / - / -	Stroke (2%). High-risk patient cohort: acute MI or unstable angina (65%); prior MI (66%); 3-vessel disease (48%)
Alexander[191] (2000)	Various	≥ 75	34,878	-	3.1 / 0.9 / -	Composite results from 6 large registries. Stroke (0.4%); results of PCI improved over time.
Ang[215] (2000)	Various	> 70 > 80	524 65	99 96	1.1 / 0.6 / 1.3 1.5 / 0 / 0	No difference in short-term risk of stroke or need for repeat PCI
Alfonso[186] (1999)	Stent	≥ 65 < 65	378 601	93 95	4.7 / 4.2 / 0 1.3 / 3.4 / 0.3	More in-hospital death and MACE (6.8% vs. 3.4%) in the elderly.
Bage[107] (1998)	Stent	> 70	87	-	4.6 / 0 / 0	EFS at 8.6 months (84%)
DeGregorio[108] (1998)	Stent	> 75 < 75	137 2551	- 	2.2 / 2.9 / 3.7 0.1 / 1.7 / 1.4	1-yr survival (91%); 1-yr EFS (54%); elderly with lower EF, more multivessel disease, and more unstable angina
Chauhan[137] (1998)	Stent	< 80 ≥ 80	5624 265	99 99	0.2 / 0.8 / - 0.8 / 1.1 / -	TLR (12.6% vs. 11.7%). More vascular and bleeding complications in the very elderly
Gaxiola[154] (1998)	Stent	< 75 ≥ 75	280 282	97 94	0.7 / 0.7 / 0.7 3.7 / 2.4 / 1.2	EFS at 6 months (81% vs. 77%)
Nasser[92] (1997)	Stent	< 65 65-74 > 75	252 258 35	97 97 97	1.0 / 0.5 / 4.0 0 / 6.5 / 4.3 0 / 0 / 0	EFS at 9 months (90% vs. 89% vs. 90%)
Fishman[19] (1995)	DCA + Stent	< 70 ≥ 70	388 116	96 91	0.8 3.5	
Movsowitz[20] (1994)	DCA	< 65 66-75 ≥ 75	222 101 50	96 88 95	5.7 10.9 9.5	Transfusion required in 17% of patients ≥ 75 years. Trend toward more groin complications in the elderly
Elliot[21] (1994)	PTCA DCA ROTA Stent	> 70 > 70 > 70 > 70	443 56 91 29	92 98 97 86	4.3 1.8 2.2 13.8	Vascular complications (13% vs. 9% vs. 14% vs. 45%)

Abbreviations: CABG = emergency coronary artery bypass grafting; D = in-hospital death; DCA = directional coronary atherectomy; EF = ejection fraction; EFS = event-free survival (without death, MI, CABG, re-PTCA); MACE = major adverse cardiac events; MI = in-hospital Q-wave myocardial infarction; PCI = percutaneous coronary intervention; PSS = Palmaz Schatz stent; ROTA = Rotablator; - = not reported
* Device + adjunctive PTCA as needed
† In-hospital complications

Table 7.5. Important Considerations for Elderly Patients Undergoing Coronary Intervention

Patient Group	Measure
All patients	Ensure euvolemia Check neurologic and peripheral vascular status Consider sedation with antihistamines rather than benzodiazepines Remove sheaths as soon as possible Promote early ambulation Remove bladder catheter early Prescribe support stockings if prolonged bedrest Simplify medical regimen and educate patient prior to discharge
EF < 40% or culprit supplies large myocardial territory	Consider angiography to evaluate peripheral vessels for IABP Consider Rotablator for calcified lesions Perform culprit vessel angioplasty and/or stent; stage remaining stenoses
Suboptimal result	Prepare for stent implantation
Acute coronary syndrome	Perform culprit vessel angioplasty and/or stent; stage remaining stenoses Consider platelet IIb/IIIa inhibitors

Abbreviations: IABP = intra-aortic balloon pump; EF = ejection fraction

E. **APPROACH.** Patients between the ages of 65-75 with symptomatic coronary artery disease should not be denied percutaneous or surgical revascularization because of age alone or concerns about excessive complications, even during acute MI.[183] Although CABG and PTCA achieve similar long-term survival rates, PTCA is associated with less in-hospital morbidity and mortality, but greater need for repeat revascularization. Patients with anatomic features unsuitable for percutaneous intervention and those with severe 3-vessel disease with LV dysfunction may have a survival advantage after CABG. Although stents have decreased the incidence of in-hospital ischemic complications, elderly patients are at higher risk for medical and vascular complications. It is important to pay special attention to volume status, contrast load, renal function, bleeding and peripheral vascular complications to minimize morbidity and mortality (Table 7.5).

VERY ELDERLY PATIENTS (AGE > 80 YEARS)

A. **BYPASS SURGERY.** In-hospital mortality is 5-10% in octogenarians undergoing CABG, and another 5% develop perioperative MI or stroke (Table 7.2). The marked decline in perioperative morbidity and mortality in the late 1990's has been attributed to better patient selection, maintenance of higher perfusion pressures, and improvements in pre- and post-operative patient care.[187] In addition to advanced age, risk factors for operative mortality include female gender, unstable angina, diabetes mellitus, smoking, poor ejection fraction, and severe angina. Five-year survival ranges from 60-85%; 30% of late deaths are due to noncardiac causes. At 1-year follow-up, up to 90% of patients are in functional Class 1 or 2.

Table 7.6. PTCA for Patients Over Age 80: Acute Outcome

Series	N	Success (%)	Complications (%) D / Q-MI / CABG
Kobayashi[208] (2001)	94 (stent)	-	0 / 0 / 0
Batchelor[214] (2000)	7472 (various devices)	84	3.8 / 1.9 / 4.4
Ang[215] (2000)	65 (various devices)	96	1.5 / 0 / 0
Thompson[197] (2000)	2968	94	3.5 / - / -
Jollis[12] (1995)	20,006*	-	7 / - / -
Weyrens[23] (1994)	26	65	23 / 4 / -
Little[14] (1993)	118	89	2 / 1 / 1
Foreman[15] (1992)	67	84	6 / 5 / 2
Santana[24] (1992)	53+	83	15 / 4 / -
Bedotto[25] (1991)	111	91	6 / 3 / 0
Jackman[26] (1991)	31	90	6 / 6 / 10
Myler[27] (1991)	74	80	1 / 0 / 4
Jeroudi[28] (1990)	54	91	4 / 4 / 0
Rizo-Patron[29] (1990)	53	83	2 / 5 / 7
Rich[30] (1988)	22	86	0 / 14 / 0
Kern[31] (1988)	21	67	19 / 0 / 14

Abbreviations: CABG = emergency coronary artery bypass grafting; D = in-hospital death; Q-MI = in-hospital Q-wave myocardial infarction (some studies did not distinguish between Q-wave and non-Q-wave MI); - = not reported
* From the Medicare Provider Analysis and Review (MEDPAR) file
+ All patients had unstable angina

B. **PERCUTANEOUS REVASCULARIZATION.** Procedural success were achieved in 65-94% of patients > 80 years old (Table 7.6),[32,188] although success rates ≥85% are expected in contemporary practice. Compared to younger patients, octogenarians have more acute complications, in-hospital mortality, and late cardiac death. Nevertheless, 87% of patients in one study were subjectively improved after PTCA, 33% were more physically active, and 55% required less medication.[28] Three-year survival rates of 80-91% have been reported,[27,28] and > 90% of long-term survivors indicated a high level of satisfaction with their quality of life and health status.[14] In anatomically suitable lesions, stent implantation may enhance the early and late outcome after intervention. Octogenarians with acute MI benefit from primary PTCA or stenting with procedural success in 98%, 30-day mortality in 16%, and 1-year event-free survival of 77%.[182]

C. **CONCLUSIONS.** When medical therapy fails to control anginal symptoms in octogenarians, PTCA, stenting, and other techniques can be performed with high success rates, but acute ischemic complications occur more often than in younger patients. Short-term follow-up reveals relief of angina, but frequent late cardiac events from serious comorbid medical problems. To minimize morbidity and mortality during percutaneous intervention, it is important to pay special attention to volume status, contrast load, renal function, bleeding, and peripheral vascular complications (Table 7.5).

FEMALE PATIENTS

A. **BACKGROUND.** Many studies suggest differences in the prevalence, manifestations, diagnosis, and prognosis of coronary artery disease between men and women.[33-35,109,151,167,168] Compared to men, women with non-Q-wave MI had more risk factors for atherosclerosis, partially explaining higher 1-year mortality in women.[165]

B. **PERCUTANEOUS REVASCULARIZATION.** Several studies suggest that females have a higher in-hospital mortality than males (Tables 7.7, 7.8). However, females were older, and had a higher prevalence of diabetes mellitus, hypertension, unstable angina, and prior MI. After accounting for these differences, gender probably has little or no independent effect on outcome,[147,161] even in the setting of primary PTCA or stenting for acute MI.[166] Females are at increased risk for major ischemic and peripheral vascular complications, possibly due to greater comorbidity and lower body surface area. Although women had more bleeding and vascular complications after abciximab than men, major bleeding in women was similar with and without abciximab.[170]

C. **CABG.** One-year occlusion rates of SVG and LIMA grafts are similar for men and women.[169]

D. FOLLOW-UP. Compared to males, females had similar survival and *better* event-free survival (freedom from death, MI, repeat PTCA, or CABG).[38,39] Mayo Clinic investigators found no difference in 5-year infarct-free survival, although females required less late CABG.[44]

E. CONCLUSIONS. In-hospital mortality is higher for women undergoing PTCA, but is largely related to older age, advanced angina class, small body habitus, and comorbid conditions. Long-term results are similar to men. PTCA and other devices should not be withheld in women who are considered good candidates for intervention because of concerns of lower success rates and more complications.[109]

AFRICAN-AMERICANS

A. BACKGROUND. African-Americans have more risk factors for coronary artery disease and higher cardiac mortality than the general population.[55] Most studies suggest that CABG is equally effective among black and white patients in reducing symptoms and improving survival,[56] although 15-year survival was lower in African-Americans in the Coronary Artery Surgery Study (CASS).[89] Although several studies suggest racial disparities in referral of patients for cardiac catheterization, percutaneous intervention, and CABG,[110-112] survival rates are similar between African-Americans and Caucasians with similar disease severity.[112] Some differences in referral may be due to greater reluctance among African-Americans to undergo invasive procedures.[110,113]

B. PERCUTANEOUS REVASCULARIZATION (Table 7.9). Despite greater comorbidity among African-Americans, results from the 1985-1986 NHLBI PTCA Registry indicate that PTCA outcome is independent of race.[57] However, other reports describing laser, atherectomy, and stents suggest higher procedure-related death among African-Americans,[58,195] which be due to a higher prevalence of comorbid conditions.[58]

C. FOLLOW-UP. One-year survival and event-free survival following percutaneous intervention were lower among African-Americans in one report[195] but not in another;[58] 5-year outcomes were similar[57] (Table 7.9). More than 80% of patients have improved anginal status and repeat PTCA is required in 20-25%, similar to the general population.

D. CONCLUSIONS. Despite more comorbidity, African-Americans have excellent results after percutaneous revascularization. Aggressive management of risk factors for atherosclerosis is mandatory (Chapter 41).

Table 7.7. Effect of Gender on PTCA Outcome

Series	Gender	N	Success (%)	Complications (Male vs. Female) (%)** D / Q-MI / CABG
Vakili[199]	Male	727[++]	-	2.3 / - / -
(2000)	Female	317[++]	-	7.9 / - / -
				MACE: In-hospital / 1 mo / 6 mo (%)
Adamian[123]	Male	2113	98	0.9 / 1.3 / 4.7
(1999)	Female	247	95	3.6 / 4.8 / 9.8
Jacobs[156]	Female (1985-6)	545	79	2.6 / 4.6 / 4.6
(1997)	Female (1993-4)	274	89	1.5 / 1.8 / 1.8
Jacobs[104]	Male	656	-	In-hospital mortality (1.2% vs. 0.8%);
(1996)	Female	248	-	5-yr mortality (14.4% vs. 14.1%)
Stone[36]	Male	145[++]	90	2.1 / 2.8 / -
(1995)	Female	50[++]	80	4.0 / 2.0 / -
Malenka[37]	Male	11,493	94	Death (0.7% vs. 1.6%); MI or CABG
(1995)	Female	5472	95	(4.5% vs. 5.0%)
Weintraub[38]	Male	7940	90	0.1 / 0.8 / 2
(1994)	Female	2845	91	0.7 / 1 / 2
Arnold[39]	Male	3726	93	0.3 / 0.4 / 4.5
(1994)	Female	1274	94	1.1 / 0.4 / 5
Cavero[40]	Male	340[†]	-	Females had higher in-hospital death but
(1994)	Female	340[†]	-	similar total and event-free survival
Peterson[8][*]	Male	129,675	-	30-day mortality (3.0% vs. 3.8%);
(1994)	Female	96,240	-	1-yr mortality (7.8% vs. 8.2%)
Kelsey[148]	Male	1590	89	0.3 / 4.3 / 3.3
(1993)	Female	546	88	2.6 / 4.6 / 4.8
Bell[42]	Male	1508	90	3.1 / 0.6 / 2.1
(1993)	Female	593	87	5.4 / 0.7 / 2.9
Kahn[43]	Male	7142	95	0.8 / 1.4 / 1.6
(1992)	Female	2033	95	1.4 / 1.7 / 1.6

Abbreviations: D = in-hospital death; MI = in-hospital Q-wave myocardial infarction; CABG = emergency coronary artery bypass grafting; MACE = major adverse cardiac events (death, MI, repeat revascularization); - = not reported
† Multivessel PTCA or CABG
* From the Medicare Provider Analysis and Review (MEDPAR) file
++ Primary PTCA for acute MI
** In-hospital complications unless otherwise stated

Table 7.8. Effect of Gender on Stent, Atherectomy, and Laser Outcomes

Series	Modality	Gender	N	Results
Dangas[209] (2001)	Various	Male Female	347*/4583 180*/1805	Compared to African American males, African American females had higher in-hospital mortality (4.1% vs. 1.0%, p = 0.006), Q-MI (1.9% vs. 0.2%, p = 0.037), and MACE (8.6% vs. 2.4%, p = 0.001). No difference in hospital outcome for Caucasion males vs. females. Female gender was an independent predictor of 1-yr mortality
Watanabe[223] (2001)	Stent/PTCA	Male Female	64,016 54,532	Females had 2-fold higher in-hospital mortality and more in-hospital CABG
Thompson[224] (2001)	Stent/PTCA CABG	Male Female Male Female	24,111 12,141 14,397 6338	After adjusting for baseline differences, females had higher in-hospital mortality after CABG (but not after stent/PTCA)
Sousa[225] (2001)	Stent	Male Female	16,905 6848	Females had higher in-hospital mortality (1.8% vs. 0.9%, p < 0.0001), even after adjusting for baseline differences
EPISTENT[190] (2000)	Stent/PTCA	Male Female	2399 (total)	30-day death, MI, or urgent revascularization (male vs. female): stent-placebo (10.5% vs. 11.7%); stent-abciximab (4.2% vs. 8.7%); PTCA-abciximab (7.6% vs. 5.1%). Females ≥ 65 years with lower 30-day composite endpoint in PTCA/abciximab vs. stent/abciximab groups (2.2% vs. 14.4%)
Ang[198] (2000)	Various	Male Female	1861 723	No differences in procedural success, death, MI, or stroke. Females required more rePTCA (2.5% vs. 1.2%) and emergency CABG (2.9% vs. 1.4%)
Weintraub[136] (1998)	Stent	Male Female	1046 410	Females had higher in-hospital mortality (1.0% vs. 0.7%), 6-month mortality (4.3% vs. 2.9%), and restenosis (27% vs. 22%)
Lansky[93] (1997)	Various	Male Female	1983 1076	Females had lower acute angiographic success (82% vs. 87%), more in-hospital CABG (3% vs. 1.6%), similar 1-yr death (~5.5%) and CABG (~11%), and less repeat PTCA (21% vs. 24%)
Mehran[91] (1997)	Stent	Male Female	836 364	Females had higher in-hospital Q-MI (1.3% vs. 0.4%) and vascular complications (9.4% vs. 3.9%), but similar clinical events at 6 months
Nasser[92] (1997)	Stent	Male Female	396 149	No difference in in-hospital events or clinical follow-up at 9 months
Hermiller[86] (1996)	Bailout stent	Male Female	606 270	Females had similar ischemic complications but more vascular complications (13% vs. 5%)
STRESS[45] (1995)	PSS	Male Female	170 35	Females had similar EFS (83% vs. 80%), restenosis (36% vs. 30%), and TLR (14%) at 8 months. Females were older, had smaller vessels, and developed more peripheral vascular complications (14% vs. 5%)

Table 7.8. Effect of Gender on Stent, Atherectomy, and Laser Outcomes

Series	Modality	Gender	N	Results
Fishman[19] (1995)	Stent or DCA	Male Female	413 91	Females had lower procedural success (89% vs. 96%), similar major complications (~1%), and greater peripheral vascular complications (25% vs. 9%)
Baumbach[46] (1994)	ELCA	Male Female	1156 365	Females had 2.5-fold increase in severe dissection and 2.4-fold increase in perforation
Combs[47] (1994)	PTCA + DCA	Male Female	982 406	Females had more acute closure (5.2% vs 2.7%). Emergency CABG and procedural success rates were equivalent
Ellis[49] (1994)	ROTA	Male Female	243 82	Females had a 2.4-fold increase in procedural failure and a 3-fold increase in ischemic complications
Casale[51] (1993)	ROTA	Male Female	1951 785	Females had lower success (93% vs. 95%) and more ischemic complication (12.5% vs 7.4%). Females were older, and had more diabetes, unstable angina, and calcified lesions
Movsowitz[54] (1994)	DCA	Male Female	281 137	Females had lower procedural success (68% vs. 80%), primarily due to inability to engage the ostium (with the guiding catheter) and the inability to cross the lesion with the device due to smaller vessel size

Abbreviations: CABG = coronary artery bypass grafting; DCA = directional coronary atherectomy; EFS = event-free survival (without death, MI, CABG, re-PTCA); GRS = Gianturco-Roubin stent; MI = myocardial infarction; PSS = Palmaz Schatz stent; ROTA = Rotablator; TLR = target lesion revascularization
* African-Americans

DIABETICS

A. **BACKGROUND.** Patients with insulin-dependent diabetes mellitus (Type I) are prone to micro- and macrovascular complications, whereas those with non-insulin dependent diabetes (Type II) are more prone to macrovascular complications.[162] The most important manifestation of macrovascular disease is coronary artery disease due to accelerated atherosclerosis, which causes nearly 50% of deaths in these patients. Compared to nondiabetics, patients with diabetes mellitus have a 2-3-fold higher rate of coronary artery disease, and are at increased risk for myocardial infarction, congestive heart failure, and death.[149,172,174] Experimental studies suggest enhanced platelet, coagulation, and vasoconstrictor activity, more endothelial dysfunction, and reduced fibrinolytic capacity in diabetics, predisposing to a hypercoagulable state and more ischemic events (Table 7.10).[153,159,172,175]

Table 7.9. Results of Coronary Intervention in African-Americans

Series	Modality	Group	N	Success (%)	Complications (%)⁺ D / Q-MI / CABG	Other (Black vs. White)
Dangas[209] (2001)	Various	Black female	180	-	4.1 / 1.9 / -	Female gender was a predictor of higher 1-yr mortality
		Black male	347	-	1.0 / 0.2 / -	
		White female	1805	-	1.2 / 0.4 / -	
		White male	4583	-	0.9 / 0.7 / -	
Dangas[195] (2000)	Various	Black	555	-	2.3 / 0.9 / 2.9	1-yr outcomes: death (11% vs. 6%); MACE (29% vs. 26%)
		White	5738	-	0.9 / 0.7 / 1.4	
Wong[127] (1999)	PTCA	Black	1137	-	0.9 / 0.4 / 0.6	
		White	20,464	-	0.9 / 0.3 / 1.5	
Scott[57] (1994)	PTCA	Black	76	76*	0 / 7 / 4	5-yr outcomes: death (11% vs. 10%); MI (13% vs. 14%); CABG (20% vs. 19%); re-PTCA (25% vs. 28%); asymptomatic (66% vs. 81%)
		White	1939	79*	1 / 5 / 4	
Chuang[58] (1994)	Various	Black	169	92	4.1 / 1.2 / 2.4	1-yr outcomes: death (1.5% vs. 1.6%); MI (0.8% vs. 1.4%); CABG (9% vs. 8%); re-PTCA (21% vs. 18%)
		White	1955	91	0.6 / 0.9 / 3.4	
Scott[59] (1993)	PTCA	Black male	337	88	0.6 / 2.1 / 4.8	No difference in survival (~ 79%) or EFS (~ 35%) at 8 years
		Black female	160	91	1.9 / 0.4 / 4.4	

Abbreviations: D = in-hospital death; MI = in-hospital Q-wave myocardial infarction (some studies did not distinguish between Q-wave and non-Q-wave MI); CABG = emergency coronary artery bypass grafting; EFS = event-free survival
* Clinical success: Final diameter stenosis < 50% without death, MI, or emergency CABG
+ In-hospital

B. BYPASS SURGERY. Compared to nondiabetics, patients with diabetes have more in-hospital death and stroke, shorter long-term survival, and more late MI, redo CABG, and PTCA (Table 7.11).[60,61] Approximately 20-25% of diabetics die within 5 years of CABG. Even after correction for differences in baseline characteristics (unstable angina, lower EF, multivessel disease, other comorbidity), diabetes mellitus remains a strong independent predictor of adverse outcome.

Table 7.10. Factors Associated with Diabetes Mellitus That Facilitate Coronary Arteriosclerosis and Adverse Outcomes[172]

Clinical Factors
Advanced age
Female gender
Obesity
Hypertension
Hyperlipidemia
Prior MI
Prior CABG

Biological Factors
Endothelial dysfunction
Reduction in coronary flow reserve
Increased platelet activity
Increased secretion of thromboxane-A_2
Increased platelet activation
Higher levels of fibrinogen and factor VII
Less antithrombin III activity
High levels of plasminogen activation inhibitor

Angiographic Factors
Small vessels, diffuse disease
Frequent multivessel and left main disease
More left ventricular dysfunction
Poor coronary collateral development
More thrombus formation

C. BALLOON ANGIOPLASTY

1. **Procedural Results (Table 7.11).** Approximately 20% of patients undergoing coronary intervention have diabetes mellitus. Most PTCA series indicate similar success rates (~ 90%) among diabetics and nondiabetics,[62-64,143] despite more unstable angina, prior MI, prior CABG, peripheral vascular disease, coronary calcification, and lower ejection fractions in diabetics.[65] Abciximab (with or without stents) improves in-hospital, 30-day, and 6-month outcomes (death, MI, revascularization), especially for insulin-dependent diabetics.[142,160]

2. **Follow-up.** Compared to nondiabetics, diabetics have shorter long-term survival, more ischemic cardiac events, and more target lesion revascularization after PTCA.[60,62,63,65,116] Potential factors include more diffuse disease, smaller vessels,[126] and more intimal hyperplasia after vessel injury.[176] Importantly, diabetics appear to have a greater propensity for plaque rupture and thrombosis, owing to increased blood viscosity, more platelet aggregation, production of procoagulant factors, decreased synthesis of prostacyclin, and impaired fibrinolysis. The impact of diabetes mellitus on restenosis was controversial, but most reports indicate higher restenosis rates.[66-71] In the Bypass

Angioplasty Revascularization Investigation (BARI) trial, diabetics treated with PTCA had higher 5-year mortality than those treated with CABG (35% vs. 19%, p = 0.0024),[60] with a relative risk of late death of 3.1.[117,118] The survival advantage with CABG was limited to diabetics who received internal mammary bypass grafts,[118] and was most pronounced in diabetics with prior MI and LV dysfunction.[171] At 7 years, the survival advantage for CABG continued to increase (mortality: 44.3% for PTCA vs. 25.6% for CABG, p < 0.001).[207] In contrast, two studies, including the nonrandomized BARI registry,[164] reported no difference in 5-year survival for diabetic patients treated by CABG vs. PTCA.[116] Differences in late mortality between studies may be partially explained by differences in case selection, glycemic control, proteinuria, and the prevalence of insulin-dependent diabetes (which seems to be associated with a worse prognosis than non-insulin dependent diabetes).[115,130,132,164] In some studies[128,145] but not in others, elevation of hemoglobin A_{1c} levels and suboptimal glycemic control were associated with a worse late outcome.[144,162] Diabetics with proteinuria had worse 2-year survival after percutaneous intervention compared to nondiabetics and diabetics without proteinuria.[163,173] The combination of diabetes and renal insufficiency identified an extremely high-risk group for 1-year death or MI (25.9%), compared to diabetics without renal insufficiency (7.8%) and nondiabetics with normal renal function (4.2%).[203] Finally, diabetics have a higher incidence of incomplete revascularization with PTCA, which is an important confounding variable when interpreting survival studies.[155]

3. **Acute MI.** In the GUSTO-IIb angioplasty substudy, primary PTCA for acute MI was equally successful in diabetics and nondiabetics, despite worse baseline clinical and angiographic characteristics in diabetics. In diabetics, primary PTCA was more effective than intravenous thrombolytic therapy.[180] In STENT-PAMI, primary PTCA or stenting for acute MI were equally effective in diabetics.[200]

D. **NON-BALLOON DEVICES.** In CAVEAT-I, compared to non-diabetics undergoing directional atherectomy, diabetics had more angiographic restenosis (60% vs. 47%) and more frequent bypass surgery (12.8% vs. 8.5%).[95] Results from STRESS I-II trials suggest that stenting may be preferred over PTCA in diabetics (Table 7.12).[98] Most studies reported higher restenosis rates after stenting and other devices in diabetics vs. nondiabetics,[96,97,99,130,131,138,141,158] although other reports found no difference.[105,125,139,140,152] Serial IVUS studies suggest more late intimal hyperplasia after all percutaneous interventions in diabetics compared to nondiabetics.[150] The BARI-II trial will randomize 2600 Type-2 diabetics with stable coronary artery disease to elective percutaneous intervention or aggressive medical therapy, and to tight glycemic control (HgbA$_{1c}$ < 7.5) with insulin or insulin-sensitizing drugs.

E. **CONCLUSIONS.** Compared to nondiabetics, diabetics undergoing PTCA have similar angiographic success but a trend toward higher in-hospital complications; long-term survival after percutaneous or surgical revascularization is reduced. Late vessel occlusion after PTCA is a common manifestation of restenosis, and may partially explain deterioration in LV function and higher mortality rates.[124] Given the high mortality rates following revascularization, aggressive risk factor modification is recommended to retard progressive disease at non-PTCA sites. Since a 1% increment in hemoglobin A_{1c} levels is associated with a 10% increase in risk of ischemic heart disease, glycemic control, antihypertensive therapy, and lipid-lowering treatment is crucial, especially in patients with Type-2 diabetes.[162] Other important risk-reduction measures, including the use of ACE inhibitors, aspirin, smoking cessation, diet, weight control, and exercise are detailed in Chapter 41.

CHRONIC DIALYSIS PATIENTS

A. **BACKGROUND.** Coronary artery disease is responsible for more than 40% of deaths among patients with end-stage renal disease. CABG is feasible for patients on dialysis, but operative mortality is increased.[72-73]

B. **BALLOON ANGIOPLASTY.** As shown in Table 7.13, residual stenosis < 50% can be achieved in 90% of cases, but major ischemic complications (particularly non-Q-wave MI) are increased, especially in those > 65 years of age.[74,161] Even mild renal insufficiency prior to percutaneous revascularization increases the risk of cardiac mortality in the years following successful intervention.[216] Despite platelet and coagulation abnormalities in patients with chromic renal insufficiency, abciximab does not appear to increase the risk of major bleeding complications.[217]

C. **STENTS.** Acute angiographic results and procedural success rates after stenting are similar for dialysis and non-dialysis patients. However, in-hospital ischemic complications and 1-year rates of death and MI are higher in dialysis patients.[161,196,202]

D. **FOLLOW-UP.** Compared to the general PTCA population, dialysis patients have a higher incidence of restenosis (50-70% vs. 20-40%) and recurrent cardiac events at 1 year (50-80% vs. 20-35%). Although perioperative mortality is higher after CABG compared to PTCA, 1- and 2-year survival is better after CABG.[134]

E. **CONCLUSIONS.** Percutaneous revascularization of chromic dialysis patients is associated with high rates of ischemic and vascular complications and restenosis. In the largest report to date, patients on hemodialysis undergoing PTCA or CABG had 2-3 fold higher mortality at 1 and 12 months compared to the general PTCA population.[74] Despite stenting, patients with renal insufficiency (on or off dialysis) have more ischemic complications and higher mortality than patients with normal renal function.[133,146]

Table 7.11. Results of PTCA in Patients with Diabetes Mellitus

Series	Group	N	Success (%)	Complications (%)[++] D / Q-MI / CABG	Comments
DESTINI[210] (2001)	PTCA Diabetic* PTCA Nondiabetic*	70 296	- -	0 / 2.9[+] / 0 0/ 3.0[+] / 0.7	Diabetics had lower EFS at 1 year (71% vs. 84%)
Sedlis[226] (2001)	PCI Diabetic CABG Diabetic	454 overall	- -	- -	Randomized trial of diabetics at high-risk for CABG (refractory unstable angina and prior CABG, MI < 7 days, LVEF < 35%, or IABP to stabilize). 3-yr survival similar (79% vs. 80%)
BARI[60,207] (2000)	PTCA Diabetic CABG Diabetic	174 183	- -	0.6 / - / - 1.2 / - / -	PTCA group had more death (44% vs. 26%), MI (9.2% vs. 5.7%), and repeat revascularization (70% vs. 11%) at 7 years
Wong[201] (2000)	PTCA Diabetic PTCA Nondiabetic	4372 18,366	- -	1.4 / 0.3 / 1.3 0.8 / 0.3 / 1.5	Diabetics had more dialysis (0.55% vs. 0.05%) and longer hospital stay (6.4 days vs. 5.5 days)
Gowda[114] (1998)	PTCA Diabetic PTCA Nondiabetic	77 299	96 97	- -	Diabetics had similar survival (92% vs. 94%) but lower EFS (55% vs. 67%) at 1 year
Weintraub[115] (1998)	PTCA Diabetic CABG Diabetic	834 1805	- -	0.4 / - / - 5.0 / - / -	Survival was similar for PTCA vs. CABG at 5 years (78% vs. 76%) and 10 years (45% vs. 48%). Survival was worse for insulin-dependent diabetics after PTCA
Van Belle[105] (1997)	PTCA Diabetic PTCA Nondiabetic	57 243	- -	- -	Diabetics had more restenosis (63% vs. 36%), late loss (0.79 mm vs. 0.41 mm), and late vessel occlusion (14% vs. 3%)
Weintraub[61] (1995)	CABG Diabetic CABG Nondiabetic	2372 10,291	- -	4.2 / - / - 1.8 / - / -	Diabetics had more stroke (3.1% vs. 1.5%), higher mortality at 5 years (26% vs. 13%) and 10 years (50% vs. 28%), and more late MI and revascularization
Stein[62] (1995)	PTCA Diabetic PTCA Nondiabetic	1133 9300	87 89	0.4 / 0.6 / 2.3 0.3 / 0.9 / 2.1	5-yr outcomes: death (17% vs. 7%); MI (19% vs. 11%); CABG (23% vs. 14%); PTCA (43% vs. 32%); EFS (36% vs. 53%)
Faxon[63] (1995)	PTCA Diabetic PTCA Nondiabetic	280 1833	85 87	3.2 / - / - 0.5 / - / -	8-yr outcomes: death (31% vs. 15%); MI (30% vs. 18%); CABG (34% vs. 26%). Diabetics had a 75% increased risk of death after controlling for baseline differences

Abbreviations: CABG = emergency coronary artery bypass grafting; D = in-hospital death; EFS = event-free survival (without death, MI, CABG, or re-PTCA); IABP = intra-aortic balloon pump; MI = in-hospital Q-wave myocardial infarction; PCI = percutaneous coronary intervention; TLR = target lesion revascularization; - = not reported
Acronyms: BARI = Bypass Angioplasty Revascularization Investigation; DESTINI = Doppler Endpoint Stenting International Investigation Coronary Flow Reserve
* Doppler-guided optimal PTCA
+ Q-wave plus non-Q-wave MI
++ In-hospital

Table 7.12. Results of Stenting in Patients with Diabetes Mellitus

Series	Group	N	Results
Abizaid[212] (2001)	Stent Diabetic Stent Nondiabetic	195 560	Elective multivessel stenting. Similar procedural success and in-hospital MACE. Diabetics had more TLR (17.7% vs. 9.1%, p = 0.004) and MACE (34.8% vs. 19.2%, p < 0.001) at 1 year
DESTINI[210] (2001)	Stent Diabetic Stent Nondiabetic	65 302	In-hospital results (diabetic vs. nondiabetic): no deaths; MI (4.6% vs. 2.3%); CABG (0% vs. 1%). 1-yr follow-up: EFS (72% vs. 79%); CABG (9.4% vs. 1.7%); rePTCA (17% vs. 17%)
CADILLAC[211] (2001)	Stent Diabetic PTCA Diabetic	184 162	Stenting vs. PTCA with and without abciximab for acute MI. Stent group had less ischemic TVR at 6 months (7.1% vs. 17.3%, p = 0.0003) vs. PTCA, but similar death, reinfarction, disabling stroke, and MACE. 6-month MACE was increased in diabetics vs. nondiabetics (17.1% vs. 12.3%, p < 0.02)
Kugelmass[227] (2001)	Stent Diabetic (male) Stent Diabetic (female)	409 314	Procedural success higher in females (92.6% vs. 87.5%, p = 0.026); no difference in in-hospital death or emergency CABG
Villareal[193] (2000)	Stent Diabetic CABG Diabetic	468 762	CABG group had more in-hospital death (5.5% vs. 0.4%) and MI (5% vs. 1.5%), but less TLR (0.4% vs. 3.2%). 2-yr survival for NIDDM better with stents
Dangas[194] (2000)	Stent Nondiabetic Stent NIDDM Stent IDDM	584 121 89	Multivessel stenting. Significant difference in 1-yr MACE (nondiabetic 24.8% vs. NIDDM 37.9% vs. IDDM 48.6%, p < 0.001) and 1-yr TVR (10.7% vs. 17.9% vs. 25.7%, p = 0.01). No difference in angiographic success or in-hospital MACE
STENT-PAMI[200] (2000)	Stent Diabetic PTCA Diabetic Stent Nondiabetic PTCA Nondiabetic	72 63 377 381	Randomized trial for acute MI. Death, recurrent MI, stroke, or ischemic TVR at 1 year: nondiabetics (stent 17% vs. PTCA 25%, p = 0.005); diabetics (stent 20% vs. PTCA 30%, p = 0.21)
Ahmed (2000)	Stent Diabetic (SVG) Stent Nondiabetic (SVG)	290 608	Diabetics had higher in-hospital mortality (2.2% vs. 0.3%, p = 0.003), 1-yr TLR (16.6% vs. 12.3%, p = 0.03), and lower 1-yr EFS (68% vs. 79%, p = 0.0003). No difference in early or late outcomes between IDDM vs. NIDDM
Pereira[204] (2000)	Stent Diabetic CABG Diabetic	44 46	Randomized trial. Similar MACE at 1 year (22.7% vs. 19.5%)
Schofer[178] (2000)	Stent Nondiabetic Stent IDDM Stent NIDDM	1439 48 177	Nondiabetics with less late loss, lower loss index, and less TLR than diabetics; no difference between IDDM and NIDDM

Table 7.12. Results of Stenting in Patients with Diabetes Mellitus

Series	Group	N	Results
Gaxiola[179] (2000)	Stent Diabetic Stent Nondiabetic	118 430	In-hospital outcomes: death (0.8% vs. 0.5%); MI (0.8% vs. 0.5%); CABG (1.7% vs. 0.5). Diabetics with more late TLR (26% vs 13%) and CABG (12% vs. 3%). Multiple stents and diabetes were independent predictors of TLR
Silva[181] (1999)	Stent Diabetic Stent Nondiabetic	28 76	Primary stenting for acute MI. MACE at 1 and 6 months were higher in diabetics than nondiabetics; EFS at 6 months was worse in diabetics (54% vs. 88%)
Joseph[177] (1999)	Stent Nondiabetic Stent IDDM Stent NIDDM	1910 58 214	In-hospital outcomes (nondiabetics vs. IDDM vs. NIDDM): death (0.8% vs. 0% vs. 0.5%); MI (1.4% vs. 0% vs. 0.5%); CABG (0.1% vs. 0% vs. 0%). Greater 1-yr survival in NIDDM vs. IDDM (97% vs. 90.7%), but similar TLR (10.5% vs. 8.2%)
Gencbay[132] (1999)	Stent Nondiabetic Stent NIDDM	96 96	Similar angiographic restenosis at 6 months (18% vs. 17%)
Alonso[131] (1999)	Stent Nondiabetic Stent Diabetic	849 134	MACE at 28 months was higher in diabetics (54% vs. 33%)
Bhaskaran[129] (1999)	Stent Diabetic PTCA Diabetic	188 570	Stent group had higher acute success (99.5% vs. 96%), higher 1-yr EFS (91% vs. 78%), and less TLR (8% vs. 16.3%)
Lansky[130] (1999)	Stent Nondiabetic Stent NIDDM Stent IDDM	386 76 102	Similar in-hospital outcomes. 1-yr TLR was highest in IDDM (27%) compared to NIDDM (10.4%) and non-diabetics (13.4%)
Carrozza[141] (1998)	Stent Diabetic Stent Nondiabetic	- -	Diabetics had more late loss, late loss index, angiographic restenosis (31% vs. 24%), and TLR (15% vs. 10%)
STRESS[98] (1997)	Stent Diabetic PTCA Diabetic	47 45	Stent group had higher acute success (100% vs. 82%), less restenosis (24% vs. 60%), and less TLR (13% vs. 31%)
Abizaid[96] (1998)	Stent Nondiabetic Stent NIDDM Stent IDDM	706 151 97	In-hospital complication rates were similar. TLR was higher in diabetics on insulin (28%) compared to those on oral therapy (18%) or nondiabetics (16%)
Elezi[97] (1997)	Stent Diabetic Stent Nondiabetic	190 991	More angiographic restenosis in diabetics (40% vs. 24%)
Yokoi[99] (1997)	Stent Diabetic Stent Nondiabetic	263 668	Acute clinical success was similar (96%), but diabetics had more restenosis (29% vs. 22%)
Van Belle[105] (1997)	Stent Diabetic Stent Nondiabetic	56 244	Similar angiographic restenosis (26%), late loss (0.78 mm), and late vessel occlusion (2%)

Abbreviations: EFS = event-free survival; IDDM = insulin-dependent diabetes mellitus; MACE = major adverse cardiac events; MI = myocardial infarction; NIDDM = non-insulin-dependent diabetes mellitus; TLR = target lesion revascularization

Table 7.13. Revascularization of Chronic Dialysis Patients

Series	Modality	Group	N	Success (%)	Complications (%) D / Q-MI / CABG	
Rinder[228] (2001)	Stent Stent	Dialysis No Dialysis	27 989	- -	MACE at 9 months (29.6% vs. 20.9%)	
Sharma[196] (2000)	ROTA/Stent ROTA/Stent	Dialysis No dialysis	157 803	96 -	Early MACE 1.8 -	Late (20 mos) 12.1 / - / TVR 28 2.8 / - / -
Beygui[202] (2000)	PTCA[++] PTCA[++]	Dialysis No dialysis	119 1328	91 91	Early 2.5 / 3.9 / - 1 / 1.5 / -	MACE (6 mos) 52 37
LeFeuvre[161] (2000)	Stent PTCA Stent PTCA	Dialysis No Dialysis Dialysis No Dialysis	27 250 60 864	96 97 85 90	Early 7 / 0 / 0 1.6 / 0.4 / 0.8 0 / 0 / 0 1.6 / 0.8 / 0.2	Late 15 / 0 / 35* 1.6 / 2 / 27* 12 / 0 / 36* 4 / 4 / 41*
Gruberg[133] (1999)	Stent Stent Stent	Dialysis CRF Normal	53 340 4018	- - -	Early 4.9 / 1.6 / 1.6 3.2 / 0.5 / 0.8 0.8 / 0.5 / 1.2	Late 34 / 0 / 16* 14 / 0.3 / 9* 4.1 / 0.4 / 14*
Dambrin[206] (1999)	Stent Stent	Dialysis No dialysis	21 211	96 97	In-hospital MACE 12 3	Late MACE/death 32 / 19 23.5 / 2
Simsir[119] (1998)	PTCA CABG	Dialysis Dialysis	19 22	- -	In-hospital mortality (5.3% vs. 4.5%)	
Chang[100] (1997)	PTCA CABG	Dialysis Dialysis	105 84	94 -	Mortality in-hospital (8.7% vs. 14.5%) and at 22 months (53% vs. 49%)	
Gradaus[101] (1997)	PTCA PTCA	Dialysis No dialysis	20 20	- -	Restenosis (60% vs. 49%)	
Koyanogi[120] (1996)	PTCA CABG	Dialysis Dialysis	20 23	76 -	EFS at 5 years (18% vs. 70%)	
Ahmed[74] (1995)	CABG PTCA PTCA	Dialysis Dialysis No dialysis	168 202 58,837	- - -	Mortality at 30 days (8.9% vs. 5.4% vs. 2.8%) and at 1 year (32% vs. 32% vs. 8%)	

Abbreviations: D = death; MI = Q-wave myocardial infarction; CABG = coronary artery bypass grafting; TLR = target lesion revascularization; TVR = target vessel revascularization; CRF = chronic renal failure; ROTA = Rotablator; MACE = death/MI/PTCA/CABG; - = not reported
* Target lesion revascularization
++ Provisional stenting

CARDIAC TRANSPLANT PATIENTS

A. **BACKGROUND.** Coronary artery disease affects 20-40% of allografts 1-5 years after transplantation, and is the leading cause of death among patients who survive more than one year. Angiographic findings of allograft arteriopathy range from focal stenoses to diffuse involvement of the entire epicardial coronary circulation. Because allograft hearts are denervated, angina pectoris is distinctly uncommon; clinical presentations typically include myocardial infarction, heart failure, or sudden death. Medical therapy consists of risk-factor modification, immunosuppressive and antiplatelet agents, diet, and exercise. Diltiazem[75] and lipid-lowering agents may retard the progression of coronary disease and are uniformly recommended, even in the absence of hyperlipidemia. Limitations of bypass surgery include early problems with wound healing and infection, and late disease progression. Re-transplantation is feasible but is associated with significant postoperative mortality and a 50% recurrence rate.

B. **PERCUTANEOUS REVASCULARIZATION (Table 7.14).** PTCA, atherectomy, and stents have been applied to small numbers of patients. Combined data show success in 95% and in-hospital mortality in 5%. Results are slightly better with stents.

C. **FOLLOW-UP.** In a multicenter report,[76] 39% of PTCA patients died or required retransplantation at 19 months, and actuarial survival at 5-years was only 30%. Restenosis rates ranged from 33-55%.

D. **CONCLUSIONS.** PTCA and stenting can be performed with acceptable success and complication rates in cardiac transplant patients with focal or tubular stenoses, although repeat intervention may be required. Data on restenosis are incomplete.

SILENT ISCHEMIA

A. **BACKGROUND.** The presence of silent ischemia increases the risk of adverse cardiac events.[45] Findings from the Asymptomatic Cardiac Ischemia Pilot (ACIP) trial suggest that compared to medical therapy alone, revascularization may improve the extent and frequency of exercise-induced ischemia,[80] anginal status, and 1-year survival.[81,82]

B. **PTCA.** Following successful PTCA, objective evidence of ischemia was alleviated in 53-93% of patients at 3-6 months;[83,84] 3-year total and infarct-free survival was 98% and 96%, respectively.[83]

C. **CONCLUSIONS.** Elective PTCA on patients with silent ischemia is safe and effective. The ACIP and other ongoing randomized trials will determine whether suppression of silent ischemia by PTCA or bypass surgery improves long-term outcome.

Table 7.14. Coronary Intervention in Cardiac Transplant Patients

Series	Modality	N	Success (%)	Complications (%) D / Q-MI / CABG	Other
Patel[121] (1997)	PTCA	10	100	-	-
	ROTA	6	100		
	CABG	5	60		
	TMR	1	100		
	CABG/TMR	1	100		
Jain[103] (1997)	Stent	10	100	0	-
Heublein[122] (1997)	Stent	27	100	0 / 0 / -	Restenosis (25%)
Wong[220] (1997)	Stent	12	100	-	Subacute thrombosis (8.3%)
					Allograft survival[†]
Halle[76] (1995)	PTCA	66	94	8 / - / -	61% at 19 months
	DCA	11	82	18 / - / -	82% at 8 months
	CABG	12	-	33 / - / -	58% at 9 months

Abbreviations: ROTA = Rotablator; TMR = transmyocardial laser revascularization; D = in-hospital death; MI = in-hospital Q-wave myocardial infarction; CABG = emergency coronary artery bypass grafting; - = not reported
† Freedom from death or re-transplantation

* * * * *

REFERENCES

1. Kahn JW, Hartzler GO. Saphenous vein graft angioplasty in a teenager. Am J Cardiol 1990;65:25-260.
2. Mehan V, Urban P, et al. Coronary angioplasty in the young: procedural results and late outcome. J Invas Cardiol 1994;6:202-208.
3. Buffet P, Colasante B, et al. Long-term follow-up after coronary angioplasty in patients younger than 40 years of age. Am Heart J 1994;127:509-513.
4. Kofflard M, van Dombur R, van den Brand M, de Jaegere P. 5-year follow-up of coronary angioplasty in patients aged 35 years or younger. Circulation 1994;88(Part II):I-218.
5. Stone GW, Ligon RW, Rutherford BD, et al. Short-term outcome and long-term follow-up following coronary angioplasty in the young patient: an 8-year experience. Am Heart J 1989;118:873-877.
6. Hannan E, and Burke J. Effect of age on mortality in coronary artery bypass surgery in New York, 1991-1992. Am Heart J 1994;128:1184-91.
7. O'Keefe J, Sutton M, et al. Coronary angioplasty versus bypass surgery in patients >70 years old matched for ventricular function. J Am Coll Cardiol 1994;24:425-430.
8. Peterson ED, Gollis JG, Bebchuk JD, DeLong ER, et al. Chances in mortality after myocardial revascularization in the elderly. The national Medicare experience. Ann Intern Med. 1994;121:919-927.
9. Mick MJ, Simpfendorfer C, et al. Early and late results of coronary angioplasty and bypass in octogenarians. Am J Cardiol 1991;68:1316-1320.
10. Lindsay J, Reddy V, et al. Morbidity and mortality rates in elderly patients undergoing percutaneous coronary transluminal angioplasty. Am Heart J 1994;128:697-702.
11. Burstein S, Sun GW, Hammer JS, Mann JD, et al. Adjusted influence of age and gender on PTCA outcomes and hospital resource consumption. J Am Coll Cardiol 1994;March Special Issue:223A.
12. Jollis JG, Peterson ED, Bebchuk JD, DeLong ER, et al. Coronary angioplasty in 20,006 patients over age 80 in the United States. J Am Coll Cardiol 1995; February Special Issue:47A.
13. Thompson RC, Holmes DR, Grill DR, Bailey KR. Changing outcome of angioplasty in elderly. J Am Coll Cardiol 1996;27:8-14.
14. Little T, Milner M, Lee K, Contantine J, Pichard AD, Lindsay JJ. Late outcome and quality of life following percutaneous transluminal coronary angioplasty in octogenarians. Cathet Cardiovasc Diagn 1993;29:261-266.
15. Foreman DE, Berman AD, McCabe CH, et al. PTCA in the elderly: the "young-old" versus the "old-old". J Am Geriatr Soc 1992;40:19-22.
16. ten Berg J, Bal E, et al. Initial and long-term results of percutaneous transluminal coronary angioplasty in patients 75 years of age and older. Cathet Cardiovasc Diagn 1992;26:165-170.
17. Thompson RC, Holmes DR, Gersh B, Mock MB. Percutaneous transluminal coronary angioplasty in the elderly: early and long-term results. J Am Coll Cardiol 1991;17:1245-1250.
18. Yokoi H, Kimur T, Sawada Y, Nosaka H, et al. Efficacy and safety of Palmaz-Schatz stent in elderly (≥ 75 years old) patients: early and follow-up results. J Am Coll Cardiol 1995; February Special Issue:47A.
19. Fishman RF, Kuntz RE, Carrozza JP, et al. Acute and long-term results of coronary atherectomy in women and the elderly. Circulation (in-press).
20. Movsowitz H, Manginas A, et al. Directional coronary atherectomy can be successfully performed in the elderly. Am J Cardiol 1994;31:261-263.
21. Elliot JM, MacIsaac AI, Lefkovits J, Horrigan MCG, Franco I, Whitlow PL. New coronary devices in the elderly: comparison with angioplasty. Circulation 1994;90:4:I-333.
22. Henson, K. D., J. J. Popma, et al. Comparison of results of rotational coronary atherectomy in three age groups (<70,70 to 79 and >80 years). Am J Cardiol 1993;71:862-864.
23. Weyrens F, Goldberg I, et al. Percutaneous transluminal coronary angioplasty in patients aged >90 years. Am J Cardiol 1994;74:397-398.
24. Santana J, Haft J, LaMarche N, Goldstein J. Coronary angioplasty in patients eighty years of age or older. Am Heart J 1992;124:13-18.
25. Bedotto JB, Rutherford BD, McConahay DR, et al. Results of multivessel percutaneous transluminal coronary angioplasty in persons aged 65 years and older. Am J Cardiol 1991;67:1051-1055.
26. Jackman JD, Navetta FI, Smith JE, et al. Percutaneous transluminal coronary angioplasty in octogenarians as an effective therapy for angina pectoris. Am J Cardiol 1991;116:119.
27. Myler RK, Webb JG, Nguyen KPV, et al. Coronary angioplasty in octogenarians: comparison to coronary bypass surgery. Cathet Cardiovasc Diagn 1991;23:3-9.
28. Jeroudi OM, Kleiman NS, Minor ST,et al. Percutaneous transluminal coronary angioplasty in octogenarians. Ann Intern Med 1990;113:423-428.
29. Rizo-Patron C, Hamad N, Paulus R, et al. Percutaneous transluminal coronary angioplasty in octogenarians with unstable coronary syndromes. Am J Cardiol 1990;66:857-858.
30. Rich JJ, Crispino CM, Saporito JJ, et al. Percutaneous transluminal coronary angioplasty in octogenarians. Am J Cardiol 1988;61:457-458.
31. Kern MJ, Deligonoul U, Galan K, et al. Percutaneous transluminal coronary angioplasty in octogenarians. Am J Cardiol 1988;61:457-458.
32. Weyrens EJ, Goldenberg I, Fishman MJ, et al. Percutaneous transluminal coronary angioplasty in patients aged > 90 years. Am J Cardiol 1994;74:397-398.
33. Lerner DJ, Kannel WB. Patterns of coronary heart disease morbidity and mortality in the sexes: a 26-year follow-up of the Framingham population. Am Heart J 1986;111:383-390.
34. Harper R, Kennedy G, DeSanctis R, et al. The incidence and pattern of angina prior to acute myocardial infarction: a study of 577 cases. Am Heart J 1979;97:178-183.
35. Weiner DA, Ryan TJ, McCabe CH, et al. Exercise stress testing: correlations among history of angina, ST-segment

response and prevalence of coronary-artery disease in the Coronary Artery Surgery Study (CASS). N Engl J Med 1979;301:230-235.

36. Stone G, Grines C, Browne K, et al. Comparison of in-hospital outcome in men versus women treated by either thrombolytic therapy or primary coronary angioplasty for acute myocardial infarction. Am J Cardiol 1995;75:987-992.

37. Malenka DJ, O'Connor GAT, Robb J, Kellett M Jr., et al. Is female gender a risk factor for adverse outcomes following PTCA? Circulation 1995;92:I-437.

38. Weintraub WS, Wenger NK, Kosinski AS, et al. Percutaneous transluminal coronary angioplasty in women compared with men. J Am Coll Cardiol 1994;24:81-90.

39. Arnold A, Mick M, et al. Gender differences for coronary angioplasty. Am J Cardiol 1994;74:18-21.

40. Cavero PG, O'Keefe JH, McCallister B, Cochran V, et al. Effect of gender on early and longterm outcome after multiple vessel revascularization with coronary bypass surgery or balloon angioplasty. J Am Coll Cardiol 1994;February Special Issue:351A.

41. Kelsey S, James M, Holubkov AL, Holubkov R. Results of percutaneous transluminal coronary angioplasty in women. 1985-1986 National Heart, Lung, and Blood Institute's Coronary Angioplasty Registry. Circulation 1993;87:720-727.

42. Bell MR, Holmes DR, Berger PB, et al. The changing in-hospital mortality in women undergoing percutaneous transluminal coronary angioplasty. JAMA 1993;269:2091-2095.

43. Kahn JK, Rutherford BD, McConahay DR, et al. Comparison of procedural results and risks of coronary in men and women for conditions other than acute myocardial infarction. Am J Cardiol 1992;69:1241-1242.

44. Bell M, Grill D, Garratt K, Berger P, Gersh B, Holmes D. Long-term outcome of women compared with men after successful coronary angioplasty. Circulation 1995;91:2876-2881.

45. Erne P, Evequoz D, Zuber M, Yoon S, Burckhardt D. Swiss interventional study on silent ischemia II (SWISSI II): Study design and preliminary results. Circulation 1995;92:I-80.

46. Baumbach A, Bittl J, Fleck E, et al. Acute complications of excimer laser coronary angioplasty: A detailed analysis of multicenter results. J Am Coll Cardiol 1994;23:1305-1313.

47. Combs WG, Rothenberg MD, Burke JA, et al. Gender does not influence the morbidity and mortality associated with diagnostic and interventional cardiac catheterization procedures. J Am Coll Cardiol 1994;February Special Issue:401A.

48. Dean LS, Voorhees WD, Sutor C, Roubin GS. Female gender: A risk factor for complications following intracoronary stenting? A Cook Multicenter Registry Report. Circulation 1994;90:4:I-620.

49. Ellis, S., J. Popma, et al. Relation of clinical presentation, stenosis morphology, and operator technique to the procedural results of rotational atherectomy-facilitated angioplasty. Circulation 1994;89:882-892.

50. Bowling BA, May M, Lichtenberg A, et al. Clinical and angiographic outcome of new interventional devices in men and women. Circulation 1994;88:I-448.

51. Casale PN, Marco J, Warth D, Buchbinder M. Women have a lower success rate and higher complication rate with percutaneous rotational atherectomy. Circulation 1994;88:I-448.

52. Henson KD, Popma JJ, Satler LF, Kent KM, et al. Late clinical outcome after new device angioplasty in women. J Am Coll Cardiol 1993;21:2:233A.

53. Mehta S, Margolis JR, Bejarano J, et al. Acute and long-term results with new devices do not demonstrate significant gender differences: Results from the NACI Registry. Circulation 1994;88:I-448.

54. Movsowitz H, Emmi R, Manginas A, et al. Does female gender affect the success rate and outcome of directional coronary atherectomy? Circulation 1994;88:I-448.

55. Sempos C, Cooper R, Kovear MD, McMullen M. Divergence of the recent trends in coronary mortality for the four major race-sex groups in the United States. Am J Public Health 1988;78:1422-1427.

56. Maynard C, Fisher LD, Passamani ER. Survival of black persons compared with white persons in the Coronary Artery Surgery Study (CASS). Am J Cardiol 1987;60:513-518.

57. Scott, N, Kelsey S, et al. Percutaneous transluminal coronary angioplasty in African-American patients (The National Heart, Lung, and Blood Institute 1985-1986 Ppercutaneous Transluminal Coronary Angioplasty Registry). Am J Cardiol 1994;73:1141-1146.

58. Chuang YC, Merritt AJ, Popma JJ, Bucher TA, et al. Do racial differences affect outcome after new device angioplasty? J Am Coll Cardiol 1994;February Special Issue:301A.

59. Scott NA, Capers Q, Weintraub WS, Liberman HA, et al. In hospital and long term outcome of PTCA in African-American women and men. Circulation 1994;88:I-448.

60. The BARI Investigators. Comparison of coronary bypass surgery with angioplasty in patients with multivessel disease. N Engl J Med 1996;335:217.

61. Uthoff K, Schuerholz T, Mugge A, Schaefers JH, et al. Coronary revascularization in renal patients—coronary angioplasty (PTCA) or coronary artery bypass grafting (CABG)? Circulation 1995;92:I-643.

62. Stein B, Weintraub W, et al. Influence of diabetes mellitus on early and late outcome after percutaneous transluminal coronary angioplasty. Circulation 1995;91:979-989.

63. Faxon DP, Kip KE, Currier JW, Yeh W, et al. Diabetics have a significantly poorer eight-year outcome after angioplasty. Circulation 1995;92:I-76.

64. Tan K, Sulke N, et al. Clinical and lesion morphologic determinants of coronary angioplasty success and complications: Current experience. J Am Coll Cardiol 1995;25:855-65.

65. Bailey WL, Westerhausen DR, Rutherford BD, McConahay DR, et al. Characteristics and long-term outcomes of diabetic patients presenting for coronary angioplasty. J Am Coll Cardiol 1993;21:2:273A.

66. Carrozza J, Kuntz R, et al. Angiographic and clinical outcome of intracoronary stenting: Immediate and long-term results from a large single-center experience. J Am Coll Cardiol 1992;20:328-337.

67. Rensing BJ, Hermans WR, Strauss BH, Serruys PW. Regional differences in elastic recoil after percutaneous

transluminal coronary angioplasty: A quantitative angiographic study. J Am Coll Cardiol 1991;17:34B.

68. Weintraub WS, Kosinski AS, Brown CL, King SB III. Can restenosis after coronary angioplasty be predicted from clinical variables? J Am Coll Cardiol 1993;21:6-14.

69. Levin GN, Leya F, Keeler G, Berdan LG, Jacobs AK. The impact of diabetes mellitus on restenosis following directional coronary atherectomy and PTCA: A report from CAVEAT-1. Circulation 1994;90:4:I-652.

70. Faxon DP. Effect of high dose angiotensin-converting enzyme inhibition on restenosis: Final results of the MARCATOR study, a multicenter, double-blind, placebo-controlled trial of cilazapril. J Am Coll Cardiol 1995;2:362-9.

71. Bourassa MG, Lesperance J, Eastwood C, et al. Clinical, physiologic, anatomic and procedural factors predictive of restenosis after percutaneous transluminal coronary angioplasty. J Am Coll Cardiol 1991;18:368-76.

72. Kahn JK, Rutherford BD, McConahay DR, et al. Short and longterm outcome of percutaneous transluminal coronary angioplasty in chronic dialysis patients. Am Heart J 1990;119:484-489.

73. Reusser LM, Osborn LA, White HJ, et al. Increased morbidity after coronary angioplasty in patients on chronic hemodialysis. Am J Cardiol 1994;73:965-6.

74. Ahmed WH, Pashos CL, Ayanian JZ, Bittle JA. 30-day and one-year mortality in hemodialysis patients undergoing coronary revascularization: results from a national cohort. Circulation 1995;92:I-75.

75. Schroeder J, Gao SZ, et al. A preliminary study of diltiazem in the prevention of coronary artery disease in heart-transplant recipients. N Engl J Med 1993;328:164-170.

76. Halle A, DiSciascio G, et al. Coronary angioplasty, atherectomy and bypass surgery in cardiac transplant recipients. J Am Coll Cardiol 1995;26:120-8.

77. Swan JW, Norell M, Yacoub M, et al. Coronary angioplasty in cardiac transplant recipients. Eur Heart J 1993;14:65-70.

78. Sandhu JS, Uretsky BF, Reddy S, et al. Potential limitations of percutaneous transluminal coronary angioplasty in heart transplant recipients. Am J Cardiol 1992;69:1234-1237.

79. Mullins PA, Shapiro LM, Aravot DA, et al. Experience of percutaneous transluminal coronary angioplasty in orthotopic transplant recipients. Eur Heart J 1991;12:1205-1207.

80. Chaitman B, Stone P, Knatterud G, et al. Asymptomatic cardiac ischemia pilot (ACIP) study: impact of anti-ischemia therapy on 12-week rest electrocardiogram and exercise test outcomes. J Am Coll Cardiol 1995;26:585-593.

81. Rogers W, Bourassa M, Andrews T, et al. Asymptomatic cardiac ischemia pilot (ACIP) study: outcome at 1-year for patients with asymptomatic cardiac ischemia randomized to medical therapy or revascularization. J Am Coll Cardiol 1995;26:594-605.

82. Bourassa M, Pepine C, Forman S, et al. Asymptomatic cardiac ischemia pilot (ACIP) study: effects of coronary angioplasty and coronary bypass graft surgery on recurrent angina and ischemia. J Am Coll Cardiol 1995;26:606-614.

83. Knatterud GL, Bourassa MG, Pepine CJ, et al. Effects of treatment strategies to suppress ischemia in patients with coronary artery disease: 12-week results of the Asymptomatic

Cardiac Ischemia Pilot (ACIP) study. J Am Coll Cardiol 1994;24:11-20.

84. Stone GW, Spaude D, Ligon RW, et al. Usefulness of PTCA in alleviating silent myocardial ischemia in patients with absent or minimal painful myocardial ischemia. Am J Cardiol 1989;64:560-564.

85. Lefevre T, Morice MC, Labrunie B, et al. Coronary stenting in elderly patients. Results from the stent without coumadin French Registry. J Am Coll Cardiol 1996;27:252A.

86. Hermiller J, Fry E, Berkompas D, et al. Effect of gender on acute outcome following intracoronary bailout stenting. J Invas Cardiol 1996;8.

87. Thompson RC, Holmes DR, Grill DE, Mock MB, Bailey KR. Changing outcome of angioplasty in the elderly. J Am Coll Cardiol 1996;27:8-14.

88. Laster SB, Rutherford BD, Giorgi LV, et al. Results of direct PTCA in octogenarians. Am J Cardiol 1996;77:10-13.

89. Taylor HA, Mickel MC, et al. Long-term survival of African Americans in the Coronary Artery Surgery Study (CASS). J Am Coll Cardiol 1997;29:2:358-64.

90. Mullany CJ, Brooks M, et al. Outcome of patients $\geq$ 65 years undergoing coronary revascularation: A report from Bypass Angioplasty Revascularization Investigation (BARI). J Am Coll Cardiol 1997;29(Suppl. A):73A.

91. Mehran R, Bucher TA, et al. Coronary stenting in women: Early in-hospital and long-term clinical outcomes. J Am Coll Cardiol 1997;29(Suppl. A):454A.

92. Nasser TK, Fry ETA, et al. Coronary stenting in women: Clinical outcomes are equivalent to men. J Am Coll Cardiol 1997;29(Suppl. A):71A.

93. Lansky AJ, Kennard E, et al. Does gender affect outcome in the new approaches to coronary intervention (NACI) registry. J Am Coll Cardiol 1997;29(Suppl. A):459A.

94. Hasdai D, Bell M, et al. Outcome $\geq$ 10 years after successful percutaneous transluminal coronary angioplasty. Am J Cardiol 1997;79:1005-1011.

95. Levine GN, Jacobs AK, et al. Impact of diabetes mellitus on percutaneous revascularization (CAVEAT-I). Am J Cardiol 1997;79:748-755.

96. Abizaid A, Kornowski R, Mintz GS, et al. The influence of diabetes mellitus on acute and late clinical outcomes following coronary stent implantation. J Am Coll Cardiol 1998;32:584-9.

97. Elezi S, Schuhlen H, et al. Stent placement in diabetic versus non-diabetic patients. Six-month angiographic follow-up. J Am Coll Cardiol 1997;29(Suppl. A):188A.

98. Savage MP, Fischman DL, et al. Coronary intervention in the diabetic patient: Improved outcome following stent implantation versus balloon angioplasty. J Am Coll Cardiol 1997;29(Suppl. A):188A.

99. Yokoi H, Nosaka H, et al. Coronary stenting in the diabetic patients: Early and follow-up results. J Am Coll Cardiol 1997;29(Suppl. A):455A.

100. Chang GL, Ghazzal ZMB, et al. Coronary revascularization in patients on chronic dialysis. J Am Coll Cardiol 1997;29(Suppl. A):180A.

101. Gradaus F, Schoebel FC, et al. High rate of restenosis following coronary angioplasty in patients with chronic renal failure. J Am Coll Cardiol 1997;29(Suppl. A):418A.

102. Nasser TK, Fry ETA, et al. In-hospital and interim clinical outcomes of coronary stents in the elderly. J Am Coll Cardiol 1997;29(Suppl. A):71A.

103. Jain SP, Zhang S, et al. Is coronary stenting a better option in palliative treatment of cardiac allograft vasculopathy? J Am Coll Cardiol 1997;29(Suppl. A):28A.

104. Jacobs AK, Kelsey SF, et al. Improved outcome for women undergoing coronary revascularization: A report from the bypass angioplasty revascularization investigation (BARI). Circulation 1996;94:I-205.

105. Van Belle E, Bauters C, Hubert E, et al. Restenosis rates in diabetic patients. A comparison of coronary stenting with balloon angioplasty in native coronary vessels. Circulation 1997;96:1454-60.

106. Ellis CJ, French JK, White HD, Ormiston JA, Whitlock RML, Webster MWI. Results of percutaneous coronary angioplasty in patients < 40 years of age. Am J Cardiol 1998;82:135-139.

107. Bage MD, Bauman WB, Gupta R, Berkovitz KE, Ormond AP Jr., Grigera F, Josephson RA. Coronary stenting in the elderly: Longitudinal results in a wide spectrum of patients treated with a new and more practical approach. Cathet Cardiovasc Diagn. 1998;44:397-404.

108. De Gregorio J, Kobayashi Y, Albiero R, Reimers B, Di Mario C, Finci L, Colombo A. Coronary artery stenting in the elderly: Short-term outcome and long-term angiographic and clinical follow-up. J Am Coll Cardiol 1998;32:577-583.

109. Hussain JMA, Estrada AQ, Kogan A, Dadkhah S, Foschi AA. Trends in success rate after percutaneous transluminal coronary angioplasty in men and women with coronary artery disease. Am Heart J 1997;134:19-27.

110. Whittle J, Conigliaro J, Good CB, Joswiak M. Do patient preferences contribute to racial differences in cardiovascular procedure use? J Gen intern Med 1997;12:267-273.

111. Gillum RF, Gillum BS, Francis CK. Coronary revascularization and cardiac catheterization in the United States: Trends in racial differences.

112. Ferguson JA, Tierney WM, Westmoreland GR, Mamlin LA, Segar DS, Eckert GJ, Zhou ZH, Martin DK, Weinberger M. Examination of racial differences in management of cardiovascular disease. J Am Coll Cardiol 1997;30:1707-1713.

113. Sedlis SP, Fisher VJ, Tice D, Esposito R, Madmon L, Sterinberg EH. Racial differences in performance of invasive cardiac procedures in a department of Veterans Affairs Medical Center. J Clin Epidemiol 1997;50:899-901.

114. Gowda MS, Vack JL, Hallas D. One-year outcomes of diabetic versus nondiabetic patients with non-Q-wave acute myocardial infarction treated with percutaneous transluminal coronary angioplasty. Am J Cardiol 1998;81:1067-1071.

115. Weintraub WS, Stein B, Kosinski A, et al. Outcome of coronary bypass surgery versus coronary angioplasty diabetic patients with multivessel coronary artery disease. J Am Coll Cardiol 1998;31:10-19.

116. Barsness GW, Peterson ED, Ohman EM, Nelson CL, DeLong ER, Reves JG, Smith PK, Anderson D, Jones RH, Mark DB, Califf RM. Relationship between diabetes mellitus and long-term survival after coronary bypass and angioplasty. Circulation 1997;96:2551-2556.

117. Chaitman BR, Rosen AD, Williams DO, Bourassa MG, Aguirre FV, Pitt B, Rautaharju PM, Rogers WJ, Sharaf B, Attubato M, Hardison RM, Srivatsa S, Kouchoukos NT, Stocke K, Sopko G, Detre K, Frye R. Myocardial infarction and cardiac mortality in the Bypass Angioplasty Revascularization Investigation (BARI) randomized trial. Circulation 1997;96:2162-2170.

118. The BARI Investigators. Influence in diabetes in 5-year mortality and morbidity in a randomized trial comparing CABG and PTCA in patients with multivessel disease. The Bypass Angioplasty Revascularization Investigation (BARI). Circulation 1997;96:1761-1769.

119. Simsir, et al. A comparison of coronary artery bypass grafting and percutaneous transluminal coronary angioplasty in patients on hemodialysis. Cardiovasc Surg 1998;6:500-505.

120. Koyanagi T, Nishida H, Kitamura M, Endo M, Koyanagi H, Kawaguchi M, Magosaki N, Sumiyoshi T, Hosoda S. Comparison of clinical outcomes of coronary artery bypass grafting and percutaneous transluminal coronary angioplasty in renal dialysis patients. Ann Thorac Surg 1996;61:1793-6.

121. Patel VS, et al. Revascularization procedures in patients with transplant coronary artery disease. Eur J Cardiothorac Surg 1997;11:895-901.

122. Heublein B, Pethig K, MaaB C, Wahlers T, Haverich A. Coronary artery stenting in cardiac allograft vascular disease. Am Heart J 1997;134:930-938.

123. Adamain M, De Gregorio J, Kobayashi N, Corvaja N, Di Francesco L, Albiero R, Moussa I, Vaghetti M, Di Mario C, Moses J, Colombo A. Coronary interventions: Is being a woman a risk factor? J Am Coll Cardiol 1999;33[suppl A]:25A.

124. Van Belle E, Abolmaali K, Bauters C, Mc Fadden EP, Lablanche JM, Bertrand ME. Restenosis, late vessel occlusion and left ventricular function 6 months after balloon angioplasty in diabetics patients. J Am Coll Cardiol 1999;33[suppl A]:25A.

125. Mattos L, Sousa JE, Stone G, Morice MC, Boura J, O'Neill W, Cox D, Garcia E, Madonna O, Grines C. Primary stentings versus PTCA in diabetic patients with acute myocardial infarction: Six months results of the stent PAMI trial. J Am Coll Cardiol 1999;33[suppl A]:33A.

126. De Gregorio J, Kobayashi N, Adamian M, Corvaja N, Moussa I, Reimers B, Linci L, DiFrancesco L, Albiero R, Di Mario C, Moses J, Colombo A. A comparison of diabetics with restenosis to diabetics without restenosis. J Am Coll Cardiol 1999;33[suppl A]:82A.

127. Wong SC, Papadakos S, Rosenberg C, O'Brien RJ, Gustafson G. Are there clinical and procedural outcome differences between African and White American undergoing percutaneous coronary interventions? J Am Coll Cardiol 1999;33[suppl A]:82A.

128. Al-Rashdan IR, Rankin JM, Elliott TG, Wong CW, Carere RG, Hilton JD, Henderon MA, Hayden RI, Spinelli JJ, Buller CE. Glycemic control and major adverse cardiac events after PTCA in patients with diabetes mellitus. J Am Coll Cardiol 1999;33[suppl A]:97A.

129. Bhaskaran A, Siegel R, Barker B, Underwood P, Breisblatt W, Nuttall A, Swanson D, Vermillion J, Santos P. Stenting during coronary intervention improves procedural and long-

term clinical outcomes in diabetics. J Am Coll Cardiol 1999;33[suppl A]:97A.

130. Lansky AJ, Mehran R, Popma JJ, Hanzel G, Kent HM, Stone GW, Breedy F, Tepordei G, Burwell N, Pichard A, Satler LF, Leon MB. Insulin treatment of diabetic women predicts a worse outcome after intracoronary stenting. Clinical results of 564 consecutive patients. J Am Coll Cardiol 1999;33[suppl A]:97A.

131. Alonso JJ, Fernandez-Aviles F, Duran JM, Ramos B, Serrado A, Garcimartin I, de la Fuente L, Munoz JC, Garci-Moran E. Influence of diabetes mellitus on the initial and long-term outcome of patients treated with coronary stenting. J Am Coll Cardiol 1999;33[suppl A]:98A.

132. Gencbay M, Degertekin M, Dinar I, Turan, F. Coronary stent implantation in patients with non-insulin dependent diabetes mellitus. J Am Coll Cardiol 1999;33[suppl A]:98A.

133. Gruberg L, Mehran R, Lansky A, Pichard AD, Peterson M, Walters CT, Murphy M, Laird JR, Satler LF, Kent KM, Stone GW, Leon MB. Stents do not improve acute and long-term clinical outcomes in patients with chronic renal failure and coronary disease. J Am Coll Cardiol 1999;33[suppl A]:28A.

134. Gradaus F, Iven K, Schoebel FC, Leschke M, Heering P, Grabensee B, Strauer BE. Comparison of coronary bypass surgery versus coronary angioplasty in patients with chronic renal failure. J Am Coll Cardiol 1999;33[suppl A]:97A.

135. Bartorelli AL, Montorsi P, Fabbiochi F, Trabattoni D, Galli S, Granchini L, Lavarra F, Ravagnani P, Cozzi S, Loaldi A. Does coronary stenting eliminate gender difference in percutaneous revascularization outcome? Circulation 1998:98[suppl I]:I-77.

136. Weintraub WS, Thompson TD, Ghazzal ZMB, Douglas JS, Morris DC, King SB. Does gender influence the outcome of coronary stenting? Circulation 1998:98[suppl I]:I-77.

137. Chauhan MS, Schmidt JM, Cutlip D. Outcome of stenting in the aged. Circulation 1998:98[suppl I]:I-78.

138. Schofe J, Rau T, Schloter M, Mathey DG. Angiographic outcome after stenting of coronary lesions in diabetic versus non-diabetic patients: A matched comparison. Circulation 1998:98[suppl I]:I-78.

139. Marso SP, Ellis SG, Bhatt DL, Sapp SK. The stenting in diabetics debate: Insight from the large GUSTO IIb exexperience with extended follow-up. Circulation 1998:98[suppl I]:I-78.

140. Rankin JM, Bullre CE, Al-Rashdan IR, Henderon MA, Hilton CD, Hayden RI, Carere RG, Spinelli JJ. Coronary angiolasty in diabetics: have outcomes improved in the stent era? Circulation 1998:98[suppl I]:I-79.

141. Carrozza JP, Neimann D, Kuntz RE, Cutlip D. Diabetes mellitus is associated with adverse 6-month angiographic and clinical outcome following coronary stenting. Circulation 1998:98[suppl I]:I-79.

142. Bhatt DL, Marso SP, Lincoff MA, et al. Abciximab Reduces Mortality in Diabetics Following Percutaneous Coronary Intervention. J Am Coll Cardiol 2000:35;931-928.

143. Moraes DL, Leopold JA, Cupples A, Moxey C, Ryan TJ, Jacobs AK. Diabetes does not influence outcome of percutaneous coronary intervention. Circulation 1998:98[suppl I]:I-147.

144. Holmes DR, Rihal CS, Garratt KN, Terzic A, Grill D. Relationship between diabetic glycemic control and outcome after percutaneous coronary intervention. Circulation 1998:98[suppl I]:I-148.

145. Bruno J, Feldrappe A, Niederst PN. Influence of current- and long-term metabolic state of PTCA-outcome in diabetics. Circulation 1998:98[suppl I]:I-148.

146. Rubenstein M, Harrell L, Bazari H, Palacios IF. Are patients with renal failure good candidates for percutaneous coronary revascularization in the new device era? Circulation 1998:98[suppl I]:I-148.

147. Bell MR, Grill DE, Garratt KN, Berger PB, Gersh BJ, Holmes DR Jr. Long-term outcome of women compared with men after successful coronary angioplasty. Circulation 1995;91:2876-2881.

148. Kelsey SF, James M, Holubkov AL, Holubkov R, Cowley MJ, Detre KM. Results of percutaneous transluminal coronary angioplasty in women. 1985-1986 National Heart, Lung, and Blood Institute's Coronary Angioplasty Registry. Circulation 1993;87:720-727.

149. Pajunen P, Nieminen MS, Taskinen MR, Syvanne M. Quantitative comparison of angiographic characteritics of coronary artery disease in patients with noninsulin-dependent diabetes mellitus compared with matched nondiabetic control subjects. Am J Cardiol 1997;80:550-556.

150. Kornowski R, Mintz GS, Kent KM, Pichard AD, Satler LF, Bucher TA, Hong MK, Popma JJ, Leon MB. Increased restenosis in diabetes mellitus after coronary interventions is due to exaggerated intimal hyperplasia. A serial intravascular ultrasound study. Circulation 1997;95:1366-1369.

151. Fetters JK, Peterson ED, Shaw LJ, Newby K, Califf RM. Sex-specific differences in coronary artery diseases risk factors, evaluation, and treatment: Have they been adequately evaluated? Am Heart J131(4):796-813.

152. Van Belle E, Bauters C, Hubert E, Bodart JC, Abolmaali K, Meurice T, McFadden EP, Lablanche, JM, Bertrand ME. Restenosis rates in diabetic patients. A comparison of coronary stenting and balloon angioplasty in native coronary vessels. Circulation 1997;96:1454-1460.

153. Silva JA, White CJ. Diabetes mellitus as a risk factor for development of vulnerable (unstable) coronary plaque: A review of possible mechanisms. J Interven Cardiol 1998;11:19-36.

154. Gaxiola E, Vlietstra RE, Browne KF, Brenner AS, Ebersole DG, Roman L, Weekes TT, Kerensky RA. Is the outcome of coronary stenting worse in elderly patients? J Interven Cardiol 1998;11:37-40.

155. Gum PA, O'Keefe JH, Borkon AM, Spertus JA, Bateman TM, McGraw JP, Sherwant K, Vacek J, McCallister BD. Bypass surgery versus coronary angioplasty for revascularization of treated diabetic patients. Circulation 1997;96:[suppl III]:II-7-II10.

156. Jacobs AK, Kelsey SF, Yeh W, et al. Documentation of decline in morbidity in women undergoing coronary angioplasty (A report from the 1993-1994 NHLBI Percutaneous Transluminal Coronary Angioplasty Registry). Am J Cardiol 1997;80:979-984.

157. Lau KW, Ding ZP, Johan A, Lim YL. Midterm angiographic outcome of single-vessel intracoronary stent placement in diabetic versus nondiabetic patients: A matched comparative

study. Am Heart J 1998;136:150-155.

158. Aoki I, Shimoyama K, Oaki N, et al. Platelet-dependent thrombin generation in patients with diabetes mellitus: Effects of glycemic control on coagulability in diabetes. J Am Coll Cardiol 1996;27:560-566.

159. Kleiman NS, Lincoff M, Kereiakes DJ, et al. Diabetes mellitus, glycoprotein IIb/IIIa blockade, and heparin. Evidence for a complex interaction in a multicenter trial. Circulation 1998;97:1912-1920.

160. Marso SP, Lincoff AM, Ellis SG, et al. Optimizing the percutaneous interventional outcomes for patients with diabetes mellitus: Results of the EPISTENT (Evaluation of Platelet IIb/IIIa Inhibitor for Stenting Trial) diabetic substudy. Circulation 1999;100:2427-2484

161. LeFeuvre C, Dambrin G, Helft G, et al. Comparison of clinical outcome following coronary stenting or balloon angioplasty in dialysis versus non-dialysis patients. Am J Cardiol 2000;85:1365-1368.

162. Laakso M. Benefits of strict glucose and blood pressure control in Type 2 Diabetes: Lessons from the UK Prospective Diabetes Study. Circulation 1999;99:461-462.

163. Marso SP, Ellis SG, Tuzcu EM, et al. The importance of proteinuria as a determinant of mortality following percutaneous coronary revascularization in diabetics. J Am Coll Cardiol 1999;33:1269-77).

164. Detre KM, Guo P, Holubkov R, et al. Coronary revascularization in diabetic patients: A comparison of the randomized and observational components of the Bypass Angioplasty Revascularization Investigation (BARI). Circulation 1999;99:633-640.

165. Gowda SM, Vacek JL, Hallas D. Gender-related risk factors and outcomes for non-Q wave myocardial infarction patients receiving in-hospital PTCA. J Invas Cardiol 1999;11:121-126.

166. Azar RR, Waters DD, McKay RG, et al. Short- and medium-term outcome differences in women and men after primary percutaneous transluminal mechanical revascularization for acute myocardial infarction. Am J Cardiol 2000;85:675-679.

167. Vaccarino V, Parsons L, Every NR, et al. Sex based differences in early mortality after myocardial infarction. N Engl J Med 1999;341:217-25.

168. Gan SC, Beaver SK, Houck PM, et al. Treatment of acute myocardial infarction and 30-day mortality among women and men. N Engl J Med 2000;343:8-15.

169. Tan E, van der Meer J, Jan de Kam P. et al. Worse clinical outcome but similar graft patency in women versus men one year after coronary artery bypass graft surgery owing to an excess of risk factors in women. J Am Coll Cardiol 1999;34:1760-8.

170. Cho L, Topol EJ, Balog C. et al. Clinical benefit of glycoprotein IIb/IIIa blockade with abciximab is independent of gender: Pooled analysis from EPIC, EPILOG, and EPISTENT trials. J Am Coll Cardiol 2000;36:381-6.

171. Detre KM, Lombardero MS, Brooks MM, et al. The effect of previous coronary artery bypass surgery on the prognosis of patients with diabetes who have acute myocardial infarction. N Engl J Med 2000;342:989-97.

172. Hammoud T, Tanguay J, Bourassa MG. Management of coronary artery disease therapeutic options in patients with diabetes. J Am Coll Cardiol 2000;36:355-65.

173. Marso SP, Ellis SG, Gurm HS, et al. Proteinuria is a key determinant of death in patients with diabetes after isolated coronary artery bypass grafting. Am Heart J 2000;139:939-44.

174. Devereux RB, Roman MJ, Paranicas M, et al. Impact of diabetes on cardiac structure and function: The strong heart study. Circulation 2000;101:2271-2276.

175. Mak K, Topol EJ. Emerging concepts in the management of acute myocardial infarction in patients with diabetes mellitus. J Am Coll Cardiol 2000;35:563-8.

176. Moreno PR, Fallon JT, Murcia AM, et al. Tissue characteristics of restenosis after percutaneous transluminal coronary angioplasty in diabetic patients. J Am Coll Cardiol 1999;34:1045-9.

177. Joseph T, Fajadet J, Jordan C. et al. Coronary stenting in diabetics: Immediate and mid-term clinical outcome. Cathet Cardiovasc Intervent 1999;47:279-284.

178. Schofer J, Schluter M, Rau, et al. Influence of treatment modality on angiographic outcome after coronary stenting in diabetic patients: A controlled study. J Am Coll Cardiol 2000;35:1554-9.

179. Gaxiola E, Vlietstra RE, Brenner AS, et al. Diabetes and multiple stents independently double the risk of short-term revascularization. J Interven Cardiol 2000;13:87-91.

180. Hasdai D, Granger CB, Srivatsa SS, et al. Diabetes mellitus and outcome after primary coronary angioplasty for acute myocardial infarction: Lessons from the GUSTO-IIb angioplasty substudy. J Am Coll Cardiol 2000;35:1502-12.

181. Silva JA, Ramee SR, White CJ, et al. Primary stenting in acute myocardial infarction: Influence of diabetes mellitus in angiographic results and clinical outcome. Am Heart J 1999;138:446-55.

182. Antoniucci D, Valenti R, Santoro GM, et al. Systematic primary angioplasty in octogenarian and older patients. Am Heart J 1999;138:670-4.

183. Baradat K, Wilkinson P, Deaner A, et al. How should age affect management of acute myocardial infarction? A prospective cohort study. Lancet 1999;353:955-59.

184. Berger AK, Radford MJ, Wang Y, Krumholz HM. Thrombolytic therapy in older patients. J Am Coll Cardiol 2000;36:366-74.

185. Holmes DR, White HD, Pieper KS, et al. Effect of age on outcome with primary angioplasty versus thrombolysis. J Am Coll Cardiol 1999;33:412-9.

186. Alfonso F, Azcona L, Perez-Vizcayna MJ, et al. Initial results and long-term clinical and angiographic implications of coronary stenting in elderly patients. J Am Coll Cardiol 1999;149:1483-87.

187. Pliam MB, Zapolanski A, Ryan CJ, et al. Recent improvement in results of coronary bypass surgery in octogenarians. J Invas Cardiol 1999;11:281-289.

188. Wennberg DE, Malenka DJ, Sengupta A, et al. Percutaneous transluminal angioplasty in the elderly: Epidemiology, clinical risk factors, and in-hospital outcomes. Am Heart J 1999;137:639-45.

189. Gravina Taddei CF, Weintraub WS, Douglas JS, et al. Influence of age on outcome after percutaneous transluminal coronary angioplasty. Am J Cardiol 1999;84:245-251.

190. Foody JM, Balog C, Cho L, et al. Older women benefit from balloon PTCA rather than stenting when combined with IIb/IIIa anti-platelet therapy: A gender specific treatment interaction from EPISTENT. J Am Coll Cardiol 35:12A.

191. Alexander KP, Malenka DJ, Hannan EL, et al. Outcomes of PCI in the aged: Results from 6 large registries. Circulation 2000;102:II-642.

192. Lindeboom WK, Disco CM, Unger F, et al. Comparison of effectiveness and cost effectiveness of CABG versus percutaneous intervention in patients with multivessel disease by age. Circulation 2000;102:II549.

193. Villareal RP, Lee V, Elayda M, Wilson JM. Survival after coronary artery bypass surgery or coronary stenting in patients with diabetes mellitus. Circulation 2000;102:II549.

194. Dangas G, Kobayashi Y, D'Agate D, et al. Long term results after multivessel stenting in diabetic patients. Circulation 2000;102:II-194.

195. Dangas G, Feldman D, D'Agate D, et al. Impact of race on clinical outcome after percutaneous coronary interventions: Results in 6945 patients. Circulation 2000;102II-479.

196. Sharma SK, Cheema AM, Andrews P, et al. Current status of percutaneous coronary intervention (PCI) in patients with chronic renal failure on hemodialysis. Circulation 2000;102:II-480.

197. Thompson TD, Veledar E, Zhang Z, et al. PTCA outcomes among very elderly patients during the stent era: Contemporary results from the national cardiovascular network (NCN). Circulation 2000;102:II-480.

198. Ang PCH, Harper RW, Meredith IT, et al. Angioplasty in women: A re-look into their clinical success and complications. J Am Coll Cardiol 2000;33:71A.

199. Vakili BA, Brown DL. Influence of gender on in-hospital outcomes of patients undergoing primary percutaneous transluminal coronary angioplasty for acute myocardial infarction; New York State experience. J Am Coll Cardiol 2000;35:72A.

200. Mattos L, Grines C, Sousa JE, et al. One year follow-up after primary coronary interventions for acute myocardial infarction in diabetic patients: STENT-PAMI trial results. J Am Coll Cardiol 2000;35:72A.

201. Wong SC, Papadakos S, Rosenberg C, et al. The impact on diabetes mellitus on in-hospital clinical outcomes post-angioplasty. J Am Coll Cardiol 2000;35:72A.

202. Beygui F, Metzger JP, Le Feuvre C, et al. Coronary angioplasty with provisional stenting in dialysis patients: In-hospital and 6 month outcomes. J Am Coll Cardiol 2000;35:202A.

203. Mehran R, Dangas G, Gruberg L, et al. The detrimental impact of chronic renal insufficiency and diabetes mellitus on late prognosis after percutaneous coronary interventions. J Am Coll Cardiol 2000;35:203A.

204. Pereira CF, Bernardi V, Martinez J, et al. Diabetic patients with multivessel disease treated with percutaneous coronary revascularization had similar outcome than those treated with surgery: One year follow up results from two Argentine randomized studies (ERACI-ERACI II). J Am Coll Cardiol 2000;35:3A.

205. Lucas FL, Mc Grath PD, Malenka DJ, et al. Long term survival following CABG and PTCA in the elderly: A study of 4993 patients in northern New England. J Am Coll Cardiol 2000;35:219A.

206. Dambrin G, LeFeuvre C, Metzger J-P, et al. Comparison of coronary stenting in hemodialysis and non-hemodialysis patients. J Am Coll Cardiol 1999;33:92A.

207. The BARI Investigators. Seven-year outcome in the Bypass Angioplasty Revascularization Investigation (BARI) by treatment and diabetic status. J Am Coll Cardiol 2000;35:1122-9.

208. Kobayashi Y, Dangas G, Mehran R, et al. Stenting elderly patients in the new millennium: Results in the year 2000. J Am Coll Cardiol 2001;1189(27):52A.

209. Dangas G, Mehran, Lansky AJ, et al. Gender and racial differences in clinical outcomes after percutaneous coronary interventions. J Am Coll Cardiol 2001;37(2):15A.

210. Moussa I, Colombo A, DiMario C, et al. Long-term outcome of patients with versus without diabetes mellitus in the DESTINI trial. J Am Coll Cardiol 2001;37(2):65A.

211. Stuckey, Grines CL, Tcheng, et al. Does stenting and glycoprotein IIb/IIa receptor blockade improve the prognosis of diabetics undergoing primary angioplasty in acute myocardial infarction: The CADILLAC trial. J Am Coll Cardiol 2001;838(2):342A.

212. Abizaid A, Dangas G, Mehran R, et al. One-year results after multivessel stenting in diabetic vs. non-diabetic patients. J Am Coll Cardiol 2001;860(4):68A.

213. Whang W, Bigger T. Diabetes and outcomes of coronary artery bypass graft surgery in patients with severe left ventricular dysfunction: Results from the CABG patch trial database. J Am Coll Cardiol 2000;36:1166-72.

214. Batchelor W, Anstrom K, Muhlbaier H, et al. Contemporary outcome trends in the elderly undergoing percutaneous coronary interventions: Results in 7,472 octogenarians. J Am Coll Cardiol 2000;36:723-30.

215. Ang P, Omar Farouque HM, Harper R,et al. Percutaneous coronary intervention in the elderly: A comparison of procedural and clinical outcomes between the eighth and ninth decades. J Invas Cardiol 2000;12:488-494.

216. Best P, Lennon R, Ting H, et al. Even mild renal insufficiency is associated with increased mortality after percutaneous coronary interventions. J Am Coll Cardiol 2001;37(2):76A.

217. Best P, Lennon R, Ting H, et al. The safety of abciximab before percutaneous coronary revascularization in patients with chronic renal insufficiency. J Am Coll Cardiol 2001;37(2):4A.

218. Moschi G, Antoniucci D, Valkenti R, et al. Primary PTCA in the elderly. Results in patients aged 80 years or above. Circulation 1998;98 (Suppl I): I-153.

219. Shawl FA, Lapetine FL, Kadra WY, et al. Stent supported carotid angioplasty (SSCA) has more favorable outcome in octogenarians compared to non-octogenarians. Circulation 1998;98 (Suppl I): I-304.

220. Wong PMT, Piamsombonn C, Mathur A, et al. Efficacy of coronary stenting in the management of cardiac allograft vasculopathy. Am J Cardiol 1998 Jul 15;82:239-41.

221. Trabattoni D, Montorsi P, Loaldi A, et al. How is the outcome of coronary stenting in the elderly compared to younger patients? J Am Coll Cardiol 2001;37(2):160A.

222. Baklanov D, Marcu CB, Chawarski C, et al. Coronary stenting is safe and effective in high risk octogenarian patient cohort. J Am Coll Cardiol 2001;37(2):161A.

223. Watanabe C, Maynard C, Ritchie JL, et al. Short-term outcomes following coronary artery stenting: Higher mortality and bypass surgery rates in women compared with men. J Am Coll Cardiol 2001;37(2):9A.

224. Thompson T, Mahoney EM, Valedar E, et al. Gender differences among patients undergoing coronary revascularization. Results from the National Cardiovascular Network (NCN). J Am Coll Cardiol 2001;37(2):16A.

225. Sousa A, Mattos L, Costa M, et al. In-hospital outcome after stenting in women compared to men. Results from the Registry of the Brazilian Society of Interventional Cardiology: CENIC. J Am Coll Cardiol 2001;37(2):16A.

226. Seldis S, Morrison DA, Sethi G, et al. Percutaneous coronary intervention versus coronary bypass graft surgery: Outcome of diabetics in the AWESOME randomized trial and registry. J Am Coll Cardiol 2001;37(2):336A.

227. Kugelmass AD, Mehta S, Simon AW, et al. Gender differences in outcomes among diabetic patients undergoing percutaneous coronary interventions. J Am Coll Cardiol 2001;37(2):65A.

228. Rinder M, Tamirisa P, Lasala J, et al. Hemodialysis and major adverse cardiac events after stenting: Results from the TOPPS trial. J Am Coll Cardiol 2001;37(2):68A.

II

Intervention by
Lesion Morphology
and Location

OVERVIEW OF INTERVENTIONAL DEVICES

Robert D. Safian, M.D.
Mark S. Freed, M.D.

Several interventional devices are now widely used for percutaneous coronary revascularization, including balloon angioplasty, atherectomy, lasers, and stents (Tables 8.1-8.4). Although non-balloon devices have been developed to address the known limitations of PTCA, with few exceptions, no clear advantage over PTCA has been demonstrated. Nevertheless, certain commercially-available devices or device combinations may have value for treating selected lesion morphologies and angiographic complications.

A. LIMITATIONS OF INTERVENTIONAL DEVICES

1. **Failure to Cross a Chronic Total Occlusion with a Guidewire.** This common and important problem precludes PTCA, atherectomy, lasers, and stenting. Potential remedies include prolonged infusions of thrombolytic drugs and investigational devices such as rotational angioplasty (ROTACS), vibrational angioplasty, therapeutic ultrasound, optical coherence reflectometry, and the excimer laser guidewire (Chapter 16). In contrast, failure to cross a subtotal occlusion is extremely rare and is usually due to severe target vessel tortuosity; these cases can usually be managed by special guidewire and guiding catheter techniques (Chapters 11, 16).

2. **Failure to Cross a Lesion with a Device.** Once the target lesion has been crossed with a guidewire, percutaneous intervention may be unsuccessful due to the inability to access the lesion with the intended device. These failures may be due to proximal vessel tortuosity (Chapter 11) or severe lesion calcification (Chapter 12), precluding passage of inflexible devices such as DCA or stents; these cases can often be managed by PTCA. At times, severe lesion rigidity or calcification precludes passage of even low-profile balloons. Such failures can often be treated by Rotablator atherectomy (Chapter 27), followed by definitive lumen enlargement with stents, PTCA, or DCA. Intravascular ultrasound (IVUS) can be used to assess the extent and distribution of calcium to guide debulking (Chapters 12, 31).

3. **Failure to Dilate or Deploy a Device.** Once a target lesion has been crossed with a guidewire and the intended device has been properly positioned, failure of intervention may be due to the inability to fully dilate or deploy the device. In some PTCA cases, extreme lesion rigidity precludes full balloon expansion despite high pressure balloons. Such failures can often be treated by the use of Rotablator (Chapter 27), excimer laser (Chapter 30), or DCA (Chapter 28). In other cases, full balloon expansion is readily achieved, but significant elastic recoil limits adequate lumen enlargement (Chapter 13); this problem can often be managed by stents (Chapter 26), Rotablator (Chapter 27), or DCA (Chapter 28).

Table 8.1. Interventional Devices

Percutaneous Transluminal Coronary Angioplasty (PTCA)*

Atherectomy Devices
    Directional coronary atherectomy (DCA)*
    Transluminal extraction catheter (TEC)*
    High-speed rotational atherectomy (Rotablator)*
    Pullback atherectomy catheter (PAC)
    Rotary atherectomy system (X-Sizer)

Lasers
    Excimer laser coronary angioplasty (ELCA)*
    Infrared laser coronary angioplasty (ILCA)
    Excimer laser guidewire

Stents
    Balloon-expandable stents
    Self-expanding stents
    Hybrid stents
    Autologous vein graft or PTFE-covered stents
    Radioactive stents
    Drug-coated stents
    Biodegradable stents

Thermal Devices
    Laser balloon angioplasty**
    Physiologic low-stress angioplasty (PLOSA)**
    Radiofrequency balloon

Other Devices
    Thrombectomy devices (AngioJet,* Hydrolyzer)
    Cutting balloon angioplasty*
    Local drug delivery systems*
    Vascular brachytherapy systems*
    Therapeutic ultrasound
    Vibrational angioplasty
    Low-speed rotational angioplasty catheter system (ROTACS)
    Distal embolic protection devices (GuardWire, others)
    Percutaneous vascular closure devices*

*   FDA-approved
**   Removed from market

Table 8.2. Coronary Atherectomy Devices: Technical Features

| | Atherectomy Method | | |
	Directional	Rotational	Extractional
Names	Directional coronary atherectomy (DCA) AtheroCath	Rotablator	Transluminal Extraction Catheter (TEC)
Description	Nonflexible housing with window on one side and balloon on other side. Cup-shaped cutter inside housing is connected to a drive cable. Hollow nosecone is tapered and acts as a specimen collection chamber	Spindle-shaped, diamond-coated brass burr connected to a flexible drive housed in 4F Teflon sheath. Compressed air turbine controls speed of rotation	Stainless steel conical cutting blades attached to a hollow torque tube. Vacuum bottle creates constant suction during cutting
Method of action	Atheroma situated in cutting window is excised and stored in nosecone collection chamber for retrieval; "Dotter" and angioplasty effects also operative	Preferential pulverization of hard atheromatous tissue and relative sparing of plaque-free wall. Particles pass through coronary microcirculation	Simultaneous excision and aspiration of particulate slurry (atheroma, clot, saline)
Rotational speed	1500-2000 rpm. Controlled by hand-held battery-powered, motor drive unit; speed not adjustable	150,000-200,000 rpm. Controlled by compressed air turbine; speed adjustable by foot pedal	750 rpm. Controlled by trigger on hand-held, battery-powered motor drive unit; speed not adjustable
Saline irrigation during device activation	No	Yes; lubricates and cools rotation system	Yes; creates particulate effluent for aspiration
Cutter movement	Rotating cutter moves forward in stationary housing; excision during cutter advancement	Rotating burr tracks through lesion over guidewire; pulverization during burr advancement	Rotating cutter tracks through lesion over guidewire; cutting during advancement
Adjunctive PTCA	70-90%	> 90%	> 90%
FDA Status	Approved	Approved	Approved

Table 8.3. Coronary Laser Systems: Technical Features

	Excimer Laser	Holmium
Description	Multi-element fiber passes over 0.014" guidewire. Short (2-3 sec) laser bursts. Adjunctive PTCA required in most cases. Tissue contact not required	Multi-element fiber passes over 0.014" guidewire. Tissue contact not required
Mechanism	Vaporization; acoustic shock or pressure waves; minimal thermal effects	Vaporization; acoustic shock or pressure waves; minimal thermal effects
Laser characteristics: Media Wavelength Mode	Xenon Chloride Ultraviolet Pulsed	Holmium:YAG Infrared Pulsed
FDA status	Approved	Investigational

Table 8.4. Intracoronary Stents: Technical Features

	NIR®/NIROYAL™ Elite (BSC)[++]	Radius™ (BSC)	Wallstent™ (BSC)	BX-Velocity™ (Cordis/J & J)
Expansion	Balloon	Self	Self	Balloon
Material	Stainless steel Gold-plated[+]	Nitinol	Platinum/cobalt	Stainless steel
Configuration	Closed cell, transformable geometry	Multisegmented slotted tube, square struts	Woven wire mesh, round wires	Curved sections and interconnected N-links
Strut thickness (mm/inch)	0.1 / 0.004	0.11 / 0.0045	0.08 / 0.003	0.14 / 0.0055
Metal surface area (%)	12 - 16	20	14	15-20
Shortening (%)	< 5	< 5	15-20	< 1.5 mm
Recoil (%)	< 0.5	0	0	0
Delivery sheath	No	Yes	Yes	No
Delivery profile (mm)	1.1 - 1.2	1.42	1.53	1-1.2
Minimum guide ID (in)	0.064	0.066	0.064	0.067
Length (mm)	9,12,15,18,25,31	14,20,31	17-48	8,13,18,23,28,33
Expanded diameter (mm)	2.5-4.0	3.0-4.0[‡]	3.5-6.0[†]	2.25-5.0
Deployment pressure (atm)	8	NA	NA	10-16
Rated burst pressure (atm)	16	NA	NA	16

AVE = Arterial Vascular Engineering; BSC = Boston Scientific Scimed; J & J = Johnson & Johnson
+   NIROYAL
†   For vessels 3.0-5.5 mm in diameter
‡   For vessels 2.75-4.25 mm in diameter
++ Manufactured by Medinol; distributed by Boston Scientific Scimed
NA = not available

Table 8.4. Intracoronary Stents: Technical Features

Multi-Link TETRA™ (Guidant)	Multi-Link ULTRA™ (Guidant)	BeStent™2 (Medtronic AVE)	S660™ (Medtronic AVE)	S670™ (Medtronic AVE)
S.T.E.P™ Balloon	Balloon	Balloon	Balloon	Balloon
Stainless steel	Stainless steel	Stainless steel	Stainless steel	Stainless steel
Slotted tube, multiple corrugated rings connected with multiple links	Slotted tube, multiple corrugated rings connected with multiple links	Laser-cut tubular stent system with Discrete Technology	Sinusoidal rings, elliptorectangular elements	Sinusoidal ring elements, elliptorectangular struts
VTS™ Technology 0.09-0.12 / 0.036-0.0049	0.13 / 0.005	0.085 / 0.033	0.13 x 0.15 / 0.005	0.13 x 0.15 / 0.005 x 0.006
14	19	12 - 17	~ 20	17 - 23
2.7	2.7	~ 0⁺	~ 1.5	3.5
< 2	1.7	< 2.2	~ 2	1.5
No	No	No	No	No
1.0-1.2	1.4-1.42	~ 1.0	1.0	1.1
0.056	0.066-0.075	0.064	0.064	0.064
8,13,18,23,28,33,38	13,18,28,38	9,12,15,18,24,30	9,12,15,18,24	9,12,15,18,24,30
2.5-4.0 Post-expansion 4.5	3.5-5.0 Post-expansion 5.5	3.0-4.5 (USA)	2.5	3.0-4.0
8 (nominal)	9 (nominal)	8	8	8
16	14	16 (3.0, 3.5 mm) 15 (4.0 mm)	16	16 15 (4.0 mm)

AVE = Arterial Vascular Engineering; BSC = Boston Scientific Scimed; J & J = Johnson & Johnson
†   For vessels 3.0-5.5 mm in diameter
‡   For vessels 2.75-4.25 mm in diameter
++ Manufactured by Medinol; distributed by Boston Scientific Scimed
NA = not available
VTS = Variable Thickness Strut

4. **Dissection and Acute Closure.** Severe dissection and abrupt closure complicate 2-10% of PTCA procedures, increasing the risk of death, MI, and emergency bypass surgery (Chapter 20). Neither laser nor atherectomy has been shown to reduce the incidence of acute closure or associated clinical complications. In contrast, the coronary stent has proven to be highly effective in treating dissection, reversing acute closure, and improving clinical outcome (Chapter 26). Intravascular ultrasound is often useful to optimize stent implantation, evaluate the cause of angiographic "haziness" after stenting (which may be due to nonobstructive plaque or occult dissection), and identify the cause of stent thrombosis (Chapters 26, 31).

5. **Thrombus and Distal Embolization.** Intraluminal thrombus reduces procedural success and increases the risk of ischemic complications after percutaneous intervention. Hydrodynamic thrombectomy devices (e.g., AngioJet, Hydrolyser) (Chapter 9), TEC atherectomy (Chapter 29), and platelet IIb/IIIa receptor antagonists (Chapter 34) may reduce CK elevation after treatment of thrombotic lesions. The GuardWire distal embolic protection device was recently shown to reduce distal embolization and ischemic complications by 50-60% during vein graft intervention in the SAFER trial (Chapter 17).

6. **Recurrent Ischemia and Restenosis.** Restenosis is the most important long-term limitation of percutaneous intervention. Stents offer the best opportunity for primary prevention of restenosis in native coronary arteries and saphenous vein grafts. Intravascular ultrasound may optimize stent results and possibly reduce target lesion revascularization, particularly in patients at high-risk for restenosis. No adjunctive therapy has clearly been shown to prevent restenosis; cilostazol, local delivery of antiproliferative drugs, vascular gene therapy, and radiation therapy show promise but require further study. Stents are also the preferred interventional device for restenotic lesions after balloon angioplasty or atherectomy. The FDA had approved the use of gamma- and beta-radiation for the treatment of in-stent restenosis, which has been shown to reduce the risk of subsequent restenosis by 30-50% (Chapter 24). Unresolved issues include the optimal dose, duration, and timing of brachytherapy; the value of adjunctive therapy (e.g., platelet receptor antagonists; debulking vs. dilating prior to brachytherapy); and the prevention of late thrombosis and edge effect ("candy-wrapper" lesions).

B. EVALUATION OF INTERVENTIONAL DEVICES (Table 8.5)

1. **Procedural Success.** The "preferred" definition of procedural success is final diameter stenosis < 50% in the absence of a major complication (death, Q-wave MI, or emergency CABG). Nevertheless, other definitions are frequently used, including angiographic success (final diameter stenosis < 50%), device success (decrease in diameter stenosis > 20%), and clinical success (procedure success without an early clinical event). It is important to verify that similar definitions are used when comparing different studies. When two devices are used in succession to treat a lesion (e.g., Rotablator followed by adjunctive PTCA for calcified stenoses), "procedural success" frequently refers to final outcome. In reality, four outcomes are possible (Figure 8.1): (1) device success and PTCA success; (2) device success and PTCA failure; (3) device failure and PTCA

success; and (4) device failure and PTCA failure.   There is ongoing debate as to whether angiographic and clinical outcomes should be reported after each device, or only from the final result.   The problem in reporting results only at the end of the procedure is that it overestimates the value of a bad device that is salvaged by a good device, and underestimates the value of a good device that is followed by a bad device.   Furthermore, prognostic information may be lost when results are not recorded after each device; even when salvaged by PTCA, abrupt closure after TEC, ELCA, or Rotablator strongly predicted subsequent ischemic complications (Chapter 20).

2.   **Assessment of Lumen Enlargement.**   Conventional measures of lumen enlargement include absolute lumen dimensions (minimal lumen diameter, reference diameter) and percent diameter stenosis.   However, use of these measures is confounded by several factors, including differences in device size, vessel size, and device "efficiency" (i.e., ratio of final lumen diameter-to-device diameter.   Available studies suggest that the efficiency of lumen enlargement for some lasers, atherectomy devices, and stents is superior to PTCA; however, the magnitude of lumen enlargement (assessed by absolute dimensions and diameter stenosis) is limited by the small sizes of devices (particularly for ELCA, TEC, and Rotablator).

3.   **Relationship Between Immediate Lumen Enlargement and Late Outcome.**   Several studies suggest an inverse relationship between post-procedural lumen diameter and angiographic restenosis (i.e., "bigger is better").   While these studies found that device type itself had little if any impact on restenosis, other studies suggest the contrary: In the ERBAC trial, a trend toward *more* restenosis was observed in the Rotablator and excimer laser groups (vs. PTCA) despite *larger* post-procedural lumen diameters (Chapter 30).   Very high (> 70%) restenosis rates were also reported after laser balloon angioplasty despite excellent initial lumen enlargement.   One study of matched lesions also suggested that DCA may result in more intimal hyperplasia than PTCA or stents.   In CAVEAT-I, despite *greater* acute gain and a larger final lumen, DCA patients had a *higher* incidence of late myocardial infarction compared to PTCA patients (Chapter 28).   Collectively, these data suggest that the final lumen diameter and possibly the device type (i.e., type of vessel injury) impact on late lumen dimensions and restenosis.   Furthermore, attainment of a larger post-procedural lumen diameter does not ensure a lower incidence of cardiac events or restenosis.

C.   **IMPORTANT CONSIDERATIONS IN USING INTERVENTIONAL DEVICES.**   Over the last 5 years, enormous experience has been achieved with newer atherectomy, laser, and stent devices.   The use of a lesion-specific, multi-device approach may optimize results and decrease complications.

1.   **Facilitated Lumen Enlargement.**   There is a growing impression among interventionalists that sequential use of two different devices may improve procedural outcome compared to using one device.   When atherectomy or laser angioplasty is followed by PTCA, this approach has been called *facilitated angioplasty*; the use of two different non-balloon devices (e.g., Rotablator, TEC, or

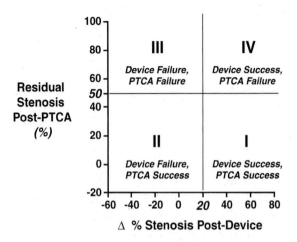

Figure 8.1 Angiographic Outcomes After Interventions with Devices and Adjunctive PTCA

ELCA followed by DCA or stent) has been called *transcatheter device synergy*. Observational studies suggest a possible role for plaque debulking with Rotablator (Chapter 27) or DCA (Chapter 28) prior to stenting for certain lesion morphologies. Facilitated lumen enlargement is only one aspect of the broader concept of "facilitated intervention," which considers the impact of two or more devices used in succession on procedural complications, late outcome, and cost.

2. **Lesion-Specific Approach to Coronary Intervention (Table 8.6).** Current studies have failed to demonstrate major differences in overall outcome between patients treated with PTCA, laser, or atherectomy. Laser and atherectomy devices appear to have fairly narrow "niche" applications (Chapters 27-29). In contrast, coronary stents have superior results compared to PTCA for a broad range of lesion morphologies and now account for 60-80% of all percutaneous interventions. Nevertheless, certain lesion subsets are more amenable to some devices than others:

   a. **Bifurcation lesions (Chapter 10).** Treatment of bifurcation lesions includes PTCA, debulking with Rotablator or DCA followed by PTCA or stenting, or primary stenting using several different technical approaches.

   b. **Calcified lesions (Chapter 12).** Focal, calcified lesions are best treated by Rotablator followed by PTCA (with a noncompliant balloon) or stenting. The ideal treatment of long, calcified lesions is unknown.

   c. **Ostial lesions (Chapter 14).** Aorto-ostial and branch ostial lesions are best managed by atherectomy (Rotablator or DCA) followed by PTCA or stenting, or by primary stenting alone. PTCA without debulking is not recommended. The cutting balloon may be useful for noncalcified ostial lesions.

d. **Long lesions and small vessels (Chapter 15).** Long lesions may be treated by PTCA with acceptable success rates, although the risk of acute closure and restenosis is increased compared to focal lesions; atherectomy offers no clear advantage over PTCA. Two stenting techniques have been used for diffuse disease: Stenting long segments of disease between normal proximal and distal vessels, or "spot stenting" more focal areas of severe disease amidst longer segments of diffuse disease; the best approach is unknown. Acceptable success and complication rates can be obtained in small vessels using PTCA, or stenting; preliminary data from randomized trials suggest a possible advantage for stents.

e. **Chronic total occlusion (Chapter 16).** Although the presence of a chronic total occlusion was once a contraindication to stenting, most randomized trials demonstrate less restenosis, reocclusion, and target vessel revascularization compared to PTCA. Stents also hold promise for the management of totally occluded vein grafts, although progressive disease at non-stented sites is a persistent cause of graft failure.

f. **Saphenous vein grafts (Chapter 17).** Vein grafts $\geq$ 3 mm in diameter are usually treated by stenting, and ostial lesions are treated by balloon-expandable stents to minimize elastic recoil. Useful adjuncts include distal embolic protection devices, AngioJet or TEC for thrombus, and IVUS. Diffusely degenerated vein grafts remain problematic for all interventional devices (Chapter 17).

3. **Adjunctive Imaging Techniques.** Intravascular ultrasound, coronary angioscopy, and the intracoronary Doppler flowire and pressure wire may have important uses as adjuncts to percutaneous intervention. Intravascular ultrasound (Chapter 31) is useful for assessing vessel dimensions prior to and following intervention, identifying the extent and distribution of calcification, and possibly optimizing stenting and DCA. Coronary angioscopy (Chapter 32) is superior to angiography in evaluating intraluminal thrombus and dissection. Doppler flow and pressure measurements (Chapter 33) may be valuable for assessing the physiologic response to catheter-based intervention and predicting complications. All of these techniques may be used to evaluate "borderline lesions" prior to intervention and suboptimal or hazy results after intervention, and assist in decision-making (e.g., device selection, need for further intervention).

Table 8.5. Efficacy and Safety of Interventional Devices

	PTCA	DCA	TEC	ROTA	ELCA	Stent
Success	≥ 90%	-	-	-	-	-
Acute Closure	4-5%	-	-	-	-	↓
Dissection	30%	↓↓	↑	↓	↑	↓↓
Spasm	1-2%	-	↑	↑	↑	↓
MI: Q-wave	1%	-	-	-	-	-
non Q-wave	1-2%	↑	-	↑	-	-
CABG	2%	-	-	-	-	-
Death	<1%	-	-	-	-	-
Perforation	0.3%	↑	↑	↑	↑	-
Restenosis	30-50%	-	-	-	-	↓
Adjunctive PTCA	NA	70-80*	90	90	90	100

Abbreviations: DCA = directional coronary atherectomy; ELCA = excimer-laser coronary angioplasty; NA = not applicable
ROTA = Rotablator; TEC = transluminal extraction catheter atherectomy
- Equivalent rate/risk
↑ Increased risk
↓ Decreased risk
* Optimal atherectomy technique

4. **Adjunctive Pharmacotherapy.** Aspirin, heparin, and clopidogrel (for stenting) are the mainstays of interventional pharmacotherapy. There are also compelling data to support the routine use of platelet glycoprotein IIb/IIIa receptor antagonists in patients with and without acute coronary syndromes undergoing percutaneous revascularization. Various combinations of IIb/IIIa inhibitors, heparin (unfractionated or low-molecular-weight), fibrinolytics, and direct thrombin inhibitors are under evaluation prior to, during, and after coronary intervention for stable and unstable ischemic syndromes (Chapter 34). Direct thrombin inhibitors (lepirudin, argatroban) are approved for procedural anticoagulation in patients with heparin-induced thrombocytopenia. Other useful therapies include intracoronary calcium antagonists, sodium nitroprusside, or adenosine for no-reflow (Chapter 21), and possibly superselective infusions of thrombolytics for chronic total occlusion (Chapter 16). Local drug delivery systems may further improve the efficacy of adjunctive medical therapy (Chapter 35). Vascular gene therapy, serotonin antagonists, thromboxane inhibitors, prostacyclin analogues, ADP antagonists and other antiplatelet agents await further investigation.

Table 8.6. Interventional Devices: Lesion-Specific Indications

Lesion Morphology	PTCA	Stent	DCA	ROTA	TEC	ELCA
Elective Use						
Eccentric	+	+	+	+	-	-
Ulcerated	+	+	+	+	-	-
Ostial	-	+	+	+	-	+
Total occlusion	+	+	-	+/-	+/-	+/-
Bifurcation	+	+/-	+	+/-	-	-
Diffuse Disease	+	-	-	+/-	-	+/-
Thrombus	-	-	-	-	+	+/-
Severe angle	+	-	-	-	-	-
Suboptimal PTCA						
Focal dissection	+/-	+	-	-	-	-
Long dissection	+/-	+	-	-	-	-
Elastic	-	+	+	+	-	-
Rigid	-	-	+	+	-	+/-

Abbreviations: DCA = directional coronary atherectomy; ELCA = excimer laster coronary angioplasty; PTCA = percutaneous transluminal coronary angioplasty; ROTA = Rotablator; TEC = transluminal extraction catheter
\+ Favorable
\- Unfavorable

C. CARDIOVASCULAR RISK REDUCTION. Proper control of dyslipidemia and hypertension reduces the risk of death, MI, and stroke by 50-80%. These and other risk reduction measures are described in Chapter 41.

* * * * *

9 INTRACORONARY THROMBUS

Daniel T. Lee, M.D.
Robert D. Safian, M.D.

Among patients undergoing PTCA for medically refractory acute coronary syndromes, the incidence of thrombus is 40% by angiography and 90% by angioscopy.[1-4] Compared to lesions without thrombus, PTCA of thrombotic lesions is associated with an increased risk of acute thrombotic occlusion, emergency bypass surgery, myocardial infarction, and death.[5-25,164] Likewise, new intraluminal filling defects left untreated after PTCA markedly increase the risk of abrupt closure (7-fold), emergency CABG (20-fold), and major adverse cardiac events (4-fold).[161] Various pharmacologic and mechanical approaches have been employed with the hope of providing safe revascularization for these patients, although optimal therapy awaits definition.

A. **DEFINITION AND DETECTION.** Since there is no uniform angiographic definition of intracoronary thrombus, the rates of intracoronary thrombus vary widely between studies. The strictest angiographic criteria require definite intraluminal globular filling defects in multiple angiographic views or, if the vessel is totally occluded, a convex margin that stains with contrast and persists for several cardiac cycles.[1-3] Angiographic assessment of thrombus is sometimes based on the "thrombus score" (0 = no thrombus; 1 = intraluminal haziness; 2 = definite thrombus < ½ vessel diameter; 3 = definite thrombus 0.5-2 vessel diameters; 4 = definite thrombus > 2 vessel diameters).[174,175] Angiography has poor sensitivity (as low as 19%) for detecting intracoronary thrombus, but specificity approaches 100% when strict definitions are used.[12-25] Predictive accuracy for visual assessment is even worse after intervention, as filling defects due to dissection or plaque separations are not readily distinguished from thrombus. Direct visualization by coronary angioscopy (Chapter 32) is the best method for detecting intraluminal thrombus, followed by intravascular ultrasound (Chapter 31) and contrast angiography.[28,168] Filling defects on angiography often corresponded to red thrombus on angioscopy, whereas hazy lesions may be white thrombus, intimal disruptions, or smooth plaque.[17]

B. **PATHOPHYSIOLOGY.** Ulceration and rupture of lipid-rich atheroma activate the extrinsic pathway of coagulation and initiate intracoronary thrombosis[29-32,38] (Chapter 40). Thrombus formation results in a spectrum of clinical manifestations ranging from silent occlusion to acute myocardial infarction or sudden death. Intimal and medial dissection after PTCA resembles the deep vascular injury of spontaneous plaque rupture and is a powerful stimulus for thrombus formation.

Table 9.1. Impact of Pre-Procedural Thrombus On PCI Outcome

Series	N	Description	Results
Cafri[142] (2001)	82 24	Thrombus-Immediate PCI Thrombus-Delayed PCI	Combined endpoint (residual thrombus, distal embolization, no-reflow, acute closure, acute stent thrombosis) higher with immediate PCI compared to delayed PCI after drug therapy (27% vs. 4.2%, $p \leq 0.018$)
Singh[177] (2000)	2406 1508	No thrombus Thrombus	Thrombus group had lower procedural success and higher in-hospital death (odds ratio 2.09, $p = 0.02$). No impact of thrombus on late survival
EPIC[129] (1998)	849 496 710	No thrombus Possible thrombus Thrombus	Angiographic thrombus had highest risk of acute closure (13% vs. 11% vs. 7.6%, $p < 0.01$), but had no impact on 30-day or 6-month clinical outcome; benefit of abciximab was similar for all groups
Giri[140] (1998)	507	Thrombus score in patients treated with PTCA for acute MI	High thrombus score was associated with more angiographic (no-reflow, distal embolization, TIMI flow < 3) and clinical complications
Shah[128] (1996)	573 4098	Unstable or post-infarct angina with thrombus Unstable or post-infarct angina without thrombus	Thrombus group had more acute closure (13.4% vs. 8.4%) and MI (5.1% vs. 3.2%)
White[20] (1996)	74	Angioscopic thrombus in 61%	Thrombus group had more in-hospital ischemia (16% vs. 10%, $p = 0.03$) and major cardiac events (14% vs. 2%, $p = 0.03$)
Mehran[39] (1995)	245	Randomized trial of IC urokinase vs. placebo	Urokinase group had more abrupt closure (15% vs. 5.9%, $p = 0.03$) and major cardiac events (17.3% vs. 6.8%, $p = 0.02$)
Hillegass[21] (1995)	238 1476 450	Unstable angina with thrombus Unstable angina; no thrombus Stable angina	Thrombus group had lower success (80%) and more acute closure (11%) and CABG (9%). PTCA outcome was similar for unstable angina without thrombus and stable angina groups
Tan[22] (1995)	46	Thrombus in 3.6% of 1248 lesions	Thrombus group had more acute closure (8.7% vs 3.1%, $p = 0.04$)
Violaris[23] (1994)	159	Thrombus in 4.5% of 3529 lesions	Thrombus group had more late reocclusion (13.8% vs 5.3%, $p < 0.001$)
Tenaglia[24] (1994)	93	Thrombus in 12% of 779 lesions	Thrombus group had more acute closure (6.1-fold)
Myler[25] (1992)	82	Thrombus in 10.5% of 779 lesions	Thrombus group had more major cardiac events (7.3% vs. 1%, $p > 0.003$). All events occurred in patients receiving urokinase

Table 9.1. Impact of Pre-Procedural Thrombus On PCI Outcome

Series	N	Description	Results
Pavlides[40] (1991)	30	IC urokinase: 250,000-500,000 over 20 min; IV urokinase: 250,000-3 MU over 30-60 min	Urokinase did not improve PTCA success, but reduced cardiac event rate (19% vs. 3%)
	27	No urokinase	
Chapekis[41] (1991)	21	Continuous IC urokinase (120,000 U bolus; 120,000 U/hr x 24 hrs). IV Heparin: 1000 U/hr.	Distal embolization (5%); no acute closure
Kiesz[42] (1991)	29	IC urokinase (250,000 U bolus every 5 min, up to 1.5 MU or until thrombus resolves)	Complete resolution of thrombus (83%); PTCA success (93%)
Mooney[8] (1990)	112	Aspirin, dipyridamole, nifedipine; intraprocedural heparin (IV 10,000 U and IC 3000 U). Balloon:artery ratio = 1.2	Acute closure (7%); nonobstructive residual thrombus (24%); emergency or elective CABG (7%)
Lasky[43] (1990)	35	Aspirin, heparin pre-PTCA	PTCA success (94% vs. 61%); acute closure (6% vs. 33%)
	18	Aspirin, no heparin pre-PTCA	
Deligonul[7] (1988)	45	Aspirin pre-procedure (84%); heparin 5-10,000 U bolus (65%)	Distal embolization and/or thrombotic occlusion (31%)
Sugrue[6] (1986)	34	Aspirin, dipyridamole, IV heparin (5-10,000 U bolus, infusion x 24 hrs)	Acute occlusion (24%)

Abbreviations: IC = intracoronary; IV = intravenous; CABG = coronary artery bypass surgery; MU = million units; MI = myocardial infarction; EPIC = Evaluation of c7E3 for the Prevention of Ischemic Complications; PCI = percutaneous coronary intervention

C. **PTCA AND THROMBOTIC LESIONS (Table 9.1).**[5-8,20-25,40-48,164] PTCA of thrombotic lesions is associated with an increased risk for acute occlusion, distal embolization, and no-reflow compared to PTCA of lesions without thrombus. The risk for ischemic complications is greatest for thrombotic vein grafts.[39] Aspirin and heparin are the mainstays of therapy, while randomized data suggest that routine use of thrombolytic agents may lead to an adverse outcome.[39] Pretreatment with abciximab has been evaluated in high-risk patients (many with thrombus) undergoing PTCA, DCA, or stenting. EPIC, EPILOG, and EPISTENT all showed highly significant reductions in early and late cardiac events,[129,167-171] particularly with respect to CK release (Chapter 34). In contrast, hirulog was not superior to heparin for thrombus-containing lesions.[164]

D. **NON-BALLOON DEVICES AND THROMBOTIC LESIONS (Tables 9.2, 9.3).** Data from the NACI Registry and others demonstrated that patients with intracoronary thrombus had more LV dysfunction, multivessel disease, prior CABG, prior MI, and unstable angina than patients without thrombus.[44] Furthermore, intracoronary thrombus was associated with a 2.8-fold higher risk of major complications, and the presence of thrombus dramatically influenced device selection: Thrombus was present in 2% of Rotablator, 5-11% of ELCA, 10% of DCA, and 41% of TEC cases. Outcome after new device interventions in vein grafts was related more to thrombus and lesion length rather than to device selection per se.[45] Recent data indicate that distal embolic protection devices may improve the safety of percutaneous revascularization for thrombotic lesions in native vessels and vein grafts (Chapters 17, 36); the SAFER trial reported 50-60% reductions in ischemic complications using the GuardWire during vein graft intervention.

1. **Directional Atherectomy (DCA) (Chapter 28).**[46-54] Early studies reported greater procedural success and fewer complications in patients with thrombus, compared to patients without thrombus.[46] More recent data indicate that thrombus, unstable angina, and recent MI increase the risk for ischemic complications and emergency CABG after DCA, so we generally avoid DCA in lesions with thrombus.

2. **Rotablator.** Intracoronary thrombus is considered a contraindication to Rotablator atherectomy due to the increased risk of distal embolization and no-reflow.

3. **Extraction Atherectomy (TEC) (Chapter 29).** TEC atherectomy is commonly used for thrombus extraction, and angioscopic studies confirm its efficacy.[55,56] Nevertheless, the presence of thrombus in native vessels or vein grafts was the strongest independent predictor for major in-hospital complications after TEC in the NACI Registry (odds ratio 3.4).[152] Furthermore, dissections are common after TEC, and no-reflow or distal embolization may occur in 8-12% of vein grafts.[57] Restenosis rates are also high. Compared to PTCA of degenerated vein grafts, one study demonstrated less CK elevation after TEC.[59] Similar results were reported in TOPIT, which randomized patients to TEC or PTCA in thrombus-containing lesions in native vessels or vein grafts (Table 9.4); the magnitude of reduction in CK elevation was similar to that seen with prophylactic use of abciximab.

4. **Excimer Laser Angioplasty (ELCA) (Chapter 30).** Although lasers have not been shown to be thrombogenic in animal models,[69,70] relatively few patients with thrombus have been treated.[74] In a report from the Excimer Laser Coronary Angioplasty Registry,[76] procedural success was 81% in thrombotic lesions and 90% in simple lesions; distal embolization occurred in 5.7%. Others have also reported lower clinical success in thrombotic lesions (58% vs. 95% for nonthrombotic lesions, p = 0.0001).[71] By multivariate analysis, the presence of thrombus was identified as the most important determinant of procedural failure. Others have reported considerable success in patients with thrombotic lesions.[132] Excimer laser usage has declined dramatically in recent years and is rarely used today.

Table 9.2. Comparison of Mechanical Techniques for Thrombotic Lesions

Device	Mechanism	Advantages	Disadvantages	Status
TEC	Cut, aspirate plaque and thrombus	Efficient extraction of fresh thrombus	Less useful for extraction of organized thrombus and plaque; frequent dissection; small diameter (1.8-2.5 mm)	FDA approved
AngioJet	Thrombus removal by Venturi effect	Removes large, fresh thrombus	Bradycardia, no-reflow; not useful for organized thrombus; temporary pacemaker recommended	FDA approved
Hydrolyzer	Thrombus removal by Venturi effect	Ease of use	Bulky, inflexible; poor for organized thrombus	Investigational
Sonicath	Ultrasound thrombolysis	Flexible	Limited experience	Investigational
Acolysis	Ultrasound thrombolysis	Flexible	Limited experience	Investigational

5. **Stents (Chapter 26).** The presence of intraluminal thrombus is no longer considered a contraindication to stent insertion.[76,127,136,148] Stent coatings with heparin, silicone carbide, and various other materials may further reduce thrombogenicity.[147] Several observational and multicenter randomized trials have confirmed the safety and efficacy of stent implantation in patients with acute myocardial infarction and unstable angina (Chapters 5, 26).

6. **AngioJet (Figure 9.1).** The AngioJet is a percutaneous rheolytic thrombectomy catheter that removes thrombus via the Venturi effect. The 5F double-lumen catheter is highly flexible, utilizes a 0.014-inch guidewire, and requires an 8F guiding catheter (internal diameter $\geq$ 0.080 inches). The AngioJet has been successfully used for thrombotic vein grafts (Chapter 17) native coronary arteries, acute MI,[130,131] and stent thrombosis. Clinical trials in Europe and the United States have been completed, and the AngioJet was recently approved by the FDA (Tables 9.5, 9.6).[80,126,132]

E. INVESTIGATIONAL TECHNIQUES (Tables 9.2, 9.5, 9.7, 9.8)
1. **Suction Thrombectomy.** First described in 1994,[78] recent results indicate successful removal of thrombus in 77% of patients, which was associated with a marked improvement in antegrade flow.[133]

2. **Hydrolyser Catheter.** Fajadet initially described vein graft thrombectomy in 7 patients utilizing a 7F Hydrolyser catheter,[79] which is a double-lumen catheter that aspirates thrombus via the Venturi effect. A 6F device was later studied in a small number of patients[149,156] but is not yet FDA approved in the United States.

Table 9.3. Impact of Non-Balloon Devices On Thrombus

Series	N	Device	Outcome
Meany[60] (1995)	183	TEC (SVG)	Angiographic success not affected by thrombus
Dooris[63] (1995)	59	TEC (SVG)	Thrombus associated with lower clinical success (69% vs. 88%) and more angiographic and clinical complications (no-reflow, Q-wave MI)
Al-Shaibi[59] (1995)	124	TEC (SVG)	Less CK elevation compared to PTCA
Moses[57] (1995)	59	TEC	Thrombus associated with distal embolization after TEC
Baumbach[72] (1994)		ELCA	Thrombus associated with a 6.4-fold decrease in procedural success
O'Neill[44] (1993)	345	Various	Thrombus associated with lower angiographic success (85% vs. 93%, p < 0.001), more embolization (6% vs. 0.6%, p < 0.001), and more cardiac events (9% vs. 3%, p < 0.001)
Emmi[47] (1993)	58	DCA	Thrombus associated with more ischemic complications (15.5% vs. 7.9%, p = 0.06) and CABG (10.3% vs. 3.9%, p = 0.03)
Estella[71] (1993)	12	ELCA	Thrombus associated with lower clinical success (58% vs. 95%, p < 0.0001)

Abbreviations: TEC = transluminal extraction catheter; SVG = saphenous vein graft; ELCA = excimer laser coronary angioplasty; DCA = directional coronary atherectomy; MI = myocardial infarction; CK = creatinine kinase; CABG = emergency coronary artery bypass surgery

3. **Ultrasound (Tables 9.2, 9.7).** Therapeutic ultrasound may ablate fresh thrombus and produce coronary vasodilation,[81-83] particularly when enhanced by perfluorocarbon (PFC) emulsions. These devices utilize a 4.2F monorail catheter (compatible with 7-8F guiding catheters and 0.014-inch guidewires) that unsheathes a solid probe connected to a piezoelectric transducer. Electrical energy is converted to mechanical motion at the probe tip, resulting in thrombus ablation. Adjunctive PTCA or stenting is usually required.[154,155] The ATLAS (Acolysis during Treatment of Lesions Affecting SVGs) trial is a multicenter randomized trial to evaluate acolysis vs. abciximab in thrombotic vein grafts; results are pending. The ATLAS MI trial is a multicenter registry evaluating acolysis in patients with acute MI and saphenous vein graft occlusion.

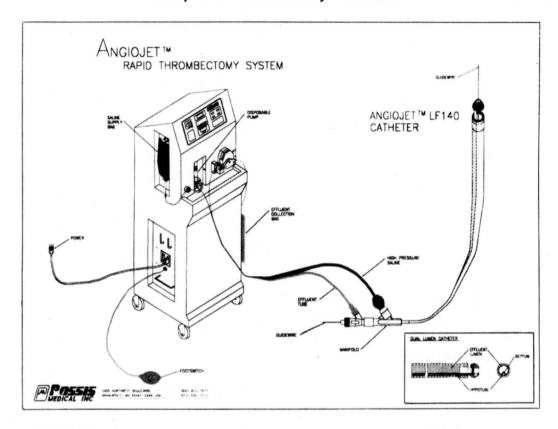

Figure 9.1. Possis AngioJet

4. **Radiofrequency-Balloon Angioplasty.** Radiofrequency energy can modify thrombus-containing lesions.[84,85] Clinical investigations are pending.

F. PHARMACOLOGIC THERAPY OF PRE-EXISTING THROMBUS (Chapters 5, 34).

1. **Heparin and Aspirin.** PTCA of thrombus-containing lesions has been associated with acute closure in up to 20% of patients;[5-7] pretreatment with a 2-14 day course of heparin and aspirin has been shown to reduce the risk of PTCA in some studies, but not in others.[32,43,86-89] Recent data suggest that high-dose intravenous heparin (ACT > 350-400 seconds) is associated with lower rates of abrupt closure. High-dose intracoronary heparin may be associated with arrhythmic complications because of its polyvalent anionic nature and should be avoided. Local delivery of heparin (4000 units) resulted in high intramural levels that persisted for several days and a 60% reduction in platelet deposition. Further studies of local drug delivery to prevent thrombotic complications are pending.

2. **Thrombolytic Therapy.** The efficacy of thrombolysis as adjunctive therapy for thrombotic lesions is controversial. Although older observational studies suggested a role for intracoronary thrombolytic therapy when thrombus was present prior to (Table 9.1) or after PTCA (Table 9.8),[9,40,41,42,90-98] systemic thrombolytic therapy has consistently failed to result in clinical benefit for patients with unstable angina and non-Q-wave MI despite modest angiographic improvement.[95] The TAUSA study showed that patients with angina at rest had similar outcomes with or without intracoronary urokinase,[96] and that urokinase administration was associated with more acute closure.[39] Similar findings were observed in other clinical trials of acute MI and unstable angina (Chapter 5). Possible explanations for the disappointing results of adjunctive thrombolysis include enhanced platelet aggregation and worsening stenosis from intramural hemorrhage after PTCA. Based on available data, we generally avoid thrombolytics during interventional procedures, although some operators use prolonged (8-24 hour), low-dose intracoronary or intragraft lytic infusions for resistant chronic total occlusions (Figure 9.2, Chapter 16). In contrast to systemic or intracoronary lytic infusions, preliminary data using pulse-infusion thrombolysis (PIT), which involves high-pressure spray injections of concentrated fibrinolytic agents directly into thrombus, suggest some benefit for reducing distal embolization and no-reflow.[143,157] The Dispatch-Urokinase Efficacy Trial (DUET) is a multicenter randomized trial designed to assess locally delivered urokinase vs. conventional therapy in thrombotic lesions; results are pending. In the United States, concerns about contamination of urokinase resulted in its withdrawal from the market. Similar lytic infusions are performed with t-PA or r-PA (Chapters 17, 39).

Table 9.4. Early Results of TOPIT Trial: TEC Or PTCA In Thrombus-Containing Lesions[176]

	TEC	PTCA	p-Value
N	131	134	
Success (%)	98	97	NS
MACE (%)	4.5	11.2	0.06
CK elevation (%)	4.5	15.4	0.03
Final diameter stenosis (%)	27	26	NS
Dissection (%)	38	29	0.04
Distal embolization (%)	2	4	NS
No-reflow (%)	5	8	NS
Perforation (%)	0	0.7	NS
Final TIMI flow < 3 (%)	2	3	NS

Abbreviations: CK = creatine kinase; MACE = major adverse cardiac events (death, MI, acute closure, rePTCA, CABG); TOPIT = Transluminal Extraction Atherectomy Or PTCA in Thrombus-Containing Lesions

3. **Antiplatelet and Antithrombotic Drugs (Table 9.9, Chapters 5, 34).** Except for abciximab,[113] results with other potent antiplatelet and antithrombin agents for bailout indications are either lacking or have been disappointing.

4. **Local Drug Delivery (Table 9.7).** [114-117,124] To improve thrombus dissolution and avoid the side effects of systemic therapy, local delivery of heparin, thrombolytics, and other agents is under continued investigation (Chapters 5, 35). A variety of catheters have been developed including the Dispatch catheter, hydrogel-coated balloon, and Transport catheter (Chapter 35).[138,165-167]

G. **POST-PTCA THROMBUS.**[60,61,113,118-123] Post-procedural thrombus is difficult to detect, since "haziness" is most often due to intimal dissection. Thrombolytic therapy has been used in several small series with equivocal results (Table 9.8), and the results of rescue abciximab in native vessels and vein grafts (by intravenous or local delivery) have been mixed (Table 9.9).[138,141,145,158,160,163] Further controlled trials are needed.

H. **STENT THROMBOSIS (Chapter 26).** Stent thrombosis is usually a manifestation of suboptimal stent deployment due to incomplete expansion, inadequate apposition, or unstented residual disease or dissection. If stent thrombosis occurs, remedial causes should be sought and corrected (Chapter 26). The AngioJet is highly effective in removing fresh thrombus in this setting. The utility of rescue abciximab requires further study.[159]

Table 9.5. Results of Mechanical Thrombectomy for Thrombotic Lesions

Series	N	Device	Outcome
Ischinger[135] (2000)	106	X-SIZER (acute coronary syndromes)	Able to reach target lesions (76%); stenosis reduction or improvement $\geq$ 1 TIMI flow grade without MACE (81% of successful deployments); adjunctive PCI (98%)
DeLago[179] (2000)	46	AngioJet (acute MI)	Procedure success (96%); TIMI 3 flow (100%); distal embolization (6%); PTCA/stenting (89%)
Nakagawa[130] (1998)	31	AngioJet (acute MI)	Procedure success (94%); angiographic restenosis (21%); adjunctive PTCA (97%)
Silva[131] (1998)	70	AngioJet (acute MI)	Clinical success at 30 days (90%); adjunctive PTCA or another device (95%)
VEGAS-2[136] (1998)	346	AngioJet vs. urokinase	Procedure success (86% vs. 80%); 30-day MACE (20% vs. 38%)
Van den Bos[149] (1997)	7	Hydrolyzer	Thrombus removal (100%); distal embolization (14%); subacute reocclusion (14%)
van Ommen[156] (1997)	31	Hydrolyzer	Thrombus removal (94%); distal embolization (6%); adjunctive PTCA, stent, or lytics (90%)

Abbreviations: MACE = major adverse cardiac events; VEGAS = Vein Graft AngioJet Study

Table 9.6. Results of Multicenter AngioJet Trials[172,173]

	VEGAS-2 Randomized Trial		Registry	
	AngioJet	**Urokinase**	**Acute MI**	**Lytic Exclusion**
No. Patients	180	169	107	105
Success (%)				
Lesion	87.6	79.6	83.0	77.9
Procedure	86.3	72.2	77.1	76.0
Device	87.4	75.3	82.9	76.9
Final Diameter Stenosis (%)	22	28	24	24
MACE (30 days) (%)				
Death	1.7	3.0	7.5	1.9
CK-MB elevation	15.6	32.5	13.1	23.8
Myocardial infarction	11.1	19.5	3.7	14.3
Q-wave	2.2	5.3	0	1.0
non-Q-wave	8.9	14.2	3.7	13.3
TLR	3.3	3.6	2.8	5.7
Acute closure	3.3	4.7	4.7	5.7
Bleeding	5.0	11.8	13.1	12.4
Vascular	4.4	17.8	12.1	9.5
Stroke	1.7	1.2	1.9	1.0
Length of Stay (days)	4.1	4.9	-	-
Cost (US dollars)				
Procedure	8669	10,520	-	-
Total	17,314	22,932	-	-

Abbreviations: MACE = major adverse cardiac events; TLR = target lesion revascularization; VEGAS = Vein Graft AngioJet Study; - = not reported

Table 9.7. Results of Mechanical Thrombolysis

Series	N	Technique	Setting	Outcome
Ishibashi[143] (1999)	43	PIT	Native (acute MI)	Compared to primary PTCA, PIT was associated with less distal embolization and no-reflow, but no difference in procedural success or reocclusion
Rosenschein[155] (1999)	20	UT	SVG	Procedural success (65%); distal embolization (5%); adjunctive PTCA or stent (100%)
Barsness[138] (1998)	58	LD (abciximab, Dispatch)	SVG	Significant improvement in thrombus score and stenosis severity, but not TIMI flow; adjunctive stent (88%)
Fajadet (1998)	100	UT	Native, SVG (Acolysis Registry)	Successful recanalization (95%); adjunctive PTCA or stent (94%)
Murakami[153] (1998)	43	AT	Acute MI	Successful reperfusion for AT + PTCA (91%), but similar to PTCA alone
Papadokos[133] (1998)	73	AT	Native, SVG	Successful aspiration of thrombus or plaque (77%); marked improvement in TIMI-flow; adjunctive stenting (100%)
Glazier[165] (1997)	95	LD (UK, HCB)	Acute MI, unstable angina	Resolution of thrombus (82%); significant improvement in thrombus score and TIMI flow abrupt closure (3.2%); distal embolization (1.1%); no-reflow (1.1%)
Glazier[166] (1997)	15	LD (UK, Dispatch)	SVG	Significant improvement in thrombus score and TIMI flow; procedural success (93%)
Hamm[154] (1997)	13	UT	Native (acute MI)	TIMI-3 flow after UT + PTCA (86%)
Stefanidis[146] (1997)	10	AVGCS	Acute MI	Immediate success (100%); subacute thrombosis (10%)
ACUTE[150] (1997)	15	UT	Native (acute MI)	TIMI-3 flow (87%); adjunctive PTCA (10%)

Abbreviations: ACUTE = Analysis of Coronary Ultrasound Thrombolysis Endpoints in Acute MI; AT = aspiration thrombectomy; AVGCS = autologous vein graft coated stent; HCB = hydrogel-coated balloon; LD = local delivery; PIT = pulse infusion thrombolysis; SVG = saphenous vein graft; UK = urokinase; UT = ultrasound thrombolysis

Table 9.8. Results of Thrombolytic Therapy for Post-Procedural Thrombus

Series	N	Adjunctive Therapy	Results
Ishibashi[143] (1999)	43	Pulsed-infusion thrombolysis (PIT) prior to PTCA for acute MI	PIT was associated with less distal embolization and no-reflow, but no difference in procedural success or reocclusion
Grines[118] (1995)	34	IC lytics during primary PTCA	Post-PTCA thrombus was not predictive of ischemic events; more ischemia after lytics (18.4% vs. 10.6%, p = 0.10)
Lincoff[120] (1992)	43	IC urokinase or t-PA for abrupt closure	PTCA success (44%) not related to lytics
Chapekis[41] (1991)	12	IC urokinase (120,000 U bolus, 120,000 U/hr x 24 hrs); IV heparin (1000 U/hr)	Acute closure (8%)
Pavlides[119] (1991)	256	Urokinase	Major cardiac events increased (21% vs 9%, p = 0.01) when UK was used for abrupt closure
deFeyter[121] (1991)	34	IC urokinase	Success (65%)
Herrmann[40] (1990)	55	IC t-PA (20 mg bolus followed by 50 mg IV infusion over 1-2 hr)	Less CABG in t-PA vs. PTCA groups (1.8% vs. 6.8%)
Schieman[9] (1990)	48	IC urokinase (100,000-250,000 units over 20-65 min); heparin infusion and aspirin for 5 days	No in-hospital re-PTCA, MI, or death
Haft[122] (1990)	36	IC urokinase or t-PA	Success (72%)
Gulba[123] (1990)	27	IC and IV t-PA	Initial success (82%); reocclusion within 36 hours (55%)

Abbreviations: IC = intracoronary; IV = intravenous; t-PA = tissue plasminogen activator; CABG = emergency coronary artery bypass surgery

Table 9.9. Results of Rescue IIb/IIIa Inhibitors and Hirulog for Thrombus

Series	N	Adjunctive Therapy	Results
ESPIRT[144] (2001)	77	Rescue eptifibatide for thrombotic complications (42%)	Bailout therapy was associated with more MI (30% vs. 7%, p = 0.01) and urgent PCI at 48 hours (14% vs. 0%, p = 0.03) compared to "no bailout"
Fuchs[137] (2000)	298	Rescue abciximab for thrombus, dissection Type $\geq$ C, no-reflow, suboptimal result, or distal embolization	Stents in 73%. In-hospital results: death (1.3%); Q-MI (0.7%); non-Q-MI (31%); TLR (4.6%). Late events: death (1.7%); MI (2.7%); TVR (15.1%); EFS at 1-yr (83%)
Velianou[139] (2000)	186	Abciximab (planned 45%; rescue for threatened or acute closure 55%)	In-hospital results (planned vs. rescue): death (1.2% vs. 1.0%); Q-MI (2.4% vs. 2.0%); non-Q-MI (7% vs. 12.9%); TLR (1.2% vs. 0%). 6-month results (planned vs. rescue): death (2.3% vs. 4.0%); MI (9.4% vs. 14.9%); TVR (4.7% vs. 20.8%, p = 0.001)
de Lemos[132] (2000)	92	Rescue abciximab (n = 29) vs. no abciximab (n = 63); TIMI 14 substudy	Abciximab group had greater ST-segment resolution 90-180 minutes after PCI
Piamsomboon[178] (1999)	73	Abciximab (planned 74%; rescue 26%) in acute coronary syndromes with thrombus-containing lesions	Death (1.4%); Q-wave MI (1.4%); non-Q-wave MI (18%). No subacute thrombosis, emergency CABG, or repeat PTCA
Ahmed (1999)	45	Rescue abciximab in degenerated SVG	No benefit on procedural success or major ischemic complications compared to "no-abciximab"; more non-Q-MI in rescue group (40.5% vs. 17.7%)
Fuchs[145] (1999)	186	Rescue abciximab for thrombus and suboptimal PTCA	Procedural success (95.3%); in-hospital MACE (4.7%); non-Q-MI (24.7%); 1-year TLR (24.9%) and EFS (71%)
Haase[163] (1999)	63	Rescue abciximab for thrombus and threatened or acute closure	Repeat PTCA 2 minutes after abciximab. Marked improvement in thrombus score and TIMI flow; MACE (2%); late TVR (15%)
Sullebarger[162] (1999)	17	Planned abciximab and TEC in SVG	Abciximab was associated with higher procedural success (100% vs. 50%) and less distal embolization/no-reflow (0% vs. 30%) compared to "no abciximab"
Barsness[138] (1998)	58	Local delivery of abciximab in thrombotic SVG	Significant improvement in thrombus score and stenosis severity, but not TIMI flow. Adjunctive stent (88%)
Garbarz[160] (1998)	138	Rescue abciximab for thrombus and suboptimal PTCA	Angiographic success in 84% (100% success for stent thrombosis); adjunctive PTCA or stent (100%); MACE (17%); bleeding and vascular complications (27%); transfusion (5%)

Table 9.9. Results of Rescue IIb/IIIa Inhibitors and Hirulog for Thrombus

Series	N	Adjunctive Therapy	Results
Grantham[141] (1998)	185	Planned and unplanned (rescue) abciximab in thrombotic SVG	Procedural success higher with planned abciximab; no impact of abciximab on angiographic (distal embolization, no-reflow) or clinical complications
Henry[159] (1998)	16	Rescue abciximab for acute stent thrombosis	Recurrent thrombosis after PTCA for stent thrombosis may respond to abciximab
Muhlestein[158] (1997)	29	Rescue abciximab for thrombus after PCI	Procedural success (97%), clinical success (93%). Significant improvement in thrombus score and TIMI flow, without distal embolization or no-reflow
Shah[164] (1997)	567	Hirulog vs. heparin for thrombus-containing lesions (Hirulog Angioplasty Study)	Thrombus-containing lesions were associated with more MI (5.1% vs. 3.2%) and abrupt closure (13.6% vs. 8.3%); no difference between hirulog and heparin in acute or late outcomes

Abbreviations: EFS = event-free survival; MACE = major adverse cardiac events; PCI = percutaneous coronary intervention; Q-MI = Q-wave myocardial infarction; SVG = saphenous vein graft; TIMI = Thrombolysis in Myocardial Infarction; TLR= target lesion revascularization

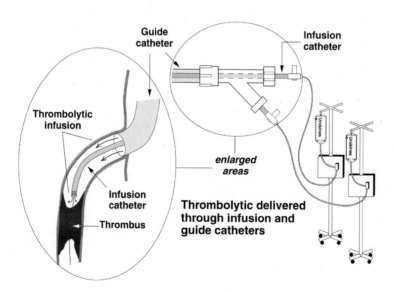

Figure 9.2. Setup for Intracoronary Thrombolytic Infusion

* * * * *

REFERENCES

1. Ambrose JA, Winters SL, Stern A, et Al. Angiographic morphology and the pathogenesis of unstable angina pectoris. J Am Coll Cardiol 1985;5:609-616.

2. Fuster V, Badimon L, Badimon J, et al. The pathogenesis of coronary artery disease and the acute coronary syndromes. N Eng J Med 1992;326:242-250.

3. Cowley MJ, DiSciascio G, Vetrovec GW. Coronary thrombus in unstable angina: Angiographic observations and clinical relevance. In Hugenholtz PG and Goldman BG (eds): Unstable Angina: Current Concepatients and Management. Schattauer Press, Stuttgart, 1985;95-102.

4. Gotoh K, Minamino T, Katoh O, et al. The role of intracoronary thrombus in unstable angina: Angiographic assessment and thrombolytic therapy during ongoing anginal attacks. Circulation 1988;77:526-534.

5. Mabin TA, Holmes DR, Smith HC. Intracoronary thrombus role in coronary occlusion complicating PTCA. J Am Coll Cardiol 1985;5:198-202.

6. Sugrue DR, Holmes DR, Smith HC. Coronary artery thrombus as a risk factor for acute vessel occlusion during PTCA: Improved results. Br Heart J 1986;53:62-66.

7. Deligonul V, Gabliani GI, Caroles DG, et al. PTCA in patients with intracoronary thrombus. Am J Cardiol 1988;62:474-476.

8. Mooney MR, Fishman-Mooney J, Goldenberg I, et al. Percutaneous transluminal coronary angioplasty in the setting of large intracoronary thrombus. Am J Cardiol 1990;65:427-431.

9. Schieman G, Cohen BM, Kozina J, et al. Intracoronary urokinase for intracoronary thrombus accumulation complicating percutaneous transluminal coronary angioplasty in acute ischemic syndromes. Circulation 1990;82:2052-2060.

10. Yanagida S, Mizuno K, Miyamolo A. Comparison of findings between coronary angiography and angioscopy. Circulation 1989;80 (Supp II):376.

11. Ramee SR, White CJ, Collins TJ, et al. Percutaneous angioscopy during coronary angioplasty using a steerable microangioscope. J Am Coll Cardiol 1991;17:100-105.

12. Mizuno K, Satumora K, Miyamoto A, et al. Angioscopic evaluation of coronary-artery thrombi in acute coronary syndromes. New Engl J Med 1992;326:287-291.

13. Mizuno K, Miyamoto A, Satomura K, et al. Angioscopic coronary macromorphology in patients with acute coronary disorders. Lancet 1991,337:809-812.

14. Mizuno K, Hikita H, Miyamoto A, Satomura K, et al. The pathogenesis of an impending infarction and its treatment - an angioscopic analysis. Jpn Circ J 1992, 56:1160-5.

15. Hombach V, Hoher M, Kochs M, Eggeling T, et al. Pathophysiology of unstable angina pectoris-correlations with coronary angioscopic imaging. Eur Heart J 1988,;9:40-5.

16. Waxsman S, Sassower M, Zarich S, et al. Angioscopy can identify lesion specific predictors of early adverse outcome following PTCA in patients with unstable angina. Circulation 1994;90:I-490.

17. Manzo K, Netso R, Sassower M, Leeman D, et al. Coronary lesion morphology by angioscopy vs angiography: The ability to detect thrombi. J Am Coll Cardiol 1994: 955-4023.

18. Annex BH, Ajluni SC, Larkin TJ, O'Neill WW, Safian RD. Angioscopic guided interventions in a saphenous vein bypass graft. Cathet Cardiovasc Diagn 1994;31:330-3.

19. den Heijer P, Foley D, Escaned J, Hillege HL, Serruys PW, Lie KI. Angioscopic versus angiographic detection of intimal dissection and intracoronary thrombus. J Am Coll Cardiol 1994;955-100.

20. White CJ, Ramee SR, Collins TJ, et al. Coronary thrombi increase PTCA risk: Angioscopy as a clinical tool. Circulation 1996:93:253-258.

21. Hillegass WB, Ohman EM, O'Hanesian MA, et al. The effect of preprocedural intracoronary thrombus on patient outcome after percutaneous coronary intervention. J Am Coll Cardiol 1995;21:94A

22. Tan K, Sulke N, Taub N, Sowton E. Clinical and lesion morphologic determinants of coronary angioplasty success and complications: Current experience. J Am Coll Cardiol 1995;25:855-65.

23. Violaris AG, Herrman JP, Melkert R, et al. Does local thrombus formation increase long-term luminal renarrowing following PTCA? A quantitative angiographic analysis. J Am Coll Cardiol 1994;February Special Issue:139A.

24. Tenaglia A, Fortin D, Califf R, Frid D, et al. Predicting the risk of abrupt vessel closure after angioplasty in an individual patient. J Am Coll Cardiol 1994;24:1004-11.

25. Myler R, Shaw R, Stertzer S, Hecht H, et al. Lesion morphology and coronary angioplasty: Current experience and analysis. J Am Coll Cardiol 1992;19:1641-52.

26. Sherman CT, Litvack F, Grundfest W, Lee M, et al. Coronary angioscopy in patients with unstable angina pectoris. N Engl J Med 1986, 315:913-9.

27. den Heijer P, van Dijk RB, Hillege HL, et al. Serial angioscopic and angiographic observations during the first hour after successful coronary angioplasty: A preamble to a multicenter trial addressing angioscopic markers for restenosis. Am Heart J 1994;128:656-63.

28. Siegel RJ, Fischbein MC, Chae JS, Helfant RH, Hickey A, Forrester JS. Comparative studies of angioscopy and ultrasound for the evaluation of arterial disease. Echocardiography 1990;7:495-502.

29. Chesebro J, Zoldhelyi P, Fuster V: Pathogenesis of Thrombosis in Unstable Angina. Am J Cardiol 1991;68:2B-10B.

30. Fuster V, Lewis A. Conner Memorial Lecture. Mechanisms leading to myocardial infarction: Insights from studies of vascular biology. Circulation 1994;90:2126-2146.

31. Kawai C. Pathogenesis of acute myocardial infarction: Novel regulatory system of bioactive substances in the vessel wall. Circulation 1994; 90:1033-1043.

32. Jang Y, Lincoff AM, Plow EF, Topol EJ. Cellular adhesion molecules in coronary artery disease. J Am Coll Cardiol 1994;24:1591-601.

33. Lefkovits J, Topol EJ. Direct thrombin inhibitors in cardiovascular medicine. Circulation 1994; 90:1522-1536.

34. Davies MJ, Thomas, AC. Plaque fissuring-the cause of acute myocardial infarction, sudden ischemic death, and crescendo

angina. Br Heart J 1985;53:363-373.

35. Falk E. Plaque rupture with severe pre-existing stenosis precipitating coronary thrombosis. Characteristics of coronary atherosclerotic plaques underlying fatal occlusive thrombi. Br Heart 1983;50:127-134.

36. Davies MJ, Bland JM, Hangartner JRW, et al. Factors influencing the presence of absence of acute coronary artery thrombi in sudden ischemic death. Eur Heart J 1989;10:203-208.

37. Badimon L, Badimon JJ, Gahez A, et al. Influence of arterial damage and wall shear forces on platelet deposition. Ex vivo study u.a. swine model. Arteriosclerosis 1986;6:312-330.

38. Fernandez-Ortiz A, Badimon JJ, Falk E, et al. Characterization of the relative thrombogenicity of atherosclerotic plaque components: implications for consequences of plaque rupture. J Am Coll Cardiol 1994;23:1562-9.

39. Mehran R, Ambrose JA, Bongu M, et al. Angioplasty of complex lesions in ischemic rest angina: Results of the thrombolysis and angioplasty in unstable angina (TAUSA) trial. J Am Coll Cardiol 1995;26:961-966.

40. Pavlides GS, Schreiber TL, Gangadharan V, et al. Safety and efficacy of urokinase during elective coronary angioplasty. Am Heart J 1991;121:731-736.

41. Chapekis AT, George BS, Candela RJ. Rapid thrombus dissolution by continuous infusion of urokinase through an intracoronary perfusion wire prior to and following PTCA: Results in native coronaries and patent saphenous vein grafts. Cathet Cardiovasc Diagn 1991;23:89-92.

42. Kiesz R, Hennecken J, Bailey S. Bolus administration of intracoronary urokinase during PTCA in the presence of intracoronary thrombus. Circulation 1991;84:II-346.

43. Laskey MAL, Deutsch E, Barnathan E, et al. Influence of heparin therapy on percutaneous transluminal coronary angioplasty outcome in unstable angina pectoris. Am J Cardiol 1990;65:1425-1429.

44. O'Neill WW, Sketch MH Jr, Steenkiste A, Detre K. New device intervention in the treatment of intracoronary thrombus: Report of the NACI registry. Circulation 1993;88:I-595.

45. Sketch MH Jr, Davidson CJ, Popma J, et al. Morphologic and quantitative predictors of acute outcome with new devices in saphenous vein grafts. J Am Coll Cardiol 1994; 90:219A.

46. Holmes DR, Ellis SG, Garratt KN. Directional coronary atherectomy for thrombus-containing lesions: Improved outcome. Circulation 1991;84:II-26.

47. Emmi R, Movsowitz H, Manginas A, Wells E, et al. Directional coronary atherectomy in lesions with co-existing thrombus. Circulation 1993;88:I-596.

48. Cowley MJ, Whitlow PL, Baim DS, et al. Directional coronary atherectomy of saphenous vein graft narrowings: Multicenter investigational experience. Am J Cardiol 1993;72:30E-34E17.

49. Cowley MJ. DiSciascio G. Experience with directional atherectomy since pre-market approval. Am J Cardiol 1993;72:12E-20E.

50. Sabri MN, Johnson D, Warner M, Cowley MJ. Intracoronary thrombolysis followed by directional atherectomy. A combined approach for thrombotic vein graft lesions considered unsuitable for angioplasty. Cathet Cardiovasc Diagn 1992;26:15-18.

51. Saito S, Arai H, Kim K, Aoki N, et al. Primary directional atherectomy for acute myocardial infarction. Cathet Cardiovasc Diagn 1994;32:44-48.

52. Topol EJ, Leya F, Pinkerton CA, et al. A comparison of directional atherectomy with coronary angioplasty in patients with coronary artery disease. N Engl J Med 1993;329:221-7.

53. Adelman AG, Cohen EA, Kimball BP, et al. A comparison of directional atherectomy with balloon angioplasty for lesions of the left anterior descending coronary artery. N Engl J Med 1993;329:228-33.

54. Abdelmeguid AE, Ellis SG, Sapp SK, et al. Directional coronary atherectomy in unstable angina pectoris. J Am Coll Cardiol 1994;24:46-54.

55. Annex BH, Larkin TJ, O'Neill WW, Safian RD. Evaluation of thrombus removal by transluminal extraction atherectomy by percutaneous coronary angioscopy. Am J Cardiol 74:606-609.

56. Kaplan B, Safian RD, Goldstein JA, Grines CL, O'Neill WW. Efficacy of angioscopy in determining the effectiveness of intracoronary urokinase and TEC atherectomy thrombus removal from an occluded saphenous vein graft prior to stent implantation. Cathet Cardiovasc Diagn 1995;36:335-337.

57. Moses J, Yeh W, Popma J, Sketch M, NACI Investigators. Predictors of distal embolization with the TEC catheter: A NACI registry report. J Am Coll Cardiol 1995;27:179A.

58. Hong M, Wong S, Popma J, et al. Favorable results of debulking followed by immediate adjunct stent therapy for high-risk saphenous vein graft lesions. J Am Coll Cardiol February Special Issue, 1996.

59. Al-Shaibi KF, Goods C, Jain S, Negus B, et al. Does transluminal extraction atherectomy reduce distal embolization in saphenous vein grafts? Circulation 1995;92:I-329.

60. Meany T, Leon M, Kramer B, Margolis J, et al. Transluminal extraction catheter for the treatment of diseased saphenous vein grafts: A multicenter experience. Cathet Cardiovasc Diagn 1995;34:112-120.

61. O'Neill WW, Kramer BL, Sketch MH et al. Mechanical extraction atherectomy. Report of the US transluminal extraction catheter investigation. Circulation 1992;86:I-79.

62. Annex BH, Larkin TJ, Safian RD. Evaluation of intracoronary thrombus by percutaneous coronary angioscopy before and after transluminal extraction atherectomy. Am J Cardiol 1994;74:606-609.

63. Dooris M, May M, Grines CL, Pavlides GS, et al. Comparative results of transluminal extraction atherectomy in saphenous vein graft lesions with and without thrombus. J Am Coll Cardiol 1995;25:1700-1705.

64. Safian RD, Grines CL, May MA, Lichtenberg A, et al. Clinical and angiographic results of transluminal extraction coronary atherectomy in saphenous vein bypass grafts. Circulation 1994;89:302-312.

65. Popma JJ, Leon MB, Mintz GS, Kent KH, et al. Results of coronary angioplasty using the transluminal extraction catheter. Am J Cardiol 1992;70:1526-32.

66. Hong MK, Popma JJ, Pichard AD, Kent et al. Clinical

significance of distal embolization after transluminal extraction atherectomy in diffusely diseased saphenous vein grafts. Am Heart J 1994;127:1496-503.

67. Moses JW, Tierstein PS, Sketch MH, et al. Angiographic determinants of risk and outcome of coronary embolus and myocardial infarction (MI) with the transluminal extraction catheter (TEC): A report from the New Approaches for Coronary Intervention (NACI) Registry. J Am Coll Cardiol 1994;February Special Issue:219A.

68. Larkin TJ, O'Neill WW, Safian RD, et al. A prospective study of transluminal extraction atherectomy in high-risk patients with acute myocardial infarction. J Am Coll Cardiol 1994;February Special Issue:226A.

69. Tomaru T, Nakamura F, Yanagisawa-Miwa A, et al. Reduced vasoreactivity and thrombogenicity with pulsed laser angioplasty: Comparison with balloon angioplasty. J Intervn Cardiol 1995;8:6:643-651.

70. Shefer A, Forrester JS, Litvack F. Recanalization of acute thrombus: Comparison of acute success and short-term patency after excimer laser coronary angioplasty, balloon angioplasty and intracoronary thrombolysis in pigs. J Am Coll Cardiol 1991;17:205A.

71. Estella P, Ryan TJ Jr, Landzberg JC, Bittl JA. Excimer laser assisted coronary angioplasty for lesions containing thrombus. J Am Coll Cardiol 1993;21:1550-6.

72. Baumbach A, Oswald H, Kvasnika J, Fleck E, et al. Clinical results of coronary excimer laser angioplasty: Report from the European Coronary Excimer Laser Angioplasty Registry. Eur Heart J 1994;15:89-95.

73. Cook Sl, Eigler NL, Shefer A, et al. Percutaneous excimer laser coronary angioplasty in lesions not ideal for balloon angioplasty. Circulation 1991;84:632-43.

74. Klein LW, Litvack F, Holmes D, et al. Prospective multicenter analysis of excimer laser coronary angioplasty (ELCA) in stenoses with complex morphology. J Am Coll Cardiol 1991:448A.

75. Chasteney EA, Ravichandran PS, Furnany AP, et al. Laser thrombolysis for bypass graft thrombosis. J Am Coll Cardiol 1994;February Special Issue:374A.

76. Grinstead WC, Kleiman NS, Marks GF, et al. Stenting of coronary arteries containing thrombus: Angiographic and clinical outcomes of 109 patients from the Gianturco-Roubin Flex-Stent™ Registry. J Am Coll Cardiol 1996.

77. Agrawal SK, Ho DSW, Liu M, Iyer S, et al. Predictors of thrombotic complications after placement of the flexible coil stent. Am J Cardiology Vol. 73; 1216-1219.

78. Dooris M, Grines CL. Successful reversal of cariogenic shock precipitated by saphenous vein graft distal embolization using aspiration thrombectomy. Cathet Cardiovasc Diagns 1994;33:267-71.

79. Fajadet J, Bar O, Jordan C, Robert G, et al. Human percutaneous thrombectomy using the new hydrolyser catheter: preliminary results in saphenous vein grafts. J Am Coll Cardiol 1994;February Special Issue:220A.

80. Ramee S, Kuntz R, Schatz R, et al. Preliminary experience with the POSSIS coronary AngioJet Rheolytic Thrombectomy Catheter in the VeGAS I Pilot Study. J Am Coll Cardiol 1996;27:69A.

81. Hartnell GG, Saxton JM, Friedl SE, Abela GS, Rosenchein U. Ultrasound thrombus ablation: in vitro assessment of a novel device for intracoronary use. J Interven Cardiol 1993;6:69-76.

82. Siegel RJ, Gunn J, Ahsan A, Fiscbein MC, et al. Use of therapeutic ultrasound in percutaneous coronary angioplasty. Experimental in vitro and initial clinical experience. Circulation 1994;89:1587-92.

83. Gal D, Monteverde C, Hogan J, et al. In vivo assessment of ultrasound angioplasty of fibrotic total occlusions. Circulation 1991;84:II-422.

84. Nardone D, Bravette B, Shi Y, et al. Effect of microwave thermal angioplasty on intracoronary thrombus. Circulation 1991;84:II-300.

85. Yamashita K, Satake S, Ohira H, Ohtomo K. Radiofrequency thermal balloon coronary angioplasty: A new device for successful percutaneous transluminal coronary angioplasty. J Am Coll Cardiol 1994;23:336-40.

86. Myler RK, Shaw NE, Stertzer SH, et al. Unstable angina and coronary angioplasty. Circulation 1990;82:88-95.

87. Hettleman BD, Aplin RA, Sullivan PR, et al. Three days of heparin pretreatment reduces major complications of coronary angioplasty in patients with unstable angina. J Am Coll Cardiol 1990;15:154A.

88. Pow TK, Varricchione TR, Jacobs AK, et al. Does pretreatment with heparin prevent abrupt closure following PTCA? J Am Coll Cardiol 1988;11:238A.

89. Lukas MA, Deutsch E, Hirshfeld JW Jr, et al. Influence of heparin therapy on percutaneous transluminal coronary angioplasty outcome in patients with coronary arterial thrombus. Am J Cardiol 1990;65:179-182.

90. Vaitkus PT, Laskey WK. Efficacy of adjunctive thrombolytic therapy in percutaneous transluminal coronary angioplasty. J Am Coll Cardiol 1994;24:1415-23.

91. Suryapranata H, DeFeyter PJ, Serruys PW. Coronary angioplasty in patients with unstable angina pectoris: Is there a role for thrombolysis? J Am Coll Cardiol 1988;12:69A-77A.

92. Goudreau E, DiSciascio G, Vetrovec GW, et al. Intracoronary urokinase as an adjunct to percutaneous transluminal coronary angioplasty in patients with complex coronary narrowings or angioplasty - induced complications. Am J Cardiol 1992;69:57-62.

93. Ambrose J, Torre S, Sharma S, et al. Adjunctive urokinase for PTCA in unstable angina. Circulation 1991;84:590.

94. Ambrose JA, Almeida OD, Sharma SK, et al. Adjunctive thrombolytic therapy during angioplasty for ischemic rest angina. Results of the TAUSA trial. Circulation 1994;90:69-77.

95. The TIMI IIIB Investigators. Effects of tissue plasminogen activator and a comparison of early invasive and conservative strategies in unstable angina and non Q wave myocardial infarction: Results of the TIMI IIIB trial. Circulation 1994;89:1545-1556.

96. The TIMI IIIA Investigators. Early effects of tissue-type plasminogen activator added to conventional therapy on the culprit coronary lesion in patients presenting with ischemic cardiac pain at rest. Results of the Thrombolysis in Myocardial Ischemia (TIMI IIIA) Trial. Circulation 1993;87:38-52.

97. Grines, C, Ajluni S, Savas V, Samyn J, Pavlides G, et al. Prolonged urokinase infusion for chronic total native coronary occlusions. J Am Coll Cardiol 1996;27

98. Hartmann JR, Mc Keever LS, Stamato NJ, et al. Recanalization of chronically occluded aortocoronary saphenous vein bypass grafts by extended infusion of urokinase: Initial results and short-term clinical follow-up. J Am Coll Cardiol 1991;18:1517-1523.

99. Taylor MA, Santoran EC, Aji J, Eldredge WJ, et al. Intracerebral hemorrhage complicating urokinase infusion into an occluded aortocoronary bypass graft. Cathet Cardiovasc Diagn 1994;31:206-210.

100. Brown DL, Topol EJ. Stroke complicating percutaneous coronary revascularization. Am J Cardiol 1993;72:1207-1209.

101. Gold GH, Gimple LW, Yasuda T, et al. Pharmacodynamic study of F (ab')2 fragments of murine monoclonal antibody 7E3 directed against human platelet glycoprotein IIb/IIIa in patients with unstable angina pectoris. J Clin Invest 1990;86:651-9.

102. Kleiman NS, Ohman EM, Ellis SG, et al. Profound inhibition of platelet aggregation with monoclonal antibody 7E3 Fab following thrombolytic therapy: Results of the TAMI 8 pilot study. Circulation 1993;86:I-260.

103. The EPIC Investigators. Use of a monoclonal antibody directed against the platelet glycoprotein IIb/IIIa receptor in high-risk coronary angioplasty. N Engl J Med 1994;330:956-61.

104. Topol EJ, Fuster V, Harrington RA, Califf RM, et al. Recombinant hirudin for unstable angina pectoris: a multicenter randomized trial. Circulation 1994;89:1557-1566.

105. Topol EJ, Bonan R, Jewitt D, Sigwart U, et al. Use of direct antithrombin, hirulog, in place of heparin during angioplasty. Circulation 1993;87:1622-1629.

106. van den Bos AA, Deckers JW, Heyndricks GR, et al. Safety and efficacy of recombinant hirudin (CGP 393) versus heparin in patients with stable angina pectoris undergoing coronary angioplasty. Circulation 1993;88:2058-2066.

107. Antmann EM, for TIMI 9A Investigators. Hirudin in acute myocardial infarction. A safety report from the Thrombolysis in Myocardial Ischemia (TIMI) 9A Trial. Circulation 1994;90:1624-30.

108. Neuhaus KL, Essen RV, Tebbe U, Jessel A, et al. Safety observations from the pilot phase of the randomized r-hirudin for improvement of thrombolysis (HIT-III) study. A study of the Arbeitsgemeinschaft Leitender Kardiologischer Krankenhausarzte (ALKK). Circulation 1994;90:1638-42.

109. The Global Use of Strategies to Open Occluded Coronary Arteries (GUSTO) II Investigators. Randomized trial of intravenous heparin versus recombinant hirudin for acute coronary syndromes. Circulation 1994;90:1631-7.

110. Lincoff AM, Topol EJ, Ellis SG. Local drug delivery systems for the prevention of restenosis. Circulation 1994;90:2070-2084.

111. Nunes GL, Hanson SR, King SB 3rd, et al. Local delivery of a synthetic antithrombin with a hydrogel-coated angioplasty balloon catheter inhibits platelet-dependent thrombosis. J Am Coll Cardiol 1994;23:1578-83.

112. McKay R, Fram DB, Hirst JA, Klernan FJ, et al. Treatment of intracoronary thrombus with local urokinase using a new, site-specific drug delivery system: The Dispatch catheter. Cathet Cardiovasc Diagn 1994;33:181-88.

113. Muhlestein JB, Gomez MA, Karagounis L, Anderson G. "Rescue ReoPro": Acute utilization of abciximab for the dissolution of coronary thrombus developing as a complication of coronary angioplasty. Circulation 1995;92:I-607.

114. Fram DB, Aretz T, Azrin MA, Mitchel JF,et al. Localized intramural drug delivery during balloon angioplasty using hydrogel-coated balloons and pressure augmented diffusion. J Am Coll Cardiol 1994;23:1570-7.

115. Plante S, Dupuis G, Mongeau CJ, Durand P. Porous balloon catheters for local delivery: Assessment of vascular damage in a rabbit iliac angioplasty model. J Am Coll Cardiol 1994;24:820-4.

116. Hong MK, Wong SC, Popma JJ, Kent KM, et al. A dual-purpose angioplasty-drug infusion catheter for treatment of intragraft thrombus. Cathet Cardiovasc Diagn 1994;32:193-5.

117. Gershony G, Glass PR. Coronary thrombosis: A novel catheter-based approach to treatment. Cathet Cardiovasc Diagn 1994;31:147-149.

118. Grines C, Brodi B, Griffin J, Donohue B, et al. Which primary PTCA patients may benefit from new technologies? Circulation 1995;92:I-146.

119. Pavlides G, Schreiber TL, Gangadharan V, et al. Safety and efficacy of urokinase during elective coronary angioplasty. Am Heart J 121:731, 1991.

120. Lincoff AM, Popma JJ, Ellis SG, et al. Abrupt vessel closure complicating coronary angioplasty: Clinical, angiographic and therapeutic profile. J Am Coll Cardiol 19:926, 1992.

121. de Feyter PJ, van den Brand M, Jaarman G, et al. Acute coronary artery occlusion during and after percutaneous transluminal coronary angioplasty. Circulation 83:927, 1991.

122. Haft JI, Goldstein JE, Homoud MK, et al. PTCA following myocardial infarction: Use of bailout fibrinolysis to improve results. Am Heart J 120:243, 1990.

123. Gulba DC, Daniel WG, Simon R, et al. Role of thrombolysis and thrombin in patients with acute coronary occlusion during percutaneous transluminal coronary angioplasty. J Am Coll Cardiol 16:563, 1990.

124. Kerensky RA, Franco EA, Bertolet BD, et al. Lysis of intravascular thrombus prior to coronary stenting using the dispatch infusion catheter. Cathet & Cardiovasc Diagn 1996;38:410.

125. van Ommen VG, van den Bos A, Pieper M, et al. Removal of thrombus from aortocoronary bypass grafts and coronary arteries using the 6Fr hydrolyser. Am J Cardiol 1997;79:1012-1016.

126. Hamburger J, Brekke M, di Mario C, et al. The Euro-ART study: An analysis of the initial European experience with the AngioJet rapid thrombectomy catheter. J Am Coll Cardiol 1997;29(Suppl. A):213A.

127. Alfonso F, Rodriguez P, Phillips P, et al. Clinical and angiographic implications of coronary stenting in thrombus-containing lesions. J Am Coll Cardiol 1997;29:725-33.

128. Shah PB, Ahmed WH, Ganz P, et al. Hirulog compared with

eparin during coronary angioplasty for thrombus-containing lesions. Circulation 1996;94:I-197.

129. Khan, MM, Ellis SG, Aguirre, FV, Weisman HF, Widermann NM. Claiff RM, Topol EJ, Kleiman NS. Does intracoronary thrombus influence the outcome of high risk percutaneous transluminal coronary angioplasty? Clinical and angiographic outcomes in a large multicenter trial. J Am Coll Cardiol 1998;31:31-36.

130. Nakagawa Y, Matsuo S, Kimura T, Yokoi H, Tamura T, Hamasaki N, Nasaka, H, Nobuyoshi M. Thromboectomy with AngioJet catheter in native coronary arteries for patients with acute or recent myocardial infarction. Am J Cardiol 1999;83:994-999.

131. Silva JA, Saucado JF, Lamoue AS, et al. Rheolytic thrombectomy using the POSSIS AngioJet catheter in patients with acute myocardial infarction presenting within eight hours of symptom onset. Circulation 1998;98:17.

132. deLemos J, Gibson M, Autman EM, et al. Abciximab improves microvascular function after rescue PCI: A TIMI 14 substudy. J Am Coll Cardiol 2000;35:40A.

133. Papadokos S, Wong C, Gustafson G. Safety and efficacy of suction thrombectomy using infusion catheters in thrombus laden coronary lesions followed by stent placement. Circulation 1998;98:17.

134. van Leeuwen T, Meertens J, Velema E, Post M, Borst C. Intraluminal vapor bubble induced by excimer laser pulse causes microsecond arterial dilation and invagination leading to extensive wall damage in the rabbit. Circulation 1993;87:1258.

135. Ischinger TA. A novel device for removal of thrombus from coronary arteries: the X-SIZER multicenter trial. J Am Coll Cardiol 2000;35:41A

136. Ramos S, Baim D, Popma J, et al. A randomized, prospective, multi-center study comparing intracoronary urokinase in rheolytic thrombectomy with the POSSIS AngioJet catheter for intracoronary thrombus: final results of the VEGAS II trial. Circulation 1998;98:17.

137. Fuchs S, Kornowski R, Mehran R, et al. Clinical outcomes following "rescue" administration of abciximab in patient undergoing percutaneous coronary angioplasty. J Invas Cardiol 2000;12:497-501.

138. Barsness GW, Butler CE, Ohmas EM, et al. Reduced thrombus burden in saphenous vein grafts with abciximab given through a local delivery catheter. Circulation 1998;98:17.

139. Velianou JL, Strauss BH, Kreatsoulas C, et al. Evaluation of the role of abciximab (Reopro) as a rescue agent during percutaneous coronary interventions: In-hospital and six-month outcomes. Cathet Cardiovasc Intervent 2000;51:138-144.

140. Giri S, Kieman JF, hirst JA, et al. Intracoronary thrombus is a marker for adverse angiographic and clinical outcomes in patients undergoing primary angioplasty. Circulation 1998;98:17.

141. Grantham JA, Mathew V, Holmes DR. Antiplatelet therapy with abciximab in percuaneous intervention of thrombus-containing bypass grafts. Circulation 1998;98:17.

142. Cafri C, Svirsky R, Gilutz H, et al. Better procedural results in coronary thrombosis are obtained with delayed percuaneous coronary intervention J Am Coll Cardiol 2001;37(2):34A.

143. Ishabushi F, J Am Coll Cardiol 1999;33:2A.

144. Cantor W, Hellkamp A, O'Shea J, et al. Bailout platelet GP II/IIIa inhibition in coronary stent implantation: Observations from the ESPRIT trial. J Am Coll Cardiol 2001;37(2):84A

145. Fuch S, Meharen R, Dangas G, et al. Clinical outcomes following "rescue" administration of abciximab in patients undergoing percutaneous coronary angioplasty. J Am Coll Cardiol 1999;33:2A.

146. Stefanadis C, Tsiamis E, Viachopoulos C, Toutouzas K, Stratos C, Kallikazaros I, Vavuranakis M, Toutouzas P. Autologous vein graft-coated stents for the treatment of thrombus-containing coronary artery lesions. Cathet Cardiovasc Diagn. 1997;40:217-222.

147. Ozbek C, Heisel A, Grob B, Bay W, Schieffer H. Coronary implantation of silicone-carbide-coated Palmaz-Schatz stents in patients with high risk of stent thrombosis without oral anticoagulation. Cathet Cardiovasc Diagn. 1997;41:71-78.

148. Alfonso F, Rodriguez P, Phillips P, Goicolea J, Hernandez R, Perez-Vizcayno MJ, Fernandez-Ortiz A, Segovia J, Banuelos C, Aragoncillo P, Macaya C. Clinical and angiographic implications of coronary stenting in thrombus-containing lesions. J Am Coll Cardiol 1997;29:725-733.

149. Van den Bos AA, van Ommen V, Corbeij HMA. A new thrombosuction catheter use: Initial results with clinical and angiographic follow-up in seven patients. Cathet Cardiovasc Diagn. 1997;40:192-197.

150. Rosenschein U, Roth A, Rassin T, Basan S, Laniado S, Miller HJ. Analysis of coronary ultrasound thrombolysis endpoints in acute myocardial infarction (ACUTE Trial). Results of the feasibility phase. Circulation 1997;95:1411-1416.

151. Braden GA, Xenopoulos NP, Young T, Utley L, Kutcher MA, Applegate RJ. Transluminal extraction catheter atherectomy followed by immediate stenting in treatment of stenting vein grafts. J Am Coll Cardiol 1997;30:657-63.

152. Sketch MH, Davidson CJ, Yeh W, Margolis JR, Matthews RV, Moses JW, Pichard AD, Safian RD, O'Neill W, Siegel RM, Baim DS. Predictors of acute and long-term outcome with transluminal extraction atherectomy: The New Approaches to Coronary Intervention (NACI) Registry. Am J Cardiol 1997;80(10A):68K-77K.

153. Murakami T, Mizuno S, Takahashi Y, Ohsato K, Moriuchi I, Arai Y, Mifune J, Shimizu M, Ohnaka M. Intracoronary aspiration thrombectomy for acute myocardial infarction. Am J Cardiol 1998;82:839-844.

154. Hamm CW, Steffen W, Terres W, de Scheerder I, Reimers J, Cumberland D, Siegel RJ, Meinertz T. Intravascular therapeutic ultrasound thrombolysis in acute myocardial infarctions. Am J Cardiol 1997;80: 200-203.

155. Rosenschein U, Gaul G, Erbel R, Amann F, Velasguez D, Stoerger H, Simon R, Gomex G, Troster J, Bartorelli A, Pieper M, Kyriakides Z, Laniado S, Miller HI, Cribier A, Fajadet J. Percutaneous transluminal therapy of occluded saphenous vein grafts. Can the challenge be met with ultrasound thrombolysis? Circulation 199;99:26-29.

156. van Ommen VG, van den Bos AA, Pieper M, den Heyer P, Thomas MR, Ozbeck S, Bar FW, Wellens HJJ. Removal of thrombus from aortocoronary bypass grafts and coronary

rteries using the 6Fr hydrolyser. Am J Cardiol 1997;79:1012-1016.

157. Saito T, Taniguchi I, Nakamura S, Oka H, Mizuno Y, Noda K, Yamashita, S, Oshima S. Pulse-spray thrombolysis in acutely obstructed coronary artery in critical situations. Cathet Cardiovasc Diagn. 1997;40:101-108.

158. Muhlestein JB, Karagounis LA, Treehan S, Anderson JL. "Rescue" utilization of abciximab for the dissolution of coronary thrombus developing as a complication of coronary angioplasty. J Am Coll Cardiol 1997;30:1729-1734.

159. Henry P, Boughalem K, Rinaldi JP, Makowski S, Khalife K, Guermonprez JL, Blanchard D. Use of anti-GP IIb/IIIa in acute thrombosis after intracoronary stent implantation. Cathet Cardiovasc Diagn. 1998;43:105-107.

160. Garbarz E, Farah B, Vuillemenot A, Andre F, Angioi M, Machecourt J, Bassand JP, Wolf JE, Danchin N, Prendergast B, Lung B, Vahanian A. "Rescue" abximab for complicated percutaneous transluminal coronary angioplasty. Am J Cardiol 1998;82:800-802.

161. Ambrose JA, Almeida OD, Sharm SK, Dangas G, Ratner DE. Angiographic evaluation of intracoronary thrombus and dissection following percutaneous transluminal coronary angioplasty (The Thrombolysis and Angioplasty in Unstable Angina [TAUSA] Trial). Am J Cardiol 1997;79:559-563).

162. Sullebarger JT, Dalton RD, Nasser A, Matar FA. Adjunctive abciximab improves outcomes during recanalization of totally occluded saphenous vein grafts using transluminal extraction atherectomy. Cathet Cardiovasc Diagn. 1999;46:107-110.

163. Haase KK, Mahrholdt H, Schroder S, Baumbach A, Oberhoff M, Herdeg C, Karsch KR. Frequency and efficacy of glycoprotein IIb/IIIa therapy for treatment of threatened or acute vessel closure in 1332 patients undergoing percutaneous transluminal coronary angioplasty. Am Heart J 1999;137:234-240.

164. Shah PB, Ahmed WH, Ganz P, Bittl JA. Bivalirudin compared with heparin during coronary angioplasty for thrombus-containing lesions. J Am Coll Cardiol 1997;30:1264-1269.

165. Glazier JJ, Hirst JA, Kiernan FJ, Fram DB, Eldin AM, Primiano CA, Mitchel JF, McKay RG. Site-specific intracoronary thrombolysis wtih urokinase-coated hydrogel balloons: Acute and follow-up studies in 95 patients. Cathet Cardiovasc Diagn. 1997;41:246-253.

166. Glazier JJ, Kiernan Fj, Bauer HH, Fram DB, Primiano CA, Michel JF, Doughterty JE, McKay RG. Treatment of thrombotic saphenous vein bypass grafts using local urokinase infusion therapy with the dispatch catheter. Cathet Cardiovasc Diagn. 1997;41:261-267.

167. Hong MK, Wong C, Popma JJ, Kent KM, Pichard AD, Satler LF, Mintz GS, Nikonow K, Leon MB. A dual-purpose angioplasty-drug infusion catheter for the treatment of intragraft thrombus. Cathet Cardiovasc Diagn. 1994;32:193-195.

168. Franzen D, Sectem U, Hopp HW. Comparison of angioscopic, intravascular ultrasonic, and angiographic detection of thrombus in coronary stenosis. Am J Cardiol 1998;82:1273-1275.

169. EPIC Investigators. Use of a monoclonal antibody directed against the platelet glycoprotein IIb/IIIa receptor in high-risk coronary angioplasty. N Eng J Med 1994;330:956-961.

170. The EPILOG Investigators. Platelet glycoprotein IIb/IIIa receptor blockade and low-dose heparin during percutaneous coronary revascularization. N Engl J Med 1997;336:1689-1696.

171. The EPISTENT Investigators. Randomized placebo-controlled trial to assess safety of coronary stenting with use of platelet glycoprotein IIb/IIIa blockade. Lancet 1998;352:87-92.

172. Cohen DJ, Cosgrove R, Berezin R, Popma JJ, Leion MB, Kuntz RE, Ramee S. Cost-effectiveness of rheolytic thrombectomy for thrombus-containing coronary lesions: Results from the VEGAS 2 Trial. J Am Coll Cardiol 1999;47A.

173. Moses JW. Mechanical thrombectomy in acute ischemic syndromes: Cutters, suckers, and busters. J Invasc Cardiol 1998;10(supplA):36A-40A.

174. Gurbel PA, Navetta FI, Bates ER, et al. Lesion-directed administration of alteplase with intracoronary heparin in patients with unstable angina and coronary thrombus undergoing angioplasty. Cathet Cardiovasc Diagn 1996;37:382-391.

175. The TIMI IIIA Investigators. Early effects of tissue-type plasminogen activator added to conventional therapy on the culprit coronary lesion in patients presenting with ischemic cardiac pain at rest. Circulation 1993;87:38-52.

176. Kaplan B. Personal communication.

177. Singh M, Ting HH, Araujo NA, et al. Influence of thrombus on the outcome of coronary interventions in the current era. J Am Coll Cardiol 2000;35:90A.

178. Piamsomboon C, Wong PMT, Mathur A, et al. Does platelet glycoprotein IIb/IIIa receptor antibody improve in-hospital outcome of coronary stenting in high-risk thrombus containing lesions? Cathet Cardiovasc Intervent 1999;46:415-420.

179. DeLago A, Papaleo R, Macina A, Chander R. Initial experience with AngoJet mechanical thrombectomy in the treatment of acute myocardial infarction. J Am Coll Cardiol 2000;35;19A.

10 BIFURCATION LESIONS

Robert D. Safian, M.D.

A. **DESCRIPTION (Figure 10.1).** A true bifurcation lesion is defined as the presence of a stenosis >50% involving both a parent vessel and the ostium of its sidebranch. Vessel bifurcations are predisposed to atherosclerosis from turbulent flow and increased shear stress.[1] Although true bifurcation lesions account for only 4-16% of interventional procedures, about 20% of parent vessel lesions have mildly diseased sidebranches.[2-5] The vast majority of bifurcation lesions involve the LAD-diagonal bifurcation. Bifurcation lesions were originally considered a contraindication to PTCA due to the increased risk of sidebranch occlusion, but PTCA and other devices are now commonly applied to a wide variety of vessel bifurcations with high success and acceptable complication rates.

B. **APPROACH TO BIFURCATION LESIONS**

1. **Need for Sidebranch Protection**. The likelihood of significant sidebranch narrowing or closure depends on whether the sidebranch originates from the primary lesion and the degree to which its ostium is narrowed (Tables 10.1, 10.2). Branch vessels which do not originate from the parent vessels are at low risk for sidebranch occlusion even if they are transiently occluded during balloon inflation.[6] For sidebranches that originate from the parent lesion, the risk of occlusion is lowest if the sidebranch contains an ostial stenosis < 50%, intermediate if the sidebranch contains a non-ostial stenosis > 50%, and highest if the sidebranch contains an ostial stenosis > 50%. In one study, the risk of progressive narrowing was 12% if the branch ostial stenosis was ≤ 50% vs. 41% if the branch ostial stenosis was > 50%.[7] When primary atheroma obstructs both the parent vessel and sidebranch ostium by > 50%, there is a high incidence of branch occlusion (14-34%) [4,6,8] or narrowing (27-41%) [7-9] unless the branch is protected by a guidewire (Figure 10.2).

Table 10.1. Parent Vessel-Sidebranch Relationships[2,4,6,8,9]

Anatomy	Risk of Sidebranch Occlusion	Technical Difficulty Wiring Occluded Branch	Protection Recommended
Branch not involved by parent vessel lesion but in jeopardy due to transient occlusion during balloon inflation	Low (< 1%)	Low	No
Branch originates from diseased parent vessel segment; branch is normal	Moderate (1-10%)	Low to moderate	Probably yes; depends on vessel size and distribution
Ostium of branch vessel > 50% stenosis	High (14-35%)	High	Yes

Predictors of sidebranch occlusion include significant branch-ostial stenosis, parent vessel dissection, and unstable angina. Factors not predictive of sidebranch occlusion include branch vessel caliber, parent vessel PTCA success, and anatomic location of the branch.[3,4,9,10] Tables 10.1 and 10.2 summarize the need for sidebranch protection.

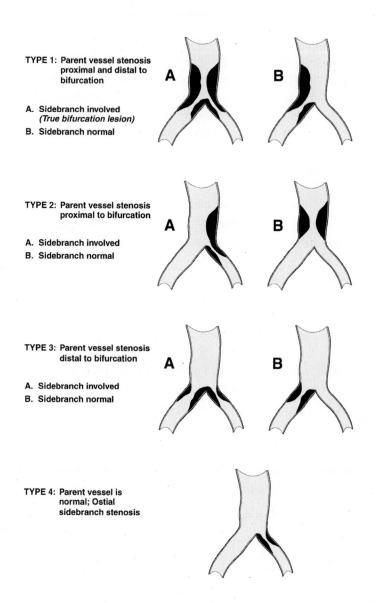

TYPE 1: Parent vessel stenosis proximal and distal to bifurcation

A. Sidebranch involved *(True bifurcation lesion)*
B. Sidebranch normal

TYPE 2: Parent vessel stenosis proximal to bifurcation

A. Sidebranch involved
B. Sidebranch normal

TYPE 3: Parent vessel stenosis distal to bifurcation

A. Sidebranch involved
B. Sidebranch normal

TYPE 4: Parent vessel is normal; Ostial sidebranch stenosis

Figure 10.1. Classification of Bifurcation Lesions

Table 10.2. Need for Sidebranch Protection

Sidebranch protection recommended	1. Any sidebranch > 2.0 mm in diameter that has an ostial stenosis ≥ 50% and originates from the parent vessel lesion (Figure 10.1; Types 1A, 2A, 3A). "True" bifurcation lesions (Figure 10.1; Type 1A) are associated with a high incidence of sidebranch occlusion and a low salvage rate when left unprotected
	2. Any sidebranch > 2 mm in diameter (without ostial stenosis) that originates from the parent vessel lesion (Figure 10.1; Type 1B). Although it is usually possible to retrieve these occluded sidebranches, their large caliber justifies protection. In such lesions, a double guidewire approach is reasonable. If sidebranch occlusion occurs, sequential PTCA or a kissing balloon technique may be employed
Sidebranch protection probably not necessary*	1. The sidebranch is normal and does not originate from the parent vessel lesion (Figure 10.1; Type 2B, 3B). Although the sidebranch may be transiently covered by the inflated balloon in the parent vessel, the risk of occlusion is low
	2. The sidebranch is < 1.5 mm in diameter and would not receive a bypass graft during CABG
	3. The sidebranch supplies a small amount of viable myocardium
	4. Isolated stenosis of the origin of the sidebranch usually does not require protection of the parent vessel (Figure 10.1; Type 4)

* In these lesions, it may be reasonable to leave the sidebranch unprotected; if sidebranch occlusion does occur, it can be retrieved by conventional PTCA or not retrieved at all, depending on the clinical situation.

   2.   PTCA Techniques (Table 10.3)

   a.   Double Guiding Catheter Technique. This outdated approach was initially recommended before the availability of low-profile balloons and large-lumen 7F and 8F guiding catheters. It involves placement of two guiding catheters (via two arterial punctures) in the aortic root, and requires separate engagement and retraction of each guide to permit sequential advancement of each guidewire and balloon system.

   b.   Single Guiding Catheter Technique. Virtually all 8F giant-lumen (internal diameter ≥ 0.084-inch) guiding catheters can accommodate most balloons and guidewires needed for bifurcation angioplasty, even when two 0.014-inch over-the-wire systems are used. Regardless of the approach (sequential or kissing balloons), a 2- or 3-way Touhy-Borst adapter can be used, although the 3-way adapter may reduce loss of blood and contrast. To minimize the risk of guidewire entanglement, parent vessel and sidebranch guidewires should be advanced simultaneously to the tip of the guide catheter, the more difficult lesion wired first, and guidewire rotation limited to < 180°. If both vessels are angulated or tortuous, the larger vessel should be wired first. Balloon diameters should be selected to match the caliber of the disease-free segment of each vessel just beyond the bifurcation; deliberate undersizing increases the risk of procedural failure, while oversizing increases the risk of complications. In general, bifurcation lesions may be approached with double guidewires and sequential PTCA or kissing balloons.

Table 10.3. Technical Approaches to Bifurcation Angioplasty

Approach	Advantages	Disadvantages
Guiding Catheter Technique		
Two-guide approach	• Large variety of balloon catheters to choose from • Excellent visualization	• Two arterial punctures • More procedural complexity • Potential ostial injury
One-guide approach	• One access site • Fewer catheter engagements; less risk of ostial injury • Less time consuming	• Limited choice of balloons, wires • Visualization may be impaired
Protection Technique		
Double-guidewire	• Maintains continuous access to both vessels • Less obstruction to coronary flow from a guidewire than a balloon • Better contrast opacification • Less expensive if the same balloon can be used for both branches	• Increased risk of wire entanglement
Double balloon on-the-wire	• Allows immediate PTCA of branch if needed • Balloon serves as a "stent" during sequential dilatations	• Increased risk of wire entanglement • Cannot upsize or exchange without giving up wire position and having to recross lesion with wire • May impair contrast opacification
Double balloon over-the-wire	• Maintains guidewire access in the parent vessel • Allows immediate PTCA of sidebranch for abrupt closure	• Increased risk of wire entanglement • May impair contrast opacification
Inflation Technique		
Sequential balloon inflation	• Requires less intracoronary hardware • Can use same balloon for both vessels	• Increased risk of wire entanglement • Does not eliminate "snow-plow" or shifting plaque • Single balloon may not match diameter of parent vessel proximal and distal to branch
Kissing balloon inflations	• Minimizes "snow-plow" and shifting plaque • Allows PTCA of large caliber proximal vessel without overdilating smaller vessel distal to bifurcation	• More complex procedure • Increased risk of wire entanglement • May overdilate parent vessel proximal to bifurcation

1. **Double Guidewire, Sequential PTCA.** This approach involves placing guidewires in both parent vessel and sidebranch before balloon inflation. The main advantage to this technique is that it maintains continuous access to both limbs of the bifurcation in the event acute closure occurs or balloon exchange is needed; it does not, however, prevent shifting-plaque or sidebranch narrowing. Monorail balloons, over-the-wire balloons, fixed wire-balloons, or any combination of the above may be used. Initial use of bare guidewires allows excellent visualization during contrast injections and is a popular approach. Once both guidewires are in place, the parent vessel and sidebranch are dilated in sequential fashion; the same balloon may be used if the bifurcation limbs are the same diameter. Fixed wire-balloon systems can be used, but the sidebranch cannot be protected if balloon upsizing becomes necessary. When a fixed-wire system is used to dilate the parent or branch, it is best to advance the balloon beyond the lesion to assess the angiographic result before removing the system. Although tapered balloons provided more uniform balloon-to-artery ratios proximal and distal to Type 1 and 2A bifurcations (Figure 10.1),[42] they are no longer manufactured.

2. **"Kissing Balloon" Technique.** Simultaneous kissing-balloon inflations are preferable to prevent shifting plaque and snow-plow injury (Figure 10.2). By performing simultaneous inflations, adequate dilatation of the proximal vessel can be achieved without oversizing the balloon relative to the smaller distal vessels (Figure 10.3).

3. **Debulking Technique.** Several studies suggest that debulking (followed by PTCA) is an alternative to PTCA alone for bifurcation lesions;[47,48] DCA, Rotablator, and other devices have been used (Table 10.4).
   a. **DCA Technique.** Bifurcation DCA can be performed using sequential or kissing guidewires (Figure 10.4).[13,16,17,18,20] Sequential intervention is recommended, using either DCA of the parent vessel and PTCA of the sidebranch, or DCA of both vessels (Chapter 28). Nitinol wires are resistant to damage during DCA and should be used for the kissing wire technique;[15] when this technique is used, the AtheroCath should be rotated < 180° to prevent wire entanglement. Predilation of sidebranches with ostial disease is sometimes recommended to reduce the risk of sidebranch occlusion during DCA of the parent vessel. Low balloon inflation pressures should be used to reduce the risk of shifting plaque.

   b. **Rotablator Technique.** Protection of a sidebranch is not feasible during Rotablator of bifurcation lesions. If both limbs of the bifurcation exceed 2.5 mm in diameter, the vessel that is more difficult to wire should be treated first. Some operators recommend gentle predilation of the sidebranch before Rotablator of the parent vessel to minimize sidebranch occlusion. If the branch origin is angulated, a conservative burr strategy is recommended using a final burr-to-artery ratio ≤ 0.6. Kissing balloons are commonly employed after Rotablator.

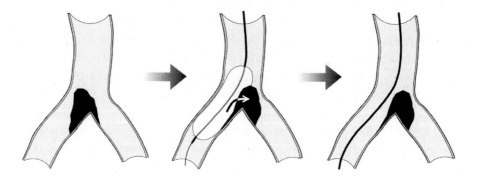

Figure 10.2. "Snow-Plow" Effect

During PTCA of the parent vessel, shifting plaque causes sidebranch narrowing. Simultaneous dilatation of both limbs of the bifurcation ("kissing-balloon" technique) is often required when the snow-plow effect complicates PTCA

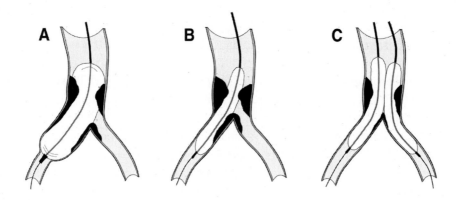

Figure 10.3. Bifurcation Stenosis Requiring Simultaneous Balloon Inflations

When the target lesion extends from a large proximal vessel segment to a smaller distal (post-bifurcation) vessel, "kissing" balloon inflations are usually necessary
A. Sizing the balloon to the proximal vessel results in overdilating the distal vessel
B. Sizing the balloon to the distal vessel results in underdilating the proximal vessel
C. Kissing balloon inflations allow adequate dilatation of both proximal and distal vessel segments

Table 10.4. Results of Debulking Bifurcation Lesions

Series	N	Success (%)	SBO (%)	MACE (%)	TVR (%)
Dauerman[47]	30 (PTCA)	73	3	6.7	1 yr: 53%
(1998)	40 (DCA or	97	22	2.5	1 yr: 28%
	Rotablator)				
Brener[48]	32 (PTCA)	-	3	3	-
(1996)	34 (DCA)	-	15	9	-

Abbreviations: SBO = sidebranch occlusion; DCA = directional coronary atherectomy; TVR = target vessel revascularization; MACE = in-hospital major adverse cardiac events (death, MI, CABG, rePTCA).

4. **Stent Technique.** Experimental data show well-preserved flow into nondiseased sidebranches after stent placement.[33] Nevertheless, stents should be used cautiously in patients with stenoses involving significant sidebranches; even though sidebranches may still be accessible by PTCA,[45] added technical expertise is required for successful salvage.   When a parent lesion requires intervention but has a sidebranch, the decision to implant a stent is based on the need for immediate revascularization of the sidebranch, the likelihood of future revascularization, the size of the sidebranch, and the amount of viable myocardium served by that branch. In general, jeopardy of acute marginal branches of the RCA, small diagonal branches of the LAD, and small obtuse marginal branches of the left circumflex artery may not represent significant contraindications to stent placement, even if the sidebranch becomes occluded. There are four different technical approaches to stenting bifurcation lesions (Table 10.5, Figure 10.5): (1) Stent and retrieve (stent parent vessel and retrieve sidebranch if necessary); (2) T-stent (stent sidebranch, then stent parent vessel); (3) Culotte stent (stent parent vessel, then stent branch through first stent); and (4) Kissing stent (double wire, kissing balloons, then kissing stents).[50-61,69]

C. PROCEDURAL RESULTS

1. **PTCA (Table 10.6).** Although successful dilation can be achieved in 87-100% of parent vessel lesions, successful sidebranch revascularization occurs less often (76-89%).[2-5,8-10] In addition to the usual risks of PTCA, bifurcation angioplasty is associated with the additional risks of sidebranch occlusion, incomplete dilation due to the snow-plow effect (Figure 10.2), and retrograde propagation of dissection from sidebranch to parent vessel. Branch occlusion may be silent, or may present with chest pain, hemodynamic instability, or malignant arrhythmias depending upon the vessel caliber, presence and adequacy of collaterals, other coronary disease, and left ventricular function. Causes of sidebranch occlusion include snow-plow injury, dissection, spasm, and thrombosis.

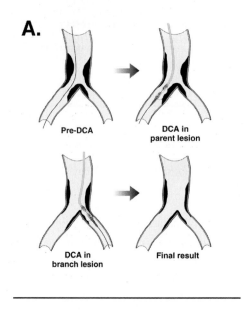

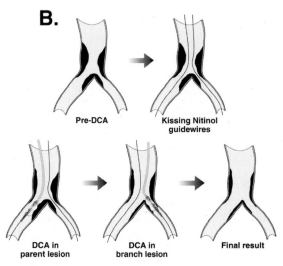

Figure 10.4. Bifurcation Lesions: DCA Techniques

A. Sequential guidewires and sequential DCA
B. Kissing nitinol guidewires and sequential DCA

Table 10.5. Comparison of Stent Techniques for Bifurcation Lesions[50]

Technique	Description	Advantages	Disadvantages
Stent and retrieve	Stent parent vessel; retrieve sidebranch if clinically indicated	Stent implantation is easy	Sidebranch retrieval is potentially challenging and may be unsuccessful
T-stent	Stent sidebranch, then stent parent vessel	Well-suited for branches that originate at 90° angles from parent vessel; good coverage of parent vessel	Technically challenging; may lead to inadequate coverage of branch ostium or excessive stent protrusion into parent vessel
Culotte stent (Y-stent)	Stent parent vessel (or most angulated vessel), then stent branch through first stent	Good stent coverage of bifurcation	Technically challenging; may not be able to pass wires easily into either branch after stenting
Kissing stent	Double wire, followed by kissing balloons and kissing stents	Good stent coverage of lesion; well-suited for large vessel and branch with mild angulation; relatively easy	Reconstruction of carina may lead to overexpansion of proximal vessel

2. **Debulking Techniques.** Several studies report significantly better immediate lumen enlargement after debulking strategies, but more frequent sidebranch compromise.[47,48]

 a. **Directional Atherectomy (DCA) (Table 10.7).** Observational studies report that sidebranch occlusion occurs in 0.7-7.7% of unselected lesions,[14,21-29] and in up to 37% of bifurcation lesions treated by DCA.[18] Fortunately, most sidebranch closures can be salvaged by PTCA. Much like PTCA, baseline narrowing of the sidebranch origin increases the risk of sidebranch occlusion during DCA.[20] In highly selected bifurcation lesions, high procedural success (91-100%) and low major complication rates (0-3%) have been reported.[14,17,18] In one study of transient sidebranch occlusion after DCA, salvage by PTCA or DCA resulted in a final diameter stenosis of 6-12% in the parent vessel and 0-17% in the sidebranch.[18] In CAVEAT-I, DCA led to higher success (88% vs. 74%, p < 0.001) and less restenosis (50% vs. 61%, p < 0.001) compared to PTCA, but more ischemic complications (9.5% vs. 3.7%, p < 0.001).[48] In a nonrandomized study, debulking with DCA resulted in less target lesion revascularization.[47]

 b. **Rotablator.** Initially considered a contraindication,[40,41] Rotablator is now often used to debulk bifurcation lesions prior to PTCA or stenting. The incidence of sidebranch occlusion with Rotablator depends on the degree of branch ostial stenosis: 42% for ostial stenosis > 50%, and 16% for ostial stenosis < 50%.[62]

3. **Stents (Table 10.8).** Stents should be used cautiously in lesions with large sidebranches (Chapter 26). Early studies with the Gianturco-Roubin and Palmaz-Schatz stents suggested acceptable success and complication rates, with sidebranch occlusion in 6-19%.[30,34,35,38,39,43,45,46,63] Predictors of sidebranch occlusion included ostial stenosis > 50% and parent vessel disease spanning the bifurcation.[63] In the randomized STARS trial, sidebranch occlusion occurred in 5% of patients after Palmaz-Schatz stenting and was associated with greater need for CABG and late TLR. In contemporary stent practice, access to occluded sidebranches has been facilitated by the availability of flexible, low-profile modified coil and tubular mesh designs. Despite several stent techniques for bifurcation lesions, none has clearly emerged as the treatment of choice and all are technically demanding (Table 10.5, Figure 10.5). In most cases, the simpler technique of "stent-and-retrieve" has been associated with fewer complications and better late outcome than more complex double-stent techniques. Acute sidebranch occlusion after stenting may be successfully salvaged by PTCA in 84% of patients,[65] and the development of ostial sidebranch stenosis late after prior stent placement ("stent-jail") may be treated by PTCA or Rotablator.[66] In general, Rotablator should not be considered unless the branch ostium was dilated immediately after stent deployment; Rotablator has been used to treat a restenotic sidebranch when the stent struts had not been reoriented by prior PTCA,[67,68] but this technique is not recommended due to the increased risk for burr entrapment.

4. **Other Devices.** The application of ELCA or TEC to true bifurcation lesions is generally not recommended because of the inability to protect diseased sidebranches and the increased risk of procedural complications and failure.[36]

5. **Retrieval of Occluded Sidebranches.** Salvage rates depend on whether the affected sidebranch contains a high-grade ostial stenosis, and whether the branch was initially protected by a second wire. Acutely occluded sidebranches without ostial stenoses can be reopened in 75-100% of cases, although salvage rates < 50% were reported when the ostium of the sidebranch contained a significant stenosis prior to occlusion.[4,8,11] In a report of 15 patients with sidebranch occlusion, 67% demonstrated spontaneous recanalization at 6-month follow-up angiography; if this phenomenon occurs early, it may explain the low incidence of myocardial infarction after sidebranch occlusion.[13]

6. **Parent Vessel Closure.** Sustained patency of the parent vessel is rarely affected by occlusion of its sidebranch; retrograde propagation of dissection from sidebranch to parent vessel is rare.[9]

7. **Myocardial Infarction, Emergency CABG, and Death.** Myocardial infarction is uncommon after sidebranch occlusion.[4-6,9] Of 167 patients with sidebranch occlusion after PTCA, chest pain occurred in 13% and Q-wave MI in 8%; septal perforator occlusion comprised 27% of all branch closures and was not associated with MI. Among patients with branch occlusion in the 1985-1986 NHLBI PTCA Registry, emergency CABG was required in 11% and death occurred in 3%.[37] When data from several large retrospective series are complied, the overall incidence of death is < 1%.

Table 10.6. Results of PTCA for Bifurcation Lesions

Series	Morphology	Sidebranch Protection	N	Success (%)	MACE (%)	Restenosis (%)
Tan[42] (1995)	Bifurcation	Yes	135	95	2.2*	-
	Bifurcation	No	52	85	3.8*	-
	Non-bifurcation		970	93	3.4*	-
CAVEAT[19] (1993)	Bifurcation		-	74	3.7	ARS (61% vs. 52%)
	Non-bifurcation		-	86	6.1	
Myler[5] (1992)	Bifurcation	Yes	17	94	0	-
	Bifurcation	No	106	89	3.8	-
	Non-bifurcation		656	95	1.4	-
Ciampricotti[4] (1992)	Bifurcation	No	22	95	0	-
Weinstein[8] (1991)	Bifurcation	Yes	35	97	0	CRS (42% vs. 6%)
	Bifurcation	No	21	76		
Renkin[2] (1991)	Bifurcation	Yes	34	97	2.9	ARS (37% overall)
	Bifurcation	No	8	88	12.5	
Thomas[11] (1988)	Bifurcation	Yes	54	87	6.0	CRS (30%)
George[3] (1986)	Bifurcation	Yes	52	98	3.8	ARS (53%); CRS(32%)

Abbreviations: ARS = angiographic restenosis; CAVEAT = Coronary Angioplasty versus Excisional Atherectomy Trial (DCA arm); CRS = clinical restenosis; MACE = major adverse cardiac events; - = not reported
* Acute closure

Table 10.7. Results of DCA for Bifurcation Lesions

Series	N	Success (%)	MACE (%)	SBO (%)
Miguel (1994)	122	-	0.8	17
CAVEAT[19] (1993)	Bifurcation 88	9.5	50	
	Non-bifurcation 90	8.2	-	
Mansour[17] (1992)	8	100	0.00	0
Hinohara[14] (1991)	22	91	4.5	-

Abbreviations: CAVEAT = Coronary Angioplasty versus Excisional Atherectomy Trial (DCA arm); MACE = in-hospital major adverse cardiac events (death, Q-wave myocardial infarction, emergency coronary artery bypass grafting); SBO = sidebranch occlusion; - = not reported

Table 10.8. Results of Stents for Bifurcation Lesions

Series	N	Stent	Technique	Results
Suwaidi[69] (2000)	77 (A)	Various	Stent in one branch; PTCA in other branch	Procedural success (89.5% in group A vs. 97.4% in group B). In-hospital MACE higher with Culotte stenting vs. T-stenting (p = 0.004). No difference in MACE at 1 year
	54 (B)	Various	T-stent, Culotte stent	
Yamashita[70] (2000)	53 (A)	-	Stent in one branch; PTCA in other branch	Acute procedural success similar. Group B had lower residual stenosis (p < 0.001) and higher in-hospital MACE (p < 0.05); 6-month TVR and MACE were similar
	39 (B)	-	Stent in both branches	
de Scheerder[57] (1999)	21	V-Flex	Culotte stent	Procedural success (100%); CK elevation (10%)
Sheiban[56] (1999)	54	Various	T-stent	Procedural success (100%); ARS (45%)
Anzuini[60] (1998)	59	Wiktor	Culotte stent, T-stent, stent-and-retrieve	Procedural success in 96% (similar for different techniques); more in-hospital MACE (43% vs. 17%) and higher restenosis (41% vs. 19%) using Culotte and T-stent vs. stent-and-retrieve
Brunel[61] (1998)	107	-	Multiple	Angiographic success (93%); higher restenosis (57% vs. 21%) and TLR (43% vs. 8%) in double-stent techniques vs. stent-and-retrieve
Carrie[52] (1998)	54	Wiktor	Culotte stent, T-stent	Clinical success (91%); sidebranch occlusion (5.5%); angiographic restenosis (25.6%)
Chevalier[51] (1998)	50	Various	Culotte stent	Clinical success (94%); non-Q-MI (6%); TLR (24%)
Lefevre[59] (1998)	161	-	Multiple	Procedural success (96%); significant learning curve suggested by lower TLR (10.9% vs. 36.7%) and less MACE (14.6% vs. 45.6%) during later experience
Pan[58] (1998)	70	-	Stent-and-retrieve, T-stent	T-stent patients had similar procedural success (91% vs. 93%) but more MACE at 15 months (39% vs. 13%)

Abbreviations: ARS = angiographic restenosis; TLR = target lesion revascularization, MACE = major adverse cardiac events (death, MI, repeat revascularization)

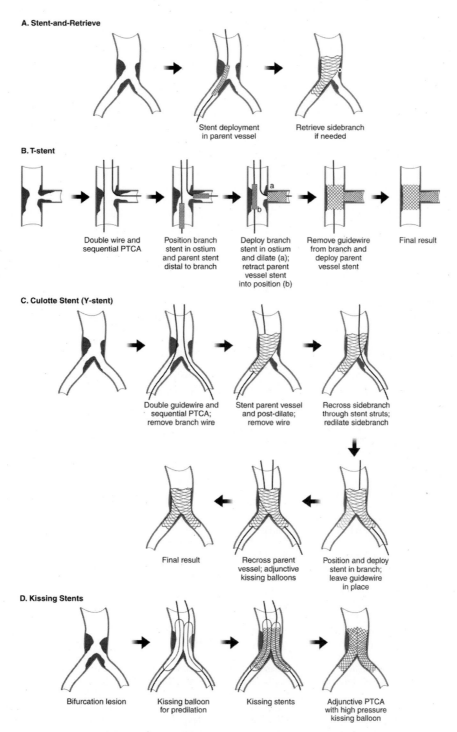

A. Stent-and-Retrieve

Stent deployment
in parent vessel

Retrieve sidebranch
if needed

B. T-stent

Double wire and
sequential PTCA

Position branch
stent in ostium
and parent stent
distal to branch

Deploy branch
stent in ostium
and dilate (a);
retract parent
vessel stent
into position (b)

Remove guidewire
from branch and
deploy parent
vessel stent

Final result

C. Culotte Stent (Y-stent)

Double guidewire and
sequential PTCA;
remove branch wire

Stent parent vessel
and post-dilate;
remove wire

Recross sidebranch
through stent struts;
redilate sidebranch

Final result

Recross parent
vessel; adjunctive
kissing balloons

Position and deploy
stent in branch;
leave guidewire
in place

D. Kissing Stents

Bifurcation lesion

Kissing balloon
for predilation

Kissing stents

Adjunctive PTCA
with high pressure
kissing balloon

Figure 10.5. Stenting Techniques for Bifurcation Lesions

REFERENCES

1. Pinkerton CA, Slack JD. Complex coronary angioplasty: A technique for dilatation of bifurcation stenosis. Angiology 1985:543-548.

2. Renkin J, Wijns W, Hanet C, et al. Angioplasty of coronary bifurcation stenoses. Cathet Cardiovasc Diagn 1991;22:167-173.

3. George BS, Myler RK, Stertzer SH, et al. Balloon angioplasty of coronary bifurcation lesions. Cathet Cardiovasc Diagn 1986;12:124-138.

4. Ciampricutti R, El-Gamol M, Van Golder B, et al. Coronary angioplasty of bifurcation lesions without protection of large sidebranches. Cathet Cardiovasc Diagn 1992;27:191-196.

5. Myler RK, Shaw RE, Stertzer SH, et al. Lesion morphology and coronary angioplasty: Current experience and analysis. J Am Coll Cardiol 1992.

6. Meier B, Gruentzig AR, King SB III, et al. Risk of side branch occlusion during coronary angioplasty. Am J Cardiol 1984;53:10-14.

7. Boxt LM, Meyeruvitz MF, Taus RH, et al. Sidebranch occlusion complicating percutaneous transluminal coronary angioplasty. Radiology 1986;161:681-683.

8. Weinstein JS, Baim DS, Sipperly ME, et al. Salvage of branch vessels during bifurcation lesion angioplasty. Cathet Cardiovasc Diagn 1991;22:1-6.

9. Vetrovec GW, Cowley MJ, Wolfgang TC, et al. Effects of percutaneous transluminal coronary angioplasty in lesion associated branches. Am Heart J 1985;109:921-925.

10. Arora RR, Raymond RE, Dimas AP, et al. Side branch occlusion during coronary angioplasty: Incidence, angiographic characteristics, and outcome. Cathet Cardiovasc Diagn 1989;18:210-212.

11. Thomas TS, Williams DO, Most AS. Efficacy of coronary angioplasty of bifurcation lesions: Immediate and late outcome. Circulation 1988;78:II-632.

12. Shiu MF, Singh A. Spontaneous recanalization of sidebranches occluded during percutaneous transluminal coronary angioplasty. Brit Heart J 1985;54:215-217.

13. Eisenhauer AC, Clugston RA, Ruiz CE. Sequential directional atherectomy of coronary bifurcation lesions. Cathet Cardiovasc Diagn 1993;Suppl 1:54-60.

14. Hinohara T, Rowe MH, Robertson GC, et al. Effect of lesion characteristics on outcome of directional coronary atherectomy. J Am Coll Cardiol 1991;17:1112-20.

15. Grassman ED, Leya FS, Lewis BE, Johnson SA, et al. Examination of common PTCA guidewires used for sidebranch protection during directional coronary atherectomy of bifurcation lesions performed in vivo and in vitro. Cathet Cardiovasc Diagn 1993; Suppl 1:48-53.

16. Safian R, Schreiber T, Baim D. Specific indications for directional coronary atherectomy: Origin left anterior descending coronary artery and bifurcating lesions. Am J Cardiol 1993;72:35E-41E.

17. Mansour M, Fishman RF, Kuntz RE, Carrozza JP. Feasibility of directional atherectomy for the treatment of bifurcation lesions. Cor Art Dis 1992;3:761-765.

18. Lewis B, Leya F, Johnson S, et al. Acute procedural results in the treatment of 30 coronary artery bifurcation lesions with a double-wire atherectomy technique for side-branch protection. Am Heart J 1994;127:1600-1607.

19. Lewis B, Leya F, Johnson S, et al. Outcome of angioplasty (PTCA) and atherectomy (DCA) for bifurcation and non-bifurcation lesions in CAVEAT. Circulation 1993;88:I-601.

20. Campos-Esteve M, Laird J, Kufs W, Wortham CD. Side-branch occlusion with directional coronary atherectomy: Incidence and risk factors. Am Heart J 1994;128:686-690.

21. Kaufmann UP, Garratt KN, Vlietstra RE, Menke KK. Coronary atherectomy: First 50 patients at the Mayo Clinic. Mayo Clin Proc 1989;64:747-752.

22. Safian R, Gelbfish J, Erny R, Schnitt S, et al. Coronary atherectomy. Clinical, angiographic, and histological findings and observations regarding potential mechanisms. Circulation 1990;82:69-79.

23. Rowe MH, Hinohara T, White NW, Robertson GC. Comparison of dissection rates and angiographic results following directional coronary atherectomy and coronary angioplasty. Am J Cardiol 1990;66:49-53.

24. Garratt K, Holmes D, Bell M, et al. Results of directional atherectomy of primary atheromatous and restenosis lesions in coronary arteries and saphenous vein grafts. Am J Cardiol 1992;70:449-454.

25. Fishman R, Kuntz R, Carrozza J, et al. Long-term results of directional coronary atherectomy: Predictors of restenosis. J Am Coll Cardiol 1992;20:1101-1110.

26. Baim D, Tomoaki H, Holmes D, et al. Results of directional coronary atherectomy during multicenter preapproval testing. Am J Cardiol 1993;72:6E-11E.

27. Cowley M, DiSciascio G. Experience with directional coronary atherectomy since pre-market approval. Am J Cardiol 1993;72:12E-20E.

28. Popma J, Mintz G, Satler L, et al. Clinical and angiographic outcome after directional coronary atherectomy: A qualitative and quantitative analysis using coronary arteriography and intravascular ultrasound. Am J Cardiol 1993;72:55E-64E.

29. Umans V, de Feyter P, Deckers J, et al. Acute and long-term outcome of directional coronary atherectomy for stable and unstable angina. Am J Cardiol 1993;74:641-646.

30. Guarneri E, Sklar M, Russo R, et al. Escape from stent jail: An in vitro model. Circulation 1995;92:I-688.

31. Nakamura S, Hall P, Maiello L, Colombo A. Techniques of Palmaz-Schatz stent deployment in lesions with a large side branch. Cathet Cardiovas Diagn 1995;34:353-361.

32. Colombo A, Gaglione A, Nakamura S. "Kissing" stents for bifurcational coronary lesion. Cathet Cardiovas Diagn. 1993;30:327-330.

33. Iniguez A, Macaya C, Alfonso F, Goicolea J. Early angiographic changes of side branches arising from a Palmaz-Schatz stented coronary segment: Results and clinical implications. J Am Coll Cardiol 1994;23:911-915.

34. Mazur W, Grinstead C, Hakim A, et al. Fate of side branches after intracoronary implantation of the Gianturco-Roubin flex-stent for acute or threatened closure after percutaneous transluminal coronary angioplasty. Am J Cardiol 1994;74:1207-1210.

35. Guarneri E, Sklar M, Russo R, Claire D, Schatz R, Teirstein P.

Escape from stent jail: An in vitro model. Circulation 1995;92:I-688.

36. Bittl JA, Sanborn TA, Tcheng JE, et al. Clinical success, complications and restenosis rates with excimer laser coronary angioplasty: The PELCA Registry. Am J Cardiol 1992;70:1533-1539.

37. Holmes DR JR, Holubkov R, Vlietstra RE, et al. Comparison of complications during percutaneous transluminal coronary angioplasty from 1977 to 1981 and from 1985 to 1986. The National Heart, Lung, and Blood Institute Percutaneous Transluminal Coronary Angioplasty Registry. J Am Coll Cardiol 1988;12:1149-1155.

38. Fischman DL, Savage MP, Leon MB, et al. Fate of lesion-related sidebranches after coronary artery stenting. J Am Coll Cardiol 1993;22:1641-6.

39. Pan M, Medina A, de Lezo JS, et al. Follow-up patency of sidebranches covered by intracoronary Palmaz-Schatz stent. Am Heart J 1995;129:436-440.

40. Whitlow PL, Cowley M, Bass T, et al. Risk of high speed rotational atherectomy in bifurcation lesions. J Am Coll Cardiol 1993;21:445A.

41. Warth DC, Leon MB, O'Neill WW, et al. Rotational atherectomy multicenter registry: Acute results, complications and 6-month angiographic follow-up in 709 patients. J Am Coll Cardiol 1994;24:641-8.

42. Tan Kim, Sulke N, Taub N, Sowton E. Clinical and lesion morphologic determinants of coronary angioplasty success and complications: Current experience. J Am Coll Cardiol 1995;25:855-865.

43. Colombo A, Maiello L, Itoh A, et al. Coronary stenting of bifurcation lesions: Immediate and follow-up results. J Am Coll Cardiol 1996; 27:277A.

44. Mehta S, Popma J, Margolis JR, et al. Complications with new angioplasty devices. Are these device specific? J Am Coll Cardiol 1996;27:168A.

45. Caputo RP, Chafizedeh ER, Stoler RC, et al. "Stent Jail" — A minimum security prison. J Invas Cardiol 1996;8.

46. Carrie D, Elbaz M, et al. "T" shaped stent placement: a technique for the treatment of coronary bifurcation lesions. J Am Coll Cardiol 1997;29(Suppl. A):16A.

47. Dauerman HL, Higgins PJ, Sparano Am, et al. Mechanical debulking versus balloon angioplasty for the treatment of true bifurcation lesions. J Am Coll Cardiol 1998;32:1845-1852.

48. Brener SJ, Leya FS, Apperson-hanse C, et al. A comparison of debulking versus dilatation of bifurcation coronary arterial narrowings (from the CAVEAT I Trial). Am J Cardiol 1996;78:1039-1041.

49. Fischell TA, Drexler H. Pullback atherectomy (PAC) for the treatment of complex bifurcation coronary artery disease. Cathet Cardiovasc Diagn. 1996;38:218-221.

50. Di Mario C, Colombo A. Trousers-stents: How to choose the right size and shape? Cathet Cardiovasc Diagn. 1997;41:197-199.

51. Chevalier B, Glatt B, Royer T, Guyon P. Placement of coronary stents in bifurcation lesions by the "Culotte" technique. Am J Cardiol 1998;82:943-949.

52. Carrie D, Elbaz M, Dambrin G, et al. Coronary stenting of bifurcation lesions using "T" or "Reserve Y" configuration with Wiktor stent. Am J Cardiol 1998;82:1418-1421.

53. Teirstein PS. Kissing Palmaz-Schatz stents for coronary bifurcation stenoses. Cathet Cardiovasc Diagn. 1996;37:307-310.

54. Lowe HC, Kumar R, Roy PR. New balloon expandable stent for bifurcation lesions. Cathet Cardiovasc Diagn. 1997;42(2):235-236.

55. Sievert H, Rohde S, Ensslen R, et al. Initial clinical experience with the new EBI (BARD-XT) flexible coronary stent: Acute results and follow-up. Cathet Cardiovasc Diagn. 1998;43:159-162.

56. Sheiban I, Albiero R, Marsico F, et al. Immediate and long-term results "T" stenting in bifurcational coronary lesions. J Am Coll Cardiol 1999;33(suppl A):91A.

57. de Scheerder I, Dens J, Desmet W, et al. Treatment of bifurcation lesions using a new tubular stent. J Am Coll Cardiol 1999;33(suppl A):97A.

58. Pan M, de Lezo JS, Romero M, et al. Simple and complex stent strategies for bifurcated coronary lesions. Circulation 1998;98(suppl I):I-638.

59. Lefevre T, Louvard Y, Morice MC, et al. Stenting of bifurcation lesions: Seven-month follow-up of a prospective study. Circulation 1998;98(suppl I):I-638.

60. Anzuini A, Raffaele S, rosanio S, et al. Implantation of the Wiktor stent in coronary bifurcation lesions: Immediate and follow-up results. Circulation 1998;98(suppl I):I-638.

61. Brunel P, Commeau P, Koning R, et al. Assessment of coronary bifurcation lesions treated with stent implantation on the parent vessel and with balloon or stent on the sidebranch. Circulation 1998;98(suppl I):I-639.

62. Walton AS, Pomerantsev EV, Oesterle SN, et al. Outcome of narrowing related side branches after high-speed rotational atherectomy. Am J Cardiol 1996;77:370-373.

63. Aliabdi D, Tilli FV, Bowers TR, et al. Incidence and angiographic predictors of side branch occlusion following high-pressure intracoronary stenting. Am J Cardiol 1997;80:994-997.

64. Caputo RP, Chafizadeh ER, Stoler RC, Lopex JJ, Cohen DJ, Kuntz RE, Carrozzar JP Jr., Baim DS. Stent jail: A minumum-security prison. Am J Cardiol 1995;77:1226-1229.

65. Dauerman HL, Cohen DJ, Carrozza JP Jr., et al. Rotational atherectomy for the treatment of restenotic ostial side branches jailed by prior stent placement. Cathet Cardiovasc Diagn. 1998;43:447-450.

66. Kini A, Vidhun R, Sharma S. Rotational atherectomy: A new treatment modality for ostial stenoses of "stent-jailed" sidebranches. J Invasc Cardiol 1998;10(3):169-172.

67. Duvvuri S, Daley-Sterling F, Sharma SK, Ambrose JA. Rotational atherectomy of a side branch through a Palmaz-Schatz stent: Is stent jail impenetrable to rotational atherectomy? J Interv Cardiol 1998;10(3):187-190.

68. Khoja A, Ozbek C, Bay W, Heisel A. Trouse-like stenting: A new technique for bifurcation lesions. Cathet Cardiovasc Diagn. 1997;41:192-196.

69. Suwaidi JA, Berger PB, Rihal CS, et al. Immediate and long-term outcome of intracoronary stent implantattion for true bifurcation lesions. J Am Coll Cardiol 2000;35:929-36.

70. Yamashita R, Nishida T, Adamian MG, et al. Bifurcation lesions: Two stents versus one stent—immediate and follow-up results. J Am Coll Cardiol 2000;35:1145-51.

11 PROXIMAL VESSEL TORTUOSITY AND ANGULATED LESIONS

Mark S. Freed, M.D.
Robert D. Safian, M.D.

PROXIMAL VESSEL TORTUOSITY

A. DEFINITION. No single definition of proximal vessel tortuosity has gained widespread acceptance. Different definitions include the presence of two or more bends ≥75° proximal to the target lesion; at least one proximal bend ≥90°; or the presence of "significant" vessel curvature proximal to the target lesion (without being more specific). Others grade proximal tortuosity according to the number of 45° bends (no/mild = 0-1 bend, moderate = 2 bends, severe = 3 or more bends).

B. PROCEDURAL OUTCOME

1. **PTCA.** In the past, balloon angioplasty in vessels with proximal tortuosity was associated with a higher incidence of acute complications and procedural failure (due to inability to cross the lesion with a guidewire and inadequate guiding catheter support) (Table 11.1).[1,2,4,5] However, our impression is that contemporary low-profile balloons, extra-support hydrophilic guidewires, and geometric guiding catheters have improved the results of PTCA in these and other challenging lesions.

2. **Non-Balloon Devices.** Severe proximal vessel tortuosity is problematic for all atherectomy devices, stents and lasers, which are more bulky, less flexible, and less trackable than balloon catheters. Although there has been little change in the flexibility and trackability of laser and atherectomy devices in the last several years,[6] dramatic improvements in stent technology now allow reliable stent delivery in most lesions (Chapter 26). DCA is virtually never considered in the setting of extreme tortuosity due to the increased risk of failure and complications,[5,7,8] even with small housing and GTO devices. The lower-profile Flexi-Cut™ DCA device can be used with 8F guiding catheters and may have better trackability, but has not yet been released.

C. TECHNICAL CONSIDERATIONS AND APPROACH

1. **Equipment.** The proper combination of guiding catheter, guidewire, and balloon catheter is critical to the success and safety of PTCA of tortuous vessels.

   a. **Guiding Catheter.** The optimal guiding catheter provides stable position, coaxial alignment, easy torque control, kink-resistance, a soft tip, and a stiff shaft to maximize "back-up" support (Figure 11.1). The choice of guiding catheter is usually determined by the orientation (take-off) of the target vessel and size of the aortic root (Table 11.2).

Table 11.1. Effect of Proximal Tortuosity on Acute PTCA Outcome

Series	N	Morphology	Success (%)	Other Results
Tan[1]	965	No tortuosity	93	Acute closure (3% vs. 4.2% vs. 6%)
(1995)	142	Moderate tortuosity	93	
	50	Severe tortuosity	84	
Ellis[2]	189	Type A lesion	92	Acute complications (2% vs. 15%)
(1990)	65	Proximal tortuosity	72	
Gossman[3]	53	No Shepherd Crook	98	Difficulty crossing lesion (13% vs.
(1988)	51	Shepherd Crook	86	33%)

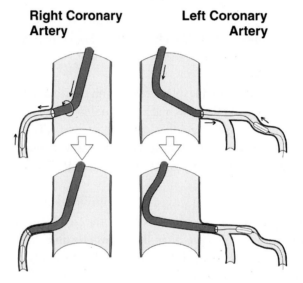

Figure 11.1. Deep-Seating Maneuver

The deep-seating maneuver can be used to increase guiding catheter support. To perform this technique, the balloon is retracted as the guide is advanced and gently rotated clockwise. The balloon is then re-advanced while gentle forward pressure is maintained on the guide. Extreme care must be taken to maintain distal guidewire position and avoid vessel trauma. Once the balloon has reached the stenosis, the guide is withdrawn to its original position.

Table 11.2. Guide Catheter Selection Based on Target Vessel Orientation

Vessel Orientation	Tip Configuration for Coaxial Alignment
Right Coronary Artery	
Superior take-off	Left Amplatz, El Gamal, Hockey Stick, IMA, or a geometric right catheter; best "back-up" may be from the left brachial approach
Marked inferior take-off	Multipurpose or Amplatz catheter. If a Judkins right catheter is used, deep vessel engagement may be required to improve back-up (Figure 11.1)
Horizontal take-off	JR4, Hockey Stick, or right Amplatz
Left Coronary Artery	Left Amplatz or a geometric left catheter

b. **Guidewire.** The choice of guidewire is largely based on operator preference.   Virtually all guidewires have a lubricious coating to enhance guidewire movement. Although 0.018" guidewires have superior flexibility and support, most have been replaced by 0.014" guidewires. For tortuous vessels, conventional 0.014" floppy guidewires may be sufficient, but in situations where the guidewire tip prolapses away from the target lesion, a tapered-core guidewire may be better. In some situations, steerability and tip-response are lost as the wire passes through multiple curves; partial advancement of the balloon catheter (or any other suitable transport catheter) may improve guidewire support, torque control, and steerability. If this maneuver fails, other options include the use of stiffer tip guidewires to improve handling characteristics, extra-support guidewires (in which the shaft rather than the tip is stiffer) to straighten vessel curves and ease guidewire movement, and hydrophilic guidewires, some of which are made of Nitinol and are extremely flexible and kink-resistant. Although heavy-duty guidewires are generally not well suited as primary guidewires because of their stiffness and poor torque control, they provide excellent support and will enhance tracking of balloons when other guidewires fail. (When heavy-duty wires are used, pseudolesions should be anticipated.) The Wiggle-wire (Guidant, Santa Clara, CA) is a unique 0.014-inch guidewire with multiple sinusoidal curves near its tip. This wire may be extremely useful during stenting of lesions in tortuous vessels; as the wire is gently advanced and retracted, the tip of the balloon is deflected in a slighly different direction, facilitating access to the target lesion.

c. **Balloon Dilatation Catheter.** As with guidewires, the choice of balloon catheters is largely dependent on operator preference. Important characteristics for negotiating tortuous vessels include deflated profile, trackability, pushability, and guidewire movement. Deflated balloon profile is the easiest to measure (and is highly marketed by balloon manufacturers), but is less important that trackability and pushability. Although technical specifications of balloon products derived from in-vitro testing are less important than its performance in the hands of the operator, certain design features are worthy of consideration. In general, over-the-wire systems are more trackable and pushable than monorail designs; they are also easier to use when guidewire exchanges are needed. By comparison, monorail catheters have lower profiles than over-the-wire systems, and fixed balloon-wire systems have the lowest profile but lack guidewire tip response and steerability.

2. **Approach.** The following approach is recommended for PTCA of lesions with proximal vessel tortuosity:

   - Place a 30-cm long introducing sheath into the femoral artery to minimize iliac artery tortuosity and enhance guiding catheter support.

   - Choose a guide catheter that maximizes stable coaxial alignment and back-up support. Further back-up support can be obtained by using larger (8-9F) guides.

   - Use a 0.014" tapered-core flexible guidewire or hydrophilic wire to cross the lesion. Added support (and ease of guidewire exchange) may be achieved by trailing a transport catheter or over-the-wire balloon several centimeters behind the guidewire tip. Be sure to advance the guidewire as far beyond the lesion as possible so the balloon tracks over the stiffer portion of the wire. In different cases, a transfer catheter may be used to exchange for a Wiggle-wire or support wire.

   - Have the patient take in a deep breath. This will occasionally straighten proximal tortuosity and facilitate guidewire and balloon advancement.

   - Try a fixed wire-balloon system when an over-the-wire or monorail system fails.

   - Consider the left brachial approach when PTCA fails from the femoral approach. Superselective guide catheter intubation may increase procedural success (Chapter 2).

ANGULATED LESIONS

A. **BALLOON ANGIOPLASTY (Table 11.3).** PTCA of angulated (> 45-60°) lesions was thought to increase the risk of procedural failure, major ischemic complications, and restenosis.[2,12,13,22,23] Nevertheless, high procedural success (85-95%) and low complication rates (< 3%) are often reported. Complications are usually due to dissection and abrupt closure, possibly from straightening the vessel during balloon inflation. Although noncompliant (PET or thin-walled polyethylene) balloons[10,14] and long balloons may result in less "straightening force," [15,16,26] one study found no difference in lumen enlargement or complications between compliant and noncompliant balloons.[27]

B.   **NON-BALLOON DEVICES.** Virtually all atherectomy and laser devices should be avoided in severely angulated lesions due to the increased risk of dissection and perforation. One study using the Rotablator reported procedural success in 85% of moderately angled lesions (45-60°), but angulation > 60° was a powerful predictor of procedural failure, major ischemic complications, and perforation.[6] In a larger report, Rotablator treatment of angulated lesions > 45° resulted in lower success (86% vs 94%), more dissection (36% vs 16%), and higher mortality (2.7% vs. 0.3%) compared to non-angulated lesions.[17] Likewise, DCA has been used with high success (91%) and low complications (3.6%) in lesions with mild angulation (≤30°),[7] but angulation ≥45° was an independent predictor of procedural failure (relative risk 4.8) and major ischemic complications (relative risk 2.7).[8] Similarly, TEC and ELCA should not be used on severely angulated lesions due to the high risk of complications.[6,18,19] Most contemporary designs have superb conformability and can be used to treat mild or moderately angulated lesions without difficulty. Stenting of highly angulated lesions is more problematic with balloon-expandable stents (although a small study suggests safety and efficacy[25]), since stenting of hinge points may result in higher restenosis rates.[24] Tissue prolapse occurs more often with coil stents than with slotted tubular or mesh stents.

C.   **APPROACH.** The easiest and safest approach to percutaneous revascularization of highly angulated lesions is PTCA with a long balloon. The choice of balloon material is less important because of the high-degree of conformability of 30-40 mm balloons. Fixed wire-balloon systems are also quite conformable (due to the lack of a catheter shaft) and can be quite useful. Severe angulation is a contraindication to laser and atherectomy devices, particularly when the bulk of atheroma is situated on the inner curve of the angled vessel segment (Figure 11.2). When complex dissections occur in severely angulated lesions, mesh stents or self-expanding stents may be preferable to coil designs to minimize tissue prolapse. Patients with severely angulated stenoses that supply large myocardial territories should be considered for bypass surgery, particularly in the presence of multivessel disease not well-suited for stenting.

Table 11.3. Effect of Lesion Angulation on Acute PTCA Outcome

Series	N	Angulation	Success (%)	MACE (%)
Tan[1]	991	< 45°	94	2.2[†]
(1995)	136	45-90°	88	8.8[†]
	30	> 90°	83	13[†]
Myler[10]	543	< 45°	94	1.3
(1992)	158	45-90°	95	2.5
	78	≥ 90°	94	2.6
Savas[11]	69*	≥ 45°	88	1
(1992)				
Ellis[2]	189	Type A	92	2
(1990)	144	≥ 45°	72	13[++]
	32	≥ 60°	53	-

Abbreviations: MACE = in-hospital major adverse cardiac events (death, MI, rePTCA, emergency CABG); - = not reported

*   All lesions ≥2 cm in length were treated with long (40-mm) balloons
†   Acute closure
++ Dissection occurred in 46% of angulated lesions compared to 8% of non-angulated lesions

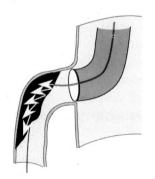   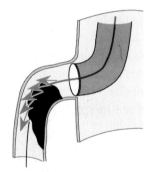

Lesion on Outer Curve: **Lesion on Inner Curve:**
Device directed into lesion   Device deflected into disease-free wall

Figure 11.2. Angulated Lesions: Impact of Lesion Location

Angulated lesions with plaque situated along the outer curve may sometimes be considered for ELCA, TEC, or Rotablator. In contrast, when plaque is situated along the inner curve, these devices may deflect away from the plaque and into the disease-free wall, increasing the risk of dissection and perforation.

* * * * *

REFERENCES

1. Tan K, Sulke N, Taub N, Sowton E. Clinical and lesion morphologic determinants of coronary angioplasty success and complications: Current experience. J Am Coll Cardiol 1995;25:855-65.

2. Ellis SG, Vandormael MG, Cowley MJ, et al. Coronary morphologic and clinical determinants of procedural outcome with angioplasty for multivessel coronary disease. Implications for patient selection. Circulation 1990;82:1193-1202.

3. Gossman DE, Tuzcu EM, Simpfendorfer C, et al. Percutaneous transluminal angioplasty for shepherd's crook right coronary artery stenosis. Cathet Cardiovasc Diagn 1989;15:189-191.

4. Flood RD, Popma JJ, Chuang YC, Salter LF, et al. Incidence, angiographic predictors, and clinical significance of coronary perforation occurring after new device angioplasty. J Am Coll Cardiol 1994;23:301A.

5. Holmes DR, Berdan L, et al. Abrupt closure: The coronary angioplasty versus excisional atherectomy trial (CAVEAT) experience. J Am Coll Cardiol 1994;23:I-585A.

6. Ellis SG, Popma JJ, Buchbinder M, Franco I, et al. Relation of clinical presentation, stenosis morphology, and operator technique to the procedural results of rotational atherectomy and rotational atherectomy-facilitated angioplasty. Circulation 1994;89:882-892.

7. Hinohara T, Rowe MH, Robertson, GC, Selmon MR, et al. Effect of lesion characteristics on outcome of directional coronary atherectomy. J Am Coll Cardiol 1991;17:1112-20.

8. Ellis SG, De Cesare NB, Pinkerton CA, Whitlow P, et al. Relation of stenosis morphology and clinical presentation to the procedural results of directional coronary atherectomy. Circulation 1991;84:644-653.

9. Torre SR, Lai SM, Schatz RA. Relation of clinical presentation and lesion morphology to the procedural results of Palmaz-Schatz stent placement: A New Approaches to Coronary Intervention (NACI) registry report. J Am Coll Cardiol 1994;23:135A.

10. Myler RK, Shaw RE, Stertzer SH, Hecht HS, et al. Lesion morphology and coronary angioplasty: Current experience and analysis. J Am Coll Cardiol 1992;19:1641-52.

11. Savas V, Puchrowicz S, Williams L, et al. Angioplasty outcome using long balloons in high-risk lesions. J Am Coll Cardiol 1992;19:34A.

12. Hermans WRM, Foley DP, Rensing BJ, Rutsch W, et al. Usefulness of quantitative and qualitative angiographic lesion morphology, and clinical characteristics in predicting major adverse cardiac events during and after native coronary balloon angioplasty. Am J Cardiol 1993;72:14-20.

13. Tenaglia AN, Zidar JP, Jackman JD, Fortin DF, et al. Treatment of long coronary artery narrowings with long angioplasty balloon catheters. Am J Cardiol 1993;71:1274-1277.

14. Ellis SG and Topol EJ. Results of percutaneous transluminal coronary angioplasty of high-risk angulated stenoses. Am J Cardiol 1990;66:932-937.

15. Barasch E, Conger JL, Janota T, Peters JJ, et al. PTCA of lesions on a bend: Effects of balloon material, balloon length, and inflation sequence. Circulation 1994;90:I-435.

16. Gray WA, Ghazzal ZMB, White HJ. The effects of balloon length and angle severity on the straightening force developed by polyethylene terephthalate (PET) angioplasty balloons. Circulation 1994;90:I-587.

17. Chevalier B, Commeau P, Favereau X, Gueri Y, et al. Limitations of rotational atherectomy in angulated coronary lesions. J Am Coll Cardiol 1994;23:285A.

18. Ghazzal ZMB, Hearn JA, Litvack F, Goldenberg T, et al. Morphological predictors of acute complications after percutaneous excimer laser coronary angioplasty. Results of a comprehensive angiographic analysis: Importance of the eccentricity index. Circulation 1992;86:820-827.

19. Bittl JA, Sanborn TA, Tcheng JE, Siegel RM, et al. Clinical success, complications, and restenosis rates with excimer laser coronary angioplasty. Am J Cardiol 1992;70:1533-1539.

20. Hong MK, Popma JJ, Wong SC, Kent KM, et al. Incidence of and factors associated with abrupt closure in patients undergoing elective, new device angioplasty in native coronary arteries. J Am Coll Cardiol 1995;25:122A.

21. Freed M, May M, Lichtenberg A, Strzelecki M, et al. Predictors of angiographic and clinical complications after new device coronary interventions. Circulation 1994;90:I-549.

22. Van Belle E, Bauters C, Lablanche JM, et al. Angiographic determinants of acute closure after coronary angioplasty: A prospective quantitative coronary angiographic study of 3679 procedures. J Am Coll Cardiol 1994;23:222A.

23. Meckel CR, Ahmed W, Ferguson JJ, Strony J, et al. Angiographic predictors of severe dissection during balloon angioplasty: A report from the Hirulog Angioplasty Study. Circulation 1994;90:I-64.

24. Phillips PS, Alfonso F, Segovia J, et al. Effects of Palmaz-Schatz stents on angled coronary arteries. Am J Cardiol 1997;79:191-193.

25. Abhyankar AD, Luyue G, Bailey BP. Stent implantation in severely angulated lesions. Cathet Cardiovasc Diagn 1997;40:261-264.

26. Barasch E, Conger JL, Kadipasaoglu KA, et al. PTCA in angulated segments: Effects of balloon material, balloon length, and inflation sequence on straightening forces in an in vitro model. Cathet Cardiovasc Diagn. 1996;39:207-212.

27. Safian RD, Hoffmann MA, Almany S, Kahn J, Reddy V, Marsalese D, Gangadharan V, Ajluni S, Friedman HZ, Schreiber TL, Grines CL, O'Neill WW. Comparison of coronary angioplasty with compliant and noncompliant balloons (The Angioplasty Compliance Trial). Am J Cardiol 1995;76:518-520.

12 CALCIFIED LESIONS

Mark S. Freed, M.D.
Robert D. Safian, M.D.

In 1988, the American College of Cardiology/American Heart Association Task Force on Assessment of Diagnostic and Therapeutic Cardiovascular Procedures published a report regarding appropriate utilization of PTCA in the treatment of patients with coronary artery disease. In that report, moderate-to-heavy calcification (Type B characteristic) was considered an important risk factor for procedural failure and acute closure. Recent data suggest that better acute outcomes can be readily achieved using a multi-device revascularization strategy.

A. **LIMITATIONS OF ANGIOGRAPHY.** Intravascular ultrasound (IVUS) has been used to evaluate the depth and extent of coronary artery calcification, and to determine the sensitivity and specificity of coronary angiography for detecting calcium.[1,2] The severity of angiographic calcium correlated with increasing arcs and lengths of calcium by IVUS (Table 12.1) and the extent of coronary atherosclerosis.[47] However, angiography has poor sensitivity for detecting mild or moderate lesion calcium, and only moderate sensitivity for detecting extensive lesion calcium (Table 12.2).[48] Surprisingly, 11% of lesions with angiographic calcium are not calcified by IVUS (i.e., false positives). A prospective comparison between IVUS- and angiography-guided therapy suggests that IVUS can be useful for assessment of calcified lesions and for guiding therapy (Chapter 31).

Table 12.1. Assessment of Lesion Calcification By Angiography and IVUS

| | Angiographic Assessment of Calcification | | |
	None/Mild	Moderate	Severe
No. lesions	715	306	134
IVUS findings			
Lesion calcium (%)	61	90	98
Arc of calcium (degrees)	71	165	238
Length of calcium (mm)	3.6	7.2	9.7

Table 12.2. Sensitivity of Angiography for Detecting Lesion Calcium

IVUS Finding		Sensitivity of Angiography (%)*
Arc of calcium (degrees):	< 90	25
	91 - 180	50
	181 - 270	60
	271 - 360	85
Length of calcium (mm):	≤ 5	42
	6 - 10	63
	≥ 11	61
Location of calcium:	Superficial only	60
	Deep only	54
	Superficial + deep	24

* Percent of calcified lesions on IVUS with calcium on angiography

B. BALLOON ANGIOPLASTY

1. **Acute Results.** The impact of lesion calcification on PTCA success is variable: One report showed that lesion calcium had an adverse impact on procedural success,[3] while another did not[4] (Table 12.3). In a third report, the presence of lesion calcium was an independent predictor of significant residual stenosis after PTCA.[5] Mechanisms of suboptimal lumen enlargement include the inability to expand the lesion and elastic recoil (Figure 12.1). The impact of lesion calcification on major ischemic complications also varies: some reports showed a correlation, while others did not (Table 12.4). Differences in these older studies probably reflect the insensitivity of angiography for identifying the depth and extent of lesion calcification.

2. **Coronary Artery Dissection.** IVUS has shown that lesion calcium plays a direct role in promoting dissection following PTCA. In patients undergoing coronary and peripheral angioplasty, both the incidence and extent of dissection was significantly higher among calcified lesions.[9] When present, dissection usually originated at the transition between calcified and noncalcified plaque, presumably due to nonuniform shear forces generated by balloon expansion. In another study of calcified lesions, the incidence of dissection increased from 22% after Rotablator to 77% after adjunctive PTCA; there was also a shift in the location of dissection from inside (after Rotablator) to outside the calcified plaque (after PTCA).

Table 12.3. Influence of Lesion Calcium on Acute Outcome After PTCA

Series	Morphology	N	Success (%)
Tan[3] (1995)	Calcified	81	74
	Noncalcified	1076	94
Myler[4] (1992)	Calcified	140	92
	Noncalcified	639	95

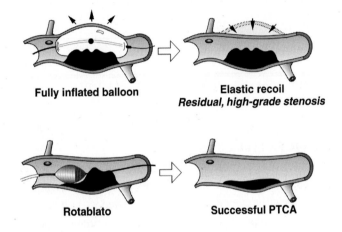

Fully inflated balloon

Elastic recoil
Residual, high-grade stenosis

Rotablato

Successful PTCA

Figure 12.1. Elastic Recoil After PTCA of Calcified Lesions

Rather than cracking the hard, calcified atheroma, PTCA causes stretching of the contralateral plaque-free wall segment and ineffective dilatation. The Rotablator appears particularly well-suited for calcified lesions.

3. **Restenosis.** Most studies fail to show any association between lesion calcium and restenosis after PTCA.

4. **Technical Requirements.** Higher inflation pressures are frequently required to dilate calcified stenoses, increasing the risk of balloon rupture and dissection. Although 89% of calcified lesions were successfully dilated with inflation pressures < 10 atm,[6] Rotablator atherectomy may increase lesion compliance, render the lesion more responsive to PTCA at low inflation pressures, and reduce the incidence of dissection. Rotablator has essentially replaced all other techniques for revascularizing calcified lesions.[11,46]

Table 12.4. Influence of Lesion Calcium on Ischemic Complications After PTCA

Series	Morphology	N	MACE (%)	Comments
Tan[3] (1995)	Calcified Noncalcified	81 1076	14* 2.5*	
Danchin[6] (1994)	Calcified Noncalcified	285 1801	4.3 3.7	
Hermans[7] (1993)	Calcified	69	-	Lesion calcium did not predict MACE
Myler[4] (1992)	Calcified Noncalcified	140 639	3.6 1.3	
Ellis[8] (1990)	Calcified	46	-	Relative risk of MACE = 1.5 for calcified lesions

Abbreviations: MACE = in-hospital major adverse cardiac events (death, MI, PTCA, CABG); - = not reported
* Acute closure

C. NON-BALLOON DEVICES (Table 12.5)

1. **Rotablator Atherectomy (Chapter 27).** Rotablator is a unique device for the management of calcified lesions. Rotablator preferentially ablates calcified atheroma,[28,29] results in larger and more concentric lumens with fewer dissections in calcified vs. noncalcified lesions,[30] and produces microfractures in calcium deposits to increase lesion compliance and responsiveness to PTCA.[29] Procedural success rates > 90% and complication rates < 5% are routinely achieved after Rotablator atherectomy of calcified stenoses.[13,15,26] In fact, Ellis et al[14] reported more procedural complications in noncalcified lesions treated with Rotablator. Conclusions regarding the impact of lesion calcium on restenosis after Rotablator have varied. In one report, restenosis was no different for calcified and noncalcified lesions (54% vs. 50%),[15] while in another report restenosis was 2-3 times more likely in calcified lesions.[27] Preliminary reports from STRATAS (Study To Determine Rotablator and Transluminal Angioplasty Strategy) suggest that aggressive debulking with larger burrs and longer ablation times does not improve immediate or late outcomes compared to more conservative debulking strategies.[45] In an IVUS study of Rotablator followed by PTCA, DCA, or stents, Rotablator plus stent (Rotastent) achieved the largest lumen and smallest residual stenosis[43] (Table 12.5)(Chapter 27). At the present time, Rotablator atherectomy is the preferred method for revascularizing calcified stenoses.

Table 12.5. Non-Balloon Devices for Calcified Lesions: Acute Outcome

Series	Device	Morphology	N	Success (%)	MACE (%)	Comments
Singh[51] (2001)	PTCA ± Stent ROTA	Calcified	2065 447	- -	10.9 13.0	Residual stenosis < 50% (93% vs. 98%, p < 0.0001)
Kobayashi[52] (2001)	Stent	No/mild Ca^{++} Mod. Ca^{++} Severe Ca^{++}	215 75 76	- - -	- - -	Final lumen CSA > 6.0 mm^2 (71% vs. 60% vs. 58%). Only 72% of severely calcified lesions by IVUS were calcified on angiography
Hoffmann[43] (1998)	ROTA/PTCA Stent ROTA/Stent	Calcified (vessel > 3mm)	147 103 56	99 98 98	1.4 3.0 3.6	FDS (27% vs. 14% vs. 4%); TLR (28% vs. 21% vs. 15%)
Moussa[44] (1997)	ROTA/Stent	Calcified	106	93	-	TLR (18%)
Ahmed[46] (1996)	ELCA	Undilatable	38	89	8	RS (45%)
Dussaillant[41] (1996)	ROTA/Stent ROTA/DCA ROTA/PTCA	Calcified (vessel ≥ 3mm)	83 120 235	- - -	0 - -	FDS (12% vs. 16% vs. 24%)
MacIssac[15] (1994)	ROTA	Noncalcified Calcified	1083 1078	95 94	3.4 4.1	RS (50% vs. 54%)
deMarchena[25] (1994)	Holmium-laser	All lesions Calcified	365 111	94 90	2.7 4.5	
Bittl[22] (1993)	ELCA	Undilatable	36	92	-	Non-Q-MI (6%)
Altmann[16] (1993)	ROTA	No/mild Ca^{++} Mod. Ca^{++}	182 378	96 96	2.1 2.8	1-yr EFS (67% vs. 75%)
Reisman[17] (1993)	ROTA	Undilatable	67	96	1.5	RS (36%)
Popma[18] (1993)	DCA	All lesions Calcified	306 60	95 94	- -	1-yr EFS (72% vs. 80%)
Bittl[23] (1992)	ELCA	Calcified	170	83	-	RS (43%)
Hinohara[19] (1991)	DCA	Type A Calcified	105 70	98 87	0 5.7	
Ellis[20] (1991)	DCA	Calcified	47	-	-	Relative risk of failure 1.98
TEC[21] database	TEC	Noncalcified Calcified	278 154	96 89	- -	

Abbreviations: AC = abrupt closure; CSA = cross-sectional area; DCA = directional coronary atherectomy; EFS = event-free survival; ELCA = excimer laser coronary angioplasty; FDS = final diameter stenosis; MACE = in-hospital major adverse cardiac events;
RS = restenosis; TEC = transluminal extraction atherectomy; TLR = target lesion revascularization; - not reported

2. **Directional Coronary Atherectomy (DCA).** DCA has a very limited ability to excise calcified plaque and should be avoided when moderate or heavy lesion calcium is present. IVUS studies clearly show that lesion calcium correlates with ineffective plaque removal after DCA,[18,31-34] although DCA may be effective after initial Rotablator.[35,42] DCA should also be avoided when there is significant calcification proximal to the target lesion because of failure to reach the target lesion. Future improvements in DCA technology and the availability of a special calcium-cutter (Flexi-Cut device) may increase the application of DCA to calcified lesions.

3. **TEC Atherectomy.** TEC should not be used for heavily calcified lesions. Because of the excellent flexibility of TEC cutters, vessel calcification proximal to the target lesion is not a contraindication to TEC atherectomy.

4. **Excimer Laser Coronary Angioplasty (ELCA) (Chapter 31).** Among 170 calcified lesions treated with ELCA, procedural success was achieved in 83%, which is slightly lower than for noncalcified stenoses.[23] Better results may be obtained by starting with small fibers and higher fluence (50-60 mJ/mm^2). Although one report found an association between lesion calcification and major complications,[23] two reports did not.[36,37] Restenosis occurs in 40-50% of lesions after ELCA and appears to be independent of lesion calcification.[23] In contrast to Rotablator atherectomy,[29] which increases lesion compliance by removing calcium, ELCA renders the lesion more responsive to PTCA by fracturing (rather than removing) calcium.[38] Like the Rotablator, ELCA is effective in treating some undilatable stenoses.[22] Nevertheless, the high predictability of success with Rotablator has rendered ELCA nearly obsolete for treating calcified lesions.

5. **Holmium Laser Angioplasty.** The Holmium Laser Coronary Registry reported lower procedural success and more ischemic complications among calcified stenoses. Nevertheless, final results were acceptable and similar to those achieved by ELCA.[25]

6. **Stents.** Heavy lesion calcium increases the risk of incomplete stent expansion[34] and restenosis.[39] When heavily calcified plaque is first modified by the Rotablator, final lumen cross-sectional area after stenting may be smaller than in lesions without calcification,[40] although it is still larger compared to Rotablator followed by PTCA[12,14] or DCA.[14] If a lesion cannot be fully dilated with a balloon, stent placement is contraindicated since incomplete stent expansion increases the risk of stent thrombosis and restenosis.

D. TECHNICAL STRATEGY (Figures 12.2, 12.3)

1. **Superficial and Deep Calcium**
   a. **Focal Lesions.** If calcification is present on angiography, IVUS may be used to guide therapy based on the depth and extent of lesion calcium and vessel size (Figure 12.3). If IVUS is not available, we recommend Rotablator atherectomy; adjunctive PTCA (with a noncompliant balloon) or stenting often results in excellent lumen enlargement without dissection.

Calcification by Angiography

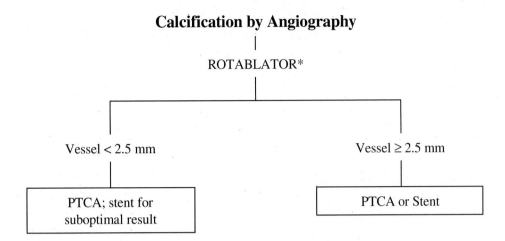

Figure 12.2. **Treatment of Calcified Lesions When IVUS is <u>NOT</u> Available**

* For angulated lesions use a burr/artery ratio of 0.5; for all other lesions use a burr/artery ratio of 0.6-0.8.

b. Long Lesions. The ideal treatment of long, calcified lesions is unknown. PTCA may be attempted using a long balloon, but the risk of dissection or suboptimal result is increased. ELCA is theoretically appealing for long lesions, but disappointing long-term outcomes have resulted in a marked decline in ELCA over the last few years. The Rotablator is effective in treating calcified stenoses, but its use in long lesions may be associated with a higher risk of no-reflow, non-Q-wave MI, and restenosis. Slow passes with a small burr ($\leq$ 1.75 mm) and a stepwise increase in burr size not to exceed 0.25 mm may result in excellent pulverization of calcium, few complications, and good angiographic results.

2. Deep Calcium Only. Unlike superficial calcium located at the intimal-lumen interface, deep calcium (at or near the medial-adventitial border) does not usually interfere with PTCA or stenting. Device selection can be based on associated lesion morphologies, with or without antecedent Rotablator.

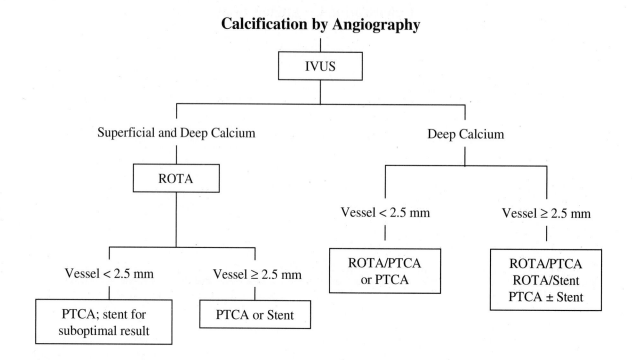

Figure 12.3. Treatment of Calcified Lesions When IVUS IS Available

ROTA = Rotablator

* * * * *

REFERENCES

1. Mintz G, Popma J, et al. Patterns of calcification in coronary artery disease. A statistical analysis of intravascular ultrasound and coronary angiography in 1155 lesions. Circulation 1995;91:1959-1965.
2. Mintz GS, Pichard AD, Kovach JA, et al. Impact of preintervention intravascular ultrasound imaging on transcatheter treatment strategies in coronary artery disease. Am J Cardiol 1994;73:423-430.
3. Tan, K., N. Sulke, et al. Clinical and lesion morphologic determinants of coronary angioplasty success and complications: Current experience. J Am Coll Cardiol 1995;25:855-65.
4. Myler RK, Shaw RE, Stertzer SH, et al. Lesion morphology and coronary angioplasty: Current experience and analysis. J Am Coll Cardiol 1992;19:1641-52.
5. Van Belle, E, Bauters C, Lablanche JM, McFadden EP, Quandalle P, Bertrand ME. Angiographic determinants of acute outcome after coronary angioplasty: A prospective quantitative coronary angiographic study of 3679 procedures. J Am Coll Cardiol 1994;March Special Issue:222A.
6. Danchin N, Buffet P, Dibon O, et al. Should specific angioplasty techniques be used to treat calcified coronary artery lesions? A retrospective study. Circulation 1994;90:I-436.
7. Hermans WR, Foley D, et al. Usefulness of quantitative and qualitative angiographic lesion morphology, and clinical characteristics in predicting major adverse cardiac events during and after native coronary balloon angioplasty. Am J Cardiol 1993;72:14-20.
8. Ellis SG, Vandormael MG, Cowley MJ, et al. Coronary morphologic and clinical determinants of procedural outcome with angioplasty for multivessel coronary disease. Implications for patient selection. Circulation 1990;82:1193-1202.
9. Fitzgerald P, Ports T, Yock P. Contribution of localized calcium deposits to dissection after angioplasty: An observational study using IVUS. Circulation 1992;86:64-70.
10. Khurana S, Bakalyar D, Schreiber T, et al. Facilitated lumen enlargement by longitudinal force focused angioplasty. J Am Coll Cardiol 1995;March Special Issue:345A.
11. Solar RJ, Meaney DF, Miller RT, et al. Enhanced lumen enlargement with new focused force angioplasty device. Circulation 1995;92:I-147.
12. Mintz GS, Dusaillant GR, Wong SC, et al. Rotational atherectomy followed by adjunct stents: The preferred therapy for calcified lesions in large vessels? Circulation 1995;92:I-329.
13. Warth D, Leon M, et al. Rotational atherectomy multicenter registry: Acute results, complications and 6-month angiographic follow-up in 709 patients. J Am Coll Cardiol 1994;24:641-648.
14. Ellis S, Popma J, et al. Relation of clinical presentation, stenosis morphology, and operator technique to the procedural results of rotational atherectomy-facilitated angioplasty. Circulation 1994;89:882-892.
15. MacIssac AI, Whitlow PL, Cowley MJ, Buchbinder M. Angiographic predictors of outcome of coronary rotational atherectomy from the completed multicenter registry. J Am Coll Cardiol 1994;March Special Issue:353A.
16. Altmann DB, Popma JJ, Kent KM, et al. Rotational atherectomy effectively treats calcified lesions. J Am Coll Cardiol 1993;21 (Part II):443A.
17. Reisman M, Devlin PG, Melikian J, Fenner J, Buchbinder M. Undilatable noncompliant lesions treated with the Rotablator: Outcome and angiographic follow-up. Circulation 1993;Speical Issue:2949.
18. Popma JJ, Mintz GS, Satler LF, et al. Clinical and angiographic outcome after directional coronary atherectomy. A qualitative and quantitative analysis using coronary arteriography and intravascular ultrasound. Am J Cardiol 1993;72:55E-64E.
19. Hinohara T, Rowe MH, Robertson GC, et al. Effect of lesion characteristics on outcome of directional coronary atherectomy. Circulation 1991;17:1112-1120.
20. Ellis SG, De Cesare NB, Pinkerton CA, et al. Relation of stenosis morphology and clinical presentation to the procedural results of directional coronary atherectomy. Circulation 1991;84:644-653.
21. IVT® Coronary TEC® Atherectomy Clinical Database Investigators Meeting. 1992.
22. Bittl JA, Sanborn TA, Tcheng JE, Watson LE. Excimer laser-facilitated angioplasty for undilatable coronary lesions: Results of a prospective, controlled study. Circulation 1993;88:I-24.
23. Bittl J, Sanborn T, et al. Clinical success, complications and restenosis rates with excimer laser coronary angioplasty. Am J Cardiol 1992;70:1533-1539.
24. Levine S, Mehta S, Krauthamer D, et al. Excimer laser coronary angioplasty of calcified lesions. J Am Coll Cardiol 1991;17(2):206A.
25. deMarchena EJ, Mallon SM, et al. Effectiveness of holmium laser-assisted coronary angioplasty. Am J Cardiol 1994;73:117-121.
26. Leon MB, Kent KM, Pichard AD, et al. Percutaneous transluminal coronary rotational angioplasty of calcified lesions. Circulation 1991;84(4):II-521.
27. Leguizamon JH, Chambre DF, Torresani EM, et al. High-speed coronary rotational atherectomy. Are angiographic factors predictive of failure, major complications or restenosis? A multivariate analysis. J Am Coll Cardiol 1995:Special Issue:95A.
28. Mintz G, Potkin B, et al. Intravascular ultrasound evaluation of the effect of rotational atherectomy in obstructive atherosclerotic coronary artery disease. Circulation 1992;86:1383-1393.
29. Kovach J, Mintz G, et al. Sequential intravascular ultrasound characterization of the mechanisms of rotational atherectomy and adjunct balloon angioplasty. J Am Coll Cardiol 1993;22 (4):1024-32.
30. Fitzgerald PJ, Stertzer SH, Hidalgo BO, Myler RK, et al. Plaque characteristics affect lesion and vessel response to coronary rotational atherectomy: An intravascular ultrasound study. J Am Coll Cardiol 1994;March Special Issue:353A.
31. De Franco AC, Tuzcu EM, Moliterno DJ, et al. "Directional"

oronary atherectomy removes atheroma more effectively from concentric than eccentric lesions: Intravascular ultrasound predictors of lesional success. J Am Coll Cardiol 1995;February Special Issue:137A.

32. Matar FA, Mintz GS, Kent KM, et al. Predictors of intravascular ultrasound endpoints after directional coronary atherectomy in 170 patients. J Am Coll Cardiol 1994;February Special Issue:302A.

33. DeLezo JS, Romero M, Medina A, et al. Intracoronary ultrasound assessment of directional coronary atherectomy: Immediate and follow-up findings. J Am Coll Cardiol 1993;21:298-307.

34. Hong MK, Chuang YC, Prunka N, Satler LF. Predictors of early and late cardiac events in patients undergoing saphenous vein graft angioplasty with PTCA and new device modalities. Circulation 1993;88:I-601.

35. Henson KD, Flood R, Javier SP, et al. Transcatheter device synergy: Use of adjunct directional atherectomy after rotational atherectomy or excimer laser angioplasty. J Am Coll Cardiol 1994;February Special Issue:220A.

36. Ghazzal Z, Hearn J, et al. Morphological predictors of acute complications after percutaneous excimer laser coronary angioplasty. Results of a comprehensive angiographic analysis: Importance of the eccentricity index. Circulation 1992;86:820-827.

37. Baumbach A, Bittl J, Fleck E, et al. Acute complications of excimer laser coronary angioplasty: A detailed analysis of multicenter results. J Am Coll Cardiol 1994;23:1305-1313.

38. Mintz GS, Kovach JA, Javier SP, et al. Mechanisms of lumen enlargement after excimer laser angioplasty: An intravascular ultrasound study. Circulation 1995;92:3408-14.

39. Tamura T, Kimura T, Nosaka H, Nobuyoshi M. Predictors of restenosis after Palmaz-Schatz stent implantation. Circulation 1994;90:I-324.

40. Goldberg SL, Hall P, Almagor Y, Maiello L, et al. Intravascular ultrasound guided rotational atherectomy of fibro-calcific plaque prior to intracoronary deployment of Palmaz-Schatz stents. J Am Coll Cardiol 1994;February Special Issue:290A.

41. Dussaillant GR, Mintz GS, Pichard AD, et al. The optimal strategy for treating calcified lesions in large vessels: Comparison of intravascular ultrasound results of rotational atherectomy + adjunctive PTCA, DCA, or stents. J Am Coll Cardiol 1996;27:153A.

42. Dusaillant GR, Mintz GS, Pichard AD, et al. Mechanisms and immediate and long-term results of adjunct directional coronary atherectomy after rotational atherectomy. J Am Coll Cardiol 1996;27:1390-7.

43. Hoffmann R, Mintz GS, Kent KM, Pichard AD, Satler LF, et al. Comparative early and nine-month results of rotational atherectomy, stents, and the combination of both for calcified lesions in large coronary arteries. Am J Cardiol 1998;81:552-557.

44. Moussa I, Di Mario C, Moses J, Reimers B, et al. Coronary stenting after rotational atherectomy in calcified and complex lesions. Angiographic and clinical follow-up results. Circulation 1997;96:128-136.

45. Bass TA, Williams DO, Ho, KKL, et al. Is an aggressive Rotablator strategy preferable to a standard Rotablator strategy in patients with heavily calcified coronary lesions? A report from the STRATAS trial. J Am Coll Cardiol 1998;71:378A.

46. Ahmed WH, Al-Anazi MM, Bittl JA. Excimer laser-facilitated angioplasty for undilatable coronary narrowings. Am J Cardiol 1996;78:1045-1047.

47. Mintz GS, Pichard AD, Popma JJ, Kent KM, et al. Determinants and correlates of target lesion calcium in coronary artery disease: A clinical, angiographic and intravascular ultrasound study. J Am Coll Cardiol 1997;29:268-74.

48. Tuzcu EM, Berkalp B, DeFranco AC, Ellis SG, et al. The dilemma of diagnosing coronary calcification: Angiography versus intravascular ultrasound. J Am Coll Cardiol 1996;27:832-838.

49. Mintz GS, Pichard AD, Kent KM, Satler LF, Popma JJ, Leon MB. Interrelation of coronary angiographic reference lumen size and intravascular ultrasound target lesion calcium. Am J Cardiol 1998;81:387-391.

50. Kiesz SR, Rozek MM, Ebersole DG, et al. Novel approach to rotational atherectomey results in low restenosis rates in long, calcified lesions: Long-term results of the San Antonio Rotablator Study (SARS). Cathet Cardiovasc Intervent 1999;48:48-53.

51. Singh M, Mathew V, Lennon RJ, et al. Comparison of rotational atherectomy versus PTCA with or without stenting in calcified lesions: In-hospital and 6-month outcome. J Am Coll Cardiol 2001;37(2):10A.

52. Kobayashi Y, Mehran R, Dangas G, et al. Effect of coronary plaque calcification on the final lumen dimensions after stenting without rotational atherectomy: An intravascular ultrasound study. J Am Coll Cardiol 2001;37(2):11A.

53. Braden GA, Herrington DM, Kerensky RA, Kutcher MA, Little WC. Angiography poorly predicts actual lesion eccentricity in severe coronary stenoses: Confirmation by intracoronary ultrasound imaging. J Am Coll Cardiol 1994;March Special Issue:413A.

13 ECCENTRIC LESIONS

Mark S. Freed, M.D.
Robert D. Safian, M.D.

A. LIMITATIONS OF ANGIOGRAPHY. Contrast angiography has poor predictive value for the detection of eccentric plaque morphology. In one report of angiographically-apparent eccentric lesions, only 63% had eccentric plaque morphology by intravascular ultrasound (IVUS), and 70% of angiographically "concentric" lesions were eccentric by IVUS.[1] In a second report, concordance between IVUS and angiography for assessment of lesion eccentricity was only 53%.[2] Eccentric stenoses have greater luminal cross-sectional area and less calcium than concentric stenoses, suggesting a less advanced form of coronary atherosclerosis. Although eccentricity is usually considered a dichotomous characteristic (i.e., present or absent), more than two-thirds of coronary stenoses have some degree of eccentricity.

B. DEFINITIONS OF ECCENTRIC LESIONS. There are several definitions of lesion eccentricity, as shown in Table 13.1.

C. BALLOON ANGIOPLASTY (Table 13.2). High success (> 90%) and low complication rates (< 3%) have been consistently reported for PTCA of most eccentric lesions.[3,4] While originally classified as an ACC/AHA "Type B" characteristic (procedural success in 60-85% and increased risk of acute closure), most data indicate that lesion eccentricity does not adversely affect procedural success or restenosis.[3-5] Observational reports suggest that compared to concentric lesions, PTCA of eccentric lesions may be associated with more elastic recoil, less effective plaque compression, more vasospasm, and suboptimal lumen enlargement.[6-8]

D. NON-BALLOON DEVICES (Table 13.2)

    1. Directional Coronary Atherectomy (DCA). DCA is highly effective for treating lesions with mild, moderate, and extreme eccentricity.[9] However, when compared to concentric lesions, eccentric lesions required more adjunctive PTCA (13% vs. 3%) and were associated with more complications (3.2% vs 0%).[10] Greater degrees of eccentricity also correlated with higher rates of restenosis after LAD atherectomy.[11]

Table 13.1. Definitions of Eccentric Lesions

Angiographic	Lumen in outer 1/4 of the apparent normal lumen
IVUS	Ratio of maximal-to-minimal plaque thickness > 2, or relative sparing of a portion of the vessel circumference (i.e., minimum plaque thickness < 0.75 mm)
Pathological	Arc of disease-free vessel wall

Table 13.2. Percutaneous Revascularization of Eccentric Stenoses

Series	Modality	Morphology	N	Success (%)	Other Results
Tan[3] (1995)	PTCA	Concentric Eccentric	491 666	93 92	AC (2.6% vs. 3.8%)
Myler[4] (1992)	PTCA	Concentric Eccentric	304 475	92 96	MACE (2.6% vs. 1.1%)
Popma[12] (1993)	DCA	Concentric Eccentric	71 235	96 94	- -
Hinohara[13] (1991)	DCA	Concentric Eccentric (mild-mod) Eccentric (extreme)	116 122 85	92 86 95	CABG (1.7% vs. 3.3% vs. 2.4)
Warth[14] (1994)	Rotablator	Concentric Eccentric	141 205	98 93	MACE (0% vs. 4.4%)
IVT Registry[15] (1992)	TEC	Concentric Eccentric	207 316	96 92	- -
AIS[16] Database (1992)	ELCA	Concentric Eccentric	135 174	92 89	- -
Leon[17] (1993)	DELCA	Concentric Eccentric	22 110	90 (overall)	Death (0.9); Q-MI (0.9); CABG (3.8); AC (3.8)
Ghazzal[18] (1993)	DELCA	Eccentric	150	91	-

Abbreviations: AC = acute closure; CABG = emergency coronary artery bypass grafting; DCA = directional coronary atherectomy; DELCA = directional ELCA; EFS = event-free survival; ELCA = excimer laser coronary angioplasty; MACE = major adverse cardiac events (in-hospital death, MI, CABG); Q-MI = Q-wave myocardial infarction; TEC = transluminal extraction atherectomy; - = not reported

Importantly, DCA outcome is highly dependent on associated lesion morphology: DCA success was 95% in eccentric lesions with irregular contour, 86% in long eccentric lesions, and only 64% in calcified eccentric lesions.[10] In another report of eccentric lesions, DCA success was 94% and 1-year event-free survival was 72%.[12] Contrary to popular belief, IVUS imaging revealed less plaque resection after DCA of eccentric lesions compared to concentric lesions (19% vs. 30%, p = 0.02). However, new DCA catheters with the capability for simultaneous ultrasound imaging and tissue excision may improve lumen enlargement and decrease complications.

2. **Rotablator.** Rotablator may be useful for rigid or calcified eccentric stenoses because of its ability to selectively ablate hard tissue (principle of differential cutting). Although Rotablator can be used to treat other types of eccentric lesions,[20,21] there is no advantage over PTCA. Lesion eccentricity (in addition to tortuousity and lesion length > 10mm) was a risk factor for coronary perforation[22] and intralesional spasm after Rotablator.[23]

3. **TEC Atherectomy.** TEC has no special value for eccentric lesions in native coronary arteries,[15] although it may be a useful adjunct for thrombotic eccentric lesions in saphenous vein grafts (Chapter 17).

4. **Excimer Laser.** Although data from the ELCA registry suggested that lesion eccentricity did not adversely affect procedural success, major complications,[24] or restenosis,[25] another angiographic analysis suggested that lesion eccentricity was a risk factor for in-hospital ischemic complications.[26] For lesions with extreme eccentricity, directional ELCA may be preferable to conventional ELCA, particularly in vessels < 3 mm in diameter. The directional ELCA system is comprised of an array of eccentrically-arranged fibers which can be directed toward eccentric plaque and away from angiographically normal vessel wall (Figure 13.1). Directional ELCA successfully treated 90% of highly eccentric lesions,[27] with significant reduction in plaque mass[17] and only 11% elastic recoil.[18] Final diameter stenosis was 24% following directional ELCA and adjunctive PTCA.

5. **Stents.** Virtually all stent designs are capable of treating eccentric lesions. Stents are unmatched in their ability to enlarge lumen dimensions, resist elastic recoil, and decrease dissection, all of which are important considerations when treating eccentric lesions. The favorable results of simplified anticoagulation regimens (i.e., without warfarin) make stents the treatment of choice for a wide range of lesions, including those with eccentric morphology.[27]

E. **TECHNICAL STRATEGY.** The approach to percutaneous revascularization of eccentric lesions is based on associated lesion morphology (Figure 13.2).

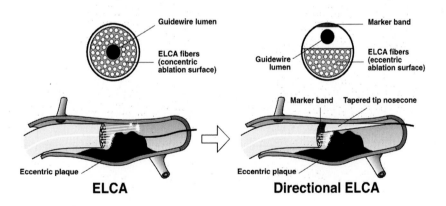

Figure 13.1. Directional ELCA of Eccentric Lesions

When using conventional ELCA for eccentric lesions, part of the concentric ablation surface fails to make contact with the plaque. In contrast, the eccentric plaque is fully exposed to the eccentric ablation surface of directional ELCA.

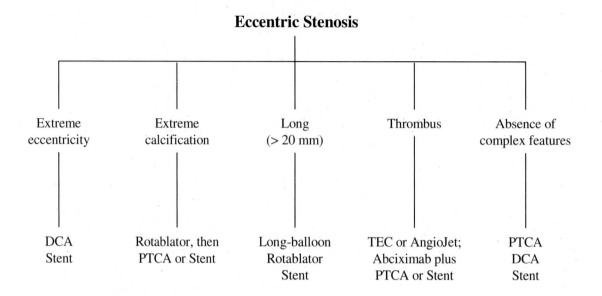

Figure 13.2. Treatment of Eccentric Lesions

Abbreviations: DCA = directional coronary atherectomy; TEC = transluminal extraction atherectomy

* * * * *

REFERENCES

1. Braden GA, Herrington DM, Kerensky RA, et al. Angiography poorly predicts actual lesion eccentricity in severe coronary stenoses: Confirmation by intracoronary ultrasound imaging. J Am Coll Cardiol 1994;Special Issue:413A.

2. Mintz GS, Popma JJ, Pichard AD, Kent KM, et al. Comparison of intravascular ultrasound and coronary angiography in the assessment of target lesion plaque distribution in coronary artery disease. TCT Meeting (Washington DC), February, 1995; Abstract.

3. Tan K, Sulke N, et al. Clinical and lesion morphologic determinants of coronary angioplasty success and complications: Current experience. J Am Coll Cardiol 1995;25:855-65.

4. Myler RK, Shaw RE, Stertzer SH, et al. Lesion morphology and coronary angioplasty: Current experience and analysis. J Am Coll Cardiol 1992;19:1641-52.

5. Ellis SG, Vandormael MG, Cowley MJ, et al. Coronary morphologic and clinical determinants of procedural outcome with angioplasty for multivessel coronary disease. Implications for patient selection. Circulation 1990;82:1193-1202.

6. Kimball BP, Eric SB, Cohen EA, et al. Comparison of acute elastic recoil after directional coronary atherectomy versus standard balloon angioplasty. Am Heart J 1992;124:1459.

7. Baptista J, diMario C, Ozaki Y, de Feyter P, et al. Determinants of lumen and plaque changes after balloon angioplasty: A quantitative ultrasound study. J Am Coll Cardiol 1994;March Special Issue:414A.

8. Fiscell TA, Bausback KN. Effects of luminal eccentricity on spontaneous coronary vasoconstriction after successful percutaneous transluminal coronary angioplasty. Am J Cardiol 1991;68:530.

9. Matar FA, Mintz GS, Kent KM, Pinnow E, et al. Predictors of intravascular ultrasound endpoints after directional coronary atherectomy in 170 patients. J Am Coll Cardiol 1994;March Special Issue:302A.

10. Ellis S, Popma J, et al. Relation of clinical presentation, stenosis morphology, and operator technique to the procedural results of rotational atherectomy-facilitated angioplasty. Circulation 1994;89:882-892.

11. Schiele TM, Marx R, Vogt M, Leschke M, et al. Eccentricity of coronary arteries is a predictor of chronic restenosis after directional coronary atherectomy. Circulation 1995;92:I-328.

12. Popma JJ, Mintz GS, Satler LF, et al. Clinical and angiographic outcome after directional coronary atherectomy. A qualitative and quantitative analysis using coronary arteriography and intravascular ultrasound. Am J Cardiol 1993;72:55E-64E.

13. Hinohara T, Vetter JW, Selmon MR, et al. Directional coronary atherectomy is effective treatment for extremely eccentric lesions. Circulation 1991;84:II-520.

14. Warth D, Leon M, et al. Rotational atherectomy multicenter registry: Acute results, complications and 6-month angiographic follow-up in 709 patients. J Am Coll Cardiol 1994;24:641-648.

15. IVT® Coronary TEC® Atherectomy Clinical Database Investigators Meeting, 1992.

16. Advanced Interventional Systems Coronary Excimer Laser Database. Goldenberg T. 1992.

17. Leon MB, Henson KD, Lavier SP, et al. Early results with directional laser angioplasty is unfavorable coronary lesions. Circulation 1993;88;I-23.

18. Ghazzal ZMB, Litvack F, Rothbaum DA, et al. The directional laser catheter: Quantitative angiographic core lab analysis from the first five centers. Circulation 1993; 88:I-23.

19. Fitzgerald PJ. Lesion composition impacts size and symmetry of stent expansion: Initial report from the STRUT Registry. J Am Coll Cardiol 1995;February Special Issue;49A.

20. MacIssac AI, Whitlow PL,. Cowley MJ, Buchbinder M. Angiographic predictors of outcome of coronary rotational atherectomy from the completed multicenter registry. J Am Coll Cardiol 1994;February Special Issue:353A.

21. Leguizamon JH, Chambre DF, Torresani EM, et al. High-speed coronary rotational atherectomy. Are angiographic factors predictive of failure, major complications or restenosis? A multivariate analysis. J Am Coll Cardiol 1995:February Special Issue:95A.

22. Hong MK, Chuang YC, Prunka N, Satler LF. Predictors of early and late cardiac events in patients undergoing saphenous vein graft angioplasty with PTCA and new device modalities. Circulation 1993;88:I-601.

23. Fitzgerald PJ, Stertzer SH, Hidalgo BO, Myler RK, et al. Plaque characteristics affect lesion and vessel response to coronary rotational atherectomy: An intravascular ultrasound study. J Am Coll Cardiol 1994;February Special Issue:353A.

24. Baumbach A, Bittl J, Fleck E, et al. Acute complications of excimer laser coronary angioplasty: A detailed analysis of multicenter results. J Am Coll Cardiol 1994;23:1305-1313.

25. Bittl J, Sanborn T, et al. Clinical success, complications and restenosis rates with excimer laser coronary angioplasty. Am J Cardiol 1992;70:1533-1539.

26. Ghazzal Z, Hearn J, et al. Morphological predictors of acute complications after percutaneous excimer laser coronary angioplasty. Results of a comprehensive angiographic analysis: Importance of the eccentricity index. Circulation 1992;86:820-827.

27. Rechavia E, Federman J, Shefer A, et al. Usefulness of a prototype directional excimer laser coronary angioplasty catheter in narrowings unfavorable for conventional excimer or balloon angioplasty. Am J Cardiol 1995;76:1144-46.

14 OSTIAL LESIONS

Mark S. Freed, M.D.
Robert D. Safian, M.D.

The presence of an ostial stenosis poses a special management problem for the interventional cardiologist, since ostial lesions are the most likely to be associated with suboptimal angiographic results due to lesion rigidity and elastic recoil. Efforts to improve lumen dimensions by aggressive PTCA frequently result in further elastic recoil, dissection, and a high incidence of restenosis. Successful treatment of ostial lesions is highly dependent on the use of non-balloon devices.

A. DEFINITIONS OF OSTIAL LESIONS

1. **Aorto-Ostial Stenosis.** A lesion that involves the junction between the aorta and the orifice of the RCA, left main, or a saphenous vein graft.

2. **Branch-Ostial Stenosis**. A lesion that involves the junction between a large epicardial vessel and the orifice of a major branch. In some studies, these are referred to as "origin" lesions.

3. **Other.** Some reports define an ostial lesion as one that is located within 3-5 mm of the vessel orifice but does not necessarily involve the ostium. The subtleties of these various definitions are important when comparing the results of different studies of ostial lesions.

B. PROCEDURAL RESULTS

1. **Balloon Angioplasty (Table 14.1).** The earliest study of PTCA of ostial RCA stenoses reported procedural success in 79% and emergency CABG in 9%.[9] These poor results were attributed to inadequate guide support, frequent lesion rigidity and elastic recoil, and ostial trauma due to high inflation pressures and guiding catheter injury. Since that time, procedural success and complication rates have improved, primarily due to technical advances in PTCA hardware and increased operator experience. More recent data indicate that highly-selected ostial lesions can be revascularized as safely as nonostial stenoses.[1,2,8] Nevertheless, even though PTCA success and complication rates have improved, quantitative angiographic studies report higher residual stenosis for ostial lesions compared to nonostial lesions (40-50% vs. 25-35%).[8] In addition, elastic recoil accounts for 50% loss in acute luminal gain even in the absence of other complex characteristics. These suboptimal angiographic results may not manifest as acute ischemic complications, but certainly account for the high incidence of restenosis and the need for repeat intervention. Atherectomy and stents are now used to revascularize ostial lesions. PTCA alone is not recommended.

Table 14.1. PTCA of Ostial Lesions: Acute Outcome

Series	Lesion	N	Success (%)	MACE (%)	Other
Keramati[45] (2001)	LAD Non-LAD	42 328	94% (overall)	14.2 1.5	Stent in 40% Stents in 25%
Inoue[37] (2000)	LAD (CB) LAD	7 7	- -	- -	Cutting balloon had more acute gain (1.7 mm vs. 0.48 mm) and less late loss (0.54 mm vs. 1.32 mm)
Muramatsu[38] (1999)	AO (CB)	37	95	0	Restenosis (43%)
Wishmeyer[30] (1999)	AO BO	73 98	97 93	- -	AC (4.1% vs. 20%); TLR (22% vs. 16%)
Jain[29] (1997)	RCA	23	88	0	TLR at 21 months (47%)
Tan[1] (1995)	Nonostial AO + BO	1080 77	93 94	- -	AC (0% vs. 3.5%)
Tan[2] (1994)	Nonostial AO BO	48 34 116	90 85 87	6 6 7	Highest residual stenosis for AO lesions
CAVEAT[3] (1995)	LAD	33	87	3	Restenosis (46%)
Sawada[4] (1994)	LAD/LCX	80	90	-	Restenosis (61%); TLR (58%)
Brown[5] (1993)	LAD	40	100	0	-
Myler[6] (1992)	AO + BO	14	93	0	-
Bedotto[7] (1991)	AO	60	85	0	-
Mathias[8] (1991)	BO	106	74	13	-
Topol[9] (1987)	AO	53	79	9.4	Restenosis (38%)

Abbreviations: AC = acute closure; AO = aorto-ostial; BO = branch-ostial; CB = cutting balloon; EFS = event-free survival (freedom from death, MI, CABG, repeat PTCA); LAD = left anterior descending coronary artery; LCX = left circumflex coronary artery; MACE = in-hospital major adverse cardiac events; TLR = target lesion revascularization; - = not reported

2. **Non-Balloon Devices.** Nonrandomized studies of ostial lesions treated with atherectomy, lasers, and stents reported procedural success rates > 90% and low complication rates (Tables 14.2,14.3). Stenting, DCA, Rotablator, and ELCA with adjunctive PTCA usually lead to better lumen enlargement than PTCA alone.[4,20-22,26] Putative mechanisms for these favorable results include the elimination of elastic recoil (stent), and the resection (DCA), pulverization (Rotablator), and ablation (ELCA) of plaque. Despite excellent acute results, restenosis rates are 40-55% for atherectomy[3,4,15,29-31] and lasers,[4,25] and 22-35% for stents.[4,22,26,28-34] In the CAVEAT-I trial, acute and long-term outcomes were similar for ostial LAD lesions randomized to DCA or balloon angioplasty (Chapter 28),[15] although the incidence of non-Q-wave MI was higher after DCA.

C. TECHNICAL CONSIDERATIONS
1. Balloon Angioplasty
a. Guiding Catheter Selection. Most ostial RCA lesions can be successfully approached with a right Judkins, left Amplatz, or Hockey Stick guide, depending on the vessel takeoff and the degree of coaxial alignment. For ostial LAD, circumflex, and branch ostial lesions, a left Judkins guide will usually suffice unless better support is needed due to vessel tortuosity. If pressure damping occurs, a sidehole catheter should be used. In general, coaxial alignment will minimize ostial injury, permit proper positioning of interventional devices, and facilitate angiographic assessment of the ostium. As long as coaxial alignment is maintained, it is usually possible to advance and center the balloon with the guiding catheter positioned just outside the ostium. Once the balloon is properly positioned, the guiding catheter can be gently retracted 1-2 cm into the aorta (Figure 14.1); gentle forward pressure on the balloon catheter or low-pressure balloon inflation (1-2 atm) may help maintain proper balloon position while the guide is retracted. The balloon should not be fully inflated inside the guiding catheter due to the risk of balloon rupture and air embolism. To ensure that the stenosis is not due to transient spasm prior to intervention, it is helpful to administer intracoronary nitroglycerin or perform a subselective contrast injection in the Sinus of Valsalva.

b. Balloon Dilatation
    1. Aorto-Ostial Stenosis. PTCA alone (without antecedent atherectomy or subsequent stenting) is rarely utilized for ostial stenoses. For calcified and noncalcified lesions, a long (30-40 mm) balloon may be preferable to shorter balloons (10-20 mm) to avoid the proximal or distal balloon migration during inflation ("watermelon seed" effect) (Figure 14.2). This problem is less common with long balloons and after pretreatment with Rotablator, DCA, or ELCA.

    2. Branch-Ostial Stenosis. When dilating a branch-ostial lesion (especially ostial LAD or circumflex lesions), the balloon should be positioned to avoid obstructing blood flow to the uninvolved vessel; proper positioning can be confirmed by a small test injection. Generally, the balloon diameter should match the diameter of the branch vessel and not the parent vessel. Other important technical considerations are detailed in Chapter 10.

Table 14.2. Results of Atherectomy and Lasers for Ostial Stenosis

Series	Device	Lesion	N	Success (%)	MACE (%)	Other Results
Motwani[39] (2000)	ROTA	RCA	119	97.5	0.8	TVR at 2 years (16%); adjunctive PTCA or stent (98%)
Waksman[10] (1995)	Various	AO (native) SVG	184 122	89 94	3 2	TLR (33% vs. 39%)
Cowley[12] (1995)	ROTA	Nonost. RCA Ostial RCA	251 109	96 93	2.4 4.6	AC (44% vs. 1.8%); RS (48% vs. 52%)
Ellis[11] (1994)	ROTA	-	68	91	-	
Commeau[13] (1994)	ROTA	AO BO	32 110	97 94	9 2.7	
Koller[14] (1994)	ROTA TEC	AO + BO AO + BO	29 72	93 90	9 5.4	AC (7% vs. 6%); RS (39% vs. 59%)
Stephan[15] (1995)	DCA	AO BO	30 73	70 92	3 0	RS (36% vs. 37%)
CAVEAT[3] (1995)	PTCA DCA	LAD LAD	33 41	87 86	3 7	RS (46% vs. 48%)
Popma[16] (1993)	DCA	AO + BO	81	98	-	EFS at 3 months (66%)
Robertson[17] (1991)	DCA	AO BO	41 75	78 92	4.9 0	RS (46% vs. 54%)
Litvack[18] (1994)	ELCA	-	280	89	7	
deMarchena[19] (1994)	ILCA	-	23	91	4	
Sawada[4] (1994)	PTCA ELCA DCA Stent	LAD + LCX	80 24 29 22	90 88 90 100	- - - -	RS (61% vs. 59% vs. 33% vs. 33%); TLR (58% vs. 47% vs. 25% vs. 18%)
Brogan[21] (1993)	ROTA ELCA DCA TEC Stent	AO + BO	101 16 58 16 11	97 94 97 95 91	2 1 1 0 0	EFS at 1 year (64%)

Abbreviations: AC = acute closure; AO = aorto-ostial; BO = branch-ostial; DCA = directional coronary atherectomy; EFS = event-free survival (freedom from death, MI, CABG, repeat PTCA); ELCA = excimer laser coronary angioplasty; ILCA = infrared laser coronary angioplasty; MACE = in-hospital major adverse cardiac events (death, MI, PTCA, CABG); ROTA = Rotablator; RS = restenosis; TEC = transluminal extraction catheter; TLR = target lesion revascularization; - not reported

Table 14.3. Results of Stents for Ostial Lesions

Series	Device	Lesion	N	Success (%)	In-hospital MACE (%)	Other Results		
Ahmed[36] (2000)	Debulk/Stent Stent	AO SVG	133 187	- -	- -	Similar 1-yr EFS and TVR (19.4% vs. 18.2%)		
Park[35] (2000)	Stent	AO LAD	111	97	4.5	ARS (26%); TLR (11.7%); 2-yr EFS (84.6%)		
Mintz[40] (2000)	Stent	Ostial vs. nonostial	-	-	-	TLR higher in ostial group (17.4% vs. 12.0% p = 0.02)		
Wishmeyer[30] (1999)						Diss(%)	AC(%)	6-mo TLR(%)
	PTCA	AO	73	97	-	22	4.1	22
	Debulk	AO	32	100	-	16	3.1	19
	Stent	AO	73	100	-	1.4	0	25
	PTCA	BO	98	93	-	15	2.0	16
	Debulk	BO	24	100	-	8.3	0	17
	Stent	BO	23	100	-	0	0	29
Peterson[41] (1999)	Stent	AO RCA	88	98	-	-		
Asakaura[31] (1998)	PSS DCA	LAD LAD	11 13	100 100	0 0	More plaque shift after stenting than DCA		
Mathur[33] (1997)	PSS GRS	BO BO	14 34	100 100	0 0	TLR (7.1% vs. 17.6%)		
Kurbaan[34] (1997)	MLS, WS	AO	11	100	0	Cutting balloon before stenting		
Jaim[29] (1997)	PTCA ROTA/DCA ELCA stent	RCA RCA RCA	23 20 54	88 77 96	0 0 2	TLR: 47% 40% 24%		
DeCesare[32] (1996)	PSS	LAD	23	87	0	RS (22%)		
Colombo[26] (1996)	Stent	AO	35	100	0	RS (23%)		
DeCesare[27] (1996)	Stent	Ostial LAD	23	100	0	RS (22%)		
Rocha-Singh[22] (1995)	Stent	AO + BO	41	93	5	RS (28%)		
Wong[43] (1995)	PSS	AO SVG	104	97	2	RS (62%)		

Abbreviations: AC = acute closure; AO = aorto-ostial; BO = branch-ostial; DCA = directional coronary atherectomy; EFS = event-free survival (freedom from death, MI, CABG, repeat PTCA); ELCA = excimer laser coronary angioplasty; GRS = Gianturco-Roubin stent; ILCA = infrared laser coronary angioplasty; MACE = major adverse cardiac events; MLS = MultiLink stent; PSS = Palmaz-Schatz stent; ROTA = Rotablator; RS = restenosis; TEC = transluminal extraction catheter; TLR = target lesion revascularization; WS = Wallstent; - = not reported

2. **Non-Balloon Devices.** The principles of guiding catheter engagement are similar to those of PTCA (see above). Coaxial alignment is an absolute requirement for all mechanical approaches to ostial lesions. Ideal visualization of the ostial lesion is essential for positioning the device properly, optimizing angiographic results, minimizing ischemia, and avoiding complications. Aggressive guiding catheter engagement should be avoided, to properly position the device, image the ostium, and reduce the risk of vessel injury. Other fluoroscopic landmarks (calcification, rib margins, vertebral bodies, shaft of the guiding catheter, pacemaker, pulmonary artery catheter) are valuable to ensure proper guide position and device placement. It is usually possible to advance and retract the device with the guiding catheter positioned just outside the ostium. Frequent test injections are required to verify that the guide tip does not inadvertently engage beyond the ostium. When DCA is performed on aorto-ostial lesions, the housing will partially extend into the aorta (Figure 14.3). When performing Rotablator, the initial burr should be small (burr/artery ratio = 0.5); further increases in burr size are guided by subsequent angiography up to a final burr/artery ratio ≤ 0.8 (Figure 14.4). This approach facilitates passage of the device and reduces the risk of dissection. Atherectomy and laser techniques are described in Chapters 27-30. In the past, stenting of aorto-ostial lesions was technically demanding, but the recent availability of flexible, low-profile, radiopaque stents has facilitated ostial stent implantation. Pretreatment of ostial lesions with debulking devices (DCA, Rotablator) and/or PTCA is recommended to ensure successful stent deployment; primary stenting of ostial lesions is not recommended. The proximal 1 mm of the stent should extend into the aorta to ensure complete coverage of the lesion. In general, slotted tubular stents are preferable to coil or self-expanding stents because of greater radial strength, less stent distortion, and less chance of guiding catheter damage to the stent. Optimal technique employs high-pressure balloons to ensure stent apposition (Figure 14.5)(Chapter 26). IVUS is very useful to accurately identify the vessel reference size and optimize stent results (Chapter 31).

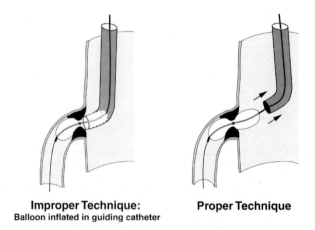

Improper Technique: **Proper Technique**
Balloon inflated in guiding catheter

Figure 14.1. Aorto-Ostial Lesions: PTCA Technique

Proper technique requires gentle retraction of the guiding catheter 1-2cm into the aorta prior to balloon inflation.

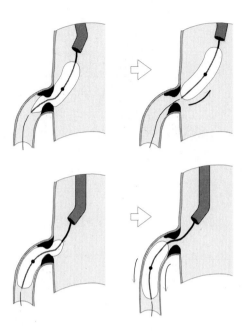

Figure 14.2. "Watermelon-Seed" Effect During Aorto-Ostial PTCA

When dilating ostial lesions, the balloon may prolapse into the aorta or distal vessel, leaving a high-grade residual stenosis. Long balloons (30-40 mm) may be useful in this situation.

D. CASE SELECTION. Because of the suboptimal results of PTCA alone, multi-device therapy based on vessel size and lesion calcification is recommended (Table 14.4, Figure 14.6). Debulking is usually recommended prior to stenting (vessels $\geq$ 2.5 mm) or PTCA (vessels < 2.5 mm); lesion calcification (particularly multiquadrant superficial calcification identified by IVUS) is a clear indication for debulking with Rotablator. Even in noncalcified ostial lesions in large vessels, Rotablator has replaced DCA in most institutions as the primary method of debulking prior to stenting. Nevertheless, DCA is suited for noncalcified ostial stenoses in vessels $\geq$ 2.5 mm, especially for eccentric or ulcerated lesions. TEC may be useful for ostial vein graft lesions with thrombus, but is contraindicated in the presence of significant calcification, marked eccentricity, extreme angulation, or dissection. Stents are often used for ostial lesions unless the lesion cannot be fully expanded with a balloon.

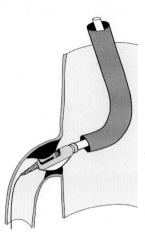

Figure 14.3. Aorto-Ostial Lesions: DCA Technique

Proper technique requires gentle retraction of the guiding catheter 2-3 cm into the aorta prior to cutter activation. It is important to establish other landmarks (rib margins, catheter shaft) to ensure precise positioning of the AtheroCath. Failure to retract the guide may result in partial excision of the tip of the guide during cutter activation.

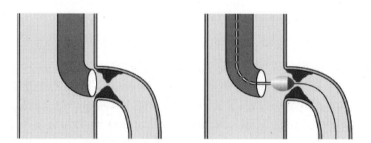

Figure 14.4. Aorto-Ostial Lesions: Rotablator Technique

Proper technique involves selection of a guiding catheter that provides ideal coaxial alignment and use of a Rotablator support guidewire. After crossing the lesion with the guidewire, allow the guide to gently "kick-out" of the ostium to facilitate ablation of the ostial lesion. The platform speed should be adjusted in the guiding catheter. Remove all slack in the guidewire to avoid kinking at the ostium.

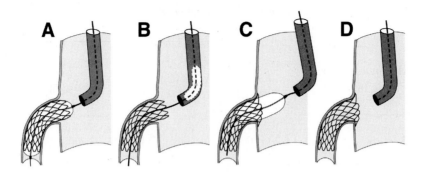

Figure 14.5. Aorto-Ostial Lesions: Stent Technique

A. Position the stent-delivery balloon so 1 mm of stent extends into the aorta. The guide must be retracted 1-2 cm before deploying the stent
B. After stent deployment, remove the delivery balloon while maintaining backward tension on the guide to prevent it from advancing into the ostium and damaging the stent
C. Perform adjunctive PTCA with a high pressure balloon; consider IVUS to ensure full stent expansion and apposition Flaring the proximal end of the stent with a slightly larger balloon is useful
D. Final result

Table 14.4. Ostial Lesion Morphology and Percutaneous Revascularization

Morphology	CB	DCA	TEC	Rotablator	ELCA	Stent
Type A	+	+	-	+	+	+
Thrombus	-	-	+	-	-	+[a]
Calcification (mod-heavy)	±	-	-	+	-	+[b]
Long segment of disease	±	-	-	±	+	+
Marked eccentricity	±	+	-	+	+[c]	+
Dissection (focal)	-	-	-	-	-	+
Ulcerated	±	+	-	+	+	+
Restenosis lesion	+	+	-	+	+	+
SVG	+	+	±	+	+	+

Abbreviations: CB = cutting balloon; DCA = directional coronary atherectomy; TEC = transluminal extraction atherectomy; ELCA = excimer laser coronary angioplasty
+ Favorable
- Unfavorable
a After thrombus removal
b May be considered after Rotablator
c Directional ELCA may have a role

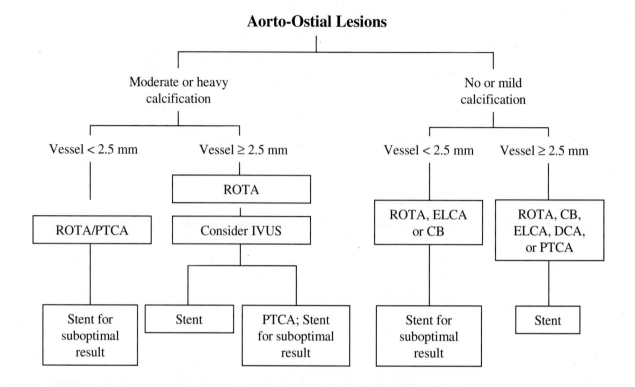

Figure 14.6. Approach to Aorto-ostial Lesions in Native Vessels and Saphenous Vein Grafts

CB = cutting balloon; DCA = directional coronary atherectomy; ELCA = excimer laser coronary angioplasty; ROTA = Rotablator

* * * * *

REFERENCES

1. Tan K, Sulke N, Taub N, Sowton E. Clinical and lesion morphologic determinants of coronary angioplasty success and complications: Current experience. J Am Coll Cardiol 1995;25: 855-65.

2. Tan K, Sulke N, Taub N, Karani S, Sowton E. Percutaneous transluminal coronary angioplasty of aorta ostial, non-aorta ostial, and branch ostial stenoses. J Am Coll Cardiol 1994;February Special Issue:351A.

3. Boehrer JD, Ellis SG, Pieper K, et al. Directional atherectomy versus balloon angioplasty for coronary ostial and nonostial left anterior descending coronary artery lesions: Results from a randomized multicenter trial. J Am Coll Cardiol 1995;25:1380-6.

4. Sawada Y, Kimura T, Shinoda E, et al. Poor outcome of balloon angioplasty (BA) for ostial left anterior descending and circumflex: Impact of new angioplasty devices. Circulation 1994;90:I-436.

5. Brown R, Kochar G, et al. Effects of coronary angioplasty using progressive dilation on ostial stenosis of left anterior descending artery. Am J Cardiol 1993;71:245-247.

6. Myler R, Shaw R, et al. Lesion morphology and coronary angioplasty: Current experience and analysis. J Am Coll Cardiol 1992;19:1641-1652.

7. Bedotto JB, McConahay DR, Rutherford BD. Balloon angioplasty of aorta coronary ostial stenoses revisited. Circulation 1991;84:II-251.

8. Mathias DW, Fishman-Mooney J, Lange HW, et al. Frequency of success and complications of coronary angioplasty of a stenosis at the ostium of a branch vessel. Am J Cardiol 1991;67:491-495.

9. Topol EJ, Ellis SG, Fishman J, et al. Multicenter study of percutaneous transluminal angioplasty for right coronary artery ostial stenosis. J Am Coll Cardiol 1987;9:1214-1218.

10. Waksman R, Ghazzal ZMB, Kennard ED, et al. Acute outcome and follow-up of ostial versus proximal lesions treated with new devices: Report of the NACI Registry. Circulation 1995;92:I-73.

11. Ellis S, Popma J, et al. Relation of clinical presentation, stenosis morphology, and operator technique to the procedural results of rotational atherectomy-facilitated angioplasty. Circulation 1994;89:882-892.

12. Cowley CA, Patterson PE, Kipperman RM, et al. Multicenter rotational coronary atherectomy registry experience in coronary artery ostial stenoses. TCT Course (Washington DC), February, 1995.

13. Commeau P, Zimarino M, Lancelin B, et al. Rotational coronary atherectomy for the treatment of aorto-ostial and branch-ostial lesions. Circulation 1994;90:I-213.

14. Koller P, Freed M, et al. Success, complications, and restenosis following rotational and transluminal extraction atherectomy of ostial stenoses. Cathet Cardiovasc Diagn. 1994;31:255-260.

15. Stephen WJ, Bates ER, Garratt KN, et al. Directional atherectomy in coronary and saphenous vein graft ostial stenoses. Am J Cardiol 1995;75:1015-1018.

16. Popma J, Mintz G, et al. Clinical and angiographic outcome after directional coronary atherectomy: A qualitative and quantitative analysis using coronary arteriography and intravascular ultrasound. Am J Cardiol 1993;72:55E-64E.

17. Robertson GC, Simpson JB, Vetter JW. Directional coronary atherectomy for ostial lesions. Circulation 1991;84:II-251.

18. Litvack F, Eigler N, Margolis J, et al. Percutaneous excimer laser coronary angioplasty: results in the first consecutive 3,000 patients. J Am Coll Cardiol 1994;23:323-9.

19. deMarchena EJ, Mallon SM, et al. Effectiveness of holmium laser-assisted coronary angioplasty. Am J Cardiol 1994;73:117-121.

20. Sabri M, Cowley, et al. Immediate results of interventional devices for coronary ostial narrowing with angina pectoris. Amer J Cardiol 1994;73:122-125.

21. Brogan WC, Popma JJ, Pichard AD, et al. A lesion-specific approach to new device therapy in ostial lesions. J Am Coll Cardiol 1993;21:233A.

22. Rocha-Singh K, Morris N, et al. Coronary stenting for treatment of ostial stenoses of native coronary arteries or aortocoronary saphenous venous grafts. Am J Cardiol 1995;75: 26-29.

23. Zampieri PA, Colombo A, et al. Results of coronary stenting of ostial lesions. Am J Cardiol 1994;73:901-903.

24. Teirstein P, Stratienko AA, Schatz RA. Coronary stenting for ostial stenosis: Initial results and six month follow-up. Circulation 1991;84:II-250.

25. Wong SC, Pompa JJ, Chuang YC, et al. Angiographic and clinical outcomes in saphenous vein graft (SVG) versus native coronary aorto-ostial lesions. J Am Coll Cardiol 1994;March Special Issue:302A.

26. Colombo A, Itoh A, Maiello L, et al. Coronary stent implantation in aorto-ostial lesions: Immediate and follow-up results. J Am Coll Cardiol 1996;27:253A

27. De Cesare NB, Galli S, Loaldi A, et al. Palmaz-Schatz stent for the treatment of left anterior descending ostial stenosis: Acute and long-term results. J Invas Cardiol 1996;8.

28. Schuhlen H, Hausleiter, et al. Coronary stent placement in ostial lesions. Six-month clinical and angiographic follow-up. J Am Coll Cardiol 1997;29(Suppl. A):16A.

29. Jain SP, Liu MW, Dean LS, et al. Comparison of balloon angioplasty versus debulking devices versus stenting in right coronary ostial lesions. Am J Cardiol 1997;79:1334-1338.

30. Wishmeyer JB, Huber KC, Johnson WJ, et al. Procedural outcomes of aorto-ostial vs. coronary ostial lesions. J Am Coll Cardiol 1999;33:82A.

31. Asakaura Y, Takagi S, Ishikawa S, et al. Favorable strategy for the ostial lesion of the left anterior descending coronary artery: Influence on narrowing of circumflex coronary artery. Cathet Cardiovasc Diag 1998;43:95-100.

32. DeCesare NB, Bartorelli AL, Galli S, et al. Treatment of ostial lesion of the left anterior descending coronary artery with Palmaz-Schatz coronary stent. Am Heart J 1996;132:716-720.

33. Mathur A, Liu MW, Goods CM, et al. Results of elective stenting of branch ostial lesions. Am J Cardiol 1997;79:472-474.

34. Kurbaan AS, Kelly PA, Sigwart U. Cutting balloon angioplasty and stenting for aorto-ostial lesions.

Heart1997;77:350-352.

35. Park SJ, Lee CW, Hong MK, et al. Stent placement for ostial left anterior descending coronary artery stenosis: Acute and long-term (2-year) results. Cathet Cardiovasc Intervent 2000;49:267-271.

36. Ahmed JM, Hong MK, Mehran R, et al. Comparison of debulking followed by stenting versus stenting alone for saphenous vein graft aortoostial lesions: Immediate and one-year clinical outcomes. J Am Coll Cardiol 2000;35:1560-8.

37. Inoue T, Hoshi K, Yaguchi I, et al. Cutting balloon angioplasty for ostial lesions of the left anterior descending artery. J Interven Cardiol 2000;13:7-14.

38. Muramatsu T, Tsukahara R, Ho M, et al. Efficacy of cutting balloon angioplasty for lesions at the ostium of the coronary arteries. J Invas Cardiol 1999;11:201-206.

39. Motwani JG, Raymond RE, Franco I, et al. Effectiveness of rotational atherectomy of right coronary artery ostial stenosis. Am J Cardiol 2000;85:563-567.

40. Mintz GS, Mehran R, Jackson M, et al. Diabetes and ostial lesion location have an additive effect on target lesion revascularization after stent implantation. J Am Coll Cardiol 2000;35:17A.

41. Peterson M, Carter A, Mehran R, et al. Can debulking prior to stenting be justified as standard treatment for right coronary artery ostial lesions? J Am Coll Cardiol 1999;33 (2 Suppl A):27A.

42. Rechavia E, Litvack F, Macko G, et al. Stent implantation of saphenous vein graft aorto-ostial lesions in patients with unstable ischemic syndromes: Immediate angiographic results and long-term clinical outcome. J Am Coll Cardiol 1995;25:866-870.

43. Wong SC, Popma J, Hong M, et al. Procedural results and long-term clinical outcomes in aorto-ostial saphenous vein graft lesions after new device angioplasty. J Am Coll Cardiol 1995;25:394A.

44. Fenton S, Fischman D, Savage M, et al. Long-term angiographic and clinical outcome after implantation of balloon-expandable stents in aortocoronary saphenous vein grafts. Am J Cardiol 1994;74:1187-1191.

45. Keramati S, Douglas J, Morris D, et al. Contemporary approach to the percutaneous revascularization of branch-ostial coronary lesions. J. Am Coll Cardiol 2001;37(2):46A.

15 LONG LESIONS AND SMALL VESSELS

Mark Freed, M.D.
Robert D. Safian, M.D.

A. BALLOON ANGIOPLASTY (Table 15.1)

1. Standard-Length (20 mm) Balloons

a. Success. Although angioplasty success declines as lesion length increases,[1,5,6] procedural success can still be achieved in most lesions > 20 mm in length (Table 15.1). Long lesions with other complex features (e.g, calcium, angulation) are often treated with long-balloons (30-40 mm) or other devices. In the randomized Amsterdam Rotterdam (AMRO) trial of ELCA vs. PTCA for long coronary lesions,[9] PTCA success was only 79%. Furthermore, intravascular ultrasound has shown that the actual residual stenosis is frequently underestimated by contrast angiography since the "normal" reference segment used to measure stenosis severity is often diseased itself (Chapter 31). It may be important to distinguish "long lesions" from "diffuse disease," which are often used interchangeably. We and others consider long lesions to be more than 10 mm in length, and diffuse disease to be the presence of three or more 50% stenoses in at least one-third of the vessel.

b. Complications. The impact of lesion length on major complications is controversial. Several reports indicate that PTCA of long lesions is associated with an increased risk for coronary artery dissection[6,10] and abrupt closure.[1,6,12-14] In these studies, the incidence of abrupt closure was 1-6% for lesions < 10 mm and 9-14% for lesions > 10 mm. In contrast, other studies failed to find a relationship between lesion length and acute closure[15] or major complications.[5,16,18,19] These divergent results may be due to differences in patient characteristics, associated lesion morphologies, the presence of multivessel disease, and the use of long (30-40 mm) balloons and other devices.

c. Restenosis. The influence of lesion length on restenosis is controversial. The Multi-Hospital Eastern Atlantic Restenosis Trial (M-HEART) demonstrated a direct relationship between lesion length and restenosis (lesion lengths of 0.3-2.9 mm, 3.0-4.6 mm, 4.7-7.0 mm, and 7.1-28.0 mm showed restenosis rates of 32%, 33%, 42%, and 49%, respectively).[20] Other reports failed to demonstrate any association.[21,22] Although long lesions may result in a greater loss in lumen diameter at 6 months, these observations do not necessarily correlate with clinical restenosis.[23]

2. Long (30-40 mm) Balloons.
Considerable clinical experience suggests that long (30-40 mm) balloons may improve acute results—increased success, fewer dissections, less acute closure[6]—by distributing inflation pressure more evenly across the diseased vessel segment and atheroma/vessel junction (Figure 15.1, Table 15.1). In fact, long-balloon angioplasty of long lesions resulted in

success and complication rates similar to those achieved with standard-length balloon angioplasty of focal stenoses.[7] In a small randomized trial comparing long- and standard-length balloons, long balloons resulted in fewer dissections (18% vs. 55%) and required fewer inflations.[24] Collectively, these data suggest that long balloons are associated with higher procedural success and fewer dissections than standard-length balloons.

3. **Tapered Balloons.** Most branching coronary arteries taper in diameter by at least 0.5 mm over 20 mm of vessel length (average taper = 0.22 mm per 10 mm of arterial length).[25] Significant tapering often poses a problem for optimal balloon sizing, especially for long lesions (Figure 15.2).[51] To address this problem, Banka et al[25] performed PTCA with a tapered balloon (0.5 mm decrement in balloon diameter over 25 mm of balloon length) to achieve procedural success in 80% and angiographic dissection in only 2% of tapered lesions. It is currently unknown whether tapered balloons offer any advantage, since most manufacturers do not market tapered balloons.

Table 15.1. Balloon Angioplasty of Long Lesions: Acute Outcome

Series	Balloon Length	Lesion Length (mm)	N	Success (%)	Complications (%) D / Q-MI / CABG	Dissection (%)	AC (%)
Appelman[9] (1996)	-	> 10	157	79	0 / 1.3 / 1.9	55	0.6
Tan[1] (1995)	20-40	< 10	959	95	-	-	1.5
		10-20	153	85	-	-	11
		> 20	45	74	-	-	16
Kaul[2] (1995)	20-40	11-20	112	96	1 / 1 / 1	24	3
		> 20	29	97	0 / 3 / 0	32	3
Cates[3] (1994)	80	> 40	54	91	- / - / 4	-	-
Mooney[4] (1993)	-	> 10	327	93	0 / 1 / 1.5	29	5
Myler[5] (1992)	-	≤ 10	365	95	2.1	-	-
		11 - 20	278	91	0	-	-
		> 20	136	89	0	-	-
Zidar[6] (1992)	20	< 10	579	95	1.2 / - / 4.8	6.6	5.9
	20	> 10	149	90	0.7 / - / 8.1	18.1	14.1
	≥ 30	> 10	90	98	1.1 / - / 3.3	8.9	5.6
Savas[7] (1992)	40	> 20	109	90	2	35	7
	40	> 20 (bend ≥ 45°)	69	88	1	20	7

Abbreviations: AC = acute closure; CABG = in-hospital coronary artery bypass surgery; D = in-hospital death; Q-MI = in-hospital Q-wave myocardial infarction; - = not reported

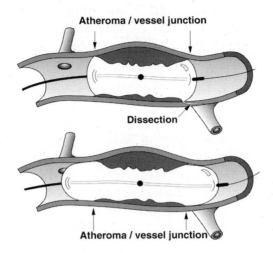

Figure 15.1. Long Lesions: PTCA Technique

Long (30-40 mm) balloons may be employed to more evenly distribute inflation pressure throughout the diseased vessel segment and limit dissection.

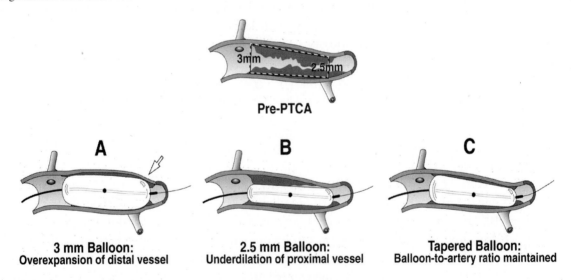

Figure 15.2. Long Lesions in Tapered Vessels: PTCA Technique

Balloon sizing is problematic for long lesions in tapered vessels:

A. Sizing the balloon to the proximal segment results in overdilating the distal segment, increasing the risk of dissection

B. Sizing the balloon to the distal segment results in underdilating the proximal segment, leaving a significant residual stenosis

C. A tapered balloon theoretically ensures better matching of balloon and vessel size

B. NON-BALLOON DEVICES (Tables 15.2, 15.3). Atherectomy, lasers, and stents are used to revascularize long lesions, but interdevice comparisons have been hampered by marked differences in baseline clinical and lesion characteristics. Long lesion length appears to independently predict acute closure[39] and coronary perforation[40] following some devices, emphasizing the importance of device selection.

1. **Atherectomy (Table 15.2)**

    a. **Rotablator Atherectomy.** Although early Rotablator success was possible in only 70% of long lesions,[29] recent studies reported success in more than 90% of lesions 16-25mm in length.[26-28,52] Nevertheless, increasing lesion length has been associated with an increased risk of MI,[26,28,29] coronary artery perforation,[41] and restenosis.[42] Despite these complications, many interventionalists believe that Rotablator atherectomy (with adjunctive PTCA as needed) is the preferred method of revascularizing long lesions, especially those with calcium. In such lesions, it is important to use slow passes with a small burr to minimize microcavitation and the generation of particulate debris, which can result in slow-flow and ischemic complications.

    b. **Directional Coronary Atherectomy (DCA).** DCA of long lesions resulted in lower success, more abrupt closure and emergency CABG, and higher restenosis rates compared to DCA of focal stenoses[30,43]. In the CAVEAT trial, lesion length (in addition to calcification) predicted DCA failure.[44] Although procedural success was reported in 97% of long lesions by making a series of longitudinal cuts through the entire length of the lesion, lesions were highly selected for favorable morphology. Most operators rarely consider DCA a practical strategy for long lesions.

    c. **TEC Atherectomy.** Although TEC atherectomy may be used to treat native coronary artery lesions, it may not have an advantage over PTCA except in the presence of thrombus. In small numbers of select long lesions, procedural success for TEC and adjunctive PTCA was > 90%.

2. **Lasers (Table 15.2)**

    a. **Excimer Laser Coronary Angioplasty (ELCA).** Data from the first 3000 patients enrolled into the ELCA Registry indicated procedural success rates of 90% for both short and long lesions.[34] Importantly, procedural success was independent of lesion length. Although dissections were more common in long lesions,[45] major ischemic complications occurred with equal frequency among short and long lesions.[34,45,46] In the Amsterdam Rotterdam (AMRO) trial, lesions ≥ 10 mm were randomized to ELCA (without saline infusion) or balloon angioplasty. No differences in procedural success, late clinical events, or functional status were observed (Table 15.2).[9,32] However there was more acute closure (8% vs. 0.8%, p = 0.005) and a trend towards more restenosis in the ELCA group (52% vs. 41%, p = 0.13);[9] ELCA was also associated with additional costs of $4476 per treated segment.[47] In the Excimer-Laser Rotablator Balloon Angioplasty for C-Lesions (ERBAC) trial, both ELCA and Rotablator resulted in better immediate lumen enlargement, but no difference in restenosis at 6 months compared to PTCA (Chapters 30)

    b. **Holmium Laser Angioplasty.** Results from the Holmium Laser Coronary Registry indicate that high procedural success ($\geq$ 90%) and low complication rates ($\leq$ 3%) can be achieved for lesions > 10 mm in length, although success rates were lower for lesions > 20 mm.[35]

3. **Stents (Table 15.3).** The use of stents for long lesions remains controversial, since there appears to be a strong relationship between lesion length and restenosis. Two stent approaches include "spot stenting" of more focal areas of severe disease amidst longer segments of diffuse disease, and stenting long segments of disease between "normal" proximal and distal vessel. The best approach is unknown (Chapter 26).

C. **APPROACH TO LONG LESIONS (Figure 15.3).** The approach to long lesions is dependent on the presence of thrombus, calcification, and vessel size. Intracoronary thrombus is best treated with adjunctive platelet glycoprotein IIb/IIIa receptor antagonists and/or mechanical thrombectomy with TEC or the AngioJet, whereas target lesion calcification is best treated with the Rotablator. Definitive lumen enlargement is usually achieved with PTCA with or without stenting. Provisional stenting is a reasonable strategy particularly in small vessels (Table 15.4): stenting may be deferred if an excellent result is achieved by PTCA alone, reserving future stenting for focal restenosis.

D. **CONCLUSIONS.** Balloon angioplasty of long lesions may be performed with acceptable procedural success rates, although the risk of acute closure and restenosis appears to be increased when compared to focal stenoses. Atherectomy and laser with or without adjunctive PTCA, have not been shown to be superior to PTCA alone, and the value of stents for long lesions awaits further definition.

Table 15.2. Results of Atherectomy and Laser for Long Lesions

Series	Device	Lesion Length (mm)	N	Success (%)	MACE (%)	Other Results
Kiesz[84] (1999)	Rotablator	≥ 15	101	98	0	RS (28%); TLR (19%)
AMRO[9,32,33] (1996)	ELCA PTCA	> 10 > 10	151 157	80 79	5.8 3.2	TLR at 6 months (26% vs. 24%); RS (52% vs. 41%)
Litvack[34] (1994)	ELCA**	< 10 10-19 20 29 ≥ 30	1832 1042 467 251	91 92 89 87	6 4.6 6.6 7.3	
Warth[26] (1994)	Rotablator	≤ 10 11-25	588 195	- 	0.2 2.1	
Ellis[27] (1994)	Rotablator	0-4 5-8 9-12 13-16	286 69 27 6	- 	4.2 10.1 18.5 50	
Reisman[28] (1993)	Rotablator	< 10 11-15 15-25	953 180 143	95 97 92	3.9 1.7 6.3	Non-Q-MI (4% vs. 5.5% vs. 6.2%)
Tierstein[29] (1992)	Rotablator	≤ 10 > 10	12 30	92 70	- -	RS (22% vs. 75%)
Mooney[4] (1993)	DCA	> 10	88	97	2	Acute closure (4.6%); dissection (19%)
Robertson[30] (1990)	DCA	< 10 10-19 ≥ 20	250 59 19	93 90 79	2 5 10	RS (33% vs. 53% vs. 62%)
Favereau[93] (1992)	Rotablator	10-20 > 20	215 73	95 84	- -	
TEC[31] Registry	TEC	< 10 10-20 > 20	266 220 38	93 93 95	- - -	
deMarchena[35] (1994)	Holmium-laser	≤ 10 11-20 > 20	123 193 49	97 94 90	2.7 3.1 0	

Abbreviations: AMRO = Amsterdam Rotterdam trial; DCA = directional coronary atherectomy; ELCA = excimer laser coronary angioplasty; MACE = in-hospital major adverse cardiac events (death, MI, rePTCA, CABG); RS = restenosis; TEC = transluminal extraction catheter; TLR = target lesion revascularization; - = not reported

Table 15.3. Results of Stents for Long Lesions

Series	Stent (lesion)	N	Success (%)	MACE (%) Early	MACE (%) Late	ARS (%)	TLR (%)
Oemrawsingh[94] (2001)	GFX XL (> 20 mm): With IVUS	48	-	-	-	18	-
	Without IVUS	52	-	-	-	36	-
ADVANCE[85] (2000)	Stent (> 20 mm)	-	-	-	19	27	-
	PTCA (> 20 mm)	-	-	-	14	42	-
Kornowski[74] (2000)	Stent (> 25 mm)	116	96	3.4	-	-	14.5
	Stent (< 20 mm)	1110	98	1.0	-	-	13.8
Hong[75] (2000)	Multiple (≥ 20 mm)	246	-	-	-	32	-
Ormiston[78] (2000)	MultiLink (25, 35 mm)	120	98		3	32	14
DeGregorio[65] (2000)	Spot stenting (IVUS)	101	-	3.0	22	26	20
	Long stent	143	-	3.5	36	38	32
Kobayashi[66] (1999)	Stent (≤ 20 mm)	565	96	-	-	24	-
	Stent (21-35 mm)	278	98	-	-	35	-
	Stent (> 35 mm)	247	92	-	-	47	-
Schalij[76] (1999)	Micro Stent II	119	98	5.4	10.1	-	-
Williams[77] (1999)	Wallstent	182	99	3.7	-	41	-
Nakagawa[71] (1999)	GFX ≤ 18	64	97	-	-	23.4	14.1
	GFX 24	56	96	-	-	35.7	21.4
	GFX 30	26	96	-	-	46.2	34.6
Kerr[86] (1998)	Various	34	94	-	-	18	24 (SAT 3%)
Rankin[67] (1998)	Stent (< 16 mm)	-	-	-	-	-	6.3
	Stent (16-32 mm)	-	-	-	-	-	13.2
	Stent (> 32 mm)	-	-	-	-	-	17.8
Kobayashi[68] (1998)	PSS	-	92	-	-	16.5	-
	Nir 16	-	93	-	-	13.3	-
	Nir 32	-	93	-	-	51.3	-
Elezi[69] (1998)	Stent (≥ 15 mm)	371	-	-	28.3	33.7	-
	Stent (< 15 mm)	1420	-	-	21.8	25.2	-
LeBreton[72] (1998)	Nir 32	187	93	3.5	19.6	-	6
Antoniucci[73] (1998)	Freedom (> 20 mm)	27	100	0	11	38	11
Akira[37] (1995)	PSS	62	-	-	-	39	-
	GRS	26	-	-	-	35	-
	Wiktor	21	-	-	-	24	-

Abbreviations: ARS = angiographic restenosis; GRS = Gianturco-Roubin stent; MACE = major adverse cardiac events (death, MI, CABG, rePTCA); PSS = Palmaz-Schatz stent; SAT = subacute thrombosis; TLR = target lesion revascularization; - = not reported

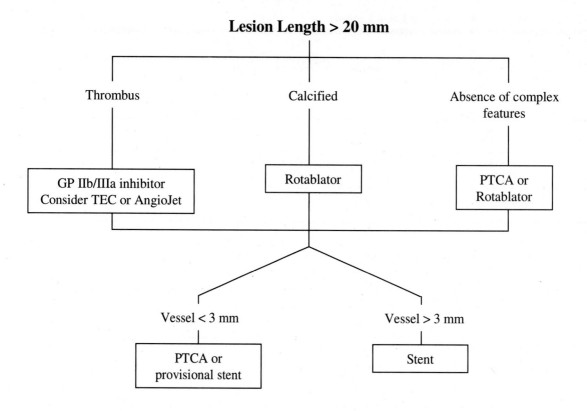

Figure 15.3. Approach to Long Lesions

Table 15.4. Results of Percutaneous Intervention in Small Vessels

Series	Device (vessel diameter)	N	Success	Early MACE	Other Results
Feres[95] (2001)	Stent (≤ 2.5mm)	397	98	-	Less TVR at 9 months for balloon diameter > 2.5mm vs. ≤ 2.5mm (12.3% vs. 21.7%, p = 0.005)
SISA[79] (2001)	PTCA BeStent	353	98 98	8.8 3.9	No difference in MACE at 6 months (23% vs. 19%) or 1 year (27% vs. 22%); similar ARS (32% vs. 28%)
RAP[96] (2001)	BeStent (2.2-2.7mm) PTCA	212 214	- -	- -	Randomized trial. Stents had less restenosis (27% vs. 37%, p < 0.05) and reocclusion (1.4% vs. 3.7%, p < 0.01), but similar MACE (11% vs. 14%) at 6 months
SISCA[97] (2001)	BeStent (2.1-3.0mm) PTCA	74 71	95 80	- -	Less MACE at 6 months after stenting (2.4% vs. 9.5%, p = 0.025)
Stankovic[98] (2001)	Final balloon < 3mm Final balloon = 3mm	124 385	- -	5.6 6.3	Late MACE, restenosis, and TLR were similar between groups. All vessels ≤ 2.8mm
Germing[88] (2000)	Stent (< 3 mm) Stent (> 3 mm)	128 92	- -	- -	No difference in hospital MACE or SAT (1.6% vs. 1.1%); more late TLR in small vessels
Briguori[89] (2000)	PTCA (< 3mm) Stent (< 3 mm)	97 12	95 97	- -	No difference in hospital or late MACE; trend towards more restenosis after PTCA; SAT after stenting (0.9%)
Caputo[80] (2000)	XT Stent PSS	178 160	- -	- -	Late MACE (18% vs. 12%); TLR (12% vs. 18%); RS (41% vs. 32%)
Al Suwaidi[81] (2000)	Stent (2.5 mm) Stent (≥3.0 mm)	108 4077	97 97	- -	Late MACE (35% vs. 21%)
Mori[82] (2000)	PTCA/stent (3.0/2.5 mm) PTCA/stent (2.5/2.5 mm)	31 53	- -	- -	RS (12% vs. 53%); TLR (10% vs. 35%)
Kastrati[83] (2000)	PTCA (diabetes) Stent (diabetes)	49 51	- -	- -	Similar death (4%), MI (4%), TLR (20% vs. 25%), and RS (44%) at 7 months
Hamasaki[64] (1999)	PTCA PSS MLS	199 1005 303	87 92 92	- - -	ARS: 56% TLR: 40% 31% 19% 23% 13%
Zidar[91] (1998)	GR II	258	99	2.4	
Adiyana[90] (1998)	Stent (≥ 3 mm) Stent (< 3 mm)	696 602	95 96	- -	No difference in in-hospital MACE or SAT; 1-yr EFS better for small vessels (71% vs. 63%, p < 0.01)

Table 15.4. Results of Percutaneous Intervention in Small Vessels

Series	Device (vessel diameter)	N	Success	Early MACE	Other Results
Shuhlen[54] (1998)	Stent	574	-	-	SAT (2.8%); ARS (38%); 1-yr TLR (24%); 1-yr MACE (26%). No difference in ARS or EFS at 6 months between high- and low-pressure inflations
Farshid[55] (1998)	BeStent	135	99	-	SAT (0.7%); ARS (12.6%)
Michael[56] (1998)	PTCA	83	84	-	TLR at 6 months (10.8% vs. 11.1%)
	Stent	54	93		
Schunkert[62] (1999)	PCI ($\leq$ 2.5 mm)	819	92	3.4	
	PCI (> 2.5 mm)	1493	96	2.0	
Deutsch[63] (1999)	Stent-DM ($\geq$3.0 mm)	10	-	-	ARS: 22%
	Stent-no DM ($\geq$3.0 mm)	88	-	-	25%
	Stent-DM (< 3.0 mm)	20	-	-	50%
	Stent-no DM (< 3.0 mm)	122	-	-	34%
Elezi[57] (1998)	Stent (< 2.8 mm)	870	-	4.5	SAT (2.4% vs. 2.5% vs. 2.0%); ARS (39% vs. 28% vs. 20%)
	Stent (2.8-3.2 mm)	866	-	3.3	
	Stent (> 3.2 mm)	866	-	2.9	
Koning[59] (1998)	Stent	50	100	2	ARS (30%); TLR (13%)
Savage[60] (1998)	PTCA	168	92	-	ARS (55% vs. 34%); 1-yr EFS (67% vs. 78%)
	Stent	163	100	-	
Waksman[61] (1998)	PTCA	148	95	-	Late MACE (31% vs. 34%); TLR (22% vs. 27%)
	Stent	284	92	-	
STRESS I-II[92] (1997)	PSS (< 3 mm)	-	-	-	ARS (35% vs. 54%); EFS (78% vs. 67%)
	PTCA (< 3 mm)	-	-	-	
Lau[58] (1997)	Stent	44	100	0	ARS (41%)

Abbreviations: ARS = angiographic restenosis; DM = diabetes mellitus; GR II = Gianturco-Roubin II stent; MACE = major adverse cardiac events (death, MI, CABG, rePTCA); MLS = MultiLink stent; PCI = percutaneous coronary intervention; PSS = Palmaz-Schatz stent; RS = restenoses; SAT = subacute stent thrombosis; TLR = target lesion revascularization; - = not reported. *Acronyms:* RAP = Restenosis en Arteries Pequenas; SISA = Stenting In Small Arteries; SISCA = Stenting In Small Coronary Arteries; STRESS = Stent Restenosis Study

* * * * *

REFERENCES

1. Tan K, Sulke N, Taub N, Sowton E. Clinical and lesion morphologic determinants of coronary angioplasty success and complications: Current experience. J Am Coll Cardiol 1995;25: 855-65.

2. hospital outcome of percutaneous transluminal coronary angioplasty for long lesions and diffuse coronary artery disease. Cathet Cardiol Diagn 1995;35:294-300.

3. Cates WU, Knopf WD, Lembo NJ, Bernstein C, et al. The 80 mm balloon: The first 95 vessel cumulative experience. J Am Coll Cardiol 1994;23:58A.

4. Mooney M, Mooney-Fishman, J, et al. Directional atherectomy for long lesions: Improved results. Cathet Cardiovasc Diagn 1993;1:26-30.

5. Myler R, Shaw R, et al. Lesion morphology and coronary angioplasty: Current experience and analysis. J Am Coll Cardiol 1992;19:1641-1652.

6. Zidar JP, Tenaglia AN, Jackman JD, et al. Improved acute results for PTCA of long coronary lesions using long angioplasty balloon catheters.   J Am Coll Cardiol 1992;19:34A.

7. Savas V, Puchrowicz S, Williams L, et al. Angioplasty outcome using long balloons in high-risk lesions. J Am Coll Cardiol 1992;19:34A.

8. Goudreau E, DiSciascio G, Kelly K, et al. Coronary angioplasty of diffuse coronary artery disease. Am Heart J 1991;121:12-19.

9. Appleman YEA, Piek JJ, Strikwerda S, et al. Randomized trial of excimer laser angioplasty vs. balloon angioplasty for treatment of obstructive coronary artery disease. Lancet 1996;347:79-84.

10. Raymenants E, Bhandari S, Stammen F, et al. Effects of angioplasty balloon material and lesion characteristics on the incidence of coronary dissection in 2150 dilated lesions. J Am Coll Cardiol 1993;21:291A.

11. Raymenants E, Bhandari S, Stammen F, De Scheerder I, et al. Effects of angioplasty balloon material and lesion characteristics on the incidence of coronary dissection in 2150 dilated lesions. J Am Coll Cardiol 1993;21:291A.

12. Ellis SG, Roubin GS, King SB III, et al. Angiographic and clinical predictors of acute closure after native vessel coronary angioplasty. Circulation 1988;77:372-379.

13. Detre KM, Holmes DR Jr, Holubkov R, et al. Incidence and consequences of periprocedural occlusion. The 1985-1986 National Heart, Lung and Blood Institute Percutaneous Transluminal Coronary Angioplasty Registry. Circulation 1990;82:739-750.

14. Tenaglia AN, Fortin DF, Califf RM, et al. Predicting the risk of abrupt vessel closure after angioplasty in an individual patient. J Am Coll Cardiol 1994;23:1004-1011.

15. de Feyter PJ, van den Brand M, Jaarman G, et al. Acute coronary artery occlusion during and after percutaneous transluminal coronary angioplasty. Frequency, prediction, clinical course, management, and follow-up. Circulation 1991;83:927-936.

16. Hermans WR, Foley D, et al. Usefulness of quantitative and qualitative angiographic lesion morphology, and clinical characteristics in predicting major adverse cardiac events during and after native coronary balloon angioplasty. Am J Cardiol 1993;72:14-20.

17. Ellis SG, Vandormael MG, Cowley MJ, et al, and the Multivessel Angioplasty Prognosis Study Group. Coronary morphologic and clinical determinants of procedural outcome with angioplasty for multivessel coronary disease. Circulation 1990;82:1193-202.

18. Savage MP, Goldberg S, Hirshfeld JW, et al, for the M-Heart Investigators. Clinical and angiographic determinants of primary coronary angioplasty success. J Am Coll Cardiol 1991;17:22-8.

20. Hirshfeld JW Jr, Schwartz JS, Jugo R, et al. Restenosis after coronary angioplasty: A multivariate statistical model to relate lesion and procedure variables to restenosis. J Am Coll Cardiol 1991;18:647-656.

21. Ellis SG, Roubin GS, King SB III, et al. Importance of stenosis morphology in the estimation of restenosis risk after elective percutaneous transluminal coronary angioplasty. Am J Cardiol 1989;63:30-34.

22. Leimgruber PP, Roubin GS, Hollman J, et al. Restenosis after successful coronary angioplasty in patients with single-vessel disease. Circulation 1986;73:710-717.

23. Foley DP, Meilkert R, Umans VA, et al. Is the relationship between luminal increase and subsequent renarrowing linear or non-linear in patients undergoing coronary interventions? J Am Coll Cardiol 1994;Special Issue:302A.

24. Brymer JF, Khaja F, and Kraft L. Angioplasty of long or tandem coronary artery lesions using a new longer balloon dilatation catheter: A comparative study. Cathet and Cardiovasc Diagn 1991;23:84-88.

25. Banka V, et al. Effectiveness of decremental diameter balloon catheters (Tapered balloon). Am J Cardiol 1992;69:188.

26. Warth D, Leon MB, O'Neill W, et al. Rotational atherectomy multicenter registry: Acute results, complications and 6-month angiographic follow-up in 709 patients. J Am Coll Cardiol 1994;24: 641-648.

27. Ellis S, Popma J, et al. Relation of clinical presentation, stenosis morphology, and operator technique to the procedural results of rotational atherectomy-facilitated angioplasty. Circulation 1994;89:882-892.

28. Reisman M, Cohen B, Warth D, et al. Outcome of long lesions treated with high speed rotational ablation. J Am Coll Cardiol 1993;21:443A.

29. Teirstein PS, Warth DC, Haq N, et al. High speed rotational coronary atherectomy for patients with diffuse coronary artery disease. J Am Coll Cardiol 1991;18:1694-1701.

30. Robertson GC, Selmon MR, Hinohara T, et al. The effect of lesion length on outcome of directional coronary atherectomy. Circulation 1990;82:III-623.

31. IVT™ Coronary TEC™ Clinical Database. Investigators Meeting 1992.

32. Appleman YE, Piek J, Redekop WK, et al. Excimer laser angioplasty versus balloon angioplasty in longer coronary lesions: A multivariate analysis. Circulation 1995;92:I-74.

33. Foley DP, Appleman YE, Piek JJ. Comparison of angiographic restenosis propensity of excimer laser coronary angioplasty and balloon angioplasty in the AMsterdam ROtterdam (AMRO) trial. Circulation 1995;92:I-477.

34. Litvack F, Eigler N, Margolis J, et al. Percutaneous excimer laser coronary angioplasty: Results in the first consecutive 3,000 patients. J Am Coll Cardiol 1994;23:323-9.

35. deMarchena EJ, Mallon SM, et al. Effectiveness of holmium laser-assisted coronary angioplasty.   Am J Cardiol

1994;73:117-121.

36. Maiello L, Hall P, Nakamura S, et al. Results of stent implantation of diffuse coronary disease assisted by intravascular ultrasound. J Am Coll Cardiol 1995;February Special Issue:156A.

37. Akira I, Hall P, Maiello L, et al. Coronary stenting of long lesions (greater than 20 mm) — a matched comparison of different stents. Circulation 1995;92:I-688.

38. Sutton JM, Ellis SG, Roubin GS, et al. Major clinical events after coronary stenting. The multicenter registry of acute and elective Gianturco-Roubin stent placement. Circulation 1994;89:1126-1137.

39. Hong MK, Popma JJ, Wong SC, et al. Incidence of and factors associated with abrupt closure in patients undergoing elective, new device angioplasty in native coronary arteries. J Am Coll Cardiol 1995;Feb Special Issue:122A

40. Flood RD, Popma JJ, Chuang YC, et al. Incidence angiographic predictors, and clinical significance of coronary perforation occurring after new device angioplasty. J Am Coll Cardiol 1994;February Special Issue:301A.

41. Cohen BM, Weber VJ, Bass TA, et al. Coronary perforation during rotational ablation: Angiographic determinants and clinical outcome. J Am Coll Cardiol 1994;February Special Issue:354A.

42. Leguizamon JH, Chambre DF, Torresani EM, et al. High-speed coronary rotational atherectomy. Are angiographic factors predictive of failure, major complications or restenosis? A multivariate analysis. J Am Coll Cardiol 1995;February Special Issue:95A.

43. Popma J, Topol E, et al. Abrupt vessel closure after directional coronary atherectomy. J Am Coll Cardiol 1992;19:1372-1379.

44. Lincoff AM, Ellis SG, Leya F, et al. Are clinical and angiographic correlates of success the same during directional coronary atherectomy and balloon angioplasty? The CAVEAT Experience. Circulation 1993;88:I-601.

45. Baumbach A, Bittl J, Fleck E, et al. Acute complications of excimer laser coronary angioplasty: A detailed analysis of multicenter results. J Am Coll Cardiol 1994;23:1305-1313.

46. Ghazzal, Z., J. Hearn, et al. Morphological predictors of acute complications after percutaneous excimer laser coronary angioplasty. Results of a comprehensive angiographic analysis: Importance of the eccentricity index. Circulation 1992;86:820-827.

47. Appleman YE, Birnie E, Piek JJ, et al. Excimer laser angioplasty versus balloon angioplasty in longer coronary lesions: A cost-effectiveness analysis. Circulation 1995;92:I-512.

48. Shaknovich A, Moses JW, Undemir C, et al. Procedural and short-term clinical outcomes in multiple Palmaz-Schatz stents (PSSs) in very long lesions/dissections. Circulation 1995;92:I-535.

49. Hall P, Nakamura S, Maiello L, et al. Factors associated with late angiographic outcome after intravascular ultrasound guided Palmaz-Schatz coronary stent implantation: A multivariate analysis. J Am Coll Cardiol 1995;February Special Issue:36A.

50. Tamura T, Kimura T, Nosaka H, Nobuyoshi M. Predictors of restenosis after Palmaz-Schatz stent implantation. Circulation 1994;90:I-324.

51. Laird JR, Popma JJ, Knopf WD, et al. Angiographic and procedural outcome after coronary angioplasty in high-risk subsets using a decremental diameter (tapered) balloon

catheter. Am J Cardiol 1996;77:561-8.

52. Reisman M, Harms V, Whitlow P, et al. Comparison of early and recent results with rotational atherectomy. J Am Coll Cardiol 1997;29:353-7.

53. Hamasaki N, Nosaka H, et al. Influence of lesion length on late angiographic outcome and restenotic process after successful stent implantation. J Am Coll Cardiol 1997;29(Suppl. A):239A.

54. Schuhlen H, Hausletter J, Herzzentrum D et al. High versus low balloon pressure for stent deployment in small (< 3 mm) coronary arteries— One-year results of a randomized trial. Circulation 1998;98(Suppl I):I-160.

55. Farshid A, Friend CA, Allan RM, et al. Favorable acute and six month follow-up results after coronary stenting using the small beStent in 2.5-3.0 mm arteries. Circulation 1998;98(Suppl I):I-639.

56. Michael L, Buller CE, Catellier D, et al. Efficacy of stenting vs. balloon angioplasty in small diameter (<3 mm) total coronary occlusions: A total occlusion study of Canada substudy. Circulation 1998;98(Suppl I):I-639.

57. Elezi S, Kastrati A, Neumann FJ, et al. Vessel size and long-term outcome after coronary stent placement. Circulation 1998;98:1875-1880.

58. Lau KW, He Q, Ding ZP, Johan A. Safety and efficacy of angiography-guided stent placement in small native coronary arteries of < 3.0 mm in diameter. Clin Cardiol 1997;20:711-716.

59. Koning R, Chan C, Eltchaninoff H, et al. Primary stenting of de novo lesions in small coronary arteries: A prospective, pilot study. Cathet Cardiovasc Diagn. 1998;45:235-238.

60. Savage MP, Fischman DL, Rake R, Leon MB, et al. Efficacy of coronary stenting versus balloon angioplasty in small coronary arteries. J Am Coll Cardiol 1998;31:307-311.

61. Waksman R, Mehran R, Saucedo JF, et al. Balloons PTCA is equivalent to stents in patients with small coronaries: A comparative retrospective matching study. J Am Coll Cardiol 1999;33(Suppl I):273A.

62. Schunkert H, Harrell L. Small coronary vessels: A suitable target for percutaneous revascularization in the new device era? J Am Coll Cardiol 1999;33(Suppl I):275A.

63. Deutsch E, Martin JL, Fischman DL, et al. The late benefit of coronary stenting in small vessels is reduced in diabetic patients. J Am Coll Cardiol 1999;33(Suppl I):275A.

64. Hamasaki N, Nosaka H, Kimura T, et al. Stenting for small vessel using new generation flexible stent-comparision of balloon angioplasty and Palmaz-Schatz stent. J Am Coll Cardiol 1999;33(Suppl I):32A.

65. DeGregorio J, Moussa I, Kobayashi Y, et al. The use of IVUS-guidid PTCA and spot stenting in the treatment of long lesions: A comparison to traditional stenting. J Am Coll Cardiol 2000;35:62A.

66. Kobayashi Y, DeGregorio J, Reimers B, et al. The length of the stented segment is an independent predictor of restenosis. J Am Coll Cardiol 1998;33(Suppl A):366A.

67. Rankin JM, Lohavanichbutr K, Carere RG, et al. Low rate of repeat revascularization despite stenting long segments. Circulation 1998;98(suppl I):I-285.

68. Kobayashi Y, DeGregorio J, Reimers B, et al. Immediate and follow-up results following implantation of the long and short NIR stent: Comparison with the Palmaz-Schatz stent. J Am Coll Cardiol 1998;33(Suppl A):312A.

69. Elezi S, Kastrati A, Wehinger A, et al. Stent placement in long (≥ 15 mm) coronary lesions. J Am Coll Cardiol

1998;33:273A.

70. Kornowski R, Mehran R, Lansky AJ, Fuchs S. Procedural results and late clinical outcomes following percutaneous interventions using long ($\geq$ 25 mm) stents. J Am Coll Cardiol 1998;33(Suppl A):69A.

71. Nakagawa Y, Yufu K, Tamura T, Tokoi H, et al. Stenting for long lesion with long GFX stent. J Am Coll Cardiol 1999;33(Suppl I):69A.

72. LeBreton H, Bedossa M, Commeau P, et al. Clinical and angiographic results of stenting for long coronary arterial atherosclerotic lesions. Am J Cardiol 1998;82:1539-1542.

73. Antoniucci D, Valenti R, Santoro GM, et al. Preliminary experience with stent-supported coronary angioplasty in long narrowings using the long freedom force stent: Acute and six-month clinical and angiographic results in a series of 27 consecutive patients. Cathet Cardiovasc Diagn. 1998;43:163-167.

74. Kornowski R, Bhargava B, Fuchs S, et al. Procedural results and late clinical outcomes after percutaneous interventions using long ($\geq$ 25 mm) versus short (< 20 mm) stents. J Am Coll Cardiol 2000;35:612-8.

75. Hong MK, Park SW, Mintz GS, et al. Intravascular ultrasonic predictors of angiographic restenosis after long coronary stenting. Am J Cardiol 2000;85:441-445.

76. Schalij MJ, Udayachalerm W, Oemrawsingh P, et al. Stenting of long coronary artery lesions: Initial angiographic results and 6-month clinical outcome of the micro stent II-XL. Cathet Cardiovasc Intervent 1999;48:105-112.

77. Williams IL, Thomas MR, Robinson NMK, et al. Angiographic and clinical restenosis following the use of long coronary wallstents. Cathet Cardiovasc Intervent 1999;48:287-293.

78. Ormiston J, Ruygrok PN, Webster M, et al. Stenting of long coronary lesions: A prospective 6-month quantitative angiographic study (STELLA trial). J Am Coll Cardiol 2000;35:62A

79. Schalij MJ, Doucet S, Hilton D., et al. The SISA study: A randomized comparison of balloon angioplasty and stent to prevent restenosis in small arteries: 6 month angiographic and 12 month clinical outcome. J Am Coll Cardiol 2001;37(2);79A.

80. Caputo RP, Giambartolomei A, Simons A, et al. Small vessel stenting—Comparison of modular vs. slotted tube design. Six month results from the EXTRA trial. J Am Coll Cardiol 2000;35:56A

81. Al Suwaidi J, Garratt KN, Rihal CS, et al. Immediate and one-year outcome of coronary stent implantation in small coronary vessels using 2.5 mm stents. J Am Coll Cardiol 2000;35:63A.

82. Mori F, Tsurumi Y, Nakamura A, et al. Stenting in small coronary vessels (<2.5mm): Impact of stent over-dilatation following initial stent deployment. Circulation 2000;102:II-641.

83. Kastrati A, Mehilli J, Dirschinger J, et al. Is stenting superior to PTCA for lesions in small coronary vessels in diabetic patients? Results from the ISAR-Smart randomized trial. Circulation 2000:102:II-387.

84. Kiesz RS, Rozek MM, Ebersole DG, et al. Novel approach to rotational atherectomy results in low restenosis rates in long, calcified lesions: Long-term results of the San Antonio Rotablator Study (SARS). Cathet Cardiovasc Intervent 1999;48:48-53.

85. Serruys PW. Presented at the XXII European Society of Cardiology, 2000.

86. Kerr AJ, Stewart RAH, Low CJS, et al. Long stenting in native coronary arteries: Relation between vessel size and outcome. Cathet Cardiovasc Diagn 1998;44:170-174.

87. Reimers B, Di Mario C, Nierop P, Pasquetto G, Camenzind E, Ruygrok P. Long-term restenosis after multiple stent implantation. A quantitative angiographic study. Circulation 1995;92:I-327.

88. Germing A, Von Dryander S, Machraoui A, et al. Coronary artery stenting in vessels with reference diameter < 3 mm. J Intervent Cardiol 2000;13:1309-314.

89. Briguori C, Nishida T, Adamian M, et al. Coronary stenting versus balloon angioplasty in small coronary artery with complex lesions. Cathet Cardiovasc Intervent 2000;50:390-397.

90. Adiyana T, Moussa I, Reiners B, et al. Angiographic and clinical outcome following coronary stenting of small vessels: A comparison with coronary stenting of large vessels. J Am Coll Cardiol 1998;32:1610-8.

91. Zidar JP, O'Shaughnessy CD, Dean LS, Holmes DR, Moore PB, Rogers EW, Fry ETA, Raizer AE, Voorhees WD, Leon MB. Elective GR II stenting in small vessels: multicenter results. J Am Coll Cardiol 1998; (??): 274A.

92. Savage MP, Fischman DL, Rake R, et al. Efficacy of coronary stenting versus balloon angioplasty in small coronary arteries. J Am Coll Cardiol 1997;31:307-311.

93. Favereaux X, Chevalier B, Commeau P, et al. Is rotational atherectomy more effective than balloon angioplasty for the treatment of long coronary lesions? SCA & I Meeting Abstracts, 92.

94. Oemrawsingh PV, Schalij MJ, van der Wall EE, et al. Guidance of long stent implantation by intravascular ultrasound has a significantly better outcome compared to implantation guided by angiography alone: Final results of a randomized study (The TULIP study). J Am Coll Cardiol 2001;37(2):20A.

95. Feres F, Costa MA, Staico R, et al. Is stent oversizing the best strategy to treat small vessels? J Am Coll Cardiol 2001;37(2):10A.

96. Garcia E, Gomez-Recio M, Moreno R, et al. Stent reduces restenosis in small vessels. Results of the RAP study. J Am Coll Cardiol 2001;37(2):10A.

97. Moer R, Myreng Y, Albertson P, et al. Stenting in small coronary arteries (SISCA): A randomized comparison of heparin coated bestent and balloon angioplasty. J Am Coll Cardiol 2001;37(2):46A.

98. Stankovic G, Nishida T, Corvaja N, et al. Effect of balloon oversizing in stenting small vessels. J Am Coll Cardiol 2001;37(2):73A.

16 CHRONIC TOTAL OCCLUSION

Mark S. Freed, M.D.
Robert D. Safian, M.D.

CORONARY ARTERY OCCLUSION

PTCA of chronic total occlusions represents 10-20% of all angioplasty procedures and poses a management dilemma for the interventional cardiologist. Although collaterals maintain myocardial viability under resting conditions, they often fail to provide sufficient blood flow during periods of increased oxygen demand, resulting in lifestyle-limiting angina. Successful revascularization improves anginal status, increases exercise capacity, and reduces the need for late bypass surgery. However, PTCA of a chronic total occlusion is associated with lower success rates, higher equipment costs, increased radiation exposure, and more restenosis compared to PTCA of nontotal occlusions. Improved guidelines for case selection, new interventional devices, and adjunctive pharmacotherapy may favorably impact these patients.

A. **PATHOPHYSIOLOGY (Table 16.1).** The success of percutaneous techniques for revascularization of total occlusions is determined by the clinical presentation, presence of collaterals, and morphology of the obstruction, which vary between acute and chronic total occlusion.

   1. **Acute Occlusion.** These patients frequently present with acute myocardial infarction and absent or poorly developed collaterals. Unless coronary flow is restored within 4-6 hours, myocardial injury is permanent. Pathologically, the obstructed lumen typically consists of ruptured plaque and fresh clot. These types of acute occlusions are readily crossed with conventional guidewires, accounting for procedural success rates exceeding 90%. The likelihood of successful recanalization decreases over the ensuing months as fresh thrombus undergoes organization, fibrosis, and calcification.

   2. **Chronic Total Occlusion.** These patients frequently present with a change in anginal status rather than acute MI. Well-developed collaterals may provide flow equivalent to a 90-95% stenosis, which helps maintain myocardial viability and prevents resting myocardial ischemia.[1] Overall contractile function may be normal, or a regional wall-motion abnormality may be present due to hibernating myocardium or non-Q-wave MI. Pathologically, the major constituent of a chronic total occlusion is fibrocalcific plaque.[112] These obstructions are often resistant to guidewire crossing, accounting for lower success rates compared to nontotal occlusions.

Table 16.1. Total Coronary Occlusion: Clinical and Pathological Features

	Acute Occlusion	Chronic Occlusion
Presentation	Acute MI	Change in anginal status; angina is usually exertional (collateral insufficiency)
Histopathology	Ruptured fibrous cap overlies soft atheroma; acute occlusive thrombus is common	Complex fibrocalcific atherosclerosis with chronic organized thrombus
Spontaneous recanalization	Occasional	Rare

Collaterals
    Intracoronary
    Intercoronary
	
	Rare
	Less common
		
		Occasional (bridging collaterals)
		Common

Myocardial viability	Uncommon unless collaterals are present	Collaterals sustain viability; wall motion may be normal
PTCA success	High	Variable; depends on duration and morphology

B. INDICATIONS AND BENEFITS OF PERCUTANEOUS REVASCULARIZATION (Table 16.2).

C. BALLOON ANGIOPLASTY

1. **Procedural Outcome.** Compared to PTCA of nontotal occlusions, revascularization rates for chronic total occlusions remain disappointingly low (Table 16.3). Older series comprising more than 4400 total coronary occlusions indicate an overall success rate of 69% (range 47-81%) (Table 16.4).   The most common reasons for procedural failure included the inability to cross the occlusion with a guidewire (80%), failure to cross the occlusion with a balloon (15%), and failure to dilate the stenosis (5%). The recent availability of several varieties of hydrophilic guidewires has improved failure to traverse total occlusions, and use of the Rotablator has decreased procedural failures due to lesion rigidity.

2. **Predictors of Success.** Case selection remains the single most important predictor of PTCA success. Depending on the presence of clinical and angiographic variables, recanalization rates range from 18-87% (Tables 16.5-16.7, Figure 16.1):

    a. **Complete vs. Functional Occlusion.** Pooled data indicate that functional occlusions (99% stenosis with delayed incomplete opacification of the distal vessel segment) are more often recanalized than complete occlusions (76% vs. 67%). It is essential to differentiate the true lumen of a functional occlusion from the perivascular channel of a bridging collateral; the former is a predictor of PTCA success, while the latter predicts PTCA failure. This distinction can usually be made by obtaining multiple angiographic projections of the occlusion, but sometimes is not apparent until attempts are made to cross the occlusion with a guidewire.

Table 16.2. Chronic Total Occlusion: Indications and Benefits of Revascularization

Indications
    Medically refractory angina
    Large area of ischemia by noninvasive studies
    Favorable angiographic appearance

Proven Benefits
    Relief of exertional angina
    Improvement in global and regional left ventricular function and exercise capacity[27,114,115,116,117]
    Reduction in the need for late CABG by 50%

Possible Benefits
    Potential source of collaterals to other vessels
    Improvement in left ventricular remodeling following MI[114]
    Improvement in event-free survival

b. **Duration of Occlusion.** The duration of occlusion is estimated as the time interval between a major ischemic event (Q-wave MI, new onset angina, abrupt worsening in anginal status) and PTCA. Successful revascularization is highest for occlusions < 1 week, intermediate for occlusions 2-12 weeks, and lowest for occlusions > 3 months. Occlusion duration alone should not preclude revascularization since procedural success for occlusions > 6 months may be as high as 50-75%.[8,12]

c. **Length of Occlusion.** While it is generally felt that occlusion lengths > 15 mm are associated with lower success rates, this characteristic alone should not preclude PTCA.

d. **Sidebranch at Point of Occlusion.** This occlusion characteristic is associated with reduced success due to the tendency of the guidewire to pass into the sidebranch.

e. **Presence of a Tapered Stump.** Funnel-shaped or tapered occlusions are associated with higher recanalization rates than occlusions with abrupt cutoffs. Tapered occlusions frequently contain small recanalized channels that escape detection by angiography but provide a potential route for successful guidewire passage.[80,112]

f. **Intracoronary "Bridging" Collaterals.** Most angioplasty series suggested that the presence of bridging collaterals was the single most important determinant of failed PTCA for chronic total occlusions. However, Kinoshita et al [9] reported equally high success rates for total occlusions with (n = 109) and without (n = 324) bridging collaterals (75% vs. 83%, p = 0.07). The authors attributed the high success rate to operator experience and aggressive use of stiff wires. Our own experience suggests that when faint bridging collaterals coexist with one or more favorable characteristics (e.g., tapered stump, short segment of occlusion), success rates may exceed 50%. However, occlusions that are associated with extensive bridging collaterals ("caput medusa") are generally considered unsuitable for PTCA due to extremely low success rates (< 20%). These networks of vessels consist of dilated vasa vasorum and neovascular channels and are very fragile and susceptible to perforation during crossing attempts.

Table 16.3. PTCA of Nontotal vs. Chronic Total Occlusion: Acute Outcome

Series	Group[+]	N	Success (%)	Complications (%) D / MI / CABG
Berger[30]* (1996)	Nontotal	1295	-	0 / 1.4 / 0
	Total	139	-	0 / 1.5 / 0.3
Jaup[125]** (1995)	Nontotal	280	84	0 / 2.1 / 0.9
	Functional	67	75	1.5 / 0 / 0
	Total	453	67	2.5 / 1.0 / 1.1
Favereau[2] (1995)	Nontotal	2065	96	1.4
	Total	292	67	1.7
Tan[3] (1995)	Nontotal	1157	93	0.4 / 0.7 / 2.1
	Total	91	66	0 / 0 / 0
Ruocco[4] (1992)	Nontotal	1429	82	0.7 / 4.8 / 3.5
	Total	271	59	1.8 / 3.6 / 3.3
Myler[5] (1992)	Nontotal	779	94	1.7
	Total	122	76	1.6
Plante[6] (1991)	Nontotal			
	Stable Angina	637	-	4
	Unstable Angina	442	-	8
	Total			
	Stable Angina	44	48	2.5
	Unstable Angina	46	65	2.0
Stone[7] (1990)	Nontotal	6950	96	0.9 / 1.5 / 1.7
	Total	905	72	0.8 / 0.6 / 0.8
Safian[8] (1988)	Nontotal	711	90	0.4 / 3 / 2
	Functional	102	78	1 / 3 / 3
	Total	169	63	0 / 0 / 2

Abbreviations: D = in-hospital death; CABG = emergency coronary artery bypass surgery; MI = in-hospital myocardial infarction; - = not reported
+ Functional total occlusion = 99% stenosis (TIMI flow = 1)
  Nontotal occlusion = 51-99% stenosis (TIMI flow $\geq$ 2)
  Total occlusion = 100% stenosis (TIMI flow = 0);
* In-hospital complication rate among successfully dilated occlusions
** Magnum wire

g. **Other Factors**. Other factors variably associated with lower success rates include lesion calcification, proximal vessel tortuosity, distal location, RCA or circumflex occlusion, diffuse proximal disease, multivessel disease, and unstable angina.[7,14,15,18,19] However, none of these factors are considered significant contraindications to PTCA in the hands of experienced operators.

Table 16.4. PTCA of Chronic Total Occlusion: Acute Outcome

Series	N	Success (%)	Complications (%) D / Q-MI / CABG
Noguchi[127] (2000)	226	59	- / 1.3 / -
Nobuyoshi[119] (1998)	1138	63	- / - / -
Berger[30] (1996)	139	-	0 / 1.4 / 2.9
Favereau[2] (1995)	367	67	1.7
Jaup[125] (1995)	453	67	2.5 / 1.0 / 1.1
Kinoshita[9] (1995)	433	81	0.3 / 0 / 0
Ishizaku[10] (1994)	111	62	0 / 1.6 / 0
Tan[11] (1993)	312	61	0.3 / - / 1.6
Shimizu[12] (1993)	468	75	- / - / -
Maiello[14] (1992)	365	64	0 / 0.6 / 0.3
Myler[5] (1992)	122	76	1.6
Ivanhoe[15] (1992)	480	66	1 / 2 / -
Ruocco[4] (1992)	271	59	2 / 1 / 2
Bell[16] (1991)	354	66	0.3 / 1.7 / 2.5
Stone[7] (1990)	971	72	0.8 / 0.6 / 0.8

Abbreviations: D = death, Q-MI = Q-wave myocardial infarction, CABG = emergency coronary artery bypass grafting; - = not reported

Table 16.5. Chronic Total Occlusion: Predictors of PTCA Outcome

Procedural Success	Procedural Failure
Functional occlusion	Total occlusion
Occlusion age < 12 weeks	Occlusion age > 12 weeks
Length < 15 mm	Length > 15 mm
Tapered stump	Abrupt cut-off
No sidebranch at point of occlusion	Sidebranch present
No bridging collaterals	Extensive bridging collaterals ("Caput Medusa")

3. **Complications.** Although PTCA of a chronic total occlusion is generally considered a "low-risk" procedure, the incidence of major complications is similar to nontotal occlusions, and the presence of a chronic total occlusion is an independent predictor of acute closure.[20,21] Major complications include acute closure (5-10%), MI (0-2%), emergency CABG (0-3%), and death (0-1%) (Table 16.4). In one report,[2] reocclusion within 24 hours of successful PTCA occurred in 8% of total occlusions compared to 1.8% of nontotal occlusions. Reocclusion was silent in 87%. In another study of chronic total occlusion, complications after PTCA occurred in 20% of patients who presented with unstable angina compared to 2.5% in those with stable angina.[6] Ischemic complications are usually due to dissection, thrombus, distal embolization, or damage to collaterals. Less common complications include coronary artery perforation[51] (relative risk 3.1[13]), reperfusion arrhythmias (including rare delayed ventricular fibrillation),[23] and guidewire entrapment and fracture. Acute reocclusion may cause ST-segment elevation and hemodynamic deterioration due to delayed recruitment of previously functioning collaterals.

4. **Late Outcome**
   a. **Anginal Status and Exercise Capacity (Table 16.7).** The majority of patients with successful PTCA are asymptomatic at follow-up. In the three largest reports, 70% of patients were asymptomatic 1-4 years after PTCA.[4,15,24] Absence of symptoms does not exclude restenosis, since 40% of patients with restenosis may be free of chest pain.[25]

   b. **Ventricular Function.** Although data are limited, successful PTCA may improve ventricular relaxation and regional wall motion.[19,26] Global ejection fraction improved in some studies,[27,114-117] but not in another.[28] Among patients with successfully recanalized occlusions, those with persistent patency and normal flow had better global function and less ventricular dilatation than patients without patent vessels.[29]

   c. **Death, MI, CABG (Tables 16.9, 16.10).** Most studies indicate that successful recanalization of a chronic total occlusion reduces the need for CABG by 50-75%. However, PTCA does not improve survival or reduce the incidence of late MI.

Table 16.6. Impact of Occlusion Duration on PTCA Outcome

Series	Occlusion Duration	N	Success (%)
Tan[3] (1995)	< 3 months	42	76
	> 3 months	49	57
Ishizaku[10] (1994)	< 1 month	11	91
	> 1 month	100	56
Myler[5] (1992)	< 1 week	99	87
	1-12 weeks	73	88
	> 3 months	49	59
Bell[16] (1992)	< 1 week	60	74
	1-4 weeks	15	93
	1-3 months	243	67
	> 3 months	45	64
Maiello[14] (1992)	< 1 month	73	89
	1-3 months	77	87
	> 3 months	110	45
Stone[7] (1990)	< 12 weeks	29	90
	> 12 weeks	39	74

   d. **Restenosis (Table 16.11).** Restenosis and complete reocclusion are very common after PTCA, with rates of 40-75% and 11-34%, respectively. Observational and randomized trials of stents vs. PTCA indicate less restenosis and target lesion revascularization with stents (Tables 16.14, 16.18).

D. EQUIPMENT SELECTION AND PTCA TECHNIQUE. PTCA of a chronic total occlusion can be technically challenging and, compared to PTCA of nontotal occlusions, is associated with more procedural time, increased cost (due to use of more guiding catheters, guidewires, and balloons), and more radiation exposure to the patient and operator (Table 16.12). Improvements in equipment have improved success and reduced complications, particularly with regard to the availability of hydrophilic guidewires.

   1. **Guiding Catheter.** It is essential to use a guiding catheter that provides good back-up support and coaxial alignment. For chronic total occlusions in native coronary arteries, a geometric or left Amplatz guide will provide excellent support. If a Judkins or Multipurpose guiding catheter is used, the "deep-seating" maneuver may be employed to provide extra back-up (Chapter 11). Deep catheter intubation from the left brachial approach may enhance support when PTCA from the femoral approach proves unsuccessful, but is rarely necessary. Occasionally, another catheter placed in the contralateral coronary artery to image the collateral flow to the occluded vessel may facilitate recanalization.

Table 16.7. Impact of Occlusion Characteristics on PTCA Outcome

Series	Success (%)			
	Length Short / Long	Occlusion Type Functional[+] / Total[++]	Tapered Stump Yes / No	Bridging Collaterals Yes / No
Noguchi[127] (2000)	67 / 40	-	-	-
Mousa[93]** (1998)	-	96 / 95	-	-
Schofer[96]*** (1998)	68 / 25	-	-	-
Kinoshita[9] (1995)	-	-	-	75 / 83
Tan[11] (1993)	-	-	69 / 43	70 / 20
Maiello[14]* (1992)	71 / 60	68 / 69	83 / 51	67 / 29
Ivanhoe[15] (1992)	-	78 / 60	73 / 60	-
Stone[7] (1990)	85 / 69	83 / 74	88 / 59	18 / 85

*   Success rate with/without sidebranch at occlusion site (61% vs. 69%)
+   Functional occlusion = faint, late antegrade filling beyond the lesion
++ Total occlusion = absence of antegrade filling beyond the lesion
** Stent trial (after guidewire crossing)
*** Laser guidewire
-    Not reported

2. **Guidewires**

    a. **Conventional Angioplasty Wires.** Serial use of progressively stiffer but flexible guidewires is a popular approach to crossing a chronic total occlusion. Some operators prefer to begin with stiff wires or glidewires, since soft-tip wires will successfully cross only 30-50% of occlusions. We frequently begin with a 0.018" gold-tip angled Glidewire, and exchange for a flexible 0.014" wire after crossing the occlusion. We avoid monorail systems for total occlusions because of inferior balloon tracking and the inability to readily exchange the guidewire. If collaterals are present, a late freeze-frame image can be used to estimate the length of the occlusion, identify the distal vessel, and help direct the guidewire through the expected lumen.[35] Extra support for the guidewire can be achieved by trailing the balloon catheter or a less expensive transfer catheter 1-2 cm behind the tip of the guidewire.

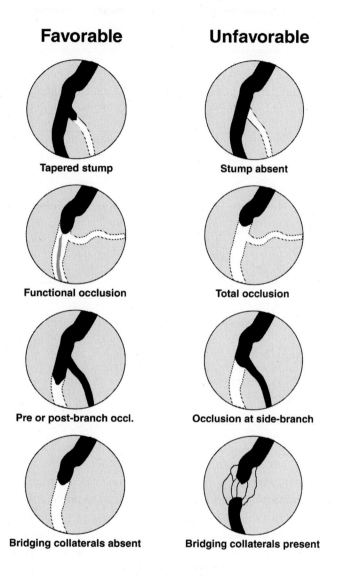

Figure 16.1. Chronic Total Occlusion: Lesion Morphology and Procedural Success

Table 16.8. Chronic Total Occlusion: Symptom Status After Percutaneous Revascularization

Series	Device	N	Follow-up (months)	Asymptomatic (%)
Sirnes[97] (1998)	Stent	59	6	57
	PTCA	57	6	24
Suttorp[95] (1998)	Stent	38	6	84
Berger[30] (1996)	PTCA	139	6	87*
Stewart[13] (1993)	PTCA	45	12	68*
Ivanhoe[15]** (1992)	PTCA	264	36	69
Ruocco[4]† (1992)	PTCA	160	24	69
Bell[16]†† (1991)	PTCA	234	32	76

*   Asymptomatic or Class I
**   Successful vs. unsuccessful PTCA: 4-year freedom from death (99% vs. 96%), death or MI (93% vs. 89%), CABG (87% vs. 64%)
†   2-year death rate in successful vs. unsuccessful PTCA groups (1.2% vs 14.3%)
††   Less need for CABG after successful PTCA. No differences in MI, death, or severe angina between successful and unsuccessful PTCA

The Ultrafuse-X catheter (Boston Scientific Scimed) is well-suited for this purpose since it allows distal contrast injection without relinquishing guidewire position. Excessive guidewire rotation should be avoided during crossing attempts to prevent tip fracture. If the guidewire buckles, it should be retracted and reoriented rather than forced into the occlusion. Once the wire crosses the occlusion, intraluminal position should be confirmed prior to balloon inflation. Clues to proper guidewire position include free guidewire rotation and easy advancement and retraction of the guidewire. Confirmation of intraluminal positioning is aided by contrast injection through the guiding catheter, central lumen of the balloon, or transfer catheter positioned distal to the occlusion. Clues to improper guidewire position include loss of free rotation, inability to advance the guidewire beyond the occlusion, or inability to advance a balloon or transport catheter through the occlusion. If these latter conditions are observed, the wire may be subintimal or in a small bridging collateral outside the lumen. In any case, balloon inflation should not be performed due to increased risk of dissection and vessel perforation.

Table 16.9. PCI of Nontotal vs. Chronic Total Occlusion: Long-Term Outcome

Series	Occlusion Type	F/U (months)	Death (%)	MI (%)	CABG (%)	PTCA (%)	Combined Event (%)
Mousa[93]	Total (stent)	8	1	3.2	5.4	15	25
(1998)	Nontotal (stent)		2.9	2.4	4.1	14	23
Elezi[98]	Total (stent)	12	-	6.1[†]	1.5	31	36*
(1998)	Nontotal (stent)		-	4.1[†]	1.8	18	23
Berger[30]	Total (PTCA)	6	1.4	2.9	-	-	21[+]
(1996)	Nontotal (PTCA)		0.5	2.4	-	-	18
Violaris[31]	Total (PTCA)	6	0	3.6	3.6	21	29*
(1995)	Nontotal (PTCA)		0.2	2.8	2.4	17	22
Ruocco[4]	Total (PTCA)	2	††	5	19	9*	25[+]
(1992)	Nontotal (PTCA)			9	15	20	30
Safian[8]	Total (PTCA)	2	-	-	14*	-	41
(1988)	Nontotal (PTCA)		-	-	8	-	28

Abbreviations: CABG = coronary artery bypass grafting; MI = myocardial infarction; PCI = percutaneous coronary intervention; PTCA = percutaneous transluminal coronary angioplasty; F/U = follow-up; - = not reported
† Combined death/MI
†† Relative risk compared to nontotal occlusion (4.39); late death for successful vs. failed PTCA of total occlusion (9% vs. 14%, $p < 0.05$)
* $p < 0.05$
+ CABG or PTCA

b. **Hydrophilic Guidewires.** The Glidewire and other hydrophilic guidewires[121,122,123] have been successfully employed for peripheral and coronary angioplasty and are popular because of their flexibility, kink-resistance, and lubriciousness. Small series suggest that the Glidewire may successfully cross 30-60% of occlusions that cannot be crossed with conventional guidewires (Table 16.3),[36-38] which is probably true of other hydrophilic guidewires from many manufacturers (Chapter 1).

c. **Magnum-Meier™ Recanalization Wire.** This ball-tipped guidewire consists of a 0.014", 0.018", or 0.021" solid-steel wire shaft, a flexible distal spring wire comprised of Teflonized® tungsten, and a 1-mm olive-shaped tip (Figure 16.2). The wire has been designed to increase pushability and reduce subintimal wire passage. The Magnarail balloon (monorail design) and Magnum-Meier over-the-wire balloon are currently the only commercially available balloons able to accommodate 0.021" wires. Results from observational studies and randomized trials have not demonstrated clear superiority over conventional PTCA guidewires.[25,39,124-126]

Table 16.10. Impact of Successful vs. Unsuccessful Revascularization of Chronic Total Occlusion on Long-Term Clinical Outcome

Series	Immediate Result	F/U (months)	Death (%)	MI (%)	CABG (%)	PTCA (%)	Combined Event (%)
Naguchi[127]	Successful (PTCA)	51	5	-	7 (11-yrs)	-	-
(2000)	Unsuccessful (PTCA)		16	-	27*	-	-
Dzavik[140]	Successful (stent)	12-36	-	-	-	-	37
(2000)	Unsuccessful (stent)		-	-	-	-	73
Stewart[13]	Successful (PTCA)	12	2.2	-	16*	13	31*
(1993)	Unsuccessful (PTCA)		4.1	-	45	16	64
Ivanhoe[15]	Successful (PTCA)	4	-	-	13*	-	7++*
(1992)	Unsuccessful (PTCA)		-	-	36	-	11
Bell[16]	Successful (PTCA)	5-7	18	11	18*	-	-
(1991)	Unsuccessful (PTCA)		25	5	58	-	-
Finci[33]	Successful (PTCA)	2	5	-	7*	-	33+*
(1990)	Unsuccessful (PTCA)		3	-	37	-	41

Abbreviations: CABG = coronary artery bypass grafting; MI = myocardial infarction; PTCA = percutaneous transluminal coronary angioplasty; F/U = follow-up; - = not reported
* p < 0.05
++ Death or MI

3. **Balloon Dilatation Catheter**

   a. **Over-The-Wire Systems.** Although a variety of low-profile on-the-wire and monorail balloon catheters are available, an over-the-wire system is preferred because it allows guidewire exchanges, balloon upsizing, and enhanced trackability. If difficulty is encountered advancing the balloon into the occlusion, maneuvers to increase guiding catheter support may be of value. Constant forward pressure on the balloon is generally more successful than aggressive tapping of the balloon against the occlusion ("jack-hammering"), which usually does not transmit additional force. If the reference vessel diameter cannot be estimated, the vessel should be predilated with a 1.5 or 2.0 mm balloon. If the reference vessel diameter is easily estimated (because of collateral filling of the distal vessel), a full-sized balloon may be used. For heavily calcified occlusions, high-pressure balloons may be preferred, but there is otherwise no specific advantage to any balloon material. The Rotablator is an important adjunct if lesion rigidity precludes balloon advancement; guidewire position in the true lumen must be ensured prior to burr activation.

   b. **Fixed Wire-Balloon Systems.** Balloon-on-the-wire catheters are generally not considered first-line systems due to their lack of pushability, trackability, and steerability. However, because of their extremely low profile, they may occasionally cross total occlusions when over-the-wire balloons fail.[48] When a fixed wire-balloon system is used, a bare guidewire may be positioned beyond the stenosis to maintain distal access while the device is removed.

Table 16.11. Late Angiographic Results After Revascularization of Chronic Total Occlusion

Series	Occlusion	Device	N	Restenosis (%)	Reocclusion (%)
Noguchi[127] (2000)	Total	PTCA	134	40	-
Buller[128]* (1999)	Total	PTCA	208	70	-
Sievert[133]* (1999)	Total	PTCA	55	62	13
		Stent	55	26	2
Hoher[131]* (1999)	Total	PTCA	43	64	24
	Total	Stent	42	32	3
Lau[137] (1999)	Total	Stent	43	33	-
	Nontotal	Stent	43	28	-
Rubartelli[102]* (1998)	Total	PTCA	97 (overall)	68	24
		Stent		32	3
Nobuyoshi[119] (1998)	Total	PTCA	413	57	28
Mori[129]* (1996)	Total	PTCA	96 (overall)	56	11
		Stent		28	7
Sirens[88]* (1996)	Total	PTCA	114 (overall)	74	26
		Stent		57	12
Berger[30] (1996)	Total	PTCA	139	49	19
	Nontotal		1295	42	7
Kinoshita[9] (1995)	Total	PTCA	433	55	15
Violaris[31]* (1995)	Total	PTCA	266	45	19
	Nontotal		3317	34	5
	Absolute	PTCA	109	45	24
	Functional		157	45	16
Ishizaku[10] (1995)	Total	PTCA	62	55	18
Bell[16] (1992)	Total	PTCA	69	59	14
Ivanhoe[15] (1992)	Total	PTCA	175	54	16
Anderson[27] (1991)	Total	PTCA	70	71	34

* Randomized trial

Table 16.12. Chronic Total Coronary Occlusion: Time, Equipment, and Cost

Series	Occlusion	Procedure Time (min)	Radiation Time (min)	Equipment Guides / Wires / Balloons	Cost ($)
Stewart[13]	Total	73	30	-	-
(1993)	Nontotal	59	18	-	-
Bell[16]	Total	74	31	2.0 / 2.7 / 1.8	1947
(1991)	Nontotal	59	18	1.5 / 1.5 / 1.3	1398

Abbreviations: - = not reported

4. **Adjunctive Thrombolytic Therapy.** Small reports (using different lytic agents and infusion regimens) suggest that prolonged intracoronary thrombolytic infusions may improve recanalization rates, coronary flow, and PTCA success (Tables 16.14, 16.15).

E. **NON-BALLOON DEVICES.** Failure to cross a chronic total occlusion with a guidewire accounts for 80% of unsuccessful procedures. This limitation is extremely important because all currently available devices (balloon, atherectomy, excimer laser, stent) require initial crossing of the occlusion with a guidewire. Preliminary data suggest that several rotational, laser, and ultrasound devices may be capable of recanalizing 30-50% occlusions resistant to PTCA guidewires (Table 16.13). Once the occlusion is crossed, conventional PTCA, atherectomy, laser, and stents can be used to improve lumen dimensions (Tables 16.15, 16.18).

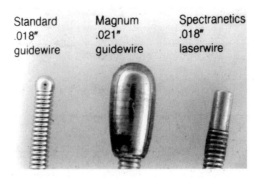

Figure 16.2. The Magnum-Meier™ Recanalization Wire and Laserwire

Table 16.13. Crossing Total Occlusions Resistant to PTCA Guidewires

Series	N	Device Success (%)*	Final Success (%)*	Other Results
Crosswire				
Kahler[134] (2000)	107	42	-	Hemopericardium (1.8%); contrast staining (4.6%)
Corcos[121] (1998)	56	79	-	Perforation (36%); tamponade (1.8%)
Serial Guidewire				
Reimers[100] (1998)	301	73	62	Tamponade (1%); contrast staining (8%)
Reimers[123] (1998)	95	71	65	Perforation, tamponade, emergency surgery in 1 patient (1.2%)
Glidewire				
Freed[36] (1993)	59	54	39	No perforations
Rees[37] (1991)	33	58	52	Non-flow-limiting dissections (52%)
Magnum Wire				
Meier[124] (1997)	50	46	-	In-hospital death (1.5%); emergency surgery (0.8%); perforation (4%)
Pande[39] (1992)	28	45	39	See Table 16.14
Haerer[25] (1991)	102	32	32	See Table 16.14
Laserwire[†]				
Oesterle[99] (1998)	179	61	56	Coronary perforation (16%); tamponade (1.7%)
Schofer[96] (1997)	66	50	47	Success 68% for lesion length $\leq$ 10 mm and 25% for lesion length 30-40 mm
Hamburger[82] (1997)	345	59	-	Coronary perforation (21%); tamponade (1.0%); non-Q-wave MI (0.9%). Predictors of success were occlusion duration < 40 weeks and length < 30 mm
Steffen[92] (1997)	59	47	-	
Shinobi Wire				
Khanna[136] (1999)	13	69	69	Stiff, torquable, Teflon-coated wire. No perforations, contrast staining, or emergency CABG
Vibrational Angioplasty				
Cannon[138] (2000)	14	71	43	Local perforation (14%); no death or emergency CABG
Rees[42] (1995)	18	89	78	
ROTACS				
Danchin[43] (1995)	50	-	66	See Table 16.14

Abbreviations: ROTACS = Rotational Angioplasty Catheter System; - = not reported
* Device success = cross occlusion with device; final success = procedural success after adjunctive PTCA or stent
† Visible entry port and visualization of distal vessel via collaterals required. PTCA guidewire crossing not attempted prior to laserwire.

Table 16.14. Randomized Trials of Percutaneous Revascularization for Chronic Total Occlusion

Trial	N	Design	1° Success (%)	Comments
Crosswire				
Lafavre[135]	46	Conventional wire	35	Crosswire required less fluoroscopy (19.2 vs. 24.3 min)
(1999)	42	Crosswire	74	and procedure time (42 vs. 57 min)
Laserwire				
TOTAL[101]	145	Laserwire	64	Similar complications; laserwire was useful when
(1998)	160	PTCA	48	conventional wires failed (58% success)
Magnum Wire				
Pande[39]	100	Magnum	45	Magnum success after PTCA failure (39%); PTCA
(1992)		PTCA	67	success after Magnum failure (12%). No difference in
				fluoroscopy time
Haerer[25]	102	Magnum	32	Magnum failures salvaged by other systems in 48%
(1991)		PTCA	68	
		Omniflex	59	
ELCA				
AMRO[45]	103	ELCA	65	No difference in 6-month clinical endpoints or
(1996)		PTCA	61	reocclusion
ROTACS				
Danchin[43]	100	ROTACS	66	No advantage for ROTACS
(1995)		PTCA	60	
STENTS				
SARECCO[132]	55	Stent	-	Stents had higher EFS at 2 years (52% vs. 26%, p <
(1999)	55	PTCA	-	0.05)
TOSCA[128,139]	202	Stent	-	Stents had less TVR (23% vs. 31%, p = 0.03) and
(1999)	208	PTCA	-	similar MACE (40% vs. 46%) at 1-3 years
Hoher[131]	42	Stent	-	Stents had less restenosis (32% vs. 64%), less
(1999)	43	PTCA	-	reocclusion (3% vs. 24%), and higher EFS (70% vs.
				45%) at 6 months
STOP[103]	48	Stent	-	Stents had less TLR at 6 months (19% vs. 39%)
(1999)	48	PTCA	-	
MAJIC[104]	87	Stent	-	Stents had less TLR at 6 months (30% vs. 63%)
(1998)	96	PTCA	-	
GISSOC[102]	56	Stent	-	Stents had less restenosis (32% vs. 68%), reocclusion
(1998)	54	PTCA	-	(8% vs. 34%), TLR (5% vs. 18%), and recurrent
				ischemia (14% vs. 46%) at 9 months
SICCO[88,97]	58	Stent	-	Stents had less restenosis (32% vs. 74%), reocclusion
(1996)	59	PTCA	-	(12% vs. 26%), and TLR at 10 months (22% vs. 42%)
				and at 2.8 years (19% vs. 48%)
Thrombolysis				
Zidar[110]	60	Intracoronary		PTCA success after lytic regimens (52-56%). More
(1996)		urokinase		bleeding, vascular complications at higher doses.
				Clinical improvement (76%); reocclusion (9%);
				restenosis (59%); target vessel revascularization (36%).

Abbreviations: EFS = event free survival; ELCA = Excimer Laser Coronary Angioplasty; ROTACS = Rotational Angioplasty Catheter System; TLR = target lesion revascularization; MACE = major adverse cardiac events (death, MI, TLR); - = not reported.
Acronyms: AMRO = Amsterdam-Rotterdam Trial; GISSOC = Gruppo Italiano di Studio Sullo Stent Nelle Occlusioni Coronariche; MAJIC = Mayo Japan Investigation for Chronic Total Occlusion; SARECCO = Stent or Angioplasty after Recanalization of Chronic Coronary Occlusions; SICCO = Stenting in Chronic Coronary Occlusion; STOP = Stents in Total Occlusion and Restenosis Prevention; TOSCA = Total Occlusion Study of Canada; TOTAL = Total Occlusions Trial with Angioplasty Using Laser Guidewire

Table 16.15. Intracoronary Thrombolysis for Occlusions Resistant to PTCA Guidewires

Series	N	Lytic	Results	Other
Zidar[47,110] (1996)	60	UK (1.6-3.2 MU x 8 hrs) via infusion wire + guide catheter	PTCA success 52-59% for all doses	Major bleeding and vascular complications were increased at higher lytic doses. Restenosis (59%) and reocclusion (9%) at 6 months
Ajluni[52] (1995)	25	UK (100,000-240,000 U/hr x 8-25 hrs) via infusion wire + guide catheter	↑ Coronary flow (28%); PTCA success (52%)	MI (8%); significant bleeding (8%); length of stay (5.1 days)
Cecena[53] (1993)	20	UK bolus (120,000 U IC) plus up to 200,000 U/hr x 24 hrs via infusion wire + guide catheter	↑ Coronary flow (90%); PTCA success (94%)	No MI or emergent CABG; blood transfusion (10%)
Vaska[54] (1991)	11	tPA (5-10 mg/hr x 6 hrs) via infusion wire	↑ Coronary flow (91%); PTCA success (82%)	No death, MI, or emergent CABG; acute closure (10%)

Abbreviations: UK = urokinase; MI = in-hospital myocardial infarction; CABG = emergency coronary artery bypass grafting; MU = million units; tPA = tissue plasminogen activator

1. **Devices for Occlusions Resistant to PTCA Guidewire Crossing (Table 16.13)**
   a. **Laserwire.** An 0.018" excimer laser guidewire (PrimaWire, Spectranetics) has been developed to recanalize chronic total occlusions that cannot be crossed with conventional guidewires (Figure 16.2). Use of this guidewire requires meticulous technique and careful patient selection to avoid severe dissection and perforation. Only a small fraction of total occlusions may be suitable for the laserwire since its use must be limited to short segments of occlusion in straight vessels, and the operator must be able to visualize the proximal and distal extent of the occlusion throughout the ablation procedure. To perform this technique safely, frequent use of orthogonal views or biplane angiography are required to ensure the laserwire is directed along the major axis of the vessel. If contralateral collaterals are present, the donor vessel should be engaged with a second guiding catheter from the contralateral femoral artery to identify the distal end of the occlusion. Even partial penetration of the occlusion may allow successful crossing with a conventional wire. Once a channel is formed, the lesion is treated with PTCA or another device. Observational and randomized trials suggest that the laserwire may have slight incremental benefit for crossing refractory total occlusions, but there is a high incidence of coronary perforation and tamponade.[82,83,92,96,99,101]

   b. **Ultrasound Probe (Figure 16.3).** Therapeutic ultrasound catheters that transmit vibrational energy via ball-tipped guidewires are now being used to recanalize total occlusions. Ongoing studies, including the multicenter European CRUSADE trial, hope to clarify the mechanism of action and define acute and long-term outcomes.

   c.   **Vibrational Angioplasty.** This technique involves the use of a guidewire attached to a motor. When activated, the motor causes rapid oscillation of the advancing guidewire. Among 18 lesions resistant to conventional techniques, vibrational angioplasty was successful in 78%.[42]

   d.   **ROTACS: Low-Speed Rotational Angioplasty Catheter System (Figure 16.4).** This battery-driven, over-the-wire catheter is comprised of several helical stainless-steel coils, a moveable polyethylene or polyolefin sheath, and a 1.3-1.8 mm olive-shaped ball-tip. Using an 8F guiding catheter, the ROTACS is advanced over a conventional angioplasty guidewire until it abuts the occlusion. After removing the guidewire, the electric motor is activated and continuous forward pressure is applied to the catheter while it rotates at 200 rpm. The central lumen of the catheter is used to deliver contrast injections and assess progress. If unsuccessful, the sheath can be advanced to increase support. If the catheter crosses the occlusion, the guidewire should be reinserted and the ROTACS system exchanged for a conventional balloon catheter. ROTACS was used to successfully recanalize about half of resistant occlusions, including vessels occluded up to 12 months.[44] The BAROCCO trial, a randomized study of ROTACS vs. PTCA in 100 chronic total coronary occlusions, revealed ROTACS success in 40% and PTCA success in 52% of lesions (p = NS).[43] PTCA was able to salvage 59% of ROTACS failures, whereas only 17% of PTCA failures could be salvaged by ROTACS. The investigators concluded that initial use of ROTACS does not offer an advantage over PTCA, but could be reserved for PTCA failures. This device is rarely used and is not available in the United States.

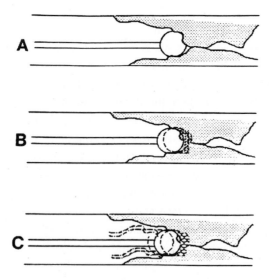

Figure 16.3. Ultrasound Angioplasty

Oscillations of the ultrasound catheter produce microcavitations resulting in fragmentation of plaque.

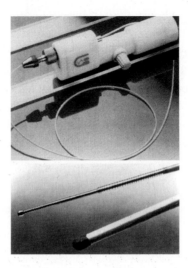

Figure 16.4. Rotational Angioplasty Catheter System (ROTACS)

---

e. **Optical Coherence Reflectometry (OCR).** The Safe-Steer Guidewire (Intraluminal Therapeutics, Inc) is a new system that is currently under evaluation for revascularization of chronic total occlusions which cannot be crossed with a guidewire. The system relies on optical reflectance to differentiate plaque, thrombus, and blood from vessel wall, facilitating guidewire advancement.

2. **Devices Used for Wire-Crossable Occlusions (Tables 16.16, 16.17)**

   a. **Lasers**. In the multicenter Amsterdam-Rotterdam (AMRO) trial, 103 patients with total occlusions were randomized to excimer laser angioplasty (ELCA) or PTCA. No differences were observed in procedural success (65%), late reocclusion (ELCA 33%, PTCA 23%), or 6-month event-free survival.[45] Most procedural failures were due to inability to cross the occlusion with a guidewire, but if the occlusion was crossed, success rates were 90%.[59,63,71] Major ischemic complications were infrequent, although restenosis rates approached 50%.[63] ELCA is rarely utilized today for chronic total occlusions.

   b. **Atherectomy (Chapters 27-29).** Among 145 total occlusions crossed with a guidewire in multicenter Rotablator Registry, procedural success was achieved in 91%.[57] Acute closure occurred in 7.2%, half of which developed after the patient left the catheterization laboratory. Rotablator may be especially useful if a rigid chronic total occlusion cannot be crossed or dilated with a balloon. Few data are available regarding the ability of DCA or TEC to recanalize chronic total occlusions. In one report, DCA was successful in 15 of 17 occlusions after crossing the occlusion with a guidewire.[55,56]

c. **Stents (Table 16.17).** Although the presence of a chronic total occlusion was once a relative contraindication to stenting, recent data indicate a definite role. Most randomized trials demonstrated less restenosis, less reocclusion, and less target lesion revascularization with stents,[88,89,97,102-104] although some did not.[107,108,120] Risk factors for restenosis are similar to those for stenting nontotal occlusions, and include final MLD, length of stent, final balloon/artery ratio, and dissection.[98,109] Older stent trials frequently used original warfarin-based strategies, which may have had an adverse impact on late outcome; more contemporary antiplatelet strategies have enhanced the safety and efficacy of stenting.

Table 16.16. Results of Atherectomy and Lasers for Chronic Total Occlusion

Device	N	Success (%)	In-hospital MACE (%)	Other
DCA				
Dick[55] (1991)	7	86	0	Occlusion duration 41 days (range 5-105 days)
Hinohara[56] (1991)	10	90	0	
Rotablator				
Braden[142] (2001)	139	-	3.2	Clinical restenosis (19%)
Levin[87] (1996)	15	100	0	Dissection (18%); acute closure (7.2%)
Omoigui[57] (1995)	145	91	5.7	
ELCA				
Schofer[111] (1996)	80	90	1.2	Minor dissection (45%); restenosis (53%, including 20% reocclusion)
Klein[59] (1994)	172 (> 3 months) 107 (< 3 months)	85 90	2.0	Acute closure (4.5% vs. 2.7%); perforation (0% vs. 0.9%)
Baumbach[61] (1993)	212	-	-	Total occlusion predictive of perforation
Holmes[62] (1993)	172	90	3.7	
Bittl[64] (1992)	127	84	-	
Holmium Laser				
deMarchena[65] (1994)	25	100	0	

Abbreviations: ELCA = excimer laser coronary angioplasty; DCA = directional coronary atherectomy; RS = restenosis; MACE = major adverse cardiac events; - = not reported

Table 16.17. Results of Stents for Chronic Total Occlusion

Series	Device	N	Results
Gruberg[133] (2000)	Debulk*/stent Stent alone	44 108	In-hospital MACE (2.3% vs. 6.5%); no difference in TLR (14.4% vs. 16.3%) or MACE (19.6% vs. 25.6%) at 14 months
Azuma[130] (2000)	Debulk+/stent Stent alone	52 224	Debulk/stent with less restenosis (odds ratio 0.38 [CI 0.19-0.78])
SARECCO[132] (1999)	PTCA Stent	55 55	Randomized trial. 2-year EFS higher with stents (52% vs. 26%, p < 0.05).
TOSCA[128,139] (1999)	PTCA Stent	202 200	Randomized trial. At 6 months, stents had a 45% reduction in clinically driven TVR. At 1-3 years, stents had less TVR (23% vs. 31%, p = 0.03) and similar MACE (40% vs. 46%)
Hoher[131] (1999)	Stent PTCA	43 42	Randomized trial. Success (95% vs. 88%); in-hospital MACE (1.5% vs. 0.5%). At 6 months, stenting was associated with less restenosis (32% vs. 64%), less reocclusion (3% vs. 24%), and higher EFS (70% vs. 45%)
STOP[103] (1999)	Stent PTCA	48 48	Randomized trial. Less TLR (19% vs. 39%) at 6 months with stents
Anzuini[94] (1998)	Stent	89	Success (98%); in-hospital MACE (5.6%); restenosis (32%) and reocclusion (4%) at 19 months; MACE at 1 year (13%) and 3 years (28%)
Suttorp[95] (1998)	Stent	38	Restenosis (40%) and reocclusion (23%) at 6 months
GISSOC[102] (1998)	Stent PTCA	56 54	Randomized trial. Stents had less restenosis (32% vs. 68%), reocclusion (8% vs. 34%), TLR (5% vs. 18%) and recurrent ischemia (14% vs. 46%) at 9 months
MAJIC[104] (1998)	Stent PTCA	87 96	Randomized trial. Stents had less TLR at 3 months (15% vs. 41%) and at 6 months (30% vs. 63%)
Yamasaki[106] (1998)	Stent PTCA	143 75	Stents with greater patency at 3 years (88% vs. 63%)
Carere[107] (1998)	Stent OPTCA SOPTCA	194 122 74	Substudy of TOSCA. OPTCA and stents with similar 6-month patency, TLR, angiographic restenosis. Both were significantly better than SOPTCA
Title[108] (1998)	Stent PTCA	54 83	Substudy of TOSCA in vessels < 3 mm. At 6 months, stents had similar restenosis (53% vs. 63%) and TLR (11% vs. 11%), more non-Q-MI (17% vs. 4%), and higher patency (98% vs. 87%)
Rau[968] (1998)	Stent	143	Restenosis (22%) and reocclusion (7%) at 4.5 months
SICCO[109] (1998)	Stent	143	Randomized trial. Stents has less restenosis (32% vs. 74%), less reocclusion (12% vs. 26%), less TLR at 10 months (22% vs. 42%) and 2.8 years (19% vs. 48%), and less MACE at 2-8 years (6% vs. 24%)
Elezi[90] (1997)	Stent (CTO) Stent (no CTO)	54 972	CTO group had more restenosis (40% vs. 26%) and reocclusion (14% vs. 3%)
Mathey[91] (1997)	Stent	143	Restenosis (28%); reocclusion (7%)

Table 16.17. Results of Stents for Chronic Total Occlusion

Series	Device	N	Results
Mori[105] (1996)	Stent PTCA	43 53	Stents had less restenosis (28% vs. 57%) and rePTCA (28% vs. 49%) at 6 months, and less MI + CABG (2.3% vs. 11%). Stenting (not PTCA) was associated with improvement in LV ejection fraction
Saito[120] (1996)	Stent PTCA	34 35	Randomized trial. Stents had similar reocclusion (6.3% vs. 11.4%), restenosis (36.7% vs. 34.4%), and TLR (20% vs. 25%)
Ozaki[86] (1996)	Stent PTCA	20 66	Similar restenosis (29% vs. 45%)
Ooka[67] (1995)	Stent PTCA	47 65	Stents had less restenosis (44% vs. 68%) and reocclusion (10% vs. 35%)
Goldberg[163] (1995)	PSS	60	Restenosis (20%); 14-month EFS (77%)

Abbreviations: TLR = target lesion revascularization; CTO = chronic total occlusion; MACE = major adverse cardiac events (death, MI, repeat revascularization); OPTCA = optimal PTCA; SOPTCA = suboptimal PTCA
Acronyms: See Table 16.14
*   DCA, ELCA, or Rotablator prior to stenting
+   DCA or Rotablator prior to stenting

SAPHENOUS VEIN GRAFT OCCLUSION

Of the more than 600,000 saphenous vein bypass grafts placed each year, 10-15% will be occluded at one year and 50% by 10 years after operation. Among the 10-20% of patients who require reoperation within 10 years, repeat bypass surgery is technically more difficult and has been associated with increased morbidity and mortality compared to the initial operation (Chapter 17).

A. PATHOLOGY. The etiology of saphenous vein graft occlusion is dependent on the time interval following bypass surgery.[73,74] In the first month, graft occlusion is almost always due to graft thrombosis from poor surgical technique (suture line stenosis, intraoperative vein trauma) or poor distal run-off. Between 1-12 months, initial hyperplasia is the most common cause. After 1 year, occlusion is caused by graft atherosclerosis, which is indistinguishable from coronary arteriosclerosis. Once graft occlusion occurs, retrograde thrombosis to the aorto-ostial junction is common.

B. PTCA. Although PTCA can successfully revascularize approximately 70% of occluded vein grafts, there is a high incidence of distal embolization (11%), late graft occlusion (40-50%), and late cardiac events (event-free survival of 54% at 1 year and 34% at 3 years).[75] When distal embolization occurs, 50% are associated with vessel closure or CK elevation.[75] Embolization may present as abrupt cutoff of distal vessels (amenable to repeat dilation or lytics), or may be inferred on the basis of no-reflow. PTCA alone is rarely utilized as sole therapy for occluded vein grafts.

C. **NON-BALLOON DEVICES.** Recanalization of occluded vein grafts using atherectomy, thrombectomy, laser, stent, and embolic protection devices is discussed in detail in Chapter 17.

D. **PROLONGED INTRAGRAFT THROMBOLYSIS.** Hartmann and associates[77] were the first to systematically study the use of prolonged urokinase infusions for chronically occluded vein grafts. In the multicenter ROBUST trial,[78] 107 patients with one occluded vein graft received intragraft urokinase for at least 24 hours. Successful recanalization was achieved in 69% of patients, but there was a high incidence of major complications (death 6.5%, Q-wave MI 5%, non-Q-wave MI 17%, emergency CABG 4%, stroke 3%). Six-month angiography revealed sustained vessel patency in only 40%. Lytic infusion through the central lumen of an inflated balloon (Balloon-Occlusive-Intravascular-Lysis-Enhanced-Recanalization; BOILER) is also feasible.[79]

CONCLUSIONS

Successful recanalization of chronic total coronary occlusions often results in marked improvements in long-term symptomatic status and exercise capacity, and reduces the need for late CABG by 50%. The benefits of revascularization may be improved by stents and contemporary antiplatelet regimens. However, the management of totally occluded saphenous vein bypass grafts remains problematic. PTCA should be abandoned as sole therapy in vein grafts due to the high incidence of acute embolization and late revascularization. Stents hold promise as a means of reducing late reocclusion and restenosis, but progressive disease at non-stented sites is a persistent cause of late graft failure. The role of mechanical and pharmacologic strategies will require further prospective, randomized evaluation. Our approach to the patient with chronic total occlusion is summarized in Figure 16.5.

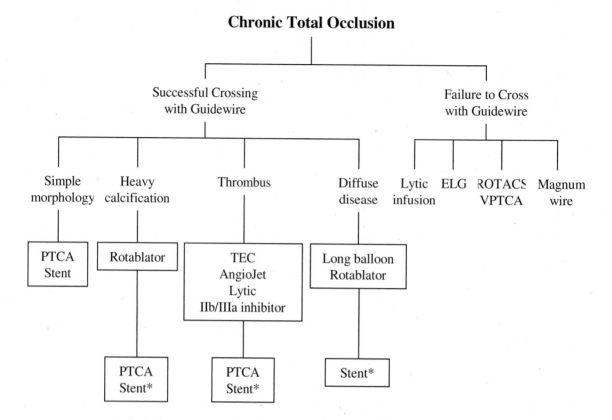

Figure 16.5. Approach to Chronic Total Coronary Occlusion

Abbreviations: ELG = excimer laser guidewire; TEC = transluminal extraction catheter; ROTACS = rotational angioplasty catheter system; VPTCA = vibrational angioplasty

* Consider provisional stenting for suboptimal PTCA (residual stenosis > 30% or dissection)

* * * * *

REFERENCES

1. Flameng W, Schwarz F, and Hehrlein FW. Intraoperative evaluation of the functional significance of coronary collateral vessels in patients with coronary artery disease. Am J Cardiol 1978;42:187-192.

2. Favereau X, Corcos T, Guerin Y, et al. Early reocclusion after successful coronary angioplasty of chronic total occlusions. J Am Coll Cardiol 1995;25:139A.

3. Tan K, Sulke N, Taub N, Sowton E. Clinical and lesion morphologic determinants of coronary angioplasty success and complications: Current experience. J Am Coll Cardiol 1995;25:855-65.

4. Ruocco NA Jr, Ring ME, Holubkov R, et al. Results of coronary angioplasty of chronic total occlusions (the National Heart, Lung, and Blood Institute 1985-1986 Percutaneous Transluminal Angioplasty Registry). Am J Cardiol 1992;69:69-76.

5. Myler R, Shaw R, Stertzer S, et al. Lesion morphology and coronary angioplasty: Current experience and analysis. J Am Coll Cardiol 1992;19:1641-1652.

6. Plante S. Laarman GJ, de Feyter PJ, et al. Acute complications of percutaneous transluminal coronary angioplasty for total occlusion. Am Heart J 1991;121:417.

7. Stone GW, Rutherford BD, McConahay DR, et al. Procedural outcome of angioplasty for total coronary artery occlusion: An analysis of 971 lesions in 905 patients. J Am Coll Cardiol 1990;15:849-856.

8. Safian RD, McCabe CH, Sipperly ME, et al. Initial success and long-term follow-up of percutaneous transluminal coronary angioplasty in chronic total occlusions versus conventional stenoses. Am J Cardiol 1988;61:23G-28G.

9. Kinoshitaw I, Katoh O, Nariyama J, Otsuji S, et al. Coronary angioplasty of chronic total occlusions with bridging collateral vessels: Immediate and follow-up outcome from a large single-center experience. J Am Coll Cardiol 1995;26:409-15.

10. Ishizaka N, Issiki T, Saeki F, et al. Angiographic follow-up after successful percutaneous coronary angioplasty for chronic total coronary occlusion: Experience in 110 consecutive patients. Am Heart J 1994;127:8.

11. Tan KH, Sulke AN, Taub NA, Watts E, Sowton E. Coronary angioplasty of chronic total occlusions: Determinants of procedural success. J Am Coll Cardiol 1993;21:76A.

12. Shimizu M, Kato O, Otsuji S, et al. Progress in initial outcome of PTCA for complete occlusion. Circulation 1993;88:I-504.

13. Stewart J, Denne L, Bowker T, et al. Percutaneous transluminal coronary angioplasty in chronic coronary artery occlusion. J Am Coll Cardiol 1993;21:1371-1376.

14. Maiello L, Colombo A, Gianrossi R, et al. Coronary angioplasty of chronic occlusions: Factors predictive of procedural success. Am Heart J 1992;124:581-584.

15. Ivanhoe RJ, Weintraub WS, Douglas JS Jr, et al. Percutaneous transluminal coronary angioplasty of chronic total occlusions. Primary success, restenosis, and long-term clinical follow-up. Circulation 1992;85:106-115.

16. Bell MR, Berger PB, Reeder GS, et al. Successful PTCA of chronic total coronary occlusions reduces the need for coronary artery bypass surgery. Circulation 1991;84:II-250.

17. Shimizu M, Kato O, Otsuji S, et al. Progress in initial outcome of PTCA for complete occlusion. J Am Coll Cardiol 1993;88:I-504.

18. Bell MR, Berger PB, Reeder GS, et al. Initial and long-term outcome of 354 patients after coronary balloon angioplasty of total coronary artery occlusions. Circulation 1992;85:1003.

19. Melchior JP, Meier B, Urban P, et al. Percutaneous transluminal coronary angioplasty for chronic total coronary arterial occlusion. Am J Cardiol 1987;59:535-538.

20. Tenaglia A, Fortin D, Califf R. Predicting the risk of abrupt closure after angioplasty in an individual patient. J Am Coll Cardiol 1994;24:1004-1011.

21. Ruocco NA, Ring ME, Holubkov R, Jacobs AK. Results of coronary angioplasty of chronic total occlusions (the National Heart, Lung, and Blood Institute 1985-1986 Percutaneous Transluminal Angioplasty Registry). Am J Cardiol 1992;69:69-76.

22. Stone GW, Rutherford BD, McConahay DR, et al. Procedural outcome of angioplasty for total coronary artery occlusion: An analysis of 971 lesions in 905 patients. J Am Coll Cardiol 1990;15:849-856.

23. Burger W, Kadel C, Keul H, Vallbracht C, Kaltenbach M. A word of caution: Reopening chronic coronary occlusions. Cathet Cardiovasc Diagn 1992;27:35-39.

24. Bell MR, Berger PB, Bresnahan JF, Reeder GS. Initial and long-term outcome of 354 patients after coronary balloon angioplasty of total coronary artery occlusions. Circulation 1992;85:1003-1011.

25. Haerer W, Schmidt A, Eggeling T, et al. Angioplasty of chronic total coronary occlusions. Results of a controlled randomized trial. J Am Coll Cardiol 1991;17:113A.

26. Meier B. Total coronary occlusion: A different animal? J Am Coll Cardiol 1991;17:50B.

27. Anderson TJ, Knudtson ML, Roth DL, et al. Improvement in left ventricular function following PTCA of chronic totally occluded arteries. Circulation 1991;84:II-519.

28. Serruys PW, Umans V, Heyndrickx GR, et al. Elective PTCA of totally occluded coronary arteries not associated with acute myocardial infarction; short-term and long-term results. Eur Heart J 1985;6:2-12.

29. Danchin N, Angiol M, Beurrie D, et al. Late recanalization of chronic total coronary occlusion: Maintained vessel patency improves global and regional left ventricular function and avoids remodeling. J Am Coll Cardiol 195;25:345A.

30. Berger PB, Holmes DR, Ohman M, et al. Restenosis, reocclusion and adverse cardiovascular events after successful balloon angioplasty of occluded versus nonoccluded coronary arteries. Results from the Multicenter American Research Trial with Cilazapril after Angioplasty to Prevent Transluminal Coronary Obstruction and Restenosis (MARCATOR). J Am Coll Cardiol 1996;27:1-7.

31. Violaris A, Melkert R, Serruys P. Long-term luminal renarrowing after successful elective coronary angioplasty of total occlusions. A quantitative angiographic analysis.

Circulation 1995;91:2140-2150.

32. Kadel C, Burger W, Hartmann A, et al. Long-term follow-up in 686 patients with attempted reopening of chronic coronary occlusions. Circulation 1993;88:I-505.

33. Finci L, Meier B, Fayre J et al. Long-term results of successful and failed angioplasty for chronic total coronary arterial occlusion. Am J Cardiol 1990;66:660.

34. Mintz G, Popma J, Pichard A, et al. Increased plaque burden affects procedural outcomes of total occlusions: An intravascular ultrasound study. J Am Coll Cardiol 1995;25:61A.

35. Sherman CT, Sheehan D and Simpson JB. Simultaneous cannulation: A technique for percutaneous transluminal coronary angioplasty of chronic total occlusions. Cathet Cardiovasc Diagn 1987;13:333-336.

36. Freed M, Boatman JE, Siegel N, et al. Glidewire treatment of resistant coronary occlusions. Cathet Cardiovasc Diagn 1993;30:201-204.

37. Rees MR, Sivananthan MV, Verma SP. The use of hydrophilic Terumo glidewires in the treatment of chronic coronary artery occlusions. Circulation 1991;84:II-519.

38. Hosny A, Lai D, Mancherje C, Lee G. Successful recanalization using a hydrophilic-coated guidewire in total coronary occlusions after unsuccessful PTCA attempts with standard steerable guidewires. J Interven Cardiol 1990;3:225-230.

39. Pande AK, Meier B, Urban P, de la Serna F. Magnum/magnarail versus conventional systems for recanalization of chronic total coronary occlusions: A randomized comparison. Am Heart J 1992;123:1182-1186.

40. Haerer W, Schmidt A, Eggeling T, et al. Angioplasty of chronic total coronary occlusions. Results of a controlled randomized trial. J Cardiol 1991;17:113A.

41. Serruys PW, Hamburger J, Fleck E, Koolen JJ, et al. Laser guidewire: A powerful tool in recanalization of chronic total coronary occlusion. Circulation 1995;92:I-76.

42. Rees M, Michalis L. Vibrational coronary angioplasty: Challenging chronic total occlusions. Preliminary clinical data. J Am Coll Cardiol 1995;25:368A.

43. Danchin N, Cassagnes J, Juilliere Y, Machescourt J. Balloon angioplasty versus rotational angioplasty in chronic coronary occlusions (the BAROCCO study). Am J Cardiol 1995;75:330-334.

44. Kaltenbach M, Vallbracht C, and Hartmann A. Recanalization of chronic coronary occlusions by low speed rotational angioplasty (ROTACS). J Interven Cardiol 1991;4:155-165.

45. Appleman Y, Koolen J, Piek JJ, et al. Longterm outcome of excimer laser angioplasty versus balloon angioplasty in functional and total coronary occlusions. Am J Cardiol 1996;78:757-762.

46. Sato Y, Nosaka H, Kimura T, Nobuyoshi M. Randomized comparison of balloon angioplasty versus coronary stent implantation for total occlusion. J Am Coll Cardiol 1996;27:152A.

47. Zidar FJ, Kaplan BM, O'Neill WW, et al. Prospective, randomized trial of prolonged intracoronary urokinase infusion for chronic total occlusions in native coronary arteries. J Am Coll Cardiol 1996;27:1406-12.

48. Höpp HW, Franzen D, Deutsch HJ, et al. New option for balloon recanalization of total coronary occlusions. Cathet Cardiovasc Diagn 1991;24:226-230.

49. Little T, Rosenberg J, Seides S, et al. Probe ™ angioplasty of total coronary occlusion using the Probing Catheter ™ technique. Cathet Cardiovasc Diagn. 1990;21:124.

50. Hamm CW, Jupper W, Kuck K, et al. Recanalization of chronic total occluded coronary arteries by new angioplasty systems. Am J Cardiol 1990;66:1459.

51. Flood RD, Popma JJ, Chuang YC, Salter LF, et al. Incidence, angiographic predictors, and clinical significance of coronary perforation occurring after new device angioplasty. J Am Coll Cardiol 1994;23:301A.

52. Ajluni S, Jones D, Zidar F, Puchrowicz S, Margulis A. Prolonged urokinase infusion for chronic total native coronary occlusions: Clinical, angiographic, and treatment observations. Cath Cardiovas Diagn. 1995;34:106-110.

53. Cecena FA. Urokinase infusion after unsuccessful angioplasty in patients with chronic total occlusion of native coronary arteries. Cath Cardiovasc Diagn. 1993;28:214-218.

54. Vaska KJ, Whitlow PL. Selective tissue plasminogen activator infusion for chronic total occlusions of native coronary arteries failing angioplasty. Circulation 1991;84:II-250.

55. Dick R, Haudenschild C, Popma J, et al. Directional atherectomy for total coronary occlusions. Cor Art Dis 1991;2:189-199.

56. Hinohara T, Rowe M, Robertson G, et al. Effect of lesion characteristics on outcome of directional coronary atherectomy. J Am Coll Cardiol 1991;17:1112-1120.

57. Omoigui N, Reisman M, Franco I, Whitlow P. Rotational atherectomy in chronic total occlusions. J Am Coll Cardiol 1995;25:97A.

58. Stertzer SH, Rosenblum J, Shaw RE, et al. Coronary rotational ablation: Initial experience in 302 procedures. J Am Coll Cardiol 1993;21:287-95.

59. Klein L, Litvack F, Holmes D, et al. Prospective multicenter analysis of excimer laser coronary angioplasty (ELCA) in stenosis with complex morphology. J Am Coll Cardiol 1994:February Special Issue 448A.

60. Litvack F, Eigler N, Margolis J, et al. Percutaneous excimer laser coronary angioplasty: Results in the first consecutive 3,000 patients. J Am Coll Cardiol 1994;23:323-329.

61. Baumbach A, Bittl J, Fleck E, Geschwind H, Sanborn T. Acute complications of excimer laser coronary angioplasty: A detailed analysis of multicenter results. J Am Coll Cardiol 1994;23:1305-1313.

62. Holmes DR, Forrester JS, Litvack F, Reeder GS, et al. Chronic total obstruction and short-term outcome: The excimer laser coronary angioplasty registry experience. Mayo Clin Proc 1993;68:5-10.

63. Buchwald AB, Werner GS, Unterberg C, et al. Restenosis after excimer laser angioplasty of coronary stenoses and chronic total occlusions. Am Heart J 1992;123:878-885.

65. deMarchena EJ, Mallon SM, Knopf WD, et al. Effectiveness of holmium laser-assisted coronary angioplasty. Am J Cardiol 1994;73:117-121.

66. Torre SR, Lai SM, Schatz RA. Relation of clinical presentation and lesion morphology to the procedural results of

Palmaz-Schatz stent placement: A new approaches to coronary intervention (NACI) registry report. J Am Coll Cardiol 1994;23:135A.

67. Ooka M, Suzuki T, Yokoya K, Hayase M, et al. Stenting after revascularization of chronic total occlusion. Circulation 1995;92:I-94.

68. Hsu Y-S, Tamai H, Ueda K, et al. Clinical efficacy of coronary stenting in chronic total occlusions. Circulation 1994;90:I-613.

69. Almagor Y, Borrione M, Maiello L, et al. Coronary stenting after recanalization of chronic total coronary occlusions. Circulation 1993;88:I-504.

70. Bilodeau L, Iyer S, Cannon A, et al. Stenting as an adjunct to balloon angioplasty for recanalization of totally occluded coronary arteries: Clinical and angiographic follow-up. J Am Coll Cardiol 1993;21:292A.

71. Rothbaum DA, Linnemeier TJ, Krauthamer D, et al. Excimer laser angioplasty in total coronary occlusions: A registry report. Circulation 1991;84:II-744.

72. Ooka M, Suzuki T, Kosokawa H, et al. Stenting vs. non-stenting after revascularization of chronic total occlusion. Circulation 1994;90:I-613.

73. Saber RS, Edwards WD, Holmes DR Jr, et al. Balloon angioplasty of aortocoronary saphenous vein bypass grafts: A histopathologic study of six grafts from five patients, with emphasis on restenosis and embolic complications. J Am Coll Cardiol 1988;12:1501-1509.

74. Waller BF, Rothbaum DA, Gorfinkel HJ, et al. Morphologic observations after percutaneous transluminal balloon angioplasty of early and late aortocoronary saphenous vein bypass grafts. J Am Coll Cardiol 1984;4:784-792.

75. Kahn J, Rutherford B, McConahay D, et al. Initial and long-term outcome of 83 patients after balloon angioplasty of totally occluded bypass grafts. J Am Coll Cardiol 1994;23:1038-1042.

76. Margolis JR, Mehta S, Kramer B, et al. Extraction atherectomy for the treatment of recent totally occluded saphenous vein grafts. J Am Coll Cardiol 1994;23:405A.

77. Hartmann JR, McKeever LS, Stamato NJ, et al. Recanalization of chronically occluded aortocoronary saphenous vein bypass grafts by extended infusion of urokinase: Initial results and short-term clinical follow-up. J Am Coll Cardiol 1991;18:1517-1523.

78. Hartmann JR, McKeever LS, O'Neill WW, White CJ, et al. Recanalization of chronically occluded aortocoronary saphenous vein bypass grafts with long-term, low dose direct infusion of urokinase (ROBUST): A serial trial. J Am Coll Cardiol 1996;27:60-6.

79. Busch UW, Weingartner F, Renner U, Neumann FJ, et al. Balloon-occlusive-intravascular-lysis-enhanced-recanalization (B-O-I-L-E-R) of thrombotic saphenous vein graft occlusions: A new technique of selective intravascular thrombolysis. J Am Coll Cardiol 1993;21:451A.80.

80. Katsuragawa M, Fujiwara H, Miyamae M, Sasayama S. Histologic studies in percutaneous transluminal coronary angioplasty for chronic total occlusion: comparison of tapering and abrupt types of occlusion and short and long occluded segments. J Am Coll Cardiol 1993;21:604-611.

81. Jaup T, Allemann Y, Urban P, et al. The Magnum wire for percutaneous coronary balloon angioplasty in 723 patients. J Invas Cardiol 1995;7:259-64.

82. Hamburger JN, Serruys PW, Scabra-Gomes, R, Simon R, et al. Recanalization of total coronary occlusions using a laser guidewire (The European TOTAL surveillance study). Am J Cardiol 1997;80:1419-1423).

83. Moussa I, DiMario C, Blengino S, et al. Coronary stenting of chronic total occlusions without anticoagulation: Immediate and long-term outcome. J Invas. Cardiol 1996;8.

84. Mehta S, Margolis JR, Bittl JA, Tcheng JE, et al. Finally, treatment of chronic total occlusions-ablation with excimer laser angiopalsty. J Invas. Cardiol 1996;8.

85. Sharma SK, Duvvuri S, Cocke T, et al. Directional coronary atherectomy (DCA) of chronic total occlusions. J Invas. Cardiol 1996;8.

86. Ozaki Y, Violaris AG, Hamburger J, et al. Short- and long-term clinical and quantitative angiographic results with the new, less shortening Wallstent for vessel reconstruction in chronic total occlusion: A quantitative angiographic study. J Am Coll Cardiol 1996;28:354-360.

87. Levin TN, Carroll J, Feldman T. High-speed rotational atherectomy for chronic total coronary occlusions. Cathet and Cardiovasc Diagn 1996;3:34-39.

88. Sirnes A, Golf S, Myreng Y, et al. Stenting in chronic coronary occlusion (SICCO): A randomized, controlled trial of adding stent implantation after successful angioplasty. J Am Coll Cardiol 1996;28:1444-51.

89. Sievert H, Rohde S, Schulze R, et al. Stent implantation after successful balloon angioplasty of a chronic coronary occlusion - A randomized trial. J Am Coll Cardiol 1997;29(Suppl. A):15A.

90. Elezi S, Schuhlen H, et al. Six-month angiographic follow-up after stenting of chronic total coronary occlusions. J Am Coll Cardiol 1997;29(Suppl. A):16A.

91. Mathey DG, Seidensticker A, et al. Chronic coronary artery occlusion: Reduction of restenosis- and reocclusion-rates by stent treatment. J Am Coll Cardiol 1997;29(Suppl. A):396A.

92. Steffen W, Hamm CW, et al. Is laserwire recanalization of chronic total occlusions associated with a greater risk than conventional recanalisation? J Am Coll Cardiol 1997;29(Suppl. A):459A.

93. Moussa I, DiMario C, Monthsses J, et al. Comparison of angiographic and clinical outcomes of coronary stenting of chronic total occlusions. Am J Cardiol 1998;81:1-6.

94. Anzuini A, Rosanio S, Legrand V, et al. Wiktor stent for treatment of chronic total coronary artery occlusions: Short- and long-term clinical and angiographic results from a large multicenter experience. J Am Coll Cardiol 1998;31:281-288.

95. Suttorp MJ, Mast EG, Plokker HWT, et al. Primary coronary stenting after successful balloon angioplasty of chronic total occlusions: A single-center experience. Am Heart J 1998;135:318-322.

96. Schofer J, Rau T, Schluter M, Mathey DG. Short-term results and intermediate-term follow-up of laser wire recanalization of chronic coronary artery occlusion: A single center experience. J Am Coll Cardiol 1197;30:1722-1728.

97. Sirnes PA, Golf S, Myreng Y, et al. Sustained benefit of stenting chronic coronary occlusion: Long-term clinical follow-

up of the stenting in chronic coronary occlusion (SICCO) study. J Am Coll Cardiol 1998;32:305-310.

98. Elezi S, Kastrati A, Wehinger A, et al. Clinical and angiographic outcome after stent placement for chronic coronary occlusion. Am J Cardiol 1998;82:803-806.

99. Oesterle SN, Bittl JA, Leon MB, et al. Laser wire for crossing chronic total occlusions: "Learning Phase" results from the U.S. TOTAL Trial. Cathet Cardiovasc Diagn. 1998;44:235-243.

100. Reimers B, Kobayashi Y, Akiyama T, et al. Mechanical approach in the recanalization of total coronary occlusions: A consecutive series of 322 lesions. J Am Coll Cardiol 1998;31:101A.

101. Serruys PW, Teunissen Y. Randomized comparison of laser guidewire and mechanical guidewires for recanalization of chronic total coronary occlusion: The TOTAL trial, final result and follow-up at 30 days. J Am Coll Cardiol 1998;30:81A.

102. Rubartelli P, Niccoli L, Verna E, et al. Stent implantation versus balloon angioplasty in chronic coronary occlusions: Results from the GISSOC trial. J Am Coll Cardiol 1998;32:90-96.

103. Lotan C, Krakover R, Turgerman Y, et al. The STOP study - a randomized multicenter Israeli study for stents in total occlusion and restenosis prevention. J Am Coll Cardiol 1999;32:28A.

104. Tamai H, Tsuchigane E, Suzuki T, et al. Interim results from MAYO Japan investigation for chronic total occlusion (MAJIC). Circulation 1998;98:I-639-I-640.

105. Mori M, Kurogane H, Hayashi T, et al. Comparison of results of intracoronary implantation of the Palmaz-Schatz stent with conventional balloon angioplasty in chronic total coronary artery occlusion. Am J Cardiol 1996;78:985-989.

106. Yamasaki K, Nakamura T, Yung-Sheng H, et al. Three-year angiographic follow-up of coronary stenting in patients with chronic total occlusion. Circulation 1998;98:I-283-I-284.

107. Carere RG, Barbeau G, Dzavik V, et al. Do superior balloon angioplasty resutls provided stent-like outcomes in coronary occlusions. Circulation 1998;98:I-284.

108. Title LM, Buller Ce, Catellier D, et al. Efficacy of stenting vs. balloon angiopaslty in small diameter (< 3 mm) total coronary occlusions: A total occlusion study of Canada substudy. Circulation 1998;98:I-639.

109. Rau T, Schofer J, Schulter M, et al. Stenting of nonacute total coronary occlusions: Predictors of late angiographic outcome. J Am Coll Cardiol 1998;31:275-280.

110. Zidar FJ, Kaplan BM, O'Neill WW, Jones DE, et al. Prospective, randomized trial of prolonged intracoronary urokinase infusion of chronic total occlusions in native coronary arteries. J Am Coll Cardiol 1996;27:1406-1412.

111. Schofer J, Kresser J, Rau T, et al. Recanalization of chronic coronary artery occlusions using laser followed by balloon angioplasty. Am J Cardiol 1996;78:836-838.

112. Srivatsa SS, Edwards WD, Boos CM, et al. Histologic correlates of angiographic chronic total coronary artery occlusions. Influence of occlusion duration on neovascular channel patterns and intimal plaque composition. J Am Coll Cardiol 1997;29:955-963.

113. Puma JA, Sketch MH Jr., Tcheng JE, et al. The natural history of single-vessel chronic coronary occlusion: A 25-year experience. Am Heart J 1997;133:393-399.

114. Danchin N, Angioi M, Cador R, et al. Effect of late percutaneous angioplasty recanalization of total coronary artery occlusion on left ventricular remodeling, ejection fraction, and regional wall motion. Am J Cardiol 1996;78:729-735.

115. Pamir G, Oral D, Omurlu K, et al. Improvement of left ventricular function and wall motion abnormalities after recanalization of total occlusion of left anterior descending coronary artery by percutaneous transluminal coronary angioplasty. J Invas Cardiol 1997;9:417-423.

116. Gottschall CAM, Trindade I, Miller V. Changes in left ventricular function after coronary recanalization by percutaneous transluminal coronary angioplasty (PTCA). J Invas Cardiol 1997;9:146-153.

117. Rambaldi R, Hamburger JN, Geleijnse ML, Oldermans D, et al. Early recovery of wall motion abnormalities after recanalization of chronic totally occluded coronary arteries: A dobutamine echocardiogarphic, prospective, single-center experience. Am Heart J 1998;136:831-836.

118. Delacretaz E, Meier B. Therapeutic strategy with total coronary artery occlusions. Am J Cardiol 1997;79:185-187.

119. Nobuyoshi M, Shizuta S. Update on percutaneous management of chronic total occlusion. J Interven Cardiol 1998;11(Suppl):S-42-S-45.

120. Sato Y, Nosaka H, Kimura T, et al. Randomized comparison of balloon angioplasty versus coronary stent implantation for total occlusion. J Am Coll Cardiol 1996;27:152A.

121. Corcos T, Favereau X, Guerin Y, et al. Recanalization of chronic coronary occlusions using a new hydrophilic guidewire. Cathet Cardiovasc Diagn. 1998;43:83-90.

122. Bahl VK, Chandra S, Goswami KC, et al. Crosswire™ for recanalization of total occlusive coronary arteries. Cathet Cardiovasc Diagn 1998;45:323-327.

123. Reimers B, Camassa N, Di Mario C, et al. Mechanical recanalization of total coronary occlusions wtih the use of a new guidewire. Am Heart J 1998;135:726-731.

124. Meier B. Chronic coronary occlusion—treatment options and results. J Invas Cardiol 1997;9:56-60.

125. Jaup T, Allemann Y, Urban P, Dorsaz PA, et al. The Magnum wire for percutaneous coronary balloon angioplasty in 723 patients. J Invas Cardiol 1995;7:259-264.

126. Allemann Y, Kaufmann UP, Meyer BJ, et al. Magnum wire for percutaneous coronary balloon angioplasty in 800 total chronic occlusions. Am J Cardiol 1997;80:634-637.

127. Noguchi T, Miyazaki S, Morii I, et al. Percutaneous transluminal coronary angioplasty of chronic total occlusions. Determinants of primary success and long-term clinical outcome. Cathet Cardiovasc Intervent 2000;49:258-264.

128. Buller CE, Dzavik V, Carere RG, et al. Primary stenting versus balloon angioplasty in occluded coronary arteries. The total occlusion study of Canada (TOSCA). Circulation 1999;100:236-242.

129. Mori M, Kurogane H, Hayashi T, et al. Comparison of results of intracoronary implantation of the Palmaz-Schatz stent with conventional balloon angioplasty in chronic total coronary arterial occlusion. Am J Cardiol 1996;78:985-9.

130. Azuma J, Tsuchikane E, Otsuji S, et al. Efficacy of plaque debulking prior to stenting for chronic coronary total occlusion. Circulation 2000;102:II-388.

131. Hoher M, Wohrle J, Grebe OC, et al. A randomized trial of elective stenting after balloon recanalization of chronic total occlusions. J Am Coll Cardiol 1999;34:722-9.

132. Sievert H, Rohde S, Utech A, et al. Stent or angioplasty after recanalization of chromic coronary occlusions? The SARECCO trial. Am J Cardiol 1999;84:386-390.

133. Gruberg L, Mehran R, Dangas G, et al. Effect of plaque debulking and stenting on short- and long-term outcomes after revascularization of chronic total occlusions. J Am Coll Cardiiol 2000;35:151-6.Kahler J, Koster R, Brockhoff C, et al. Initial experience with a hydrophilic-coated guidewire for recanalization of chronic coronary occlusions. Cathet Cardiovasc Intervent 2000;49:45-50.

134. Lefevre T, Louvard Y, Loubeyre C, et al. A randomized study comparing two guidewire strategies for angioplasty of chronic total coronary occlusion. Am J Cardiol 2000;85:1144-48.

135. Khanna A, Roubin GS, Iyer SS, et al. Use of the Shinobi wire in chronic coronary occlusions. Cathet Cardiovasc Intervent 1999;48:100-104.

136. Lau KW, Ding ZP, Johan A, et al. Angiographic restenosis rate in patients with chronic total occlusions and subtotal stenoses after initially successful intracoronary stent placement. Am J Cardiol 1999;83:963-966.

137. Cannon L, Siegel R, Greenberg J, et al. Recanalization of total coronary occlusions using a the Sonicross low frequency ultrasound catheter. J Am Coll Cardiol 2000;33:41A.

138. Buller CE, Teo KK, Carere RG, et al. 3-year clinical outcome from the total occlusion study of Canada (TOSCA) trial. Circulation 2000;102:II-387.

139. Dzavik V, Carere RG, Catellier DJ, et al. Clinical outcomes in relation to long-term patency status: Observations from the total occlusion study of Canada. Circulation 2000;102:II-388.

140. Azuma J, Tsuchikane E, Otsuji S, et al. Efficacy of plaque debulking prior to stenting for chronic coronary total occlusions. Circulation 2000;102:II-388.

141. Braden GA, Kutcher MA, Rankin KM, et al. Debulking using rotational atherectomy of chronic total coronary occlusion leads to high initial success and very low restenosis rates. J Am Coll Cardiol 2001;37(2):46A.

17 CORONARY ARTERY BYPASS GRAFTS

Mark Dooris, M.B.B.S.
Robert D. Safian, M.D.

SAPHENOUS VEIN GRAFTS

A. DEFICIENCIES OF CORONARY ARTERY BYPASS SURGERY. Coronary artery bypass surgery (CABG) is an established form of revascularization. Despite its ability to relieve angina and prolong survival,[1] deficiencies exist:

1. **Recurrent Ischemia.** After CABG, ischemia recurs in 17% of patients at one year and 63% of patients at 10 years. Ischemia may be due to new disease in vessels not previously bypassed, progressive disease in native vessels beyond the graft anastomosis, or disease in the bypass grafts themselves. In patients presenting with unstable angina more than 5 years after CABG, 85% have culprit lesions in a vein graft.[214]

2. **Vein Graft Failure.** The rate of saphenous vein graft (SVG) failure is 8% at 1 year, 38% at 5 years, and 75% at 10 years after CABG.[2] In asymptomatic patients, silent occlusion occurs in 28% at 1-3 years, 32% at 4-6 years, and 35% at 7-11 years after CABG.[3] Factors strongly associated with graft atherosclerosis include cigarette smoking and hyperlipidemia, followed in importance by native vessel diameter < 1.5 mm, female gender, and elevated lipoprotein (a). Although diabetes and hypertension are strong risk factors for late mortality, data about promoting vein graft atherosclerosis are inconsistent. Native vessel location and severity of native vessel stenosis do not have a strong impact on late graft failure. Levels of homocysteine, fibrinogen, and other hemostatic factors are important risk factors for coronary atherosclerosis, but their influence on graft atherosclerosis has not been defined.[1] Current recommendations for prevention of graft atherosclerosis include aspirin (325 mg/d) starting no later than the first postoperative day, smoking cessation, and lipid-lowering therapy. Aspirin may not affect graft patency after one year, but is maintained indefinitely to reduce overall cardiac morbidity and mortality. Clopidogrel is indicated in patients intolerant of aspirin; combination therapy with clopidogrel plus aspirin vs. aspirin alone is currently under investigation. Sulfinpyrazone, dipyridamole, and warfarin have not been shown to prevent graft atherosclerosis. Recently, aggressive lowering of LDL-cholesterol to < 100 mg/dL by intensive medical therapy resulted in delayed progression of SVG atherosclerosis,[271] which applied to all patients irrespective of age, gender, or risk factors.[272] At present, the only way to avoid vein graft atherosclerosis and degeneration is to leave it in the leg!

3. **Repeat Revascularization.** Repeat CABG or PCI is required in 4% of patients at 5 years, 19% at 10 years, and 31% at 12 years after initial CABG. Compared to CABG patients treated percutaneously between 1979-1994, those treated from 1995-1998 were older, and had more LV

dysfunction and complex target lesion morphology. Despite these adverse characteristics, procedural success and long-term outcomes (death, repeat revascularization, recurrent angina) were better, coinciding with more aggressive risk factor modification, improvement in technique, and widespread availability of stents.

B. TREATMENT OPTIONS FOR VEIN GRAFT DISEASE

1. **Repeat CABG.** The risks of repeat CABG are 2- to 4-fold higher than initial CABG, with periprocedural death in 2-5% and MI in 2-8% of patients.[4-10] Five- and 10-year survival rates are 84-94% and 75%, respectively,[11-18] but 5-year event-free survival (freedom from death, MI, PTCA, or CABG) and angina-free survival are only 64% and 50%.[12,13] These immediate and long-term results reflect the technical difficulty of reoperation and the frequency of unfavorable patient characteristics. Risk factors for perioperative morbidity and mortality after repeat surgery include left main disease, anginal class III or IV, age > 60 years, diabetes mellitus, ejection fraction < 40%, and incomplete revascularization.[9] Some patients are not suitable candidates for reoperation because of small target vessels, poor LV function, serious comorbid medical problems, or limited availability of suitable conduits. In addition, the risk of injury to a patent internal mammary graft is 5-38% at less experienced surgical centers.[19-22] Three nonrandomized studies comparing PTCA vs. repeat CABG demonstrated less in-hospital death and MI after PTCA, but more complete revascularization and less target lesion revascularization (TLR) at 4 years after repeat CABG.[213,215,194]

2. **Balloon Angioplasty.** The technique of PTCA in vein grafts is similar to that in native coronary arteries. Proper guiding catheter selection is important to ensure adequate back-up and coaxial alignment. The configuration of the guiding catheter depends on target vessel takeoff from the ascending aorta (Figures 17.1, 17.2), and the size of the curve depends on the diameter of the aorta. For lesions involving the distal body of the graft, distal anastomosis, or native vessel beyond the anastomosis (Figure 17.3), short (90 cm) guiding catheters or PTCA balloon catheters with long shafts (140-150 cm) may be useful.

   a. **Success and Major Complication Rates.** PTCA of saphenous vein grafts can be performed with procedural success rates of 78-97% and in-hospital complication rates of 0-12% (Table 17.1).[23-42] Contemporary series indicate that despite higher risk patients (advanced age, LV dysfunction, multivessel coronary disease), PTCA can be performed without an increased risk of major ischemic complications compared to earlier studies.[43] Clinical complications are usually associated with one or more of the angiographic complications described in the next section.

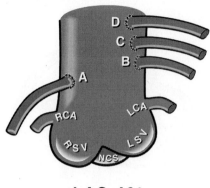

LAO 40°

Figure 17.1. Usual Arrangement of Saphenous Vein Bypass Grafts From the Ascending Aorta

Abbreviations: LAD = left anterior descending coronary artery; LAO = left anterior oblique; LCA = left coronary artery; LSV = left Sinus of Valsalva; NCS = noncoronary sinus; RCA = right coronary artery; RSV = right Sinus of Valsalva

From proximal to distal:

A. Grafts to the distal RCA or distal left circumflex (left dominant system)

B. Grafts to the LAD

C. Grafts to the diagonal branches

D. Grafts to the obtuse marginal branches or ramus

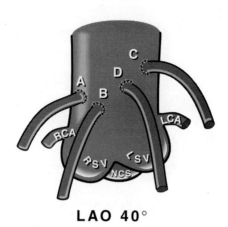

LAO 40°

Figure 17.2. Origin of Saphenous Vein Grafts: Guiding Catheter Selection

Abbreviations: LAD = left anterior descending coronary artery; LAO = left anterior oblique; LCA = left coronary artery; LSV = left Sinus of Valsalva; NCS = noncoronary sinus; RCA = right coronary artery; RSV = right Sinus of Valsalva

A.   Usual orientation of vein grafts to the distal RCA from the lateral wall of the aorta above the right Sinus of Valsalva
B.   More anterior origin of vein grafts to the distal RCA
C.   Usual orientation of vein grafts to the left coronary artery from the anterior wall of the aorta above the left Sinus of Valsalva
D.   More anterior orientation of vein grafts to the left coronary artery

Guiding Catheter Selection:

Primary	*Alternate*
A. Multipurpose	JR, AL, right Bypass
B. AL	JR, Multipurpose, Hockey Stick
C. JR, Hockey Stick	AL, left bypass, Multipurpose
D. AL, Hockey Stick	JR, left bypass, Multipurpose

Table 17.1. Results of PTCA in Saphenous Vein Grafts

Series	N	Graft Age (months)	Success (%)	Complications (%) D / MI / CABG	Restenosis (%)
Hanekamp[227] (2000)	72	-	89	9.7 (MACE)	35.6
Dharmadhikari[226] (2000)	31	-	-	3.2 / 6.4 / 3.2	12-mo EFS (48%)
Gruberg[260] (1999)	182	-	96	1 / 11.5 / 0	25
Winters[256] (1999)	82	-	88	-	-
Tan[23] (1994)	50	50	86	- / - / -	39
Morrison[24] (1994)	89	98	93	3 / 3 / 1	51
Unterberg[25] (1992)	55	46	89	- / - / -	-
Miranda[26] (1992)	409	>12	94	- / - / -	-
Meester[27] (1991)	59	56	86	1.2 / 8.3 / 2.4	-
Plokker[28] (1991)	454	67	90	0.7 / 2.8 / 1.3	-
Douglas[29] (1991)	672	≤ 120	90	1.2 / 2.3 / 3.5	-
Jost[30] (1991)	49	40	94	0	-
Webb[31] (1990)	168	66	85	0	50
Dorros (1989)[32]	241	-	91	2.3 / 5.2 / 1.4	-
Platko[33] (1989)	107	50	92	2 / 5.9 / 2	61
Pinkerton[34] (1988)	100	60	93	- / - / -	-
Cote[35] (1987)	83	51	86	0	23
Ernst[36] (1987)	33	-	97	0	31

Abbreviations: D = death; MI = myocardial infarction; CABG = emergency coronary artery bypass surgery; - = not reported

b. **Angiographic Complications**

1. **Distal Embolization.** Distal embolization causing abrupt vessel cutoff during PTCA occurs in 2-15% of vein grafts > 3 years old, especially those with soft, friable intraluminal material ("rat-bite" appearance by angiography).[1,32,33,44,46] Independent predictors of distal embolization include diffuse degeneration and large plaque volume, but not thrombus or ulceration.[45] An angioscopy study also found that vein graft friability rather than thrombus was the strongest predictor of distal embolization and no-reflow.[47] When elevated CK-MB is used as a marker for distal embolization, rates up to 20% have been reported for PTCA, DCA, TEC, and stents; independent predictors included angiographic thrombus and large vessel diameter, but not device type.[46] Although some data suggest that abciximab may reduce distal embolization and non-Q-wave MI during vein graft intervention, other observational studies suggest limited benefit (Table 17.2). In contrast to native vessels, abciximab has not been shown to impact 6-month outcome after vein graft intervention.[48] It is important to distinguish distal embolization leading to abrupt cutoff of a distal branch from no-reflow; distal embolization is treated by gentle guidewire manipulation, repeat PTCA, infusion of thrombolytic drugs, or emergency CABG (refractory cases), whereas no-reflow is more responsive to intragraft pharmacologic agents (Chapter 21).

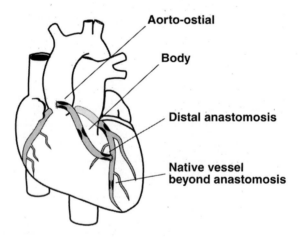

Figure 17.3. Target Lesion Location in Post-CABG Patients

Table 17.2. Abciximab for Thrombus in Vein Grafts

Series	N	Adjunctive Therapy	Results
Ahmed (1999)	45	Rescue abciximab in degenerated SVG	No benefit in procedural success or major ischemic complications compared to "no-abciximab"; more non-Q-wave MI in rescue group (40.5% vs. 17.7%)
Sullebarger[193] (1999)	17	Planned abciximab and TEC in SVG	Abciximab was associated with higher procedural success (100% vs. 50%) and less distal embolization/no-reflow (0% vs. 30%) compared to no abciximab
Mathew[278] (1999)	210 133	No abciximab Planned abciximab	No difference in hospital or late MACE, procedural success, or distal embolization
Barsness[232] (1998)	58	Local delivery of abciximab in thrombotic SVG	Abciximab associated with significant improvement in thrombus score and stenosis severity, but not TIMI flow. Adjunctive stents in 88%
Grantham[235] (1998)	185	Planned and unplanned (rescue) abciximab in thrombotic SVGs	Procedural success was higher with planned abciximab; no impact of abciximab on angiographic (distal embolization, no-reflow) or clinical complications
Mak[209] (1997)	101	Vein graft intervention in EPIC trial	Compared to placebo, abciximab was associated with less distal embolization (2% vs. 18%), less non-Q-wave MI (2% vs. 12%), and similar MACE at 30 days and 6 months

Abbreviations: MACE = major adverse cardiac events; SVG = saphenous vein graft; TEC = transluminal extraction catheter

2. **No-Reflow.** The etiology of no-reflow is uncertain, but may be secondary to microvascular embolization and/or spasm (Chapter 21). True no-reflow does not respond to lytic therapy, repeat PTCA, or CABG, but may respond to intracoronary nitroprusside or calcium antagonists.[49] The incidence of no-reflow following vein graft intervention is 5-15%, and is more frequent in old (>3 years) and degenerated grafts.[33,44,50] Distal embolic protection devices have been shown to prevent macro- and microembolization during vein graft intervention (see below).

3. **Abrupt Closure.** Abrupt closure complicates 1-2% of vein graft interventions, which is lower than the 2-12% incidence following native vessel PTCA.[23-42] Abrupt closure is usually caused by severe dissection, and is best managed by stenting (Chapter 20). Emergency redo CABG is also feasible, but is associated with mortality rates up to 15% due to other serious comorbidities, technical difficulties in harvesting conduits, and potential delays in achieving satisfactory cardiopulmonary bypass.[49,51,53]

4. **Perforation.** Although coronary artery and vein graft perforation are rare complications after PTCA, the incidence is higher following atherectomy or laser angioplasty.[54,55] Cardiac tamponade is unusual after vein graft perforation due to the extrapericardial course of vein grafts and post-pericardiotomy fibrosis. The management of vein graft perforation is similar to that of native vessel perforation (Chapter 22).

c. **Restenosis.** The major limitation of PTCA in saphenous vein grafts is restenosis, which occurs in 23-73% of patients within 6 months (Table 17.1). Clinical recognition is often difficult because of coexistent multivessel disease and collaterals, which limit the interpretation of myocardial perfusion studies and recurrent symptoms. Independent predictors of restenosis include proximal, ostial, or diffuse disease, vein grafts > 3 years of age, small vessels, and chronic total occlusions. The presence of diabetes, shown to adversely effect long-term outcome after native vessel PTCA (Chapter 3), is also associated with reduced long-term event-free survival after vein graft intervention.[56]

3. **Non-Balloon Devices.** In busy interventional practices, more than 75% of vein grafts are treated by devices other than PTCA. These devices have allowed more patients with advanced age, LV dysfunction, and extensive coronary disease to undergo catheter-based intervention without increasing the incidence of major complications.[43]

a. **Transluminal Extraction Catheter (TEC) Atherectomy (Chapter 29)**

1. **Overall Results.** TEC received FDA-approval in 1993 and has been advocated as a potential treatment for degenerated vein grafts. As shown in Table 17.3, procedural success rates are 80-90% for nonoccluded vessels and 60-75% for occluded vessels.[57-60] The frequent development of angiographic complications, including distal embolization (2-17%),[57-62] no-reflow (8.8%),[57] and abrupt closure (2-5%)[57-60] reflect the application of TEC to complex lesions, many of which are poorly suited for other devices. Major clinical complications including Q-wave MI (0.7-3.7%) and death (0-10.3%) have not been reduced by TEC. Angiographic follow-up suggests restenosis in 60-70%, including late vessel occlusion in 30% in one study.[57] Because TEC relies on cutting and aspiration, it should be well-suited for thrombus-containing lesions; angioscopy studies demonstrate partial or complete thrombus removal in 75%,[63,64] although intimal flaps are extremely common.[65] In the TOPIT trial of TEC or PTCA in thrombus-containing lesions, there was less procedure-related CK elevation after TEC (Table 17.4). An emerging competitive technology is the distal embolic protection device. The PercuSurge GuardWire has been shown to markedly reduce distal embolization, no-reflow, CK elevation, and in-hospital mortality; other devices are under investigation (see below).

Table 17.3. In-hospital Results of TEC Atherectomy in Saphenous Vein Grafts

	Bejarano[218] (1997)	Meany[59] (1995)	Twidale[60] (1994)	Safian[57] (1994)	Popma[58] (1992)
No. lesions	106	650	88	158	29
Adjunctive PTCA (%)	100	74	95	91	86
Success (%)	87	89	86	84	82
Complications (%)					
Myocardial infarction	6.6	0.7	3.4	2.0	3.7
Death	2.0	3.2	0	2.0	10.3
Acute closure	4.7	2.0	5.0	5.0	-
Distal embolization	11.8	2.0	4.5	11.9	17
No-reflow	0	-	-	8.8	-

Abbreviations: - = not reported

Table 17.4. TOPIT Trial: TEC or PTCA in Thrombotic Lesions[237]

	TEC*	PTCA	p-value
No. lesions	131	134	
Success (%)	98	97	NS
Ischemic complications+ (%)	4.5	11.2	0.06
CK elevation (%)	4.5	15.4	0.03
Final diameter stenosis (%)	27	26	NS
Dissection (%)	38	29	0.04
Distal embolization (%)	2	4	NS
No-reflow (%)	5	8	NS
Perforation	0	0.7	NS
Final TIMI flow < 3	2	3	NS

Abbreviations: CK = creatine kinase; NS = not statistically significant; TOPIT = Transluminal Extraction Atherectomy or PTCA in Thrombus-Containing Lesions
+ Death, MI, acute closure, rePTCA, or CABG
* Adjunctive intervention required in majority of causes for definitive lumen enlargement

Table 17.5. Comparison of Mechanical Techniques for Thrombotic Lesions

Device	Mechanism	Advantages	Disadvantages	Status
TEC	Cut, aspirate plaque and thrombus	Efficient extraction of fresh thrombus	Less useful for extraction of organized thrombus and plaque; frequent dissection; small diameter (1.8-2.5 mm)	FDA-approved
AngioJet	Thrombus removal by Venturi effect	Removes large, fresh thrombus	Bradycardia; no-reflow; not useful for organized thrombus	FDA-approved
Hydrolyzer	Thrombus removal by Venturi effect	Ease of use	Bulky; inflexible; poor for organized thrombus	Investigational
Sonicath	Ultrasound thrombolysis	Flexible	Limited experience	Investigational
Acolysis	Ultrasound thrombolysis	Flexible	Limited experience	Investigational

2. **Thrombotic Vein Grafts.** There are a variety of mechanical techniques for removal of thrombus (Table 17.5). Compared to vein grafts without thrombus treated by TEC, the presence of thrombus increased the risk of angiographic failure (25% vs. 11%), clinical failure (31% vs. 12%), angiographic complications (27% vs. 11%), and clinical complications (13.3% vs 2.4%) (Table 17.6).[66,67] Using CK-MB as a biochemical marker of distal embolization, one study reported a lower incidence of distal embolization after TEC compared to PTCA (7% versus 22%, $p < 0.02$).[68] In the multicenter NACI Registry, distal embolization occurred in 7.4% of lesions, resulted in a 6-fold increase in hospital mortality and a 5-fold increase in MI, and correlated with myocardial infarction, "stand-alone" TEC, vein graft thrombus, and large vessel diameter.[69] Several studies have suggested a synergistic role ("device synergy") for TEC followed by stenting for degenerated and/or thrombotic vein grafts;[64,70,71] some reports suggest that stent deferral (1-2 months after TEC) may reduce distal embolization and major clinical complications, although the incidence of silent graft occlusion during the waiting period may be as high as 15%.[70] Because of the relatively high risk of graft occlusion during this waiting period, we empirically stage definitive stenting 2-3 weeks after initial TEC. During this interval, we recommend antiplatelet therapy with aspirin and clopidogrel, as well as subcutaneous injections of heparin (5,000-10,000 U SQ BID) or enoxaparin (20-30 mg SQ BID).

b. **Directional Coronary Atherectomy (DCA) (Chapter 28).** Morphologic characteristics favorable for vein graft DCA include large caliber, lack of tortuosity, and absence of heavy calcification. When used in focal complex lesions in large grafts, procedural success was 85-97% with major complications in 0-7% (Tables 17.3, 17.8);[72-78] success rates were lower in ostial lesions and long (> 20 mm) lesions.[72] Restenosis after DCA has been reported in 31-63%,[72-75,77] and was lower in de novo lesions (38%) compared to restenotic lesions (75%).[76,79]

Table 17.6. Impact of TEC Atherectomy on Thrombus in Saphenous Vein Grafts

Series	N	Outcome
Misumi[217] (1996)	163	Less distal embolization after TEC vs. PTCA (3.9% vs. 16.7%, p < 0.01)
Meany[59] (1995)	183	Angiographic success not affected by thrombus
Dooris[67] (1995)	59	Thrombus associated with decreased clinical success (69% vs. 88%) and increased angiographic and clinical complications (no-reflow, Q-wave MI)
Al-Shaibi[68] (1995)	124	Less CK elevation after TEC vs. PTCA

Abbreviations: TEC = transluminal extraction catheter; MI = myocardial infarction; CK = creatinine kinase

In CAVEAT-II (Coronary Angioplasty versus Excisional Atherectomy Trial), DCA had higher procedural success rates and better luminal enlargement compared to PTCA, but there was a higher incidence of complications, mostly related to non-Q-wave MI.[80] At 6 months, there was no difference in angiographic restenosis but a trend toward less target lesion revascularization after DCA (Table 17.9).[80] In general, DCA offers little advantage compared to PTCA alone. Debulking with DCA prior to stenting is currently under investigation.

c. **Excimer Laser Angioplasty (ELCA) (Chapter 30).** Although saphenous vein grafts represent up to 15% of vessels treated with ELCA, there are relatively few published data about the immediate and long-term results (Table 17.10).[81-84] In a study of 545 vein graft lesions, procedural success was 92% after adjunctive PTCA, which was required in 91% of lesions.[82] Angiographic complications included acute vessel closure (4%), distal embolization (3.3%), and perforation (1.3%). At least one major complication occurred in 6.1% of patients including death (1%), Q-wave MI (2.4%), non-Q-wave MI (2.2%), and CABG (0.6%). Lesion length > 10 mm was an independent predictor of procedural failure, major complications, and restenosis, while ostial location and vessel diameter < 3 mm were associated with fewer major complications.[82] Angiographic and clinical follow-up revealed a high incidence of late cardiac events, including angiographic restenosis in 52% (late vessel occlusion in 24%) and 1-year event-free survival in only 48%.[81] In a comparative study of ELCA vs. PTCA using quantitative angiography and matched lesions, there were no differences in immediate angiographic results or cardiac events at 1 year.[211] Results using the infrared Holmium laser appear similar.[84] When applied to vein graft patients with diffuse in-stent restenosis, ELCA resulted in a high incidence of in-hospital complications (death 1%, CABG 2%, Q-wave MI 1%, non-Q-wave MI 14%) and 1-year ischemic events (death 11%, non-Q-wave MI 8%, TLR 32%).[279]

Table 17.7. In-hospital Results of Directional Atherectomy in Saphenous Vein Grafts

Series	No. Lesions	Success (%)	Major Complications (%)*
NACI[238] (1997)	209	86	2.2
Holmes[80] (1995)	149	89	4.7
Stephan[127] (1995)	57	86	0
Cowley[72] (1993)	363	85	2.5**
Garratt[76] (1992)	26	96	3.8
Pomerantz[75] (1992)	35	94	0
DiScasio[74] (1992)	96	97	1.4
Ghazzal[78] (1991)	286	87	2.1
Selmon[77] (1991)	87	91	2.6
Kaufmann[73] (1990)	14	93	7

*   Death, myocardial infarction, or emergency coronary artery bypass surgery
** DCA Registry: vascular repair 3.5%; non-Q-wave MI 3%; restenosis rate 57% (38% for de novo lesions; 75% for restenosis lesions)

d. Stents (Chapter 26). The randomized SAVED (Saphenous Vein De Novo) trial demonstrated superior lumen enlargement, higher procedural success, and less MACE after Palmaz-Schatz stenting than PTCA for focal de novo lesions in vein grafts.[87,190,203] Bleeding and vascular complications were more frequent after stenting due to the older warfarin-based anticoagulation regimens (Table 17.11). The randomized WINS (Wallstent in Saphenous Vein Grafts) trial demonstrated equivalence of the coronary Wallstent to the Palmaz-Schatz stent in de novo and restenotic lesions in vein grafts (Table 17.12). The WINS Registry also demonstrated the efficacy of the Wallstent in large (4.0-5.5 mm) vein grafts (Table 17.12), which is now FDA-approved for native vessel and vein graft revascularization. In high-risk patients (poor left ventricular function, unstable angina, recent or acute MI), stenting can be accomplished with procedural success rates > 90% and major complication rates < 5%; in one study, total and event-free survival at 4-years were 79% and 29%, respectively. Graft age > 10 years and baseline LV dysfunction were predictors of adverse outcome.[208] Numerous observational studies show that

Table 17.8. Angiographic Complications After DCA of Saphenous Vein Grafts

Series	N	Vessel	Complications (%)		
			Acute Closure	DE or No-reflow	Perforation
NACI[238] (1997)	1329	N, SVG	1.1	1.4	1.0
Stephan[127] (1995)	160	N, SVG	4.0	4.0	-
Fortuna[239] (1995)	396	N, SVG	3.6	-	-
Popma[240] (1993)	306	N, SVG	2.3	1.3	0.3
Cowley[72] (1993)	318	SVG	1.9	7.2	0.6
Baim[241] (1993)	1032	N, SVG	3.9	1.8	0.6
Pomerantz[75] (1992)	35	SVG	0.00	2.9	0.00
Fishman[242] (1992)	225	N, SVG	3.2	0.00	0.5
Popma[243] (1992)	1140	N, SVG	4.2	-	0.6
Garratt[76] (1992)	165	N, SVG	-	2.0	-
Hinohara[244] (1991)	382	N, SVG	3.7	2.1	0.8
Safian[245] (1990)	76	N, SVG	1.5	1.5	0.00
Kaufmann[73] (1989)	50	N, SVG	4.0	4.0	0.00

Abbreviations: DCA = directional coronary atherectomy; N = native vessel; SVG = saphenous vein graft; DE = distal embolization; - = not reported

Table 17.9. CAVEAT-II Trial: DCA vs. PTCA for Saphenous Vein Grafts[80]

	DCA	PTCA	p-Value
No.	149	156	-
Graft age (years)	9.5	9.9	-
Lesion Location (%)			
Aorto-ostial	14.8	9.0	-
Proximal body	28.2	36.5	-
Mid-body	38.3	33.3	-
Distal body	18.8	27.6	-
Distal anastomosis	5.4	4.5	-
Lesion length (mm)	10.9	11.0	-
In-hospital Results (%)			
Success	89.2	79.0	< 0.05
Final diameter stenosis	31.5	37.6	< 0.001
Acute closure	4.7	2.6	NS
Distal embolization	13.4	5.1	< 0.01
Perforation	0.7	0.00	NS
Q-wave MI	1.3	1.9	NS
Non-Q-wave MI	16.1	9.6	< 0.10
CABG	0.7	1.3	NS
Death	2.0	1.9	NS
Composite endpoint	20.1	12.2	< 0.10
Follow-up Results (%)			
Angiographic restenosis	46	51	NS
Event-free survival	60	56	NS
Target lesion revascularization	19	26	< 0.10

Abbreviations: CABG = emergency coronary artery bypass grafting; CAVEAT-II = Coronary Angioplasty Versus Excisional Atherectomy Trial for Patients with Saphenous Vein Bypass Grafts; DCA = directional coronary atherectomy; MI = myocardial infarction

Table 17.10. In-hospital Results of ELCA for Saphenous Vein Grafts

Series	No. Lesions	PTCA (%)	Success (%)	Complications (%)*
Strauss[81] (1995)	125	83	89	3.7
DeMarchena[84†] (1994)	34	-	100	0
Bittl[82] (1994)	545	91	92	6.1
Litvack[83] (1994)	480	-	92	-

Abbreviations: ELCA = excimer laser coronary angioplasty; PTCA = adjunctive balloon angioplasty; - = not reported
* Death, myocardial infarction, or emergency coronary artery bypass surgery
† Holmium laser

a variety of stents can be deployed in vein grafts with high success rates (95-100%), a low incidence of stent thrombosis (0-8%) and major clinical complications (0-4%), and a possible reduction in restenosis compared to other devices (Table 17.13)[88-101] Restenosis rates appear higher for ostial and restenotic lesions (30-60%) compared to other vein graft sites and *de novo* lesions (17-39%). Compared to DCA of aorto-ostial vein graft lesions, stenting resulted in better immediate angiographic results and less late target lesion revascularization; event-free survival at 1-year was only 42% for DCA and 53% for stents.[102] Despite high procedural success and low complication rates, vein graft stenting has been associated with significant attrition in late outcome; event-free survival was 75% at 6 months, 67% at 12 months, and only 55% at 24 months, mostly due to progressive disease in nonstented vessels.[103,104] Although the greatest need for TLR after vein graft intervention is within the first 8 months, the risk of TLR continues to rise for 18-24 months suggesting that, unlike native vessel angioplasty, patients need to be followed closely for "delayed" restenosis after vein graft intervention.[273,276] Compared to patients undergoing stenting of native coronary arteries, patients undergoing vein graft stenting had lower 5-year survival (70.5% vs 93.4%) and event-free survival (21.1% vs 63.3%).[191] These observations were also confirmed in SAVED, WINS, and other trials in which 30-50% of late cardiac events were due to death, MI, or revascularization of sites other than the original target lesion.[216] These data are in stark contrast to stenting in native vessels, in which 90% of late cardiac events are due to revascularization of the original target lesion. In a large study of vein graft stenting in 1000 patients, diabetics had more in-hospital MACE and death compared to nondiabetics despite similar procedural success, no-reflow, and distal embolization.[259] At 1 year, total survival and event-free survival were lower in diabetics despite less target vessel revascularization. In-hospital and 1-year outcomes were similar for insulin-dependent and non-insulin-dependent diabetics (Table 17.14).

Table 17.11. SAVED Trial: PTCA vs. Palmaz-Schatz Stent for Saphenous Vein Grafts [203]

	PSS (n = 108)	PTCA (n = 107)	p-Value
Baseline Characteristics			
Ejection fraction (%)	5.3	52	-
Graft age (years)	10.1	9.4	-
Thrombus	6	8	-
In-hospital Outcome (%)			
Final diameter stenosis	12	32	< 0.001
Angiographic success	97	86	< 0.01
Procedural success	92	69	< 0.001
Crossover	-	7	NS
MACE	6	11	NS
Bleeding/vascular events	17	5	< 0.01
6-month Outcome (%)			
Diameter stenosis	46	51	< 0.05
Angiographic restenosis	36	47	NS
MACE	26	39	< 0.05
TLR	17	26	NS

Abbreviations: MACE = major adverse cardiac events (death, MI, CABG, PTCA); PSS = Palmaz-Schatz stent; SAVED = Saphenous Vein De Novo; angiographic success = final diameter stenosis < 50%; procedural success = final diameter stenosis < 50% without crossover or in-hospital complications; TLR = target lesion revascularization (CABG, PTCA)

Table 17.12. WINS Trial: Wallstent in Saphenous Vein Grafts [223,224]

	WINS Randomized Trial		WINS Registry
	Wallstent	Palmaz-Schatz Stent	Wallstent
N (patients/lesions)	139/156	129/141	210/236
In-hospital Outcome (%)			
Procedure success	98	99	95
Final diameter stenosis	5.4	8.5	7.9
Stent thrombosis	0.7	0.8	2.4
MACE + stroke	8.6	7.8	16.7
Transfusion	5.0	3.9	6.7
Vascular complications	6.5	6.2	9.0
6-month Outcome (%)			
Diameter stenosis	42	46	39
Angiographic restenosis	33	33	28
TLR	13	12	8
MACE + stroke	28	23	27

Abbreviations: MACE = major adverse cardiac events (death, MI, rePTCA, CABG); TLR = target lesion revascularization (rePTCA or CABG)

Table 17.13. Results of Observational Studies of Stents for Saphenous Vein Grafts

Series	Stent	Lesions (N)	Success (%)	SAT (%)	Complications (%) D / MI / CABG	VSR/XF (%)	RS (%)
Roffi[285]	Stent	206	-	-	-	-	30-day MACE
(2001)	No stent	72	-	-	-	-	(20% vs. 18%)
Leon[281]	Symbiot	25	-	-	-	-	6.7
(2001)	(PTFE-coated)						
Ahmed[285]	PSS (diabetic)	290	95	1.2	2.2 / 1.3 / 1.3		1-yr EFS
(2000)	PSS (nondiabetic)	618	92	1.6	0.3 / 1.2 / 0.6	-	(67% vs. 79%)
Hanekamp[227]	Wiktor	78	91	-	9	-	21.9
(2000)	PTCA	72	89	-	9.7	-	35.6
Choussat[277]	Wall++	126	-	-	3.2 / 8.7 / 0	-	44
(2000)							
Nishida[257]	Multiple	129	97	-	1 / 10.9 / 2	-	21
(2000)							
Horlitz[258]	Multiple	30	90	3.3	0 / 3.3 / 6.6	-	38.5
(2000)	(ostial)						
Briguori[262]	PTFE Stent	25	96	0	0 / 4 / 0	-	31
(2000)	Stent	62	97	0	0 / 12 / 1.6	-	39
Bhargava[254]	Single	649	99	0.7	1.3 / 17.1 / 0.9		23.2
(2000)	Multiple	70	98	0	2.8 / 30.8 / 0		20.9
Stoerger[225]	PTFE stent	70	99	3.2	1.6 / 1.6 / -	-	22
(2000)							
Dharmadhikari[226]							12-mo EFS:
(2000)	PTFE stent	30	-	-	3.2 / 0 / 0	-	73
	Stent	125	-	-	0 / 8.8 / 0	-	56
	PTCA	31	-	-	32. / 6.4 / 3.2	-	48
Scavetta[265]	Multiple	92	95	3.3	3.3 / 8 / 0	2.2 / 9.8	-
(1999)							
Gruberg[260]	PTCA+	182	96	0	1 / 11.5 / 0	6	25
(1999)	Stent+	77	99	0	0 / 12.0 / 1	4	14
Safian[255]	Wall	139	-	0.7	-	-	38.6
(1999)	PSS	130	-	0.8			40.8
Winters[256]	TEC	85	99	-	-	-	-
(1999)	Stent	127	99	-			
	PTCA	82	88	-			
Safian[252]	PSS	114	100	-	-	-	32
(1998)	Wall	101	95	-			13
Al-Mubarak[253]	TEC (<15mm)	18	-	0	0 / 0 / 0	-	-
(1998)	Wall (>15mm)	21	-	4.7	0 / 0 / 0		
SAVED[203]	PSS	108	97	-	6	17	36
(1997)	PTCA	107	86	-	11	5	47

Table 17.13. Results of Observational Studies of Stents for Saphenous Vein Grafts

Series	Stent	Lesions (N)	Success (%)	SAT (%)	Complications (%) D / MI / CABG	VSR/XF (%)	RS (%)
Frimerman[208] (1997)	PSS, B	186	97.3	1.6	1.1 / 1.1 / 0/5	4.8 / 8.0	45
deJaegere[202] (1996)	PSS, Wall	62	89	3.0	3 / 3 / 5	12.9 / 9.8	30**
Wong[88] (1995)	PSS	624	98.8	1.4	1.7 / 0.3 / 0.9	8.0 / 6.3	30
Rechavia[89] (1995)	PSS,B	29	100	0	0.00	3.4 / 6.8	-
Wong[90] (1995)	PSS,B	309	95.3	1.7	1.3 / 0.9 / 0.4	8.4 / 25	-
Denardo[91*] (1995)	PSS,B	300	93.3	6.7	0	16.7	-
Piana[92] (1994)	PSS,B	200	98.5	0.6	- / 0.6 / 0	8.5 / 14.0	0

Abbreviations: Success = procedural success (some studies do not distinguish between angiographic vs. clinical success); RS = restenosis; SAT = subacute thrombus; MI = in-hospital myocardial infarction (some studies do not distinguish between Q-wave vs. non-Q-wave MI); CABG = emergency coronary artery bypass surgery; VSR/XF = vascular surgery repair/blood transfusion; Wall = Wallstent; Wik = Wiktor stent; PSS = Palmaz-Schatz stent; B = biliary stent; GRS = Gianturco-Roubin stent; - = not reported
*　Thrombotic vein grafts; adjunctive urokinase infusion for 20.5 hrs.
** 5-year event-free survival (no death, MI, TLR)
+　Distal anastomotic lesions
++ Diffusely degenerated grafts

e.　**Covered Stents (Chapter 26).** Stents covered with autologous vein or PTFE have been used to treat perforations and to cover segments of disease in vein grafts to minimize distal embolization, no-reflow, and restenosis. Preliminary studies suggest that covered stents may be associated with less CK elevation than non-covered stents, but their impact on restenosis and recurrent ischemic events has not been compelling.[200,201,219,222,264,280,238]

f.　**Rotablator Atherectomy (Chapter 27).** Rotablator is contraindicated in degenerated vein grafts and thrombus-containing lesions due to the risk of distal embolization, no-reflow, and myocardial infarction. Rotablator has been used successfully in some aorto-ostial, mid-body, and distal anastomotic vein graft lesions,[105,106,195,210,261,268] but it has no proven benefit for treatment of in-stent restenosis.

Table 17.14. Results of Saphenous Vein Graft Stenting in Diabetics[259]

	Nondiabetics	Diabetics		IDDM	NIDDM	
	(n = 618)	(n = 290)	p-Value	(n = 101)	(n = 189)	p-Value
Graft age (months)	110	90	NS	87	92	NS
Lesion Characteristics (%)						
Thrombus	14.7	7.5	0.03	7.4	7.4	NS
Degeneration	39.1	38.2	NS	56.5	32.1	0.001
In-hospital Complications (%)						
Abrupt closure	0.5	0	NS	0	0	NS
No-reflow	1.4	2.8	NS	4.4	1.3	NS
Distal embolization	2.7	2.6	NS	2.9	2.7	NS
In-hospital Outcomes (%)						
Procedural success	98	95	NS	95	96	NS
MACE	2.2	4.7	0.02	4.9	4.4	NS
Death	0.3	2.2	NS	2.0	2.4	NS
Q-wave MI	1.2	1.3	NS	1.8	1.1	NS
Non-Q-wave MI	17.8	15.2	NS	13.6	16.1	NS
CABG	0.6	1.3	NS	1.8	1.0	NS
RePTCA	1.2	1.6	NS	2.7	1.0	NS
Subacute thrombosis	1.6	1.2	NS	1.5	1.0	NS
1-year Follow-up (%)						
Death	5.0	12.3	0.001	13.4	11.7	NS
Q-wave MI	1.8	2.5	NS	3.6	1.9	NS
TLR	16.6	12.6	0.03	3.3	3.2	NS
TVR	22.6	17.2	0.04	23.1	21.4	NS
Event-free survival	79	67	< 0.001	69	66	NS

Abbreviations: IDDM = insulin-dependent diabetes mellitus; MACE= major adverse cardiac events (death, MI, rePTCA, CABG); MI = myocardial infarction; NIDDM = non-insulin-dependent diabetes mellitus; NS = not statistically significant; TLR = target lesion revascularization; TVR = target vessel revascularization

    g. Hydrodynamic Thrombectomy Devices. Hydrodynamic thrombectomy devices such as the Cordis Hydrolyzer and Possis AngioJet rely on the Bernouille principle for aspiration of thrombus and debris, and have been used to "clean-up" degenerated, friable, and thrombotic vein grafts prior to definitive revascularization. Earlier clinical studies suggested benefit,[107,108,188,212] although in-hospital MACE occurred in almost 14% of patients.[246] The multicenter randomized VEGAS-2 (Vein Graft AngioJet Study) trial compared intracoronary urokinase infusion to the AngioJet (Table 17.15) in thrombotic lesions, many of which were

Table 17.15. Results of VEGAS-2: AngioJet vs. Urokinase for Thrombotic Lesions[228,229]

	AngioJet	Urokinase
No.	180	169
Success (%)		
Lesion	87.6	79.6
Procedure	86.3	72.2
Device	87.4	75.3
Final Diameter Stenosis (%)	22	28
30-day MACE (%)		
Death	1.7	3.0
CK-MB elevation	15.6	32.5
Myocardial infarction	11.1	19.5
Q-wave	2.2	5.3
Non-Q-wave	8.9	14.2
Target lesion revascularization	3.3	3.6
Abrupt closure	3.3	4.7
Bleeding	5.0	11.8
Vascular complications	4.4	17.8
Stroke	1.7	1.2
Length of Stay (days)	4.1	4.9
Cost (US Dollars)		
Procedural	8669	10,520
Total	17,314	22,932

Abbreviations: MACE = major adverse cardiac events; Vegas-2 = Vein Graft AngioJet Study

in vein grafts.[228,229] Compared to urokinase, the AngioJet was associated with less CK elevation (presumably due to less distal embolization) and fewer bleeding and vascular complications; these data supported FDA-approval of the AngioJet.

h. **Prolonged Urokinase Infusion for Occluded Saphenous Vein Grafts (Chapter 16).** PTCA may be performed on totally occluded vein grafts, but angiographic success is only 70% and 3-year event-free survival is only 34%.[109] Several studies suggested that intragraft urokinase was a useful adjunct to balloon angioplasty,[110,111] directional atherectomy,[112] and stenting[91,113] for occluded vein grafts, but urokinase is no longer available in the United States. Although lytic infusions may increase the chance of immediate success, early complications included MI,[110,114,115] bleeding,[110,116] and hematoma formation;[110] 6-month patency was only 25% for occlusions at the distal anastomosis and 50% for occlusions in the body of the graft.[117] A randomized trial of low-dose (125,000 U/hr) vs. high-dose (350,000 U/hr) intragraft infusion of recombinant urokinase (rUK) demonstrated more bleeding complications (especially access site bleeding) in the high-dose group, and similar procedural success rates. Importantly, in-hospital mortality was 2% in both groups (due to fatal intracranial hemorrhage), and other severe bleeding complications occurred in 12% of patients.[275] As an alternative to prolonged infusions, some advocate use of a "pulse-spray" mini-dose infusion, which may decrease the dose and duration of lytic infusion and minimize bleeding and vascular complications.[118] Since urokinase is no longer available in the United States, continuous t-PA infusion has been used in its place. A common strategy is to administer a bolus (10-20 mg) of t-PA into the graft, followed by an infusion of 0.5-2.0 mg/hr for 12-24 hours. When considering intragraft lytic therapy, it is important to consider the risk of early bleeding complications and the likelihood of long-term benefit. For many patients, the benefit does not justify the risk.

i.   Mechanical Thrombolysis. "Mechanical" thrombolysis using therapeutic ultrasound has been used in small number of patients with thrombotic occlusions in saphenous vein grafts; procedural success was achieved in 65% of patients using the Acolysis System.[192,281] Other techniques for mechanical thrombolysis including aspiration thrombectomy and local drug delivery (Table 17.16), which will compete with other approved devices (TEC, AngioJet) as adjuncts to stents for revascularization of vein grafts, but are unlikely to achieve more than a "niche" role. Randomized trials comparing ultrasound thrombolysis to abciximab are currently in progress.

Table 17.16. Results of Mechanical Thrombolysis for Saphenous Vein Grafts

Series	N	Technique	Setting	Outcome
Rosenschein[192] (1999)	20	UT	SVG	Procedural success (65%); distal embolization (5%); adjunctive PTCA or stent (100%)
Papadokos[230] (1998)	73	AT	Native, SVG	Successful aspiration of thrombus or plaque (77%); marked improvement in TIMI flow; adjunctive stenting (100%)
Fajadet (1998)	100	UT	Native, SVG (Acolysis Registry)	Successful recanalization (95%); adjunctive PTCA or stent (94%)
Barsness[232] (1998)	58	LD (abciximab, Dispatch)	SVG	Significant improvement in thrombus score and stenosis severity but not TIMI flow; adjunctive stent (88%)
Glazier[233] (1997)	15	LD (UK, Dispatch)	SVG	Significant improvement in thrombus score and TIMI flow; procedural success (93%)

Abbreviations: AT = aspiration thrombectomy; UT = ultrasound thrombolysis; LD = local delivery; UK = urokinase; native = native coronary artery; SVG = saphenous vein graft

Table 17.17. Devices for Distal Protection*

Balloon Occlusion Devices
  PercuSurge GuardWire**

Filter Devices
  Cordis Angioguard
  Guidant Accunet
  EPI Filter
  Medtronic distal protection filter
  Bard device
  Mednova filter
  Microvena TRAP
  Intratherapeutics Intraguard
  Boston Scientific Captura Wire

Catheter Occlusion Devices
  Parodi Guiding KJ
  Coppi Invatec Guiding KT
  Kachel catheter

---

*   Courtesy of Dr. Max Amor and Dr. Michel Henry
** SAFER trial demonstrated a marked reduction in ischemic complications in vein grafts (Chapter 17); CAFÉ and
     SHELTER trials are in progress

> **j. Glycoprotein IIb/IIIa Receptor Antagonists.** Data are limited on the role of abciximab during vein graft intervention (Table 17.2). In the EPIC trial, pretreatment with abciximab was associated with less distal embolization than placebo, but the incidence of major cardiac events at 30 days and 6 months was similar.[209] The value of locally delivered GP IIb/IIIa inhibitors and "rescue" therapy awaits definition.
>
> **k. Distal Embolic Protection Devices.** A variety of new devices are under evaluation to prevent distal embolization during vein graft and other vascular interventions (Tables 17.17, 17.18). These devices rely on the use of balloon or catheter occlusion or filter devices to trap and remove debris during intervention.[221] In the recent SAFER (Saphenous Vein Free of Emboli Randomized) trial, 800 patients undergoing saphenous vein graft intervention were randomized to standard interventional therapy with the PercuSurge GuardWire vs. no distal protection (Figure 17.4). The trial was interrupted after 551 patients because of marked therapeutic benefit of distal protection, including a 50-60% reduction in hospital and 30-day MACE (Table 17.19) irrespective of the use of IIb/IIIa inhibitors. Randomized trials of other devices are in progress.

Table 17.18. Distal Embolic Protection Devices*

	Advantages	Disadvantages
Balloon occlusion devices	• Easy to use • Compatible with devices • Aspirate large and small particles • Reliably trap debris	• No antegrade flow • 5-8% are intolerant • Balloon-induced injury • Not as steerable as PTCA wires • Difficult to image during the procedure
Filter devices	• Preserve antegrade flow • Contrast imaging is possible throughout the procedure	• May not capture all debris • Difficult to evaluate retrieval of debris during the procedure • Filters may clog • Delivery catheters may cause embolization before filter deployment
Catheter occlusion devices	• Transient reversal of flow in internal carotid artery	• More cumbersome to use than other devices

* Courtesy of Dr. Max Amor and Dr. Michel Henry

C. **APPROACH TO THE PATIENT WITH PREVIOUS BYPASS SURGERY**. For patients in whom percutaneous revascularization seems warranted, available data suggest that a lesion-specific, multi-device approach may be preferred (Table 17.20). Graft age, lesion location, and lesion morphology may influence immediate and long-term results (Figure 17.5). However, once distal embolic protection devices become available for routine use, the approach to these patients may be simplified to PTCA and stent using embolic protection.

1. **Graft Age.** The cause of postoperative graft failure is influenced by the time interval from operation, including acute thrombosis within the first month (PTCA during this has been associated with higher restenosis rates[121,122]), fibrointimal hyperplasia between 1-12 months, and varying degrees of complex atherosclerosis after 12 months.[119] Many interventionalists believe that older grafts greatly increase the risk of procedural failure and complications, although several studies suggest that lesion morphology and graft degeneration are more important than graft age per se.[120,123,124] The optimal strategy for old degenerated vein graft lesions is unknown. Repeat bypass surgery may be the preferred in some patients.

2. **Lesion Location.** In general, intervention on aorto-ostial and proximal vein graft lesions is associated with less angiographic success, fewer procedural complications, and more restenosis than lesions in the body of the graft.

   a. **Proximal and Aorto-Ostial Lesions.** PTCA of proximal and ostial lesions appears to have lower success rates (86% vs. 93%) and higher restenosis rates (up to 80%) compared to other vein graft sites. All atherectomy devices can be applied to aorto-ostial vein graft lesions with acceptable success and complication rates, but adjunctive angioplasty is required for definitive lumen enlargement. There are no data to suggest lower restenosis rates compared to PTCA alone.[102,107,126,127] Independent predictors of restenosis after vein graft intervention include final lumen diameter and ostial location, but not device type; restenosis occurred in 42% of ostial lesions but only 17% of nonostial lesions.[128]

b. **Lesions in the Body of the Graft.** Focal stenoses can be treated with PTCA or stenting with success rates > 90% and complication rates < 5%, although stenting is frequently preferred because of improvement in late outcome (Table 17.11). DCA is also effective, but the incidence of non-Q-wave MI is higher compared to PTCA.[102]

c. **Distal Anastomotic Lesions.** Distal anastomotic stenoses can be safely and effectively treated with PTCA, which is probably the device of choice for lesions at this location. Stenting is also feasible, but may be challenging because of differences in diameter between the vein graft and native vessel. Procedural success and complications are similar for PTCA and stents, although TLR is somewhat lower with stents.[260]

Table 17.19. The SAFER Trial: Impact of Distal Protection on Vein Graft Intervention[286]

	GuardWire (n = 273)	No GuardWire (n = 278)
Baseline Characteristics		
Age (yrs)	68	69
Angina class III-IV (%)	75	75
Ejection fraction (%)	48	47
Thrombus (%)	39	38
Lesion length (mm)	15.8	17.4
Procedural Results (%)		
Technical success	93	-
Procedural success	90.5	82
No-reflow	3.4	8.0**
Final TIMI-3 flow	98.1	94.2**
In-hospital Outcome (%)		
TLR	0.4	0.7
Any MI	8.4	16.5
Q-wave MI	1.1	2.2
Non-Q-wave MI	7.3	14.4
Death	0.7	1.1
Any MACE	8.8	17.3*
30-day MACE	9.9	19.8*

Abbreviations: MACE = major adverse cardiac events (death, MI, TLR); MI = myocardial infarction; SAFER = Saphenous Vein Free of Emboli Randomized; TLR = target lesion revascularization
* $p < 0.001$
** $p < 0.05$

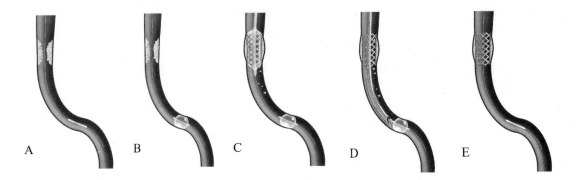

Figure 17.4. The PercuSurge GuardWire Distal Embolic Protection Device

A. Lesion is crossed with the GuardWire.
B. Distal protection balloon is inflated.
C. Stenting is performed under distal protection.
D. Export aspiration catheter is advanced and embolic debris is aspirated.
E. Protection balloon is deflated and the final result is evaluated.
Courtesy of PercuSurge.

Table 17.20. Lesion-Specific Indications in Saphenous Vein Grafts

Lesion	PTCA	STENT	DCA	ROTA	TEC	ELCA
Concentric	+	+++	+	-	++	++
Eccentric	+	+++	+	-	++	++
Ulcerated	+	+++	+	-	+	++
Ostial	±	+++	++	+	±	++
Total Occlusion	±	++	-	-	++	+
Thrombus	-	+	-	-	++	+
Diffuse Degeneration	-	-	-	-	±	-

Abbreviations: DCA = directional coronary atherectomy; ROTA = Rotablator; TEC = transluminal extraction catheter; ELCA = excimer laser coronary angioplasty; + = limited value; ++ = reasonable alternative; +++ = first-line treatment; ± = limited value, may be associated with higher incidence of complications than other devices; - = should be avoided;

3. **Lesion Morphology**
   a. **Vein Grafts > 3 mm.** Because of the favorable impact of stents on late outcome, we believe that stenting is the treatment of choice for vein grafts ≥ 3 mm in diameter. At our institution, single or multiple balloon- or self-expanding stents (vessel diameter 3.0-5.5 mm), biliary stents (vessel diameter 4.0-7.0 mm), and peripheral Wallstents (vessel diameter 6.0-9.0 mm) are used for focal or tubular lesions in the body of vein grafts. Ostial lesions are always treated with

balloon-expandable stents to minimize elastic recoil. If clot is suspected on clinical or angiographic grounds, useful adjuncts include TEC atherectomy or the AngioJet (to excise and aspirate atherothrombotic debris), and distal embolic protection devices (to reduce ischemic events). IVUS may also be useful to assess vessel size and optimize results.

b. **Vein Grafts < 3 mm.** For focal or tubular lesions in vein grafts < 3 mm, many devices are feasible, but none have been shown to be superior to PTCA. IVUS should be strongly considered to assess vessel size and optimize results, especially with stents (Chapter 31).

c. **Degenerated Grafts and Chronic Total Occlusions.** Diffusely degenerated vein grafts and chronic total occlusions remain problematic for all catheter-based interventions. In one study, treatment of degenerated grafts was the strongest independent predictor of in-hospital (odds ratio 7.7) and late (odds ratio 1.9) MACE.[257] Wallstents can be used in degenerated grafts, but in-hospital MACE occurred in 10.3%, and 3-year event-free survival was only 43%.[277] In selected cases, multiple peripheral, biliary, or coronary stents can be implanted with acceptable short-term outcome,[130] but long-term data on graft patency are not available. Total endovascular reconstruction using coronary or peripheral Wallstents is also feasible; in-hospital complications and mid-term clinical results appear to be acceptable, although long-term patency has not been well-defined.[207,220] Another interventional strategy involves intragraft infusion of t-PA (to establish patency),[91] followed by TEC atherectomy (to debulk residual thrombus), 3-4 weeks of anticoagulation (to "clean up" the graft), and stenting within 4-6 weeks (for definitive lumen enlargement) (Chapter 26). As previously described, this deferred stent strategy may reduce distal embolization and major clinical complications, but silent interim graft occlusion occurs in 15%.[70,131] In the near future, concerns about distal embolization may be attenuated when distal embolic protection devices are available. Although protection devices may reduce in-hospital ischemic complications, they are unlikely to have much impact on late restenosis or target lesion revascularization.

4. **Acute Myocardial Infarction.** There are limited data on percutaneous revascularization of vein grafts for acute MI.[136,137,263,267] These studies suggest a larger burden of thrombus in culprit vein grafts compared to coronary arteries, which is commonly refractory to intravenous thrombolytic therapy. More effective reperfusion may be achieved by percutaneous techniques,[135] albeit at a greater risk of embolic complications compared to native vessels.[263] However, the National Registry of Myocardial Infarction-2 reported no difference in hospital death or stroke for post-CABG patients treated with lytic therapy or PTCA.[270] In patients in the PAMI-2 study who developed acute MI after CABG, the infarct-related vessel was a bypass graft in 55% and a native vessel in 45%. PTCA was less likely to be performed when the infarct-related vessel was a vein graft, and these patients had more flow impairment and higher in-hospital (9.4% vs. 2.6%, p = 0.02) and 6-month (14.3% vs. 4.1%, p = 0.001) mortality.[267] Compared to acute MI during native vessel revascularization, acute MI due to graft occlusion has a lower frequency of ST elevation and Q-waves on ECG, less CK elevation, and worse in-hospital outcome.[198]

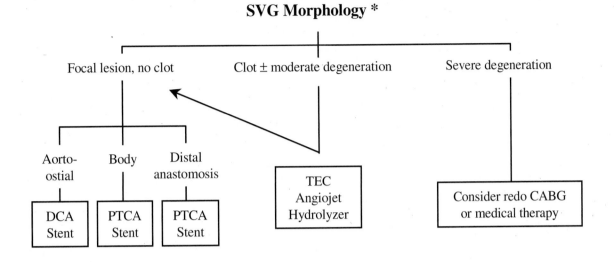

Figure 17.5. Approach to Saphenous Vein Graft Intervention

* Extent of degeneration is estimated by angiography. This approach may be simplified (PTCA, stent) when distal embolic protection devices are available

---

INTERNAL MAMMARY ARTERY

The internal mammary artery (IMA) is the conduit of choice for CABG.[136,137] Compared to saphenous vein grafts, IMA grafts demonstrate better flow, less atherosclerosis, and higher 10-year patency rates (95% vs. 30%). Despite excellent long-term patency, recurrent ischemia may occur secondary to stenosis in either the IMA or native vessel beyond the anastomosis. PTCA of the left IMA can be performed with success rates of 80-100% and a low incidence of abrupt closure, distal embolization, acute MI, and emergency surgery (Table 17.21).[138-147] Procedural failures are largely due to failure to cross the lesion with the guidewire or balloon, or inability to reach the stenosis due to vessel tortuosity. Overall restenosis rates are < 20%, and restenosis rates are lower for lesions at the distal anastomosis compared to the body of the graft.[138] PTCA and stenting of both IMAs is now readily accomplished without difficulty.[148-152,266] Rotablator atherectomy has also been successfully applied to distal anastomotic lesions and to native vessels via the LIMA graft.[269]

A. TECHNICAL CONSIDERATIONS DURING IMA INTERVENTION

1. **Subclavian Artery Tortuosity.** Difficulty may be encountered in cannulating the subclavian artery due to vessel tortuosity. When this occurs, it is easier to enter the left subclavian artery (or brachiocephalic artery) in the 60° LAO projection, which elongates the aortic arch and allows

excellent visualization of the great vessels. In this projection, the left subclavian artery usually originates just distal to the left edge of the tracheal air stripe; gentle counter-clockwire rotation of the catheter will result in rapid engagement of the left subclavian artery in most patients. The innominate artery usually originates just proximal to the right edge of the tracheal air stripe in the 60° LAO projection, and similar counter-clockwire rotation usually works nicely. If the subclavian artery cannot be entered with a preformed IMA guiding catheter, a right Judkins catheter may be used and later exchanged for an IMA guide. If tortuosity of the subclavian artery precludes tracking of the guiding catheter into the IMA, an ipsilateral brachial or radial approach may be used.[153,154]

2. **IMA Engagement.** The IMA is often readily engaged in the AP projection, but if difficulty is encountered, a shallow (20-30°) RAO (for the LIMA) or LAO (for the RIMA) projection will facilitate engagement. Caution should be taken to avoid forceful engagement with the guiding catheter since the IMA is prone to dissection and vasospasm. If the IMA is small, a 6-7F guiding catheter (with or without sideholes) may provide adequate support without pressure damping. Patients should be adequately pretreated with nitroglycerin and calcium blockers; selective bolus injections of nitroglycerin (100-300 mcg) should be used liberally.

3. **Equipment Selection.** The IMA is frequently very tortuous, and low-profile balloons are usually necessary. Equipment selection and technical approaches to PTCA of tortuous vessels are discussed in Chapter 11. Due to the length and redundancy of the IMA, a balloon with a long (150-cm) shaft may be required. Alternatively, short (90-cm) guiding catheters may be used or fashioned (by cutting 10-15 cm from the proximal end of the guide catheter and replacing the hub with an appropriately sized introducing sheath).

B. **CORONARY STEAL AND THE IMA.** After IMA grafting, myocardial perfusion depends on blood flow through the subclavian artery. The coronary-subclavian steal syndrome results from stenosis in the subclavian artery proximal to the IMA, which compromises myocardial blood flow.[155-164] Clinical manifestations include angina or myocardial infarction, variably associated with signs and symptoms of subclavian artery stenosis, such as arm claudication, vertebrobasilar insufficiency, blood pressure difference between arms, a supraclavicular bruit, or diminished ipsilateral brachial and radial pulses. Potential treatment strategies include carotid-subclavian bypass,[164-166] PTA,[164,167-171] directional atherectomy,[172] and stenting,[164-173] but we strongly favor stenting (Chapter 36). Occasionally, coronary steal may be due to an unligated large internal mammary artery sidebranch;[174] in this situation, coil embolization can relieve signs and symptoms of myocardial ischemia.[168,174,175,205]

Table 17.21. Results of Percutaneous Revascularization of the Internal Mammary Artery

Series	Device	No. Lesions	Success (%)	Restenosis (%)
Gruberg[266] (2000)	Stent PTCA	39 174	97 97	15.4 5.4
Hearne[138] (1998)	PTCA	68	88	19
Devlin[197] (1997)	PTCA	82	84	34
Crowley[206] (1996)	PTCA	20	75	10
Sketch[139] (1992)	PTCA	14	93	8
Popma[140] (1992)	PTCA	20	80	-
Dimas[141] (1991)	PTCA	31	90	14
Bell[142] (1989)	PTCA	7	100	0
Hill[143] (1989)	PTCA	11	82	-
Shimshak[144] (1988)	PTCA	26	92	13
Pinkerton[145] (1987)	PTCA	13	92	-

Abbreviations: PCI = percutaneous coronary intervention; - = not reported

REVASCULARIZATION OF OTHER ARTERIAL CONDUITS

The gastroepiploic artery, which may be used as an in-situ graft (gastroduodenal-to-coronary artery) or as a free arterial graft,[177-181] has long-term patency rates similar to the left internal mammary artery.[179] The in-situ conduit poses a number of technical challenges for imaging and percutaneous revascularization due to complex anatomy and tortuosity.[182,183] Since the celiac axis gives rise to the common hepatic artery, which gives rise to the gastroduodenal artery, which in 80-90% of cases ultimately gives rise to the gastroepiploic artery, selective cannulation of the gastroduodenal artery is required to adequately opacify the conduit. In

10-20% of cases, the gastroepiploic artery arises from the superior mesenteric artery, which increases the length and tortuosity of the conduit.[183] Adequate opacification can be achieved in only 50% of in-situ conduits, thereby limiting the success of percutaneous intervention. Among gastroepiploic artery grafts that can be cannulated and adequately opacify, PTCA success is 70-80%.[184-186] Stenting is feasible in selected cases.[199] Vasospasm is common during gastroepiploic intervention, so pretreatment with nitrates and/or calcium antagonists is recommended. PTCA of radial artery bypass grafts has also been reported.[196]

REVASCULARIZATION OF NATIVE VESSELS VIA BYPASS GRAFTS

Following CABG, recurrent ischemia may be due to new disease in native vessels distal to the graft anastomosis. The approach to percutaneous revascularization of these lesions is similar to bypass graft intervention (in terms of guiding catheter selection) and native vessel intervention (in terms of device selection and sizing). PTCA and stenting may be performed via vein grafts or IMA grafts as clinically indicated. Success rates exceed 90%,[187] and immediate results and complications are similar to PTCA of native coronary arteries. Rotablator of native vessels has also been performed via SVG or IMA grafts.

* * * * *

REFERENCES

1. Morwani JG, Topol EJ. Aortocoronary saphenous vein graft disease pathogenesis, predispositions, and prevention. Circulation 1998;97:916-931.

2. Campeau L, Enjalbert M, Lesperance J, et al. The relation of risk factors to the development of atherosclerosis in saphenous-vein bypass grafts and the progression of disease in the native circulation. N Engl J of Med 1984;311:1329-1332.

3. White C, Campeau L, Knatterud G, Probstfield J, Investigators at PCCT. Patency of saphenous vein bypass grafts following elective angiography: Preliminary results from the POST CABG Clinical Trial. J Am Coll Cardiol 1993;21:18A.

4. Reul GJ, Cooley DA, Ott DA, et al. Reoperation for recurrent coronary artery disease. Arch Surg 1979;114:1269-1275.

5. Schaff HV, Orszulak TA, Gersh BJ, et al. The morbidity and mortality of reoperation for coronary artery disease and analysis of late results with use of actuarial estimate of event-free interval. J Thorac Cardiovasc Surg 1983;85:508-515.

6. Foster ED, Fisher LD, Kaiser GC, et al. Comparison of operative mortality and morbidity for initial and repeat coronary artery bypass grafting: The coronary artery surgery study (CASS) registry experience. Ann of Thoracic Surg 1984;38:563-570.

7. Pidgeon J, Brooks N, Magee P, et al. Reoperation for angina after previous aortocoronary bypass surgery. Br Heart J 1985;53:269-75.

8. Laird-Meeter K, VanDomBurg R, Vanden Brand MJBM, et al. Incidence, risk, and outcome of reintervention after aortocoronary bypass surgery. Br Heart J 1987;57:427-35.

9. Lytle BW, Loop FD, Cosgrove DM, et al. Fifteen hundred coronary reoperations: results and determinants of early and late survival. J Thorac Cardiovasc Surg 1987;93:847-859.

10. Verheul HA, Moulign AC, Hondema S, et al. Late results of 200 repeat coronary artery bypass operations. Am J of Cardiol 1991;67:24-30.

11. Noyez L, van der Werf T, Janssen D, Klinkenberg T. Early results with bilateral internal mammary artery grafting in coronary reoperations. Am J Cardiol 1992;70:1113-1116.

12. Verheul H, Moulijn A, Hondema S, Schouwink M. Late results of 200 repeat coronary artery bypass operations. Am J Cardiol 1991;67:24-30.

13. Lytle B, Loop F, Cosgrove D, Taylor P. Fifteen hundred coronary reoperations. J Thorac Cardiovasc Surg. 1987;93:847-859.

14. Loop F, Lytle B, Cosgrove D, et al. Reoperation for coronary

atherosclerosis. Changing practice in 2509 consecutive patients. Ann Surg 1990;212:378-386.

15. Lamas G, Mudge G, Collins J, et al. Clinical response to coronary artery operation. J Am Coll Cardiol 1986;8:274-279.

16. Pidgeon J, Brook N, MaGee P, Pepper JR. Reoperation of angina after previous aortocoronary bypass surgery. Br Heart J 1985;53:269-275.

17. Foster E, Fisher L, Kaiser G, Meyers W, CASS atPIo. Comparison of operative mortality and morbidity for initial and repeat coronary artery bypass grafting: The CASS Registry Experience. Ann Thorac Surg 1984;38:563-570.

18. Schaff H, Orszulak T, Gersh B, Piehler J. The morbidity and mortality of reoperation for coronary artery disease and analysis of late results with use of actuarial estimate of event-free interval. J Thorac Cardiovasc Surg. 1983;85:508-515.

19. Lytle BW, McElroy D, McCarthy P, Loop FD, et al. Influence of arterial coronary bypass grafts on the mortality in coronary reoperations. J Thorac Cardiovasc Surg 1994;107:675-82

20. Ivert TS, Ekestrom S, Petriffy A, Weiti R. Coronary artery reoperations. Early and late results in 101 patients. Scand J Thoracic Cardiovasc Surg 1988;22:111-8

21. Perrault L, Carrier M, Cartier R, Leclerc Y, Hebert Y, Diaz OS, Pelletier C. Morbidity and mortality of reoperation for coronary artery bypass grafting: significance of atheromatous vein grafts. Can J Cardiol 1991;7:427-30

22. Gonzalez-Santos JM, Ennabli K, Grondin C. Repeat coronary artery bypass grafting in patients with patent atherosclerotic grafts: a special challenge. Thorac Cardiovasc Surg (West Germany) 1984;32:346-9.

23. Tan K, Henderson R, Sulke N, Cooke R. Percutaneous transluminal coronary angioplasty in patients with prior coronary artery bypass grafting: ten years' experience. Cath Cardiovasc Diagn 1994;31:11-17.

24. Morrison D, Crowley S, Veerakul G, Barbire C, Grover F, Sacks J. Percutaneous transluminal angioplasty of saphenous vein grafts for medically refractory unstable angina. J Am Coll Cardiol 1994;23:1066-1070.

25. Unterberg C, Buchwald A, Wiegand V, Kreuzer H. Coronary angioplasty in patients with previous coronary artery bypass grafting. J Vasc Dis 1992:653-659.

26. Miranda CP, Rutherford BD, McConahay DR, et al. Angioplasty of older saphenous vein grafts continues to be a sound therapeutic option. J Am Coll Cardiol 1992;19, 3:350A.

27. Meester BJ, Samson M, Suryapranata H, et al. Long-term follow-up after attempted angioplasty of saphenous vein grafts: The Thoraxcenter Experience 1981-1988. Eur Heart J 1991;12:648-653.

28. Plokker HWT, Meester BH, Serruys PW. The Dutch experience in percutaneous transluminal angioplasty of narrowed saphenous veins used for aortocoronary arterial bypass. Am J Cardiol 1991;67:361-366.

29. Douglas JS, Weintraub WS, Liberman HA, et al. Update of saphenous graft (SVG) angioplasty: Restenosis and long-term outcome. Circulation 1991; 84: II-249.

30. Jost S, Gulba D, Daniel WG, Amende I. Percutaneous

transluminal angioplasty of aortocoronary venous bypass grafts and effect of the caliber of the grafted coronary artery on graft stenosis. Am J Cardiol 1991;68:27-30.

31. Webb JG, Myler RK, Shaw RE, et al. Coronary angioplasty after coronary bypass surgery: Initial results and late outcome in 422 patients. J Am Coll Cardiol 1990;16:812-820.

32. Dorros G, Lewin RF, Mathiak LM. Coronary angioplasty in patients with prior coronary artery bypass surgery: all prior coronary artery bypass surgery patients and patients more than 5 years after coronary bypass surgery. Cardiol Clin 1989;7:791-803.

33. Platko WP, Hollman J, Whitlow PL, et al. Percutaneous transluminal angioplasty of saphenous vein graft stenosis: long-term follow-up. J Am Coll Cardiol 1989;14:1645-1650.

34. Pinkerton CA, Slack JD, Orr CM, et al. Percutaneous transluminal angioplasty in patients with prior myocardial revascularization surgery. Am J Cardiol 1988;61:15G-22G.

35. Cote GC, Myler RK, Stertzer SH, et al. Percutaneous transluminal angioplasty of stenotic coronary artery bypass grafts: 5 years' experience. J Am Coll Cardiol 1987;9:8-17.

36. Ernst S, van der Feltz T, Ascoop C, et al. Percutaneous transluminal coronary angioplasty in patients with prior coronary artery bypass grafting. J Thorac Cardiovasc Surg 1987;93:268-275.

37. Douglas J, Robinson K, Schlumpf M. Percutaneous transluminal angioplasty in aortocoronary venous graft stenoses: Immediate results and complications. Circulation 1986;74:II-363.

38. Reeder G, Bresnahan J, Holmes DJ, et al. Angioplasty for aortocoronary bypass graft stenosis. Mayo Clin Proc 1986;61:14-19.

39. Corbelli J, Franco I, Hollman J, et al. Percutaneous transluminal coronary angioplasty after previous coronary artery bypass surgery. Am J Cardiol 1985;56:398-403.

40. Gamal M, Bonnier H, Michels R, Heijman J, Stassen E. Percutaneous transluminal angioplasty of stenosed aortocoronary bypass grafts. Br Heart J 1984;52:617-620.

41. Block P, Cowley M, Kaltenbach M, Kent K, Simpson J. Percutaneous angioplasty of stenoses of bypass grafts or of bypass graft anastomotic sites. Am J Cardiol 1984;53:666-668.

42. Douglas JS, Gruentzig AR, King SB, et al. Percutaneous transluminal coronary angioplasty in patients with prior coronary bypass surgery. J Am Coll Cardiol 1983;2:745-754.

43. Douglas J, Weintraub W, King SI. Changing perspectives in vein graft angioplasty. J Am Coll Cardiol 1995;25:78A.

44. Guzman LA, Villa AE, Whitlow P: New atherectomy devices in the treatment of old saphenous vein grafts: Are the initial results encouraging? Circulation 1992;86:I-780.

45. Liu MW, Douglas JS, Lembo NJ, King SBI. Angiographic predictors of a rise in serum creatine kinase (distal embolization) after balloon angioplasty of saphenous vein coronary artery bypass grafts. Am J Cardiol 1993;72:514-517.

46. Altmann D, Popma J, Hong M, et al. CPK-MB elevation after angioplasty of saphenous vein grafts. J Am Coll Cardiol

1993;21:232A.

47. Tilli FV, Kaplan BM, Safian RD, Grines CL, O'Neill WW. Angioscopic plaque friability: a new risk factor for procedural complications following saphenous vein graft interventions. J Am Coll Cardiol 1996 (in-press).

48. Challapalli RM, Eisenberg MJ, Sigmon K, Lemberger J. Platelet glycoprotein IIb/IIIa monoclonal antibody (c7E3) reduces distal embolization during percutaneous intervention of saphenous vein grafts. Circulation 1995;92:I-607.

49. Abbo KM, Dooris M, Glazier S, O'Neill WW, et al. No-reflow after percutaneous coronary intervention: Clinical and angiographic characteristics, treatment, and outcome. Am J Cardiol 1995;75:778-782.

50. de Feyter PJ, Serruys PW, van den Brand M, Meester H, Beatt K, Surypanyata H. Percutaneous transluminal angioplasty of totally occluded venous bypass grafts: a challenge that should be resisted. Am J Cardiol 1989;64:88-90.

51. Weintraub WS, Cohen CL, Curling PE, et al. Results of coronary surgery after failed elective coronary angioplasty in patients with prior coronary surgery. J Am Coll Cardiol 1990;16:1341-1347.

52. Kahn JK, Rutherford BD, McConahay DR, Johnson WL, Giorgi LV, Shimshak TM, Hartzler GO. Outcome following emergency coronary artery bypass grafting for failed elective balloon angioplasty in patients with prior coronary bypass. Am J Cardiol 1990;66:285-8

53. Lemmer JH, Ferguson DW, Rakel BA, Rossi NP. Clinical outcome of emergency repeat coronary artery bypass surgery. J Cardiovasc Surg (Torino) 1990;31:429-7

54. Ellis SG, Ajluni S, Arnold AZ, Popma JJ, Bittl JA, Eigler NL, Cowley MJ, Raymond RE, Safian RD, Whitlow PL. Increased coronary perforation in the new device era: incidence, classification, management and outcome. Circulation 1994;90:2725-2730

55. Ajluni SC, Glazier S, Blankenship L, O'Neill WW, Safian RD. Perforations after percutaneous coronary interventions: Clinical, angiographic, and theapeutic observations. Cathet Cardiovasc Diagn 1994;32:206-212.

56. Douglas J, King SI. Ten year follow-up of patients undergoing vein graft angioplasty. Circulation 1994;90:I-333.

57. Safian RD, Grines CL, May MA, Lichtenberg A, Juran N, Schreiber TL, Pavlides GS, Meany TB, Savas V, O'Neill WW. Clinical and angiographic results of transluminal extraction coronary atherectomy in saphenous vein bypass grafts. Circulation 1994;89:302-312.

58. Popma JJ, Leon MB, MIntz GS, Kent KH, Satler LF, Garrand TJ, Pichard AJ. Results of coronary angioplasty using the Transluminal Extraction Catheter. Am J Cardiol 1992;70:1526-32

59. Meany T, Leon MB, Kramer B, et al. A multicenter experience of atherectomy of transluminal extraction in catheter for the treatment of diseased of saphenous vein grafts. Cathet Cardiovasc Diagn 1995;34:112-120.

60. Twidale N, Barth CW, Keperman RM, et al. Acute results and long-term outcome of transluminal extraction catheter atherectomy for saphenous vein graft stenoses. Cathet Cardiovasc Diagn 1994;31:187-191.

61. Hong MK, Popma JJ, Pichard AD, Kent KH, Satler LF, Chuang YC, Mintz GS, Keller MB, Leon MB. Clinical significance of distal embolization after Transluminal Extraction Atherectomy in diffusely diseased saphenous vein grafts. Am Heart J 1994;127:1496-503

62. Kramer B. Optimal therapy for degenerated saphenous vein graft disease. J Invas Cardiol 1995;7:14D-20D.

63. Annex B, Larkin T, O'Neill W, Safian R. Evaluation of thrombus removal by transluminal extraction coronary atherectomy by percutaneous coronary angioscopy. Am J Cardiol 1994;74:606-609.

64. Kaplan BM, Safian RD, Grines CL, Goldstein JA, et al. Usefulness of adjunctive angioscopy and extraction atherectomy before stent implantation in high-risk aortocoronary saphenous vein grafts. Am J Cardiol 1995;76:822-826.

65. Moses J, Lieberman S, Knopf W, et al. Mechanism of transluminal extraction catheter (TEC) atherectomy in degenerative saphenaous vein grafts (SVG). An angioscopic observational study. J Am Coll Cardiol 1993;21:442A.

66. Moses J, Tierstein P, Sketch M, et al. Angiographic determinants of risk and outcome of coronary embolus and myocardial infarction (MI) with the transluminal extraction catheter (TEC): A report from the New Approaches to Coronary Intervention (NACI) Registry. J Am Coll Cardiol 1994;23:220A.

67. Dooris M, Hoffmann M, Glazier S, et al. Comparative results of transluminal extraction coronary atherectomy in saphenous vein graft lesions with and without thrombus. J Am Coll Cardiol 1995;25:1700-5.

68. Al-Shaibi, KF, Goods CM, Jain SP, et al. Does transluminal extraction atherectomy reduce distal embolization in saphenous vein grafts? Circualtion 1995;92:I-329.

69. Moses JW, Yeh W, Popma JJ, Sketch MH. Predictors of distal embolization with the TEC catheter: A NACI Registry Report. Circulation 1995;92:I-329.

70. Hong M, Pichard A, Kent K, et al. Assessing a strategy of stand-alone extraction atherectomy followed by staged stent placement in degenerated saphenous vein graft lesions. J Am Coll Cardiol 1995;25:394A.

71. Parks JM. TEC before stent implantation. J Invas Cardiol 1995;7:10D-13D.

72. Cowley MJ, Whitlow PL, Baim DS, Hinohara T, Hall K, Simpson JB. Directional coronary atherectomy of saphenous vein graft narrowings: multicenter investigational experience. Am J Cardiol 1993;72:30E-34E.

73. Kaufmann UP, Garratt KN, Vliestra RE, Holmes DR. Transluminal atherectomy of saphenous vein aortocoronary bypass grafts. Am J Cardiol 1990:65:1430-1433

74. DiScascio G, Cowley MJ, Vetrovec CW, et al. Directional coronary atherectomy of saphenous vein graft lesions unfavorable for balloon angioplasty: Results of a single-center experience. Cathet Cariovasc Diagn 1992;26:75.

75. Pomerantz RM, Kuntz E, Carozza JP, Fishman RF, Mansour M, Schnitt SJ, Safian RD, Baim DS. Acute and long-term outcome of narrowed saphenous venous grafts treated by endoluminal stenting and directional atherectomy. Am J Cardiol 1992;70:161-167

76. Garratt KN, Holmes DR Jr, Bell MR, Berger PB, Kauffmann UP, Bresnahan JF, Vliestra RE. Results of directional atherectomy of primary atheromatous and restenosis lesions in coronary arteries and saphenous vein grafts. Am J Cardiol 1992;70:449-454.

77. Selmon MR, Hinohara T, Robertson GC, Rowe MH, Vetter JW, Bartzokis TC, Braden IJ, Simpson JB. Directional coronary atherectomy for vein graft stenoses. J Am Coll Cardiol 1991;17:23A

78. Ghazzal ZMB, Douglas JS, Holmes DR, Ellis SG, Kereiakes DJ, Simpson JB, KIng SB, and the Directional Atherectomy Multicenter Investigational Group. Directional coronary atherectomy of saphenous vein grafts: recent multicenter experience. J Am Coll Cardiol 1991;17:219A

79. Hinohara T, Robertson GC, Selmon MR, Vetter JW, Rowe MH, Braden LJ, McAuley BJ, Sheehan DJ, Simpson JB. Restenosis after directional coronary atherectomy. J Am Coll Cardiol 1992;20:623-632

80. Holmes D, Topol E, Califf R, et al. A multicenter, randomized trial of coronary angioplasty versus directional atherectomy for patients with saphenous vein bypass graft lesions. Circulation 1995;91:1966-1974.

81. Strauss BH, Natarajan MK, Batchelor WB, Yardley DE, et al. Early and late quantitative angiographic results of vein graft lesions treated by excimer laser with adjunctive balloon angioplasty. Circulation 1995;92:348-356.

82. Bittl JA, Sanborn TA, Yardley DE, Tcheng JE, Isner JM, Choksi SK, Strauss BH, Abela GS, Walter PD, Scmidhofer M, Power JA for the Percutaneous Excimer Laser Coronary Angioplasty Registry. Predictors of outcome of percutaneous excimer laser coronary angioplasty of saphenous vein bypass graft lesions. Am J Cardiol 1994;74:144-148

83. Litvack F, Eigler N, Margolis J, Rothbaum, D, et al. Percutaneous excimer laser coronary angioplasty: Results in the first consecutive 3,000 patients. J Am Coll Cardiol 1994;23:323-329.

84. De Marchena EJ, Mallon SM, Knopf WD, et al. Effectiveness of Holmium laser-assisted coronary angioplasty. Am J Cardiol 1994;73:117-121.

85. Serruys PW, de Jaegere P, Kiemeneij F, et al. A comparison of balloon-expandable stent implantation with balloon angioplasty in patients with coronary artery disease. N Engl J Med 1994;331: 489-95

86. Fischman DL, Leon MB, Baim DS et al. A randomized comparison of coronary stent placement and balloon angioplasty in the treatment of coronary artery disease. N Engl J Med 1994;331:496-501.

87. Savage M, Douglas J, Fischman D, et al. Coronary stents versus balloon angioplasty for aorto-coronary saphenous vein bypass graft disease: Interim results of a randomized trial. J Am Coll Cardiol 1995;25:79A.

88. Wong SC, Baim D, Schatz R, et al. Immediate results and late outcomes after stent implantation in saphenous vein graft lesions: The multicenter US Palmaz-Schatz Stent experience. J Am Coll Cardiol 1995;26:704-712.

89. Rechavia E, Litvack F, Macko G, Eigler N. Stent implantation of saphenous vein graft aorto-ostial lesions in patients with unstable ischemic syndromes: Immediate angiographic results and long-term clinical outcome. J Am Coll Cardiol 1995;25:866-870.

90. Wong SC, Popma J, Pichard A, Kent K. Comparison of clinical and angiographic outcomes after saphenous vein grafts angioplasty using coronary versus "biliary" tubular slotted stents. Circulation 1995;91:339-350.

91. Denardo SJ, Morris NB, Rocha-Singh, KJ, et al. Safety and efficacy of extended urokinase infusion plus stent deployment for treatment of obstructed, older saphenous vein grafts. Am J Cardiol 1995;76:776-780.

92. Piana RN, Moscucci M, Cohen DJ, Kugelmass AD, Senerchia C, Kuntz RE, Baim DS, Carozza JP Jr. Palmaz-Schatz stenting for treatment of focal vein graft stenosis: immediate results and long-term outcome. J Am Coll Cardiol 1994;23:1296-30.

93. Eeckhout E, Goy JJ, Stauffer JC, Vogt P, Kappenberger L. Endoluminal stenting of narrowed saphenous vein grafts: long-term clinical and angiographic follow-up. Cathet Cardiovasc Diagn 1994;32:139-46

94. Keane D, Buis B, Reifart N, Plokker TH. Clinical and angiographic outcome following implantation of the new less shortening wallstent in aortocoronary vein grafts: Introduction of a second generation stent in the clinical arena. J Interven Cardiol 1994;7:557-564.

95. Fenton S, Fischman D, Savage M, et al. Long-term angiographic and clinical outcome after implantation of balloon-expandable stents in aortocoronary saphenous vein grafts. Am J Cardiol 1994;74:1187-1191.

96. Leon MB, Wong SC, Pichard A. Balloon expandable stent implantation in saphenous vein grafts. In Hermann HC, Hirschfeld JW (Eds). Clinical Use of the Palmaz Schatz Intracoronary Stent. Futura Publishing Company Inc. 1993; 111-121.

97. Fortuna R, Heuser R, Garratt K, Schwartz R, Buchbinder M. Wiktor intracoronary stent: Experience in the first 101 vein graft patients. Circulation 1993;88:I-309.

98. Bilodeau L, Iyer S, Cannon A, et al. Flexible coil stent (Cook, Inc.) in saphenous vein grafts: clinical and angiographic follow-up. J Am Coll Cardiol 1992;19:264A.

99. Strauss B, Serruys P, Bertrand M, Puel J. Quantitative angiographic follow-up of the coronary wallstent in native vessel and bypass grafts European experience-March 1986 to March 1990). Am J Cardiol 1992;69:475-481.

100. deScheerder I, Strauss B, deFeyter P, Beatt K. Stenting of venous bypass grafts: a new treatment modality for patients who are poor candidates for reintervention. Am Heart J 1992;123:1046-1054.

101. Urban P, Sigwart U, Golf S, Kaufmann U, Sadeghi H, Kappenberger L. Intravascular stenting for stenosis of aortocoronary venous bypass grafts. J Am Coll Cardiol 1989;13:1085-1091.

102. Wong SC, Popma J, Hong M, et al. Procedural results and longterm clinical outcomes in aorto-ostial saphenous vein graft lesions after new device angioplasty. J Am Coll Cardiol 1995;25:394A.

103. Wong C, Popma J, Chuang Y, et al. Economic impact of reduced anticoagulation after saphenous vein graft stent placement. J Am Coll Cardiol 1995;25:80A.

104. Sketch M, Wong C, Chuang Y, et al. Progressive deterioration in late (2-year) clinical outcomes after stent implantation in saphenous vein grafts: The Multicenter JJIS experience. J Am Coll Cardiol 1995;25:79A.

105. Bass T, Gilmore P, Buchbinder M. Coronary rotational atherectomy (PTCRA) in patients with prior coronary revascularization: A registry report. Circulation 1992;86:I-653.

106. Freed M, Niazi K, O'Neill W. Percutaneous coronary rotational atherectomy: The William Beaumont Hospital experience. p.297. In Restenosis After Intervention With New Mechanical Devices. ed. Dordrecht, The Netherlands: Kluwer Academic, 1992.

107. van Ommen V, Veen Mat Daemen E, Habets J, Wellens H. In vivo evaluation of the safety to the vessel wall of the hydrolyser (a hydrodynamic thrombectomy catheter). J Am Coll Cardiol 1994;23:406A.

108. Fajadet J, Bar O, Jordan C, Robert G, Laurent J, Callard J, Cassagneau B, Marco J. Human percutaneous thrombectomy using the new Hydrolyser catheter: preliminary results in saphenous vein grafts. J Am Coll Cardiol 1994;220A

109. Kahn J, Rutherfors B, McConahay D, et al. Initial and long-term outcome of 83 patients after balloon angioplasty of totally occluded bypass grafts. J Am Coll Cardiol 1994;23:1038-1042.

110. Hartmann JR, McKeever LS, Stamato NJ, et al. Recanalization of chronically occluded aortocoronary saphenous vein bypass grafts by extended infusion of urokinase: Initial results and short-term clinical follow-up. J Am Coll Cardiol 1991;18, 6:1517-1523.

111. Hartmann J, McKeever L, Teran J. Prolonged infusion of urokinase for recanalization of chronically occluded aortocoronary bypass grafts. Am J Cardiol 1988;61:189-191.

112. Sabri MN, Johnson D, Warner M, Cowley MJ. Intracoronary thrombolysis followed by directional coronary atherectomy: a combined approach for thrombotic vein graft lesions considered unsuitable for angioplasty. Cathet Cardiovasc Diagn 1992;26:15-18

113. Eagan J, Strumpf R, Heuser R. New treatment approach for chronic total occlusions of saphenous vein grafts: thrombolysis and intravascular stents. Cathet Cardiovasc Diagn 1993;29:62-69101.

114. Blankenship JC, Modesto TA, Madigan NP. Acute myocardial infarction complicating urokinase infusion for total saphenous vein graft occlusion. Cath Cardiovasc Diagn 1993;28:39-43.

115. Gurley JC, MacPhail BS. Acute myocardial infarction due to thrombolytic reperfusion of chronically occluded saphenous vein coronary bypass grafts. Am J Cardiol 1991;68:274-276.

116. Taylor MA, Santoran EC, Aji J, Eldredge WJ, Cha SD, Dennis CA. Intracerebral hemorrhage complicating urokinase infusion into an occluded aortocoronary bypass graft. Cathet Cardiovasc Diagn 1994;31:206-210.

117. Hartmann J, McKeever L, O'Neill W, White C, Whitlow P, Enger E. Recanalization of chronically occluded bypass grafts: The effect of angioplasty site following extended urokinase infusion on 6-month patency. J Am Coll Cardiol 1995;25:149A.

118. Torre S, Marotta C, Blum M, Banas J. "Pulse Spray" mini-urokinase infusion for recanalization of recently occluded saphenous vein grafts. J Am Coll Cardiol 1995;25:94A.

119. de Feyter PJ, van Suylen RJ, de Jaegere PPT, Topol EJ, Serruys PW. Balloon angioplasty for the treatment of saphenous vein bypass grafts. J Am Coll Cardiol 1993;21:1539-49.

120. Bredlau CE, Roubin GS, Leimgbruber PP, et Al. In-hospital morbidity and mortality in patients undergoing elective coronary angioplasty. Circulation 72;5:1044-1052.

121. Dorogy ME, Highfill WT, Davis RC. Use of angioplasty in the management of complicated perioperative infarction following bypass surgery. Cathet Cardiovasc Diagn 1993;29:279-82.

122. Kahn JK, Rutherford BD, McConahay DR, Giorgi LV, Johnson WL, Shimshak TM, Hartzler GO. Early postoperative balloon coronary angioplasty for failed coronary artery bypass grafting. Am J Cardiol 1990;66:943-6

123. Abdelmeguid A, Ellis S, Whitlow P, et al. Lack of graft age dependency for success of directional coronary atherectomy and Palmaz-Schatz stenting. J Am Coll Cardiol 1993;21:31A.

124. Abdelmeguid A, Ellis S, Whitlow P, et al. Discordant results of extraction atherectomy in old and young saphenous vein grafts: The NACI experience. J Am Coll Cardiol 1993;21:442A.

125. Koller PT, Freed M, Grines CL, O'Neill WW. Success, complications and restenosis following rotational and transluminal extraction atherectomy of ostial stenoses. Cathet Cardiovasc Diagn 1994;31:255-260.

126. Abdelmeguid AE, Whitlow PL, Simpfendorfer C, Sapp SK, et al. Percutaneous revascularization of ostial saphenous vein graft stenoses. J Am Coll Cardiol 1995;26:955-960.

127. Stephan W, Bates E, Garratt K, Hinohara T, Muller D. Directional atherectomy of coronary and saphenous vein graft ostial stenoses. Am J Cardiol 1995;75:1015-1018.

128. Hong M, Popma J, Chuang Y, et al. Predictive model of target-lesion revascularization after balloon and new device saphenous vein graft angioplasty. J Am Coll Cardiol 1994;23:139A.

129. Glazier, Keiman FJ, Bauer JF, Mitchel DB, et al. Treatment of thrombotic saphenous vein graft stenoses/occlusions with

local urokinase delivery with the dispatch catheter-initial results. Circulation 1995;92:I-671.

130. Kaul U, Agarwal R, Mathur A, Wasir HS. Intracoronary stent placement in thrombus containing vein graft lesions. J Invas Cardiol 1995;7:248-250.

131. Heuser R. Treatment alternatives for chronically occluded saphenous vein grafts. J Invas Cardiol 1995;7:94-96.

132. Grines CL, Booth DC, Nissen SE, Gurley JC, Bennett KA, O,Connor WN, De Maria AN. Mechanisms of acute myocardial infarction in patients with prior coronary artery bypass grafting and therapeutic implications. Am J Cardiol 1990;66:1292-6

133. Santiago P, Vacek JL, Rosamond TL, Kramer KH, Crouse LJ, Beauchamp GD. Comparison of results of coronary angioplasty during acute myocardial infarction with and without prior coronary bypass surgery. Am J Cardiol 1993;72:1348-1351

134. Kahn JK, Rutherford BD, McConahay DR, Johnson W, Giorgi VL, Ligon R, Hartzler GO. Usefulness of angioplasty for acute myocardial infarction in patients with prior coronary artery bypass grafting. Am J Cardiol 1990;65: 698-702

135. Kaplan BM, Larkin T, Safian RD, O'Neill WW, et al. A propsective study of extraction atherectomy in patients with acute myocardial infarction. J Am Coll Cardiol 1996;27:365A.

136. Spencer FC. The internal mammary artery: The ideal coronary bypass graft? N Engl J Med 1986;314:50-51.

137. Loop FD, Lytle BW, Cosgrove DM, et al. Influence of internal mammary-artery graft on 10 year survival and other cardiac events. N Engl J Med 1986;314:1-6.

138. Hearne S, Davidson CJ, Zidar JP, Phillips HR, Stack RS, Sketch MH Jr. Internal mammary artery graft angioplasty: Acute and long-term outcome. Cathet Cardiovasc Diagn 1998;44:153-156.

139. Sketch MH Jr., Quigley PJ, Perez JA et al. Angiographic follow up after internal mammary artery angioplasty. Am J Cardiol 1992;70:401.

140. Popma JJ, Cooke RH, Leon MB et al. Immediate procedural and long-term clinical results in internal mammary artery angioplasty. Am J Cardiol 1992;69:1237

141. Dimas AP, Arora RR, Whitlow PL, et al. Percutaneous transluminal angioplasty involving internal mammary artery grafts. Am Heart J 1991;122:423

142. Bell MR, Vliestra RE, et al. Percutaneous transluminal angioplasty of left internal mammary artery grafts: Two years experience with a femoral approach. Br Heart J 1989;61:417

143. Hill DM, McAuley BJ, Sheehan DJ et al. Percutaneous transluminal angioplasty of left internal mammary artery bypass grafts. J Am Coll Cardiol 1989;13:221A

144. Shimshak TM, Giorgi LV, Johnson WL et al. Application of percutaneous transluminal coronary angioplasty to the internal mammary artery graft. J Am Coll Cardiol 1988;12:1205

145. Pinkerton CA, Slack JD, Orr CM, Van Tassel JW. Percutaneous transluminal angioplasty involving internal mammary artery bypass grafts: a femoral approach. Cathet Cardiovasc Diagn 1988;13:414

146. Cote G, Myler RK, Stertzer SH et al. Percutaneous transluminal angioplasty of stenotic coronary artery bypass grafts. J Am Coll Cardiol 1987;9:8

147. Singh S,. Coronary angioplasty of internal mammary artery graft. Am J Med 1987,82:361

148. Steffenino G, Meier B. Finci L, von Segesser L, Velebit V. Percutaneous transluminal angioplasty of right and left internal mammary artery grafts. Chest 1986;90:849-51

149. Brown RI, Galligan L, Penn IM, Weinstein L. Right internal mammary artery graft angioplasty through a right brachial approach using a new custom guide catheter: a case report. Cathet Cardiovasc Diagn 1992;25:42-5

150. Almagor Y, Thomas J, Colombo A. A balloon expandable stent at the origin of the left internal mammary artery graft: a case report. Cathet Cardiovasc Diagn 1991;24:256-258

151. Bajaj RK, Roubin GS. Intravascular stenting of the right internal mammary artery. Cathet Cardiovasc Diagn 1991;24:252-255

152. Hadjimiltiades S, Gourassas J, Louridas G, Tsifodimos D. Stenting the distal anastomotic site of the left internal mammary artery graft: a case report. Cathet Cardiovasc Diagn 1994;32:157-161

153. Dorros G, Lewin RF. The brachial artery method to transluminal internal mammary artery angioplasty. Cathet Cardiovasc Diagn 1986;12:341-346

154. Salinger M, Drummer B, Furey K, et al. Percutaneous angioplasty of internal mammary artery graft stenosis using the brachial approach: a case report. Cathet Cardiovasc Diagn 1986;12:261-5

155. Ishi K, Hirota Y, Kawamura K, Suma H, Takeuchi A. Coronary-subclavian steal corrected with percutaneous transluminal angioplasty. J Cardiovasc Surg (Torino) 1191;32:275-7

156. Laub GW, Muralidharan S, Naidech H, Fernandez H, Adkins M, McGrath LB. Percutaneous transluminal subclavian angioplasty in a patient with postoperative angina. Ann Thorac Surg 1991;52:850-1

157. Belz M, Marshall JJ, Cowley MJ, Vetrovec GW. Subclavian balloon angioplasty in the management of the coronary-subclavian steal syndrome. Cathet Cardiovasc Diagn 1992;25:161-3

158. Soulen MC, Sullivan KL. Subclavian artery angioplasty proximal to a left internal mammary coronary artery bypass graft: case report. Cardiovasc Intervent Radiol 1991;14:355-7

159. Feld H, Nathan P, Raninga D, Shani J. Symptomatic angina secondary to coronary-subclavian steal syndrome treated successfully by percutaneous transluminal angioplasty of the subclavian artery. Cathet Cardiovasc Diagn 1992;26:12-4

160. Holmes JR, Crane R. Coronary steal through a patent internal mammary artery graft: treatment by subclavian angioplasty. Am Heart J 1993;125:1166-7

161. Shapira S, Braun SD, Puram B, Patel G, Rotman H. Percutaneous transluminal angioplasty of proximal subclavian

artery stenosis after left internal mammary to left anterior descending artery bypass surgery. J Am Coll Cardiol 1991;18:1120-3

162. Perrault LP, Carrier M, Hudon G, Lemarbre L, Hebert Y, Pelletier LC. Transluminal angioplasty of the subclavian artery in patients with internal mammary artery grafts. Ann Thorac Surg 1993,56:927-30

163. Motarjeme A, Gordon GI. Percutaneous transluminal angioplasty of the brachiocephalic vessels: guidelines for therapy. Int Angiol 1993;12:260-9

164. Rabah MM, Gangadharan V, Brodsky M, Safian RD. Unstable coronary ischemic syndromes due to coronary subclavian steal: Case reports and review of the literature. Am Heart J 1996;131:374-378.

165. Ziomek S, Quinones-Baldrich WJ, Busuttil RW. The superiority of synthetic arterial grafts over autologous veins in carotid-subclavian bypass. J Vasc Surg 1986;3:140-5.

166. McIvor ME, Williams GM, Brinker J. Subclavian coronary steal through a LIMIA-to LAD bypass graft. Cathet Cardiovasc Diagn 1988;14:100-104.

167. Ishii K, Hirota Y, Kitz Y, Kawamura K, et al. Coronary-subclavian steal corrected with percutaneous transluminal angioplasty. J Cardiovasc Surg 1991;32:275-277.

168. Benzuly K, Kaplan B, Bowers T, Safian RD. Coronary-subclavian steal due to fistulae from the left internal mammary artery to the pulmonary artery: Treatment by coil embolization. Cathet Cardiovasc Diagn (in-press).

169. Laub GW, Muraldharan S, McGrath LB. Percutaneous transluminal subclavian angioplasty in a patient with postoperative angina. Ann Thorac Surg 1991;52:850-1.

170. Perrault LP, Carrier M, Hudon G, Pelletier LC. Transluminal angioplasty of the subclavian artery in patients with internal mammary grafts. Ann Thorac Surg 1993;56:927-930.

171. Dorros G, Lewin RF, Jamnadas P, Mathiak LM. Peripheral transluminal angioplasty of the subclavian and innominate arteries utilizing the brachial approach: acute outcome and follow-up. Cathet Cardiovasc Diagn 1990;19:71-76.

172. Breall JA, Grossman W, Stillman IE, Gianturco LE, Kim D. Atherectomy of the subclavian artery for patients with symptomatic coronary-subclavian steal syndrome. J Am Coll Cardiol 1993;21:1564-1570.

173. Breall JA, Kim D, Baim DS, Skillman JJ, Grossman W. Coronary-subclavian steal; and unusual cause of angina pectoris after successful internal mammary-coronary artery bypass grafting. Cathet Cardiovasc Diagn 1991;24:274-276.

174. Sbarouni E, Corr L, Fenech A. Microcoil embolization of large intercostal branches of internal mammary artery grafts. Cathet Cardiovasc Diagn 1994;31:334-336

175. Mishkel GJ, Willinsky R. Combined PTCA and microcoil embolization of a left internal mammary artery graft. Cathet Cardiovasc Diagn 1192;27:141-6

176. Fischell TA, Haddad N, Baskerville S, Foster MT. Ultrasound thrombolysis for the treatment of thrombotic occlusion of degenerated saphenous vein grafts. Cathet Cardiovasc Intervent 2000;50:90-95.

177. Lytle BW, Cosgrove DM, Ratliff NB, Loop F. Coronary artery bypass grafting with the right gastroepiploic artery. J Thorac Cardiovasc Surg 1989;97:826-31

178. Verkkala K, Jarvinen A, Keto P, Virtanen K, Lehtola A, Pellinen T. Right gastroepiploic artery as a coronary bypass graft. Ann Thorac Surg 1989, 47:719-9

179. Grandjean JG, Boonstra PW, den Heyer P, Ebels T. Arterial revascularization with the right gastroepiploic artery and internal mammary arteries in 300 patients. J Thorac Surg 1994,107:1309-1315

180. Perrault LP, Carrier M, Hebert Y, Hudon G, Cartier R, Leclerc Y, Pelletier LC. Clinical experience with the right gastroepiploic artery in coronary bypass grafting. Ann Thorac Surg 1993;56:1082-4

181. Suma H, Wanibuchi Y, Terada Y, Fukuda S, Takayama T, Furuta S. The right gastroepiploic artery graft. Clinical and angiographic midterm results in 200 patients.

182. Tanimoto Y, Matsuda Y, Fujii B, Kobayashi Y, Hatashi K, Takashiba K, Hamada Y, Hanazono S, Ando K, Hashimoto T. Angiography of the right gastroepiploic artery for coronary artery bypass graft. Cathet Cardiovasc Diagn 1989;16:35-8

183. Ishiki T, Yamaguchi T, Nakamura M, et al. Postoperative angiographic evaluation of gastroepiploic artery grafts: technical considerations and short-term patency. Cathet Cardiovasc Diagn 1991;21:233-8

184. Komiyama N, Nakanishi S, Yanagashita Y, Nishiyama S, Seki A, Watanabe Y, Konishi T, Fuse K. Percutaneous transluminal coronary angioplasty of gastroepiploic artery graft. Cathet Cardiovasc Diagn 1990;21:177-9

185. Watson LE, Schoolar EJ. PTCA of Gastroepiploic Bypass. Cathet Cardiovasc Diagn 1991;22:193-196.

186. Ishiki T, Yamaguchi T, Tamura T, Saeki F, Furuta Y, Ikari Y, Chiku N, Suma H. Percutaneous angioplasty of stenosed gastroepiploic artery grafts. J Am Coll Cardiol 1993, 22:727-32

187. Bartlett JC, Tuzcu M, Simpfendorfer C, Dorosti K. Percutaneous transluminal coronary angioplasty of native coronary arteries via saphenous vein grafts. J Invas Cardiol 1991;3:62-65.

188. Ramee S, Kuntz R, Schatz R, et al. Preliminary experience with the POSSIS coronary angiojet rheolytic thrombectomy catheter in the VEGAS 1 pilot study. J Am Coll Cardial 1996;27:69A.

189. Hong M, Wong S, Popma J, et al. Favorable results of debulking followed by immediate adjunct stent therapy for high risk saphenous vein graft lesions. J Am Coll Cardial 1996;27:179A.

190. Douglas J, Savage M, Bailey S, et al. Randomized trial of coronary stent and balloon angioplasty in the treatment of saphenous vein graft stenosis. J Am Coll Cardial 1996;27:178A.

191. Laham RJ, Carrozza JP, Berger C, et al. Long-term (4-6 year) outcome of Palmaz-Schatz stenting: Paucity of late clinical stent-related problems. J Am Coll Cardiol 1996;28:820-6.

192. Rosenschein U, Gaul G, Erbel R, Amann F, Velasguez D,

Stoerger H, Simon R, Gomex G, Troster J, Bartorelli A, Pieper M, Kyriakides Z, Laniado S, Miller HI, Cribier A, Fajadet J. Percutaneous transluminal therapy of occluded saphenous vein grafts. Can the challenge be met with ultrasound thrombolysis? Circulation 1999;99:26-29.

193. Sullebarger JT, Dalton RD, Nasser A, Matar FA. Adjunctive abciximab improves outcomes during recanalization of totally occluded saphenous vein grafts using transluminal extraction atherectomy. Cathet Cardiovasc Diagn. 1999;46:107-110.

194. Stephan WJ, O'Keefe JH, Piehler JM, McCallister BD, Dahiya RS, Shimshak TM, Ligon RW, Hartzler GO. Coronary angioplasty versus repeat coronary artery bypass grafting for patients with previous bypass surgery. J Am Coll Cardiol 1996;28:1140-1146.

195. Cardenas JR, Strumpf RK, Heuser RR. Rotational atherectomy in restenosis lesions at the distal saphenous vein graft anastomosis. Cathet Cardiovasc Diagn 1995;36:53-57.

196. Blanchard D, Ztot S, Pagny JY, Boughalem K, et al. Percutaneous transluminal angioplasty of radial artery grafts. Cathet Cardiovasc Diagn 1998;45:400-404.

197. Devlin G, Schwartz L, Drouin K, Lima VC, Marquis JF. The short- and long-term outcome of left internal mammary artery angioplasty. J Interven Cardiol 1997;10:301-305.

198. Moreno R, Lopez de Sa E, Lopez-Sendon J, Rubio R, Babadilla JF, Garcia EJ, Delcan JL. Determining whether acute myocardial infarction in patients with previous coronary bypass grafting is the result of narrowing of a bypass conduit or of a native coronary artery. Am J Cardiol 1997;79:670-671.

199. Roriz R, de Gevigney GD, Howarth N, Revel D. Case of successful percutaneous stenting of an in situ gastroepiploic-coronary bypass graft. Cathet Cardiovasc Diagn 1998;45:67-69.

200. Gurbel PA, Criado FJ, Curnutte EA, Patten P, Secada-Lovio J. Percutaneous revascularization of an extensively diseased saphenous vein bypass graft with a saphenous vein-covered Palmaz stent. Cathet Cardiovasc Diagn 1997;40:75-78.

201. Stefanadis C, Toutouzas K, Tsiamis E, Vlachopoulos C, Kallikazaros I, Stratos C, Toutouzas P. Total reconstruction of a diseased saphenous vein graft by means of conventional and autologous tissue-coated stents. Cathet Cardiovasc Diagn 1998;43:318-321.

202. deJaegere PP, van Domburg RT, de Feyter PJ, Ruygroik PN, van der Giessen WJ, can den Brand MJ, Serruys PW. Long-term clinical outcome after stent implantation in saphenous vein grafts. J Am Coll Cardiol 1996;28:89-96.

203. Savage MP, Douglas JS, Fischman DL, Pepine CJ, King SB III, Werner JA, Bailey SR, et al. Stent placement compared with balloon angioplasty for obstructed coronary bypass grafts. N Engl J Med 1997;337:40-47.

204. Weintraub WS, Jones EL, Craver JM, Guyton RA. Frequency of repeat coronary bypass or coronary angioplasty after coronary artery bypass surgery using saphenous venous grafts. Am J Cardiol 1994;73:103-112.

205. Eisenhauser MD Maj, Mego DM Ltc, Cambier PA Maj.

Coronary steal by IMA bypass graft side-branches: A novel therapeutic use of a new detachable embolization coil. Cathet Cardiovasc Diagn 1998;45:301-306.

206. Crowley ST, Bies RD, Morrison DA, Barbiere CC. Percutaneous transluminal angioplasty of internal mammary arteries in patients with rest angina. Cathet Cardiovasc Diagn. 1996;38:256-262.

207. Kelly PA, Kurbaan AS, Clague JR, Sigwart U. Total endovascular reconstruction of cocluded saphenous vein grafts using coronary or peripheral wallstents. J Invas Cardiol 1997;9:513-517.

208. Frimerman A, Rechavia E, Eigler N, et al. Long-term follow-up of a high risk cohort after stent implantation in saphenous vein grafts. J Am Coll Cardiol 1997;30:1277-1283.

209. Mak KH, Challapalli R, Eisenber MJ, Anderson KM, Califf RM, Topol EJ. Effect of platelet glycoprotein IIb/IIIa receptor inhibition on distal embolization during percutaneous revascularization of aortocoronary saphenous vein grafts. Am J Cardiol 1997;80:985-988.

210. Baron SB, Arthur A. Rotational atherectomy for resistant anastomotic saphenous vein bypass graft stenosis. J Invasc Cardiol 1996;8(2):120-122.

211. Natarajan MK, Bowman KA, Chisholm RJ, Adelman AG, Isner JM, Chokshi SK, Strauss BH. Excimer laser angioplasty vs. balloon angioplasty in saphenous vein bypass grafts: Quantitative angiographic comparison of matched lesions. Cathet Cardiovasc Diagn 1996;38:153-158.

212. van Ommen CG, van den Bos AA, Pieper M, den Heyer P, Thomas MR, Ozbeck S, Bar FW, Wellens HJJ. Removal of thrombus from aortocoronary bypass grafts and coronary arteries using the 6 FR hydrolyser. Am J Cardiol 1997;79:1012-1016.

213. Weintraub WS, Jones EL, Morris DC, King SB III, Guyton RA, Craver JM. Outcome of reoperative coronary bypass surgery versus coronary angioplasty after previous bypass surgery. Circulation 1997;95:868-877.

214. Chen L, Theroux P, Lesperance J, Shabani F, Thibault B, de Guise P. Angiographic features of vein grafts versus ungrafted coronary arteries in patients with unstable angina and previous bypass surgery. J Am Coll Cardiol 1996;28:1493-1499.

215. Brener SJ, Loop FD, Lytle BW, Ellis SG, Cosgrove DM, Topol EJ. A profile of candidates for repeat myocardial revascularization implications for selection of treatment. J Thorac Caridovasc Surg 1997;114:153-163.

216. Ellis SG, Brener SJ, DeLuca S, Tuzcu EM, Raymond RE, Whitlow PL, Topol EJ. Late myocardial ischemic events after saphenous vein graft intervention — importance of initially "nonsignificant" vein graft lesions. Am J Cardiol 1997;79:1460-1464.

217. Misumi K, Matthews RV, Sun GW, Mayeda G, Burstein S, Shook TL. Reduced distal embolization with tranlsuminal extraction atherectomy compared to balloon angioplasty for saphenous vein graft disease. Cathet Cardiovasc Diagn 1996;39:246-251.

218. Bejarano J, Margolis J, Kramer B. Extraction atherectomy for recently occluded saphenous vein grafts: A retrospective study. J Invasc Cardiol 1997;9:263-269.

219. Dechene HA, Radke PW, Schwarz ER, Hoffmann R, et al. Acute and 6-month long-term results with an endoluminal polytetrafluoroethylene stent graft in patients with in-stent restenosis and venous coronary artery bypass grafts. Am J Cardiol 1999; 84(Suppl 6A):12P.

220. Choussat RP, Black AJ, Bossi I, Joseph T, Fajadet J, et al. Long-term clinical outcome after endoluminal reconstruction of diffusely degenerated saphenous vein grafts with less-shortening wallstents. Am J Cardiol 1999; 84(Suppl 6A):49P.

221. Grube E, Webb J. The SAFE Study, multicenter evaluation of a protection catheter system for distal embolization in coronary venous bypass grafts (SVG's). J Am Coll Cardiol 1999;33(2):37A.

222. Baldus S, Zeiher A, Reimers J, Elsner M, Schaps KP, et al. Reduction of restenosis in venous bypass graft lesions after implantation of a covered graft stent. J Am Coll Cardiol 1999;33(2):37A.

223. Safian RD, Kaplan B, Schreiber T, Waters J, Moses J, et al. Final results of the randomized Wallstent endoprosthesis in saphenous vein graft trial (WINS). J Am Coll Cardiol 1999;33(2):37A.

224. Safian RD, Kaplan B, Schreiber T, Waters, Moses J, Leon MH. Final results of the Wallstent endoprosthesis in large saphenous vein grafts (WINS Registry). J Am Coll Cardiol 1999;33(2):51A.

225. Stoerger H, Haase J, Hofmann M, Schwarz F. Implantation of coronary PTFE-grafts in degenerated saphenous vein grafts: Acute and intermediate term results. Circulation 2000;102:II-642.

226. Dharmadhikari A Di Mario C, Tzifos V, et al. Comparison of procedural and one-year outcome with only balloon angioplasty, covered stents and non-covered stents in saphenous vein grafts. J Am Coll Cardiol 2000;35:26A

227. Hanekamp CEE, Koolen JJ, Den Heyer P, et al. A randomized comparison between balloon angioplasty and elective stent implantation in venous bypass grafts; the Venestent study. J Am Coll Cardiol 2000;35:9A.

228. Cohen DJ, Cosgrove R, Berezin R, Popma JJ, Leon MB, Kuntz RE, Ramee S. Cost-effectiveness of rheolytic thrombectomy for thrombus-containing coronary lesions: Results from the VEGAS 2 Trial. J Am Coll Cardiol 1999;47A.

229. Moses JW. Mechanical thrombectomy in acute ischemic syndromes: Cutters, suckers, and busters. J Invasc Cardiol 1998;10(supplA):36A-40A.

230. Papadokos S, Wong C, Gustafson G. Safety and efficacy of suction thrombectomy using infusion catheters in thrombus laden coronary lesions followed by stent placement. Circulation 1998;98:17.

231. Meany T, Leon M, Kramer B, Margolis J, et al. Transluminal extraction catheter for the treatment of diseased saphenous vein grafts: A multicenter experience. Cathet Cardiovasc

Diagn 1995;34:112-120.

232. Barsness GW, Butler CE, Ohmas EM, et al. Reduced thrombus burden in saphenous vein grafts with abciximab given through a local delivery catheter. Circulation 1998;98:17.

233. Garbarz E, Farah B, Vuillemenot A, Andre F, Angioi M, Machecourt J, Bassand JP, Wolf JE, Danchin N, Prendergast B, Lung B, Vahanian A. "Rescue" abciximab for complicated percutaneous transluminal coronary angioplasty. Am J Cardiol 1998;82:800-802.

234. Baim DS, on behalf of the SAFER Investigators. Presented at TCT-2000.

235. Grantham JA, Mathew V, Holmes DR. Antiplatelet therapy with abciximab in percuaneous intervention of thrombus-containing bypass grafts. Circulation 1998;98:17

236. Hartmann JR, McKeever LS, O'Neill WW, et al. Recanalization of chronically occluded aortocoronary saphenous vein bypass grafts with long-term, low dose direct infusion of urokinase (ROBUST): A serial trial. J Am Coll Cardiol 1996;27:60-6.

237. Kaplan B. Personal communication, 2000.

238. Waksman R, Popma JJ, Kenneard ED, et al. Directional coronary atherectomy (DCA): A report from the New Approaches to Coronary Intervention (NACI) Registry. Am J Cardiol 1997;80(10A):50K-59K.

239. Fortuna R, Walston D, Hansell H, Schulz G. Directional coronary atherectomy: Experience in 310 patients. J Invas Cardiol 1995;7:57-64.

240. Popma J, Mintz G, Satler L, et al. Clinical and angiographic outcome after directional coronary atherectomy: A qualitative and quantitative analysis using coronary arteriography and intravascular ultrasound. Am J Cardiol 1993;72:55E-64E.

241. Baim D, Tomoaki H, Holmes D, et al. Results of directional coronary atherectomy during multicenter preapproval testing. Am J Cardiol 1993;72:6E-11E.

242. Fishman R, Kuntz R, Carrozza J, et al. Long-term results of directional coronary atherectomy: Predictors of restenosis. J Am Coll Cardiol 1992;20:1101-1110.

243. Popma J, Topol E, Hinohara T, et al. Abrupt vessel closure after directional coronary atherectomy. J Am Coll Cardiol 1992;19:1372-1379.

244. Hinohara T, Rowe MH, Robertson GC, et al. Effect of lesion characteristics on outcome of directional coronary atherectomy. J Am Coll Cardiol 1991;17:1112-20.

245. Safian R, Gelbfish J, Erny R, Schnitt S, Schmidt D, Baim D. Coronary atherectomy. Clinical, angiographic, and histological findings and observations regarding potential mechanisms. Circulation 1990;82:69-79.

246. Dohad S, Parris TM, Unwala A, et al. AngioJet rheolytic thrombectomy improves procedural success and outcome in high-risk patients: VEGAS II Registry final results. Am J Cardiol 1999;84(suppl 6a):48P.

247. Zimer S, Kusleika, Finander B, et al. Use of a new distal protection device during PTCA and stenting. Am J Cardiol 1999;84(suppl 6a):108P.

248. Carlino M, et al. Prevention of distal embolization during saphenous vein graft lesion angioplasty. Experience with a

new temporary occlusion and aspiration system. Circulation 1999;99:3221-3223.

249. Gerckens U, Muller R, Rowold S, et al. The angioguard. First evaluation of a new protection catheter device for distal embolization in native coronaries, SVGs, renal arteries, and carotid arteries. Am J Cardiol 1999;84(Suppl 6A):45P.

250. Grube E, Gerckens U, Muller R, et al. The SAFE study: Multicenter evaluation of a protection catheter system for distal embolization in coronary venous bypass grafts (SVGs). Am J Cardiol 1999;84(Suppl 6A):19P.

251. Hong MK, Mehran R, Satler LF, Wu H, Slack S, Greenberg A, Abizaid AS, Kent KM, Leon MB. Long-term clinical results and predictors after successful stent implantation in saphenous vein grafts. Circulation 1998; 98 (Suppl I): I-286.

252. Safian RD, Kaplan B, Schreiber T, Waters J, Moses J. Interim results of the wallstent endoprothesis in saphenous vein graft trial (WINS). Circulation 1998; 98 (Suppl I): I-662.

253. Al-Mubarak NA, Liu MW, Al-Saif SM, Al-Shaibi KF, Mufti S, Chapman GD, Dean LS. Combined transluminal extraction atherectomy (TEC) and wallstents for treatment of saphenous vein graft disease.Circulation 1998; 98 (Suppl I): I-717.

254. Bhargava B, Kornowski R, Mehran R, et al. Procedural results and intermediate clinical outcomes after multiple saphenous vein graft stenting. J Am Coll Cardiol 2000;35:389-97.

255. Safian RD, Kaplan B Schreiber T, Waters J, Moses J, Leon MH. Final results of the randomized wallstent endoprosthesis in saphenous vein graft trial. J Am Coll Cardiol 1999; 33 (2 Suppl A): 37A.

256. Winters KJ, Taniuchi M, Smith SC, Kurz HI, Lasala JM. Myocardial infarctions after saphenous vein graft revascularization: comparison of angioplasty, stenting, and transluminal extraction catheter atherectomy. J Am Coll Cardiol 1999; 33 (2 Suppl A): 51A.

257. Nishida T, Colombo A, Briguori C, et al. Contemporary percutaneous treatment of saphenous vein graft stenosis: Immediate and late outcomes. J Invas Cardiol 2000;12:505-512.

258. Horlitz M, Amin FR, Sigwart U, Clague JR. Coronary stenting of aorto-ostial saphenous vein graft lesions. J Intervent Cardiol 2000;13:303-8.

259. Ahmed JM, Hong MK, Mehran R, et al. Influence of diabetes mellitus on early and late clinical outcomes in saphenous vein graft stenting. J Am Coll Cardiol 2000;36:1186-93

260. Gruberg L, Hong MK, Mehran R, et al. In-hospital and long-term results of stent deployment compared with balloon angioplasty for treatment of narrowing at the saphenous vein graft distal anastomosis site. Am J Cardiol 1999;84:1381-1384.

261. Benrey J, Mesa A, Jain S, Garcia-Gregory A. Successful rotational atherectomy of mid-saphenous vein graft lesions. J Interven Cardiol 1999;12:205-208.

262. Briguori C, DeGregorio J, Nishida T, et al. Polytetrafluoroethylene-covered stent for the treatment of narrowings in aortocoronary saphenous vein grafts. Am J Cardiol 2000;86:343-346.

263. Watson PS, Hadjipetrou P, Cox SV, et al. Angiographic and clinical outcomes following acute infarct angioplasty on saphenous vein grafts. Am J Cardiol 1999;83:1018-1021.

264. Baldus S, Koster R, Reimers J, Hamm CW. Membrane-covered stents for the treatment of aortocoronary vein graft disease. Cathet Cardiovasc Interven 2000;50:83-88

265. Scavetta K, Oh C, Caldron R, et al. Results of saphenous vein graft stent implantation: Single center results from use of oversized balloon catheters. Angiography 1999;50:891-899.

266. Gruberg L, Dangas G, Mehran R, et al. Percutaneous revascularization of the internal mammary artery graft: Short- and long-term outcomes. J Am Coll Cardiol 2000;35:944-8.

267. Stone GW, Brodie BR, Griffin JJ, et al. Clinical and angiographic outcomes in patients with previous coronary artery bypass graft surgery treated with primary balloon angioplasty for acute myocardial infarction. J Am Coll Cardiol 2000;35:6.5-11.

268. Thomas WJ, Cowley MJ, Vetrovec GW, et al. Effectiveness of rotational atherectomy in aortocoronary saphenous vein grafts. Am J Cardiol 2000;86:88-91.

269. Thomas WJ, Cowley MJ, Vetrovec GW, et al. Effectiveness of rotational atherectomy in narrowed left internal mammary artery grafts to the left anterior descending coronary artery. Am J Cardiol 2000;86:86-82.

270. Peterson LR, Chandra NC, French WJ, et al. Reperfusion therapy in patients with acute myocardial infarction and prior coronary artery bypass graft surgery (National Registry of Myocardial Infarction-2). Am J Cardiol 1999;84:1287-1291.

271. Campeau L, Knatterud GL, Domanski M, et al. The effect of aggressive lowering of low-density lipoprotein cholesterol levels and low-dose anticoagulation on obstructive in saphenous vein bypass grafts. N Engl J Med 1997;336:153-62.

272. Campeau L, Hunninghake DB, Knatterud GL, et al. Aggressive cholesterol lowering delays saphenous vein graft atherosclerosis in women, the elderly, and patients with associated risk factors. Circulation 1999;99:3241-3247.

273. Hong MK, Mehran R, Dangas G, et al. Comparison of time course of target lesion revascularization following successful saphenous vein graft angioplasty versus successful native coronary angioplasty. Am J Cardiol 2000;85:256-258.

274. Mathew V, Clavell AL, Lennon RJ, et al. Percutaneous coronary interventions in patients with prior coronary artery bypass surgery: Changes in patient characteristics and outcome during two decades. Am J Med 2000;108:127-135.

275. Teirstein PS, Mann T, Cundey PE, et al. Low- versus high-dose recombinant urokinase for the treatment of chronic saphenous vein graft occlusion. Am J Cardiol 1999;83:1623-1628.

276. Le May MR, Labinaz M, Marquis J, et al. Predictors of long-term outcome after stent implantation in a saphenous vein graft. Am J Cardiol 1999;83:681-686.

277. Choussat R, Black AJR, Bossi I, et al. Long-term clinical outcome after endoluminal reconstruction of diffusely degenerated saphenous vein grafts with less-shortening Wallstents. J Am Coll Cardiol 2000;36:387-94.1

278. Mathew V, Grill DF, Scott CG, et al. The influence of abciximab use on clinical outcome after aortocoronary vein graft interventions. J Am Coll Cardiol 1999;34:1163-9.

279. Dangas G, Mehron R, Lansky AJ, et al. Acute and long-term results of treatment of diffuse in-stent restenosis in aortocoronary saphenous vein grafts. Am J Cardiol 2000;86:777-780.

280. Baldus S, Koster R, Elsner M, et al. Treatment of aortocoronary vein graft lesions with membrane-covered stents. A multicenter surveillance trial. Circulation 2000;102:2024-2027.

281. Leon M, Strumpf R, Buchbinder M, et al. Preliminary findings using a PTFE-coated stent in patients with saphenous vein graft disease. J Am Coll Cardiol 2001;37(2):2A.

282. Ahmed J, Hong M, Mehran R, et al. Influence of diabetes mellitus on early and late clinical outcomes in saphenous vein graft stenting. J Am Coll Cardiol 2000;37(2):36A.

283. Savage MP, Douglas JS, Fischman DL, et al. Stent placement compared with balloon angioplasty for obstructed coronary bypass grafts. Saphenous Vein *De Novo* Trial Investigators. N Engl J Med 1997;337:740-7.

284. Leon, M Strumpf R, Buchbinder M, et al. Preliminary findings using a PTFE-coated stent in patients with saphenous vein graft disease. J Am Coll Cardiol 2001;37(2):2A.

285. Roffi M, Chan A, Chew DP, et al. Stents and glycoprotein IIb/IIIa inhibitors do not improve 30-day outcome in bypass graft percutaneous interventions: A retrospective registry - based analysis. J Am Coll Cardiol 2001;37(2):77A.

286. Baim D. On behalf of the SAFER Investigators. Presented at Transcatheter Cardiovasuclar Therapeutics meeting, September 2000, Washington D.C.

18

INTERVENTIONAL APPROACHES TO ADULT CONGENITAL HEART DISEASE

Lisa W. Forbess, M.D.
Thomas M. Bashore, M.D.

In recent years, improvement in cardiovascular surgical techniques and medical care has allowed most children with congenital heart disease to survive into adulthood. These patients often have residual cardiovascular disease or develop late complications that require further intervention, many of which are amenable to catheter-based intervention. The American Heart Association Scientific Statement on Pediatric Therapeutic Cardiac Catheterization recommends that these procedures be performed in institutions with appropriate facilities and personnel, who meet specific credentialing criteria. Radiographic equipment must include high-resolution imaging, steep angulation, and biplane fluoroscopy/cineangiography. The institution must also have cardiovascular surgical services for immediate treatment of emergencies that might occur during therapeutic interventions. A variety of percutaneous interventional procedures are considered in the adult patient with congenital heart disease (Table 18.1), including vascular occlusion (patent ductus arterioses, aortopulmonary collaterals, systemic-to-pulmonary artery shunts, arteriovenous malformations), balloon valvuloplasty (pulmonic valve stenosis, aortic stenosis, membranous subaortic stenosis), angioplasty/stenting (stenosis of prosthetic conduits, pulmonary artery branch stenosis, coarctation of the aorta, systemic venous stenosis), closure of septal defects (ASD, VSD), and miscellaneous techniques.

Table 18.1. Percutaneous Interventional Procedures for Adult Congenital Heart Disease

Procedure	Indications
Vascular occlusion	Patent ductus arteriosus (PDA) Aortopulmonary collaterals Surgical systemic-to-pulmonary artery shunts Arteriovenous malformations
Balloon valvuloplasty	Valvular pulmonic stenosis Aortic stenosis Membranous subaortic stenosis Mitral stenosis
Angioplasty/stenting	Stenosis of prosthetic conduits Branch pulmonary artery stenosis Coarctation of the aorta Systemic venous stenosis
Closure of septal defects	Atrial septal defects (ASD) Ventricular septal defects (VSD)
Miscellaneous	Fontan fenestration Balloon atrial septostomy

A. **VASCULAR OCCLUSION.** Vascular occlusion techniques using coil embolization are most often
    considered for patients with patent ductus arteriosus (PDA). Occlusion techniques for aortopulmonary
    collaterals, systemic-to-pulmonary artery shunts, and pulmonary arteriovenous (AV) malformations are
    similar but less frequently employed.

1. **Vascular Occlusion Coils (Table 18.2, Figure 18.1).** A large variety of coils can be used for
    vascular occlusion.[2] Coil selection is dependent on the diameter and length of the vessel to be
    occluded, vessel tortuosity, and presence of an end-vessel (vessel which tapers progressively into
    a capillary bed). Most coils consist of a stainless steel or platinum wire covered with Dacron fiber.
    The wire is wound tightly into primary coils, and then more loosely into secondary helical coils
    after delivery; the nominal coil diameter is determined by the "effective" diameter of the extended
    coil (the primary coils and Dacron feathers). In general, platinum coils are smaller, more flexible,
    and more radiopaque than steel coils. When released, the coil shortens by forming the secondary
    helical coils. The catheter used for coil delivery must be large enough to accommodate the nominal
    diameter of the coil. Standard embolization coils are available in a variety of nominal diameters,
    coil lengths (length of extended wire), and coiled diameters (helical diameter after delivery). The
    package generally provides 3 numbers: The first is the diameter in hundredths of inches, the second
    is the number of coils, and the third is the diameter of the coil loop. For example, 35-5-3 means
    a 0.035-inch diameter coil with 5 loops with a coil loop diameter of 3 mm.

2. **General Coil Embolization Techniques.** Coil embolization may be accomplished using a 4 or
    5-French sheath in the femoral artery or vein. The mechanism of vascular occlusion is thrombus
    formation, leading to organization and eventually endothelialization;[3,4] heparin is still administered
    since it does not inhibit thrombosis.[2] Initially, an angiogram is performed to identify the target
    lesion, and prophylactic antibiotics are administered (cefazolin for 18 hours). End-hole steerable
    catheters, such as the Judkins right coronary, are best for selective angiography and coil delivery;

Table 18.2. Coils for Vascular Occlusion*

Type	Company	Material	Nominal Diameter (inch)	Coil Length (cm)	Coil Diameter (mm)
Gianturco coils	Cook	Steel wire; Dacron feathers	0.025, 0.035, 0.038, 0.052	1.2,2,2.5,3,4,5, 8,10,15	2,3,4,5,8,10, 12,15,20
Small Gianturco coils	Cook	Platinum wire; Dacron feathers	0.018	1,1.5,2.1,3	2,3,4,5,6,7
Detachable embolization coils	Cook	Platinum or steel	0.035, 0.038	3,5,8,9,10	3,4,5,7,8,9,10,12

* *Definitions*: nominal diameter = diameter of wrapped wire; coil length = extended length of wire; coil diameter =
diameter of coil loop once deployed

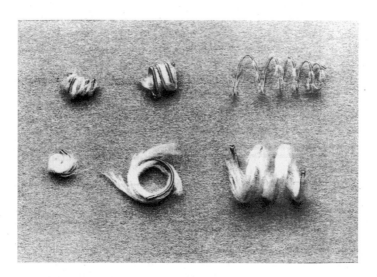

Figure 18.1. Representative Coils Used for Coil Occlusion[86]

polyurethane catheters and catheters with sideports are not recommended as coils may become jammed. Using a flexible tip guide wire, the catheter tip should be positioned at the proximal end of the structure for embolization. In end-vessels, coils are chosen with a helical diameter 20% larger than the average vessel diameter.[2] The large diameter results in a non-orderly orientation and prevents straightening of the coil within the vessel, thereby promoting occlusion. The length of the coil depends on the length of the target vessel. For a single coil, vessel length should be greater than or equal to the number of helical coil loops times the helical coil diameter.[2] In structures that are not end-vessels (such as arteriovenous malformations), care must be taken to ensure the coils do not pass through the arterial structure into the venous side. In such structures, a coil with a helical diameter approximately twice the minimal vessel diameter should be selected.[2] If additional coils are needed for occlusion, smaller coils may be selected since they will be trapped by the initial large coil.

For delivery of coils, the catheter tip should be placed well into the vessel. The coil is then loaded into the catheter with the stiff end of a pusher wire. The soft tip is used to advance the coil into the vessel. It is important to use a flexible wire to avoid pulling the catheter tip out of the desired delivery site during deployment. Completion of delivery may be accomplished by high-pressure injection of saline via a small syringe. One should not attempt to remove the catheter with a partially delivered coil, as the coil may embolize during catheter withdrawal. Improperly positioned coils should be retrieved using a bioptome or loop snare retrieval device; coils that embolize into the distal pulmonary artery circulation may be left in place. Platinum mini-coils may be delivered via a 3-French Tracker (Target Therapeutics, Freemont, CA). A 5-French guide catheter supports the 3-French delivery catheter, and a 0.015-inch flexible guidewire enables penetration into small, tortuous structures. This system is particularly useful when conventional delivery catheters cannot be advanced safely. Detachable coils allow more accurate and controlled coil delivery (Figure 18.2).

3.   **The Gianturco-Grifka Vascular Occlusion Device (GGVOD)** (Cook Inc, Bloomington, Ind)[5] (Figure 18.3) has been used for occlusion of patent ductus arteriosus (Figure 18.4), aortopulmonary collateral vessels, intrapulmonary arteriovenous fistulae, left superior vena cava connection to the left atrium, Glenn shunt, and accessory pulmonary venous connections to the inferior vena cava. The GGVOD consists of a flexible nylon sack and an occluding wire. The sack is attached to an end-hole catheter, and a modified spring guidewire is advanced through the end-hole catheter into the sack. Once inside the sack, the wire coils and fills the sack, occluding the vessel. Finally, the coil-filled sack is released from the catheter. If the sack's position is suboptimal, the filler wire can be pulled out of the sack, the sack repositioned, and the filler wire reinserted. The sack is manufactured in 3, 5, 7, and 9 mm diameters; all are delivered through an 8F Mullins sheath. To provide sufficient radial pressure, the sack should be 0.5 to 1.0 mm larger than the diameter of the vessel to be occluded.

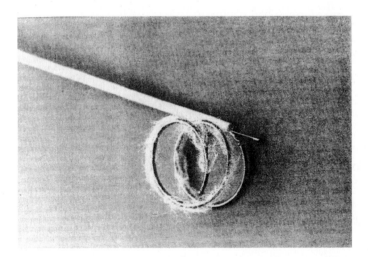

Figure 18.2. Detachable Coil

A ball near the end of the coil interlocks with the straight coil within the catheter, which allows deployment without detaching the coil until ideal positioning is certain. Advancing the straight wire out of the catheter results in coil detachment.[86]

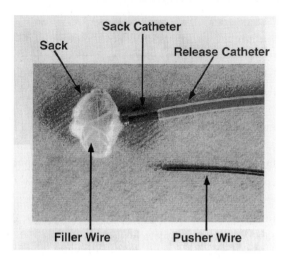

Figure 18.3. Gianturco-Grifka Coils (sacks)[87]

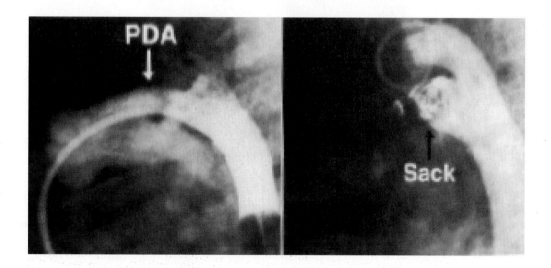

Figure 18.4. Sack Occlusion of PDA

Left panel: Patent ductus arteriosus. Right panel: Occluded ductus using Gianturco-Grifka occluder sacks.[87]

4. **Occlusion of Patent Ductus Arteriosus (PDA).** Transcatheter PDA closure was first reported in 1967[6]. Rashkind and colleagues reported their results using a small hooked umbrella occluder device,[7] and then using a double-umbrella, non-hooked occluder (Figures 18.5 and 18.6), which evolved from the early umbrella design. The Rashkind device (12 mm and 17 mm) is approved for PDA closure in all major countries except the United States and Japan. Residual shunting occurs in 38% at 1 year and 8% at 40 months using Duplex untrasound.[8,9] The Sideris Buttoned Device (Figure 18.7) and the Botalloccluder have similar outcomes.[10,11] Cambier et al described the technique of coil embolization for small PDAs in 1992 (Figure 18.8),[12] which has become the treatment of choice at many institutions. Coil occlusion provides effective therapy for more than 90% of restrictive PDAs with minimum angiographic diameters < 4 mm.[13] A new biconical spiral DuctOcclud Spiral Coil (Mepro, Nonnweiler, Germany) (Figure 18.9) has been used in a European multicenter study for PDAs with a minimum internal diameter less than 3.5 mm. Initial results show a 95% occlusion rate at 6 months (n=172).[14] More recently, the Amplatzer Duct Occluder (ADO) has been used for closure of moderate and large PDAs.[15]

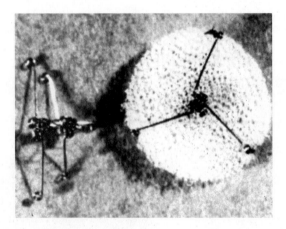

Figure 18.5. Rashkind PDA Occluder

The original occluder with Dacron disk and occluder arms.[88]

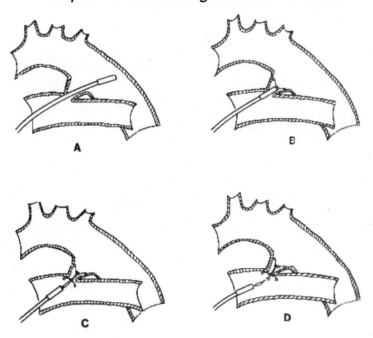

Figure 18.6. Rashkind Occluder in PDA

The disk is opened on the aortic side of the ductus and the second set of occluder arms expands on the pulmonary side.[88]

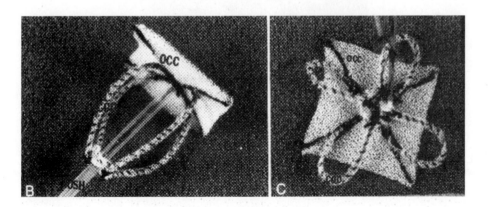

Figure 18.7. Sideris Occluder Device[89]

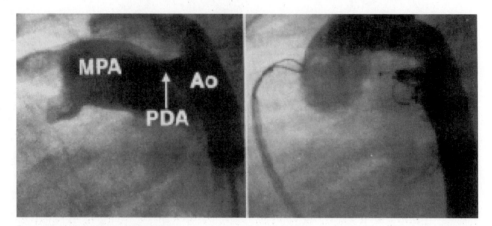

Figure 18.8. Coil Occlusion of PDA

Left panel: Patent ductus arteriosus. Right panel: Closed ductus using large occluder coils.

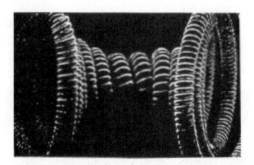

Figure 18.9. Spiral Duct Occluder[90]

5. **Technique for Coil Occlusion of PDA.** Once complete right and left heart catheterization is performed to rule out other cardiac defects, biplane angiography in the anteroposterior and lateral views is used to determine the shape, diameter, and length of the PDA. A descending aortogram or preferably a direct injection into the ductus is performed to provide a roadmap for the procedure and to measure the diameter of the aortic ampulla, as well as the minimal diameter, widest diameter, and length of the PDA. The choice of coil length and diameter is critical to minimize coil embolization and to obtain complete occlusion: *Coil diameter* should be at least twice the PDA minimal diameter;[16] however, excessively large coils may protrude into the left pulmonary artery and/or aorta (causing turbulence and possible stenosis) and direct blood flow through the center of the coil (preventing thrombosis and occlusion). *Coil length* should be sufficient to provide one-half to one full loop of coil in the main pulmonary artery and at least 2 loops of coil in the aortic ampulla.[16] We prefer to place the coil from the aortic side of the PDA, but inadvertent coil embolization during deployment occurs in up to 15% of the patients.[17] A snare advanced to the pulmonary side of the ductus can be used to prevent embolization. The Cook Detachable Embolization Coil has improved the technique of coil positioning and delivery.[17-22]

   A follow-up angiogram should be performed 10 minutes after coil release to assess residual shunting, since residual shunting across a PDA leaves the patient at risk for subacute bacterial endocarditis. While positioning a second coil, one should be careful not to dislodge the first coil. If repeat angiography demonstrates residual shunting, a third coil can be placed. Complications related to PDA coil occlusion include a persistent residual shunt in 5-10% of cases, embolization of a coil to the pulmonary or systemic artery requiring catheter retrieval, femoral artery injury, and hemolysis.

6. **Occlusion of Aortopulmonary Collaterals.** Patients with limited pulmonary blood flow may develop bronchial collaterals (typically tetralogy of Fallot and pulmonary atresia) arising from the descending thoracic aorta. Such collaterals may be embolized with coils if there is dual circulation to the pulmonary segment (Figure 18.10), leading to complete occlusion in 90%.[23-25]

7. **Occlusion of Coronary Artery Fistulas.** Coronary artery fistulas can be effectively treated using coil occlusion techniques. Coronary artery fistulas may arise from the left or right coronary artery and communicate with the right atrium, right ventricle, or pulmonary artery. Coil occlusion is most successful when a single large fistula is present. Complications include incomplete occlusion of the fistula with residual shunting, myocardial ischemia if a more distal coronary artery is inadvertently occluded, and coil embolization to the right heart or pulmonary artery.

8. **Occlusion of Pulmonary Arteriovenous Malformations.** Coil embolization has been used to close intrapulmonary arteriovenous malformations. Such vascular malformations can be hereditary (Osler-Weber Rendu syndrome) or acquired (following a Glenn procedure or a modified Fontan operation). Diffuse malformations are not amenable to coil embolization, but localized malformations are readily treated.

9. **Occlusion of Anomalous Venovenous Connections.** Patients who have undergone a Glenn shunt or modified Fontan procedure may develop right-to-right shunting and arterial hypoxemia as a manifestation of anomalous pulmonary veno-venous connections from the azygous vein or hemiazygous vein to the inferior vena cava. Coil embolization as well as the Gianturco-Grifka Vascular Occlusion device have been used for such anomalous venous connections. [26]

B. BALLOON DILATION OF CARDIAC VALVES

1. **Pulmonic Valve Stenosis.** For pulmonic stenosis, surgical valvotomy has been replaced by percutaneous balloon valvuloplasty.[27-30] Complications are rare, and pulmonary regurgitation is usually mild and inconsequential. A transpulmonic valve gradient greater than 50 mmHg is a typical indication for valvuloplasty. Doppler-estimated mean gradients correlate well with catheter-measured peak gradients. The effective balloon diameter should be 1.2-1.4 times the measured pulmonic valve annulus (usually measured by a cardiomarker catheter). When 2 balloons are used, the formula is $(D1 + D2 + 3.14 [R1 + R2]) / 3.4$, where D1 = diameter of first balloon one, D2 = diameter of second balloon, R1 = radius of first balloon, and R2 = radius of second balloon. For example, one 20 mm balloon plus one 18 mm balloon gives an effective diameter of 31.1 mm. Balloon valvuloplasty often leads to a dramatic reduction in the gradient (Figure 18.11), although dynamic infundibular obstruction may lead to a residual gradient[31] and may rarely cause RV failure after an apparently successful valvuloplasty (Figure 18.12). Infundibular hypertrophy tends to regress over time, and the residual gradient often decreases over several months.[32,33] Calcium antagonists and beta-blockers can minimize dynamic infundibular obstruction.[34] Balloon dilatation is not useful for infundibular pulmonic stenosis or dysplastic pulmonary valves since the results are suboptimal.

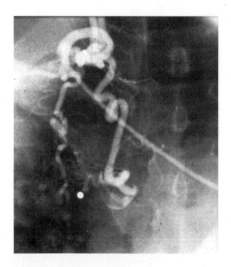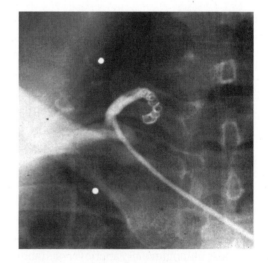

Figure 18.10. Bronchial Collateral

Left panel: A large bronchial collateral arises from the right internal mammary artery. Right panel: Coil occlusion of the bronchial collateral.

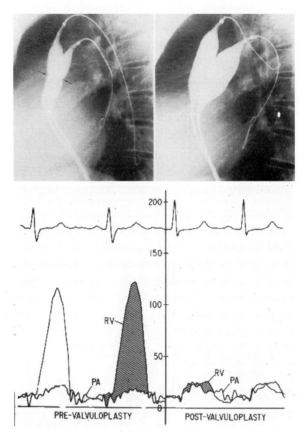

Figure 18.11. Results of Pulmonic Valvuloplasty

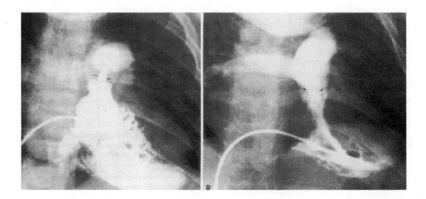

Figure 18.12. Dynamic Right Ventricular Outflow Obstruction

Following pulmonic valvuloplasty, relief of the gradient sometimes results in subpulmonic muscular (infundibular) obstruction. Left panel: Pulmonic stenosis prior to valvuloplasty. Right panel: Subpulmonic obstruction after valvuloplasty.

2. **Aortic Stenosis and Membranous Subaortic Stenosis.** Balloon aortic valvuloplasty is most useful for treatment of unicuspid or bicuspid aortic stenosis in the neonatal period, infancy, and childhood. In pediatric patients, medium and long-term results are favorable.[35,36] There have been a few reports of successful balloon dilatation for discrete membranous subaortic stenosis; however, the long-term efficacy remains unknown and surgery is generally preferred.[37,38] Fibromuscular or tunnel-like subaortic stenosis and supravalvular aortic stenosis are not amenable to balloon dilatation.

3. **Mitral Valve Stenosis.** Balloon dilatation for congenital mitral stenosis may be considered in an attempt to delay surgery or in a non-surgical candidate.[39] Since commissural fusion is not a major component of congenital mitral stenosis, balloon dilatation would not be expected to relieve obstruction.

C. ANGIOPLASTY AND STENTING

1. **Branch Pulmonary Artery Stenosis.** Pulmonary artery (PA) stenosis can occur at the main PA bifurcation or at more distal sites in the right (RPA) and/or left pulmonary artery (LPA). Branch PA stenosis is frequently associated with other congenital heart defects, especially Tetralogy of Fallot, and surgical repair of distal pulmonary artery stenosis may be difficult. Balloon dilatation of pulmonary arteries has not been very successful due to elastic recoil,[42] but stents have been successfully deployed in the pulmonary circulation with good results (Figure 18.13). The intimal proliferation seen with coronary stenting is not typical in the pulmonary artery. We recommend empiric aspirin for six months after stent placement.

2. **Stenosis of Prosthetic Conduits.** Successful reduction of gradients across stenotic prosthetic conduits has been reported.[40] The success of the procedure depends on the etiology of the obstruction: Discrete obstruction at the insertion of the conduit into the pulmonary artery is more amenable to balloon dilatation, whereas compression of the conduit between the sternum and the heart, intimal peel formation, and obstruction at the ventricular egress of the conduit are less likely to respond to balloon dilatation.[41] Stent placement may be quite effective in some of these latter situations.

3. **Systemic Venous Stenosis.** In adult congenital heart disease, one may encounter stenosis of the SVC or IVC limb of an intra-atrial baffle in patients who have undergone the Senning or Mustard operation, or obstruction of the SVC-to-pulmonary artery connection in a Glenn shunt. Surgical treatment of venous stenoses is difficult and often leads to early restenosis, whereas stenting may provide effective therapy in many situations (Figure 18.14).[43,44]

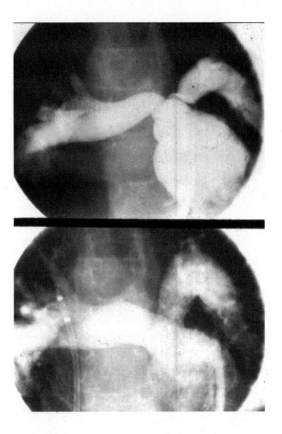

Figure 18.13. Stenting in Branch Pulmonary Artery Stenosis

Upper panel: Branch pulmonary artery stenosis. Lower panel: Initial result after stenting.

4. **Coarctation of the Aorta**

   a. **Native Coarctation.** Indications for intervening in native coarctation include hypertension proximal to the coarctation with a resting systolic pressure gradient > 20 mmHg across the narrowed segment or demonstration of an angiographically severe coarctation associated with extensive collaterals. The mechanism of relief of coarctation with balloon angioplasty involves tearing of the intima and media of the aorta;[45] intravascular ultrasound enables the operator to identify the extent of dissection and assess the adequacy of the procedure. Treatment for native coarctation of the aorta is controversial, and results of balloon dilatation with or without stent implantation are mixed. Balloon angioplasty of native coarctation is successful (residual gradient less than 20 mmHg) in 77-91% of patients.[46-48] Most complications are related to arterial injury in small patients, and aneurysms have been reported in 2-6%. Most series involving neonatal and infant coarctation show a fairly high incidence of recurrent coarctation, suboptimal results, and procedure-related morbidity and mortality. Restenosis is due to a combination of elastic recoil, intimal hyperplasia and arterial remodeling.[45] For neonatal and infant coarctation, we strongly recommend surgical repair with resection and end-to-end anastomosis; the need for reintervention has been reported as high as 70% in patients under 7 months of age.[46] For older children and adults, we prefer balloon dilatation with stent implantation if a large stent is available.

   b.   Recurrent Coarctation. For recurrent coarctation of the aorta (restenosis after surgical repair of native coarctation of the aorta), surgical treatment is often difficult because of adhesions and potential injury to spinal arteries and phrenic/recurrent laryngeal nerves. Balloon dilatation without stent implantation has been successful in 78-86% of patients.[49,50] Complications include femoral artery injury (8.5%), aortic dissection, and death. Late false aneurysm formation can occur in 4-40%.[50-52] Stent implantation may improve early and late results.[53,54]

5.   Techniques for Stent Placement. The delivery of stents is similar for both the branch pulmonary arteries and systemic veins. Typically, balloon-expandable Palmaz iliac stents (Johnson & Johnson Interventional Systems, Warren, New Jersey) are used in the pulmonary artery tree. Occasionally, smaller biliary stents are used for distal pulmonary arteries or systemic veins. The self-expanding Wallstent may have a role in more easily expandable lesions. Complications of stent implantation include balloon rupture and malposition or embolization of the stent. If the stent embolizes to the distal pulmonary artery tree, it is usually safe to leave the stent in place. Occasionally, a stented lung segment may develop pulmonary edema from increased blood flow. Diuretics are usually sufficient to treat this condition. Vessel rupture with acute hemothorax, hemoptysis, and hemodynamic collapse are rare; should this occur, coil embolization can be life-saving.

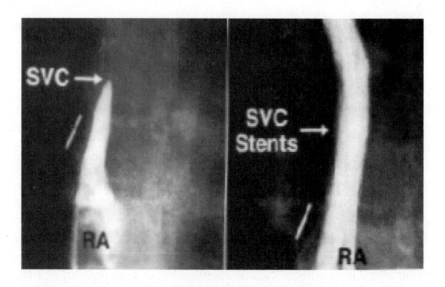

Figure 18.14. Stenting an Occluded Superior Vena Cava

Left panel: Occluded SVC. Right panel: Results after stenting.

D. CLOSURE OF SEPTAL DEFECTS (Table 18.3)

1. **Transcatheter ASD Closure.** All of the devices for secundum ASD closure must be placed against a remnant of the atrial septum; therefore, it is important that the devices are larger than the ASD itself, and precise positioning of the device is essential if the septal rim is not large. Transesophageal echocardiography generally underestimates the defect, but is always used to ensure precise placement. None of the devices are intended for closure of sinus venosus defects or primum ASDs, since the rim of septum needed to anchor the device is inadequate. Associated abnormalities of the pulmonary veins or atrioventricular valves may also require surgical correction. Complications include residual shunts (especially with large ASDs with balloon stretch diameters > 20 mm), device embolization due to undersizing or suboptimal positioning, and small leaks immediately after occlusion. At this time, no ASD closure device is commercially available in the United States. In 1976, King et al. reported the first application of a double-umbrella device in humans,[61] but because of the large (23F) complex delivery system, the device never achieved routine clinical use. In 1987, Rashkind described a single, self-expandable umbrella with barbed hooks,[62] but the device could not be reliably repositioned or retrieved, and clinical trials were stopped because of the low success rate. In 1989, Lock developed the Clamshell double umbrella device (USCI, Billerica, MA),[63] which was implanted with very high procedural success rates. However, 1-year follow-up demonstrated umbrella fracture in up to 84% of patients, associated with small fibrotic masses on the atrial wall, hemodynamically significant residual shunts, and late device embolization.[62,64] Further investigation demonstrated that the metal in the device was brittle and unable to resist flexion forces in the beating heart, so it was withdrawn from the market in 1991. Several other devices are in pre-clinical or clinical trials.

   a. **CardioSEAL.** This is a second-generation double umbrella device designed to resist metal fatigue (Figure 18.15). A multicenter randomized trial comparing the CardioSEAL to surgery is ongoing in the United States. Devices are available in 17, 23, 28, 33, and 40 mm diagonal dimension and a long 11F delivery sheath is used for deployment. An important feature is the ability to reposition or retrieve the device: If only the left atrial arms of the CardioSEAL are deployed, the device can be withdrawn into the sheath without destruction. If both sides of the device have been deployed, it can be withdrawn into the sheath but its integrity is destroyed. If the device embolizes, catheter retrieval is possible using a 14F sheath. In the North American multicenter trial,[65] ASD (6-20 mm in diameter) closure was successful in 98.5% of 132 patients. At discharge, 63% had trivial residual shunts and 37% had larger residual shunts. Device fracture was detected in 8% at 6 months, without sequelae.

   b. **Buttoned Device.** The Buttoned device (Custom Medical Devices, Amarillo, Texas) (Figure 18.15)[66] has three components: a polyurethane foam occluder, a counter-occluder, and a loading wire. This device has the least rigidity and strength of the ASD closure devices. The foam occluder is easily folded into the delivery catheter by compressing the sides of the square, and resumes its square shape when advanced out of the delivery catheter into the left atrium. The occluder remains attached to a nylon thread looped through a hollow loading wire that extends out of the end of the delivery catheter. If the occluder is positioned correctly, the

Table 18.3. Devices for Closure of Septal Defects

Device	Description	Comments
Rashkind device	Double-umbrella device (independent umbrellas with manual expansion)	Large, complex delivery system; never achieved routine application
Rashkind occluder	Single self-expanding umbrella with barbed hooks	Positioned in left atrium and anchored in position across atrial septum; unreliable deployment; never reached market
Clamshell device	Double-umbrella	High success rates for early deployment; late metal fractures led to residual shunts, device embolization; withdrawn from market in 1991
CardioSEAL	Double-umbrella device; redesigned successor to Clamshell device, with improved support to resist metal fatigue	Can be repositioned or retrieved; successful deployment in 98.5%, but significant residual shunts in 37% at discharge. Device fracture 8% at 6-months; ongoing clinical trials
Buttoned device	Consists of an occluder (polyurethane foam supported by two arms), counter-occluder, and a loading wire	Least rigid of all devices; useful for large defects; major limitation was late device embolization, but latest design has better results (device embolization <1%, residual shunt 19% at 1 year)
Angel wings device	Self-centering double-disk-device; made of super-elastic nitinol and Dacron-like material	Designed to overcome the limitations of other devices; best suited for ASDs $\leq$ 20 mm; successful occlusion in 96%, residual shunts in 4.2%. Device is being redesigned because of concerns about ease of retrieval and possible vessel injury
Atrial septal defect occluder system device (ASDOS)	Double-umbrella device made of nitinol and polyurethane	Pre-clinical trials in Europe; requires venous and arterial access. Successful occlusion in 87%. Residual shunts in 8% at discharge and 2% at 1 year
Amplatzer device	Nitinol wires tightly woven into 2 flat disc occluders, connected by a short waist	Most recent design of occluder devices; preliminary data are encouraging; may be simpler than other technique, and have better results

counter-occluder is then advanced over the loading wire and "buttoned" onto a knotted loop attached to the center of the occluder. The counter-occluder wire and the higher left atrial pressure prevent the occluder from migrating into the left atrium. The device is released by cutting one side of the nylon thread loop and pulling the thread out of the loading wire. A modified version of the device with a centering mechanism has also been described,[66] and an "inverted " device has been used in a small number of patients with right-to-left shunts. The Buttoned device has been used in hundreds of patients with ASDs up to 30 mm in diameter. The incidence of residual shunting is 34%, 28%, and 20% at 6, 12, and 24 months, respectively.[68] The major limitation of the Buttoned device is unbuttoning and device embolization,[69] but the incidence of unbuttoning has decreased from 11.1% with the first-generation device to 0.8% with the fourth generation device.[70,71] There were no cases of endocarditis or thromboembolism in 350 patient-months of follow-up.

c.   **Angel Wings Device.** To overcome some of the perceived limitations of the Clamshell and Buttoned devices, Das and colleagues developed the Angel Wings device (Microvena Corp, White Bear Lake, Minnesota), a self-centering double-disk device made of super-elastic nitinol and Dacron-like material (Figure 18.15).[72] The device has a custom delivery system connected to an 11-13F delivery catheter. The unique feature of this device is its ability to self-center on deployment, and to closely approximate the edges of the defect and tightly occlude the atrial septum. This device is best suited for defects with balloon stretch diameter $\leq$ 20 mm, but a second version of the device may be used to close larger defects. The initial results of the multicenter pilot study have been encouraging:[73] In 104 patients, septal occlusion was successful in 96%. Follow-up at 1-17 months showed a minor residual shunt in 4.2%. There were no strokes or endocarditis. Despite these encouraging results, there is concern that the stiff wire frame may perforate or lacerate the atrial wall or vena cava, especially during catheter retrieval. The device is being redesigned with a goal of easier retrievability.

d.   **Atrial Septal Defect Occluder System Device (ASDOS).** The atrial septal defect occluder system (ASDOS) (Osypka Corporation, Rheinfelden, Germany) (Figure 18.15)[74] is a double-umbrella device made of nitinol and polyurethane. For deployment, simultaneous venous and arterial access is necessary, which adds to the complexity of the procedure. The device has been used to close defects $\geq$ 30 mm in diameter. The multicenter European trial[75] reported successful occlusion in 87%; embolization or surgical retrieval was necessary in 13%. A large residual shunt persisted in 8% at discharge and in 2% at 1 year.

e.   **Amplatzer Device.** The most recently developed device is the Amplatzer septal occluder (AGA Medical Corp., Golden Valley, MN) (Figure 18.16),[76] which is comprised of 0.004-0.005 inch Nitinol wires tightly woven into two flat discs with a 4-mm connecting waist. The device diameter is dictated by the diameter of the waist, and is available from 4-26 mm with 1-mm increments. The left atrial disc is 12-14 mm larger than the waist diameter, and the right atrial disc is 8-10 mm larger than waist diameter. The prosthesis is filled with polyester threads to enhance thrombogenicity, and requires a 7F delivery catheter. The unique feature of this device is its ability to be repositioned after deployment, prior to device release. Initial experience in 30 patients with ASDs 7-19 mm is encouraging, and the device may also be used for closure of multiple ASDs in the same patient.[77] Comparisons of the Amplatzer occluder to other devices suggest better and more durable occlusion, shorter procedure time, and fewer complications.[78,79]

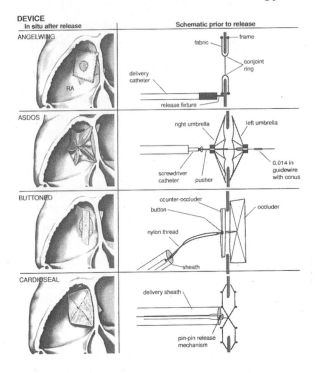

Figure 18.15. ASD Closure Devices

A schematic of popular ASD occlusion devices and their release mechanisms.

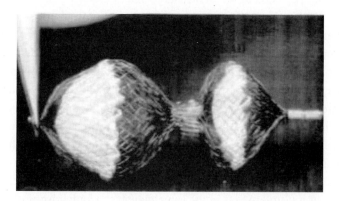

Figure 18.16. Amplatzer Septal Occluder

2. **Devices for Closure of Ventricular Septal Defects.** In adult cardiology, it is rare to encounter a patient with an untreated congenital ventricular septal defect (VSD) that requires intervention. In contrast, muscular defects in children are difficult to repair, due to the heavy trabeculations of the right ventricle and the poor outcomes with left ventriculotomy. Therefore, transcatheter techniques for VSD closure have been advocated. The CardioSEAL device, the Rashkind double-umbrella port device, the Buttoned device, and the Amplatzer VSD occluder have been used to close muscular and/or perimembranous VSD with variable success.[80-83] Most feel that apical and midmuscular VSDs are most suitable for transcatheter device closure. Since the defects are low on the septum and usually located away from the semilunar valves, atrioventricular valves, and chordal apparatus, an approach from the internal jugular vein and superior vena cava is preferred. An 11F delivery sheath is placed from the internal jugular vein, across the VSD, into the left ventricle. The entire system is then withdrawn until the distal umbrella opens partially on the left ventricular side of the defect, with proper location confirmed by angiography and transthoracic echocardiography. The device should be fixed in place and the sheath carefully withdrawn to deploy the device in the right ventricle. Passage of a catheter from the right ventricle through a muscular VSD into the left ventricle is challenging; a snare can be used to cross the defect from the left ventricle and create a "through and through" wire system. In adults, post-infarction VSDs are generally unsuitable for device closure, and surgical repair is usually recommended. Successful transcatheter VSD closure has been described for post-infarction ventricular septal defects[84,85] in patients with prohibitive surgical risk or residual shunting after surgical repair.[82]

E. OTHER PROCEDURES

1. **Creating a Fontan Fenestration.** Patients who develop protein-losing enteropathy after Fontan procedure may benefit from creation of a Fontan fenestration.[55,56] Stent placement is often needed to maintain patency of the fenestration, since balloon/blade septostomy is often ineffective due to elastic recoil and early occlusion.

2. **Balloon Atrial Septostomy.** Balloon atrial septostomy was first described by Rashkind and Miller in 1966 as a palliative procedure for transposition of the great arteries, to enhance mixing of pulmonary and systemic venous blood.[57] Blade atrial septostomy was first described by Park et al in 1975[58] and has been shown to be safe and effective, even in adult patients. For patients with severe pulmonary hypertension and right heart failure, balloon septostomy with or without blade septostomy can be a life-saving procedure.[59] The procedure may be complicated by transient atrial tachyarrhythmias, perforation of the heart, balloon rupture, embolization, laceration of the atrioventricular valves and systemic/pulmonary veins, and air embolism.[60]

F. ENDOCARDITIS PROPHYLAXIS.
We recommend a short course of periprocedural antibiotics for placement of intracardiac and intravascular prosthetic devices such as stents, coils, buttons, umbrellas, or other occlusive devices. We prescribe a cephalosporin prior to device implantation and then every 6 to 8 hours for a total 3 doses. Following device implantation, endocarditis prophylaxis is usually recommended before certain dental and surgical procedures for at least 6 months (until

endothelialization occurs).[1]   When closure of ASDs, VSDs, and PDAs is associated with residual shunting, we recommend lifelong endocarditis prophylaxis prior to invasive procedures.

* * * * *

REFERENCES

1. Allen HD, Beekman RH, Garson A, Hijazi Zm, Mullins C, O'Laughlin MP, Tauber KA. Pediatric therapeutic cardiac catheterization: a statement for healthcare professionals from the council on cardiovascular disease in the young, American Heart Association. Circulation 1998;97:609-25.
2. Moore JW, Cambier PA. Transcatheter occlusion of patent ductus arteriosus. J Intervent Cardiol 1995;l8:517-531.
3. White RI, Strandberg JV, Gross GS, Barth KH. Therapeutic embolization with long-term occluding agents and their effects on embolized tissues. Radiology 1977;125:677-87.
4. Moore JW and Berdjis F. Coil occlusion of congenital vascular malformation and surgical shunts. Progress in Pediatric Cardiology 1996;6:149-159.
5. Grifka RG, Mulins CE, Vincent JA, McMahon WS, Nihill MR, O'Laughlin MP, Slack MC, et al. New Gianturco-Grifka vascular occlusion device. Initial studies in a canine model. Circulation 1995;91:1840-1846.
6. Portsman W, Wierny L, Warnke H, Gerstberger G, Romaniuk PA. Catheter closure of patent ductus arteriosus. 62 cases treated without thoracotomy. Radiol Clin North Am 1971;9:203-18.
7. Rashkind WJ, Cuaso CC. Transcatheter closure of patent ductus arteriosus: successful use in a 3.5-kilogram infant. Pediatr Cardiol 1979;1:3-7.
8. Hosking MCK, Benson LN, Musewe N, Dyck JD, Freedom RM. Transcatheter occlusion of the persistently patent ductus arteriosus: forty-month follow-up and prevalence of residual shunting. Circulation 1991;84:2313-2317.
9. Latson LA, Hofschire PJ, Kugler JD, Cheatham JP, Gumbiner CH, Danford DA. Trancatheter closure of patent ductus arteriosus in pediatric patient. J Pediatr 1989;115:549-553.
10. Rao PS, Sideris EB, Haddad J, Rey C, Hausdorf G, Wilson AD, Smith PA, Chopra PS. Transcatheter occlusion of patent ductus arteriosus with adjustable Buttoned device: initial clinical experience. Circulation 1993;88:1119-26.
11. Verin Ve, Saveliev Vs, Kolody SM, Prokubovski VI. Results of transcatheter closure of the patent ductus arteriosus with the Botalloccluder . J Am Coll Cardiol 1993;22:1509-1514.
12. Cambier PA, Kirby WC, Wortham DC, Moore JW. Percutaneous closure of the small (<2.5 mm) patent ductus arteriosus using coil embolization. Am J Cardiol 1992;69:815-16.
13. Shim D, Fedderly RT, Beekman RH III, Ludomirsky A, Young ML, Schork MA, Lloyd TR. Follow-up of coil occlusion of patent ductus arteriosus. J Am Coll Cardiol 1996;28:207-11.
14. Moore JW. Transcatheter Devices for Congenital Heart Disease meeting. Minneapolis, Minnesota. August 1997.
15. Grifka RG. Transcatheter intervention for the treatment of congenital cardiac defects. Tex Heart Inst J 1997;24:293-300.
16. Masura J, Walsh KP, Thanopoulous B, Chan C, Bass J, Gousous Y, Gavora P, Hijazi ZM. Catheter closure of moderate-to-large -sized patent ductus arteriosus using the new Amplatzer duct occluder: immediate and short-term results. J Am Coll Cardiol 1998;31:878-82.
17. Johnston TA, Stern HJ, and O'Laughlin MP. Transcatheter occlusion of the patent ductus arteriosus: use of the retrievable coil device. Cathet Cardiovasc Intervent 1999;46:434-37.
18. Uzun OM, Hancock S, Parsons JM, Dickinson DF, Gibbs JL. Transcatheter occlusion of the arterial duct with Cook detachable coils: early experience. Heart 1996;76;269-73.
19. Ometzki AJP, Arnold R, Peart I, Sreeram N, Abdulhamed JM, Godman MJ, Pael RG, Kichiner DJ, Bu'Lock FA, Walsh KP. Transcatheter occlusion of the patent ductus arteriosus with Cook detachable coils. Heart 1996;76:531-535.
20. Akagi T, Hashino K, Sugimura T, Ishii M, Eto G, Kato H. Coil occlusion of patent ductus arteriosus with detachable coils. Am Heart J 1997;41:396-91.
21. Podnar T, Masura J. Percutaneous closure of patent ductus arteriosus using special screwing detachable coils. Cathet Cardiovasc Diagn 199741:386-91.
22. Celiker A, Qureshi SA, Bilgic A, Carminati M, Kirk R, Rosenthal E, Alehan D, Giusti, S, Baker EJ, Tynam E. Transcatheter closure of patent arterial ducts using controlled-release coils. Eur Heart J 1997;18:450-54.
23. Lois JF, Gomes AS, Smith DC, Laks H. Systemic-to-pulmonary collateral vessels an shunts; treatment with embolization. Radiology 1988;169:671-76.
24. Perry SSB, Radtke W, Fellows KE, Keane JF, Lock JE. Coil embolization to occlude aortopulmonary collateral vessels and shunts in patients with congenital heart disease. J Am Coll Cardiol 1989;13:100-108.
25. Rothman A, Tong AD. Percutaneous coil embolization of superfluous vascular connections in patients with congenital heart disease. Am Heart J 1993;126:206-13.
26. Forbess LW, O'Laughlin MP, Harrison JK. Partially anomalous pulmonary venous connection: demonstration of dual drainage allowing nonsurgical correction. Cathet Cardiovasc Diagn 1998;44:330-335.
27. Semb BKJ, Tjonneland S, Stake G, Aabyholm G. 'Balloon valvulotomy' of congenital pulmonary valve stenosis with tricuspid valve insufficiency. Cardiovasc Radiol 19792:239-41.
28. Kan JS, Whie RI Jr, Mitchell Se, Gardner TJ. Percutaneous balloon valvuloplasty: a new method for treating congenital pulmonary valve stenosis. N Engl J Med 1982;307:540-42.
29. Kaul UA, Singh B, Yagi S, Bhargava M, Arora R, Khalilullah M. Long-term results after balloon pulmonary valvuloplasty in adults. Am Heart J 1993;126:1152-5.

30. Mendelsohn AM, Banerjee A, Meyer RA, Schwartz DC. Predictors of successful pulmonary balloon valvuloplasty: 10-year experience. Cathet Cardiovasc Diagn 1996;39:236-43.

31. Brock RC. Control mechanisms in outflow tract of the right ventricle in health and disease. Guys Hosp Rep 1955;104:356-60.

32. Fawzy ME, Gala O, Dunn B, Shaikh A, Sriram R, Furan CMG. Regression of infundibular pulmonary stenosis after successful balloon pulmonary valvuloplasty in adults. Cathet Cardiovasc Diagn 1990;1:77-81.

33. Eagle MA, Holswade GR, Goldberg HP, Lukas DS, Glenn F. Regression after open valvotomy of infundibular stenosis accompanying severe pulmonic stenosis. Circulation 1958;17:862-873.

34. Fontes VS, Esteves CA, SousaJE, Silva MVD, Bembom MCB. Regression of infundibular hypertrophy after pulmonary valvuloplasty for pulmonic stenosis. Am J Cardiol 1988;62:977-79.

35. Moore P, Egio E, Mowrey H, Perry SB, Lock JE, Keane JF. Midterm results of balloon dilation of congenital aortic stenosis: Predictors of success. J Am Coll Cardiol. 196;27:1257-1263.

36. Sandhu SK, Silka MJ, Reller MD. Balloon aortic valvuloplasty for aortic stenosis in neonates, children and young adults. J Int Cardiol 1995;8:477-86.

37. Lababidi Z, Weinhaus L, Soeckle H Jr, Walls JT. Transluminal balloon dilatation for discrete subaortic stenosis. Am J Cardiol 1987;59:423-25.

38. Suarez de Lezo J, Pan M, Medina A, Romero M, Melian F, Segua J, Hernandez E, Pavlovic D, Morales J, Vivancos R, et al. Immediate and follow-up results of transluminal balloon dilation for discrete subaortic stenosis. J Am Coll Cardiol 1991;18:1309-1315.

39. Grifka RG, O'Laughlin MP, Nihill MR, Mullins CE. Double-transeptal, double-balloon valvuloplasty for congenital mitral stenosis. Circulation 1992;85:123-129.

40. Ensing G, Hagler DJ, Seward JB, Julsrud PR, Mair DD. Caveats of balloon dilation of conduits and conduit valves. J Am Coll Cardiol 1989;14:397-400.

41. Hoskin MC, Benson LN, Nakanishi , Burrows PE, Williams WG, Freedom RM. Intravascular stent prosthesis for right ventricular outflow obstruction. J Am Coll Cardiol 1992;20:373-80.

42. Lock JE, Niemi T, Einzig S, Amplatz K, Burke B, Bass JL. Transvenous angioplasty of experimental branch pulmonary artery stenosis in newborn lambs. Circulation 1981;64:886-93.

43. Ward CJB, Mullins CE, Nihill MR, Grifka RG, Vick GW III. Use of intravascular stents in systemic venous and systemic venous baffle obstructions; short-term follow-up results. Circulation 1995;91:2948-2954.

44. Dodds GA III, Harrison JK, O'Laughlin MP, Wilson JS, Kisslo KB, Bashore TM. Relief of superior vena cava syndrome due to fibrosing mediastinitis using the Palmaz stent. Chest 1994;106:315-318.

45. Ino T, Ohkubo M. Dilation mechanism, causes of restenosis and stenting in balloon coarctation angioplasty. Acta Paediatr 1997;86:367-71.

46. Fletcher SE, Nihill MR, Grifka RG, O'Luahglin MP, Mullins CE. Balloon angioplasty of native coarctation of the aorta: midterm follow-up and prognostic factors. J Am Coll Cardiol 1995;25:730-4.

47. Shaddy RE, Boucek MM, Sturtevant JE, Rutenberg HD, Jaffe RB, Tani LY, Judd VE, Veasy LG, McGough EC, Orsmond GS. Comparison of angioplasty and surgery for unoperated coarctation of the aorta. Circulation 1993;87:793-799.

48. Johnson MC, Caner CE, Strauss AW, and Spray TL. Repair of coarctation of the aorta in infancy: comparison of surgical and balloon angioplasty. Am Heart J 1993;125:464.

49. Hellenbrand We, Allen HD, Golinko RJ, Hagler DJ, Lutin W, Kan J. Balloon angioplasty for aortic recoarctation: results of valvuloplasty and Angioplasty of Congenital Anomalies Registry. Am J Cardiol 1990;65:793-97.

50. Giovanni JV, Lip GYH, Osman K, Mohan M, Ismail FI, Jayant G, Watson RDS, Singh SP. Percutaneous Balloon dilatation of aortic coarctation in adults. Am J Cardiol 1996;77:435-438.

51. Ritter SB. Coarctation and balloons: inflated or realistic? J Am Coll Cardiol 1989;13:696-699.

52. Guvendik L, Sarkar K, Dye J, Aber C. Aortic rupture and false aneurysm formation following balloon angioplasty of coarctation in an adult: successful treatment by urgent surgery. Cardiovasc Surg 1994;2:467-469.

53. Ebeid MR, Prieto LR, Latson LA. Use of balloon-expandable stents for coarctation of the aorta: initial results and intermediate-term follow-up. J Am Coll Cardiol 1997;30:1847-52.

54. Rao PS. Stents in treatment of aortic coarctation. J Am Coll Cardiol 1997;30:1853-55.

55. Warnes CA, Fledt RH, Hagler DJ. Protein-losing enteropathy after the Fontan operation: successful treatment by percutaneous fenestration of the atrial septum. May Clin Proc 1996;71:378-379.

56. Miga DE, Clark JM, Coart KS, Radtke WA. Transcatheter fenestration of hemi-Fontan baffles after completion of Fontan physiology using balloon dilatation and stent placement. Cathet Cardiovasc Diagn 1998;43:429-32.

57. Rashkind WJ, Miller WW. Creation of atrial septal defect without thoracotomy: a palliative approach to complete transposition of the great arteries. JAMA 1966;196:991-92.

58. Park SC, Zuberbuhler JR, Neches WH, Lenox CC, Zoltun RA. A new atrial septostomy technique. Cathet Cardiovasc Diagn. 1975;124:428-35.

59. Rich S, Lam, W. Atrial septostomy as palliative therapy for refractory primary pulmonary hypertension. Am J Cardiol 1983;511560-1561.

60. Ali Khan MA, Bricker JT, Mullins CE, al Yousef S, Nihill MR, Vargo TA. Blade atrial septostomy: experience with the first 50 procedures. Cathet Cardiovasc Diagn 1991;23:257-262.

61. King D, Thompson SL, Steiner C, Mills NL. Secundum atrial septal defect: nonoperative closure during cardiac catheterization. JAMA 1976;235:2506-2509.

62. Latson LA. Per-catheter ASD closure. Pediatr Cardiol 1998;19:86-93.

63. Lock JE, Rome JJ, Davis R, Van Praagh S, Perry SB, Ban Praagh R, Keane JF. Transcatheter closure of atrial septal

defectrs: experimental studies. Circulation 1989;79:1091-1099.

64. Jenkins KJ, Newburger JW, Faherty C, Hollesen A, Wise J, Swyer M, Woolsey L, Lock JE. Midterm follow-up using the original Bard clamshell septal occluder. Complete experience at one center. Circulation 1995;92(suppl 1):I-308. Abstract.

65. Moore P, Benson LN, Berman Jr W, Cetta F, Hellenbrand WE, Latson LA, Lock JE, Mulliins CE, Orsmond GS, Rome J, Zahn E. CardioSEAL device closure of secundum ASDs: how effective is it? Circulation 1998;98:(suppl I-754)3955. Abstract

66. Sideris EB, Sideris SE, Fowlkes JP, Ehly RL, Smith JE, Gulde RE. Transvenous atrial septal defect occlusion in piglets with a Buttoned double disk device. Circulation 1991;81:312-318.

67. Sideris EB, Leung M, Yoon JH, Chen CR, Lochan R, Worms AM, Rey C, Meier B. Occlusion of large atrial septal defects with a centering Buttoned device:; early clinical experience. Am Hear J. 1996;131:356-359.

68. Rao PS, Sideris EB. Follow-up results of transcatheter occlusion of secundum atrial septal defects with the Buttoned device. Cathet Cardiovasc Diagn 1996;38:112. Abstract.

69. Arabia F, Rosado LJ, Lloyd R, Sehi GK. Management of complications of Sideris transcatheter devices for atrial septal defect closure. J Thorac Cardiovasc Surg 1993;106:886-888.

70. Syamasundar-Rao P, Berger F, Rey C, Walsh K, de Lezo JS, Haddad J, Chander JS, Lloyd TR, Sideris EB. Transcatheter closure secundum atrial septal defects with fourth generation Buttoned device: immediate and short-term results. Circulation 1998;98(suppl I-414)2179.

71. Lloyd TR, Syamasundar R, Beekman RH, Mendelsohn AM, Sideris EB. Atrial septal defect occlusion with the Buttoned device (a multi-institutional U. S. Trial). Am J Cardiol 1994;73:286-291.

72. Das GS, Voss G, Jarvis G, Wyche K, Gunher R, Wilson RF. Experimental atrial septal defect closure with a new, transcatheter, self-centering device. Circulation 1993;88(p 1):1754-1764.

73. Das Gs, Hijazi ZM, O'Laughlin MP, Mendelsohn AM. Initial results of the US PFO/ASD closure trial. J Am Coll Cardiol 1996;27(Suppl A):119A. Abstract

74. Sievert H, Babic UU, Ensslen R, Schere D,Spies H, Wiederspahn T, Seplin HE. Transcatheter closure of large atrial septal defects with the Babi system. Cathet Cardiovasc Diagn 1995;36:232-240.

75. Sievert H, Babic UU, Hausdorf G, Schneider M, Hopp HW, Pfeiffer D, Pfisterer M, Friedli B, Urban P. Transcatheter closure of atrial septal defect and patent foramen ovale with ASDOS device (a multi-institutional European trial). Am J Cardiol 1998;82:1405-13.

76. Masura J, Gavora P, Formanek A, Hijazi ZM. Transcatheter closure of secundum atrial septal defects using the new self-centering Amplatzer Septal occluder: initial human experience. Cathet Cardiovasc Diagn 1997;42:388-93.

77. Cao Q-L, Hijazi ZM, Berger F, Lange PE, Radtke W, Fontes V, Pazzanesse D, Walsh KP. Transcatheter closure of multiple atral septal defects (ASD) using two Amplatzer Septal Occluder (ASO) devices: initial results. Circulation 1998;98(suppl I-414)2177. Abstract

78. Formigari R, Santoro Giuseppe, Rossetti L, Rinelli G, Guccione P, Ballerini L. Comparison of three different atrial septal defect occlusion devices. Am J Cardiol 1998;82:690-92.

79. Walsh KP, Tofeig M, Kichiner DJ, Peart I, Arnold R. Comparison of the Sideris and Amplatzer septal occlusion devices. Am J Cardiol 1999;83:933-36.

80. Kumar K, Lock JE, Geva T. Apical muscular ventricular septal defects between the left ventricle and the right ventricular infundibulum. Diagnostic and interventional considerations. Circulation 1997;95:1207-13.

81. Murzi B, Bonanomi GL, Giusti S, Luisi VS, Bernabei M, Carminati M, Vanini V. Surgical closure of muscular ventricular septal defects using double umbrella devices (intraoperative VSD device closure). Eur J Cardiothorac Surg 1997;12:450-55.

82. Sideris EB, Walsh KP, Haddad JL, Chen CR, Ren SG, Kulkarni H. Occlusion of congenital ventricular septal defects by the Buttoned device. "Buttoned device" Clinical Trials International Register. Heart 1997 77;276-9.

83. Thanopoulos BD, Tsaousis GS, Konstadopoulou GN, Zarayelyan AG. Transcatheter closure of muscular ventricular septal defects with the Amplatzer ventricular septal defect occluder: initial clinical applications in children. J Am Coll Cardiol 1999;33:1395-1399.

84. Landzberg MJ, Lock JE. Transcatheter management of ventricular septal rupture after myocardial infarction. Semin Thorac Cardiovasc Surg 1998;10:128-32.

85. Benton JP, Barker KS. Transcatheter closure of ventricular septal defect: a nonsurgical approach to the care of the patient with acute ventricular septal rupture. Heart Lung 1992;21:356-64.

86. Moore JW, Berdjus F. Coil occlusion of congenital vascular malformation and surgical shunts. Prog Pediatric Cardiol 1996;6:149-159.

87. Grifka RG. Transcatheter intervention for the treatment of congenital cardiac defects. Tex Heart Inst J 1997,24:293-300.

88. Rashkind WJ, Mullins CE, Hellenbrand WE, et al. Nonsurgical closure of patent ductus arteriosus: clinical application of the Rashkind PDA occluder system. Circulation 1987;75:583-592.

89. Sideris EB, Leung M, Yoon JH, et al. Occlusion of large artrial septal defects with a centering buttoned device and early clinical experience. Am Heart J 1996;131:356.

90. Moore JW. In: Transcatheter Devices for Congenital Heart Disease. 1997. Symposium. Minneapolis MN.

III

Complications

19 CORONARY ARTERY SPASM

Mark S. Freed, M.D.

A. BALLOON ANGIOPLASTY

1. **Intralesional Spasm.** Coronary artery spasm has been reported in 1-5% of balloon angioplasty procedures.[1,2] Predisposing factors include noncalcified lesions,[1,3] eccentric lesions,[4] and younger patients, but not variant angina.[5,6] Intravascular ultrasound may be useful in cases where it is difficult to distinguish refractory spasm from dissection. Fortunately, most cases can be successfully treated by intracoronary nitrates and/or calcium antagonists; repeat PTCA at low inflation pressures is effective, but is rarely necessary.

2. **Distal Epicardial Spasm.** Spasm of the distal vessel is common after percutaneous intervention.[7-9] Distal epicardial spasm can be reversed by intracoronary nitroglycerin or prevented by continuous intravenous nitroglycerin. Serotonin released from circulating platelets plays an important pathogenic role; ketanserin, a selective serotonin$_2$-receptor antagonist, can blunt distal epicardial spasm after PTCA.[9,10] Pretreatment with aspirin does not reliably prevent distal spasm.[8]

3. **Microvascular Spasm.** In contrast to epicardial spasm, spasm of the microvascular bed rarely responds to nitrates. The incidence, risk factors, and management of this condition are reviewed in the chapter on "no-reflow" (Chapter 21).

4. **Post-Procedural Spasm.** The PTCA site remains susceptible to spasm for several months after the procedure; ergonovine[11] and acetylcholine[12] can induce vasospasm after PTCA in 15% and 46% of patients, respectively. Spontaneous episodes of spasm may cause angina in the weeks or months following PTCA.[6,11]

B. PATHOPHYSIOLOGY.

Percutaneous devices result in coronary endothelial denudation and loss of nitric oxide, which increases sensitivity to local vasoconstrictors (e.g., serotonin from aggregating platelets) and decreases sensitivity to local vasodilators (e.g., prostacyclin, prostaglandin E$_2$).[13] Other putative mechanisms include increased production or impaired degradation of norepinephrine or platelet-derived vasoconstrictors (thromboxane, serotonin, platelet-activating factor), altered arachidonic acid metabolism (resulting in the overproduction of vasoconstricting prostanoids and leukotrienes), release of endothelium-derived contractile factor (EDCF), local adrenergic nerve dysfunction, and stimulation of stretch-dependent myogenic tone.[7-10,14-16] A decrease in forearm bloodflow and an increase in vascular resistance have been observed after coronary angioplasty; these changes were abolished by pretreatment with phentolamine (α-blocker) or verapamil,[17] suggesting the presence of a generalized neural or hormonal mechanism.[18]

C. **NON-BALLOON DEVICES.** Compared to PTCA, coronary artery spasm after other devices appears to occur with equal or greater frequency.[19-27] Spasm has been reported in 4-36% of Rotablator cases,[16,24,28,29,37] but severe spasm resulting in abrupt occlusion requiring repeat PTCA or CABG is less common (< 2%).[19] Spasm was reported in 1.2-16% of laser procedures but is very uncommon with current saline infusion techniques (Chapter 30).[21,22,25-27,30] Coronary spasm following these devices responds to intracoronary nitrates.

D. **MANAGEMENT (Figure 19.1)**

1. **Nitrates.** Coronary artery spasm usually resolves promptly to intracoronary nitroglycerin (200-300 mcg), but higher doses may be needed in some patients. Patients receiving IV, oral, or transdermal nitroglycerin without a nitrate-free interval may not respond to intracoronary nitroglycerin (or may require a higher dose), due to nitrate tolerance.

2. **Removal of Interventional Hardware.** If intralesional spasm is evident, the guidewire should remain across the lesion to maintain vascular access while nitroglycerin is administered. If spasm occurs distal to the target lesion, partial or complete removal of the guidewire may be required for the spasm to resolve.

3. **Calcium Antagonists.** Intracoronary verapamil (100 mcg/min up to 1.0-1.5 mg)[31] or intracoronary diltiazem (0.5-2.5 mg over 1 minute, up to 5-10 mg)[32] may reverse coronary spasm refractory to intracoronary nitroglycerin. A temporary transvenous pacemaker should be readily available, although the risk of AV block, bradycardia, and hypotension is low.

4. **Repeat Balloon Dilatation.** If intralesional spasm persists despite nitrates and intracoronary calcium antagonists, a prolonged (2-5 minute) low-pressure (1-4 atm.) inflation using a balloon matched to the reference segment is frequently successful at "breaking" the spasm. In fact, the vast majority of episodes of spasm respond to nitrates and repeat PTCA. "Refractory spasm" is probably due to dissection and should respond to stenting.

5. **Anticholinergics.** Acetylcholine may induce paradoxical vasoconstriction in de-endothelialized arteries,[33] presumably due to a local loss of nitric oxide and a direct vasoconstrictor effect on vascular smooth muscle. Therefore, if spasm is accompanied by hypotension and bradycardia, atropine may be administered (0.5 mg IV every 5 minutes to a total of 2.0 mg).

6. **Systemic Circulatory Support.** A rare management dilemma may arise when severe spasm is associated with ischemia and hypotension, since administration of nitrates or calcium antagonists may exacerbate hypotension and lead to further clinical deterioration. In this setting, it is best to proceed with intracoronary nitrates or calcium antagonists while preparing to support the systemic circulation with IABP. Alpha-adrenergic drugs (phentolamine) may exacerbate vasospasm and should be avoided, but inotropes such as dobutamine can be used if needed.

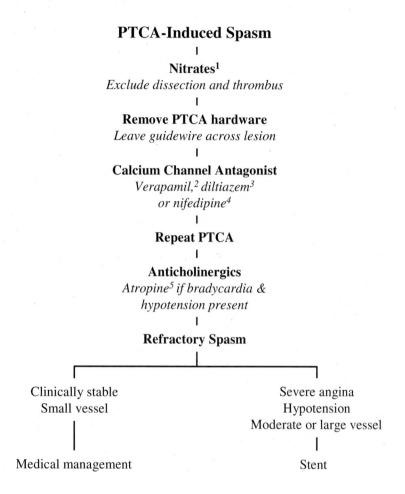

PTCA-Induced Spasm
|
Nitrates[1]
Exclude dissection and thrombus
|
Remove PTCA hardware
Leave guidewire across lesion
|
Calcium Channel Antagonist
Verapamil,[2] diltiazem[3]
or nifedipine[4]
|
Repeat PTCA
|
Anticholinergics
Atropine[5] if bradycardia &
hypotension present
|
Refractory Spasm

Clinically stable   Severe angina
Small vessel   Hypotension
                           Moderate or large vessel

Medical management   Stent

Figure 19.1. Management of Intraprocedural Spasm

1. Nitroglycerin 100-300 mcg IC bolus + intravenous infusion (20 mcg/min)
2. Verapamil 100 mcg/min IC up to 1.5 mg; temporary pacemaker on standby
3. Diltiazem 0.5-1 mg IC over 1 min up to 2.5-5.0 mg as needed; temporary pacemaker on standby
4. Nifedipine 10 mg sublingual
5. Atropine 0.5 mg IV; may repeat every 5 min up to 2.0 mg

7. **Stents.** Intracoronary stenting has been used successfully for refractory spasm, but should be reserved for situations in which all other nonoperative alternatives have failed. Most such cases of "refractory" spasm are probably dissections, which should respond to stenting.

8. **Superimposed Coronary Dissection and Thrombus.** Multiple angiographic views of the target lesion should be obtained to exclude superimposed dissection and/or thrombus. Intravascular ultrasound may help clarify the nature of the lesion and guide further therapy.

E. PREVENTION. A continuous intravenous infusion of nitroglycerin (10-50 mcg/min) may prevent distal spasm and is used routinely at our institution for most patients undergoing coronary intervention.

PTCA FOR VARIANT ANGINA

Patients with variant (Prinzmetal's) angina present with unpredictable bouts of effort angina or rest pain and ST-segment changes due to spontaneous coronary vasospasm. Dynamic obstruction of coronary blood flow may occur in angiographically normal coronary arteries, but is more common in vessels with moderate or severe fixed stenoses.[34] Although medical management alone is effective in the majority of cases, some patients continue to have disabling symptoms rarely leading to MI or sudden death. The prognosis is worse when tachy- or bradyarrhythmias occur during episodes of pain, and when spasm is superimposed on fixed lesions.[34] Compared to patients undergoing surgery for classic angina pectoris, coronary artery bypass grafting with or without sympathetic denervation is associated with a higher incidence of post-operative MI, early graft closure, and recurrent angina.[35] PTCA and stenting have occasionally been applied to patients with spasm superimposed on fixed lesions.[39] Small observational reports suggest a number of general conclusions (Table 19.1).[5,6,36,38]

Table 19.1. Results of PTCA for Organic Stenoses in Variant Angina

A high technical success rate can be achieved

Procedural complications, including PTCA-induced coronary artery spasm, are no more frequent than during PTCA for other types of coronary disease

Recurrent spasm and rest angina are not uncommon following PTCA; pharmacologic therapy with nitrates and calcium antagonists may reduce their frequency and severity

Restenosis rates are approximately 50%

Many patients derive symptomatic benefit, although the impact on event-free survival (compared to medical therapy or CABG) has not been evaluated

The role of other interventional devices is unknown

REFERENCES

1. Cowley M, Dorros G, Kelsey S, Van Raden M, Detre K. Acute coronary events associated with percutaneous transluminal coronary angioplasty. Am J Cardiol 1984;53:12C-16C.

2. Holmes DJ, Holubkov R, Vlietstra R, et al. Comparison of complications during percutaneous transluminal coronary angioplasty from 1977 to 1981 and from 1985 to 1986: The National Heart, Lung, and Blood Institute Percutaneous Transluminal Coronary Angioplasty Registry. J Am Coll Cardiol 1988;12:1149-1155.

3. Fitzgerald PJ, Stertzer SH, Hidalgo BO, et al. Plaque characteristics affect lesion and vessel response to coronary rotational atherectomy: An intravascular ultrasound study. J Am Coll Cardiol 1994:March Special Issue:353A.

4. Fischell T, and Bausback K. Effects of luminal eccentricity on spontaneous coronary vasoconstriction after successful percutaneous transluminal coronary angioplasty. Am J Cardiol 1991;68:530-534.

5. Corcos T, David PR, Bourassa MG, et al. Percutaneous transluminal coronary angioplasty for the treatment of variant angina. J Am Coll Cardiol 1985;5:1046-1054.

6. David PR, Waters DD, Scholl M, et al. Percutaneous coronary angioplasty in patients with variant angina. Circulation 1982;66:695-702.

7. Indolfi C, Piscione F, Esposito G, et al. Mechanisms of coronary vasoconstriction after successful single angioplasty of the left anterior descending artery. J Am Coll Cardiol 1993:February Special Issue:340A.

8. Fischell T, Derby G, Tse T, Stadius M. Coronary artery vasoconstriction routinely occurs after percutaneous transluminal coronary angioplasty. A quantitative arteriographic analysis. Circulation 1988;78:1323-1334.

9. Golino P, Piscione F, Benedict CF, et al. Local effect of serotonin released during coronary angioplasty. N Engl J Med 1994;330:523-8.

10. Tousoulis D, Tentolouris C, Apostolopoulos T, Toutouzas P. Effects of intracoronary ketanserin in proximal and distal segments post angioplasty. J Am Coll Cardiol 1993:February Special Issue:341A.

11. Hollman J, Austin GE, Gruentzig AR, et al. Coronary artery spasm at the site of angioplasty in the first two months after successful percutaneous transluminal coronary angioplasty. J Am Coll Cardiol 1983;2:1039-1045.

12. Kirigaya H, Aizawa T, Ogasaware K, et al. Enhanced vasospastic activity to acetylcholine of the coronary arteries undergoing previous balloon angioplasty. J Am Coll Cardiol 1993:February Special Issue:341A.

13. Cohen RA, Shepherd JT, and Vanhoutte PM. Inhibitory role of endothelium in the response of isolated coronary arteries to platelets. Science 1983;221:273-274.

14. Lam JT, Chesebro JH, Steele PM, et al. Vasospasm related to platelet deposition? Relationship in a porcine preparation of arterial injury in vivo. Circulation 1987;75:243-248.

15. Cohen RA, Zitany KM and Weisbrod RM. Accumulation of 5-hydroxy-tryptamine leads to dysfunction of adrenergic nerves in canine coronary artery following intimal damage in vivo. Circulation 1987;61:829-833.

16. Gregorini L, Marco J, Fajadet J, Brunel, P, et al. Urapidil (α 1-sympathetic blocker) attenuates post-rotational ablation "elastic recoil". Circulation 1995;92:I-94.

17. Ceravolo R, Piscoine F, Malone A, Stingone AM, et al. Reflex forearm vasoconstriction after successful angioplasty of the left anterior descending coronary artery. Circulation 1995;92:I-323.

18. Ceravolo R, Indolfi C, Piscione F, et al. Coronary and limb vascular vasoconstriction after successful single angioplasty of the left anterior descending coronary artery. J Am Coll Cardiol 1995;February Special Issue:108A.

19. Warth D, Leon M, et al. Rotational atherectomy multicenter registry: Acute results, complications and 6-month angiographic follow-up in 709 patients. J Am Coll Cardiol 1994;24:641-648.

20. deMarchena EJ, Mallon SM, et al. Effectiveness of holmium laser-assisted coronary angioplasty. Am J Cardiol 1994;73:117-121.

21. Bittl J, Sanborn T, et al. Clinical success, complications and restenosis rates with excimer laser coronary angioplasty. Am J Cardiol 1992;70:1533-1539.

22. Ghazzal Z, Hearn J, et al. Morphological predictors of acute complications after percutaneous excimer laser coronary angioplasty. Results of a comprehensive angiographic analysis: Importance of the eccentricity index. Circulation 1992;86:820-827.

23. Hinohara T, Rowe M, et al. Effect of lesion characteristics on outcome of directional coronary atherectomy. J Am Coll Cardiol 1991;17:1112-1120.

24. Safian R, Niazi K, et al. Detailed Angiographic Analysis of High-Speed Mechanical Rotational Atherectomy in Human Coronary Arteries. Circulation 1993;88:961-968.

25. Litvack F, Eigler N, et al. Percutaneous excimer laser coronary angioplasty: Results in the first consecutive 3,000 patients. J Am Coll Cardiol 1994;23:323-9.

26. Baumback A, Bittl J, Fleck E, et al. Acute complications of excimer laser coronary angioplasty: A detailed analysis of multicenter results. J Am Coll Cardiol 1994;23:1305-1313.

27. Mehta S, Popma JJ, Margolis JR, et al. Angiographic complications after new device angioplasty in native coronary arteries: A NACI Angiographic Core Laboratory Report. TCT Meeting (Washington DC),February, 1995.

28. Bertrand M, Lablanche J, Leroy F, Bauters C. Percutaneous transluminal coronary rotary ablation with Rotablator (European experience). Am J Cardiol 1992;69:470-474.

29. Teirstein PS, Warth DC, Haq N, et al. High-speed rotational coronary atherectomy for patients with diffuse coronary artery disease. J Am Coll Cardiol 1991;18:1694-1701.

30. Initial results of the European Multicenter Registry on Coronary Excimer Laser Angioplasty. European Study Group. Circulation 1991;84:II-362.

31. Babbitt DG, Perry JM, and Forman MB. Intracoronary verapamil for reversal of refractory coronary vasospasm during percutaneous transluminal coronary angioplasty. J Am Coll Cardiol 1988;12:1377-1381.

32. McIvor ME, Undemir C, Lawson J, Reddinger J. Clinical effects and utility of intracoronary diltiazem. Cathet Cardiovasc Diagn. 1995;35:287-291.

33. Ludmer PL. Selwyn AP, Shook TL, et al. Paradoxical vasoconstriction induced by acetylcholine in atherosclerotic coronary arteries. N Engl J Med 1988;315:1046-1051.

34. Waters DD, Miller DD, Szlachcic J, et al. Factors influencing the long-term prognosis of treated patients with variant angina. Circulation 1983;63:258-265.

35. Gaasch WH, Lufshanowski R, Leachment RD, et al. Surgical management of Prinzmetal's variant angina. Chest 1974;66:614-621.

36. Bertrand ME, LaBlanche JM, Thieuleux FA, et al. Comparative results of percutaneous transluminal coronary angioplasty in patients with dynamic versus fixed coronary stenosis. J Am Coll Cardiol 1986;8:504-508.

37. Mehta S, Popma J, Margolis JR, et al. Complications with new angioplasty devices. Are these device-specific? J Am Coll Cardiol 1996;27:168A.

38. Marzilli M, Sabbadini G, et al. Coronary stenting for Prinzmetal's angina. Circulation 1996;94:I-454.

39. Kaul U, Singh B, Fotedar J, Shyamsunder N. Coronary stenting for refractory coronary vasospasm of proximal left anterior descending artery. J Invas Cardiol 1998;10(2):95-97.

20 DISSECTION AND ACUTE CLOSURE

Mark S. Freed, M.D.
William W. O'Neill, M.D.
Robert D. Safian, M.D.

Prior to widespread use of coronary stents, dissection leading to acute coronary occlusion was the major cause of in-hospital death, myocardial infarction, and emergency CABG following percutaneous intervention. In contemporary practice, dissection leading to acute closure is extremely unusual, since virtually all significant dissections are treated by coronary stents, clearly the most important mechanical tool for treating dissection, reversing acute closure, and reducing the risk of subsequent ischemic complications.[139] Dissection is still an important cause of ischemic complications, but usually occurs as a manifestation of edge dissections following stenting, which may predispose to stent thrombosis.

A. **CLASSIFICATION.** Acute coronary occlusion has often been classified according to angiographic appearance and coronary flow after percutaneous intervention:
   - **Acute closure:** Total occlusion with TIMI 0-1 flow.
   - **Imminent closure:** Acute worsening of stenosis severity with TIMI 2 flow
   - **Threatened closure:** Angiographic appearance of dissection or thrombus causing > 50% residual stenosis post-intervention with normal (TIMI 3) flow.

B. **INCIDENCE AND TIMING OF ACUTE CLOSURE.** In the pre-stent era, acute closure occurred in 2-11% of elective PTCAs;[1-4] 50-80% occurred while the patient was still in the catheterization laboratory, and the rest usually occurred within 6 hours of case completion.[5-7] Late acute closure (more than 24 hours after PTCA) was more common after primary PTCA for acute MI and after PTCA for chronic total occlusion. The incidence of acute closure after laser or atherectomy was similar to or greater than that after PTCA,[9-20,14,21,38,104,107] and delayed occlusion 1-2 days after intervention was not unusual.[14,21,38] In contrast to other devices, stents have reduced the incidence of acute closure to < 1%.[106] Although subacute stent thrombosis occurred in 2.5% of patients 2-11 days after stenting using older warfarin-based regimens, the incidence of subacute stent thrombosis has declined dramatically with the use of current antiplatelet strategies (Chapter 26).

C. **CAUSES OF ACUTE CLOSURE.** Histopathological studies confirmed that dissection was the most common cause of acute closure after PTCA, followed by elastic recoil, spasm, and vessel thrombosis.[140]
   1. **Coronary Artery Dissection.** Small intimal dissections are frequent after PTCA, laser, and atherectomy devices, but are usually associated with a benign course. In contrast, untreated complex dissections may cause acute closure, and are virtually always treated with stents. The ideal treatment for dissections not associated with vessel closure or impaired flow is unknown, but most operators rely on stents to stabilize the lumen and prevent acute closure, particularly when dissection types C-F are observed (Table 20.1).

a. **Classification.** Coronary artery dissection is usually defined angiographically by the NHLBI criteria (Table 20.1). Types A and B are considered "minor" dissections since they do not adversely impact procedural outcome. In contrast, types C - F are considered "major" dissections and were associated with a 5-10-fold higher risk of myocardial infarction, emergency CABG, or death prior to the availability of stents.[128] Dissections that are long (> 10 mm) or result in > 50% residual stenosis also increase the risk of ischemic complications and represent reasonable indications for stenting even in the absence of flow impairment.

b. **Incidence of Dissection.** Following balloon angioplasty, coronary dissection is detected by angiography in 20-40% of cases[2,23-26] and by intravascular ultrasound (IVUS) and angioscopy in 60-80% of cases.[27,28] Non-flow-limiting dissections should be not necessarily be considered a complication, since the mechanism of lumen enlargement for PTCA involves stretching of the vessel wall and cracking of plaque, which manifest as dissection. Commonly, PTCA results in a hazy appearance by angiography which frequently underestimates the extent of dissection and residual stenosis (Chapter 31). Other interventional devices may also cause dissection, although the saline infusion technique has reduced the high incidence of dissection after ELCA[103] (Chapter 30), and dissection after Rotoblator is unusual if proper technique is employed (Chapter 27).

In some situations, angiography may suggest the presence of a dissection when none exists. Weak contrast injections may cause dye streaming and give false impression of an intimal tear. These "pseudo-dissections" are readily identified by better contrast injections to fully opacify the lumen. In addition, deep guide catheter intubation may deform the proximal vessel and suggest the presence of a stenosis or dissection. Repositioning the guide will often correct this problem, and intracoronary nitroglycerin (100-200 mcg) may be useful to relieve associated spasm. Finally, PTCA may cause *pseudolesions*, which manifest angiographically as segmental shelf-like deformities due to excessive straightening and invagination of the vessel wall from extra-support guidewires. Pseudolesions can be very disturbing and easily confused with vessel injury from balloons or other devices. It is important to consider a pseudolesion when a new stenosis appears remote from the target lesion, particularly when stiff guidewires are employed in tortuous vessels or used for tracking new interventional devices. Because of the uncertainty created by pseudolesions, it is generally best to exchange for a flexible guidewire. If the pseudolesion does not improve or resolve, it may be necessary to completely remove the guidewire to ensure that a true stenosis is not present.

Table 20.1. Coronary Artery Dissection: NHLBI Classification System

Type	Description	Angiographic Appearance	Acute Closure (%)
A*	Minor radiolucencies within the lumen during contrast injection with no persistence after dye clearance		-
B*	Parallel tracts or double lumen separated by a radiolucent area during contrast injection with no persistence after dye clearance		3
C	Extraluminal cap with persistence of contrast after dye clearance from the lumen		10
D	Spiral luminal filling defects		30
E**	New persistent filling defects		9
F**	Non-A-E types that lead to impaired flow or total occlusion		69

Abbreviations: NHLBI = National Heart, Lung, and Blood Institute; - = not reported
* No increase in morbidity and mortality when compared to patients without dissections
** May represent thrombus

c. **Pathophysiology of Dissection.** The mechanism of lumen enlargement after PTCA is plaque fracture, intimal splitting, and localized medial dissection. These simple or "therapeutic" dissections may escape detection by angiography or give the appearance of minor intraluminal radiolucencies or haziness. In contrast, complex dissections are characterized by deep medial tears which may create long or spiral dissections. These complex dissections often give the angiographic appearance of either an extraluminal "cap," contrast staining, or residual stenosis > 50%. Complex dissections also expose collagen and tissue factor to circulating platelets and other blood elements, increasing the risk of thrombosis, acute closure, and major ischemic complications. Complex dissections usually require stenting.

1. **Influence of Lesion Calcium.** Dissections after PTCA frequently occur at the junction between calcified and non-calcified plaque, and may be due to nonuniform transmission of dilating force across vessel segments of differing elastic properties.[35] Among calcified lesions treated by Rotablator and adjunctive PTCA, IVUS documented dissection within the plaque after Rotablator, but at the junction of normal vessel wall and calcified atheroma after PTCA.[27]

2. **Laser-Induced Dissection.** Absorption of excimer laser energy produces acoustic shock waves, which may generate pressures of 100 atm and induce vessel trauma manifest as dissection, acute closure, or perforation.[36] The saline infusion technique attenuates acoustic injury and decreases the risk of dissection (Chapter 30).[37,103]

d. **Risk Factors for Dissection after Balloon Angioplasty**. As summarized in Tables 20.2 and 20.3, angiographic, clinical, and procedural variables impact the risk of dissection. All of these studies were performed in the pre-stent era, and although their value for predicting dissection remains, the consequences of dissection have been dramatically reduced by widespread use of stents.

e. **Prognosis After Dissection**
   1. **Ischemic Complications.** Prior to the availability of coronary stents, severe dissection increased the risk of ischemic complications (death, MI, emergency CABG) more than 5-fold.[16,24,61,62] Certain clinical and angiographic features were shown to increase the risk of ischemic complications after untreated dissections (Table 20.4), suggesting that high-risk dissections should by treated by stents, even if antegrade flow is not impaired.[2,22,60,63-65]

   2. **Healing and Restenosis (Table 20.5).** The majority of balloon-induced dissections not resulting in acute ischemic complications disappear with time.[57,58] Follow-up angiography indicates that 4-16% of dissections disappear within 24 hours and 63-93% disappear by 3-6 months.[14,58,59] While small earlier studies suggested a lower incidence of restenosis with dissection, large reports indicate that dissection has no impact on restenosis rates.[25,58,59] Nevertheless, because of the uncertainty about predicting the behavior of dissections after intervention, most operators rely on stents to stabilize the lumen if dissections are observed.

Table 20.2. Angiographic and Clinical Predictors of Dissection after PTCA

Calcified lesions[26,38]

Eccentric lesions[25,38]

Long lesions[26]

Intermediate lesion length[25]

Diffuse disease[26]

Complex lesion morphology (Type B or C)[9]

Vessel curvature[25]

Absence of unstable angina[25]

Table 20.3. Impact of Balloon Angioplasty Design and Technique on Coronary Dissection Rates

Parameter	Effect on Dissection Rate ↑	↓	—	Comments
Balloon catheter design			x	Choice of catheter type (over-the-wire, on-the-wire, monorail) should be based on operator preference.
Balloon material (compliant vs. noncompliant)			x	Compliant balloons have been associated with higher,[40] equal,[41,42] and lower dissection rates,[25] but randomized trials show no difference in clinical outcome.[43,44] High-pressure inflations using compliant balloons for resistant lesions may cause "dog-boning" and increase the risk of dissection.
Balloon sizing	x			Balloon oversizing (balloon-to-artery ratio > 1.2) is a powerful independent predictor of dissection.[26] Attempt to match the balloon diameter to the disease-free distal reference segment (balloon-to-artery ratio = 1.0)
Inflation pressure (high vs. low)			x	Studies are small or retrospective. Most operators use nominal pressure and reserve high-pressure inflations for significant residual stenosis. Inflations exceeding rated burst pressure increase the risk of balloon rupture and vessel dissection. High-pressure inflations using compliant balloons may result in overstretching and dissection.
Duration of inflation (long vs. short)		x		Randomized studies comparing 3 inflations at 1 minute vs. 4-5 minutes demonstrated fewer and less severe dissections with prolonged inflations.[45] Whether multiple short inflations are comparable to fewer long inflations is unknown. Stents negate the value of these observations.
Inflation speed (slow vs. fast)		x		Two randomized studies reported fewer dissections with gradual inflations,[46,47] while no effect was seen in another.[48] Studies also suggest a benefit for gradual, prolonged inflations.[49,50] Stents negate the value of these observations.
Oscillating inflations		x		A nonrandomized study reported major dissections in 0.3% of lesions using this technique.[51] When combined with gradual balloon deflation, more dissections occurred.[52]
Deflation speed (slow vs. fast)	x		.	Gradual deflation resulted in more major dissections in two randomized trials.[52,53] Stents negate the value of these observations.
Predilatation		x		A nonrandomized study reported major dissections in only 1.3% of patients,[54] while no effect was seen in a small randomized study.[55] Use of a dual-balloon catheter (distal balloon to predilate, proximal balloon for final dilatation) resulted in a low dissection rate.[56]
Long-balloon for long lesions		x		See Chapter 15
Noncompliant long-balloon for angled lesions		x		See Chapter 11
Noncompliant balloon for calcified lesions		x		See Chapter 12
Tapered balloon for tapered lesions		x		See Chapter 15

↑ = possible increase; ↓ = possible decrease; — = no effect

Table 20.4. Risk Factors for Major Ischemic Events in the Presence of a Dissection[22,60]

Dissection length > 15 mm

NHLBI dissection types C-F (Table 20.1)

Residual diameter stenosis > 30%

Residual cross-sectional area < 2 mm^2

Transient in-lab occlusion

Unstable angina

Chronic total occlusion

D. RISK FACTORS FOR ACUTE CLOSURE

1. **Acute Closure.** Of the many clinical, angiographic, and procedural variables reported to increase the risk of acute closure (Tables 20.6, 20.7), the most powerful predictor is the presence of a complex dissection (relative risk ~ 6). The need for a scoring system to predict the risk of acute closure has been reduced by the widespread availability of stents (Table 20.8, Figure 20.1).

2. **Cardiac Death After Acute Closure**. Clinical and angiographic variables may identify patients at increased risk of cardiac death after acute closure (Table 20.9). The most powerful predictors are the *jeopardy score* (which estimates net ventricular dysfunction) and blood pressure (Figure 20.2, Table 20.10).[80] However, rapid and reliable stent deployment has improved the ability to revascularize patients with LV dysfunction, treat severe dissections, and reverse acute closure.

E. PREVENTION OF ACUTE CLOSURE

1. **Antiplatelet Agents**
   a. **Aspirin.** Preprocedural aspirin reduces the risk of acute closure by 50-75%.[71] Although the optimal dose and timing are unknown, equivalent reductions in ischemic complications were seen for patients randomly assigned to low-dose (80 mg/day) or high-dose (1500 mg/day) therapy.[81] (Since aspirin absorption may be impaired when coadministered with antacids or H$_2$ blockers, our bias is to avoid low-dose aspirin). Elective intervention should be postponed if the patient has not received aspirin for at least one day prior to the procedure. The addition of dipyridamole to aspirin offers no additional advantage.[133] When urgent intervention is required, the patient should be given chewable aspirin (324 mg). Ticlopidine, clopidogrel, and platelet receptor IIb/IIIa antagonists may also be administered, but their value in patients who are not on aspirin has not been thoroughly evaluated. Further studies are required to determine the role of combined or alternative antiplatelet agents for aspirin-resistant patients, which affects 9% of patients with coronary artery disease.[154]

Table 20.5. Fate of PTCA-Induced Coronary Artery Dissection

Healing[57-59]	The majority of dissections not resulting in acute ischemic complications disappear with time
Restenosis[25,58,59]	The presence of a dissection has no impact on restenosis.
Ischemic[128] complications	The risk of an acute ischemic complication is greatest with dissection type C-F and with post-procedural thrombus

    b. Platelet Receptor IIb/IIIa Inhibitors. GP IIb/IIIa receptor antagonists inhibit platelet aggregation, limit endovascular thrombosis, and improve acute and long-term outcome following coronary intervention (Chapters 5, 34). A controversial issue is the unplanned use of these agents for "rescue" after the development of acute or threatened closure (Tables 9.6, 20.11). In general, nonrandomized trials of rescue abciximab demonstrate a high incidence of early and late ischemic complications, which would not be unexpected in this high-risk group of patients. The strategy of planned vs. provisional use of platelet receptor antagonists awaits clarification.

    c. Clopidogrel, Ticlopidine, Dipyridamole, Dextran (Chapter 34). Clopidogrel has replaced ticlopidine as an adjunct to stenting because of its better safety profile (less neutropenia, hepatitis, skin rash), more rapid onset of action (hours vs. days), and ease of use (once a day vs. twice a day). Clopidogrel is usually given as a single 300 mg oral dose, followed by 75 mg daily for 2-4 weeks. Dextran is no longer used because of the risk of volume overload and anaphylaxis, and the availability of more effective antiplatelet agents. There are conflicting data about the value of dipyridamole, but most studies show no benefit.[125,133] We empirically administer clopidogrel to patients with a previous anaphylactic reaction to aspirin, or when urgent PTCA is required and the patient has not been receiving aspirin. The role of clopidogrel (with and without oral loading dose) plus aspirin is under evaluation for percutaneous intervention (CREDO trial) and acute coronary syndromes (COMMIT trial); results of CURE have recently been reported (Table 34.32, p 779).

 2. Anticoagulants

    a. Heparin. Heparin has been shown to decrease the risk of acute closure after PTCA.[134] However, 10,000 units of heparin results in suboptimal prolongation of the activated clotting time (ACT) in 5% of patients with stable angina and 15% of patients with unstable angina.[82] Since a low ACT is a powerful predictor of acute closure,[79,135,141,142] we recommend repeat ACTs every 30 minutes during the procedure once a therapeutic ACT has been achieved. Patients undergoing successful percutaneous revascularization should be managed without post-procedural heparin. In patients receiving prolonged heparin infusions, heparin should be discontinued slowly or tapered over 6-24 hours to prevent rebound thrombosis.[83] A controversial management issue is the use of post-procedural heparin in patients with high-risk or suboptimal stenting. In the ATLAST trial, more than 1000 patients were randomized to enoxaparin (plus aspirin and ticlopidine) vs. aspirin and ticlopidine after high-risk stenting (Table 20.12). In general, the risk of stent thrombosis and ischemic complications were lower than anticipated, and there was no observed benefit for enoxaparin. Other uses of low-molecular-weight heparins are discussed in Chapter 34.

b. **Hirudin**. Unlike heparin, hirudin is a direct and potent inhibitor of both freely circulating *and* clot-bound thrombin. Hirulog, a synthetic analog of hirudin, was substituted for heparin in 291 patients undergoing elective PTCA. Patients received a bolus dose of 0.45-0.55 mg/kg followed by a continuous infusion of 1.8-2.2 mg/kg/hr for 4 hours; an additional infusion of 0.2 mg/kg/hr was administered for up to 20 hours for periprocedural dissection, haziness, thrombus, or clinical signs of ischemia. Hirulog was associated with rapid onset, minimal bleeding complications, and acute closure in only 3.9%.[76] Studies suggest that hirudin and hirulog are no more effective than heparin in preventing acute ischemic complications, although bleeding complications may be less frequent.[136,137] Hirulog may provide more consistent dosing than heparin, and may offer reliable prevention of acute closure without the need to monitor ACT levels.[142]

Table 20.6. Risk Factors for Acute Closure After Elective PTCA*

Series	Procedures (n)	AC (%)	Risk Factors for Acute Closure	
			Preprocedural	Procedural
Tenaglia[74] (1994)	658	8.1	Thrombus Length > 5 mm Branch-point stenosis RCA location Total occlusion	-
deFeyter[6] (1991)	1423	7.3	Multivessel disease Unstable angina Eccentric or irregular	-
Ellis[73] (1988)	4722	4.4	Multivessel disease Length > 2 lumen diameters Angle > 45° Branch-point stenosis Thrombus	Dissection Residual stenosis > 30% Final pressure gradient > 20 mmHg Prolonged heparin
Other[71,72,79]			No aspirin	Inadequate heparin Balloon-to-artery ratio > 1.0

Abbreviations: AC = acute closure; RCA = right coronary artery
* Prior to widespread availability of stents

Table 20.7. Risk Factors for Acute Closure*

Clinical	Angiographic	Procedural
Female gender[6,14,38]	Bend > 45 degrees[2,3,23,42,73]	PTCA technique (Table 20.4)
Age[42]	Branch point[73,74]	Dissection[2,23,61,67,73]
Diabetes mellitus[66]	Multilesion[67,73]	Residual stenosis > 35%[73]
Unstable angina[6,61,64,67]	Long lesion[2,42,61,73,75]	Prolonged post-PTCA heparin[73]
I.C. urokinase during PTCA[68]	Thrombus[67,73-75]	Final translesional pressure
Dissection or thrombus on 15-min	Multivessel[6,61,67,73]	gradient $\geq$ 20 mmHg[73]
angiogram[69]	Eccentric[61,73]	Transient in-lab closure
Heparin < 24 hrs prior to PTCA	Vessel supplies collaterals[67]	
Myocardial infarction[77]	Tandem lesions[42]	
High-risk for CABG[67]	RCA location[74]	
Inadequate antiplatelet therapy[71,72]	LCA location[3]	
	Eccentric or irregular border[6]	
	Severe stenosis[2,3,67]	
	Type B_2 or C lesion[2,66]	
	Chronic total occlusion[72,74,75,78]	
	Calcified lesion[2,61]	
	Inadequate anticoagulation[79]	

* These risk factors were established prior to the availability of stents.

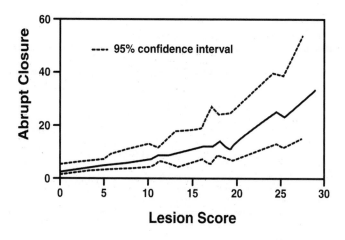

Figure 20.1. Lesion Score for Prediction of Acute Closure

See Table 20.8 for calculation of the lesion score. Dashed lines indicate 95% confidence intervals.

Table 20.8. Scoring System for Prediction of Acute Closure*[74]

Occlusion Type	Characteristic	Points
Nontotal Occlusions	Branch location	
	Yes	13
	No	0
	Length (mm)	
	> 10	10
	5 - 10	5
	< 5	0
	Thrombus score	
	2	12
	1	6
	0	0
	Right coronary artery	
	Yes	6
	No	0
Total Occlusions	Total occlusion	19
	Right coronary artery	
	Yes	6
	No	0

Individual lesion score is sum of points for all adverse characteristics present. Scores are calculated differently for total and nontotal occlusions because morphologic characteristics cannot be graded in the presence of a total occlusion. Figure 20.1 predicts the risk of acute closure based on the lesion score.
* Prior to the availability of stents

Table 20.9. Risk Factors for Cardiac Death After Acute Closure*[5,80]

Cause of Death	Risk Factors
LV failure	Female gender
	Multivessel disease
	Jeopardy score
	Collaterals originating from target vessel
	PTCA of proximal RCA
RV failure	PTCA of proximal RCA
Left main dissection	None

Abbreviations: LV = left ventricular; RV = right ventricular; RCA = right coronary artery
* These studies were conducted prior to the availability of stents

Table 20.10. Correlation of the Jeopardy Score with Systolic Blood Pressure and Risk of Death After Acute Closure*[80]

Jeopardy Score**	Systolic Blood Pressure (mmHg)		Mortality (%)
	Men	Women	
≤ 2.0	113 ± 20	109 ± 15	2.3
2.5-3.0	117 ± 13	81 ± 24	10.0
3.5-4.5	96 ± 7	65 ± 4	11.5
5.0-6.0	75 ± 5	68 ± 13	33.3

*   This study was conducted prior to the availability of stents
**   See Figure 20.2 for calculation of the jeopardy score

3. **Intra-Aortic Balloon Pump (IABP).** The role of IABP for preventing acute closure after primary PTCA for acute MI is controversial. One study reported less occlusion and in-hospital ischemic events,[77] but another showed no difference at 1- and 6-months in high-risk patients.

4. **PTCA Technique.** Balloon-to-artery ratios > 1.1 and slow balloon deflation may increase the risk of severe coronary dissection. Long balloons and noncompliant balloons may reduce the risk of acute closure in long lesions and angulated lesions. There is divergence of opinion regarding the impact of other technical considerations on dissection rate, including the number of inflations, inflation speed, duration of inflation, and the use of oscillating inflations (Table 20.3). Most of these technical nuances have been obviated by the frequent use of stents.

F. **RECOGNITION OF ACUTE CLOSURE.** Acute coronary occlusion typically presents with the sudden onset of chest pain (90%) and ST-segment elevation (75%). Less common presentations include hypotension (20%) and sudden death from heart block or ventricular fibrillation (1-10%). The clinical consequences of acute closure depend on the myocardial distribution of the target vessel, the presence and adequacy of collaterals, the extent of associated coronary disease, and baseline ventricular function. The ability to triage and manage patients with recurrent chest pain at our institution has been facilitated by comparing 12-lead ECG changes and chest pain characteristics after intervention to those induced during balloon inflation ("ischemic fingerprint"). As outlined in Figure 20.3, if chest pain develops outside the catheterization laboratory, an ECG is promptly obtained. The patient is immediately returned to the angioplasty suite for persistent ST segment changes, hemodynamic instability, nitrate-resistant symptoms, or repeated episodes of nitrate-responsive pain.

Table 20.11. Rescue IIb/IIIa Inhibitors and Hirulog for Thrombus

Series	N	Adjunctive Therapy	Results
ESPIRT[159] (2001)	77	Rescue eptifibatide for thrombotic complications (42%)	Bailout therapy was associated with more MI (30% vs. 7%, p = 0.01) and urgent PCI at 48 hours (14% vs. 0%, p = 0.03) compared to "no bailout"
Fuchs[155] (2000)	298	Rescue abciximab for thrombus, dissection Type ≥ C, no-reflow, suboptimal result, or distal embolization	Stents in 73%. In-hospital results: death (1.3%); Q-MI (0.7%); non-Q-MI (31%); TLR (4.6%). Late events: death (1.7%); MI (2.7%); TVR (15.1%); EFS at 1-yr (83%)
Velianou[156] (2000)	186	Abciximab (planned 45%; rescue for threatened or acute closure 55%)	In-hospital results (planned vs. rescue): death (1.2% vs. 1.0%); Q-MI (2.4% vs. 2.0%); non-Q-MI (7% vs. 12.9%); TLR (1.2% vs. 0%). 6-month results (planned vs. rescue): death (2.3% vs. 4.0%); MI (9.4% vs. 14.9%); TVR (4.7% vs. 20.8%, p = 0.001)
de Lemos[157] (2000)	92	Rescue abciximab (n = 29) vs. no abciximab (n = 63); TIMI 14 substudy	Abciximab group had greater ST-segment resolution 90-180 minutes after PCI
Piamsomboon[158] (1999)	73	Abciximab (planned 74%; rescue 26%) in acute coronary syndromes with thrombus-containing lesions	Death (1.4%); Q-wave MI (1.4%); non-Q-wave MI (18%). No subacute thrombosis, emergency CABG, or repeat PTCA
Ahmed (1999)	45	Rescue abciximab in degenerated SVG	No benefit on procedural success or major ischemic complications compared to "no-abciximab"; more non-Q-MI in rescue group (40.5% vs. 17.7%)
Fuchs[160] (1999)	186	Rescue abciximab for thrombus and suboptimal PTCA	Procedural success (95.3%); in-hospital MACE (4.7%); non-Q-MI (24.7%); 1-year TLR (24.9%) and EFS (71%)
Haase[161] (1999)	63	Rescue abciximab for thrombus and threatened or acute closure	Repeat PTCA 2 minutes after abciximab. Marked improvement in thrombus score and TIMI flow; MACE (2%); late TVR (15%)
Sullebarger[162] (1999)	17	Planned abciximab and TEC in SVG	Abciximab was associated with higher procedural success (100% vs. 50%) and less distal embolization/no-reflow (0% vs. 30%) compared to "no abciximab"
Barsness[163] (1998)	58	Local delivery of abciximab in thrombotic SVG	Significant improvement in thrombus score and stenosis severity, but not TIMI flow. Adjunctive stent (88%)
Garbarz[164] (1998)	138	Rescue abciximab for thrombus and suboptimal PTCA	Angiographic success in 84% (100% success for stent thrombosis); adjunctive PTCA or stent (100%); MACE (17%); bleeding and vascular complications (27%); transfusion (5%)

Table 20.11. Rescue IIb/IIIa Inhibitors and Hirulog for Thrombus

Series	N	Adjunctive Therapy	Results
Grantham[165] (1998)	185	Planned and unplanned (rescue) abciximab in thrombotic SVG	Procedural success higher with planned abciximab; no impact of abciximab on angiographic (distal embolization, no-reflow) or clinical complications
Henry[166] (1998)	16	Rescue abciximab for acute stent thrombosis	Recurrent thrombosis after PTCA for stent thrombosis may respond to abciximab
Muhlestein[167] (1997)	29	Rescue abciximab for thrombus after PCI	Procedural success in 97%, clinical success in 93%. Significant improvement in thrombus score and TIMI flow, without distal embolization or no-reflow
Shah[168] (1997)	567	Hirulog vs. heparin for thrombus-containing lesions (Hirulog Angioplasty Study)	Thrombus-containing lesions were associated with more MI (5.1% vs. 3.2%) and acute closure (13.6% vs. 8.3%); no difference between hirulog and heparin in acute or late outcomes

Abbreviations: EFS = event-free survival; MACE = major adverse cardiac; PCI = percutaneous coronary intervention; Q-MI = Q-wave myocardial infarction; SVG = saphenous vein graft; events; TIMI = Thrombolysis in Myocardial Infarction; TLR= target lesion revascularization

Table 20.12. The ATLAST Trial for High-Risk Stenting[152]

	Enoxaparin (n = 553)	Placebo (n = 549)
30-day Clinical Events (%)		
Any event	1.8	2.7
Death	0.5	0.6
MI	0.4	1.6*
Target vessel revascularization	1.1	1.8
30-day Bleeding Complications (%)		
Any bleeding	28.0	6.7**
Minor bleeding	24.8	5.1**
Major bleeding	3.3	1.6
6-month Clinical Events (%)		
Any event	16.6	19.8
Death/MI	8.6	9.1

ATLAST = Antiplatelet Therapy vs. Lovenox plus Antiplatelet therapy for patients with an increased risk of Stent Thrombosis
* p < 0.05
** p < 0.001

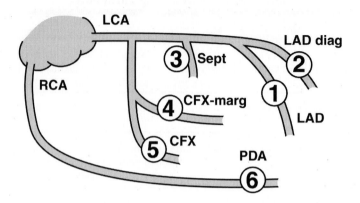

Figure 20.2. Jeopardy Score

Six arterial segments are used to calculate the jeopardy score, which considers the total region of jeopardized myocardium (supplied by the target vessel and providing collaterals to other regions) and the degree of baseline LV dysfunction. LCA = left coronary artery; RCA = right coronary artery; LAD = left anterior descending coronary artery; LAD diag = diagonal branch of LAD; Sept = 1st septal perforator; CFX = left circumflex coronary artery; CFX-marg = marginal branch of CFX; PDA = posterior descending coronary artery.

Scoring system:
- 1 point for each myocardial region supplied by the target lesion.
- 1 point for each myocardial region supplied by a vessel with diameter stenosis $\geq$ 70%.
- 0.5 point for each myocardial region that is hypokinetic at baseline and not supplied by a vessel with significant stenosis.
For example, if the target lesion is in the proximal LAD just beyond the 1st septal perforator, and there is a 70% stenosis in the CFX-marg, the jeopardy score = 2 + 1 = 3.

G. **MANAGEMENT OF ACUTE CLOSURE (Figure 20.4).** Stents represent the most important advance in the mechanical treatment of acute closure (Table 20.13).

1. **Initial Management.** Once acute closure is recognized, intracoronary nitroglycerin (100-200 mcg) should be administered to reverse superimposed spasm and an ACT > 300 seconds should be confirmed. In the pre-stent era, the standard approach to acute closure included redilatation for at least 5 minutes with a balloon matching the diameter of the adjacent reference vessel; conventional, long, or perfusion balloons were chosen depending on the extent of ischemia and the length of dissection. However, the availability of low-profile flexible stents of various lengths and diameters has virtually eliminated the need for prolonged inflations and perfusion balloons. Routine thrombolytic therapy for acute closure caused by dissection may prevent adherence of the intimal flap to the underlying vessel wall and is not recommended.[84] Several observational studies suggested benefit for "rescue" abciximab for suboptimal PTCA caused by dissection or thrombus;[130-132,138] other studies reported no benefit (Table 20.11).

2. **Poor Results After Repeat PTCA**

    a. **Vessels ≥ 2.5 mm.** If repeat PTCA is performed and results are suboptimal (final diameter stenosis > 30%, flow-limiting dissection, or progressive deterioration in the angiographic result over 10 minutes), further intervention is warranted. In vessels ≥ 2.5 mm, focal dissections or simple plaque separations are best managed by stenting, which is more effective than prolonged perfusion balloon inflations (Table 20.14). It is mandatory to identify the distal extent of dissection, since failure to cover the entire dissection with stents may predispose to stent thrombosis and acute MI.[150] The choice of stent is largely dependent on the operator, and virtually all stents have been used with high procedural success rates. Occasionally, multiple overlapping stents may be required for severe recoil or tissue protrusion through stent struts. DCA has been used for focal dissections[89-91] (Chapter 28), but stent implantation is easier and more reliable. Extensive spiral dissections should be treated with multiple tandem stents.[92] Persistent suboptimal results (flow impairment, > 50% residual stenosis) after stenting should be treated with a bailout catheter, IABP (for TIMI flow < 3, labile hemodynamics, or a large risk territory), and CABG.

    b. **Vessels < 2.5 mm.** For acute closure in vessels < 2.5 mm, prolonged balloon inflations may be employed for 10-30 minutes. Although routine use of oversized balloons (balloon/artery ratio > 1.1) is not recommended because of the chance of extending the dissection and converting a focal dissection to a long, spiral dissection, larger balloons may be considered in small vessels if intravascular ultrasound (IVUS) suggests that a larger balloon is appropriate. Stenting is now a viable approach and may be preferred to prolonged balloon inflations, since small stents are readily available. IVUS should be strongly considered in small vessels to ensure optimal stenting, since suboptimal stenting is associated with poor long-term results (Chapters 26, 31).

3. **Refractory Acute Closure.** The indications for emergency CABG after failed PTCA have changed dramatically over the last 4 years. As stent utilization increases, the need for emergency CABG for refractory acute closure has decreased to < 1% in most centers. Current indications for emergency CABG include inability to stabilize a long dissection by stents, injury to the left main coronary artery, and coronary artery perforation (Chapter 23). Perfusion balloon catheters may be useful in these situations, particularly as a bridge to emergency surgery.[151]

4. **In-hospital Management After Successful Reversal of Acute Closure.** For most patients with transient in-lab acute closure promptly treated by stenting, post-procedural management is similar to that of elective stenting. Longer periods of in-hospital management are usually recommended for patients with hospital courses complicated by myocardial infarction, hemodynamic or electrical instability, or unsuccessful revascularization. Post-procedural heparin is not recommended unless the patient has other indications for uninterrupted anticoagulation (Table 20.12).

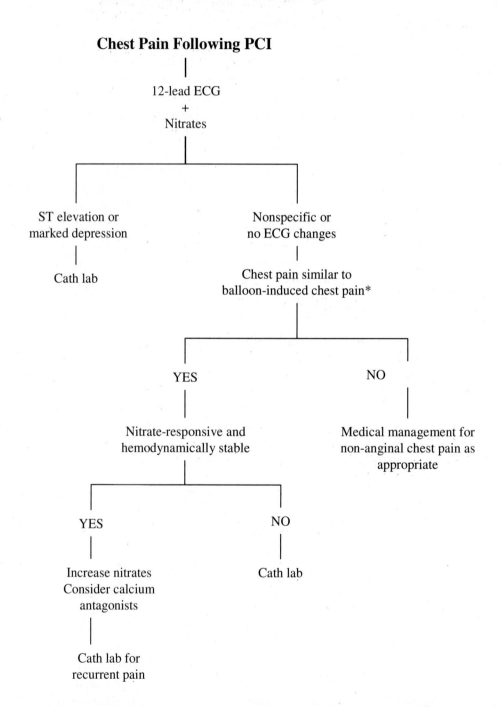

Figure 20.3. Triage of Patients with Chest Pain Following Percutaneous Revascularization

PCI = percutaneous coronary intervention
* If PCI was performed on a chronic total occlusion, these patients should return to the cath lab for repeat angiography

H. OTHER MANAGEMENT ISSUES

1. **Non-Flow-Limiting Dissection.** The majority of small intimal disruptions (residual stenosis < 30%, length < 10 mm, normal flow) may not require further mechanical or drug therapy;[88,149] however, many operators will treat such dissections with stents because of the simplicity of this approach. In situations where stenting is likely to be extremely challenging, most of these minor dissections can be treated by prolonged balloon inflations or left alone, since the risk of early ischemic complications and restenosis is low.[149] The majority of interventionalists stent non-flow-limiting dissections with high-risk features to avoid out-of-lab acute closure (Table 20.4).

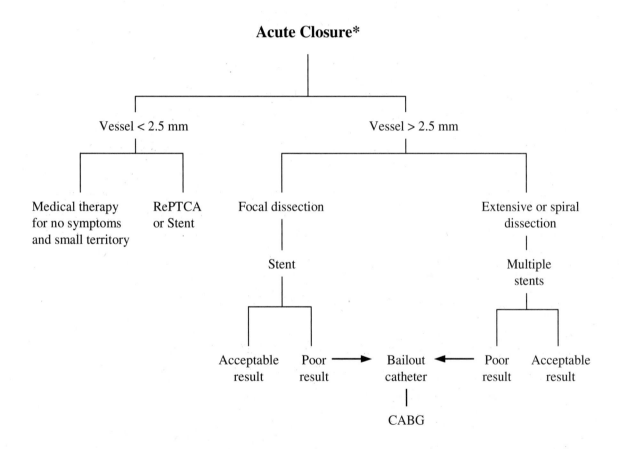

Figure 20.4. Management of Acute Closure

* Consider IVUS to guide optimal stenting (Chapter 31)

Table 20.13. In-hospital Outcome After "Bail-Out" Stenting*

Series	N	In-hospital Complications (%)	
		Stent Thrombosis	D / MI /CABG
Linnemeier[169] (1998)	173	-	0.6 / 0.6 / 1.2
Steffenino[170+] (1997)	150	6.6	5.3 / - / 2.7
Glatt[171+] (1997)	266	2.3	4.9 / 0.8 / 1.1
Spaulding[172+] (1997)	124	0.8	6.5 / 0 / 3.2
Monassier[173+] (1996)	134	3	6.8 / 4.5 / 4.5
Schomig[113] (1994)	339	6.9	1.3 / 4.0 / 9
Sutton[117] (1994)	415	-	3 / 5 / 12
Agrawal[118] (1994)	240	7	-
George[119] (1993)	518	8.7	2.2 / 5.5 / 4.3
Roubin[120] (1992)	115	7.6	1.7 / 16 / 4.2
Vrolix[121] (1994)	180	13.3	3.3 / 12 / 16.5
Garratt[122] (1994)	308	3	3.7 / 2.7 / 8.7

Abbreviations: CABG = emergency coronary artery bypass surgery; D = death; MI = myocardial infarction
* Limited to studies with N $\geq$ 100
+ Acute MI

2.   **Primary Thrombotic Closure.** Compared to vessel dissection, primary thrombosis is a much less common cause of acute closure (except for DCA, where primary thrombosis may account for $\geq$ 50% of cases). The most effective form of therapy for primary thrombosis is unknown. Potential treatment options include intracoronary thrombolysis[93,94,98](urokinase 100,000-250,000 units i.c. over 30 minutes;[93] streptokinase 0.25-1.5 million units i.c. over 60 minutes;[95] or r-tPA 20 mg i.c. over 5 minutes or 40-60 mg IV over 60-120 minutes.[96,97]), local drug delivery (Chapter 35), thrombectomy (AngioJet), repeat PTCA, and stenting (Tables 9.7, 9.8).   The use of platelet

receptor antagonists[99] ("rescue" abciximab) is controversial (Table 20.11), and is discussed in Chapters 9 and 34. TEC atherectomy has been used to aspirate thrombus, but is contraindicated in vessels < 3.0 mm or when a dissection is present. Other measures include the use of a continuous overnight superselective infusion of urokinase (80,000 units per hour through an end-hole infusion wire just proximal to the clot, and 40,000 units per hour through the guiding catheter) (Chapter 9).[98]

I. **PROGNOSIS.** As shown in Table 20.15, the prognosis of acute closure has improved over time.[38] In the pre-stent era, acute closure was associated with a 5-fold increase in periprocedural death and a 10-25-fold increase in periprocedural MI and emergency CABG (Table 20.16). The effect of successfully-treated acute closure on long-term outcome was controversial, with some reports suggesting higher restenosis and ischemic complications rates.[70,100] Among 250 patients with uncomplicated reversal of acute closure by repeat PTCA, ischemic events (death, MI, or repeat revascularization) at 6 months occurred in 45% compared to only 20% of patients without acute closure (p < 0.001).[101] In contrast, among 88 patients with transient in-lab closure responding to additional intervention, there was no adverse effect on long-term prognosis unless there was a significant elevation in CK-MB.[102] In the EPIC trial, abciximab reduced the morbidity (in-hospital and 30-day rates of MI and repeat PTCA) associated with acute closure.[126] Finally, stenting and current antiplatelet regimens have significantly reduced the risk of ischemic complications after acute closure (Chapter 26).

Table 20.14. Prolonged Perfusion Balloon (PPB) Inflations vs. Stenting for Acute Closure

Series	Design	Stent	N	Results
TASC II[85] (1995)	Randomized	-	22 PPB 22 Stent	Stent with greater success (91% vs. 46%), able to salvage 83% of PPB failures, and lower restenosis (22% vs. 50%). CABG avoided in 91%; stent thrombosis resulting in MI in 11%.
de Muinck[86] (1994)	Retrospective, non-randomized	PSS	61 PPB 36 Stent	Stent with less residual stenosis, better restoration of normal flow (94% vs. 70%), less emergency CABG (0% vs. 21%), and more subacute thrombosis (22% vs. 0%). No difference in acute closure, restenosis, or event-free survival at 3 months.
Barberis[87] (1994)	Retrospective	PSS	36 PPB 37 Stent	Stent with greater success (95% vs. 72%), more subacute thrombosis (13% vs. 0%), and able to salvage 90% of PPB failures.
Lincoff[88] (1993)	Matched case-control	GRS	61 PPB* 61 Stent	Stent with less residual stenosis (26% vs. 49%), better restoration of TIMI 3 flow (97% vs. 72%), and reduced need for emergency surgery (9% vs. 27%). No clinical benefit for stenting patients with threatened closure (dissection with normal flow).

Abbreviations: GRS = Gianturco-Roubin stent, PSS = Palmaz-Schatz stent; TASC = Trial of Angioplasty versus Stents in Canada; - = not reported
*   Prolonged inflations ± perfusion balloon

Table 20.15. Time Period of Acute Closure and Incidence of Complications*[99]

Time Period	In-hospital Complications (%)	
	Q-MI	CABG
1980-84	27	63
1985-88	16	42
1989-92	8	32

Abbreviations: Q-MI = Q-wave myocardial infarction; CABG = emergency coronary artery bypass grafting
* Pre-stent era

Table 20.16. Risk of Adverse Events for Patients With and Without Acute Closure*

Event	Incidence of Ischemic Complications (%)	
	Acute Closure	No Acute Closure
Death	5	1
MI	10 - 50	2
Emergency CABG	25 - 60	3
Perioperative death	5 - 10	-
Perioperative MI	40	-

Abbreviations: MI = myocardial infarction; CABG = emergency coronary artery bypass grafting; - = not reported
* Pre-stent era; excludes patients with acute MI

* * * * *

REFERENCES

1. Ramee SR, White CJ, Jain A, et al. Percutaneous coronary angioscopy versus angiography in patients undergoing coronary angioplasty. J Am Coll Cardiol 1991;17:125A.

2. Tan K, Sulke N, Taub N, Sowton E. Clinical and lesion morphologic determinants of coronary angioplasty success and complications: Current experience. J Am Coll Cardiol 1995;25:855-65.

3. Van Belle E, Bauters C, Lablanche J-M, McFadden E, Bertrand M. Angiographic determinants of acute outcome after coronary angioplasty: A prospective quantitative coronary angiographic study of 3679 procedures. J Am Coll Cardiol 1994:223A.

4. Lincoff AM, Popma JJ, Ellis SG, Hacker J. Abrupt vessel closure complicating coronary angioplasty: Clinical, angiographic, and therapeutic profile. J Am Coll Cardiol 1992;19:926-935.

5. Ellis S, Roubin G, King S, et al. In-hospital cardiac mortality after acute closure after coronary angioplasty: Analysis of risk factors from 8,207 procedures. J Am Coll Cardiol 1988;11:211-216.

6. de Feyter PJ, van den Brand M, Jaarman G, van Domburg R. Acute coronary artery occlusion during and after percutaneous transluminal coronary angioplasty. Frequency, prediction, and clinical course, management, and follow-up. Circulation 1991;83:927-936.

7. The Bypass Angioplasty Revascularization Investigation (BARI): Five year mortality and morbidity in a randomized study comparing CABG and PTCA in patients with multivessel coronary disease. The BARI Investigators. N Engl J Med 1996;335:217.

8. Simpfendorfer C, Belardi J, Bellamy G, Galan K. Frequency, management and follow-up of patients with acute coronary occlusions after percutaneous transluminal coronary angioplasty. Am J Cardiol 1987;59:267-269.

9. Bansal A, Choksi NA, Levine AB, et al. Determinants of arterial dissection during PTCA: Lesion type versus inflation rate. J Am Coll Cardiol 1989;12:229A.

10. Popma JJ, Topol EJ, Pinkerton CA, et al. Abrupt closure following directional coronary atherectomy: Clinical, angiographic and procedural outcome. J Am Coll Cardiol 1991;17:23A.

11. Bertrand M, Lablanche J, Leroy F, Bauters C. Percutaneous transluminal coronary rotary ablation with Rotablator (European experience). Am J Cardiol 1992;69:470-474.

12. Safian R, Lai S, Buchbinder M, Sanbron T, Sketch M. Incidence and management of abrupt closure after new device interventions. Report from the NACI Registry in 2988 lesions. Circulation 1993;88(Suppl.):I-585.

13. Mehta S, Popma J, Margolis J, et al. Angiographic complications after new device angioplasty in native coronary arteries: A NACI Angiographic Core Laboratory Report. TCT Meeting (Washington DC), February, 1995.

14. Popma J, Topol E, Hinohara T, et al. Abrupt vessel closure after directional coronary atherectomy. J Am Coll Cardiol 1992;19:1372-1379.

15. Hinohara T, Rowe M, Robertson G, et al. Effect of lesion characteristics on outcome of directional coronary atherectomy. J Am Coll Cardiol 1991;17:1112-1120.

16. Warth D, Leon M, O'Neill W, et al. Rotational atherectomy multicenter registry: Acute results, complications and 6-month angiographic follow-up in 709 patients. J Am Coll Cardiol 1994;24:641-648.

17. Ellis S, Popma J, Buchbinder M, et al. Relation of clinical presentation, stenosis morphology, and operator technique to the procedural results of rotational atherectomy and rotational atherectomy--facilitated angioplasty. Circulation 1994;89:882-892.

18. Safian R, Niazi K, et al. Detailed angiographic analysis of high-speed mechanical rotational atherectomy in human coronary arteries. Circulation 1993;88: 961-968.

19. Litvack F, Eigler N, Margolis J, et al. Percutaneous excimer laser coronary angioplasty: Results in the first consecutive 3,000 patients. J Am Coll Cardiol 1994;23:323-329.

20. Painter J, Popma J, Pichard A, et al. A comparison of early and late clinical outcomes in patients undergoing concentric and directional laser coronary angioplasty. TCT Meeting (Washington DC), February, 1995.

21. Chevalier B, Meyer P, Corcos T, et al. Delayed acute closure after rotational atherectomy: A multicenter registry. Circulation 1994;90:I-213.

22. Huber M, Mooney J, Madison J, Mooney M. Use of a morphologic classification to predict clinical outcome after dissection from coronary angioplasty. Am J Cardiol 1991;68:467-471.

23. Hermans WR, Foley DP, Rensing BJ, Rutsch W. Usefulness of quantitative and qualitative angiographic lesion morphology, and clinical characteristics in predicting major adverse cardiac events during and after native coronary balloon angioplasty. Am J Cardiol 1993;72:14-20.

24. Bailey S, Ricci D, Kiesz S, et al. Incidence and clinical impact of dissections after PTCA and stent placement: Results from the randomized stent restenosis study. TCT Meeting (Washington DC), February, 1995.

25. Hermans WR, Rensing BJ, Foley DP, Deckers JW. Therapeutic dissection after successful coronary balloon angioplasty: No influence on restenosis or on clinical outcome in 693 patients. J Am Coll Cardiol 1992;20:767-780.

26. Sharma SK, Israel DH, Kamean JL, Bodian CA. Clinical, angiographic, and procedural determinants of major and minor coronary dissection during angioplasty. Am Heart J 1993;126:39-47.

27. Kovach J, Mintz G, Pichard A, et al. Sequential intravascular ultrasound characterization of the mechanisms of rotational atherectomy and adjunct balloon angioplasty. J Am Coll Cardiol 1993;22:1024-32.

28. den Heijer P, Foley D, Escaned J, Hillege H. Angioscopic versus angiographic detection of intimal dissection and intracoronary thrombus. J Am Coll Cardiol 1994;24:649-654.

29. Ghazzal Z, Hearn J, Litvack F, et al. Morphological predictors of acute complications after percutaneous excimer laser coronary angioplasty. Results of a comprehensive angiographic analysis: Importance of the eccentricity index. Circulation 1992;86:820-827.

30. Baumbach A, Bittl J, Fleck E, Geschwind H, Sanborn T.

Acute complications of excimer laser coronary angioplasty: A detailed analysis of multicenter results. J Am Coll Cardiol 1994;23:1305-1313.

31. Dussaillant G, Popma J, Pichard A, et al. Rotational atherectomy vs. excimer laser angioplasty: A multivariable analysis of early and late procedural outcome. J Am Coll Cardiol 1995;25:330A.

32. Brown D, Giordano F, Buchbinder M. Coronary dissection following rotational atherectomy: Clinical characteristics, angiographic predictors and acute outcomes. J Am Coll Cardiol 1995;25:123A.

33. Popma J, Knopf W, Davidson C, et al. Angiographic outcome after "cutting" balloon angioplasty. J Am Coll Cardiol 1995;25:268A.

34. Knopf W, Yakubov S, Satler L, et al. Angiographic and procedural outcome after coronary angioplasty using a decremental diameter (tapered) balloon catheter. TCT Meeting (Washington DC), February, 1995.

35. Fitzgerald PJ, Ports TA, Yock PG. Contribution of localized calcium deposits to dissection after angioplasty. An observational study using intravascular ultrasound. Circulation 1992;86:64-70.

36. van Leeuwen T, Meertens J, Velema E, Post M, Borst C. Intraluminal vapor bubble induced by excimer laser pulse causes microsecond arterial dilation and invagination leading to extensive wall damage in the rabbit. Circulation 1993;87:1258.

37. Tcheng J, Wells L, Phillips H, Deckelbaum L, Golobic R. Development of a new technique for reducing pressure pulse generation during 308-nm excimer laser coronary angioplasty. Cathet Cardiovas Diagn. 1995;34:15-22.

38. Scott N, Weintraub W, Liberman H, Morris D, Douglas J, King S. Outcome after acute closure syndrome following coronary angioplasty. Circulation 1993;88:I-299.

39. Popma J, Painter J, Pichard A, et al. Incidence, predictors, prognostic significance of coronary dissections after excimer laser coronary angioplasty (ELCA). TCT Meeting (Washington DC), February, 1995.

40. Berry K, Drew T, McKendall G, et al. Balloon material as a risk factor for coronary angioplasty procedural complications. Circulation 1991;84:II-130.

41. Mooney MR, Fishman-Mooney J, Longe TF, Brandenburg RO. Effect of balloon material on coronary angioplasty. Am J Cardiol 1992;69:1481-1482.

42. Raymenants E, Bhandari S, Stammen F, De Scheerder I, Desmet W, Piessens J. Effects of angioplasty balloon material and lesion characteristics on the incidence of coronary dissection in 2150 dilated lesions. J Am Coll Cardiol 1993;21:291A.

43. Talley JD, Blankenship S, Spokojny WA, Anderson HV, et al. Does the type of balloon material used in elective PTCA make a difference in clinical complications? Results from the CRAC study. Circulation 1995;92:I-74.

44. Safian RD, Hoffmann MA, Almany S, et al. Comparison of coronary angioplasty with compliant and noncompliant balloons (The Angioplasty Compliance Trial). Am J Cardiol 1995;76:518-520.

45. Cribier A, Elchaninoff H, Chan C, et al. Comparative effects of long (> 12 min) versus standard (<3 min) sequential balloon inflations in PTCA. Preliminary results of a prospective randomized study: Immediate results and restenosis rates. J Am Coll Cardiol 1994;23:58A.

46. Remetz MS, Cabin HS, McConnell S, Cleman M. Gradual balloon inflation protocol reduces arterial damage following percutaneous transluminal coronary angioplasty. J Am Coll Cardiol 1988;11:131A.

47. Ilia R, Cabin H, McConnell S. et al. Coronary angioplasty with gradual versus rapid balloon inflation. Cathet Cardiovasc Diagn 1993;29:199-202.

48. Bansal A, Choksi N, Levein AB, et al. Determinants of arterial dissection after PTCA: lesion type versus inflation rate. J Am Coll Cardiol 1989;13:229A.

49. Tenaglia AN, Quigley PJ, Kereiakes DJ, et al. Coronary angioplasty performed with a gradual and prolonged inflation using a perfusion balloon catheter: procedural success and restenosis rate. Am Heart J 1992;124:585-589.

50. Farcot JC, Berland J, Stix A, et al. Gradual, low-pressure and prolonged (10 minutes) protected inflations decreased complications and improved results of proximal LAD angioplasty. Eur Heart J 1991;12:263.

51. Shawl F, Dougherty K, Hoff S. Does inflation strategy influence acute outcome and long-term results? Circulation 1993;88:I-587.

52. Blankenship J, Ford A, Henry S, Frey C. Coronary dissection resulting from angioplasty with slow oscillating vs. rapid inflation and slow vs. rapid deflation. Cath Cardiovasc Diagn. 1995;34:202-209.

53. Foster C, Teskey R, Kells C, et al. Does the speed of balloon deflation affect the complication rate of coronary angioplasty? J Am Coll Cardiol 1993;21:290A.

54. Banka V, Kochar G, Maniet A, Voci G. Progressive coronary dilation: An angioplasty technique that creates controlled arterial injury and reduces complications. Am Heart J 1993;125:61-71.

55. McKeever LS, O'Donnell MJ, Stamato NJ, et al. The effect of predilatation on coronary angioplasty-induced vessel wall injury. Am Heart J 1991;122:1515-1518.

56. Banka VS, Fail PS, Kochar GS, Maniet AR. Dual-balloon progressive coronary dilatation catheter: Design and initial clinical experience. Am Heart J. 1994;127:430-435.

57. Nobuyhshi M, Kimura T, Nosaka H, et al. Restenosis after successful percutaneous transluminal coronary angioplasty: Serial angiographic follow-up of 229 patients. J Am Coll Cardiol 1988;12:616-623.

58. Cappelletti A, Margonato A, Berna G, Chierchia S. Spontaneous evolution of nonocclusive coronary dissection after PTCA: A 6-month angiographic follow-up study. J Am Coll Cardiol 1995;25:345A.

59. Savage M, Dischman D, Bailey S, et al. Vascular remodeling of balloon-induced intimal dissection: Long-term angiographic assessment. J Am Coll Cardiol 1995;25:139A.

60. Bell M, Berger PB, Reeder GS, et al. Coronary dissection following PTCA: Predictors of major ischemic complications. Circulation 1991;84:II-130.

61. Bredlau CE, Roubin GS, Leimgruber PP, Douglas JS. In-hospital morbidity and mortality in patients undergoing elective coronary angioplasty. Circulation 1985;72:1044-1052. 71.

62. Foley D, Hermans W, Rensing B, Serruys P. Predictability of major adverse cardiac events after balloon angioplasty from clinical data and quantitative and qualitative angiographic analysis. J Am Coll Cardiol 1993;21:339A.

63. Ellis SG, Gallison L, Grines CL, et al. Incidence and predictors of early recurrent ischemia after successful percutaneous transluminal coronary angioplasty for acute myocardial infarction. Am J Cardiol 1989;63:263-268.

64. Roubin GS, Lin S, Niederman A, et al. Clinical and anatomic descriptors for a major complication following PTCA. J Am Coll Cardiol 1987;9:20A.

65. Ferguson J, Bittl J, Strony J, Adelman B. The relationship of dissection and thrombus after PTCA to in-hospital outcome: Results of a prospective multicenter study. Circulation 1993;88:I-217.

66. Ellis S, Vandormael M, Cowley M, et al. Coronary morphologic and clinical determinants of procedural outcome with angioplasty for multivessel coronary disease. Circulation 1990;82:1193-1202.

67. Detre KM, Holmes DR, Holubkow R, Cowley MJ. Incidence and consequences of periprocedural occlusion. The 1985-1986 National Heart, Lung, And Blood Institute Percutaneous Transluminal Coronary Angioplasty Registry. Circulation 1990;82:739-750.

68. Ambrose J, Almeida O, Sharma S, Torre S. Adjunctive thrombolytic therapy during angioplasty for ischemic rest angina. Results of the TAUSA Trial. Circulation 1994;90:69-77.

69. Ambrose J, Sharma S, Almeida O, et al. Delayed views post PTCA predict acute and in-hospital complications in patients with unstable angina. J Am Coll Cardiol 1995;25:392A.

70. Tenaglia AN, Fortin DF, Frid DJ, Gardener LH. Long-term outcome following successful reopening of abrupt closure after coronary angioplasty. Am J Cardiol 1993;72:21-25.

71. Barnathan E, Schwartz J, Taylor L, et al. Aspirin and dipyridamole in the prevention of acute coronary thrombosis complicating coronary angioplasty. Circulation 1987;76:125-134.

72. Schwartz L, Bourassa MG, Lesperange J, Aldridge HE. Aspirin and dipyridamole in the prevention of restenosis after percutaneous transluminal coronary angioplasty. N Engl J Med 1988;318:1714-1719.

73. Ellis S, Roubin G, King S, et al. Angiographic and clinical predictors of acute closure after native vessel coronary angioplasty. Circulation 1988;77:372-379.

74. Tenaglia A, Fortin D, Califf R. Predicting the risk of abrupt closure after angioplasty in an individual patient. J Am Coll Cardiol 1994;24:1004-1011.

75. Myler R, Shaw R, Stertzer S, et al. Lesion morphology and coronary angioplasty: Current experience and analysis. J Am Coll Cardiol 1992;19:1641-1652.

76. Topol E, Bonan R, Jewitt D, et al. Use of a direct antithrombin, hirulog, in place of heparin during coronary angioplasty. Circulation 1993;87:1622.

77. Ohman E, George B, White C, et al. Use of aortic counterpulsation to improve sustained coronary artery patency during acute myocardial infarction (Results of a randomized trial). Circulation 1994;90:792-799.

78. Favereau X, Corcos T, Guerin Y, et al. Early reocclusion after successful coronary angioplasty of chronic total occlusions. J Am Coll Cardiol 1995;25:139A.

79. Dougherty KG, Marsh KC, Edelman SK et al. Relationship between procedural activated clotting time and in-hospital post-PTCA outcome. Circulation 1990;82:111-189.

80. Ellis SG, Myler RK, King SB, Douglas JS. Causes and correlates of death after unsupported coronary angioplasty: Implications for use of angioplasty and advanced support techniques in high-risk settings. Am J Cardiol 1991;68:1447-1451.

81. Mufson L, Black A, Roubin G, et al. Randomized trial of aspirin in PTCA: Effect of high versus low dose aspirin on major complications and restenosis. J Am Coll Cardiol 1988;11:236A.

82. Ogilby JD, Kopelman HA, Klein LW, et al. Adequate heparinization during PTCA: Assessment using activated clotting time. J Am Coll Cardiol 1988;11:237A.

83. Gabliani G, Deligonul U, Kern M, Vandermael M. Acute coronary occlusion occurring after successful percutaneous transluminal coronary angioplasty: Temporal relationship to discontinuation of anticoagulation. Am Heart J 1988;116:696-700.

84. Spielberg C, Schnitzer L, Linderer T, et al. Influence of catheter technology and adjunct medication on acute complications in percutaneous coronary angioplasty. Cathet Cardiovasc Diagn 1990;21:72-76.

85. Ricci HR, Ray S, Buller CE, O'Neill B, et al. Six month follow-up of patients randomized to prolonged inflation of stent for abrupt occlusion during PTCA—Clinical and angiographic data: TASC II. Circulation 1995;92:I-475.

86. de Muinck E, den Heijer P, van Dijk R. Autoperfusion balloon versus stent for acute or threatened closure during percutaneous transluminal coronary angioplasty. Am J Cardiol 1994;74:1002-1005.

87. Barberis P, Marsico F, De Servi S, et al. Treatment of failed PTCA with perfusion balloon versus intracoronary stent: A short-term follow-up. J Am Coll Cardiol 1994:136A.

88. Lincoff M, Topol E, Chapekis A, et al. Intracoronary stenting compared with conventional therapy for abrupt vessel closure complicating coronary angioplasty: A matched case-control study. J Am Coll Cardiol 1993;21:866-875.

89. Bier J, Cannistra A, Mukherjee S, et al. Histopathologic findings following directional coronary atherectomy performed for failed balloon angioplasty. Circulation 1994;90:I-63.

90. Berdan L, Holmes D, Davidson-Ray L, Lam L, Talley D, Mark D. Economic impact of abrupt closure following percutaneous intervention: The CAVEAT Experience. J Am Coll Cardiol 1994;23:434A.

91. Movsowitz H, Emmi R, Manginas A, et al. Directional coronary atherectomy for failed balloon angioplasty: Outcome depends on the underlying pathology. Circulation 1993;88:I-601.

92. Shaknovich A, Moses JW, Undemir C, Cohen NT, et al. Procedural and short-term clinical outcomes of multiple Palmaz-Schatz stents (PSSs) in very long lesions/dissections. Circulation 1995;92:I-535.

93. Schieman G, Cohen BM, Kozina J, Erickson JS. Intracoronary urokinase for intracoronary thrombus

accumulation complicating percutaneous transluminal coronary angioplasty in acute ischemic syndromes. Circulation 1990;82:2052-2060.

94. Pavlides GS, Schreiber TL, Gangadharan V, et al. Safety and efficacy of urokinase during elective coronary angioplasty. Am Heart J 1991;121:731-737.

95. Haft JL, Goldstein JE, Homoud MK, et al. PTCA following myocardial infarction: Use of bailout fibrinolysis to improve results. Am Heart J 1990;120:243-247.

96. Hermann G, Zahorsky R, Meissner A, et al. Effects of acute rt-PA thrombolysis during PTA in patients with impending coronary occlusion. Eur Heart J 1990;11:23A.

97. Gulba DC, Daniel WG, Simon R, Jost S. Role of thrombolysis and thrombin in patients with acute coronary occlusion during percutaneous transluminal coronary angioplasty. J Am Coll Cardiol 1990;16:563-568.

98. Chapekis A, George B, Candela R. Rapid thrombus dissolution by continuous infusion of urokinase through an intracoronary perfusion wire prior to and following PTCA: Results in native coronaries and patent saphenous vein grafts. Cathet Cardiovasc Diagn 1991;23:89-92.

99. Muhlestein JB, Gomez, MA, Karagounis LA, Anderson JL. "Rescue ReoPro": Acute utilization of abciximab for the dissolution of coronary thrombus developing as a complication of coronary angioplasty. Circulation 1995;92:I-607.

100. Tenaglia AN, Fortin FD, Frid DJ, et al. Restenosis and long-term outcome following successful treatment of abrupt closure during and after angioplasty: Stabilization using a guidewire. Cathet Cardiovasc Diagn 1987;13:391-393.

101. Piana RN, Ahmed WH, Ganz P, Dodge T Jr., et al. The legacy of uncomplicated abrupt vessel closure during coronary angioplasty: Increased ischemic events after hospital discharge. Circulation 1995;92:I-75.

102. Abdelmeguid AE, Whitlow PL, Sapp SK, et al. Long-term outcome of transient, uncomplicated in-laboratory coronary artery closure. Circulation 1995;91:2733-2741.

103. Deckelbaum LI, Natarajan MK, Bittl JA, et al. Effect of intracoronary saline infusion on dissection during excimer laser coronary angioplasty: A randomized trial. J Am Coll Cardiol 1995;26:1264-9.

104. Holmes DR, Simpson JB, Berdan LG, et al. Abrupt closure: The CAVEAT I Experience. J Am Coll Cardiol 1995;26:1494-500.

105. Zidar JP, Kruse KR, Thel MC, et al. Integrelin for emergency coronary artery stenting. J Am Coll Cardiol 1996;March Special Issue.

106. Mehta S, Popma J, Margolis JR, et al. Complications with new angioplasty devices. Are these device specific? J Am Coll Cardiol 1996;March Special Issue.

107. Popma JJ, Baim DS, Kuntz RE, et al. Early and late quantitative angiographic outcomes in the Optimal Atherectomy Restenosis Study (OARS). J Am Coll Cardiol 1996;March Special Issue.

108. Ortiz-Fernandex A, Goicoles MJ, Perex-Vizcayno M, et al. Late clinical and angiographic outcome of bailout coronary stenting. A comparison study between Gianturco-Roubin and Palmaz-Schatz stents. J Am Coll Cardiol 1996;March Special Issue.

109. Appleman YEA, Piek JJ, Strikwerda S, et al. Randomized trial of excimer laser angioplasty versus balloon angioplasty for treatment of obstructive coronary artery disease. Lancet 1996;347:79-84.

110. Goy JJ, Eeckhout E, Stauffer J-C, Vogt P, Kappenberger L. Emergency endoluminal stenting for abrupt vessel closure following coronary angioplasty: A randomized comparison of the Wiktor and Palmaz-Schatz stents. Cathet Cardiovasc Diagn. 1995;34:128-132.

111. Urban P, Chatelain P, Brzostek T, Jaup T, Verine V, Rutishauser W. Bailout coronary stenting with 6F guiding catheters for failed balloon angioplasty. Am Heart J 1995;129:1078-83.

112. Metz D, Urban P, Camenzind E, Chatelain P, Hoang V, Meier B. Improving results of bailout coronary stenting after failed balloon angioplasty. Cathet Cardiovasc Diagn. 1994;32:117-124.

113. Schomig A, Kastrati A, Mudra H, et al. Four-year experience with Palmaz-Schatz stenting in coronary angioplasty complicated by dissection with threatened or present vessel closure. Circulation 1994;90:2716-2724.

114. Kiemeneij F, Laarman G, van der Wieken R, Suwarganda J. Emergency coronary stenting with the Palmaz-Schatz stent for failed transluminal coronary angioplasty: results of a learning phase. Am Heart J 1993;126:23-31.

115. Reifart N, Haase J, Preusler W, Schwartz F, Storger H. Randomized trial comparing two devices: The Palmaz-Schatz stent and the Strecker stent in bail-out situations. J Interven Cardiol 1994;7:539-547.

116. Chan C, Tan A, Koh T, Koh P. Intracoronary stenting in the treatment of acute or threatened closure in angiographically small coronary arteries (<3.0 mm) complicating percutaneous transluminal coronary angioplasty. Am J Cardiol 1995;75:23-25.

117. Sutton J, Ellis S, Roubin G, et al. Major clinical events after coronary stenting. The multicenter registry of acute and elective Gianturco-Roubin stent placement. Circulation 1994;89:1126-1137.

118. Agrawal S, Ho D, Liu M, et al. Predictors of thrombotic complications after placement of the flexible coil stent. Am J Cardiol 1994;73:1216-1219.

119. George B, Voorhees W, Roubin G, et al. Multicenter investigation of coronary stenting to treat acute or treated closure after percutaneous transluminal coronary angioplasty: Clinical and angiographic outcomes. J Am Coll Cardiol 1993;22:135-143.

120. Roubin G, Cannon A, Agrawal S, et al. Intracoronary stenting for acute and threatened closure complicating percutaneous transluminal coronary angioplasty. Circulation 1992;85:916-927.

121. Vrolix MC, Rutsch W, Piessens J, Kober G, Wiegand V. Bail-out stenting with Medtronic Wiktor: Results from the European stent study group. J Interven Cardiol 1994;7:549-555.

122. Garratt K, White C, Buchbinder M, Whitlow P, Heuser R. Wiktor stent placement for unsuccessful coronary angioplasty. Circulation 1994;90:I-279.

123. Ozaki Y, Keane D, Ruygrok P, de Feyter P, Stertzer S, Serruys P. Acute clinical and angiographic results with the

new AVE micro coronary stent in bailout management. Am J Cardiol 1995;76:112-116.

124. Garratt KN, Grill D, Bell MR, et al. Clinical, angiographic and technical correlates of early abrupt vascular closure during coronary intervention. J Am Coll Cardiol 1997;29(Suppl. A):276A.

125. Heidland UE, Heintzen MP, Klimek WJ, et al. Prevention of abrupt vessel closure following PTCA by intracoronary dipyridamole. A prospectively randomized trial in 1094 consecutive interventions. J Am Coll Cardiol 1997;29(Suppl. A):395A.

126. Aguirre FV, Topol EJ, Leimberger J, et al. Incidence and clinical outcome of abrupt vessel closure among patients receiving abciximab during high-risk percutaneous coronary intervention: EPIC trial results. J Am Coll Cardiol 1997;29(Suppl. A):394A.

127. Brown DL, Buchbinder M. Incidence, predictors, and consequences of coronary dissection following high-speed rotational atherectomy. Am J Cardiol 1996;78:1416-1419.

128. Ferguson JJ, Barasch E, Wilson JM, Strony J, et al. The relation of clinical outcome to dissection and thrombus formation during coronary angioplasty. J Invas Cardiol 1995;7:2-10.

129. De Scheerder IK, Wang K, Kostopoulos K, et al. Treatment of long dissections by use of a single long or multiple short stents: Clinical and angiographic follow-up. Am Heart J 1998;136:345-351.

130. Garbaraz E, Farah B, Vuillemenot A, et al. "Rescue" abciximab for complicated percutaneous transluminal coronary angioplasty. Am J Cardiol 1998;82:800-802.

131. Muhlestein JB, Karagounis LA, Treehan S, Anderson JL. "Rescue" utilization of abciximab for the dissolution of coronary thrombus developing as a complication of coronary angioplasty. J Am Coll Cardiol 1997;30:1729-34.

132. Brener JJ, Deluca SA, Rouse LC, Juran NC, et al. Planned versus "rescue" abciximab during angioplasty: in-hospital outcomes (abstr). Circulation 1996;94(suppl I):I-375.

133. Lembo Nj, Black AJR, Roubin GS, et al. Effect of pretreatment with aspirin versus aspirin plus dipyridamole on the frequency and type of acute complications of percutaneous transluminal coronary angioplasty. Am J Cardiol 1990;65:422-426.

134. Laskey MA, Deutsch E, Barnathan E, Laskey WK. Influence of heparin therapy on percutaneous transluminal coronary angioplasty outcome in unstable angina pectoris. Am J Cardiol 1990;65:1425-1429.

135. Ferguson JJ III. Conventional antithrombotic approaches. Am Heart J 1995;130:651-657.

136. Bittle JA, Strony J, Brinker JA, et al. Treatment with bivalirudin (hirulog) as compared with heparin during coronary angioplasty for unstable or postinfarction angina. Hirulog Angioplasty Study Investigators. N Engl J Med 1995;333:764-769.

137. Serruys PW, Herrman JP, Simon R, Rutsch W, Bode C, Larrman GJ, et al for the Helvetica Investigators. A comparison of hirudin with heparin in the prevention of restenosis after coronary angioplasty. N Engl J Med 1995;333:757-763.

138. Anderson HV, Revana M, Rosales O, et al. Intravenous administration of monoclonal antibody to the platelet GP IIb/IIIa receptor to treat abrupt closure during coronary angioplasty (PTCA). Circulation 1994;90:I-258.

139. Bergelson BA, Fishman RF, Tommaso CL. Abrupt vessel closure: Changing importance, management, and consequences. Am Heart J 1997;134:362-381.

140. Waller BF, Fry ETA, Peters TF, et al. Abrupt (<1 day), acute (< 1 weeks), and early (< 1 month) vessel closure at the angiographic site. Morphologic observations and causes of closure in 130 necropsy patients undergoing coronary angioplasty. Clin Cardiol 1996;19:857-868.

141. Narins CR, Hillegass WB Jr., Nelson CL, et al. Relation between activated clotting time during angioplasty and abrupt closure. Circulation 1996;93:667-671.

142. Bittl JA, Ahmed WH. Relation between abrupt vessel closure and the anticoagulant response to heparin or bivalirudin during coronary angioplasty. Am J Cardiol 1998;82:50P-56P.

143. Fernandez-Ortiz A, Goicolea J, Perez-Vizcayno M, et al. Six-month follow-up of successful stenting for acute dissection after coronary angioplasty: Comparison between slotted tube (Palmaz-Schatz) and flexible coil (Gianturco-Roubin) stent designs. J Interven Cardiol 1998;11:41-47.

144. Dean LS, George CJ, Roubin GS, Kennard ED, et al. Bailout and corrective use of Gianturco-Roubin flex stents after percutaneous transluminal coronary angioplasty. J Am Coll Cardiol 1997;29:934-940.

145. Chauhan A, Zubaid M, Buller CE, et al. Comparison of bailout versus elective stenting: Time to reassess our benchmarks of outcome. Cathet Cardiovasc Diagn 1997;41:40-47.

146. Fuchs S, Kornowski R, Mehran R, et al. Clinical outcomes following "rescue" administration of abciximab in patient undergoing percutaneous coronary angioplasty. J Invas Cardiol 2000;12:497-501.

147. Velianou JL, Strauss BH, Kreatsoulas C, et al. Evaluation of the role of abciximab (Reopro) as a rescue agent during percutaneous coronary interventions: In-hospital and six-month outcomes. Cathet Cardiovasc Intervent 2000;51:138-144.

148. Amin FR, Yousufuddin M, Stables R, et al. Non-elective intra-coronary stenting: Are the clinical outcomes comparable to elective stenting at 6 months? Inter J Cardiol 1999;71:121-127.

149. Cappelletti A, Margonato A, Rosano G, et al. Short- and long-term evolution of unstented nonocclusive coronary dissection after coronary angioplasty. J Am Coll Cardiol 1999;34:1484-8.

150. Farb A, Lindsay J, Virmani R. Pathology of bailout coronary stenting in human beings. Am Heart J 1999;137:621-31.

151. Kipshidze N, Chawla PS. Role of autoperfusion balloon in endovascular interventions. J Interv Cardiol 1999;12:329-337.

152. Zidar JP, Batchelor W, Berger PB, et al. Does the low-molecular-weight enoxaparin reduce stent thrombosis in high-risk stent patients? Results from ATLAST trial. Enoxaparin plus antiplatelet therapy vs. antiplatelet therapy alone in patients at increased risk of stent thrombosis. Circulation 1999;100:I-380.

153. Haase KK, Mahrholdt H, Schroder S, et al. Frequency and

efficacy of glycoprotein IIb/IIIa therapy for treatment of threatened or acute vessel closure in 1332 patients undergoing percutaneous transluminal coronary angioplasty. Am Heart J 1999;137:234-40.

154. Gum PA, Kottke-Marchant K, Poggio ED, et al. Profile and prevalence of aspirin resistance among patients with heart disease: A prospective, comprehensive assessment. Circulation 2000;18:II-418.

155. Fuchs S, Kornowski R, Mehran R, et al. Clinical outcomes following "rescue" administration of abciximab in patient undergoing percutaneous coronary angioplasty. J Invas Cardiol 2000;12:497-501.

156. Velianou JL, Strauss BH, Kreatsoulas C, et al. Evaluation of the role of abciximab (Reopro) as a rescue agent during percutaneous coronary interventions: In-hospital and six-month outcomes. Cathet Cardiovasc Intervent 2000;51:138-144.

157. de Lemos J, Gibson M, Autman EM, et al. Abciximab improves microvascular function after rescue PCI: A TIMI 14 substudy. J Am Coll Cardiol 2000;35:40A.

158. Piamsomboon C, Wong PMT, Mathur A, et al. Does platelet glycoprotein IIb/IIIa receptor antibody improve in-hospital outcome of coronary stenting in high-risk thrombus containing lesions? Cathet Cardiovasc Intervent 1999;46:415-420.

159. Cantor W, Hellkamp A, O'shea J, et. al. Bailout platelet GP IIb/IIIa inhibition in coronary stent implantation: Observations from the ESPRIT trial. J Am Coll Cardiol 2001;:885(3):84A.

160. Fuch S, Meharen R, Dangas G, et al. Clinical outcomes following "rescue" administration of abciximab in patients undergoing percutaneous coronary angioplasty. J Am Coll Cardiol 1999;33:2A.

161. Haase KK, Mahrholdt H, Schroder S, Baumbach A, Oberhoff M, Herdeg C, Karsch KR. Frequency and efficacy of glycoprotein IIb/IIIa therapy for treatment of threatened or acute vessel closure in 1332 patients undergoing percutaneous transluminal coronary angioplasty. Am Heart J 1999;137:234-240.

162. Sullebarger JT, Dalton RD, Nasser A, Matar FA. Adjunctive abciximab improves outcomes during recanalization of totally occluded saphenous vein grafts using transluminal extraction atherectomy. Cathet Cardiovasc Diagn. 1999;46:107-110.

163. Barsness GW, Butler CE, Ohmas EM, et al. Reduced thrombus burden in saphenous vein grafts with abciximab given through a local delivery catheter. Circulation 1998;98:17.

164. Garbarz E, Farah B, Vuillemenot A, Andre F, Angioi M, Machecourt J, Bassand JP, Wolf JE, Danchin N, Prendergast B, Lung B, Vahanian A. "Rescue" abxicimab for complicated percutaneous transluminal coronary angioplasty. Am J Cardiol 1998;82:800-802.

165. Grantham JA, Mathew V, Holmes DR. Antiplatelet therapy with abciximab in percuaneous intervention of thrombus-containing bypass grafts. Circulation 1998;98:17.

166. Henry P, Boughalem K, Rinaldi JP, Makowski S, Khalife K, Guermonprez JL, Blanchard D. Use of anti-GP IIb/IIIa in acute thrombosis after intracoronary stent implantation. Cathet Cardiovasc Diagn. 1998;43:105-107.Muhlestein JB, Karagounis LA, Treehan S, Anderson JL. "Rescue" utilization of abciximab for the dissolution of coronary thrombus developing as a complication of coronary angioplasty. J Am Coll Cardiol 1997;30:1729-1734.

167. Shah PB, Ahmed WH, Ganz P, Bittl JA. Bivalirudin compared with heparin during coronary angioplasty for thrombus-containing lesions. J Am Coll Cardiol 1997;30:1264-1269.

168. Szto G Y, Linnemeier T J, Lewis S J, et al. Safety of 10 days of ticlopidine after coronary stenting-a randomized comparison with 30 days: strategic alternatives with ticlopidine in stenting study (SALTS). J Am Coll Cardiol 1998;352A.

169. Steffenino G, Chierchia S, Fontanelli A, et al. Use of stents during emergency coronary angioplasty in patients with high-risk acute myocardial infarction: In-hospital results from the Italian multicenter registry (RAI). Eur Heart J 1997;18:272

170. Glatt B, Stratiev V, Guyton B, et al. Two years experience of primary stenting in unselected acute myocardial infarction: One month follow-up. Eur Heart J 1997;18:274.

171. Spaulding C, Cador R, Benhamda K, et al. One-week and six-month angiographic controls of stent implantation after occlusive and nonocclusive dissection during primary balloon angioplasty for acute myocardial infarction. Am J Cardiol 1997;79:1592-1595.

172. Monassier Monassier J, Elias J, Raynaud J, et al. STENTIM I: The French registry of stenting in acute myocardial infarction. J Am Coll Cardiol 1996;27:279A.

21 NO-REFLOW

Robert D. Safian, M.D.

A. **DEFINITION.** The no-reflow phenomenon was originally observed in experimental models of acute myocardial infarction (MI) and was described as a failure to restore normal myocardial blood flow despite removal of the coronary obstruction.[1,2] Since that time, no-reflow has been shown to complicate thrombolytic therapy and percutaneous revascularization with PTCA and other devices.[3-9] Defined angiographically, no-reflow manifests as an acute reduction in coronary flow (TIMI grade 0-1) in the absence of dissection, thrombus, spasm, or high-grade residual stenosis at the original target lesion. Lesser degrees of flow impairment (TIMI grade 2) are generally referred to as "slow-flow." However, studies of acute MI patients have reported that scintigraphic evidence for no-reflow may occur in the *absence* of angiographic slow-flow, suggesting that microvascular injury may be angiographically inapparent in some patients.[23] Using the Doppler Flowire, flow velocity patterns of no-reflow in patients with acute MI include systolic retrograde flow, diminished systolic antegrade flow, and rapid deceleration of diastolic flow.[24]

B. **ETIOLOGY.** The mechanisms and mediators responsible for no-reflow remain speculative, but the end result appears to be severe microvascular dysfunction. Potential mechanisms of microvascular dysfunction include vasospasm, distal embolization of thrombus or other debris, oxygen free radical-mediated endothelial injury, capillary plugging by erythrocytes and neutrophils, and intracellular/interstitial edema with intramural hemorrhage.[1,2,33]

C. **INCIDENCE.** The reported incidence of no-reflow or slow-flow after percutaneous intervention ranges from 0.6-42%, depending on the definition used and the clinical setting (Table 21.1).[4,5,7,11,12,19,21,25,26,40] Among 2318 patients undergoing contemporary percutaneous intervention, TIMI-flow $\leq$ 2 was present in 5.8%.[40] No-reflow is more common after mechanical revascularization of thrombus-containing lesions (i.e., acute MI) and degenerated vein grafts containing friable debris. Among mechanical devices, no-reflow is highest after Rotablator atherectomy (1.2-9.0%) (Table 21.2), correlates with total burr activation time,[13-15] and is reversible in > 60% of episodes; the frequent response to intracoronary calcium antagonists is strongly suggestive of microvascular spasm.[7] Other risk factors for slow-flow after Rotablator include lesion length (odds ratio 33.3), recent unstable angina (odds ratio 15.8), and use of ß-blockers within 24 hours (odds ratio 3.3).[19] In contrast, no-reflow after TEC atherectomy is frequently irreversible,[7] suggesting microembolization with vessel debris and capillary plugging. While the use of TEC correlated with persistent flow impairment,[7] these results may have been biased by its use in situations known to be associated with no-reflow (degenerated vein grafts, salvage revascularization after failed thrombolytic therapy for acute MI).

D. **CLINICAL MANIFESTATIONS AND PROGNOSIS.** In the catheterization laboratory, no-reflow usually manifests as ECG changes and chest pain.[7] However, depending on the myocardial territory,

Table 21.1. No-Reflow After Percutaneous Intervention: Incidence and Outcome

Series	Incidence	Definition	Clinical Setting	Comments
Wainstein[41] (2001)	135/4264 (3.1%)	–	All devices	No-reflow was associated with a 4-fold increase in MACE (18.1% vs. 4.6%, p < 0.001). Neither intracoronary sodium nitroprusside (SNP) nor verapamil improved outcome, despite angiographic improvement in blood flow with SNP
Leopold[40] (2000)	134/2318 (5.8%)	TIMI $\leq$ 2	All devices	No-reflow was associated with more in-hospital death (1.5% vs. 0.14%), CK elevation (14.9% vs. 5.9%), and MACE (15.7% vs. 7.0%). Predictors of no-reflow included thrombus, emergency procedure, prior MI, and prior CABG
Diez[25] (1998)	12/140 (8.6%)	TIMI $\leq$ 2	Rotablator	Nearly 4-fold reduction in the incidence of slow-flow after pretreatment with abciximab
Tsubokawa[26] (1998)	13/99 (13%)	TIMI $\leq$ 2	Rotablator	Less slow-flow with IC infusion of nicorandil (2.7%) than verapamil (16.1%)
TOPIT[42] (1997)	11/134 (8.2%)	No-reflow	TEC for thrombus	Randomized trial. Incidence of no-reflow after PTCA (5%)
Sharma[19] (1997)	22/225 (10%)	TIMI $\leq$ 2	Rotablator	Predictors of slow-flow were lesion length, recent unstable angina, and use of ß-blockers
Kaplan[21] (1996)	15/36 (42%)	TIMI $\leq$ 2	Vein grafts	No response to NTG; all responded to verapamil
Abbo[7] (1995)	66/10,767 (0.6%)	TIMI $\leq$ 1	All devices; patients with and without acute MI	Best response to verapamil (67%); worst response to urokinase (10%); high rate of adverse outcome (death 15%, MI 31%)
Wyrens[11] (1995)	24/614 (4%)	TIMI $\leq$ 1	All devices	Excellent response to diltiazem (96%)
Safian[43] (1994)	14/158 (8.8%)	No-reflow	TEC for SVG	
Piana[5] (1994)	39/1919 (2%)	TIMI $\leq$ 2	PTCA, DCA	Excellent response to verapamil (95%)
Shani[12] (1992)	11/90 (12.2%)	"slow-flow"	PTCA for acute MI	All 6 patients treated with verapamil had improvement in flow
Wilson[4] (1989)	5/370 (1.3%)	"slow-flow"	PTCA; patients with and without acute MI	No response to NTG, papaverine, or lytics

Abbreviations: DCA = directional coronary atherectomy; MI = myocardial infarction; MACE = death, MI, stroke, or repeat revascularization; NTG = nitroglycerin; PTCA = percutaneous transluminal coronary angioplasty; SVG = saphenous vein graft; TEC = transluminal extraction catheter

baseline ventricular function, and the presence of other coronary artery disease, no-reflow may be clinically silent, or induce a spectrum of ischemic manifestations including conduction disturbances, hypotension, myocardial infarction, cardiogenic shock, and death.[3,5,7] No-reflow was associated with a 10-fold higher incidence of death and myocardial infarction compared to patients without no-reflow (even after excluding patients with acute MI).[7,40]

E. **PROPHYLAXIS.** Prophylaxis against no-reflow has not been systematically studied. Some Rotablator operators add a cocktail of nitroglycerin (4 mcg/ml) and either verapamil (10 mcg/ml), diltiazem, or adenosine to the heparinized (20 units/ml) Rotablator flush solution[20,34] (Chapter 27). Pretreatment with calcium antagonists for high-risk lesions is currently under evaluation. Distal protection devices are currently under evaluation for preventing distal embolization and no-reflow, especially in vein grafts.[27,35-37] In the recent multicenter randomized SAFER trial, distal protection with the GuardWire (PercuSurge) resulted in 50-60% reduction in in-hospital death and major ischemic events (Chapter 17).[39]

Table 21.2. No-Reflow or Slow-Flow After Rotablator Atherectomy

Series	Type*	Incidence
Kini[44] (1999)	Slow-flow	90/1000 (9%)
STRATAS[45] (1998)	Slow-flow	12/104 (11.3%)
DART[46] (1997)	Slow-flow	35/442 (8.0%)
Sharma[19] (1997)	Slow-flow	22/225 (10%)
Ellis[14] (1994)	Slow-flow	28/308 (9.1%)
Warth[15] (1994)	No-reflow	9/743 (1.2%)
Safian[13] (1993)	No-reflow	7/116 (6.1%)

DART = Dilatation vs. Ablation Revascularization Trial; STRATAS = Study To Determine Rotablator and Transluminal Angioplasty Strategy
* Slow-flow = TIMI-2 flow; no-reflow = TIMI flow ≤ 1

F. MANAGEMENT (Figures 21.1, 21.2). The optimal treatment of no-reflow is unknown. Since it occurs in a variety of clinical settings and is likely to have more than one mechanism, it is unlikely that a single definitive treatment will be appropriate for all cases. It is important to remember that no-reflow is a diagnosis of exclusion: High-grade residual stenosis due to flow-limiting dissection, thrombus, and spasm should be systematically excluded since their treatment and outcome are generally more favorable than those of no-reflow. Pullback angiography and distal pressure gradient measurement may be useful to distinguish no-reflow (no angiographic lesion, no pressure gradient) from distal dissection or stenosis (distal lesion by angiography with pressure gradient).[31] Although mild degrees of flow impairment may improve spontaneously, active therapy is always recommended for no-reflow, as summarized in Figure 21.1 and detailed here:

1. **Reverse Superimposed Spasm.** Intracoronary nitroglycerin (200-800 mcg) rarely has any effect on no-reflow but may reverse superimposed spasm.[4,7] Since its use is not associated with unnecessary delay or enhanced risk, it should be used in all cases.

2. **Exclude Coronary Dissection.** Multiple angiographic views should be obtained to exclude a flow-limiting dissection. Even following "successful" PTCA, angioscopy often demonstrates intimal disruptions or frank dissections that are underestimated by angiography.[10,16] Pullback angiography with or without pressure gradient measurements may also be useful.[31] If contrast stains at the PTCA site, a flow-limiting dissection and/or thrombus is likely, and further treatment (PTCA or stent for dissection, thrombectomy for thrombus) should be performed. Caution should be used in stenting lesions with no-reflow since poor distal runoff may increase the likelihood of stent thrombosis.

3. **Administer Intracoronary Calcium Antagonists.** The most important strategy in the treatment of no-reflow is the use of intracoronary calcium antagonists. Intracoronary administration of verapamil (100-200 mcg, total dose up to 1.0-1.5 mg) or diltiazem (0.5-2.5 mg bolus, total dose up to 5-10 mg) has been shown to reverse no-reflow in 65-95% of cases.[5,7] In one report, resolution of no-reflow was 3-4 times more likely if verapamil was administered.[7] These agents should be administered through the central lumen of the balloon or transfer catheter to facilitate drug delivery to the distal vascular bed;[3,4,11] drug administered through the guiding catheter may not reach the distal vessel. Although high-degree AV block is unusual following intracoronary calcium antagonists, a temporary pacemaker should be readily available. Hypotension caused by no-reflow is not a contraindication to intracoronary calcium blockers—adjunctive therapy with pressors, inotropes, and IABP should be used as needed to support the systemic circulation while the calcium antagonist is administered. Despite the use of intracoronary calcium antagonists, ischemic complications remain higher than normal.[41]

4. **Consider Platelet Glycoprotein IIb/IIIa Inhibitors (Chapter 34).** The use of potent platelet receptor antagonists for preventing or reversing no-reflow is controversial. While some studies suggest benefit, other studies in vein grafts do not.[29] In EPIC, abciximab was associated with less distal embolization in vein grafts, but no difference in final TIMI flow.[30]

5. **Treat Distal Embolization.** If no-reflow persists despite these measures, especially following intervention on a thrombus-containing lesion, an intracoronary thrombolytic agent may be considered for presumed distal embolization (e.g., urokinase 100,000-500,000 units over 5-30 minutes or tPA 5-20 mg). However, in several clinical and experimental studies, urokinase alone was ineffective in reversing no-reflow, so its risks should be carefully weighed against its benefits.[4,7,17,18]

6. **Clear Microvascular Plugging.** A rapid and moderately forceful injection of intracoronary saline or contrast may help clear microvascular plugging due to damaged endothelial cells, erythrocytes, neutrophils or thrombus.

7. **Increase Coronary Perfusion Pressure.** Although intra-aortic balloon counter pulsation (IABP) may augment coronary perfusion pressure, promote clearance of vasoactive substances, and limit infarct size, it has not been shown to reverse no-reflow. We recommend an IABP for patients with ongoing ischemia, hemodynamic compromise, or final TIMI flow < 3. For patients with hemodynamic collapse, percutaneous cardiopulmonary bypass may provide circulatory support during sustained periods of no-reflow.

8. **Coronary Artery Bypass Surgery.** Unfortunately, CABG is not beneficial for no-reflow, since the epicardial coronary artery is widely patent and the obstruction to coronary flow is at the capillary level.

9. **Triage to ICU.** Because of the adverse outcome associated with no-reflow, patients who do not respond immediately to treatment should be monitored in an intensive care unit. Serial cardiac enzymes should be measured and a noninvasive assessment of LV function should be obtained. If myocardial infarction ensues, routine post-MI care should be administered.

10. **Other Approaches.** Potent coronary vasodilators such as papaverine, sodium nitroprusside,[41] and adenosine[22,28,38] have been used in some cases of refractory no-reflow. Intracoronary adenosine (10-20 mcg) is theoretically attractive because it inhibits neutrophil function and decreases neutrophil-mediated free-radical formation and endothelial injury. We have had favorable experience with intracoronary sodium nitroprusside (10-50 mcg), particularly when no-reflow occurs in the setting of acute MI or vein graft intervention. Antioxidants such as superoxide dismutase and allopurinol (to decrease reperfusion injury) and mannitol (to reduce myocardial edema) have been studied in experimental MI, but their value for no-reflow is unknown.

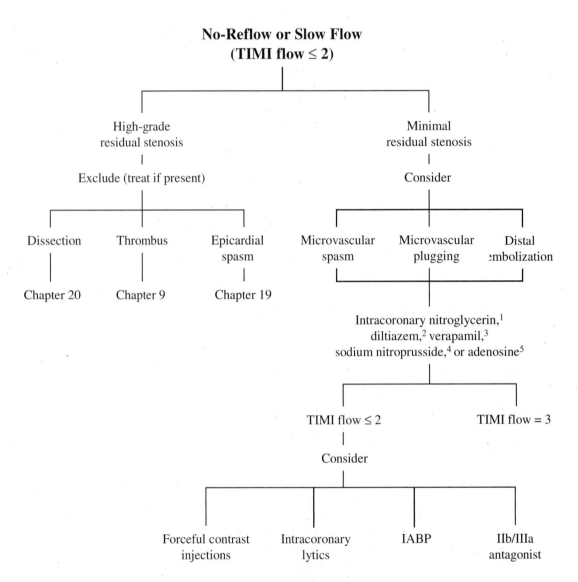

Figure 21.1. Management of Impaired Flow After Intervention

1.   Nitroglycerin 200-800 mcg IC to reverse superimposed spasm; little effect on no-reflow
2.   Diltiazem 0.5-2.5 mg IC over 1 min up to 5-10 mg as needed; temporary pacemaker on standby; limited clinical experience
3.   Verapamil 100 mcg/min IC up to 1-1.5 mg; temporary pacemaker on standby
4.   Sodium nitroprusside 10-50 mcg IC as needed
5.   Adenosine 10-20 mcg IC as needed

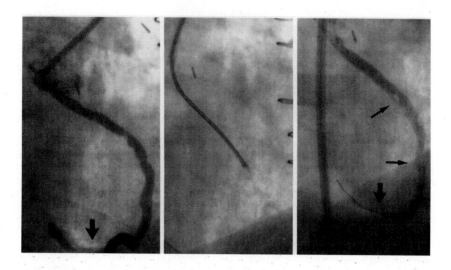

Figure 21.2. No-reflow After TEC Atherectomy

TEC atherectomy (middle panel) is performed on this degenerated saphenous vein graft (left panel), but is complicated by chest pain, ST elevation, and no-reflow (TIMI-1 flow) (right panel). Operators who perform percutaneous interventions on saphenous vein grafts should always anticipate the possibility of no-reflow, keeping a consistent treatment strategy in mind. It is of paramount importance to clearly distinguish no-reflow from abrupt closure of the target vessel, since treatment strategies are totally different. There are no prospective randomized trials comparing treatments of no-reflow, although several observational studies permit reasonable recommendations. First and foremost is the observation that many cases of no-reflow can be reversed by intracoronary calcium antagonists, sodium nitroprusside, or adenosine. Most experience is with verapamil (100-250 mcg bolus every 2-4 minutes up to 2 mg as needed), but diltiazem is also effective (1-2 mg bolus every 2-4 minutes, not to exceed 10 mg). It is very important to ensure drug delivery to the distal capillary bed: If there is TIMI flow ≤ 1, drug administered through the guiding catheter (particularly those with sideholes) will never reach the distal capillary bed. In these circumstances, it is best to advance a deflated balloon catheter, infusion catheter, or any suitable transfer catheter into the distal vessel, and administer an intracoronary calcium antagonist through the central lumen. If there is "slow-flow" (TIMI flow = 2), a calcium antagonist can be delivered through the guiding catheter. Intracoronary nitroglycerin has not been shown to effectively reverse no-reflow and should not be used as sole therapy. However, since it is not deleterious, may reverse associated epicardial spasm, and is not associated with any delays, intracoronary nitroglycerin is a reasonable adjunct. Intracoronary lytics are potentially useful for distal embolization of thrombus to epicardial vessels, but they are much less useful for the distal microembolization characteristic of no-reflow; in our experience, intracoronary urokinase restores flow in < 10% of no-reflow cases and increases the risk of bleeding and femoral vascular injury. The value of intraaortic balloon pump counterpulsation is a matter of debate; it is clearly useful when there is hemodynamic compromise, possibly useful in milder degrees of "slow-flow," and probably not useful for true no-reflow. Limited anecdotal experience with abciximab is positive, but further study is needed. Finally, conventional approaches to acute closure (prolonged balloon inflations, stents, emergency bypass surgery) have no role in the treatment of no-reflow.

* * * * *

REFERENCES

1. Kloner RA, Ganote CE, Jennings RB. The "no-reflow" phenomenon after temporary coronary occlusion in the dog. J Clin Invest 1974;54:1496-1508.

2. Kloner RA. No-reflow revisited. J Am Coll Cardiol 1989;14:1814-1815.

3. Kitazume H, Iwama T, Kubo H, et al. No-reflow phenomenon during percutaneous transluminal coronary angioplasty. Am Heart J 1988;116:211-215.

4. Wilson RF, Lesser JR, Laxson DD, et al. Intense microvascular constriction after angioplasty of acute thrombotic coronary arterial lesions. Lancet 1989:801-811.

5. Piana RN, Paik GY, Moscucci M, et al. Incidence and treatment of no-reflow after percutaneous coronary intervention. Circulation 1994;89:2514-2518.

6. Ellis SG, Popma JJ, Buchbinder M, et al. Relation of clinical presentation, stenosis morphology, and operator technique to the procedural results of rotational atherectomy and rotational atherectomy-facilitated angioplasty. Circulation 1994;89:882-892.

7. Abbo KM, Dooris M, Glazier S, et al. No-reflow after percutaneous coronary intervention: Clinical and angiographic characteristics, treatment and outcome. Am J Cardiol 1995;75:778-782.

8. Feld H, Schulhoff N, Lichstein E, et al. Direct angioplasty as primary treatment for acute myocardial infarction resulting in the no-reflow phenomenon predicts a high mortality rate. Circulation 1992;86 (suppl):I-135.

9. Pomerantz RM, Kuntz RE, Diver DJ, et al. Intracoronary verapamil for the treatment of distal microvascular spasm following PTCA. Cathet and Cardiovasc Diagn 1991;24:283-288.

10. Ritchie JL, Hansen D, Johnson C, et al. Combined mechanical and chemical thrombolysis in an experimental animal model: Evaluation by angiography and angioscopy. Am Heart J 1990;119-164.

11. Wyrens FJ, Mooney J, Lesser J, Mooney MR. Intracoronary diltiazem for microvascular spasm after interventional therapy. Am J Cardiol 1995;75:849-850.

12. Shani J, Feld H, Frankel R, Hollander G. Clinical cardiology: percutaneous transluminal coronary angioplasty in ischemic syndromes. Circulation 1992;86:I-852.

13. Safian RD, Niazi KA, Strzelecki M, et al. Detailed angiographic analysis of high-speed mechanical rotational atherectomy in human coronary arteries. Circulation 1993;88:961-968.

14. Ellis SG, Popma JJ, Buchbinder M, et al. Relation of clinical presentation, stenosis morphology, and operator technique to the procedural results of rotational atherectomy and rotational atherectomy-facilitated angioplasty. Circulation 1994;89:882-892.

15. Warth DC, Leon MB, O'Neill WW, et al. Rotational atherectomy multicenter registry: Acute results, complications and 6-month angiographic follow-up in 709 patients. J Am Coll Cardiol 1994;24:641-8.

16. Ramee SR, White CJ, Jain A, et al. Percutaneous coronary angioscopy versus intravascular ultrasound in patients undergoing coronary angioplasty. J Am Coll Cardiol 1991;17:125A.

17. Kloner RA, Alker KJ. The effect of streptokinase on intramyocardial hemorrhage, infarct size, and the "no-reflow" phenomenon during coronary reperfusion. Circulation 1984;70:513-521.

18. Kloner RA, Alker K, Campbell C, et al. Does tissue-type plasminogen activator have direct beneficial effects on the myocardium independent of its ability to lyse intracoronary thrombi? Circulation 1989;79:1125-1136.

19. Sharma SK, Dangas G, Mehran R, et al. Risk factors for the development of slow flow during rotational coronary atherectomy. Am J Cardiol 1997;80:219-222.

20. Cohen BM, Weber VJ, Blum RR, et al. Cocktail attenuation of rotational ablation flow effects (CARAFE) Study: Pilot. Cathet Cardiovasc Diagn 1996;Suppl 3:69-72.

21. Kaplan BM, Benzuly KH, Kinn JW, Bowers TR, et al. Treatment of no-reflow in degenerated saphenous vein graft interventions: Comparison of intracoronary verapamil and nitroglycerin. Cathet Cardiovasc Diagn 1996;39:113-118.

22. Fischell TA, Carter AJ, Foster MT, et al. Reversal of "no reflow" during vein graft stenting using high velocity boluses of intracoronary adenosine. Cathet Cardiovasc Diagn 1998;45:360-365.

23. Kondo M, Nakano A, Saito D, Shimono Y. Assessment of "microvascular no-reflow phenomenon" using technetium-99m macroaggregated albumin scintigraphy in patients with acute myocardial infarction. J Am Coll Cardiol 1998;32:898-903.

24. Iwakura K, Ito H, Takiuchi S, Taniyanma Y, et al. Alternation in the coronary blood flow velocity pattern in patients with no reflow and reperfused acute myocardial infarction. Circulation 1996;94:1269-1275.

25. Diez JG, Fish RD, Croitoru M, et al. The slow-flow, no-flow phenomena during rotational atherectomy: Does abciximab help? Circulation 1998;98(suppl I):I-558.

26. Tsubokawa A, Ueda K, Iwase T, et al. Efficacy of intracoronary nicorandil infusion of preventing no-reflow and slow flow during rotational atherectomy. Circulation 1998;98(suppl I):I-351.

27. Grube E, Webb J. The SAFE study. Multicenter evaluation of a protection catheter systems for distal embolization in coronary venous bypass grafts (SVG's). J Am Coll Cardiol 1999;33(supplA):37A.

28. Fischell TA, Carter AJ, Foster MT, et al. Pharmaco-hydraulic reversal of "no reflow" during stenting of degenerated saphenous vein grafts using intracoronary adenosine. Circulation 19998:98(suppl I):I-120.

29. Grantham JA, Hasdai D, Holmes DR. Antiplatelet therapy with abciximab in percutaneous intervention of thrombus-containing bypass grafts. Circulation 1998:98 (suppl I):I-572.

30. Mak KH, Challapalli R, Eisenberg MJ, et al. Effect of platelet glycoprotein IIb/IIIa receptor inhibition on distal embolization during percutaneous revascularization of aortocoronary saphenous vein grafts. Am J Cardiol 1997;80:985-988.

31. Sherman JR, Anwar A, Bret JR, Schreibfeder MM. Distal vessel pullback angiography and pressure gradient measurement: An innovative diagnostic approach to evaluate the no-reflow phenomenon. Cathet Cardiovasc Diagn

1996;39:1-6.

32. Rawitscher D, Levin TN, Cohen I, Feldman T. Rapid reversal of no-reflow using abciximab after coronary device intervention. Cathet Cardiovasc Diagn 1997;42:187-190.

33. Erbel R, Heusch G. Coronary microembolization. J Am Coll Cardiol 2000; 36: 22-24.

34. Hanna GP, Yhip P, Fujise K, et al. Intracoronary adenosine administered during rotational atherectomy of complex lesions in native coronary arteries reduces the incidence of no-reflow phenomenon. Cathet Cardiovasc Interv 1999; 48: 275-278.

35. Oesterle SN, Hayase M, Baim DS, et al. An embolization containment device, Cathet Cardiovasc Intervent 1999; 47: 243-250.

36. Carlino M, De Gregorio J, Di Mario C, et al. Prevention of distal embolization during saphenous vein graft lesion angioplasty. Experience with a new temporary occlusion and aspiration system. Circulation 1999; 99: 3221-3223.

37. Belli G, Pezzano A, De Biase AM, et al. Adjunctive thrombus aspiration and mechanical protection from distal embolization in primary percutaneous intervention for acute myocardial infarction. Cathet Cardiovasc Intervent 2000; 50: 362-370.

38. Tiede DJ, Brady PA, Garratt KN, Holmes DR. Resolution of the "no-reflow" phenomenon with intracoronary administration of adenosine. J Interven Cardiol 2000; 13: 15-18.

39. Baim, D. On behalf of the SAFER Investigators. Presented at TCT meeting, October 2000, Washington D.C.

40. Leopold JA, Berger CJ, Cupples LA, et al. No-reflow during coronary intervention: observations and implications. Circulation 2000;102:II-644.

41. Wainstein M, Frederic F, Lee M, et al. Lack of clinical efficacy of pharmacologic treatment of the no-reflow phenomenon despite significant angiographic improvement. J Am Coll Cardiol 2001;37(2):83A.

42. Kaplan B. Personal communication 2000.

43. Safian RD, Grines CL, May MA, Lichtenberg A, Juran N, Schreiber TL, Pavlides GS, Meany TB, Savas V, O'Neill WW. Clinical and angiographic results of transluminal extraction coronary atherectomy in saphenous vein bypass grafts. Circulation 1994;89:302-312.

44. Kini A, Marmur JD, Duvvuri S, et al. Rotational atherectomy: improved procedural outcome with evolution of technique and equipment. Single center results of first 1000 patients. Cathet Cardiovasc Intervent 1999;46:305-311.

45. Bass TA, Williams DO, Ho KKL, et al. Is an aggressive Rotablator strategy preferable to a standard Rotablator strategy in patients with heavily calcified coronary lesions? A report from the STRATAS Trial. J Am Coll Cardiol 1998;31:378A.

46. Reisman M, Buchbinder M, Sharma SK, et al. A multicenter randomized trial of rotational atherectomy vs PTCA: DART. Circulation 1997;96:I467A.

22 CORONARY ARTERY PERFORATION

Daniel T. Lee, M.D.
Robert D. Safian, M.D.

A. INCIDENCE AND CLASSIFICATION. Coronary artery perforation is a rare but important complication of percutaneous revascularization. Angiographic evidence for perforation has been reported in 0.1% of lesions treated with PTCA and 0.5-3.0% of lesions treated with Rotablator, DCA, TEC, or ELCA (Table 22.1).[1-7] At our institution, perforations are classified angiographically as free perforations (free contrast extravasation into the pericardium), contained perforations (localized rounded crater of contrast outside the contrast-filled lumen), or other unclassified perforations (Figure 22.1). In one report, the relative proportion of these types of perforation was 31%, 50%, and 19%, respectively; perforation was caused by a balloon or new device in 74%, a guidewire in 20%, and an indeterminate cause in 6%.[1] Most operators recognize that there has been an increased incidence of coronary artery perforation in the last 10 years, which is probably related to greater lesion complexity, and use of atherectomy devices, high-pressure PTCA after stenting, stiff and/or hydrophilic guidewires, and potent platelet glycoprotein receptor antagonists.[15,23]

B. MECHANISMS AND RISK FACTORS. During PTCA, perforation may occur as a consequence of guidewire advancement, balloon advancement, balloon inflation, or balloon rupture.[8-14] Since PTCA results in dissection and stretching of the vessel wall, oversized balloons (balloon/artery ratio >1.2) may extend these dissections through the adventitia, resulting in vessel perforation. Balloon rupture, particularly those associated with pinhole leaks (as opposed to longitudinal tears), may create

Table 22.1. Incidence of Perforation After Percutaneous Intervention

Series	N	Perforation (%)						
		All devices	PTCA	DCA	ROTA	TEC	ELCA	Stent
Gruberg[32] (2000)	30,746	0.3	-	0.5	0.4	-	0.3	-
Lansky[4] (1995)	708	2.0	-	3.2	-	2.0	1.7	1.1
Ajluni[1] (1994)	8932	0.4	0.1	0.3	0	1.3	2.0	0
Ellis[2] (1994)	12,900	0.5	0.1	0.7	1.3	2.1	1.9	-
Flood[3] (1994)	2426	0.7	0.6	0.3	0.4	0	1.7	0.2

Abbreviations: PTCA = percutaneous transluminal coronary angioplasty; DCA = directional coronary atherectomy; ROTA = Rotablator; TEC = transluminal extraction catheter, ELCA = excimer laser coronary angioplasty; - = not reported

high-pressure jets that increase the risk of dissection and perforation. Devices that alter the integrity of the vascular wall may also lead to perforation by tissue removal (TEC, DCA), pulverization (Rotablator), or ablation (ELCA).[1-6] With Rotablator, morphologic features associated with perforation include lesion eccentricity, lesion length > 10 mm, and vessel tortuosity.[16] Oversized devices, especially when used to treat bifurcation lesions and lesions located in severely angulated vessel segments, substantially increase the risk of perforation. Intracoronary stenting can also lead to perforation from use of stiff guidewires, oversized compliant balloons (for stent delivery), high-pressure balloons (for optimal stent expansion), or from subintimal passage of the stent into a vessel with severe dissection. Regardless of the device, the risk of perforation is increased when complex lesion morphology is present (chronic total occlusion, vessel bifurcation, severe tortuosity or angulation).[6] In our experience, guidewire perforations (such as those that might occur during attempted revascularization of chronic total occlusion) virtually never lead to cardiac tamponade, except in instances when patients have been pretreated with platelet receptor antagonists.[31]

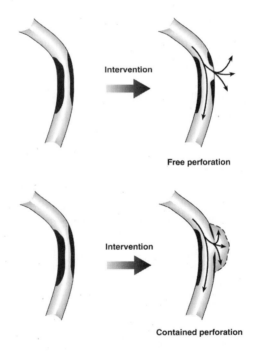

Intervention

Free perforation

Intervention

Contained perforation

Figure 22.1. Types of Coronary Artery Perforation

C. **OUTCOME.** Coronary artery perforation can result in pericardial hemorrhage and cardiac tamponade (17-24% of patients),[1,2,5] fistulae to the left or right ventricle, [9,10] or coronary arteriovenous fistulae. Clinically, coronary perforation is associated with a high incidence of death (0-9%), MI (4-26%), emergency surgery (24-36%), and blood transfusion (34%) (Table 22.2).[1,2,5,6,23] If perforation does occur, the risk of death was 2-fold higher if the patient was receiving a IIb/IIIa inhibitor during the intervention.[33] Some perforations are angiographically inapparent and may go undetected during the interventional procedure, only to manifest 8-24 hours later with the sudden appearance of cardiac tamponade.[1,2,22] Bypass graft perforation may result in chest or mediastinal hemorrhage, but cardiac tamponade is unusual due to partial pericardiectomy during bypass surgery, pericardial adhesions, and the location of most bypass grafts outside the pericardium.[1,12]

D. **PREVENTION**

1. **Guidewire Positioning.** During all percutaneous interventions, the tip of the guidewire should advance smoothly beyond the stenosis and retain torque-response. If there is buckling of the guidewire, restricted tip movement, or resistance to guidewire advancement, the wire may be subintimal and should be withdrawn and repositioned. If there is any concern that the balloon

Table 22.2. Clinical Outcome After Coronary Artery Perforation

Series	Device(s)	No. Perforations (Incidence)	In-hospital Complications (%)		
			CABG	MI	Death
Gruberg[32] (2000)	Various	88 (0.29%)	39	34	10
Bajzer[33] (1999)	Various (abciximab 31%)	75 (1.4%)	-	-	12
Cohen[16] (1996)	ROTA	22 (0.7%)	41	45.5	9
Ellis[2] (1995)	Various (except stent)	62 (0.5%)	24	19	0
Ajluni[1] (1994)	Various (except stent)	35 (0.4%)	37	26	5.6
Flood[3] (1994)	Various	9 (0.7%)	33	5.6	5.9
Holmes[6] (1994)	ELCA	36 (1.3%)	36.1	16.7	4.8
Bittl[5] (1993)	ELCA	23 (3.0%)	34.7	4.3	9

Abbreviations: CABG = emergency coronary artery bypass surgery, DCA = directional coronary atherectomy; ELCA = excimer laser coronary angioplasty; MI = myocardial infarction; PTCA = percutaneous transluminal coronary angioplasty; ROTA = Rotablator; TEC = transluminal extraction catheter

catheter may have entered a false lumen, a gentle contrast injection may be delivered through central lumen of the balloon after removing the guidewire. Persistent contrast staining indicates that a false channel has been entered, and requires withdrawal and repositioning of both the guidewire and balloon, since balloon inflation within a false lumen may result in coronary artery rupture and rapid clinical deterioration.

2. **Device Sizing.** In some studies, oversized devices (device-to-artery ratio ≥ 0.8 for TEC, ELCA and Rotablator; balloon-to-artery ratio >1.2 for PTCA) were important correlates of angiographic perforation.[1,5] Therefore, high-risk lesions (e.g., bifurcations, angulated stenoses, total occlusion) are best approached using balloon-to-artery ratios of 1.0 for PTCA, and device-to-artery ratios of 0.5-0.6 for lasers, TEC, and Rotablator. When these latter devices are used, it may be prudent to achieve further lumen enlargement by adjunctive PTCA (balloon-to-artery ratio = 1) rather than upsizing to a larger device.

3. **Other Device Considerations.** DCA is not recommended for treatment of dissections, due to the risk of perforation and the reliability and effectiveness of stents. Stent-related perforations may be avoided by meticulous attention to balloon sizing and stent position. Stents should not be used when the distal extent of a dissection cannot be identified angiographically.

E. **MANAGEMENT (Figure 22.2).** In general, guidewire perforations rarely result in adverse sequelae,[1] except in some patients who are pretreated with platelet IIb/IIIa receptor antagonists. In contrast, perforations caused by balloons, atherectomy devices, or lasers may result in hemopericardium and hemodynamic collapse,[1,2] particularly if the pericardium is normal. Regardless of the cause, initial management should focus on sealing the perforation nonoperatively and stabilizing the patient hemodynamically. The cardiac surgeons should be notified immediately and the operating room prepared for possible emergency surgery.

1. **Nonoperative Management of Coronary Perforation**
   a. **Prolonged Balloon Inflation**. A balloon (balloon-to-artery ratio = 0.9-1.0) should be immediately positioned at the site of contrast extravasation—even prior to pericardiocentesis, placement of an IABP, or CPR—and inflated to 2-6 atm for at least 10 minutes. If sealing is incomplete, a second low-pressure inflation should be performed for 15-45 minutes, using a perfusion balloon catheter if possible to prevent distal myocardial ischemia. Additional heparin should not be given. Prolonged balloon inflations (and pericardiocentesis if needed) may avoid the need for surgery in 60-70% of patients who develop coronary perforation during percutaneous intervention.[1,2,5,6]

   b. **Stents.** In some cases, stent-vein allografts[18,20,24,25] or PTFE-covered stents[21,26-28] have been used to seal perforations and pseudoaneurysms (Figure 26.15). However, preparation of a stent-vein allograft is technically demanding and may not be appropriate for patients with profound hemodynamic collapse. PTFE-covered stents are attractive for stabilizing perforations, and may soon be approved for use in the United States.

c. **Pericardiocentesis.** Echocardiography should be performed at the first sign of perforation, if possible. If pericardial hemorrhage is evident, immediate pericardiocentesis is performed. If hemodynamic collapse occurs secondary to perforation, pericardiocentesis should be performed immediately after positioning the inflated balloon across the perforated segment. As nonoperative attempts proceed to treat the perforation, the pericardiocentesis needle should be exchanged for a multiple sidehole catheter, allowing continuous aspiration and monitoring of pericardial blood.

d. **Reversal of Anticoagulation.** Initial efforts to seal the perforation should occur while the patient remains anticoagulated (to prevent vessel thrombosis). However, most interventionalists recommend immediate administration of protamine to partially reverse the effects of systemic heparinization when free perforation occurs after atherectomy or laser devices. If contrast extravasation persists despite prolonged balloon inflations, incremental doses of protamine should be administered (as guided by ACT measurements) while repeat balloon inflations are attempted. Vessel closure may be an acceptable alternative to pericardial hemorrhage if bypass surgery is not feasible or if perforation occurs in a small sidebranch. Platelet IIb/IIIa receptor antagonists should be discontinued once perforation occurs; abciximab effects can be reversed by platelet transfusions (6-10 units), but there is no antidote for eptifibatide or tirofiban. Although stent-vein allografts have been used to seal coronary pseudoaneurysms, they may be less useful for acute perforations and hemodynamic collapse because of delayed delivery to the target lesion.

e. **Embolization.** Coil embolization is a reasonable therapeutic strategy in selected cases of coronary artery perforation,[18,29,30,34] such as persistent perforation in poor candidates for surgical repair (due to small vessel or distal location, limited myocardial territory in jeopardy, initial chronic total occlusion, or other clinical situations precluding surgery). Guidewire-induced perforation of the distal coronary artery may also be treated by Gelfoam injected via an infusion catheter.[31]

f. **Monitoring Following Successful Nonoperative Management.** All patients require careful observation in a monitored unit. Continuous monitoring of the right atrial pressure will allow early detection of ongoing pericardial hemorrhage. If pericardiocentesis was performed during PTCA, the drainage catheter should remain in place for 6-24 hours. Serial echocardiography should be performed every 6-12 hours to detect reaccumulation of pericardial effusion. If bleeding persists or recurs, the patient should be referred for emergency surgery.

2. **Operative Management.** If the perforation is large, associated with severe ischemia, or if hemodynamic instability or perforation persists despite nonoperative measures, emergency surgery should be performed to control hemorrhage, repair the perforation or ligate the vessel, and bypass all vessels containing significant stenoses. If possible, a perfusion balloon catheter should be positioned and inflated at low pressure while the operating room is being prepared; intermittent

flushing of the central lumen with heparinized saline will prevent clotting and ensure antegrade blood flow. Operative management may be required in 30-40% of patients who develop perforation.[1,2,5,6] However, the need for surgery may decrease once PTFE-covered stents become available.

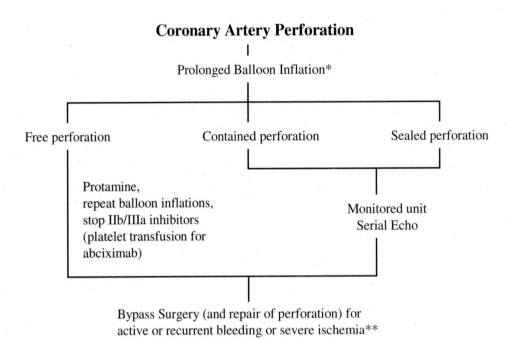

Coronary Artery Perforation

Prolonged Balloon Inflation*

Free perforation

Contained perforation

Sealed perforation

Protamine,
repeat balloon inflations,
stop IIb/IIIa inhibitors
(platelet transfusion for
abciximab)

Monitored unit
Serial Echo

Bypass Surgery (and repair of perforation) for
active or recurrent bleeding or severe ischemia**

Figure 22.2. Management of Coronary Artery Perforation

*   PTFE-covered stent is reasonable if available; vein-covered stent can be used if the patient is hemodynamically stable
**   Coil occlusion may be a reasonable alternative to CABG for small vessels

* * * * *

REFERENCES

1. Ajuni SC, Glazier S, Blankenship L, et al. Perforations after percutaneous coronary interventions: clinical, angiographic, and therapeutic observations. Cathet Cardiovasc Diagn. 1994;32:206-212.

2. Ellis SG, Ajluni S, Arnold AZ, et al. Increased coronary perforation in the new device era. Incidence, classification, management, and outcome. Circulation 1994;90:2725-2730.

3. Flood RD, Popma JJ, Chuang, Ya Chien, et al. Incidence, angiographic predictors, and clinical significance of coronary perforation occurring after new device angioplasty. J Am Coll Cardiol 1994;23:301A.

4. Lansky A, Popma JJ, Baim DS, et al. Angiographic outcome after new devices saphenous vein graft Angioplasty. Abstract from Transcatheter Cardiovascular Therapeutics, 1995.

5. Bittl JA, Ryan TJ, Keaney JF, et al. Coronary artery perforation during excimer laser coronary angioplasty. J Am Coll Cardiol 1993;21:1158-1165.

6. Holmes DR, Reeder GS, Ghazzai ZM, et al. Coronary perforation after excimer laser coronary angioplasty: the excimer laser coronary angioplasty registry experience. J Am Coll Cardiol 1994;23:330-335.

7. Cowley MJ, Dorros G, and Kelsey SF. Acute coronary events associated with percutaneous transluminal coronary angioplasty. Am J Cardiol 1984;53:12C-16C.

8. Saffitz JE, Rose TE, Oaks JB, et al. Coronary arterial rupture during coronary angioplasty. Am J Cardiol 1983;51:902-904.

9. Kimbiris DM, Iskandrian AS, Goel I, et al. Transluminal coronary angioplasty complicated by coronary artery perforation. Cathet Cardiovasc Diagn 1982;8:481-487.

10. Iannone LA and Iannone DP. Iatrogenic left coronary artery fistula-to-left ventricle following PTCA: A previously unreported complication with nonsurgical treatment. Am Heart J 1990;120:1215-1217.

11. Cherry S and Vandormael M. Rupture of a coronary artery and hemorrhage into the ventricular cavity during coronary angioplasty. Am Heart J 1990;113:386-388.

12. Teirstein PS and Hartzler GO. Nonoperative management of aortocoronary saphenous vein graft rupture during percutaneous transluminal coronary angioplasty. Am J Cardiol 1987;60:377-378.

13. Meier B. Benign coronary perforation during percutaneous transluminal coronary angioplasty. Br Heart J 1985;54:33-35.

14. Grollier G, Bories H, Commeau P, et al. Coronary artery perforation during coronary angioplasty. Clin Cardiol 1986;9:27-29.

15. Von Sohsten R, Kopistansky C, Cohen M, et al. Cardiac tamponade in the "new device" era: evaluation of 6999 consecutive percutaneous coronary interventions. Am Heart J 2000; 140: 279-283.

16. Cohen BM, Weber VJ, Reisman M, Casale A, Dorros G. Coronary perforation complicating rotational ablation: The U.S. multicenter experience. Cathet Cardiovasc Diagn. 1996;3:55-59.

17. Mehta S, Popma J, Margolis JR, Moore L, et al. Complications with new angioplasty devices. Are these device specific? J Am Coll Cardiol 1996;27 (supplement A):168A.

18. Dorros G, Jain A, Kumar K. Management of coronary artery rupture: Covered stent or microcoil embolization. Cathet Cardiovasc Diagn. 1995;36:148-154.

19. Kaplan BM, Stewart RE, Sakwa MP, et al. Repair of a coronary pseudoaneurysm with percutaneous placement of a saphenous vein allograft attached to a biliary stent. Cathet Cardiovasc Diagn. 1996;37:208-212.

20. Gruberg L, Roguin A, Beyar R. Percutaneous closure of a coronary aneurysm with a vein-coated stent. Cathet Cardiovasc Diagn. 1998;43:308-310.

21. Ramsdale DR, Mushahwar SS, Mooris JL. Repair of coronary artery perforation after rotastenting by implantation of the Jostent covered stent. Cathet Cardiovasc Diagn 1998;45:310-313.

22. Abhyakar AD, England D, Bernstein L, Harris PJ. Delayed appearance of distal coronary perforation stent implantation. Cathet Cardiovasc Diagn. 1998;43:311-312.

23. Wong CM, Mak GY, Chung DTW. Distal coronary artery perforation resulting from the use of hydrophilic coated guidewire in tortuous vessels. Cathet Cardiovasc Diagn 1998; 44: 93-96.

24. Colon PJ, Ramee SR, Mulingtapang R, et al. Percutaneous bailout therapy of a perforated vein graft using a stent-autologous vein patch. Cathet Cardiovasc Diagn 1996; 38: 175-178.

25. Caputo RP, Amin N, Marvasti M, et al. Successful treatment of a saphenous vein graft perforation with an autologous vein-covered stent. Cathet Cardiovasc Intervent 1999; 48: 382-386.

26. Campbell PG, Hall JA, Harcombe AA, et al. The Jomed covered stent graft for coronary artery aneurysms and acute perforation: a successful device which needs careful deployment and may not reduce restenosis. J Invas Cardiol 2000;12:272-276.

27. Casella G, Werner F, Klauss V, et al. Successful treatment of coronary artery perforation during angioplasty using a new membrane-coated stent. J Invas Cardiol 1999;11:622-626.

28. Bosmans JM, Claeys MJ, Dilling D, et al. Unsuccessful long-term outcome after treatment of a vein graft false aneurysm with a polytetrafluoethylene-coated Jostent. Cathet Cardiovasc Intervent 2000; 50: 105-108.

29. Thomas WJ, Moskowitz WB, Freedman A, et al. Therapeutic embolization for unusual iatrogenic complications related to coronary revascularization. Cathet Cardiovasc Intervent 46: 457-462, 1999.

30. Gaxiola E, Browne KF. Coronary artery perforation repair using microcoil embolization. Cathet Cardiovasc Diagn 1998; 43: 474-6.

31. Dixon SR, Webster MWI, Ormiston JA, et al. Gelfoam embolization of a distal coronary artery guidewire perforation. Cathet Cardiovasc Intervent 2000; 49: 214-217.

32. Gruberg L, Pinnow E, Flood R, et al. Incidence, management and outcome of coronary artery perforation during percutaneous coronary intervention. Am J Cardiol 2000;86:680-682.

33. Bajzer CT, Whitlow PL, Lincoff AM, et al. Coroanry perforation and pericardial tamponade risk in the abciximab era. J Am Coll Cardiol 1999;33:72A

34. Aslam MS, Messersmith RN, Gilbert J, et al. Successful management of coronary artery perforation with helical platinum microcoil embolization. Cathet Cardiovasc Intervent 2000;51:320-322.

23

EMERGENCY BYPASS SURGERY FOR FAILED PTCA

Francis L. Shannon, M.D.
Marc P. Sakwa, M.D.

A. **INTRODUCTION.** The role of the cardiac surgeon in managing the acute complications of percutaneous coronary procedures continues to change. Increasing use of stents has resulted in less need for emergency coronary artery bypass surgery for dissection and acute closure. However, emergency CABG is still required for refractory acute closure, injury to the left main coronary artery, coronary artery perforation, and hemodynamic collapse. Anticipating the need for emergency CABG for high-risk patients is important.

1. **Levels of Surgical Back-Up for Percutaneous Interventions.** Historically, PTCA has been a "joint venture" between interventional cardiologists and cardiac surgeons. As Andreas Gruntzig related to Joseph Craver at Emory University in 1978: "For a successful coronary angioplasty program, good cardiology is important, but superior cardiac surgery is essential."[1] Since that time, the incidence of emergency CABG for failed PTCA has decreased from 7% to less than 1% because of the use of stents for dissection.[2] In the United States, nearly all interventional cardiology programs have on-site surgical capabilities to perform emergency surgery,[3] but many European programs rely on off-site surgical "back-up."[4-6] Among programs with on-site surgical capability, the degree of support ranges from a strict "stand-by" arrangement, in which an open operating room and surgical team are immediately available, to a "back-up" arrangement in which emergency cardiac surgery is performed in the next available operating room.[7] Overall procedural mortality rates and average time intervals to surgical revascularization are similar when comparing these two strategies.[8,9] The scheme adopted by any interventional cardiology program depends on the risk profile of its patient population, technical expertise of its cardiologists, and elective case volume of its cardiac surgical team. For our institution, in which 7000 percutaneous interventions and 2000 cardiac surgical procedures are performed each year, the surgical approach described below is the safest and most efficient.

2. **Surgical Consultation Before PTCA.** Prior to percutaneous intervention, we perform a detailed risk assessment in patients with multiple or complex coronary lesions, poor left ventricular function, severe associated medical problems, previous CABG, or lack of adequate bypass conduits. This appraisal is used to identify and inform patients in whom emergency cardiac surgery is not a therapeutic option. In all other patients, a cardiac surgical team and appropriate operating room facilities are made ready for urgent management of specific PTCA complications on a "next available" basis. Optimal surgical back-up is facilitated by scheduling high-risk percutaneous interventions during times when the cardiac surgical suites are available. For patients who ultimately require emergency CABG, autoperfusion catheters and intra-aortic balloon pumps (IABP) attenuate myocardial ischemia while the operating room is being prepared, if stents cannot

be utilized successfully. Interventional complications requiring emergency CABG after hours and on weekends are supported by an off-site "on call" cardiac surgical team that is ready to initiate operation within 60 minutes of notification. On average, there is a delay of 100 minutes between identification of refractory ischemia in the cath lab and initial myocardial reperfusion in the operating room. This period includes approximately 30 minutes for placement of cardiopulmonary monitoring lines and internal mammary artery mobilization for patients stabilized by autoperfusion catheters and/or IABP. In catastrophic situations, surgical revascularization has been performed within 30 minutes of lethal myocardial ischemia.

B. INCIDENCE. The incidence of failed PTCA requiring emergency cardiac surgery within 24 hours has decreased from 7% to 2% in the 1990's, to less than 1% today.[1,11-13] This trend is due to more experienced interventional cardiologists, better patient selection, liberal use of stents for unstable dissections, and medical management of acute closure of small vessels or vessels supplying nonviable myocardium. Application of percutaneous revascularization to higher-risk patients (multivessel disease, poor LV function, advanced age, evolving MI) has resulted in greater risk for operative morbidity and mortality after emergency CABG.

C. EVALUATION AND INDICATIONS FOR EMERGENCY CABG. Once summoned to the cardiac cath lab, the surgeon performs an initial patient evaluation for pertinent comorbid conditions, hemodynamic status, and coronary anatomy.

1. **Important Associated Conditions**

   a. **Age.** Octogenarians who require emergency CABG have the highest mortality of all age subgroups. At our institution, patients > 80 years with cardiogenic shock have perioperative mortality rates exceeding 90% after emergency CABG for failed PTCA. Careful selection for emergency CABG is therefore required.

   b. **Mental Status.** Patients who have suffered cardiac arrest prior to or during percutaneous intervention should be examined closely. Recent stroke, prolonged cardiopulmonary arrest, and an unresponsive state are relative contraindications to emergency CABG.

   c. **Conduit Availability.** Patients with prior removal of greater saphenous veins for cosmetic reasons or previous vascular surgical procedures (CABG or fem-pop bypass) are poor candidates for emergency CABG. Myocardial ischemic time is increased because of the additional time necessary to mobilize arterial or lesser saphenous venous conduits. Cryopreserved human saphenous veins may be used in these circumstances, but one-year patency is less than 50%.[14]

   d. **Previous Cardiac Surgery.** In patients requiring emergency repeat CABG, myocardial ischemic time may be prolonged by difficulties in cannulation and exposure. The risk of graft atheroembolization may be increased by the cardiac manipulation necessary to establish urgent cardiopulmonary bypass.

e. Thrombolytic and Antiplatelet Agents. Prior infusion of thrombolytic, antithrombin, or antiplatelet agents as adjuncts to percutaneous intervention increases the tendency for coagulopathy but is not a contraindication to emergency surgery. Judicious use of clotting factors, platelet concentrates, and cryoprecipitate usually reduces total blood loss and delayed hemorrhage. Patients receiving platelet GP IIb/IIIa receptor antagonists should be treated by immediate discontinuation of the drug (abciximab, eptifibatide, tirofiban) and platelet transfusions (abciximab).

2. **Indications for Emergency Cardiac Surgery**
   a. **Acute Occlusion of a Major Coronary Artery.** Acute occlusion due to dissection accounted for 70% of operations in the pre-stent era, but has decreased markedly due to widespread availability of stents. Refractory acute closure must be differentiated from "no-reflow" (Chapter 21), which is not amenable to bypass surgery.

   b. **Suboptimal Angioplasty With Refractory Myocardial Ischemia.** In patients with residual dissection, ongoing ischemia, and stenosis > 70% after percutaneous intervention, intracoronary nitroglycerin and IABP will usually relieve myocardial ischemia and permit urgent surgical revascularization within 24 hours.

   c. **Coronary Artery Perforation With Pericardial Tamponade.** Initial management of coronary artery perforation in all patients includes immediate balloon inflation at the site of perforation and notification of the cardiac surgeons in case surgery is required. Although older reports considered coronary perforation an absolute indication for emergency surgery, this problem can be managed by prolonged balloon inflations (up to 30 minutes), on-table echocardiographic assessment of pericardial fluid accumulation, and pigtail catheter drainage of large pericardial effusions. In some cases, PTFE- or vein-covered stents can successfully seal persistent perforations (Chapter 22). Using this selective approach, we have performed emergency CABG and arterial repair for 40% of patients with coronary perforations. Primary indications for emergency surgery in this group include persistent hemodynamic compromise or uncontrolled hemorrhage despite prolonged balloon inflations, or inability to tolerate prolonged balloon inflations because of ischemia or hemodynamic instability. The caliber, location, and distribution of the perforated vessel are important considerations. Focal perforations in small vessels with small myocardial distributions can often be treated by coil embolization, whereas perforations in unprotected left main coronary arteries usually require surgery.

   d. **Left Main Coronary Injury or Occlusion.** Although infrequent, injury to the left main can result from direct trauma from guiding catheters, intracoronary devices, or retrograde propagation of a large dissection. Cardiovascular collapse is usually precipitous. Immediate surgery should be undertaken, particularly if stents fail to stabilize the patient. Mortality is high.

e. **Retained Intracoronary Foreign Bodies With or Without Obstruction.** Fractured fragments of balloon catheters, devices, and guidewires that remain trapped in a proximal coronary artery are potential causes of mechanical or thrombotic occlusion. Misplaced or incompletely deployed stents in native coronary arteries or saphenous vein grafts can usually be managed percutaneously by additional stenting or PTCA. We usually attempt to extract foreign bodies to prevent distal embolization and thrombosis of coronary arteries; bypass distal to the obstruction is sufficient to avert distal migration of retained hardware and maintain distal perfusion.

D. **CONTRAINDICATIONS TO EMERGENCY SURGERY.** There are few absolute criteria to deny a dying patient a chance to survive with emergency surgery. Nevertheless, the following factors may preclude successful operative outcome:
1. Acute cerebral injury from hypoxia, vascular emboli, or cerebrovascular insufficiency
2. Metastatic or untreated malignancy
3. Acquired Immunodeficiency Syndrome
4. End-stage lung disease (FEV_1 < 1.0 liters/minute or baseline pO_2 < 45 mmHg)
5. Inoperable diffuse coronary artery disease
6. Multiple previous cardiac operations with no available bypass conduits
7. Irreversible left ventricular failure
8. Cardiogenic shock with inability to wean from percutaneous cardiopulmonary support (CPS)
9. Age > 80 years with cardiogenic shock

E. **PREPARATION FOR SURGERY.** All possible interventions to minimize systemic and myocardial ischemia should be employed while the operating room is being prepared. These measures fall into the following categories:
1. **Restoration of Adequate Oxygen Delivery to the Heart and Systemic Circulation.** Airway management (endotracheal intubation and ventilation) and maintenance of adequate systemic perfusion pressure (IABP, vasopressors, inotropes) are essential, as reducing preoperative oxygen debt reduces the risk of emergency CABG (particularly in patients who are subclinically hypoxemic from the cumulative effects of sedative drugs, low cardiac output, and acute blood loss).

2. **Maintenance of Distal Coronary Blood Flow.** In the presence of acute occlusion, passage of a guidewire across the obstruction usually restores flow and permits placement of an autoperfusion catheter, particularly if stents fail. However, once the decision has been made to perform emergency surgery, further percutaneous manipulations to open the artery should be abandoned if the operating room is ready.

3. **Pharmacologic Coronary Vasodilation.** Coronary perfusion can be enhanced by intravenous nitrates if the patient is not hypotensive.

4. **Managing Cardiac Arrest.** Among patients who suffer cardiac arrest, preparation for surgery is condensed to initiating CPR and transporting the patient to the operating room. Placement of an IABP is the best use of femoral arterial access, rather than attempting to traverse the occluded coronary artery. Initiation of percutaneous CPS is considered only if an operating room is not immediately available. Initiation of cardiopulmonary bypass within 30 minutes of cardiac arrest has yielded survival rates > 90% at our institution.

F. **SURGICAL TECHNIQUES.** If the patient is hemodynamically stable and has no signs of myocardial ischemia, surgical techniques are similar to those employed during elective CABG. Radial arterial and central venous monitoring lines are placed, and the left internal mammary artery is mobilized. All other patients undergo anesthetic induction and full cardiopulmonary bypass (CPB) while saphenous veins are harvested for bypass. The immediate goals in surgical resuscitation of the unstable patient are decompression of the left ventricle on full CPB (so global myocardial oxygen demand is reduced) and restoration of effective systemic perfusion. Off-pump bypass is rarely utilized for emergency surgical revascularization.

1. **Conduit Selection.** Use of the internal mammary artery is determined by the hemodynamic stability of the patient, coronary anatomy, ability to adequately protect the ischemic zone, and maintenance of adequate distal perfusion. We are able to use the LIMA for emergency revascularization of the LAD in more than 50% of patients. For all other coronary lesions, saphenous veins are used because of dependable patency rates, versatility in patching and bypassing complex coronary injuries, and ease of harvesting in crisis situations. Cryopreserved human saphenous vein is an option in older patients with good LV function and no autologous venous conduits.

2. **Myocardial Protection.** Initial reperfusion of the ischemic zone with blood cardioplegia is a critical component of successful myocardial salvage. In most circumstances, we use antegrade cardioplegia (via the aortic root) to assure global cardiac arrest and retrograde cardioplegia (via a catheter in the coronary sinus) to achieve perfusion of myocardial zones supplied by critically narrowed or totally occluded coronary arteries. We have selectively used Buckberg's protocol of "warm induction cardioplegia" without substrate enhancement for patients with cardiogenic shock or large ischemic territories.[17] In theory, induction of diastolic cardiac arrest at an infusion temperature of 36° C allows replenishment of depleted myocardial stores of ADP and ATP prior to aortic cross-clamping. After initial warm induction, we deliver sufficient volumes of cold blood cardioplegia both antegrade and retrograde to achieve a myocardial septal temperature < 15° C. While the aorta is cross-clamped, we reinfuse cold blood cardioplegia with low potassium concentration (15 meq/L) every 15-20 minutes. We generally do not deliver a "hot shot" of antegrade cardioplegia before removal of the aortic cross clamp, but allow full cardiac reperfusion on bypass for at least 20-30 minutes before attempting to wean the patient from full support. Using this method of myocardial reperfusion and protection, we have been able to separate most patients from cardiopulmonary bypass if the cardiac index is at least 1.8 L/min/m^2.

3. **Coronary Arterial Repair and Revascularization.** One of the most challenging aspects of emergency CABG involves the need to bypass long segments of stented coronary arteries and repair long spiral dissections. The challenge relates to delivery of distal perfusion while maintaining antegrade flow to proximal branches. For long dissections, we recommend long-patch angioplasty with saphenous veins, first achieving good distal flow and then attempting to re-attach the intima proximally to establish antegrade perfusion. When long stents are used, we attempt to use the LIMA if it will reach the distal vessel. If not, venous conduits are used. We also use variations of the saphenous vein patch-angioplasty technique for distal perforations. Direct coronary arterial repair is not anatomically feasible for perforations of the proximal LAD and circumflex, so we perform distal coronary bypass and oversew the suspected perforation with pledgetted mattress sutures to prevent further bleeding. These approaches to the injured coronary artery are not standardized, but constitute our solutions to preserve as much myocardium as possible.

4. **Special Considerations.** Once the coronary arterial injury is treated, the secondary goal of complete myocardial revascularization is addressed. Decision-making in this phase of the operation has become more complex because most patients have coexistent multivessel coronary disease or previous percutaneous procedures involving other epicardial arteries. In general, the number of bypasses depends on the condition of the patient prior to operation, the adequacy of myocardial protection during surgery, and the severity of associated coronary disease. If the patient is stable and the operation is proceeding well, we place venous bypass grafts to all coronary arteries > 1.5 mm in diameter with proximal diameter stenoses exceeding 70%. In addition, we prophylactically bypass coronary arteries successfully revascularized within one month of percutaneous intervention to prevent postoperative ischemia due to restenosis.

5. **Operative Adjuncts.** Emergency surgery for failed PTCA often requires extraordinary measures to separate the patient from cardiopulmonary bypass. Pharmacologic support includes inotropes, pressors, and correction of acidosis. Blood replacement is aggressively initiated before the chest is closed to maintain a hemoglobin concentration > 9 gm/dL. Clotting factors are used to reverse the coagulopathy created by cardiopulmonary bypass and preoperative antiplatelet or thrombolytic therapy. Single or biventricular support devices are considered for patients < 65 years of age who have suffered massive, but potentially reversible myocardial injury. The chest is left open and the heart is covered with a sterile barrier when massive cardiac swelling from fluid resuscitation, myocardial edema, or epicardial hematoma preclude sternal closure (causing extrinsic compression of the heart). Among survivors, these measures are associated with a surprisingly low rate of wound and other infectious complications.

G. RESULTS OF EMERGENCY CABG

1. **Mortality.** From 1980 to 1987, fifteen studies comprising 548 patients requiring emergency CABG for PTCA failure reported an average operative mortality of 9% (range 0-17%).[8,9,18-28] While these studies have little relevance to the current era, they provide a benchmark for analyzing

current results with high-risk patients. From 1985-1992, three studies reported overall operative mortality rates of 5.7%-12.5%, and mortality rate of 40% for patients in cardiogenic shock.[1,10,12] Data from the Society of Thoracic Surgeons (1990-1993) reported operative mortality in 5.6% of 3,975 patients requiring emergency CABG within 6 hours of PTCA.[29]

2. **Perioperative Myocardial Infarction.** The rate of perioperative MI in the early multicenter studies was 42% (range 28-63%),[8,9,18-28] but most of these patients underwent emergency CABG prior to widespread use of perfusion catheters, retrograde cardioplegia, and modified surgical reperfusion described by Buckberg. These measures have reduced the incidence MI to 12.5%.[30]

3. **Low Cardiac Output State.** During the initial 24 hours following operation, cardiac index < 2.0 L/min/m^2 is associated with multisystem organ dysfunction and death.

4. **Noncardiac Morbidity.** Nonoliguric renal failure and prolonged mechanical ventilation are the most important noncardiac complications of emergency CABG and occur in 5-10% of patients. Although most patients recover from these complications, they remain susceptible to recurrent pulmonary edema, ventricular dysrhythmias, pulmonary embolism, and sepsis, which can result in late death despite meticulous postoperative care.

* * * * *

REFERENCES

1. Craver JM, Weintraub WS, Jones EL, et. al. Emergency coronary artery bypass surgery for failed percutaneous coronary angioplasty. An Surg 1992; 215:425-433.

2. Vogel JH. Changing trends for surgical standby in patients undergoing percutaneous transluminal coronary angioplasty. Am J Cardiol. 1992; 69:25F-35F.

3. Cameron DE, Stinson DC, Greene PS, et al. Surgical standby for percutaneous coronary angioplasty: A survey of patterns of practice. Ann Thorac Surg 1990;50:35-39.

4. Iniguez A, Macaya C, Hernandez R, et al. Comparison of results of percutaneous transluminal coronary angioplasty with and without selective requirement of surgical standby. Am J Cardiol 1992; 69:1161-1165.

5. Klinke WP and Hui W. Percutaneous transluminal angioplasty without on-site surgical facilities. Am J Cardiology 1992;70:1520-1525.

6. Richardson SG, Morton P, Murtagh JG, et al. Management of acute coronary occlusion during percutaneous coronary angioplasty: Experience of complications in a hospital without on-site facilities for cardiac surgery. British Med J 1990;300:355-358.

7. Meier B. Surgical standby for PTCA. In Textbook of Interventional Cardiology, E. Topol (Ed) WB Saunders 1994; p. 565-575.

8. Feyter PJ, Jaegere PP, Murphy ES, et al. Abrupt coronary artery occlusion during percutaneous transluminal coronary angioplasty. Am Heart J 1992;123:1633-1642.

9. Scott NA, Weintraub WS, Carlin SF, et al. Recent changes in the management and outcome of acute closure after percutaneous transluminal coronary angioplasty. Am J Cardiol 1993;71:1159-1163.

10. Lazar HL, Faxon DP, Paone G, et al. Changing profiles of failed coronary angioplasty patients: Impact on surgical results. Ann Thorac Surg 1992;53:269-273.

11. Greene MA, Gary LA, Slater D, et al. Emergency aortocoronary bypass after failed angioplasty. Ann Thorac Surg 1991;51:194-199.

12. Taylor PC, Boylan MJ, Lytle BW, et al. Emergent coronary bypass for failed PTCA: A 10-year experience with 253 patients. J Invasive Cardiol 1994;6:97-98.

13. Carey JA, Davres SW, Balcon R, et al. Emergency surgical revascularization for coronary angioplasty complications. Br Heart J 1994; 72:428-435.

14. Glick DB, Liddicoat JR, Karp RB. Alternative conduits for coronary artery bypass grafting. Advances in Cardiac Surgery. RB Karp (Ed) Mosby Year Book 1990 p;191-201.

15. Piana RN, Paik GY, Moscucci M, et al. Incidence and treatment of no-reflow after percutaneous coronary intervention. Circulation 1994;89:2514-2518.

16. Denny TL, Magovern JA, Kao RL, et al. Resuscitation of injured myocardium with adenosine and biventricular assist. Ann Thorac Surg 1993;105:864-884.

17. Allen BS, Buckberg GD, Fontain RM, et al. Superiority of controlled surgical reprfusion versus percutaneous transluminal coronary angioplasty in acute coronary occlusion. J Thorac Cardiovasc Surg 1993;105:864-884.

18. Lazar HL, Haan CK. Determinants of myocardial infarction following emergency coronary artery bypass for failed percutaneous coronary angioplasty. Ann Thorac Surg 1987;44:646-650.

19. Pelletier LC, Pardini A, Renkin J, et al. Myocardial revascularization after failure of percutaneous transluminal coronary angioplasty. J Thorac Cardiovasc Surg 1985;90:265-271.

20. Brediau CE, Roubin GS, Leimgruber PP, et al. In-hospital morbidity and mortality in patients undergoing elective coronary angioplasty. Circulation 1985;72:1044-1052.

21. Acinapura AJ, Cummingham JN Jr, Jacobowitz IJ, et al. Efficacy of percutaneous transluminal coronary angioplasty compared with single-vessel bypass. J Thorac Cardiovasc Surg 1985;89:35-41.

22. Killen DA, Hamaker WR, Reed WA. Coronary artery bypass following percutaneous transluminal coronary angioplasty. Ann Thorac Surg 1985;40:133-138.

23. Golding LA, Loop FD, Hollman JL, et al. Early results of emergency surgery after coronary angioplasty. Circulation 1986;74:, III-26.

24. Parsonnet V, Fisch D, Gielchinsky I, et al. Emergency operation after failed angioplasty. J Thorac Cardiovasc Surg 1988; 96:198-203.

25. Naunheim KS, Fiore AC, Fagan D et al. Emergency coronary artery bypass grafting for failed angioplasty: Risk factors and outcome. Ann Thorac Surg 1989;47:816-823.

Stark KS, Satler LF, Krucoff MW, et al. Myocardial salvage after failed coronary angioplasty. J Am Coll Cardiol 1990;15:78-82.

27. Kahn JK, Rutherford BD, McConahy DR, et al. Outcome following emergency coronary artery bypass grafting for failed elective balloon coronary angioplasty in patients with prior coronary bypass. Am J Cardiol 1990; 66:285-288.

28. Barner HB, LEA IV JW, Naunheim KS, et al. Emergency coronary bypass not associated with pre-operative cardiogenic shock in failed angioplasty, after thrombolysis for acute myocardial infarction. Circulation Suppl. I 1989;79:I152-I159.

29. Clark RE, Acinapura J, Anderson RD, et al. Data analysis of the Society of Thoracic Surgeons. National Cardiac Surgery Database. 1994, p. 78.

30. Boerher JD, Kereiakes DJ, Maveita FL, et al. Effects of profound platelet inhibition with c7E3 before coronary angioplasty and complications of coronary bypass surgery. Am J Cardiol 1994;74:1166-1170.

RESTENOSIS

24

George Dangas, M.D., Ph.D.
Michael A. Peterson, M.D.
Mark S. Freed, M.D.
Robert D. Safian, M.D.

Since the introduction of PTCA in 1977,[1] advances in catheter technology, operator experience, and adjunctive pharmacotherapy have improved early outcomes after percutaneous revascularization; procedural success > 90% and complication rates < 5% are readily achieved.[2,3] Despite these advances, long-term outcome is still limited by restenosis, and more than 150,000 patients each year require repeat target lesion revascularization. Better understanding of the mechanisms of restenosis has led to new mechanical and pharmacologic approaches.

RESTENOSIS AFTER PTCA AND ATHEROABLATIVE TECHNIQUES

A. **DEFINITIONS OF RESTENOSIS.** Restenosis may be defined angiographically or clinically. Angiographic definitions use continuous or binary angiographic variables such as minimal lumen diameter and percent diameter stenosis, while clinical definitions use clinical events such as death, MI and repeat target lesion revascularization.

1. **Angiographic Restenosis**
   a. **Dichotomous Events.** Many definitions view restenosis as a dichotomous event (i.e., present or absent). The most common definition is diameter stenosis > 50% at follow-up,[8] which was based on early studies showing impaired coronary flow reserve in such lesions.[9] Depending on which definition is chosen (Table 24.1), restenosis rates can vary widely (Figure 24.1).[10]

   b. **Continuous Outcomes.** "Restenosis" occurs to a variable extent in virtually all lesions,[11] with changes in lumen diameter following a Gaussian distribution.[12] By expressing lumen diameter and diameter stenosis as a cumulative frequency curve, restenosis rates can be determined for any dichotomous definition (Figure 24.2). Cumulative distribution curves give a better visual estimate of changes in lumen diameter following percutaneous therapy, and allow more effective comparisons between different interventions.

   c. **Comparative Measurements.** Important insights into understanding mechanisms of restenosis come from the relationship between lumen diameter at baseline, immediately after intervention, and during follow-up, expressed as acute gain and late loss (Figure 24.3). *Acute gain*, defined as the difference in lumen diameter before and immediately after intervention, is due to plaque

Table 24.1. Angiographic Definitions of Restenosis

EMORY	Diameter stenosis $\geq$ 50% at follow-up
NHLBI I	Increase in diameter stenosis $\geq$ 30% at follow-up (compared to immediately after intervention)
NHLBI II	Residual diameter stenosis < 50% after PTCA increasing to $\geq$ 70% at follow-up
NHLBI III	Increase in diameter stenosis at follow-up to within 10% of the diameter stenosis before PTCA
NHLBI IV	> 50% loss of the initial gain achieved after PTCA
THORAXCENTER IIA	$\geq$ 0.72 mm loss in lumen diameter at follow-up

Abbreviations: NHLBI = National Heart, Lung, and Blood Institute

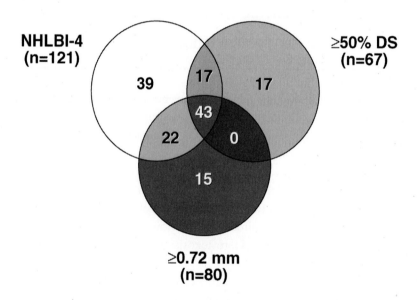

Figure 24.1. Number of Lesions with Restenosis Using Three Different Definitions

Adapted from Beatt et al,[10] with permission.

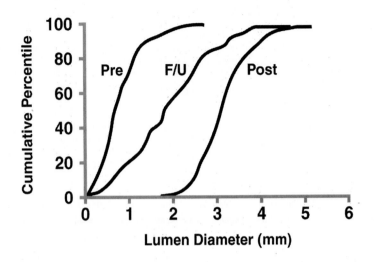

Figure 24.2. Cumulative Frequency Distribution Analysis

Cumulative distribution of baseline minimal lumen diameter (PRE), post-intervention minimal lumen diameter (POST), and follow-up minimal lumen diameter (F/U).

removal and/or arterial expansion. *Late loss,* defined as the difference in lumen diameter after intervention and at follow-up,[13] reflects the net effects of intimal hyperplasia, elastic recoil, and vascular remodeling.[14] Several studies have shown that the relationship between acute gain and late loss is constant irrespective of the device:[15] for every 1 mm of acute gain in lumen diameter, 0.5 mm is lost over 3-6 months (i.e., 50% of the initial gain is lost).[16,17] The *loss index* is the ratio of late loss to acute gain;[33] a typical loss index is 0.5. At present, the only technique which has been shown to favorably impact the loss index is brachytherapy (see below).

2. **Clinical Restenosis.** Although angiographic analyses offer insight into the mechanisms of restenosis and permit quantitative comparisons between devices, the impact on clinical outcome (recurrent angina, need for repeat PTCA or CABG, myocardial infarction, death) is more important. In fact, the correlation between quantitative angiography and symptoms is poor, particularly in the presence of a moderate (50-70%) stenosis (Table 24.2). Target lesion revascularization, defined as "clinically-driven" (recurrent symptoms and a positive stress test) revascularization of the original target lesion, has been used as a surrogate for restenosis.[20-22] Repeat revascularization of a residual stenosis > 50% in the absence of objective evidence of ischemia ("oculostenotic reflex") is *not* considered clinical restenosis. Symptomatic restenosis usually manifests as recurrent angina rather than acute MI or sudden death. Restenotic lesions consist primarily of intimal hyperplasia and fibrous tissue, and are less prone to rupture and acute thrombosis than *de novo* lesions.

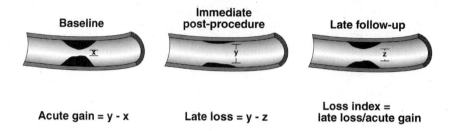

Baseline   Immediate post-procedure   Late follow-up

Acute gain = y - x   Late loss = y - z   Loss index = late loss/acute gain

Figure 24.3. Mathematical Relationship Between Acute Gain, Late Loss, and Loss Index

B. INCIDENCE OF RESTENOSIS. Restenosis rates vary depending upon patient, lesion, and device characteristics. Routine PTCA of Type A lesions commonly result in angiographic restenosis rates of 40-50%, and clinical restenosis rates are typically half the angiographic rate.[124]

C. MECHANISMS OF RESTENOSIS. Restenosis is due to varying degrees of elastic recoil, intimal thickening, and vascular remodeling (Figure 24.4).

1. **Elastic Recoil** is defined as the difference between the inflated balloon diameter and minimal lumen diameter after balloon deflation. The degree of elastic recoil depends on plastic changes in the atherosclerotic plaque and elastic characteristics of the arterial wall. Most elastic recoil occurs within 30 minutes after balloon deflation (but may occur up to 24 hours later), and can result in a 50% decrease in cross-sectional area.[23] Elastic recoil is more common after PTCA of eccentric and ostial lesions, and is greatest after PTCA, intermediate after DCA,[112] and lowest after stenting. Angiographic analysis suggests that early recoil is associated with a higher incidence of restenosis;[24,25] elimination of elastic recoil may partially explain the reduction in angiographic restenosis and repeat revascularization after stenting.[22]

2. **Intimal Thickening** is a generalized response to vessel injury caused by PTCA and other devices. Activation of the coagulation cascade and inflammatory cells results in the production of chemotactic and growth factors, which lead to thrombus formation, intimal hyperplasia (smooth muscle cell migration and proliferation), and accumulation of connective tissue matrix. Atherectomy specimens support the proliferative nature of restenosis; *de novo* lesions are usually hypocellular, whereas restenotic lesions are typically hyperplastic with smooth muscle cells.[26,27] While the angiographic relationship between acute gain and late loss supports a general correlation between the extent of arterial injury and the amount of intimal thickening, some data suggest that the type of injury may be important as well, especially with debulking therapies. Laser-balloon angioplasty

Table 24.2. Correlation Between Angiographic Findings and Clinical Symptoms After Intervention

Presentation	Correlation
Angiographic restenosis	• The stenosis may not be "functionally" significant; patients are often asymptomatic
No angiographic restenosis	• Single vessel disease: symptoms are rare • Multivessel disease: if symptoms are present, they may be due to incomplete revascularization and/or progressive disease at sites other than the original target lesion
Recurrent angina	• Single vessel disease: angiographic restenosis is likely • Multivessel disease: angiographic restenosis is not necessarily present; symptoms may be due to incomplete revascularization and/or progressive disease at sites other than the original target lesion[18]
Absence of recurrent symptoms	• Angiographic restenosis is unlikely, unless the original target lesion was a chronic total occlusion[18,19]

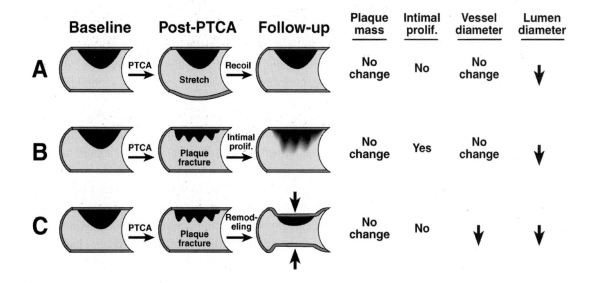

Figure 24.4. Mechanisms of Restenosis

A. *Elastic recoil.* After PTCA, there is stretching of the arterial wall, which simply returns to its original dimensions
B. *Intimal proliferation.* After PTCA, there is plaque fracture; the vessel heals by intimal proliferation
C. *Remodeling.* After PTCA, there is plaque fracture; remodeling of the vessel wall leads to a decrease in the normal vessel diameter
These mechanisms are not mutually exclusive, and may occur together in a given patient

(thermal injury), rotational atherectomy and possibly DCA may induce more intimal hyperplasia than other devices. Multiple trials using lipid-lowering drugs, vitamins, anticoagulants, IIb/IIIa antagonists, anti-inflammatory drugs, and some antiproliferative agents have failed to reduce intimal thickening. However, newer pharmacologic approaches and local brachytherapy offer some hope for reducing intimal hyperplasia (see below).

3. **Arterial Remodeling.** Experimental studies[28,29] and serial intravascular ultrasound imaging in humans[30] demonstrate a "constriction" or shrinkage of the vessel and loss in luminal diameter after coronary interventions without stenting. This "negative" arterial remodeling is the most important determinant of restenosis after PTCA and DCA, accounting for up to 85% of late lumen loss,[113,114] suggesting that pharmacologic trials to prevent restenosis after angioplasty by inhibiting intimal hyperplasia may have been targeting the wrong mechanism.[115] These observations may also partially explain the value of stents for reducing restenosis, since stents prevent negative remodeling. In contrast to restenosis after PTCA, in-stent restenosis is mostly due to neointimal hyperplasia, suggesting that pharmacologic interventions may reduce in-stent restenosis even if they were ineffective after PTCA.

D. **TIME COURSE OF RESTENOSIS.** Restenosis after PTCA is uncommon in the first month, peaks by 1-3 months, reaches a plateau within 3-6 months, and is unusual after 12 months.[31,32] A serial angiographic study showed a reduction in stenosis severity from 9 months to 5 years after PTCA.[123] The time course of restenosis after laser, directional and rotational atherectomy is similar to PTCA.

E. **PREDICTORS OF RESTENOSIS**
1. **Geometric Factors.** Several studies indicate an inverse relationship between post-procedural lumen diameter and restenosis (i.e., "bigger is better"),[13,15,20,37,38] independent of the type of device. Other studies suggested the contrary: In the ERBAC trial, a trend toward *more* restenosis was observed in the Rotablator and excimer laser groups (vs. PTCA) despite *larger* post-procedural lumen diameters.[39] Very high (> 70%) restenosis rates were also reported after laser balloon angioplasty despite excellent initial lumen enlargement,[40] leading to withdrawal of this device from the market. Finally, DCA resulted in more late loss than PTCA[41] and stents[105] despite similar acute gains. Collectively, these studies suggest that the final lumen diameter and possibly the device type (i.e., type of vessel injury) impact on late lumen dimensions and restenosis. Recent DCA data suggest that deep wall excision is not associated with higher restenosis rates.[42,43,106]

2. **Clinical and Angiographic Factors**. As shown in Table 24.3, certain clinical and angiographic variables have been identified as risk factors for restenosis;[44-58] most notorious are aorto-ostial lesions, chronic total occlusions, and diabetes. Recently, baseline "positive adaptive" remodeling—enlargement of the external elastic membrane at the target lesion by IVUS—was identified as an independent predictor of clinical restenosis after PTCA and atherectomy.[116]

Table 24.3. Risk Factors for Primary Restenosis

	YES*	MAYBE	NO**
CLINICAL			
Variant angina	X		
Recent onset angina (<2-6 mos)	X		
Unstable angina	X		
IDDM	X		
Chronic dialysis	X		
Tobacco use (continued)		X	
Primary PTCA in acute MI		X	
Hypercholesterolemia		X	
Male gender		X	
Previous MI			X
Hypertension			X
Age			X
Previous restenosis			X
ANGIOGRAPHIC			
Long lesion (> 20mm)	X		
Multivessel/Multilesional+	X		
SVG (proximal & body lesions)	X		
Chronic total occlusion	X		
Collaterals to dilated vessel	X		
Ostial stenosis	X		
Angulation (> 45° angle)	X		
LAD stenosis		X	
Eccentricity			X
Calcification			X
Bifurcation lesion			X
Thrombus			X
Proximal location			X
LIMA			X
SVG (distal anastomosis)			X
PROCEDURAL			
Positive remodeling on baseline IVUS	X		
Pressure gradient > 20mmHg	X		
Residual stenosis > 30%	X		
No dissection present			X
Balloon inflation variables			
Number of inflations			X
Inflation time			X
Maximum inflation pressure			X
Balloon material			X
Inflation technique			X

IDDM = insulin-dependent diabetes mellitus; LAD = left anterior descending coronary artery; LIMA = left internal mammary artery; MI = myocardial infarction; SVG = saphenous vein graft

* Majority of studies demonstrate an association

** Majority of studies do not demonstrate an association

+ Although multivessel/multilesional PTCA leads to an increased probability that at least one lesion will restenose when compared to single lesion PTCA, the overall rate is lower than predicted based on cumulative probabilities

F.   PREVENTION OF RESTENOSIS

1. **Pharmacologic Interventions.** Over the last decade, there have been numerous clinical trials of fish oil, corticosteroids, cytostatic agents, calcium channel blockers, lipid lowering agents, ACE inhibitors, low-molecular-weight heparin, antioxidants, and somatostatin analogues. One metanalysis suggest that calcium channel blockers and fish oil had beneficial effects on restenosis after PTCA (Figure 24.5).[59] However, the randomized CART trial did not demonstrate a benefit for fish oil,[126] and initial excitement for calcium channel blockers was tempered by negative reports from several randomized trials.[127,128] Amlodipine (10 mg/d for 2 weeks prior and 4 weeks after PTCA) decreased ischemic complications at 4 months but failed to reduce restenosis in the randomized CAPARES trial.[152] Small randomized trials of cilostazol, a phosphodiesterase III inhibitor used for claudication, have shown reductions in restenosis after PTCA and stenting[150,151]; further trials are pending. HMG Co-A reductase inhibitors (statins) have several potential mechanisms of action that could decrease restenosis, although studies thus far have been disappointing.[129] Two randomized trials suggested that abciximab and angiopeptin (somatostatin analog) significantly decreased clinical restenosis after PTCA;[60,61] however, quantitative volumetric ultrasound analysis after stenting failed to show a reduction in initial hyperplasia with abciximab,[117] and there was no difference in angiographic restenosis in the angiopeptin trial. Probucol, given one month prior to PTCA and continued for at least 6 months, showed benefit in two randomized studies,[130,131] but pretreatment for one month is impractical in most patients. Data from TREAT and TREAT-2 suggest a possible benefit effect for tranilast after angioplasty.[110] Despite initial promise, trapidil failed to decrease restenosis in the randomized TRAPIST study.[118] Trials of local delivery of alcohol and other antiproliferatives show early promise, but to date, no pharmacologic therapy has clearly been shown to reduce restenosis. Because of the differing mechanisms of restenosis after PTCA and stenting, conclusions of efficacy after PTCA do not necessarily apply to stenting.

2. **Mechanical Interventions.** The stent is the only device that has been shown to reduce the incidence of restenosis compared to PTCA. Randomized trials (STRESS, BENESTENT) have conclusively demonstrated a decrease in restenosis for *de novo* lesions in native coronary arteries. In addition, multiple observational studies strongly suggest lower restenosis rates for stents in saphenous vein grafts.[66,67] Results of the randomized SAVED trial (Stenting or Angioplasty in Vein Graft Disease) found that stents reduced clinical (but not angiographic) restenosis when compared to PTCA alone. Other atheroablative devices have been disappointing for preventing restenosis. In ERBAC,[39] despite a larger post-procedural lumen diameter, restenosis rates were higher after Rotablator and excimer laser compared to PTCA. Studies of directional atherectomy (OARS, BOAT)[68,69] reported less angiographic restenosis using "optimal atherectomy," but there was no late benefit for target vessel revascularization or major adverse cardiac events (Chapter 27).

3. **Radiation Therapy.** Limited data suggest a potential role for radiation therapy in the prevention of restenosis following balloon angioplasty in previously untreated coronary arteries. Beta-radiation reduced target lesion revascularization (6% vs. 24%, $p < 0.05$) and restenosis (8% vs.

39%, p = 0.012) in PREVENT,[148] and low restenosis rates (15% and 4%) were achieved in two other studies.[153,154] In a dose ranging study of beta-radiation after PTCA (without stents), restenosis rates after 9-Gy, 12-Gy, 15-Gy, and 18-Gy were 28.1%, 16.7%, 16.1%, and 3.9% respectively.[154] Patients receiving a stent had more thrombosis or late occlusion than patients treated by PTCA alone (14.3% vs. 3.3%). Results of other randomized trials are pending. The use of vascular brachytherapy for stent restenosis is discussed below.

G. DETECTION OF RESTENOSIS

1. **Patient Symptoms.** Recurrent symptoms have low positive predictive value for restenosis. In contrast, lack of symptoms in previously symptomatic patients is good evidence for the absence of restenosis.[72]

2. **Functional Testing (Table 24.4).** While exercise testing without perfusion imaging can provide useful information about symptomatic status, functional capacity, and the presence of myocardial ischemia, it has low sensitivity for detecting restenosis.[72-74] Stress testing using myocardial scintigraphy has better sensitivity (for detection) and specificity (for exclusion), and is often used to evaluate patients with symptoms suggestive of restenosis. Exercise radionuclide angiography is reliable for excluding restenosis after a negative test, but does not reliably identify restenosis in patients with an abnormal study. Finally, the sensitivity and specificity of exercise and dobutamine echocardiography are similar to thallium-201 scintigraphy.[73] It is important to emphasize that functional testing performed within 4 weeks of PTCA is frequently associated with false positive results,[75] which may be due to local vasoconstriction, myocardial stunning, or hibernating myocardium. Therefore, functional testing should be deferred for at least 6 weeks after PTCA unless the patient presents with early recurrence of symptoms or has disease in another vascular territory being considered for revascularization. Routine serial evaluations after PTCA are usually not recommended,[76] but may be useful in patients with atypical symptoms, silent ischemia, or extensive areas of myocardium at risk.[74,76]

H. CLINICAL FOLLOW-UP OF THE PTCA PATIENT.

The use of noninvasive testing and repeat cardiac catheterization depends on symptomatic status, the amount of viable myocardium supplied by the dilated vessel, the extent of associated coronary artery disease, and ventricular function. Routine early (< 6 months) noninvasive testing is not recommended in all patients. However, if the dilated vessel supplies a large amount of viable myocardium, an exercise test may be performed at 4-6 weeks; repeat angiography is reasonable for a markedly positive test regardless of symptomatic status.[76] If the dilated vessel supplies a small area, asymptomatic individuals may be followed clinically. A stress test is recommended for recurrent angina, and repeat cardiac catheterization may be performed for either recurrent angina or a positive stress test. Some interventionalists perform an exercise test at 4-6 months after PTCA to screen for restenosis, particularly in patients who were asymptomatic before PTCA or who had large caliber target vessels.

I. **MANAGEMENT OF RESTENOSIS.** The management of patients with restenosis depends on patient characteristics, myocardium at risk, lesion morphology, extent of coexisting coronary artery disease, and LV function. Repeat PTCA can be performed with high procedural success (> 95%) and low complication rates (< 3-5%),[51-53] and is frequently the procedure of choice for focal restenosis after stenting.[77] Early registry data suggested higher restenosis rates for stenting of restenotic lesions compared to *de novo* lesions,[78] which has been confirmed in late studies.[145] More recently, however, compared to patients with restenotic lesions treated by PTCA, those treated by stenting had fewer late cardiac events (4.8% vs. 20%).[17,80] Directional atherectomy can be used to treat restenosis after PTCA, but restenosis rates tend to be higher for restenotic compared to *de novo* lesions.[57] In a study of 1,087 restenotic lesions treated by PTCA, DCA or stents, procedural success was achieved in 94-96%; despite better initial lumen enlargement for DCA and stents, in-hospital complications, recurrent restenosis, and 3-year event-free survival were similar for all 3 devices.[81]

J. **RECOMMENDATIONS.** Stents offer the best opportunity for immediate lumen enlargement and primary prevention of restenosis in native coronary arteries and saphenous vein grafts. Intravascular ultrasound may optimize stents results and reduce target lesion revascularization, particularly in patients at high-risk for restenosis (see below). No adjunctive therapy has been clearly shown to prevent restenosis; cilostazol, local delivery of antiproliferative agents, and radiation therapy show promise but require further study. Stenting should be utilized for restenotic lesions after balloon angioplasty or atherectomy. Bifurcation lesions, long lesions, and small vessels still represent theapeutic challenges. The treatment of in-stent restenosis is discussed in the next section.

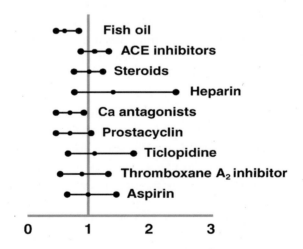

Figure 24.5. Metanalysis of Clinical Restenosis Trials

Restenosis as defined by a follow-up diameter stenosis > 50% (odds ratio and 95% confidence intervals). Data entries < 1 indicate benefit for restenosis. Adapted from Hillegass et al. [59]

Table 24.4. Detection of Restenosis

	Positive Predictive Value[+]	Negative Predictive Value[++]
Exercise treadmill		
Without thallium[91-99]	57 ± 2%	75 ± 1%
With thallium[93-97,100-102]	66 ± 2%	81 ± 2%
Radionuclide angiography[91,93,96,103,104]	39 ± 4%	85 ± 2%

+   The probability of restenosis being present when the test is positive
++   The probability of restenosis being absent when the test is negative

STENT RESTENOSIS

As the major limitation of the dominant modality in percutaneous intervention, stent restenosis has become an important practical issue. Stents were deployed in approximately 80% of 800,000 interventions in the year 2000. Assuming an average restenosis rate of 20%, more than 125,000 cases of stent restenosis may occur each year.

A. **DEFINITIONS.** As with PTCA restenosis, stent restenosis may be defined angiographically (diameter stenosis ≥50%) or clinically (target lesion revascularization, MI, or cardiac death). New proliferative lesions within 5 mm of each stent margin are generally considered part of the "treated segment," although significant stenoses in this location do not strictly qualify as "in-stent" restenosis (see below). The incidence of stent restenosis increases by 10% when the "treated segment" is considered along with the "in-stent" segment.[109]

B. **PREVENTION OF STENT RESTENOSIS BY IVUS-GUIDED STENTING.** Intravascular ultrasound studies demonstrate less restenosis after IVUS-guided stenting than angiography-guided stenting.[70,71] Arteries which appear small by angiography are often larger by IVUS, allowing the use of larger stents and balloons. IVUS can also identify poor stent expansion (pseudorestenosis), edge dissection and plaque prolapse, and can ensure a large final lumen cross-sectional area, which is the best predictor of restenosis. In the CRUISE study, operators changed therapy after viewing the IVUS images in 48% of patients;[70,71] restenosis at 1 year was < 10% if the final IVUS cross-sectional area exceeded 9.0mm^2. IVUS-guided PTCA and stenting is described in Chapter 31.

C. **MECHANISMS OF STENT RESTENOSIS**
    1. **Intimal Hyperplasia.** For stents deployed using optimal technique, subsequent restenosis is entirely due to intimal hyperplasia. Contemporary stent designs virtually eliminate negative remodeling and elastic recoil.[132]

2. **Pseudorestenosis.** Suboptimal stenting may not be recognized during deployment without IVUS. Failure to cover the entire lesion, plaque protrusion, and stent underexpansion are important causes of recurrent ischemia after stenting, and are often referred to as "pseudorestenosis," since they are not nesessarily associated with excessive intimal proliferation (Chapters 26, 31).

3. **Edge Remodeling.** The vessel wall immediately proximal and distal to the stent edge undergoes negative remodeling, which contributes to late lumen loss.

D. **TIME COURSE FOR STENT RESTENOSIS.** As with PTCA, restenosis after stenting is uncommon in the first month, peaks by the third month, reaches a plateau within 3-6 months, and is unusual after 12 months.[31,32] Several angiographic studies have shown a further increase in lumen diameter 6 months to 3 years after stent implantation, suggesting that 6-month angiography may underestimate the benefit of stenting.[34,35,36]

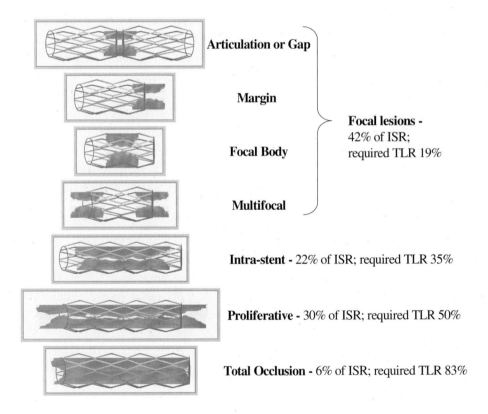

Articulation or Gap

Margin

Focal Body   **Focal lesions -** 42% of ISR; required TLR 19%

Multifocal

Intra-stent - 22% of ISR; required TLR 35%

Proliferative - 30% of ISR; required TLR 50%

Total Occlusion - 6% of ISR; required TLR 83%

Figure 24.6. Patterns of In-Stent Restenosis

Angiographic classification of 282 lesions confirmed by IVUS[134]
ISR = in-stent restenosis; TLR = target lesion revascularization at 1 year

E. PATTERNS OF STENT RESTENOSIS. One classification during the Palmaz-Schatz stent era considered stent restenosis as focal (lesion length < 10 mm) or diffuse.[134] Focal lesions accounted for 42% of stent restenosis and generally had favorable outcomes after repeat intervention, including late target lesion revascularization (TLR) in 19%. Focal lesions were further classified as articulation or gap lesions (reflecting widespread use of the Palmaz-Schatz stent), margin lesions at the stent edge, focal lesions in the body of the stent, or short, multifocal lesions (Figure 24.6). Diffuse lesions were classified as in-stent lesions in 22% (repeat TLR in 35%), diffuse "proliferative" lesions extending beyond the stent margins in 30% (repeat TLR in 50%), or total occlusion in 6% (repeat TLR in 83%).

F. PREDICTORS OF STENT RESTENOSIS (Table 24.5). The strongest predictors of stent restenosis are the pattern of restenosis (Figure 24.6), lesion length, diabetes, total plaque burden, and final lumen cross-sectional area after stenting (by IVUS)[122,132-134,136,138] The number and length of stents reflect total plaque burden, and are important predictors of stent restenosis. However, the presence of overlapping stents is not a predictor of restenosis.

G. MANAGEMENT OF STENT RESTENOSIS (Table 24.6)

   1. Angioplasty, Debulking, Restenting. IVUS studies demonstrated that PTCA for stent restenosis provided additional stent expansion and tissue extrusion out of the stent, accounting for 56% and 44% of net gain, respectively.[136] PTCA did not achieve the same dimensions as the original stent because of reintrusion of intimal tissue.[137,138] The combination of debulking (Rotablator, DCA, or laser) and adjunctive PTCA may not have benefit over PTCA alone, despite initially promising results (Table 24.7).[143,144] In the large, randomized ARTIST trial, Rotablator for diffuse stent restenosis was associated with higher in-lab complications, more late clinical events, and smaller dimensions at 6 months compared to PTCA alone,[139-142] but in ROSTER, 6-month TLR was lower after Rotablator.[167] A metanalysis of PTCA, DCA, Rotablator, laser, and restenting for stent restenosis reported a 6-month TLR of 30% regardless of the device. Although IVUS studies suggest that restenting eliminates intimal reintrusion associated with PTCA and other devices,[13] this effect is not sufficient to prevent recurrent restenosis.[119]

Table 24.5. Predictors of Stent Restenosis[122,132-134,136,138]

Major
Pattern of restenosis (i.e., focal, diffuse, proliferative, total occlusion)
Lesion length
Diabetes mellitus
Minor
Final post-procedure lumen dimensions
Total plaque burden

2. **Ionizing Radiation.** At the present time, no pharmacologic or mechanical intervention can reliably treat stent restenosis. However, brachytherapy holds real promise for inhibiting intimal proliferation and decreasing the incidence of stent restenosis.

    a. **Sources for Vascular Brachytherapy (Table 24.8).** The two systems now FDA-approved for vascular brachytherapy are the Novoste Beta-Cath system (beta-source) and the Cordis Checkmate system (gamma-source). Both beta and gamma sources can deliver the appropriate dose to limit intimal proliferation in the coronary arteries, which is estimated to be 14-20 Gray. Isotopes used for brachytherapy are shown in Table 24.9. Advantages of beta-sources include rapid attenuation of radiation (which minimizes exposure to physicians and staff), reduced shielding requirements, and shorter dwell times (Table 24.10). However, rapid attenuation increases the need for centering of the source and limits application to relatively small vessels (i.e., coronary arteries rather than iliac or femoral arteries).

Table 24.6. Treatment Strategies for Stent Restenosis

Technique	Comment
Mechanical Approaches	
PTCA	Success rates exceed 90%; restenosis rates vary from 30-80% depending on pattern of stent restenosis and nature of target lesion
Debulking (DCA, Rotablator, ELCA)	Despite initial enthusiasm, randomized trials show no benefit compared to PTCA (Table 24.7)
Stenting ("stent-wich")	Achieves the best immediate angiographic results; long-term outcomes are uncertain (Chapter 26)
Cutting balloon	May facilitate immediate lumen enlargement but further study is needed
Pharmacologic Approaches	
Anti-sense DNA	No benefit (ITALICS trial)
Abciximab	No benefit (ERASER trial)
Trapidil	TRAPIST trial pending
Tranilast	Trials pending
Brachytherapy	Shows the most promise for inhibition of intimal proliferation; efficacy of beta- and gamma-radiation are established. Residual issues include edge effect, delayed thrombosis, and unknown late effects

Table 24.7. Results of Debulking Strategies for Stent Restenosis

Series	Device	N	Comments
ROSTER[167] (2001)	ROTA PTCA	100 100	Randomized trial. ROTA had similar 30-day MACE (2% vs. 3%), but less TLR (32% vs. 45%, p = 0.04)
LARS	ELCA PTCA	160 160	Prospective multicenter randomized trial (pending)
ARTIST[168] (2000)	PTCA ROTA	146 152	Randomized trial for diffuse in-stent restenosis; ROTA had similar success (89% vs. 88%), but higher MACE (14.5% vs. 6.8%, p < 0.05), ARS (65% vs. 51%, p < 0.05), and TLR (48% vs. 36%) at 6 months
Mehran[155] (2000)	ELCA ROTA	158 161	Success (100%); compared to ROTA, ELCA had similar late MACE and 1-year TLR (28% vs 26%)
Koster[156] (2000)	ELCA	96	Poor outcomes at 6 months: ARS (54%); TLR (49%)
Haase[157] (1999)	ELCA	440	Success (92%); in-hospital MACE (6.4%). Non-randomized LARS trial
Lauer[158] (1999)	ELCA ROTA PTCA	78 83 124	Immediate lumen enlargement was better for ELCA and ROTA than PTCA, but at 6 months ROTA results were better than ELCA and PTCA
Mehran[159] (1999)	PTCA ELCA ROTA Stent	314 250 126 131	Immediate lumen enlargement was best for stenting, but no difference in 1-year TLR (PTCA 26.6%, ELCA 31%, ROTA 23.1%, stent 27%); device was not a predictor of TLR
Koster[160] (1998)	ELCA	90	Low incidence of complications
Haase[161] (1998)	ELCA PTCA	47 49	Randomized trial. ELCA had similar success (98%), in-hospital complications (8%), late MACE (25% vs. 30%), and ARS (52% vs. 47%)
Dauerman[163] (1998)	PTCA ROTA or DCA	40 40	Success in both groups (100%); better final diameter stenosis after debulking (18% vs. 26%, p = 0.01); TLR at 1 year was lower after debulking (28% vs. 46%, p = 0.18). Predictors of restenosis were diabetes, long lesion length, and smaller final MLD
Sharma[164] (1998)	ROTA	100	Success (100%); ARS (28%); TVR (26%). Predictors of re-restenosis were burr/artery ratio <0.6%, ostial lesion, stent for a restenotic lesion, and diffuse in-stent restenosis
Lee[165] (1998)	ROTA PTCA	36 45	Clinical restenosis was lower after ROTA (2.5% vs. 47%, p < 0.05) and angina-free survival was higher (72% vs. 49%, p = 0.02) at 6 months
Mehran[166] (1997)	ELCA PTCA	54 44	ELCA was associated with greater lumen gain and a trend toward less TLR (21% vs. 38%, p = 0.08)

Abbreviations: ARS = angiographic restenosis; ARTIST = Angioplasty vs. Rotational Atherectomy for Treatment of Diffuse In-Stent Restenosis; ELCA = excimer laser coronary angioplasty; LARS = Laser Angioplasty for Restenosed Stents; MACE = major adverse cardiac events; MLD = minimum lumen diameter ROTA = Rotablator; TLR = target lesion revascularization

Table 24.8. Intravascular Brachytherapy Systems

System	Company	Isotope/Source	Description
Checkmate™	Cordis	^{192}Ir/gamma	Catheter-based delivery system; FDA-approved; source ribbon is advanced through a closed-ended source lumen
Beta-Cath™	Novoste	^{90}Sr-Y/beta	Catheter-based delivery system; FDA-approved; hydraulic fluid design positions sealed radioactive sources through a source lumen within the delivery catheter
Galileo™	Guidant	^{32}P/beta	Centering catheter, ^{32}P source wire, and an automated source delivery unit
Isostent™	Cordis	^{32}P/beta	Radioactive stent; short shelf-life

b. **Studies of Radiation for Stent Restenosis (Tables 24.11, 24.12).** Results from the randomized SCRIPPS, WRIST, PREVENT, Gamma-One, START and other trials indicated 25-65% reduction in recurrent restenosis and target lesion revascularization at 6-12 months in patients treated with brachytherapy; beneficial effects persisted at 3 years in SCRIPPS.[146] Importantly, among patients treated by restenting, the incidence of late thrombosis and myocardial infarction may be increased after radiation therapy: A review of randomized and observational brachytherapy studies found a 4.5-fold increase in late thrombosis among patients who received intracoronary radiation therapy after restenting compared to those who did not (9% vs. 2%).[149] Possible explanations included delayed endothelialization of the stent struts or radiation-induced endothelial dysfunction. In Gamma-One, all cases of late thrombosis occurred in patients who had new stents placed within the previously stented target lesion at the time of brachytherapy, and no cases of late thrombosis occurred while patients were receiving ticlopidine or clopidogrel.[147] Increased late thrombosis has not been a problem with PTCA or atheroablative techniques following radiation therapy.

c. **Pitfalls of Vascular Brachytherapy.** Although brachytherapy is the only therapy which has demonstrated clear efficacy for preventing stent restenosis, there are several unresolved issues and limitations. First, optimal doses have not been established. Second, long-term follow-up studies are still pending. Third, the value of adjunctive therapies (such as platelet receptor antagonists or debulking vs. dilating prior to brachytherapy) has not yet been established. Fourth, the timing of brachytherapy (during first intervention vs. subsequent repeat revascularization) has not been defined. Finally, brachytherapy introduces a new set of clinical problems (Table 24.13, Figure 24.7), each of which requires special prevention, treatment, and evaluation.

Table 24.9. Isotopes for Vascular Brachytherapy

Isotope	Emmision	Half-life	Delivery system
^{192}Ir	Gamma	74 days	Catheter
^{32}P	Beta	14 days	Catheter, stent
^{90}Sr	Beta	28 years	Catheter
^{90}Y	Beta	64 hours	Catheter
^{188}Re	Beta	17 hours	Liquid-filled balloon
^{186}Re	Beta	90 hours	Liquid-filled balloon

    d. Recommendations. The FDA had approved the use of gamma- and beta-radiation for the treatment of stent restenosis in native coronary arteries. Brachytherapy after treatment of *de novo* lesions, brachytherapy 4-6 weeks after successful therapy of stent restenosis with PTCA, and other types of adjunctive intracoronary radiation therapy are being studied but do not have regulatory approval at this time.

H. RECOMMENDATIONS. Our recommendations are based upon available data and clinical experience. Focal stent restenosis that is contained within the stent is often successfully managed with balloon angioplasty. Focal stenoses in gaps between stents or at the margins may be stented. Diffuse lesions should be considered for intracoronary brachytherapy after PTCA or atheroablation, without additional stents. If additional stents are required at the time of brachytherapy, clopidogrel and aspirin should be given for 9-12 months, until further studies demonstrate the optimal duration of therapy.

Table 24.10. Comparison of Beta and Gamma Sources for Vascular Brachytherapy

	Beta	Gamma
Logistic Issues		
Radiation attenuation	Rapid	Minimal
Potential exposure	Low	High
Shielding requirements	Minimal	Extensive
Dwell times	2-4 minutes	10-30 minutes
Technical Issues		
Need for centering	Yes	No
Suitable for large vessels	No	Yes

Table 24.11. Results of Gamma-Radiation Trials

Trial	Isotope/System	Setting and 1⁰ Endpoint	Characteristics (placebo vs. radiation)	Results (placebo vs. radiation)	Comments
GAMMA I (n = 250)	Iridium 192 IVUS dosing; aspirin + clopidogrel or ticlopidine x 4 weeks	ISR; restenosis and TVR at 9 months	Ref: 2.73 vs. 2.69 mm LL: 20.3 vs. 19.01 mm DM: 31.3 vs. 31.4% New stents: 84.7%	Restenosis: 55% vs. 32% (p = 0.01) TLR: 42.1% vs. 24.4% (p < 0.01) TVR: 46.3% vs. 31.3% (p = 0.01) Stent thrombosis: 0.8% vs. 5.3% (p = 0.07)	Gamma radiation with IR-192 is safe and effective based on IVUS dosing
GAMMA II (n = 125)	Iridium 192 fixed dosing; aspirin + clopidogrel or ticlopidine x 4 weeks	ISR; restenosis and TVR at 9 months	Ref: 2.7 mm LL: 19.08 mm DM: 36.8% New stents: 70.4%	Restenosis: 56% vs. 34% (p = 0.01) TLR: 44.6% vs. 24.4% (p = 0.01) Stent thrombosis: 2.5% vs. 6.4% (p < 0.05)	Fixed Ir-192 dosing as effective as IVUS based dosing
SCRIPPS (n = 66)	Iridium 192 IVUS dosing	ISR; restenosis and TLR at 6 months	Ref: 2.93 vs. 2.71 mm LL: 13.1 vs. 11.7 mm New stents: >80%	Restenosis: 54% vs. 17% (p = 0.01) TLR: 44.8% vs. 11.7% (p = 0.01)	Radiation better than placebo with sustained results after 3 years (TLR = 48% vs. 15.4%, p = 0.01)
SCRIPPS III (n = 361 of 500; interim analysis)	Iridium 192; aspirin + clopidogrel x 6 months (no stent) or 12 months (with stent)	ISR; stent thrombosis at 9 months	New stents: 22%	Stent thrombosis: 0%	Less stent thrombosis with reduced stent use and prolonged antiplatelet therapy
WRIST (n = 130)	Iridium 192 fixed dosing; aspirin + clopidogrel or ticlopidine x 4 weeks	ISR; restenosis and TVR at 6 months	Ref: 2.71 vs. 2.72 mm LL: 19.9 vs. 21.0 mm DM: 39% New stents: 80%	Restenosis: 60% vs. 22% (p = 0.001) TLR: 63.1% vs. 13.8% (p = 0.01) TVR: 67.6% vs 26.1% (p = 0.01) Stent thrombosis: 3.5% vs. 7.6% (p > 0.05)	Radiation better than placebo with sustained results at 12 months (TLR = 15.4%; TVR = 38.5%)
WRIST Plavix (n = 120 of 500; interim analysis)	Iridium 192; aspirin + clopidogrel x 6 months	ISR; stent thrombosis at 9 months	New stents: 28%	Stent thrombosis: 0.8%	Less stent thrombosis with reduced stent use and prolonged antiplatelet therapy

Abbreviations: DM = diabetes mellitus; ISR = in-stent restenosis; IVUS = intravascular ultrasound; LL = lesion length; ref = reference vessel diameter; TLR = target lesion revascularization; TVR = target vessel revascularization
Courtesy of Alexandra J. Lansky, M.D.

Table 24.12. Results of Beta-Radiation Trials

Trial	Isotope/System	Setting and 1⁰ Endpoint	Characteristics (placebo vs. radiation)	Results (placebo vs. radiation)	Comments
BERT	Sr-90 Novoste 12, 14, 16 Gy dose ranging at 2mm from center of source	De novo and ISR; restenosis and TVR at 6 months	Ref: 2.88mm LL: 9.0mm DM: 15%	TLR: 17.7%	Sr-90 is safe and feasible
BETA CATH (n = 2455)	SR-90 Novoste	De novo and restenotic lesions	NA	NA	Study in progress; PTCA alone or provisional stent +/- prolonged antiplatelet therapy
Beta WRIST (n = 50)	Y-90 BSC/Schneider 20 Gy at 1mm into vessel wall	ISR; restenosis and TVR at 6 months	Ref: 2.73mm LL: 17.3mm DM: 22% New stents: 37%	Restenosis: 66% vs. 16% (p < 0.001) TLR: 66% vs. 28% (p = 0.001) TVR: 72% vs. 34% (p = 0.001) Stent thrombosis: 10% vs. 3.5%	Compared to the placebo arm of the WRIST trial, Y-90 delivered using the BSC/Schneider system is safe and effective
BETTER (n = 81 of 125; interim analysis)	P-32 Radiance Balloon 20 Gy at 1mm into vessel wall	De novo and ISR; restenosis and TVR at 6 months	Ref: 2.81mm LL: 12.34mm	TVR: 19.8% (23.3% for de novo vs. 9% for ISR) Stent thrombosis: 1.2% (1.7% for de novo vs. 0% for ISR)	Preliminary results with the Radiance Balloon demonstrate safety and feasibility
BRIE (n = 152 of 350; interim analysis)	Sr-90 Novoste	De novo, ISR, multilesion, multivessel	NA	Restenosis: PTCA arm 7% vs. stent arm 11.7%	69.5% reduction in total occlusion with prolonged antiplatelet therapy
BRITE I (n = 27)	P-32 Radiance Balloon 20 Gy at 1 mm into vessel wall	ISR; restenosis and TVR at 6 months	NA	NA	Preliminary results with the Radiance Balloon demonstrate safety and feasibility for treatment of ISR
BRITE II (n = 500)	P-32 Radiance Balloon 20 Gy at 1 mm into vessel wall	ISR; restenosis and TVR at 9 months	NA	NA	Study in progress
GENEVA (n = 154)	Y-90 BSC/Schneider 9,12,15, 18 Gy at 1mm into vessel wall	De novo; restenosis at 6 months	New stents: 19%	Restenosis: 27.5% at 9 Gy 15.8% at 12 Gy 17.5% at 15 Gy 8.3% at 18 Gy (p = 0.04 for 9 vs. 18 Gy)	A greater reduction in restenosis with 18 vs. 9 Gy was noted among patients treated with PTCA only (4.2% vs. 26.1%)

Table 24.12. Results of Beta-Radiation Trials

Trial	Isotope/System	Setting and 1⁰ Endpoint	Characteristics (placebo vs. radiation)	Results (placebo vs. radiation)	Comments
INHIBIT (n = 332)	P-32 Guidant 20 Gy at 1 mm into lumen	ISR; restenosis and TVR at 9 months	Ref: 2.7 vs. 2.7mm LL: 18 vs. 17mm DM: 28 vs. 32% New stents: 27%	Restenosis: 52% vs. 26% ($p = 0.003$) TLR: 29% vs. 11% ($p = 0.001$) TVR: 31% vs. 20% ($p = 0.033$) Stent thrombosis: 0.6% vs. 1.8% ($p = NS$)	P-32 delivery using the Guidant system is safe and effective for ISR. Tandem positioning in 39% with 49% reduction in TVR
INHIBIT Galileo (n = 125)	P-32 Guidant Galileo 20 Gy at 1mm into lumen	ISR; restenosis and TVR at 9 months	NA	NA	Registry using the Galileo system; results pending
PREVENT (n = 105)	P-32 Guidant 16, 20, 24 Gy at 1mm into vessel wall vs. placebo	De novo and ISR; restenosis and TVR at 6 months	Ref: 2.97 vs. 2.99mm DM: 21% vs. 20% New stents: 61%	Restenosis: 50% vs 22% ($p < 0.05$) TLR: 24% vs. 6% ($p < 0.005$) TVR: 32% vs. 21% ($p = NS$) Stent thrombosis: 0% vs. 8%	P-32 delivery using the Guidant system is safe and feasible
RENO (n = 110 of 1000; interim analysis)	Sr-90 Novoste	De novo and ISR; restenosis and TVR at 6 months	Ref: 3.1mm LL: 18.2 mm DM: 21.4% New stents: 37.7%	Restenosis: 28% TVR: 21.4%	Sustained results in high risk population
START (n = 476)	Sr-90 Novoste 16 Gy (for ref 2.7-3.3mm) or 20 Gy (for ref > 3.3 mm) at 2mm from center of source. Aspirin + clopidogrel x 3 months	ISR; restenosis and TVR at 9 months	Ref: 2.77 vs. 2.76 mm LL: 16 vs. 16.3 mm DM: 32.2 vs. 30.7% New stents: 20.7 vs. 21.7%	Restenosis: 45.2% vs. 28.8% ($p = 0.001$) TLR: 22.4% vs. 13.1% ($p = 0.008$) TVR: 24.1% vs. 16% ($p = 0.026$) Stent thrombosis: 0% vs. 0%	Sr-90 resulted in a reduction in restenosis by 36%. No stent thrombosis with longer antiplatelet therapy
START 40/20 (n = 210)	Sr-90 Novoste 16 Gy (for ref 2.7-3.3mm) or 20 Gy (for ref > 3.3 mm) at 2mm from center of source. Aspirin + clopidogrel x 3 months	ISR; restenosis and TVR at 6 months	Ref: 2.77 vs. 2.76 mm LL: 16 vs. 17.2 mm DM: 32 vs. 30.7% New stents: 20%	Restenosis: 45.2% vs. 21.9% ($p < 0.05$) TLR: 22.4% vs. 11.1% ($p = 0.002$) TVR: 24.1% vs. 16% ($p = 0.033$) Stent thrombosis: 0% vs. 0%	In a population matched for lesion length and arterial injury, use of a 40mm source train was as effective as a 30mm train but did not further reduce restenosis
SVG BRITE (n = 50)	P-32 Radiance Balloon 20 Gy at 1 mm into vessel wall	Saphenous vein graft; restenosis and TVR at 9 months	NA	NA	Study in progress

Abbreviations: DM = diabetes mellitus; ISR = in-stent restenosis; IVUS = intravascular ultrasound; LL = lesion length; NA = not available; ref = reference vessel diameter; TLR = target lesion revascularization; TVR = target vessel revascularization
Courtesy of Alexandra J. Lansky, M.D.

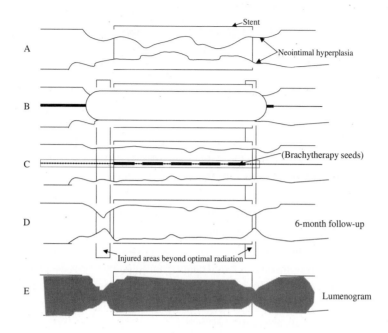

Figure 24.7. Geographic Miss and the "Candy-Wrapper" Effect

a. Diffuse, proliferative in-stent restenosis
b. PTCA enlarges the lumen by intimal extrusion
c. Intravascular brachytherapy is applied, but note that the entire segment of balloon-injury is not treated by brachytherapy ("geographic miss")
d. At follow-up, there is no intimal proliferation within the irradiated segment, but the areas "missed" by radiation have resulted in edge restenosis
e. The angiographic "lumenogram" of this lesion resembles a "candy-wrapper"

Table 24.13. Limitations of Vascular Brachytherapy

Limitation	Description	Treatment
Edge effect ("candy-wrapper" lesion)	After brachytherapy, restenosis occurs at the margins of the irradiated segment, leading to a so-called "candy-wrapper" lesion (Figure 24.7)	This lesion is probably due to a "geographic miss" or failure to treat the entire injured segment with brachytherapy. Edge effect may be prevented by careful recording of the entire zone of treatment, to ensure that it is completely irradiated
Late thrombosis	Stent thrombosis 1-9 months after brachytherapy; not due to progressive intimal proliferation. Frequently associated with acute MI. Incidence 7-10% without prolonged antiplatelet therapy	May be caused by delayed endothelialization of new stents implanted at the time of brachytherapy and can probably be avoided by prolonged (9-12 month) antiplatelet therapy

FUTURE DIRECTIONS

A. **LOCAL DELIVERY.** Site-specific pharmacologic[82] and molecular approaches[83] may prove useful in suppressing intimal hyperplasia and preventing restenosis. Some studies suggest that local drug delivery may be useful for treating thrombus,[84] although inhibition of intimal hyperplasia after balloon injury has not been demonstrated. Studies of local delivery of alcohol and other antiproliferatives are underway.[135] Very near-field ultrasound sonotherapy after stenting is also under study.[169]

B. **GENE THERAPY.** Several experimental studies suggest a role for vascular gene therapy [85-88] (in which a particular gene is overexpressed), and for antisense oligonucleotides[89-90] (which inhibit cell proliferation by preventing gene expression). Difficulties in the identification of the precise target and fundamental safety considerations have slowed eagerly anticipated progress in this field.[121] Currently, in-stent restenosis is considered the closest pure model of restenosis due to neointimal hyperplasia; the APPRAISE trial is investigating the utility of the *c-myc* antisense oligonucleotide in this setting. Several other gene therapy trials are being planned.

C. **SMART STENTS.** A new generation of coated stents is under investigation for the reduction of restenosis. These coatings involve "static" antithrombotic surfaces such as heparin, phosphenylcholine, or turbostatic carbon, as well as "active" antiproliferative agents like paclitaxel (taxol) and rapamycin. Paclitaxel inhibits microtuble formation necessary for smooth muscle cell replication and migration; rampamycin inhibits progression from G1 to S1 phase of cell replication. Preliminary data from small clinical studies of paclitaxel and rapamycin-coated stents are promising.[170,171] Studies of other "smart" stents that can be heated, cooled, dissolve over a few weeks, or deliver radiation are underway.

D. **ESTABLISHMENT OF RADIATION AS PRIMARY THERAPY FOR STENT RESTENOSIS.** Intracoronary radiation has been shown to reduce recurrence after treatment of stent restenosis. The many ongoing trials testing various radiation devices, delivery catheters, and dosimetry schemes will hopefully provide some answers for the difficult task of managing this important problem.

* * * * *

REFERENCES

1. Gruentzig AR. Transluminal dilatation of coronary artery stenoses. Lancet 1978;1:263.
2. Baim DS (ed): A symposium: Interventional Cardiology-1987. Am J Cardiol 1988;61:1g-117g.
3. Detre K, Holubkov R, Kelsey S, et al. Percutaneous transluminal coronary angioplasty in 1985-1986 and 1977-1981. The National Heart, Lung and Blood Institute Registry. N Engl J Med 1988;318:265-270.
4. Gruentzig AR, King SB III, Schlumpf M., et al. Long-term follow-up after percutaneous transluminal coronary angioplasty. The early Zurich experience. N Engl J Med. 1987;316:1127-1132.
5. Parisi AF, Folland ED, Hartigan P. A comparison of angioplasty with medical therapy in the treatment of single vessel coronary disease. Veterans Affairs ACME Investigators. N Engl J Med 1992;326:10-16.
6. Goy JJ, Eeckhout E, Burnand B et al. Coronary angioplasty versus left internal mammary artery grafting for isolated proximal left anterior descending artery stenosis. Lancet 1994;343:1449-1453.
7. Coronary angioplasty versus coronary artery bypass surgery: the Randomized Intervention Treatment of Angina (RITA) trial. Lancet 1993;341:573-380.
8. Roubin G, King SI, Douglas J, JR. Restenosis after percutaneous transluminal coronary angioplasty: The Emory University Hospital experience. Am J Cardiol 1987;60:39B-43B.
9. Gould K, Lipscomb K, Hamilton G. Physiological basis for assessing critical coronary stenosis: instantaneous flow response and regional distribution during coronary hyperemia as measures of coronary flow reserve. Am J Cardiol 1974;33:87-97.
10. Beatt KJ, Serruys PW, Renseing BJ, Hugenoltz PG. Restenosis after coronary angioplasty: New standards for clinical studies. J Am Coll Cardiol 1990;15:491-498.
11. Beatt KJ, Luijten H, de Feyter P, van den Brand M, Reiber J, Serruys P. Change in diameter of coronary artery segments adjacent to stenosis after percutaneous transluminal coronary angioplasty: Failure of percent diameter stenosis measurement to reflect morphologic changes induced by balloon dilation. J Am Coll Cardiol 1988;12:315-323.
12. Rensing BJ, Hermans WM, Deckers JW, deFeyter PJ. Lumen narrowing after percutaneous transluminal coronary balloon angioplasty follows a near gaussian distribution: A quantitative angiographic study in 1,445 successfully dilated lesions. J Am Coll Cardiol 1992;19:939-945.
13. Kuntz R, Safian R, Levine M, Reis G, Diver D, Baim D. Novel approach to the analysis of restenosis after the use of three new coronary devices. J Am Coll Cardiol 1992;19:1493-1499.
14. Gordon PC, Gibson M, Cohen DJ, Carrozza J, Kuntz R, Baim D. Mechanisms of restenosis and redilation within coronary stents-quantitative angiographic assessment. J Am Coll Cardiol 1993;21:1166-1174.
15. Kuntz RE, Gibson CM, Nobuyoshi M, Baim DS. Generalized model of restenosis after conventional balloon angioplasty, stenting and directional atherectomy. J Am Coll Cardiol 1993;21:15-25.
16. Schwartz R, Huber K, Murphy J, et al. Restenosis and the proportional neointimal response to coronary artery injury: Results in a porcine model. J Am Coll Cardiol 1992;19:267-274.
17. Beatt KJ, Serruys PW, Luijten HE, et al. Restenosis after coronary angioplasty: The paradox of increased lumen diameter and restenosis. J Am Coll Cardiol 1992;19:258-266.
18. Holmes D, Vlietstra R, Smith H, et al. Restenosis after percutaneous transluminal coronary angioplasty (PTCA): a report from the PTCA Registry of the NHLBI. Am J Cardiol 1984;53:77C-81C.
19. Gruentzig AR, King SB III, Schlumpf M, et al. Long term follow-up after percutaneous transluminal coronary angioplasty. The early Zurich experience. N Engl J Med 1987;316:1127-1132.
20. Fischman D, Leon M, Baim D. A randomized comparison of coronary stent placement and balloon angioplasty in the treatment of coronary artery disease. N Engl J Med 1994;331:496-501.
21. Serruys P, deJegere P, Kiemeneij F, et al. A comparison of balloon expandable stent implantation with balloon angioplasty in patients with coronary artery disease. N Engl J Med 1994;331(8):489-495.
22. Rodriguez A, Santaera O, Larribau M, et al. Coronary stenting decreases restenosis in lesions with early loss in luminal diameter 24 hours after successful PTCA. Circulation 1995;91:1397-1402.
23. Rensing BJ, Hermans WRM, Beatt KJ, et al. Quantitative angiographic assessment of elastic recoil after percutaneous transluminal coronary angiography. Am J Cardiol 1990;66:1039-1044.
24. Rodriguez A, Lassileau M, Santaera O, et al. Early decreases in minimal luminal diameter after PTCA are associated with higher incidence of late restenosis. J Am Coll Cardiol 1993;21:34A.
25. LaBlanche JM on behalf of the FACT Investigators. Recoil twenty-four hours after coronary angioplasty: A computerized angiographic study. J Am Coll Cardiol 1993;21:34A.
26. Johnson DE, Hinohara T, Selmon MR, Braden LJ. Primary peripheral arterial stenoses and restenoses excised by transluminal atherectomy: A histopathologic study. J Am Coll Cardiol 1990;15:419-425.
27. Garratt K, Edwards W, Kaufmann U, Vlietstra R, Holmes D. Differential histopathology of primary atherosclerotic and restenotic lesions in coronary arteries and saphenous vein bypass grafts: Analysis of tissue obtained from 73 patients by directional atherectomy. J Am Coll Cardiol 1991;17:442-448.
28. Post M, Borst C, Kuntz R. The relative importance of arterial remodeling compared with intimal hyperplasia in lumen renarrowing after balloon angioplasty (A study in the normal rabbit and the hypercholesterolemic Yucatan micropig). Circulation 1994;89:2816-2821.

29. Lafont A, Guzman L, PLW. Restenosis after experimental angioplasty. Intimal, medial and adventitial changes associated with constrictive remodeling. Circ Res 1995;76:996-1002.

30. Mintz G, Kovach J, Javier S, Ditrano C, Leon M. Geometric remodeling is the predominant mechanism of late lumen loss after coronary angioplasty. Circulation 1993;88:I-654.

31. Serruys PW, Luijten HE, Beatt KJ, et al. Incidence of restenosis after successful coronary angioplasty: a time-related phenomenon. A quantitative angiographic study in 342 consecutive patients at 1, 2, 3, and 4 months. Circulation 1988;77:361-371.

32. Nobuyoshi M, Kimura T, Nosaka H, Mioka S. Restenosis after successful percutaneous transluminal coronary angioplasty: Serial angiographic follow-up of 229 patients. J Am Coll Cardiol 1988;12:616-623.

33. Guidance for the Submission of Research and Marketing Applications for Interventional Cardiology Devices: PTCA Catheters, Atherectomy Catheters, Lasers, Intravascular Stents. Interventional Cardiology Devices Branch, Division of Cardiovascular, Respiratory and Neurology Devices, Office of Device Evaluation, US Food and Drug Administration, May 1993:29.

34. Kimura T, Yokoi H, Tamura T, Nakagawa Y, Nosaka H, Nobuyoshi M. Three years clinical and quantitative angiographic follow-up after the Palmaz-Schatz coronary stent implantation. J Am Coll Cardiol 1995;25:375A.

35. Hermiller J, Fry E, Peters T, et al. Late lesion regression within the Gianturco-Roubin Flex stent. J Am Coll Cardiol 1995;25`:375A.

36. Kimura T, Nosaka H, Yokoi H, Iwabuchi M. Serial angiographic follow-up after Palmaz-Schatz stent implantation: Comparison with conventional balloon angioplasty. J Am Coll Cardiol 1993;21:1557-1563.

37. Kuntz R, Safian R, Carrozza J, Fishman R, Mansour M, Baim D. The importance of acute luminal diameter in determining restenosis after coronary atherectomy or stenting. Circulation 1992;86:1827-1835.

38. Topol E, Leya F, Pinkerton C, et al. A comparison of directional atherectomy with coronary angioplasty in patients with coronary artery disease. N Engl J Med 1993;329:221-227.

39. Vandormael M, Reifart N, Preusler W, et al. Comparison of excimer laser angioplasty and rotational atherectomy with balloon angioplasty for complex lesions: ERBAC study final results. J Am Coll Cardiol 1994;57A.

40. Spears JR, Reyes VP, Wynne J, et al. Percutaneous coronary laser balloon angioplasty: Initial results of a multicenter experience. J Am Coll Cardiol 1990;16:293-303.

41. Umans VAWM, Keane D, Foley D, et al. Optimal use of directional coronary atherectomy is required to ensure long-term angiographic benefit: A study with matched procedural outcome after atherectomy and angioplasty. J Am Coll Cardiol 1994;24:1652-1659.

42. Garratt KN, Holmes DR, Bell MR, et al. Restenosis after directional coronary atherectomy: differences between primary atheromatous and restenosis lesions and influence of subintimal tissue resection. J Am Coll Cardiol 1990;16:1665-1671.

43. Kuntz RE, Hinohara T, Safian RD, et al. Restenosis after directional coronary atherectomy: Effects of luminal diameter and deep wall excision. Circulation 1992;86:1394-1399.

44. Carrozza JR, Kuntz RE, Fishman RF, Baim DS. Restenosis after arterial injury caused by coronary stenting in patients with diabetes mellitus. Ann Intern Med. 1993;118(5):344-349.

45. Simons M, Leclerc G, Safian RD, Isner JM. Relation between activated smooth-muscle cells in coronary artery lesions and restenosis after atherectomy. N Engl J Med 1993;328:608-613.

46. Kuntz RE, Hinohara T, Robertson GC, et al. Influence of vessel selection on the observed restenosis rate after endoluminal stenting or directional coronary atherectomy. Am J Cardiol 1992;70:1101-1108.

47. Hirshfeld JW, Schwartz JS, Jugo R, et al. Restenosis after coronary angioplasty: A multivariate statistical model to relate lesion and procedure variables to restenosis. J Am Coll Cardiol 1991;18:647-656.

48. Hermans WR, Rensing BJ, Kelder JC, et al. Postangioplasty restenosis rate between segments of the major coronary arteries. Am J Cardiol 1992;194-200.

49. Violaris A, Melkert R, Serruys P. Influence of serum cholesterol and cholesterol subfractions on restenosis after successful coronary angioplasty. A quantitative angiographic analysis of 3336 lesions. Circulation 1994;90:2267-2279.

50. Fishman RF, Kuntz RE, Carrozza JP, Miller MJ, et al. Long-term results of directional coronary atherectomy: Predictors of restenosis. J Am Coll Cardiol 1992;20:1101-1110.

51. Williams DO, Gruentzig A, Kent K, Detre K, Kelsey S, To T. Efficacy of repeat percutaneous transluminal coronary angioplasty for coronary restenosis. Am J Cardiol 1984;53:32C-35C.

52. Dimas AP, Grigera F, Arora RR, et al. Repeat coronary angioplasty as treatment for restenosis. J Am Coll Cardiol 1992;19:1310-1314.

53. Meier B, King SBI, Gruentzig AR. Repeat coronary angioplasty. J Am Coll Cardiol 1984;4:463-466.

54. Moscucci M, Piana R, Kuntz R, Kugelmass A, et al. The effect of prior coronary restenosis on the risk of subsequent restenosis after stent placement or directional atherectomy. Am J Cardiol 1994;73:1147-1153.

55. Glazier J, Varricchione T, Ryan T. Factors predicting recurrent restenosis after percutaneous transluminal coronary balloon angioplasty. Am J Cardiol 1989;63:902-905.

56. Quigley P, Hlatky M, Hinohara T. Repeat percutaneous transluminal coronary angioplasty and predictors of recurrent restenosis. Am J Cardiol 1989;63:409-413.

57. Hinohara T, Robertson G, Selmon M, et al. Restenosis after directional coronary atherectomy. J Am Coll Cardiol 1992;20:623-632.

58. Teirstein P, Hoover C, Ligon R. Repeat coronary angioplasty: Efficacy of a third angioplasty for a second restenosis. J Am Coll Cardiol 1989;13:291-296.

59. Hillegass WB, Ohman ME and Califf RM. Restenosis: The Clinical Issues. In Topol EJ (ed). *Textbook of Interventional Cardiology*, 2nd Edition, Philadelphia, WB Saunders Company, 1993; 415-435.

60. Topol E, Califf R, Weisman H, et al. Randomized trial of

coronary intervention with antibody against platelet IIb/IIIa integrin for reduction of clinical restenosis: results at six months. Lancet 1994;343:881-86.

61. Emanuelsson H, Beatt K, Bagger J. Long-term effects of angiopeptin treatment in coronary angioplasty. Reduction of clinical events but not of angiographic restenosis. European Angiopeptin Study Group. Circulation 1995;91:1689-1696.

62. Safian RD, Hoffmann MA, Almany S, et al. Comparison of coronary angioplasty with compliant and noncompliant balloons (The Angioplasty Compliance Trial). Am J Cardiol 1995;76:518-520.

63. DiSciascio G, Vetrovec GW, Lewis SA, et al. Clinical and angiographic recurrence following PTCA for nonacute total occlusions: comparisons of one versus five minute inflations. Am Heart J 1990;120:529-532.

64. Ohman EM, Marquis JF, Ricci DR, et al. A randomized comparison of the effects of gradual prolonged versus standard primary balloon inflation on early and late outcome. Results of a multicenter clinical trial. Perfusion Balloon Catheter Study Group. Circulation 1994;89:1118-1125.

65. Roubin GS, Douglas JS, King SB, et al. Influence of balloon size on initial success rate, acute complications, and restenosis after PTCA. Circulation 1988;78:557-565.

66. Piana R, Moscucci M, Cohen D, et al. Palmaz-Schatz stenting for treatment of focal vein graft stenosis: Immediate results and long-term outcome. J Am Coll Cardiol 1994;23:1296-304.

67. Wong SC, Baim DS, Schatz RA, et al. Immediate results and late outcomes after stent implantation in saphenous vein graft lesions: the multicenter U.S. Palmaz-Schatz stent experience. J Am Coll Cardiol 1995;26:704-712.

68. Simonton CA, Leon MB, Baim DS, et al. Optimal directional coronary atherectomy: final results of the Optimal Atherectomy Restenosis Study (OARS). Circulation 1998;97(4):332-9.

69. Baim DS, Cutlip DE, Sharma SK, et al. Final results of the Balloon vs Optimal Atherectomy Trial. Circulation 1998;97:322-31.

70. Fitzgerald PJ, Hayase M, Mintz GS, et al. CRUISE: Can routine intravascular ultrasound influence stent expansion? Analysis of outcomes. J Am Coll Cardiol 1998;31(Suppl A):396A

71. Hayase M, Oshima A, Zidar JP, et al. Comparison of ultrasound vs angiographic guidance for stenting in the CRUISE study. Circulation 1998;98 (Suppl I):I-222.

72. Bengston J, Mark D, Honan M. Detection of restenosis after elective percutaneous transluminal angioplasty using the exercise treadmill test. Am J Cardiol 1990;65:28-34.

73. Hecht H, DeBord L, Shaw R. Usefulness of supine bicycle stress echocardiography for the detection of restenosis after percutaneous transluminal coronary angioplasty. Am J Cardiol 1993;71:293-296.

74. Pfisterer M, Rickenbacher P, Klowski W, Muller-Brand J. Silent ischemia after percutaneous transluminal coronary angioplasty: Incidence and prognostic significance. J Am Coll Cardiol 1993;22:1446-1454.

75. Manyari D, Knudtson M, Kloiber R. Sequential thallium-201 myocardial perfusion studies after successful percutaneous transluminal coronary angioplasty: delayed resolution of exercise-induced scintigraphic abnormalities. Circulation 1988;77:86-95.

76. Miller D, Verani M. Current status of myocardial perfusion imaging after percutaneous transluminal coronary angioplasty. J Am Coll Cardiol 1994;24:260-266.

77. Baim D, Levine M, Leon M, Levine S, Ellis S, Schatz R. Management of restenosis within the Palmaz-Schatz coronary stent (the U.S. multicenter experience). Am J Cardiol 1993;71:364-366.

78. Ellis SG, Savage M, Fischman D, et al. Restenosis after placement of Palmaz-Schatz stents in native coronary arteries. Initial results of a multicenter experience. Circulation 1992;86:1836-1844.

79. Colombo A, Ferraro M, Itoh A, et al. Results of coronary stenting for restenosis. J Am Coll Cardiol 1996;28:830-6.

80. Penn I, Ricci D, Almond DG, et al. Stenting results in increased early complications and fewer late reinterventions: Final clinical data from the Trial of Angioplasty and Stents in Canada (TASC) I. Circulation 1995;92:I-475.

81. Waksman R, Weintraub WS, Ziyad MB, Douglas JS, Shen Y, King SB. Balloon angioplasty, Palmaz-Schatz stent, and directional coronary atherectomy for restenotic lesions: Retrospective comparison in a single center. J Am Coll Cardiol 1995;25;330A.

82. Muller DWM. Restenosis: Site-specific Therapy. In Topol EJ (ed). *Textbook of Interventional Cardiology*, 2nd Edition, Philadelphia, WB Saunders Company, 1993; 436-448.

83. Muller DWM. Gene therapy for cardiovascular disease. Br Heart J 1994;71:309-311.

84. Mitchell JR, Arzin MA, Fram DB, et al. Inhibition of platelet deposition and lysis of intracoronary thrombus during balloon angioplasty using urokinase-coated hydrogel balloons. Circulation 1994;90:1979-1988.

85. Ohno T, Gordon D, San H, et al. Gene therapy for vascular smooth muscle cell proliferation after arterial injury. Science 1994;265:781-784.

86. von der Leyen HE, Gibbons GH, Morishita R, et al. Gene therapy inhibiting neointimal vascular lesion: in vivo transfer of endothelial cell nitric oxide synthase gene. Proc Natl Acad Sci USA 1995;92:1137-1141.

87. Change MW, Barr E, Seltzer J, et al. Cytostatic gene therapy for vascular proliferative disorders with a constitutively active form of the retinoblastoma gene product. Science 1995;267:518-522.

88. Asahara T, Bauters C, Pastroe C, et al. Local delivery of vascular endothelial growth factor accelerates reendothelialization and attenuates intimal hyperplasia in balloon-injured rat carotid artery. Circulation 1995;91:2793-2801.

89. Simons M, Edelman ER, Dekeyser JL, et al. Antisense c-myb oligonucleotides inhibit intimal arterial smooth muscle cell accumulation in vivo. Nature 1992;359:67-70.

90. Morhisita R, Gibbons GH, Ellison KE, et al. Initimal hyperplasia after vascular injury is inhibited by antisense cdk2 kinase oligonucleotides. J Clin Invest 1994;93:1458-1464.

91. O'Keefe JH, Lapeyre AC, Holmes DR, et al. Usefulness of early radionuclide angiography for identifying low-risk patients for late restenosis after percutaneous transluminal

coronary angioplasty. Am J Cardiol 1988;61:51-54.

92. El-Tamimi H, Davies GJ, Hackett D, et al. Very early prediction of restenosis after successful coronary angioplasty: Anatomic and functional assessment. J Am Coll Cardiol 1990;15:259-264.

93. Wijns W, Serruys P, Reiber J, et al. Early detection of restenosis after successful percutaneous transluminal coronary angioplasty by exercise-redistribution thallium scintigraphy. Am J Cardiol 1985;55:357-361.

94. Wijns W, Serruys PW, Simoons ML, van den Brand M, de Feyter PJ, Reiber JH, Hugenholtz PG. Predictive value of early maximal exercise test and thallium scintigraphy after successful percutaneous transluminal coronary angioplasty. Br Heart J 1985;53:194-200.

95. Scholl JM, Chaitman BR, David PR, et al. Exercise electrocardiography and myocardial scintigraphy in the serial evaluation of the results of percutaneous transluminal coronary angioplasty. Circulation 1982;66:380-390.

96. Ernst SMPG, Hillebrand FA, Kelin B, et al. The value of exercise tests in the follow-up of patients who underwent transluminal coronary angioplasty. Int J Cardiol 1985;7:267-279.

97. Rosing DR, Van Raden MJ, Mincemoyer RM, et al. Exercise, electrocardiographic and functional responses after percutaneous transluminal coronary angioplasty. Am J Cardiol 1984;53:36C-41C.

98. Honan MB, Bengtson JR, Pryor DB, et al. Exercise treadmill testing is a poor predictor of anatomic restenosis after angioplasty for acute myocardial infarction. Circulation 1989;80:1585-94.

99. Hillegass WB, Ancukiewicz M, Bengtson JR, et al. Does follow-up exercise testing predict restenosis after successful balloon angioplasty? Circulation 1992;I-137.

100. Hardoff R, Shefer A, Gips S, et al. Predicting late restenosis after coronary angioplasty by very early (12 to 24 h) thallium-201 scintigraphy: implications with regard to mechanisms of late coronary restenosis. J Am Coll Cardiol 1990;15:1486-1492.

101. Jain A, Mahmarian JJ, Borges-Neto S, et al. Clinical significance of perfusion defects by thallium-201 single photon emission tomography following oral dipyridamole early after coronary angioplasty. J Am Coll Cardiol 1988;11:970-976.

102. Lam JYT, Chaitman BR, Byers S, et al. Can dipyridamole thallium imaging predict restenosis after coronary angioplasty? Circulation 1987;76:373.

103. DePuey EF, Leatherman RD, Dear WE, et al. Restenosis after transluminal coronary angioplasty detected with exercise-gated radionuclide ventriculography. J Am Coll Cardiol 1984;4:1103-1113.

104. DePuey EG, Boskovic D, Krajcer Z, et al. Exercise radionuclide ventriculography in evaluating successful transluminal coronary angioplasty. Cathet Cardiovasc Diagn 1983;9:153-166.

105. Umans VA, Melkert R, Foley DP, Serruys PW. Clinical and angiographic comparison of matched patients with successful directional coronary atherectomy or stent implantation for primary coronary artery lesions. J Am Coll Cardiol 1996;28:637-644.

106. Holmes DR, Garratt KN, Isner JM, et al. Effect of subintimal resection on initial outcome and restenosis for native coronary lesions an saphenous vein graft disease treated by directional coronary atherectomy: A report from the CAVEAT I and II investigators. J Am Coll Cardiol 1996;28:645-651.

107. Condado JA, Popma JJ, Lanksy AJ, et al. Effect of intracoronary Iridium[192] on late quantitative angiographic outcomes after PTCA. J Am Coll Cardiol 1997;29(Suppl. A):418A.

108. Mintz GS, Massullo V, Popma JJ, et al. Transcatheter Iridium-192 irradiation reduces in-stent neointimal tissue proliferation: A serial volumetric intravascular ultrasound analysis from the SCRIPPS trials. J Am Coll Cardiol 1997;29(Suppl. A):60A.

109. Teirstein PS, Massullo V, Jani S, et al. A double-blinded randomized trial of catheter-based radiotherapy to inhibit restenosis following coronary stenting. N Engl J Med 1997;336:1697.

110. Tamai H, Katou K, Hayakawa H, et al. The impact of tranilast on restenosis following coronary angioplasty the second tranilast restenosis following angioplasty trial (TREAT-2). Circulation 1996;94:I-620.

111. Tardif JC, Cote G, Lesperance J, et al. Probucol and multivitamins in the prevention of restenosis after coronary angioplasty. N Engl J Med 1997;337:365-72.

112. Dangas G, Cocke TP, Sharma SK, Duvvuri S, Kakarala V, Ambrose JA. Early changes in minimal luminal diameter after balloon angioplasty and directional coronary atherectomy. J Invas Cardiol 1998;10:372-375.

113. Mintz GS, Popma JJ, Pichard AD, et al. Arterial remodeling after coronary angioplasty. A serial intravascular ultrasound study. Circulation 1996;94:35-43.

114. Kimura T, Kaburagi S, Tamura T, et al. Remodeling of human coronary arteries undergoing coronary angioplasty and atherectomy. Circulation 1997;96:475-483.

115. Dangas G, Fuster V. Management of restenosis after coronary intervention. Am Heart J 1996;132:428-436.

116. Dangas G, Mintz GS, Mehran R, Lansky AJ, Kornowski R, Pichard AD, Satler LF, Kent KM, Stone GW, Leon MB. Preintervention arterial remodeling as an independent predictor of target lesion revascularization after non-stent coronary intervention. An analysis of 777 lesions with intravascular ultrasound imaging. Circulation 1999;99:3149-3154.

117. The ERASER Investigators. Acute platelet inhibition with abciximab does not reduce in-stent restenosis (ERASER study). Circulation 1999;100:799.

118. Serruys PW, Pieper M, Bos AA, et al. TRAPIST study: a randomized double blind study to evaluate the efficacy of trapidil on restenosis after successful elective coronary stenting. Circulation 1999;98(Suppl I):I-362.

119. Mehran R, Dangas G, Mintz GS, et al. In-stent restenosis: "The Great Equalizer" Disappointing clinical outcomes with all interventional strategies. J Am Coll Cardiol 1999;33 [Suppl A]:63A.

120. Waksman R, White RL, Chan RC, et al. Intracoronary gamma radiation therapy after angioplasty inhibits recurrences in patients with in-stent restenosis. Circulation 2000;101:360-5.

121. Waksman R, Bhargava B, White L, et al. Intracoronary beta-

radiation therapy inhibits recurrence of in-stent restenosis. Circulation 2000;101:1895.

122. Mehran R, Dangas G, Mintz G, et al.. Treatment of in-stent restenosis with excimer laser coronary angioplasty vs. rotational atherectomy. Circulation 2000;101:2484.

123. Ormiston JA, Stewart FM, Roche AH, et al. Late regression of the dilated site after coronary angioplasty: A 5-year quantitative angiographic study. Circulation 1997;96:468.

124. Detre K, Holubkov R, Kelsey S, et al. Percutaneous transluminal coronary angioplasty in 1985-1986 and 1977-1981. The National Heart, Lung, and Blood Institute Registry. N Engl J Med 1988;318:265.

125. King SB, Williams DO, Chougule P, et al. Endovascular beta-radiation to reduce restenosis after coronary balloon angioplasty: results of the beta energy restenosis trial (BERT). Circulation;97:2025.

126. Johansen O, Brekke M, Seljeflot I, et al. Omega-3 fatty acids do not prevent restenosis after coronary angioplasty: Results from the CART study. J Am Coll Cardiol 1999;33:1619.

127. Whitworth HB, Roubin GS, Hollman J, et al. Effect of nifedipine on recurrent stenosis after percutaneous transluminal coronary angioplasty. J Am Coll Cardiol 1986;8:1271.

128. Corcos T, David PR, Val PG, et al. Failure of diltiazem to prevent restenosis after percutaneous transluminal coronary angioplasty. Am Heart J 1985;109:926.

129. Weintraub WS, Boccuzzi SJ, Klein JL, et al. Lack of effect of lovastatin on restenosis after coronary angioplasty. N Engl J Med 1994;331:1331.

130. Tardif JC, Cote G, Lesperance J, et al. Probucol and multivitamins in the prevention of restenosis after coronary angioplasty. N Engl J Med 1997;337:365.

131. Yokoi H, Daida H, Kuwabara Y, et al. Effectiveness of an antioxidant in preventing restenosis after percutaneous transluminal coronary angioplasty: The Probucol Angioplasty Restenois Trial. J Am Coll Cardiol 1997;30:855.

132. Hoffman R, Mintz GS, Dussaillant GR. Patterns and mechanisms of in-stent restenosis: a serial intravscular ultrasound study. Circulation 1996;94:1247-1254.

133. Mintz GS, Hoffmann R, Mehran R. In-stent restenosis: The Washington Hospital Center experience. 1998;81:7E-13E.

134. Mehran R, Dangas G, et al. Angiographic patterns of in-stent restenosis: classification and implications for long-term outcome. Circulation 1999;100:1872-78.

135. Curran MJ, Fry JA, Grines CL, et al. Initial human experience with intramural ethyl alcohol for treatment of in-stent restenosis: The Beaumont Alcohol Restenosis Study (BARS). Am J of Cardiol 2000;86:25i.

136. Mehran R, Mintz GS, Popma JJ, et al. Mechanisms and results of balloon angioplasty for the treatment of in-stent restenosis. Am J Cardiol 1996;78:718-622.

137. Gorge G, Konorza E, Voegle E, et al. Incomplete restoration of luminal dimensions after PTCA in restenotic stented segments: an intravascular ultrasound analysis. J Am Coll Cardiol 1997;29:311A.

138. Reimers B, Moussa I, Akiyama T, et al. Long-term clinical follow-up after successful repeat percutaneous intervention for stent restenosis. J Am Coll Cardiol 1997;30:186.

139. Lee, et al. Am J Cardiol 1998;82:140-143.

140. Dauerman, et al. Am J Cardiol 1998;82:277-284.

141. Ferguson JJ. Meeting highlights: The 21ˢᵗ Congress of the European Society of Cardiology. Circulation 1999;100:e126.

142. Vom Dahl K. Presentation at The 21ˢᵗ Congress of the European Society of Cardiology, 1999.

143. Pattan, et al. J Am Coll Cardiol 1997;29:68A.

144. Mehran et al. Circulation 1997;96:2183-2189.

145. Gruberg L, Hong MK, Mintz GS, et al. Optimally deployed stents in the treatment of restenotic versus de novo lesions. Am J Cardiol 2000;85:333-7.

146. Teirstein PS, Massullo V, Jani S, et al. Three-year clinical and angiographic follow-up after intracoronary radiation: Results of a randomized clinical trial. Circulation 2000;101:360-5.

147. Leon MB, Teirstein PS, Moses JW, et al. Localized intracoronary gamma-radiation therapy to inhibit the recurrence of restenosis after stenting. N Engl J Med 2001;344:250-6.

148. Raizner AE, Oesterle SN, Waksman R, et al. Inhibition of restenosis with beta-emitting radiotherapy: Report of the Proliferation Reduction with Vascular Energy Trial (PREVENT). Circulation 2000;102:951-8.

149. Waksman R, Bhargava B, Mintz GS, et al. Late total occlusion after intracoronary brachytherapy for patients with in-stent restenosis. J Am Coll Cardiol 2000;36:65-8.

150. Tsuchikane E, et al. Circulation 1999;100:21-26.

151. Yamasaki M, et al. Cathet Cardiovasc Diag 1998;44:387-391.

152. Jorgensen B, et al. J Am Coll Cardiol 2000;35:592-9.

153. King SB, Williams DO, Chougule P, et al. Endovascular beta-radiation to reduce restenosis after coronary balloon angioplasty: Results of the Beta Energy Restenosis Trial (BERT). Circulation 1998;97:2025-30.

154. Verin V, Popwoski Y, de Bruyne B, et al. Endoluminal beta-radiation for the prevention of coronary restenosis after balloon angioplasty. N Engl J Med 2001;344:243-9.

155. Mehran R, Dangas G, Mintz GS, et al. Excimer laser vs. rotational atherectomy for the treatment of diffuse in-stent restenosis: acute and long-term results. J Am Coll Cardiol 1999;33(Suppl A):I-62A.

156. Koster R, Kahler J, Terres W, et al. Six-month clinical and angiographic outcome after successful excimer laser angioplasty for in-stent restenosis. J Am Coll Cardiol 2000;36:69-74.

157. Haase J, Storger H, Hoffmann M, Schwarz F. Excimer laser angioplasty with adjunctive balloon dilation versus balloon dilation alone for the treatment of in-stent restenosis: Results of a randomized single-center study. J Intervent Cardiol 1999;12:513-518.

158. Lauer B, Schmidt E, Ambrosch H, et al. Optimal treatment of in-stent-retenosis: Excimer laser-angioplasty, rotational atherectomy or conventional angioplasty? J Am Coll Cardiol 1999;33(Suppl A):I-62A.

159. Mehran R, Dangas G, Mintz GS, et al. In-stent restenosis: "The Great Equalizer" - disappointing clinical outcomes with ALL interventional strategies. J Am Coll Cardiol 1999;33(Suppl A):I-63A.

160. Koster R, Hamm CW, et al. Treatment of in-stent coronary restenosis by excimer laser angioplasty. Am J Cardiol

1998;80(11):1424-1428.

161. Hasse J, Reifart N, Schwart F, et al. Is excimer laser angioplasty superior to balloon dilatation for the treatment of in-stent restenosis? Results of prospective single center study. J Am Coll Cardiol 1998;31(Suppl C):400C.

162. Popma JJ. Oral presentation: ACC meeting, Anaheim, CA, 2000.

163. Dauerman HL, Baim DS, Cutlip DE, Sparano AM, et al. Mechanical debulking versus balloon angioplasty for the treatment of diffuse in-stent restenosis. Am J Cardiol 1998;82:277-284.

164. Sharma SK, Duvvuri S, Dangas G, Kini A, et al. Rotational atherectomy for in-stent restenosis: Acute and long-term results of the first 100 cases. J Am Coll Cardiol 1998;32:1358-1365.

165. Lee SG, Lee CW, Cheong SS, Hong MK, et al. Immediate and long-term outcomes of rotational atherectomy versus balloon angioplasty alone for treatment of diffuse in-stent restenosis. Am J Cardiol 1998;82:140-143.

166. Mehran R, Mintz GS, Satler LF, Pichard AD, et al. Treatment of in-stent restenosis with excimer laser coronary. Circulation 1997;96 (7):2183-9.

167. Sharma SK, Kini AS, King T, et al. Multivariate predictors of target lesion revascularization in the randomized trial of PTCA versus rotablator for diffuse in-stent restenosis (ROSTER). J Am Coll Cardiol 2001;37(2):2A

168. Vom Dahl J, Silber S, Niccoli SE, et al. Angioplasty versus rotational atherectomy for treatment of diffuse in-stent restenosis: clinical and angiographic results from a randomized multicenter trial (ARTIST Study). J Am Coll Cardiol 2000;35(Suppl A):7A.

169. Kuntz RE, Moses JW, Abizaid A, et al. Intravascular sonotherapy in human coronary arteries: First results of a feasibility trial. J Am Coll Cardiol 2001;37(2):45A.

170. Rensing B, Vos J, Smits P, et al. Coronary restenosis prevention with a rapamycin coated stent. J Am Coll Cardiol 2001;37(2):47A.

171. Feres F, Costa MA, Abizaid A, et al. Comparison between sirolimus-coated and noncoated stent implantation in human coronary arteries. J Am Coll Cardiol 2001;37(2):47A .

MEDICAL AND PERIPHERAL VASCULAR COMPLICATIONS

25

Kenneth Rosenfield, M.D.
James A. Goldstein, M.D.
Robert D. Safian, M.D.

RENAL INSUFFICIENCY

Depending upon the etiology, renal insufficiency after percutaneous revascularization may be transient and quickly respond to medical measures, or may progress to oliguric renal failure with volume overload, electrolyte and acid-base disturbances, and frank uremia. The most common manifestations include decreasing urine output and a rising serum creatinine in the first 2-5 days after PTCA. Early recognition, diagnosis, and treatment may prevent progression to overt renal failure.

A. **ETIOLOGY (Table 25.1).** Contrast-induced renal dysfunction is the most common cause of renal insufficiency, but the incidence varies widely depending on the definition (Table 25.2).[1] Using a rise in serum creatinine > 25% within 48 hours of contrast exposure, the incidence varies from < 1% in normal patients to approximately 50% in the highest risk groups.[2,3,87] Older purported mechanisms for contrast-induced renal dysfunction included a direct reduction in renal perfusion, secondary reduction in renal perfusion due to myocardial depression, direct tubular injury, and a hypersensitivity reaction leading to immune-mediated intraluminal obstruction.[2,3] However, it is now recognized that the renal medulla is extremely vulnerable to ischemic injury, and that intense contrast-induced medullary vasoconstriction is the most likely cause of contrast nephropathy.[199] Patients with pre-existing renal insufficiency are the most susceptible to contrast nephropathy, particularly those with diabetic renal disease.[1] In patients with or without diabetes and baseline creatinine clearance > 60 cc/min, the risk of progressive renal failure requiring dialysis is negligible. However, when baseline creatinine clearance is < 50 cc/min, the risk of end-stage renal failure is much higher in diabetics (Table 25.3). Other risk factors for contrast nephropathy in high-risk patients include large contrast volume, hypovolemia, and impaired left ventricular (LV) function (Table 25.4). Once renal dysfunction develops, creatinine levels generally peak at 3-5 days and remain elevated for 1-2 weeks.[3,4] Oliguria occurs in 30% of patients. Although recovery is most common, some patients develop profound renal failure requiring temporary or permanent dialysis, which is associated with high in-hospital mortality and poor long-term survival.[1] Other causes of renal insufficiency after percutaneous intervention include renal ischemia from angiotensin converting enzyme (ACE) inhibitors, atheroembolism, aortic dissection, a malpositioned intra-aortic balloon pump, and post-renal obstruction from prostatism or anticholinergic drug administration. Regardless of the cause, renal insufficiency may be exacerbated by hypovolemia due to dehydration, contrast-induced diuresis, and procedural blood loss.

Table 25.1. Causes of Acute Renal Insufficiency in the PTCA Patient

Etiology	Comments
PRE-RENAL CAUSES	

Volume depletion
   NPO status
   Contrast-induced diuresis
   Blood loss
	Oliguria usually responds quickly to fluids or blood as needed

Diminished cardiac output
   Contrast-induced myocardial depression
   Myocardial ischemia
	May need vasodilators and/or diuretics instead of volume expansion; use pulmonary artery catheter to guide volume replacement, if necessary

RENAL CAUSES	
Contrast-induced Renal ischemia Atheroembolism	*Contrast-induced*: Peak creatinine in 3-5 days, followed by slow recovery (days) and post-azotemia diuresis. Oliguria in 30%. Hydration and diuretics (for patients with heart failure) may be of benefit. *Renal ischemia, atheroembolism:* Look for signs of embolic phenomenon (e.g., livedo reticularis). Consider renal artery stenosis
PERI-RENAL CAUSES	
Aortic dissection Malposition of IABP Drugs	Check position of IABP Discontinue nephrotoxic drugs
POST-RENAL CAUSES (Obstruction)	
Ureteral obstruction Bladder outlet (prostatism, anticholinergic drugs)	Keep well-hydrated; avoid atropine; insert Foley catheter if necessary

Abbreviations: IABP = intra-aortic balloon pump

B. **PREVENTION (Table 25.5).** Patients with pre-existing renal insufficiency, diabetic nephropathy, or a history of prior contrast nephropathy are at increased risk for renal failure. Maintenance of optimal intravascular volume and urine flow are the most important goals of therapy.

1. **Intravenous Fluids.** The administration of intravenous fluids (100-150 cc/hr) for 8-12 hours prior to PTCA is recommended in high-risk groups; patients with left ventricular dysfunction may require diuretics and invasive hemodynamic monitoring (with a pulmonary artery catheter) to avoid pulmonary edema and guide fluid management. In a randomized study, isotonic saline hydration prior to elective PTCA resulted in less contrast nephropathy (rise in serum creatinine ≥ 0.5 mg/dL within 48 hours) compared to hydration with half-isotonic saline (0.6% vs. 2.7%, p = 0.02).[219]

2. **Nonionic Contrast.** Nonionic contrast is associated with less volume overload than ionic contrast but does not decrease the risk of contrast nephropathy.[5,6] However, iohexol reduced the rate of severe renal failure from 28% to 12% in a randomized trial of diabetic patients with renal dysfunction, and is recommended in this high-risk subset.[89]

3. **Nephrotoxic Drugs.** In addition to optimizing intravascular volume, avoidance of potentially nephrotoxic drugs (e.g., nonsteroidal anti-inflammatory agents) is reasonable.

4. **Loop Diuretics.** Loop diuretics do not protect against contrast-induced nephropathy, and prophylactic furosemide has deleterious effects on renal function due to volume depletion.[7]

5. **Mannitol.** Mannitol (12.5-25 gm IV) may increase solute excretion in patients with intravascular hemolysis, hemoglobinuria, and extreme hyperuricemia, but is contraindicated in patients with heart failure. Two prospective randomized trials reported that mannitol failed to reduce the risk of contrast nephropathy.[90,92] In fact, mannitol-induced dehydration may have similar deleterious effects as loop diuretics.

6. **Dopamine.** Dopamine increases renal blood flow, sodium excretion, and glomerular filtration rate, but the benefits in preventing contrast nephropathy are unclear. One study reported benefit in non-diabetics, but there was a greater incidence of contrast nephropathy in diabetics.[8] In another report, renal-dose dopamine (2 mcg/kg/min) plus saline provided no advantage over saline alone in preventing contrast nephropathy, and dopamine resulted in a significant increase in serum creatinine in patients with peripheral vascular disease.[191]

7. **Forced Diuresis.** Two prospective randomized trials[90,92] reached different conclusions about the value of forced diuresis in preventing progressive renal failure: One showed no benefit of furosemide or mannitol compared to saline hydration,[92] whereas another showed modest benefit.[90] In PRINCE (Prospective Randomized Trial of Prevention Measures in Patients at High Risk for Contrast Nephropathy), patients with baseline renal insufficiency (creatinine $\geq$ 2.5 mg/dL) undergoing cardiac catheterization had a modest reduction in progressive renal failure by forced diuresis (to maintain urine flow > 150 cc/hr) with crystalloids, furosemide, and dopamine.[90]

Table 25.2. Incidence of Acute Renal Failure After Coronary Intervention By Definition[87]

Definition	Incidence (%) (n = 1826 patients)
Rise in Cr > 25%	14.5
Rise in Cr > 50%	3.9
Rise in Cr > 100%	1.8
Rise in Cr > 1 mg/dL	2.4
Post-procedure Cr > 5 mg/dL or dialysis	1.3

Abbreviations: Cr = serum creatinine

Table 25.3. Probability of Renal Failure Requiring Dialysis After Coronary Intervention[87]

Subset	Baseline Creatinine Clearance (cc/min*)				
	50	**40**	**30**	**20**	**10**
Diabetes (%)	0.2	2	10	43	84
No diabetes (%)	0.04	0.3	2	12	48

* Baseline creatinine clearance prior to intervention is based on the Cockcroft-Gault formula:
  Ccr = ([140 - age] x [wt (kg)])/(serum Cr x 72). Multiply by 0.85 for females.

8. **Theophylline.** Endogenous intrarenal adenosine has been implicated in the pathogenesis of contrast nephropathy. A recent study demonstrated that contrast-induced renal dysfunction was exacerbated by dipyridamole (which potentiates adenosine's effects), and attenuated by theophylline (2.9 mg/kg PO every 12 hrs x 4, starting one hour before contrast).

9. **N-acetylcysteine.** In a small randomized trial of patients with renal insufficiency (baseline serum creatinine ≥2.5 mg/dL) undergoing CT scans with nonionic contrast, the oral antioxidant N-acetylcysteine (600 mg BID for 2 days) resulted in a 10-fold reduction in contrast nephropathy compared to placebo (2% vs. 21%, p = 0.01).[198] The prospective randomized PORCINE trial (Prevention of Radiographic Contrast-Induced Nephropathy after Coronary Angiography) is evaluating intravenous hydration vs. N-acetylcysteine (Mucomyst) for preventing contrast nephropathy after coronary intervention.

10. **Fenoldopam.** Experimental studies indicate that fenoldopam, a dopamine-1 receptor agonist, increases renal cortical and medullary blood flow, attenuates contrast-induced vasoconstriction, and prevents contrast nephropathy in high-risk patients.[200-204] Mild degrees of fenoldopam-induced hypotension are generally well-tolerated and rarely require premature termination of the drug. Important advantages of fenoldopam include its short half-life (5 minutes), rapid effect on renal blood flow (< 30 minutes), and efficacy even in the absence of fluid loading (which may be beneficial in patients with LV dysfunction). Other advantages include ease of dose titration to achieve a balance between renal medullary vasodilation (dose ≥ 0.01 mcg/kg/min) and lowering of systemic vascular resistance and blood pressure (dose ≥ 0.1 mcg/kg/min), and short treatment interval (infusion starts 1 hour before procedure and ends 4 hours after procedure). The striking benefit of fenoldopam, in contrast to the variable impact of dopamine, is due to its highly predictable physiologic effects (Table 25.6).

C. **MANAGEMENT.** Serum creatinine should be routinely obtained 12-24 hrs following intervention. If the creatinine is elevated, follow-up measurements should be obtained and medical measures instituted until renal function has stabilized. For decreasing urine output and/or rising serum creatinine after intervention:

Table 25.4. Risk Factors for Contrast-Induced Nephropathy

Definite	Possible
Baseline Cr > 1.5 mg/dL or Ccr < 60 cc/min*	Hypertension
Diabetic nephropathy	Proteinuria
Heart failure, class III-IV	Advanced age
Large contrast volume**	
Prior contrast nephropathy	
Intravascular volume depletion	

Abbreviations: Cr = creatinine; Ccr = calculated creatinine clearance
* Most important risk
** Recommendations for a "safe" contrast limit: 5cc of contrast x body weight (kg)/Cr (mg/dL); maximum = 300 cc[91] or ratio of contrast volume/Ccr ≤ 6[93]

1. **Exclude Bleeding and Bladder Outlet Obstruction.** On occasion, retroperitoneal hemorrhage, GI bleeding, or bladder obstruction (particularly in males with prostate enlargement) may first manifest as diminished urine output. These conditions must be excluded early, since they are readily reversible and their treatment is different from that of contrast nephropathy.

2. **Maintain Adequate Hydration and Urine Output.** After intervention, hydration (100-150 cc of intravenous crystalloid for 6-12 hours or 1-2 L of water orally) helps maintain a stable blood pressure and urine output, thus facilitating excretion of contrast. A helpful "rule of thumb" is to match urine output with IV fluids during the first 8-10 hours after the procedure. If the urine output falls below 40-60 cc/hr, intravenous fluids are increased. If the patient has adequate intravascular volume and baseline LV dysfunction, diuretics (furosemide 20-80 mg IV over 1-2 minutes) will frequently augment urine flow.[90] Loop diuretics and metolazone—in contrast to other diuretics—are effective in patients with impaired glomerular filtration rates (GFR) and are recommended for circulatory congestion. When heart failure and severe oliguria coexist, the combination of furosemide and metolazone may be superior to either agent alone because of sequential nephron blockade.[9] Dopamine may provide additional benefit and is commonly used in low doses (5 mcg/kg/min IV). Right heart catheterization and hemodynamic monitoring should be considered in all oliguric patients if volume status is uncertain.

3. **Consult a Nephrologist.** Progressive or persistent renal dysfunction should prompt consultation with a nephrologist. Additional noninvasive tests (e.g., renal scan, ultrasound, magnetic resonance angiogram) or initiation of dialysis should be performed as necessary.

Table 25.5. Prevention of Contrast-Induced Nephropathy

Definite Benefit	No Benefit or Harmful
Fenoldopam	Mannitol
Saline hydration*	Dopamine
Nonionic contrast**	Loop diuretics
N-acetylcysteine	Calcium antagonists
	Atrial natriuretic peptide

*   Saline hydration should be used cautiously in patients with heart failure; adjunctive treatment with furosemide may be necessary.
** Clear benefit has been demonstrated in high-risk patients with diabetes and renal insufficiency, but not in other high-risk subsets.

Table 25.6. Comparison of Dopamine and Fenoldopam

	Dopamine	Fenoldopam
Receptor Effects		
Dopamine-1 receptor	+++	+++
Dopamine-2 receptor	+++	-
Alpha receptor	++	-
Beta-1 receptor	+++	-
Beta-2 receptor	+	-
Physiologic Effects*		
Blood pressure (hypertensive)	↑	↓
Blood pressure (normotensive)	NC or ↑	NC or mild ↓
Renal cortical blood flow	↑	↑
Renal medullary blood flow	↓	↑
Glomerular filtration	NC or ↓	NC or ↑
Direct natriuresis, diuresis	NC	↑
Coronary blood flow	NC or ↓	↑
Chronotropic effects	NC or ↑	NC
Inotropic effects	NC or ↑	NC
Mesenteric blood flow	NC	↑
Pulmonary vascular resistance	NC	↓
Cerebral perfusion	NC or ↑	NC

*   Because of complex interactions with dopamine, beta, and alpha receptors, the physiologic effects of dopamine are unpredictable in a given patient. In contrast, fenoldopam is a selective dopamine-1 receptor agonist, with predictable effects on the coronary, mesenteric, and renal circulation.
NC = no change
- No effect on receptor
+ to +++ = increasing receptor agonism
↑ Increased effect
↓ Decreased effect

CONTRAST REACTIONS

A. TYPES OF CONTRAST AGENTS

1. **High-Osmolar Contrast Media.** These ionic agents are salts which consist of three iodine atoms bound to a fully-substituted benzene ring, and a methylglucamine and/or sodium ion. In the aqueous phase, these ionic agents consist of two osmotically-active particles. Most ionic agents have an osmolarity which is 5-8 times higher than blood (1400-2400 mOsm/L vs. 275 mOsm/L), a sodium content 1-7 times higher than plasma, and contain additives which bind ionized calcium.

2. **Low Osmolar Contrast Media**
   a. **Ionic Media.** Ioxaglate (Hexabrix) is an ionic dimer consisting of two osmotically-active particles for every 6 iodine atoms, and 50% less osmolality compared to high-osmolar ionic agents.

   b. **Nonionic Media.** Nonionic agents consist of 3 iodine atoms bound to a fully-substituted, uncharged benzene ring. These agents are not salts and enter the aqueous phase as a single osmotically-active compound (i.e., one osmotically-active particle for every 3 iodine atoms). These agents provide equivalent radiodensity at half the osmotic load, and do not bind ionized calcium.

B. ADVERSE REACTIONS TO RADIOGRAPHIC CONTRAST.
Despite excellent overall tolerance, contrast media can result in undesirable reactions, ranging from mild nausea to life-threatening anaphylaxis. Mortality attributable to contrast administration during coronary angiography is 4-23 deaths per million patients.[10,11] Life-threatening allergic reactions are usually described as "anaphylactoid" reactions (IgG-mediated), to distinguish them from allergic "anaphylactic" reactions (IgE-mediated); treatment recommendations are identical. Patients with a previous history of an adverse dye reaction are at highest risk for a subsequent reaction, and previous anaphylaxis recurs in 40% of patients who are not premedicated.[12] Asthmatics—especially those with nasal polyps—represent another high-risk group, and are 6-9 times more likely to develop a contrast reaction compared to non-asthmatics.[13]

1. **Hemodynamic Effects.** Transient myocardial depression and hypotension are due to calcium-binding properties and vasodilation of radiographic contrast, and are more common following administration of high-osmolar agents.

2. **Electrophysiologic Effects.** Bradycardia, AV block, ST segment and T wave changes, prolonged QT interval, and ventricular tachycardia/fibrillation have been attributed to the calcium-chelating properties of the preservatives and buffers in radiographic contrast. Ionic agents differ in their ability to bind calcium: additives in Renografin-76 (sodium EDTA, sodium citrate) chelate more calcium than Hypaque and Angiovist (calcium EDTA), which explains the greater incidence of

hemodynamic and electrophysiologic alterations with Renografin-76.[14] Nonionic agents have little if any calcium binding activity. In a randomized prospective study among patients undergoing PTCA, there was a trend toward less contrast-induced ventricular tachycardia or fibrillation with the nonionic agent iopamidol (Isovue-370) compared to the high-osmolar ionic agent meglumine sodium diatrizoate (Renografin-76).[15]

3. **Minor Reactions.** In a study of 337,647 patients, the five most frequent symptoms following intravenous contrast administration (nausea, urticaria, itching, heat sensation, vomiting) were reduced by low-osmolar contrast.[16] Low-osmolar contrast also results in less patient discomfort during internal mammary and peripheral arteriography.

4. **Severe Reactions.**   Severe reactions (dyspnea or hypotension requiring therapy, loss of consciousness, cardiac arrest) were less frequent after low-osmolar agents.[16] In patients with a previous reaction to high-osmolar agents, no reaction was observed in 95% of patients given low-osmolar contrast.[17]

5. **Thrombosis (Table 25.7).** Routine use of nonionic contrast media remains controversial in patients with acute coronary syndromes undergoing percutaneous intervention, as in-vitro and in-vivo studies demonstrated that ionic contrast has greater anticoagulant and antiplatelet activities (prolongation of PTT and clotting time, inhibition of platelet aggregation and degranulation, reduced time to thrombolysis). In earlier prospective PTCA trials, ionic contrast was associated with less in-lab acute closure, no-reflow, and recurrent ischemia compared to nonionic contrast.[18-20,81,84] The EPIC trial reported less abrupt closure, Q-wave MI, and death with ionic contrast in patients with recent MI, unstable angina, or high-risk morphology, suggesting that preexisting thrombus or hypercoagulable state contributes to the deleterious effects of nonionic contrast.[20-23] However, two recent prospective randomized trials in patients with stable and unstable angina showed no difference between nonionic and ionic contrast.[94,95] In summary, nonionic and ionic contrast may be used in patients with acute coronary syndromes. The low-osmolar ionic agent ioxaglate or low-osmolar nonionic agents should be used in patients with hemodynamic instability or serious arrhythmias.

6. **Nephrotoxicity.** Among patients with baseline renal insufficiency, no difference in contrast nephropathy was observed for high-osmolar and nonionic agents.[24,25] However, low-osmolar agents are preferred for patients with renal insufficiency requiring large contrast volumes, to minimize the volume load. Nonionic agents are preferred in high-risk patients with renal insufficiency and diabetes.[89]

7. **Cost.** Low-osmolar agents cost 15-20 times more than high osmolar agents (e.g., $100 vs $5 per 100cc). It has been estimated that routine use of low-osmolar agents for coronary angiography would increase the annual cath lab budget for contrast by $100 million in the U.S. alone.

Table 25.7. Risk of Thrombosis with Ionic and Nonionic Contrast

Study	N	Design	Results
Shrader[94] (1999)	2000	Randomized trial in elective PTCA	No difference in acute closure, repeat PTCA, or major ischemic events
Malekianpour[95] (1998)	210	Randomized trial in unstable angina	No difference in thrombus, acute closure, or repeat PTCA
Aguirre[20] (1995)	1930	Retrospective review of EPIC	Ionic contrast reduced the risk of acute closure (7% vs 10%), Q-wave MI (1.9% vs. 7%), and death (0.4% vs. 1.5%)
Piessens[18] (1993)	500	Randomized trial	Ionic contrast reduced the risk of acute thrombosis (8% vs. 18%)
Grines[19] (1993)	211	Randomized trial in unstable angina and MI patients requiring PTCA	Ionic contrast reduced the risk of recurrent ischemia requiring repeat angiography (3% vs. 11.4%), rePTCA in-hospital (1% vs. 5.8%), and rest angina at 1 month (0% vs. 5.9%)

C. **RECOMMENDATIONS.**   Low-osmolar agents can be reserved for patients most likely to derive significant clinical benefit, since these agents are costly. Although data are conflicting and opinions vary, our recommendation is to use a low-osmolar (ionic or nonionic) agent for patients with hemodynamic or electrophysiologic instability, decompensated heart failure, moderate or severe renal dysfunction, or prior history of a severe contrast reaction. In addition, patients undergoing internal mammary artery angiography will experience less discomfort when a low-osmolar agent is used. Due to unresolved issues and conflicting data about thrombotic complications, we recommend ionic agents for patients with acute myocardial infarction, post-infarction angina, or unstable angina, unless other factors favor the use of nonionic contrast

D. **PREVENTION.** The best approach for preventing contrast reactions is to plan ahead: Obtain a history of previous contrast reaction; define other risk factors; premedicate individuals with a known contrast allergy (see below); minimize contrast volume; and have equipment, medications, and personnel ready to treat life-threatening reactions.

1. **Identify Patients at Risk.** The recommendations for prophylaxis against contrast reactions during cardiac catheterization are extrapolated from the radiology literature. Shehadi[26] reported adverse reactions in 5.6% of 112,000 patients, including severe reactions in 0.02% and death in 0.007%. Another study of 302,083 patients reported any reaction in 4.7%, severe reactions in 0.07%, and death in 0.006%.[27] Patients at greatest risk for contrast reaction were those with a prior reaction, severe asthma, or multiple allergies. A history of hay fever and allergies doubled the risk of a contrast reaction, and a prior contrast reaction tripled the risk of subsequent adverse reactions.[27] Low-osmolar contrast resulted in a lower incidence of severe adverse reactions compared to high-osmolar contrast.[28,29]

2. **Pharmacologic Prophylaxis (Table 25.8).** Pretreatment with corticosteroids decreases the risk of contrast reactions, though patients pretreated for < 12 hours before exposure had no benefit compared to untreated patients.[29,30]

Table 25.8. Premedication Protocol for Prevention of Contrast Allergy*

Drug	Comment
Prednisone	40 mg PO every 6 hours, starting 12-18 hours prior to contrast exposure (Solumedrol 40 mg IV for emergency procedures)
Diphenhydramine	50 mg PO or IV before procedure
H$_2$ receptor antagonist	H$_2$ receptor antagonist is optional—no clear data to support its use. (Consider ranitidine 150 mg or cimetidine 300 mg PO before procedure)
Low-osmolar contrast	Use low-osmolar contrast to reduce the risk of reactions

* Regimens vary, and no regimen is fully protective

Table 25.9. Contrast Reactions: Presentation, Onset, and Treatment*

Type	Presentation	Onset	Treatment
Minor	Mild urticaria, pruritus, erythema	Usually occur within minutes of exposure	Occasionally requires intervention. Treatment is supportive, including observation and cool compresses; oral diphenhydramine is sometimes useful.
Moderate	Angioedema, bronchospasm, laryngeal edema	Usually occur within minutes to hours of exposure	Usually requires intervention. Treatment includes diphenhydramine (50 mg IV), steroids (e.g., hydrocortisone 100 mg IV). Anaphylactoid reactions are also treated with epinephrine (0.1-0.5cc of a 1:1,000 dilution [0.1-0.5 mg] subcutaneously every 5-15 minutes as needed). Bronchodilator treatments (e.g., albuterol aerosol 2.5 mg nebulized mist every 1-2 hours) might be of benefit.
Severe	Anaphylaxis (cardiovascular collapse or profound hypotension)	May occur immediately with a single contrast injection	Life-threatening and requires aggressive attention. Epinephrine (1-5cc of a 1:10,000 solution [0.1-0.5 mg] via IV or endotracheal tube every 5 minutes as needed), steroids (e.g., hydrocortisone 100 mg IV or solumedrol 125 mg IV), diphenhydramine (50 mg IV), and possible intubation.

* Common side effects (chemotoxic effects) to radiographic contrast, such as nausea, vomiting, and vasovagal reactions, should not be considered "allergic" manifestations. Immediate treatment, if necessary, includes centrally-acting antiemetics (compazine 2-5 mg IV) for nausea/vomiting and atropine (0.5-1.0 mg IV) for vasovagal reactions. Pretreatment with corticosteroids is not useful for these reactions, but low-osmolar or nonionic contrast will reduce the incidence and severity of these side effects. The dose for epinephrine is the same for moderate or severe contrast reactions; the dilution, injected volume, and route of administration are different.

PERIPHERAL VASCULAR COMPLICATIONS RELATED TO VASCULAR ACCESS

Percutaneous coronary interventional procedures are associated with a variety of important peripheral vascular complications.[135,139,141,144]

A. LOCAL BLEEDING AND HEMATOMA

1. **Background and Definitions.** Most complications of percutaneous interventional procedures are related to vascular access. There are numerous classifications of bleeding, but none are uniformly accepted. A commonly published classification was used by the EPIC investigators, which considers the site of hemorrhage (all intracranial hemorrhages are classified as major bleeding events), and the fall in hemoglobin concentration or hematocrit (Table 25.10). At least 50% of all bleeding complications after percutaneous intervention involve the arterial access site.[209] A hematoma is defined as a space-occupying collection of blood that is initially localized adjacent to the vessel, and ultimately spreads into the surrounding tissues. Although some hematomas are associated with an underlying pseudoaneurysm, most are not (Table 25.11).

2. **Incidence.** Hematomas are typically classified as small, moderate, or large. Since a precise definition is lacking, the true incidence of hematomas is not known; reports vary widely from 0.5 to 7%,[32,55,121-124] but may be higher. In one study of 2107 consecutive patients,[55] blood transfusion was required in 7.3% due to bleeding at the access site (5.8%), retroperitoneal bleeding (0.9%), gastrointestinal bleeding, and unknown etiology. Factors associated with bleeding complications included female gender, low body weight, advanced age, urgent procedure, low baseline hemoglobin, long procedure duration, larger sheath size, increased heparin dose, thrombolytic agents, and multivessel disease. These and others data suggest that the underlying severity of patient illness is the greatest predictor of bleeding complications.[56-62,135] In the past, coronary stenting was associated with an increased risk of bleeding complications due to aggressive anticoagulation,[61] but vascular complications have decreased with current antiplatelet regimens. Use of glycoprotein IIb/IIIa receptor antagonists and low-dose heparin with early sheath removal was not associated with increased major bleeding events in EPILOG and subsequent interventional trials (Table 25.12). Avoidance of post-procedural heparin in patients with stable or unstable ischemic syndromes[63] has markedly decreased the incidence of bleeding and vascular complications, without increasing the risk of ischemic events. Available data suggest it is important to discontinue heparin immediately after intervention in patients with good results. Although suboptimal results may increase the risk of subsequent ischemic complications, these are not prevented by prolonged heparin or enoxaparin, which only increase the risk of bleeding complications.[225]

3. **Diagnosis.** The presence of an enlarging mass surrounding the puncture site is the cardinal sign of a hematoma. Slowly expanding hematomas—including those from venous sites—can be dangerous because of their insidious nature and the risk of significant blood loss by the time the

hematoma is recognized. In obese patients, significant blood loss may occur without apparent hematoma. Bleeding may cause hypotension, a vasovagal reaction, tachycardia, or nerve palsy[125] (median nerve for brachial access; femoral nerve for femoral access). Nerve compression is more likely to occur with a pseudoaneurysm, and should be suspected when pain is out of proportion to the size of the hematoma. Interestingly, even a small hematoma or pseudoaneurysm can cause significant motor or sensory impairment.

4. **Prevention.** The key to avoiding bleeding complications is meticulous attention to the access site, recognition of predisposing factors (Table 25.11), and avoidance of post-procedural heparin. The skin nick should be larger than the sheath diameter to facilitate external expression of blood loss. Sheaths should be removed when the ACT falls to subtherapeutic levels to minimize patient discomfort and prolonged immobility. Several developments over the past several years show promise for reducing access site bleeding, including low profile equipment,[126,127,137] techniques for transradial intervention,[128-133] and arterial closure devices.

5. **Management.** Therapy depends on the extent of bleeding, size of the hematoma, degree of hemodynamic instability, and the need for uninterrupted anticoagulation. Stabilization of hemodynamic status and control of hemorrhage are the immediate priorities. The access site should be treated by direct manual compression, pneumatic compression (Femostop), or mechanical clamp. If a large hematoma is present, manual compression can help dissipate blood into the surrounding tissues and "soften" the area, which may facilitate compression and resolution of the hematoma. Rapid volume replacement (crystalloid and blood) and careful monitoring of vital signs and hemoglobin concentration are imperative. Sedative-narcotics should be administered to ease patient discomfort, and atropine or pressors should be administered, if needed. If the patient is hypertensive, blood pressure should be lowered with nitrates or vasodilators. The possibility of an underlying pseudoaneurysm should be considered (see below), although this does not alter initial management. If bleeding cannot be controlled, urgent surgical exploration may be required.

Table 25.10. Bleeding Classification in Trials of Glycoprotein IIb/IIIa Inhibitors[209]

Classification	Definition
Major bleeding	Intracranial hemorrhage Fall in hemoglobin > 5 gm/dL Fall in hematocrit > 15
Minor bleeding	Gross hematuria or hematemesis Fall in hemoglobin > 3 gm/dL with bleeding source Fall in hemoglobin > 4 gm/dL without bleeding source Fall in hematocrit > 10 with bleeding source Fall in hematocrit > 12 without bleeding source
Mild bleeding	All other observed bleeding

Table 25.11. Factors Predisposing to Vascular Access-Site Bleeding

Anatomic Factors

    Calcified (inelastic) vessels

    Elderly patient

    Obese patient

    Female patient

    Patient movement

Procedural Factors

    "Through-and-through" backwall puncture

    High puncture (above inguinal ligament)

    Low puncture (profunda or superficial femoral artery)

    Multiple punctures

    Large sheath size

    Kinking of sheath due to acute angulation

    Prolonged procedure time (higher heparin doses)

    Prolonged indwelling sheath time (higher ACT levels)

Hemodynamic Factors

    Increased pulse pressure (aortic insufficiency or non-compliant vessels)

    Severe hypertension

Hematologic Factors

    Multiple platelet antagonists (aspirin, clopidogrel, IIb/IIIa receptor antagonists)

    Antithrombotic agents (heparinoids, warfarin)

    Thrombolytic agents (tPA, SK)

    Underlying coagulopathy or thrombocytopenia

Human Factors

    Inexperience

    Inability to gain "control" of site upon sheath removal

    Short duration of pressure applied to obtain hemostasis

B. RETROPERITONEAL HEMORRHAGE

    1. Definition and Etiology. Retroperitoneal hemorrhage may occur if femoral artery access is proximal to the inguinal ligament, since effective vessel compression after sheath removal may not be possible. Since the inguinal ligament serves are a natural barrier between pelvic and infrainguinal spaces, bleeding above the inguinal ligament tracks posteriorly into the retroperitoneum, or rarely into the rectus sheath. Less commonly, retroperitoneal hemorrhage is a result of inadvertent guidewire perforation of a small pelvic vein or arteriole. Finally, spontaneous retroperitoneal bleeding from lumbar or other arteries[122] may rarely occur in association with anticoagulation and antiplatelet therapy, even in the absence of vascular procedures.

Table 25.12. Bleeding Complications in Trials of Glycoprotein IIb/IIIa Inhibitors[208]

Trial	Agent	Bleeding (%)		Transfusion (%)
		Major	Minor	
TARGET	Tirofiban	1.2	3.5	-
(n = 4802)	Abciximab	1.0	5.6	-
	p-value	_NS_	_NS_	
EPISTENT	Stent - placebo	2.2	1.7	2.2
(n = 2399)	Stent - abciximab	1.5	2.9	2.8
	PTCA - abciximab	1.4	2.9	3.1
	p-value	_NS_	_NS_	_NS_
EPILOG	Abciximab - SH	3.5	7.4	3.3
(n = 2792)	Abciximab - LH	2.0	4.0	1.9
	Placebo	3.1	3.7	3.9
	p-value	_NS_	_< 0.001_	_NS_
CAPTURE	Abciximab	3.8	4.8	7.1
(n = 1265)	Placebo	1.9	2.0	3.4
	p-value	_0.04_	_< 0.01_	_< 0.01_
EPIC	Abciximab B/I	14.0	16.9	15.0
(n = 2099)	Abciximab B	11.1	15.4	13.0
	Placebo	6.6	9.8	7.0
	p-value	_< 0.001_	_< 0.001_	_< 0.01_
ESPRIT	Eptifibatide	1.4	2.8	-
(n = 2064)	Placebo	0.4	1.8	-
	p-value	_NS_	_NS_	-
IMPACT-II	Eptifibatide (135/0.5)*	5.1	11.7	5.6
(n = 4010)	Eptifibatide (135/0.75)*	5.2	14.2	5.9
	Placebo	4.8	9.3	5.2
	p-value	_NS_	_NS_	_NS_
RESTORE	Tirofiban	2.4	-	-
(n = 2139)	Placebo	2.1	-	-
	p-value	_NS_		

Abbreviations: B = bolus; B/I = bolus + infusion; SH = standard heparin; LH = low-dose heparin
* Bolus (mcg/kg) + infusion (mcg/kg/min) dose

2. **Incidence.** The reported incidence of retroperitoneal hematoma is less than 1% after interventional procedures.[55,123]

3. **Diagnosis.** Detection of retroperitoneal hemorrhage may be difficult. Presenting symptoms range from sudden onset of pain, hypotension and abdominal distention, to vague abdominal or back pain. Often, the diagnosis is first suspected after an asymptomatic drop in hemoglobin concentration. Abdominal pain occurs in 60% of patients, and back and flank pain in 25%.[48,49] Abdominal pain is generally vague in two-thirds of cases, though occasionally it is localized over the hematoma. In addition to hypotension and tachycardia, the physical exam may reveal abdominal

distension, an abdominal mass, or a perirectal mass. The classic description of discoloration over the flank or abdomen (Grey Turner sign) is infrequent. If the hematoma is adjacent to the psoas muscle, the patient may be incapable of hip flexion, which may be the initial manifestation of retroperitoneal bleeding. A large hematoma may displace the ipsilateral ureter and kidney or mimic acute appendicitis, with right lower quadrant pain, fever, and an "acute" abdomen.[138] CT scanning is the most reliable method for establishing the presence and extent of hemorrhage, although the diagnosis may also be suggested by ultrasound or plain abdominal x-rays (psoas shadow in 30%; abdominal mass in 5%; paralytic ileus in 8%).

4. **Prevention.** Careful placement of the sheath in the common femoral artery below the inguinal ligament is essential to prevent retroperitoneal hemorrhage. Fluoroscopic localization of the intended entry site is useful (Chapter 1). Knowledge of inguinal anatomy and landmarks is crucial; the goal is to access the common femoral artery in its middle third, corresponding to the vascular segment overlying the medial third of the femoral head. The surface anatomy, particularly the inguinal crease, is an unreliable marker for deep vascular anatomy and should not be used as a landmark, particularly in obese patients. In one study,[142] the inguinal crease was an inaccurate landmark in 72% of patients. A more reliable landmark was the site of the strongest femoral pulse, which correctly identified the mid-common femoral artery in 93% of patients. Other measures to prevent retroperitoneal hemorrhage include careful guidewire manipulation, avoidance of excessive anticoagulation, and use of single anterior wall arterial punctures.

5. **Management.** Retroperitoneal hemorrhage can be fatal. Bleeding often stops spontaneously after 3-4 units of blood loss. Hypotension, hemodynamic collapse, renal failure, shock liver, and disseminated intravascular coagulopathy can occur with severe, retroperitoneal hemorrhage. If retroperitoneal hemorrhage is suspected on clinical grounds or confirmed by CT scan, heparin and platelet receptor blockers should be discontinued immediately. Removal of vascular sheaths and prolonged compression of the access site is mandatory. Fluid, blood replacement, and pressors should be initiated immediately as indicated, and vital signs must be closely monitored, since the patient can deteriorate suddenly. Rarely, progressive decline in hemoglobin concentration and hemodynamic instability warrant urgent surgical exploration. When abciximab is used, its antiplatelet effects should be reversed by immediate platelet transfusion (6-10 units). There is no antidote for eptifibatide or tirofiban, but their antiplatelet effects wear off after 6 hours.

C. PSEUDOANEURYSM

1. **Background and Definition.** A pseudoaneurysm is an encapsulated hematoma which communicates with an artery because of incomplete sealing of the media. The principal causes of pseudoaneurysm are inadequate compression following sheath removal and impaired hemostasis. Low vascular access in the superficial or profunda femoral artery increases the likelihood of pseudoaneurysm, since their deep location is less amenable to compression.

2. **Incidence.** The incidence of pseudoaneurysm formation after arterial cannulation varies from 0.03% to 0.4%, and was reported as high as 11% in stent patients treated with the older Coumadin regimen.[32,34,140,143] Factors increasing the risk of pseudoaneurysm include severe peripheral vascular disease, large sheaths, prolonged sheath time, prolonged anticoagulation, impaired platelet function, and premature ambulation.

3. **Diagnosis.** A pseudoaneurysm is frequently difficult to distinguish from an expanding hematoma. A leaking pseudoaneurysm may reside beneath a hematoma and be the cause of hematoma expansion. Any patient with a large or painful hematoma should be evaluated for a pseudoaneurysm, which can develop anytime from one day to one year (or longer) following arterial access. The classic finding is a tender, pulsatile mass with a systolic bruit; associated femoral or brachial nerve palsy may occur.[152] Pseudoaneurysms may rupture in 3.8% of patients,[153] leading to sudden massive swelling and severe pain. Confirmation of the diagnosis is by Duplex ultrasonography; angiography is unnecessary.

4. **Prevention.** Pseudoaneurysms can usually be avoided by careful sheath placement in the common femoral artery, use of small sheaths, prompt sheath removal, avoidance of post-procedural anticoagulation, treatment of hypertension at the time of sheath removal, and meticulous groin compression. The risk of pseudoaneurysm formation may be reduced by pneumatic compression devices (Femostop),[136,143] vascular closure devices, and radial intervention.[129,145,146]

5. **Management.** Treatment of a pseudoaneurysm is dependent on size, expansion, and the need for anticoagulation. Although hematomas generally resolve spontaneously, pseudoaneurysms may require compression or surgical repair. Pseudoaneurysms < 3 cm can often be followed clinically; follow-up ultrasound 1-2 weeks after initial diagnosis often demonstrates spontaneous thrombosis and obviates the need for repair. However, spontaneous thrombosis is less likely when the pseudoaneurysm is > 3 cm on initial ultrasound evaluation. If the pseudoaneurysm persists beyond two weeks or expands, surgical repair or ultrasound compression is recommended to reduce the risk of rupture. Ultrasound-guided compression is remarkably effective for closing pseudoaneurysms, but requires that the pseudoaneurysm be readily visualized. Success is 92-98% when the pseudoaneurysm has a long, thin neck and when further anticoagulation is unnecessary. Those receiving anticoagulation have success rates of 54-86%.[33,36,37,82] Ultrasound-guided compression usually requires systemic and/or local analgesia. There are no randomized trials comparing ultrasound compression to surgical repair, but the noninvasive approach has become the standard initial therapy in patients with suitable anatomy, even in the face of anticoagulation. A pneumatic compression device (Femostop) with or without ultrasound guidance can also be used as an alternative to surgery.[195] For patients with unfavorable anatomy, other non-surgical techniques include insertion of coils,[147] ultrasound-guided direct thrombin injection,[151,196] and covered stents.[186,197] Using direct-thrombin injection, 75% thrombosed within 15 seconds.[151] The major advantage of this technique is avoidance of patient discomfort and need for analgesia.[148-150] Surgical repair is reserved for failed ultrasound compression or femoral nerve involvement.[153]

D. ARTERIOVENOUS (AV) FISTULA

1. **Definition.** During vascular access, the Seldinger needle may puncture the femoral artery and overlying vein, creating an AV fistula after sheath withdrawal. The risk of AV fistula is increased by multiple passes to obtain femoral access, low puncture, high puncture (involving the common femoral artery and lateral femoral circumflex vein), and impaired clotting. Therefore, meticulous attention to the proper technique of arterial and venous access is imperative to minimize local complications.

2. **Incidence.** The incidence of AV fistula formation following diagnostic and therapeutic cardiac catheterization is 0.1-1.5%.[21,32,135]

3. **Diagnosis.** Clinical manifestations include a continuous bruit at the access site, distal arterial insufficiency ("steal phenomenon"), and a swollen, tender extremity due to venous dilatation. Color flow Doppler imaging and ultrasonography are used to confirm the diagnosis.

4. **Management.** A small AV fistula with a continuous bruit may be detected during follow-up. In patients with low-volume arteriovenous flow by Duplex, conservative therapy is reasonable, since many of these will close spontaneously.[123] In contrast, for large or symptomatic AV fistulae, surgical repair is recommended to prevent accelerated atherosclerosis, high-output heart failure, and progressive swelling and tenderness. Surgical repair involves division or excision of the fistula, or synthetic grafting of the involved vessels in unusual cases. Ultrasound-guided compression has been attempted for small fistulae,[33] but experience is limited. Endovascular stent grafting may ultimately offer a less invasive alternative to surgical repair.[186,197]

E. THROMBOTIC OCCLUSION

1. **Incidence.** Local thrombosis of the access site occurs in < 1% of patients after intervention. Risk factors include advanced age, cardiomyopathy, peripheral vascular disease, hypercoagulable states (lupus anticoagulant, Protein C or S deficiency, thrombocytosis or polycythemia, myeloma, or paraneoplastic syndrome), small body habitus, and small-caliber vessels. Small-caliber vessels are at greatest risk, which may partially explain why the brachial artery is more prone to thrombosis than the femoral artery. In the absence of other predisposing factors, vessel dissection and spasm often contribute to arterial thrombosis. In patients with pre-existing severe arterial occlusive disease, arterial thrombosis after cardiac catheterization may lead to late complications, including symptomatic ischemia (21%), amputation (11%), and death (2%).[38]

2. **Diagnosis.** Most arterial thromboses occur in the common femoral artery[39] (due to operator preference for the femoral approach), although the risk is 4-fold greater with the brachial approach (0.96% vs 0.22%; p < 0.001).[40] Manifestation of arterial occlusion include sudden or progressive pain, numbness, cyanosis, pallor, absence of a distal pulse, and a cool extremity. Physical examination and duplex scans are used to make the diagnosis, and arteriography may be necessary for confirmation and to guide therapy.

3. **Prevention.** Use of smaller sheaths is preferred in high-risk patients with peripheral vascular disease, small vessels, or hypercoagulable states. Elderly females with small body habitus are at highest risk; adequate anticoagulation, regular flushing of the arterial sheath, and timely sheath removal are essential. If an indwelling sheath is necessary, systemic anticoagulation is recommended, in addition to pressurized heparinized saline infusion through the sheath. A brachial access protocol which ensures that "downstream" blood is heparinized *prior* to catheter insertion may reduce the risk of brachial artery thrombosis. One method is to administer heparin *after* placing the guidewire in the artery, but *before* advancing the (potentially occlusive) sheath, or to give heparin directly into the sheath before inserting the catheters. Prophylactic nitroglycerin through the sheath at the beginning of the case may prevent spasm, which can promote brachial artery thrombosis.

4. **Management.** Due to the potential consequences of arterial thrombosis, heparinization and urgent thrombectomy are usually indicated. In addition to Fogarty catheter thrombectomy, bypass grafting and thromboendarterectomy are sometimes needed. Percutaneous rheolytic thrombectomy (Possis AngioJet) may be useful to treat acute peripheral vessel thrombosis; further study is needed.

F. ARTERIAL PERFORATION

1. **Background.** When advancing guidewires, catheters or other devices, the spectrum of vessel damage can range from minor endothelial injury to vessel perforation and acute hemorrhage.[41]

2. **Incidence and Diagnosis.** The incidence of arterial perforation remote from the puncture site is <0.1%.[42] Perforation should be suspected when the patient complains of acute pain at the moment of guidewire or catheter manipulation. Contrast injections may confirm extravasation of blood, but may not be diagnostic if the perforation is small; digital subtraction angiography may be more sensitive for diagnosis. For *catheter perforations*, symptoms are usually dramatic and rapid in onset, and include acute pain and hypotension. Catheter withdrawal may paradoxically lead to more discomfort, as extravasation increases when the defect becomes exposed. Bleeding from guidewire perforation may be less obvious, since the defect is usually small and extravasation is slow.

3. **Prevention.** The key to preventing perforation is to observe the entire path of guidewire and catheter advancement by fluoroscopy at all times, and to always lead with the guidewire. Tactile feedback is important: When encountering resistance to advancement, the operator should withdraw, redirect, or otherwise ensure that the wire or catheter is in correct position. Hydrophilic guidewires do not provide much tactile feedback, and must be used cautiously under fluoroscopic guidance by experienced operators.

4. **Management.** Recognition of a perforation, especially when associated with blood loss, is essential. The operator should assess ongoing extravasation; in such instances, anticoagulation should be reversed, and therapeutic coil embolization, prolonged balloon inflation, deployment of

a stent graft, and surgery are all possible solutions depending on the location and extent of perforation. Fortunately, most guidewire-induced peripheral arterial perforations are benign; spontaneous closure and insignificant blood loss are typical. Perforation into a visceral organ (e.g., renal parenchyma), whether guidewire or catheter-induced, is of major concern, since parenchymal hemorrhage and hematoma can jeopardize tissue viability. Management is organ-specific: In the case of the kidney, bleeding usually stops as anticoagulation is reversed; if not, embolization of the appropriate branch (if it can be identified) usually stops the bleeding. Appropriate volume and blood replacement are crucial. Finally, late consequences of vessel or organ perforation can include pseudoaneurysm formation, so patients should be followed closely.

G. DISSECTION

1. **Incidence.** The incidence of recognized dissection ranges from 0.01% to 0.4%,[43-47] but the true frequency is probably higher. Unrecognized local dissection at the access site contributes to the development of pseudoaneurysm, hematoma, and thrombosis. Patients with peripheral arterial occlusive disease are more prone to dissection, but propagation of dissection is more likely in a normal vessel. Remarkably, serious consequences from iatrogenic dissection during cardiac catheterization are rare. Dissections of the ascending aorta have been reported as a consequence of intervention on the RCA ostium;[178,182] once initiated, this type of aortic dissection may lead to cardiac tamponade or stroke.

2. **Prevention.** The same principles to prevent perforation also apply to dissection. Non-hydrophilic, soft-tip or J-tip guidewires are least likely to cause dissection, and may be the best choice for arterial access and catheter exchanges. Hydrophilic wires, while extremely useful in certain situations, are more likely to cause dissection, and should be employed with caution and only under fluoroscopic guidance. Dilators and sheaths should always be advanced over a leading guidewire to keep them off the arterial wall. Catheter exchanges should be performed with long (140-180 cm) wires, rather than crossing the iliac circulation each time with a shorter guidewire.

3. **Management.** Most dissections occur during retrograde advancement of the catheter or wire; therefore, antegrade blood flow will usually "tack down" the flap without further therapy. The need for surgical or percutaneous treatment depends on the severity of the dissection, involvement of major arch or visceral branches, distal flow impairment, and the presence of end-organ ischemia. For renal or iliac dissection, PTA and stenting can quickly remedy the situation; surgery is rarely necessary.

H. MISCELLANEOUS VASCULAR PROBLEMS.
Table 25.13 outlines the management of other frequently encountered vascular problems during PTCA procedures.

Table 25.13. Management of Common Vascular Problems in the PTCA Patient

Problem	Solution
Difficult access	• Choose alternate site (see Chapter 2) • Use Doppler-guided arterial puncture (Smart Needle)
Fibrotic groin or femoral bypass graft	• Dilate with progressively larger 5-9F dilators as needed
Difficulty negotiating tortuous iliac vessels	• Inject contrast through small dilator • Advance Glidewire, Wholey wire, TAD wire, or Magic-Torque wire • Insert long sheath
Sheath or catheters kink due to sharp bends	• Insert firm sheath (Terumo or Daig) over heavy-duty wire (Amplatz) • Use Amplatz or 0.063-inch wire
Bleeding around sheath	• Insert dilator (distal 1/3 cut off) to prevent kinks • Exchange for larger sheath • Apply prolonged pressure over groin • Remove sheath and compress

MEDICAL COMPLICATIONS NOT RELATED TO VASCULAR ACCESS

A. ATHEROEMBOLISM

1. **Background and Etiology.** Atheroembolism is one of the most feared complications of catheter-based procedures because it is unpredictable, difficult to treat, and associated with substantial morbidity and mortality. The clinical presentation of cholesterol embolization may be insidious and therefore easily overlooked in the aftermath of percutaneous intervention. In most cases, the etiology is catheter- or guidewire-induced mechanical disruption of friable atherosclerosis in the abdominal aorta. Complex aortic lesions, frequently unrecognized by angiography but detectable by transesophageal echocardiography (TEE), have more embolic potential.[156,157] Distal embolization may occur to the lower extremities,[50] abdominal viscera (spleen, liver, kidney, pancreas),[155,175,180] and brain.[159,161,178] Most acute occlusions of major visceral or peripheral arteries result from macroembolization of cholesterol and thrombotic debris. Microemboli may also occur, and generally result from release of cholesterol crystals and microscopic debris from ulcerated atheromatous plaque; clinical manifestations depend on the volume of debris and its ultimate destination. Showers of microemboli may result in microvascular glomerular obstruction (renal failure),[155] cutaneous tissues (livedo reticularis or necrotizing fasciitis), and the peripheral vascular bed ("blue-toe" syndrome). Even small amounts of debris can have severe consequences if embolized to the viscera or brain.[177,178]

2. **Incidence.** Clinically-recognized atheroembolization after cardiac catheterization is infrequent; one study reported retrieval of atheromatous debris from 0.5% of 7,621 patients.[186] Debris retrieval was more frequent with 8F catheters, and consisted of foam cells, cholesterol crystals, and amorphous debris. The true incidence may be as high as 10%,[51,52] but the insidious manifestations of cholesterol embolization make it difficult to diagnose. While it is impossible to predict the risk of atheroembolism in a given patient, severe peripheral vascular disease, aortic aneurysm, and mobile plaque by TEE[178] increase the risk of distal embolization and influence the approach.[130,131,133,155,176] Use of Judkins and Voda left, Multipurpose, and Judkins right guiding catheters was associated with retrieval of atherosclerotic debris in 65%, 60%, and 24% of patients, respectively.[85,158]

3. **Diagnosis.** Atheroembolic disease is diagnosed primarily from the history and physical exam. Blue-toe syndrome or livedo reticularis involving the extremities and trunk is the cardinal manifestation of peripheral microemboli, whereas the chief manifestation of macroembolic disease is acute arterial ischemia. The most extreme but rare consequence of distal embolization is ischemic ulceration and gangrene. Renal failure is also a manifestation of embolic disease;[155] generally, it is insidious over weeks to months after intervention. The peak effect of renal cholesterol embolization is usually between 4 and 8 weeks, and renal failure may be permanent; in comparison, contrast-induced renal failure usually peaks within the first week and is usually reversible. Other signs of cholesterol embolization include peripheral eosinophilia and accelerated or episodic hypertension.[53,54]

4. **Prevention.** All patients should be approached as if they are at increased risk for atheroembolization, particularly if there is known aortic atherosclerosis or aneurysmal disease. Utilization of long guidewire (260 cm) exchanges is recommended, and back-bleeding from guiding catheters (once the wire is removed) allows removal of debris. Advancement and removal of catheters should occur over a guidewire to straighten the catheter and minimize contact with the aortic wall. Brachial and radial access can minimize embolization from the abdominal aorta, but not from the ascending aorta or arch.

5. **Management.** The majority of microembolic complications are managed conservatively without specific treatment;[160] peripheral manifestations resolve over days to weeks in most patients. Use of anticoagulants is unproven and is not recommended. When renal atheroembolism is suspected, adequate hydration, maintenance of urine output, and control of hypertension are essential. Surgical management includes embolectomy for macroembolic complications, and some advocate surgical elimination of the source of atheroembolic material (e.g., abdominal aortic aneurysm).[53] Late consequences of peripheral embolization include painful ulceration of the toes, which is difficult to treat and may require amputation. Importantly, atheroembolization during previous procedures places the patient at increased risk for recurrent embolization.

B. NEUROLOGIC COMPLICATIONS

1. **Etiology.** In patients undergoing cardiac catheterization and coronary arteriography, the incidence of neurologic events is 0.07%.[31,77-79,174,177,178] Common etiologies include cardiac emboli (thrombus, calcium, vegetation), air embolus, and embolism from the aorta or carotid arteries due to guidewire or catheter manipulation. Intracranial bleeding is infrequent. Patients undergoing PTCA have a higher incidence of neurologic events (0.1-0.5%) due to the incremental risk imposed by longer procedures, emboli from guiding catheters, use of high-dose heparin and/or fibrinolytic agents, and cerebral hypoperfusion due to hypotension.[77,79,80] Patients with peripheral vascular disease have a 2-fold higher risk of major complications and stroke after percutaneous revascularization or CABG compared to patients without peripheral vascular disease.[192] In patients receiving eptifibatide in the PURSUIT trial, the risk of stroke (hemorrhagic or non-hemorrhagic) was similar to placebo.[205]

2. **Management.** A patient who sustains an intraprocedural neurologic event should undergo neurology consultation and an emergency CT scan to rule out intracranial hemorrhage. Reversible causes of altered mental status include sedative effects of drugs, hypoventilation, hypoperfusion, and metabolic abnormalities, which should be sought and corrected. In stable patients without critical coronary disease, heparin is reversed with protamine (10 mg/1,000 units of heparin IV over 5-15 minutes) prior to obtaining the CT scan. In patients with unstable angina and critical coronary disease, the decision to reverse anticoagulation must be individualized. In the absence of intracranial hemorrhage by CT scan, anticoagulation is continued. If the CT scan demonstrates hemorrhage, heparin, GP IIb/IIIa receptor antagonists, and thrombolytic infusions should be immediately discontinued. Circulating heparin should be neutralized by protamine, thrombolytics neutralized by cryoprecipitate (10 units IV) and fresh frozen plasma (2 units), and abciximab reversed by platelet transfusion (6-10 units).[80] There is no antidote to eptifibatide or tirofiban, and although the antiplatelet effects wear off within 4-6 hours of drug discontinuation, this delay may be unacceptable in patients with intracranial hemorrhage. We and others[185,206] have successfully treated procedure-related embolic stroke with catheter-directed thrombolysis and angioplasty. While only anecdotal at this time, this strategy may ameliorate one of the most devastating complications of cardiac catheterization.

C. INFECTION.
During the course of vascular intervention, the introduction of antigenically active substances into the peripheral bloodstream (proteins, endotoxin, etc.) may evoke a pyrogenic reaction.[73] Local infection at the site of arterial puncture, phlebitis, and fever occur in less than 1% of patients following interventional procedures.[83]

1. **Clinical Manifestations.** Pyrogenic reactions following cardiac catheterization generally occur within 60 minutes of the procedure, and manifest as fevers, chills, rigors, and lethargy. Local reactions (such as phlebitis) at the access site consist of erythema, painful induration, and rarely exudative drainage.

2. **Etiology and Management.** Therapy for infections following invasive procedures can be divided into systemic and local treatments. Blood cultures and a complete blood count should be obtained in all patients.

   a. **Local.** Phlebitis responds to hot soaks and elevation of the affected limb. Exudative drainage or cellulitis require antibiotics.

   b. **Systemic.** Fever and/or rigors following invasive procedures suggests transient bacteremia. It is imperative to remove indwelling catheters and sheaths and obtain blood cultures from several sites. Urine, sputum, and other cultures should be obtained as indicated. The results of these cultures and imaging studies (chest x-ray) are important to determine the course of antibiotic therapy. Fever and bacteremia often resolve after removal of indwelling lines, but empiric antibiotics are recommended in debilitated patients and those at high risk for endocarditis. The most common pathogens causing post-procedure fever are *Staphylococcus aureus* and *epidermidis*.[74-76] Approximately 50% of all *S. epidermidis* and 20-30% of *S. aureus* species are methicillin-resistant; first line antibiotic therapy is intravenous vancomycin. In the absence of endocarditis, a 7-day course of antibiotics is generally sufficient, and oral antibiotics are not necessary after discharge. Bacteremia due to gram-negative bacilli or *Candida* is rare; antimicrobial treatment directed against these organisms is not routinely recommended in the absence of culture confirmation. Continued fever and leukocytosis warrant continued antibiotics and a meticulous investigation to determine the cause. Repeat blood cultures, infectious disease consultation, and initiation of alternative antibiotic regimens should be considered depending on the clinical circumstances.

VASCULAR CLOSURE DEVICES

A. **BACKGROUND.** Several vascular closure devices have been used to achieve hemostasis after percutaneous procedures (Table 25.14). These devices offer the potential advantage of predictable closure of the arteriotomy without interrupting antiplatelet or anticoagulant therapy, and may improve patient comfort, allow early ambulation, and decrease bleeding complications. Some operators have employed vascular sealing devices to facilitate same-day discharge after coronary stenting.[211,214]

B. **DEVICES AND RESULTS.** Many vascular closure devices have been developed, but most fall into one of five categories: collagen plugs, biosealants, arterial "sandwich," percutaneous sutures, and compression girdles.

   1. **Collagen Plugs.** Biodegradable collagen insertion plugs (Vasoseal, Datascope, Inc.) have had equivocal results: One study reported bleeding complications in 33% despite initial success in 97%,[64] with more bleeding after use of sheaths ≥ 8F. Another study reported hematomas in 20% of patients while on full anticoagulation.[65] A randomized study of 150 angioplasty patients found

no difference in bleeding complications between conventional sheath removal vs. collagen plug (34% vs. 25%).[66] Other studies reported no differences in bleeding and vascular complications for the Vasoseal compared to manual or pneumatic compression,[66,67,134,179] although patients with collagen plugs perceived less discomfort. In summary, collagen plugs may improve patient comfort and allow for sheath removal while on anticoagulation,[179] but they have not been shown to significantly reduce bleeding complications.

2. **Biosealants.** Other closure devices (Duet, BioSeal) employ a thrombin-containing gel, which is delivered to the tissue surrounding the arteriotomy.[183,184] During delivery of the biosealant, a balloon is inflated within the artery to prevent leakage of thrombogenic material into the vessel. Randomized studies are pending.

3. **Vascular Sandwich with Polymer Anchor and Collagen.** The Angio-Seal™, like Vasoseal, employs bovine collagen to promote hemostasis. However, prior to delivery of the collagen plug, a biodegradable polymer anchor is delivered inside the vascular lumen, and then pulled back against the endoluminal surface of the artery with a connecting suture. The collagen ribbon is then advanced over the suture to the arterial wall, effectively "sandwiching" the arteriotomy between the anchor (inside the vessel) and the collagen (outside the vessel). The efficacy, safety, and reliability of this device have been demonstrated in several clinical trials.[162,166,168,173] Bleeding and vascular complication rates were significantly lower in patients treated with Angio-Seal, even with ongoing anticoagulation. While Angio-Seal seems to be effective and is technically easy to use, there were a few anecdotal reports of arterial thrombosis within the first 24-48 hours requiring rheolytic thrombectomy (AngioJet) or surgical repair. Factors which predisposed to serious bleeding and vascular complications following Angio-Seal included interventional procedures utilizing sheaths $\geq$ 8F (odds ratio 10.1), post-procedural heparin (odds ratio 3.2), and body size mass index < 28 (odds ratio 2.8).[215] The "learning curve" seemed to be about 50 cases.

4. **Percutaneous Suture.** Percutaneous suture-mediated closure of the access site immediately following intervention is possible with the Perclose device (Redwood City, CA). This device utilizes a catheter that deploys two (6F Techstar version) or four (8F, 10F Prostar version) needles with sutures from inside the arteriotomy, which are then delivered through the subcutaneous tissue and tied. Using a pushing device, a knot is delivered to the artery wall, thus suturing the arteriotomy to achieve immediate hemostasis. In a pilot study involving 91 patients, the device achieved immediate hemostasis despite full anticoagulation (ACT > 300 seconds) in 90%.[68] Preliminary reports from prospective, randomized trials[169,171,172] demonstrate a markedly reduced time to hemostasis, ambulation, and discharge using Techstar/Prostar Plus, with no increase in access site complications. Another randomized study confirmed these findings, and also reported fewer vascular complications in patients undergoing diagnostic cardiac catheterization (4.4% vs. 12.1%, p < 0.05), but not percutaneous revascularization (8.4% vs. 9.6%, p = NS).[217] Despite these excellent results, there is a significant learning curve,[170] and certain anatomic features preclude its use, including severe calcification, puncture below the common femoral artery bifurcation, small

caliber common femoral artery, inguinal scarring, and significant peripheral vascular disease. Technical difficulties which may lead to device failure and bleeding include suture breakage, inability to apply the knot tightly to the artery, and failure of the needles to catch the edges of the arteriotomy.

5. **Compression Girdles.** Pelvic girdle devices apply direct pressure to the femoral artery access site and are actually compression, rather than closure, devices. The prototype is the Femostop, which utilizes pneumatic pressure to achieve hemostasis. Studies with this device have shown variable but generally favorable results.[69,70] In one small study in patients receiving bolus plus infusion abciximab, the Femostop was superior to the Vasoseal and Perclose devices for vascular sealing, although differences in ACT levels and selection bias make interpretation difficult.[212] In another study, the Femostop was used for successful compression of pseudoaneurysms.[148] Other hemostasis devices include C-clamps, sandbags, and pressure bandages.[71,72,171,181]

Table 25.14. Vascular Closure Devices

Device	Classification	Description	Comments
Vasoseal[105-112]	Collagen plug	Biodegradable bovine collagen plug	Improves patient comfort; allows early sheath removal; no difference in bleeding or hematoma compared to manual compression
Duet[112,218,222]	Biosealant	Thrombin-containing biosealant gel	Feasibility trial suggests safety and efficacy in diagnostic and interventional procedures; randomized trials are underway
BioSeal[112]	Biosealant	Thrombin-containing biosealant gel	Feasibility trial suggests safety and efficacy in diagnostic and interventional procedures; randomized trials are underway
Angio-Seal[112-117,213]	Vascular "sandwich"	Biodegradable polymer, anchor, and collagen plug	Significant decrease in bleeding and hematoma compared to manual compression; improves patient comfort and allows early sheath removal and ambulation
Perclose[112,118,119]	Percutaneous suture	Percutaneous closure of arteriotomy using sutures to achieve hemostasis	Excellent hemostasis, but significant learning curve; allows early ambulation and improves patient comfort
Femostop[120]	Compression girdle	Pneumatic compression device (not closure) to achieve hemostasis	Safe alternative to manual compression

C. **CURRENT USE OF VASCULAR CLOSURE DEVICES.** There is no doubt that closure devices will play an increasingly important role in the cardiac catheterization laboratory.[165-167] At present, these devices cost $75-250, and for this reason, may be limited to patients who are at high risk for access site bleeding or require ongoing anticoagulation after sheath removal or early mobilization. Large-scale randomized comparisons between these closure techniques are not available, and there appears to be a learning curve with all of them. Studies thus far have failed to demonstrate major reductions in bleeding and vascular complications,[216] but patient comfort and the hope of early discharge are compelling. A relatively minor but annoying problem with virtually all closure devices is persistent oozing of blood around the closure site, particularly in patients receiving uninterrupted anticoagulation or GP IIb/IIIa inhibitors. In most cases, this is readily treated by a subcutaneous injection of 0.1-0.2 cc of 1:10,000 epinephrine. There is growing interest in the application of vascular closure devices to patients undergoing percutaneous intervention with adjunctive GP IIb/IIIa inhibitors, but in one large study, vascular closure devices were associated with more retroperitoneal hemorrhage than manual compression (0.9% vs. 0.1%, p = 0.01) and no difference in overall vascular and bleeding complications.[221] In contrast, percutaneous suture devices such as Perclose may improve outcomes in patients undergoing aortic or mitral valvuloplasty with 10-14F vascular sheaths.[220]

HEMATOLOGIC COMPLICATIONS

In addition to the well-known bleeding and thrombotic complications associated with percutaneous intervention, there are a variety of hematologic problems that may arise as complications of drugs used as adjuncts for intervention. The most common hematologic problems are drug-induced thrombocytopenia and neutropenia.

A. **DRUG-INDUCED THROMBOCYTOPENIA**
1. **Heparin-Induced Thrombocytopenia (Table 25.15).** Heparin-induced thrombocytopenia (HIT) is the most frequent drug-induced thrombocytopenia. Antibodies, usually of the IgG class, bind to multimolecular complexes of soluble platelet proteins (usually platelet factor 4 [PF4] and heparin).[99,101] These IgG-PF4 complexes may cause platelet activation and endothelial dysfunction, leading to clinical syndromes characterized by thrombocytopenia with or without thromboembolic complications.[99,100,101] There are two distinct clinical syndromes: Type I, a non-immune-mediated direct platelet activation leading to mild thrombocytopenia and a benign clinical course; and Type II, an immune-mediated platelet activation with moderate or severe thrombocytopenia and thromboembolic complications. The pathophysiology, clinical manifestations, and management of these syndromes differ markedly.
    a. **Heparin-Induced Thrombocytopenia Type I (HIT-I).** HIT-I is a benign clinical disorder characterized by a mild drop in platelet count (< 10% from baseline; rarely < 100,000/mm³), which typically develops 1-4 days after receiving standard systemic heparin therapy. HIT-I is

observed in 10-20% of patients receiving heparin, but is not associated with hemorrhagic or thromboembolic complications. Platelet counts typically return to normal within 1-2 days following cessation of heparin, and may normalize while therapy continues. Discontinuation of heparin is not necessary, but close monitoring of platelet counts is essential to assure that profound thrombocytopenia does not develop. HIT-I may be more frequent with unfractionated heparin; low-molecular-weight heparins may be useful in patients with HIT-I who require systemic heparinization.

b. **Heparin-Induced Thrombocytopenia Type II (HIT-II).** HIT-II is a potentially life-threatening disorder characterized by thrombocytopenia and potentially devastating thromboembolic complications due to immune-mediated (typically IgG, but also IgA and IgM) platelet activation and endothelial dysfunction. The diagnosis should be considered in any patient receiving heparin in whom the relative platelet count falls to < 50% of baseline, or an absolute platelet count of 40-60,000/mm^3. Some patients with HIT-II develop thromboembolic complications even when platelet counts are normal or only mildly decreased. Rarely, the earliest manifestations of HIT-II include skin necrosis at the site of heparin injection, an acute febrile illness similar to a transfusion reaction, increasing heparin resistance, and hemorrhage.[101] HIT-II typically manifests 5-14 days after initiating heparin; the incidence ranges from 0.5-5% of heparin-treated patients. Patients previously exposed to heparin may develop the syndrome abruptly, suggesting an amnestic response, even after "innocent" heparin exposure such as heparinized flush solutions or heparin-coated catheters. The clinical course of HIT-II is variable; immune thrombocytopenia and thromboembolic complications occur in up to 30% of affected patients within 2 weeks.[101,193] Thromboembolic complications may involve the arterial and venous circulations, resulting in venous thrombosis, lower extremity ischemia, limb amputation, stroke, and myocardial infarction. Ischemic complications are associated with a 30% mortality! The risk of thromboembolic complications is proportional to the degree of thrombocytopenia; hemorrhagic complications are unusual and platelet transfusions are not beneficial. In contrast to HIT-I, HIT-II is not associated with specific forms of heparin and may be provoked by unfractionated heparin, low-molecular-weight heparins, and various heparinoids. All forms of heparin (including flush solutions) must be immediately discontinued; platelet counts typically normalize within 3-5 days, but in some patients remain depressed for 2 weeks.

c. **Laboratory Evaluation of HIT.** Although HIT is a clinical syndrome characterized by thrombocytopenia (HIT-I, HIT-II) and thromboembolism (HIT-II), laboratory evaluation is useful for confirming the clinical diagnosis, particularly when isolated mild thrombocytopenia occurs. It is important to emphasize that early recognition of HIT-II is imperative to minimize patient morbidity and mortality; *if suspected on clinical grounds, the decision to discontinue heparin should not be delayed while awaiting further laboratory evaluation.* Several laboratory studies are potentially useful (Table 25.16): The serotonin release assay has been

Table 25.15. Heparin-Induced Thrombocytopenia (HIT)

	HIT-I	HIT-II
Mechanism	Direct platelet activation (non-immune mechanism)	IgG-antibodies to PF4 and other proteins cause platelet activation and endothelial dysfunction (immune mechanism)
Platelet count	< 10% fall from baseline; usually > 100,000/mm^3	> 50% fall from baseline; usually 40-60,000/mm^3
Clinical syndrome	Usually no clinical sequelae	High risk for thromboembolic complications; may have inflammation and necrosis at heparin injection site; bleeding is uncommon
Evaluation	(-) HIPA, (-) ELISA in non-immune cases; (+) HIPA and mild decrease in platelet count identifies patients at high-risk for HIT-II if heparin is continued	(+) HIPA identifies IgG antibodies to PF4; ELISA identifies antibodies (IgG, IgA, IgM) to PF4 and other proteins. Tests are complementary; 20% have (-) HIPA, (+) ELISA
Treatment and outcome	Platelet count may normalize despite continuation of heparin; stop heparin if not needed or if (+) HIPA	Discontinuation of <u>all</u> heparin is mandatory; platelet transfusions are not useful

Abbreviations: PF4 = platelet factor 4; HIPA = heparin-induced platelet aggregation; ELISA = enzyme-linked immunoadsorbent assay
(-) = negative test
(+) = positive test

the "gold-standard," although it may soon be replaced by other less demanding techniques (HIPA, ELISA)[96,97] with similar sensitivity and specificity. A positive HIPA test in a patient with mild thrombocytopenia may identify patients at higher risk for full-blown HIT-II if heparin is continued. Twenty percent of patients with HIT-II may have a negative HIPA; in these patients, ELISA may be positive, suggesting the presence of non-PF4 platelet antibodies.

  d. **Alternatives to Heparin in Patients with HIT.** Some patients with HIT require systemic anticoagulation for unstable angina, percutaneous intervention, or cardiac surgery. In the United States, lepirudin and argatroban are FDA-approved for anticoagulation in patients with HIT-II (Table 25.17). Although lepirudin is associated with a 30% reduction in serious thromboembolic complications compared to untreated patients, one-third of lepirudin-treated patients may experience a thromboembolic complication and almost half experience bleeding complications.[193] A few patients with HIT have received plasma exchange or high-dose intravenous IgG to reverse the heparin-associated platelet aggregation abnormality. Although re-exposure of HIT-II patients to heparin is not recommended, heparin-induced aggregation usually disappears within 2-4 weeks, and may permit brief re-exposure to heparin to allow safe CABG, when no other options are available.[101]

Table 25.16. Laboratory Studies for HIT-II and Heparin-Dependent Platelet Antibodies

Test	Rationale	Comments
Platelet aggregation test (PAT)	Measures aggregation of normal donor platelets by patient's serum or plasma, in presence of heparin	Widely used; simple, inexpensive; results available in 2-3 hrs; specificity ~ 90%, sensitivity 30-50%
Serotonin release assay (SRA)	Uses ^{14}C-serotonin-radiolabeled washed reactive donor platelets; test is positive if ^{14}C-serotonin release occurs at low (0.1 U/ml) but not high (100 U/ml) heparin concentration	Current reference standard for laboratory diagnosis of HIT; technically demanding but very sensitive and specific
Heparin-induced platelet aggregation (HIPA)	Similar to PAT, but uses washed normal donor platelets instead of platelet-rich plasma	Equal sensitivity to SRA and easier to perform; readily identifies IgG antibodies to PF4
Enzyme-linked immunoadsorbent assay (ELISA)	Uses immobilized PF4 and other platelet proteins bound to heparin as a target for HIT antibody	May be as sensitive as serotonin release assay and HIPA; may identify IgA, IgM, and IgG antibodies to PF4 and other platelet proteins

2. **Thrombocytopenia Associated With Glycoprotein IIb/IIIa Inhibitors (Chapter 34, Tables 25.18-20).** In patients receiving bolus plus infusion abciximab during high-risk PTCA, moderate thrombocytopenia (< 100,000/mm^3) developed in 5.2% of patients and severe thrombocytopenia (< 50,000/mm^3) developed in 1.6% of patients.[103] The risk of thrombocytopenia may be higher after re-exposure to abciximab, and unlike HIT-II, abrupt thrombocytopenia occurs within 6-24 hours. While the mechanism is unclear, thrombocytopenia is associated with excess bleeding and adverse clinical outcomes. Recently, a patient with acute abciximab-induced thrombocytopenia suffered fatal intracranial hemorrhage.[189] It is important to distinguish true thrombocytopenia from "pseudothrombocytopenia," which accounts for at least one-third of low platelet counts observed during treatment with abciximab[190] and may be due to in-vitro platelet clumping. Pseudothrombocytopenia is not associated with adverse clinical outcome; in-vivo platelet counts are normal and cessation of abciximab therapy is not required. A potential approach to thrombocytopenia after percutaneous intervention is shown in Figure 25.1.[207] Reports in small numbers of patents suggest benefit from platelet transfusions and possibly immunoglobulin (IgG).[104] Compared to placebo, there does not appear to be a higher incidence of thrombocytopenia in patients treated with eptifibatide[188] or tirofiban. These small- molecule antagonists may be used safely in patients requiring percutaneous intervention who develop abciximab-induced thrombocytopenia once platelet counts normalize.[223]

Table 25.17. Alternative Forms of Anticoagulation in HIT Patients[101]

Agent	Comments
Low-molecular weight heparins	May be useful in HIT-I; contraindicated in HIT-II
Heparinoids[210]	May be useful in HIT-I; contraindicated in HIT-II; none are FDA-approved in US
Platelet IIb/IIIa inhibitors	May be useful in patients with acute coronary syndromes and prior HIT-I or HIT-II; has not been evaluated as sole therapy during percutaneous intervention or cardiac surgery
Hirudin	Direct thrombin inhibitor; under evaluation for patients with HIT-II
Argatroban (Acova)[102]	Synthetic direct thrombin inhibitor; FDA-approved for systemic anticoagulation in patients with HIT-II
Lepirudin (Refludan)	Recombinant hirudin; FDA-approved for systemic anticoagulation in patients with HIT-II
Warfarin	Useful in patients with venous thromboembolic disorders and HIT
Ancrod[98]	Purified fibrinogenase derived from pit viper venom; has been used for anticoagulation for stroke, venous thrombosis, peripheral PTA, PTCA, and CABG; monitored by sequential fibrinogen levels
Iloprost	Stable prostacyclin analogue; blocks heparin-dependent platelet activation and aggregation in-vitro; has permitted safe heparin administration during vascular surgery and CABG in patients with HIT-II; not available in US

Abbreviations: HIT = heparin-induced thrombocytopenia; PTA = percutaneous transluminal angioplasty; PTCA = percutaneous transluminal coronary angioplasty; CABG = coronary artery bypass surgery

3. **Thrombotic Thrombocytopenia Purpura (TTP).** Rare cases of TTP have been reported with ticlopidine (0.02%; 50-fold higher than in the general population), and more recently with clopidogrel.[224] TTP usually presents with thrombocytopenia, bleeding, or neurologic abnormalities (headache, confusion, aphasia, focal weakness), that may wax and wane. The full-blown syndrome consists of thrombocytopenia, microangiopathic hemolytic anemia, altered mental status, renal failure, and fever. Platelet aggregates can occur and cause small vessel occlusion, and early mortality exceeds 20%. Examination of the blood typically reveals red blood cell fragments, and laboratory evaluation shows reticulocytosis, elevated bilirubin, negative Coombs test, and a normal PT/PTT. Unfortunately, limiting ticlopidine or clopidogrel therapy to 2-4 weeks after intervention does not necessarily prevent TTP. Immediate diagnosis and large-volume plasmapheresis are required for survival.[194] Isolated thrombocytopenia without TTP has also been reported after clopidogrel, which responded to discontinuation of drug and intravenous immunoglobulin.[220]

B. **DRUG-INDUCED NEUTROPENIA.** Ticlopidine is associated with neutropenia (absolute neutrophil count < 1200/mm^3) in 0.8-2.4% of patients, within 1-4 weeks of initiation of therapy. The mechanism of neutropenia is unknown. Associated pancytopenia and thrombocytopenia are extremely rare. Fortunately, neutrophil counts typically return to normal within 2 weeks of discontinuation of therapy, but occasionally remain depressed for several months. Patients receiving ticlopidine should have a complete blood count every 2 weeks for the first 3 months of therapy.

Table 25.18. Definitions of Drug-Induced Thrombocytopenia[207]

Definition	Platelet Count (x 10^3 per mm³)
Severity	
Normal	> 150
Mild	100-149
Moderate	50-99
Severe	20-49
Profound	< 20
Time of onset	
Acute	< 24 hours
Delayed	> 24 hours

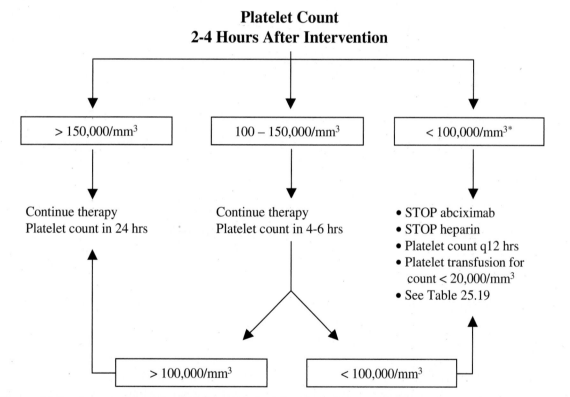

**Platelet Count
2-4 Hours After Intervention**

Figure 25.1. Approach to Thrombocytopenia After Percutaneous Intervention with GP IIb/IIIa Receptor Antagonists**

*   Aspirin and clopidogrel may be continued if the platelet count is > 50,000/mm³ and there is no bleeding, but should be stopped if the platelet count is < 50,000/mm³

** These recommendations apply to abciximab, but are reasonably applied to eptifibatide and tirofiban. The product insert recommends obtaining a platelet count 6 hours after instituting tirofiban (as opposed to 2-4 hours above); no specific recommendations are made for eptifibatide

Table 25.19. Evaluation of Thrombocytopenia After Percutaneous Intervention*

Possible Cause	Evaluation	Treatment
Pseudothrombocytopenia	Review peripheral blood smear; repeat platelet count in citrated-blood	Continue therapy as clinically indicated
Glycoprotein IIb/IIIa inhibitor	See Figure 25.1	See Figure 25.1
Heparin	See Table 25.16	See Table 25.17; stop heparin
Other medications (quinine derivatives, sulfa derivatives, phenytoin)	Obtain drug-induced platelet antibodies	Stop drug(s)
DIC, TTP	Review peripheral blood smear; measure prothrombin time, fibrinogen, D-dimer; obtain blood cultures	Plasmapheresis (TTP); stop ticlopidine or clopidogrel (TTP); treat sepsis (DIC)
ITP	Obtain platelet antibody screen	Remove or treat offending agent; steroids
Primary bone marrow disorder	Review peripheral blood smear, bone marrow biopsy	Treat as indicated

Abbreviations: DIC = disseminated intravascular coagulation; ITP = idiopathic thrombocytopenia; TTP = thrombotic thrombocytopenic purpura
* Platelet count < 100,000/mm³ any time after intervention

LATEX ALLERGY

A. **ETIOLOGY.** Hypersensitivity reactions to latex are more frequently recognized now than in the past. Finished latex for medical products is manufactured by a complex process using rubber (commercially harvested from trees), latex (a natural organic gum found in hundreds of plants), and numerous chemicals and other additives; allergic reactions may be directed against any of these components. Two general types of latex hypersensitivity reactions include Type I (IgE-dependent) and Type IV (contact dermatitis). Manifestations and treatment of latex reactions are similar to those for iodinated contrast, although contrast reactions are rarely IgE-dependent.

B. **CLINICAL MANIFESTATIONS.** The clinical manifestations of latex allergy are similar to those for iodinated contrast (Table 25.21), except that coagulopathy has not yet been reported as a manifestation of latex allergy. The risk of an allergic reaction is 0.8% for the general population, but may be as high as 5-10% in health care workers who frequently wear latex gloves or other high-risk groups (Table 25.22).[88]

Table 25.20. Thrombocytopenia in Trials of GP IIb/IIIa Inhibitors[207]

Trial	Agent	Platelet count (x 10^3/mm³)	Incidence Drug	Incidence Placebo	p-Value
— INTERVENTIONAL TRIALS —					
EPIC (n = 2099)	Abciximab	< 100	5.2	3.3	NS
		< 50	1.6	0.7	NS
EPILOG (n = 2792)	Abciximab	< 100	2.5	1.5	NS
		< 50	0.4	0.4	NS
CAPTURE (n = 1265)	Abciximab	< 100	5.6	1.3	< 0.001
		< 50	1.6	0	0.001
IMPACT (n = 4010)	Eptifibatide	< 100	2.6	2.4	NS
		< 50	0.2	0.6	NS
RESTORE (n = 2141)	Tirofiban	< 90	1.1	0.9	NS
		< 50	0.2	0.1	NS
— TRIALS OF UNSTABLE ANGINA AND NON-Q-WAVE MI —					
PRISM (n = 3231)	Tirofiban	< 90	1.1	0.4	0.04
		< 50	0.4	0.1	0.04
PRISM-PLUS (n = 1815)	Tirofiban	< 90	1.9	0.8	NS
		< 50	0.5	0.3	NS
PARAGON (n = 2282)	Lamifiban	< 100	1.9* / 0.8**	1.1	NS
PURSUIT (n = 10,948)	Eptifibatide	< 100	4.9	4.9	NS
		< 50	0.5	0.4	NS
		< 20	0.1	0.04	NS

* Lamifiban
** Lamifiban + heparin
See Table 34.31 for acronyms

C. RECOGNITION AND MANAGEMENT. Identification of latex allergy prior to intervention is as important as identifying a prior history of reactions to drugs and contrast agents. The FDA recommends that patients be asked about prior reactions to latex gloves or toy balloons, and prior occupational exposure. If latex hypersensitivity is suspected, pre-procedural skin testing is feasible; however, skin-testing has not been standardized, and may itself induce a serious reaction in sensitive individuals. The radioallergoabsorbent test (RAST) is specific for detecting anti-latex IgE antibodies, but has low sensitivity. Since a simple, sensitive screening test is not available, identification of latex allergy is often based on a high index of suspicion. If latex allergy is suspected, the following protocol is reasonable:

• Premedicate patient using the same regimen for contrast allergy
• Prepare cath lab the night before procedure by removing all latex-containing products (Table 25.23)

- Schedule the patient as first case of the day
- Instruct health care workers to use non-latex gloves when treating latex-sensitive patients

If an allergic reaction occurs after inadvertent patient exposure, the treatment is identical to that for contrast reactions (see above). Commercially available balloons for angioplasty are not made of latex, and pose no hazard to patients with a history of latex allergy.

Table 25.21. Clinical Manifestations of Latex Allergy

Cardiovascular	Respiratory	Cutaneous
Hypotension	Bronchoconstriction (wheezing)	Urticaria
Circulatory collapse	Upper airway obstruction (stridor)	Rash, flushing
Anaphylaxis		Angioedema
Life-threatening arrhythmia (VT, VF)		
Pulmonary hypertension		

Abbreviations: VT = ventricular tachycardia; VF = ventricular fibrillation

Table 25.22.   Groups at High-Risk for Latex Allergy

Patients with multiple exposures during manufacturing process
Health-care workers who frequently wear latex gloves
Known allergies to bananas, avocados, kiwi, or chestnuts
Occupational exposure during manufacturing process

Table 25.23. Latex-Containing Products and Substitutes in the Cardiac Catheterization Laboratory

Product	Substitute
Rubber tourniquet	Cloth tourniquet
Latex gloves	Vinyl gloves
IV tubing injection ports	Plastic stopcocks
Blood pressure cuff (bladder, cables)	Cover cuff00 with stockinet or Kerlix
Syringes	Glass syringes
Multipurpose medication vials (stopper)	Use single-dose glass ampules

REFERENCES

1. McCullough PA, Wolyn R, Rocher LL, Levin RN, O'Neill, WW. Acute renal failure after coronary intervention: Incidence, risk factors, and relationship to mortality. Am J Med 1997;103:368-375.

2. Cronin RE. Renal failure following radiologic procedures. Am J Med Sci 1989;298:342-356.

3. Porter GA. Contrast-associated nephropathy. Am J Cardiol 1989;64:22E-26E.

4. Manske CL, Sprafka JM, Strong JT, et al. Contrast nephropathy in azotemic diabetic patients undergoing coronary angiography. Am J Med 1990;89(5):615-620.

5. Davidson CJ, Hiatky M, Morris KG, et al. Cardiovascular and renal toxicity of a nonionic radiographic contrast agent after cardiac catheterization. A prospective trial. Ann Intern Med 1989;110:119-124.

6. Jeunikar AM, Finnie KJ, Dennis B, et al. Nephrotoxicity of high-and-low-osmolality contrast media. Nephron 1988;48:300-305.

7. Weinstein JM, Heyman S, Brezis M. Potential deleterious effect of furosemide in radiocontrast nephropathy. Nephron 1992;62:413-5.

8. Weisberg LS, Kurnid PB, Kurnid BRC. Risk of radiocontrast nephropathy in patients with and without diabetes mellitus. Kidney Int 1994;45:259-65.

9. Opie LH. Drugs for the Heart. W.B. Saunders Ca, Philadelphia, PA.

10. Ansell G, Tweedie MCK, West CR, et al. The current status of reactions to intravenous contrast media. Invest Radiol 1980;15:532-539.

11. Bilazarian SD, Mittal S, Mills RM. Recognizing the extrarenal hazards of intravascular contrast agents. J Crit Illness 1991;6:859-869.

12. Lasser EC, et al. Pre-treatment with corticosteroids to alleviate reactions to intravenous contrast material. N Engl J Med 1987;317:845-849.

13. Lang DM, Alpern MB, Visintainer PF, et al. Increased risk for anaphylactoid reaction from contrast media in patients on ß-adrenergic blockers or with asthma. Ann Intern Med 1991;115:270-276.

14. Zuckerman LS, Friehling TD, Wolf NM, et al. Effect of calcium-binding additives on ventricular fibrillation and repolarization changes during coronary angiography. J Am Coll Cardiol 1987;10:1249-1253.

15. Lembo NJ, King SB III, Roubin GS, et al. Effects of nonionic versus ionic contrast media on complications of percutaneous transluminal coronary angioplasty. Am J Cardiol 1991;67:1046-1050.

16. Katayama H, Yamaguchi K, Kozuka T, et al. Adverse reactions to ionic and nonionic contrast media. Radiology 1990;175:621-628.

17. Fischer HW, Spataro RF. Use of low-osmolality contrast media in patients with previous reactions. Radiology 1988;23:I186-I188.

18. Piessens, et al. Effects of an ionic versus a nonionic low osmolar contrast agent on the thrombotic complications of coronary angioplasty. Cathet Cardiovasc Diagn 1993;28:99-105.

19. Grines CL, Zidar F, Jones D, et al. A randomized trial of ionic vs. nonionic contrast in myocardial infarction or unstable angina patients undergoing coronary angioplasty. Circulation 1993;88:1886.

20. Aguirre FV, Topol EJ, Donohue TJ, et al. Impact on ionic and non-ionic contrast media on post-PTCA ischemic complications: results from the EPIC trial. J Am Coll Cardiol 1995;March, Special Issue:8A.

21. Bonan R, Lesperance J, Gosselin G, et al. Recoil 15 minutes post-coronary angioplasty and contrast media: A randomized double-blind comparative study. Circulation 1994;90:I488.

22. Lembo NJ, King SB III, Roubin GS, et al. Effects of nonionic versus ionic contrast media on complications of percutaneous transluminal coronary angioplasty Am J Cardiol 1991;67:1046-50.

23. Schwab SJ, Hlatky MA, Pieper KS, et al. Contrast nephrotoxicity: A randomized controlled trial of a nonionic and an ionic radiographic contrast agent. N Engl J Med 1989;320:149-153.

24. Taliercio CP, Vlietstra RE, Ilstrup DM, et al. A randomized comparison of the nephrotoxicity of Iopamidol and diatrizoate in high risk patients undergoing cardiac angiography. J Am Coll Cardiol 1991;17:384-390.

25. Shehadi WH. Adverse reactions to intravascularly administered contrast media: a comprehensive study based on prospective survey. Am J Radiol 1975;124:145-52.

26. Shehadi WH, Toniolo G. Adverse reactions to contrast media. Radiology 1980;137:299-302.

27. Palmer FJ, The RACR survey of intravenous contrast media reactions: a preliminary report. Australas Radiol 1988;32:8-11.

28. Katayama H. Report of the Japanese committee on the safety of contrast media. Presented at the Radiological Society of North America Meeting, November, 1988.

29. Lasser EC, Berry CC, Talner LB, et al. Pretreatment with corticosteroids to alleviate reactions to intravenous contrast material. N Engl J Med 1987;317:845-9.

30. Greenberg MA, Levine B, Menegus MA, et al. Single dose pre-treatment prevents adverse events associated with the use of ionic contrast agents. J Am Coll Cardiol 1995;March, Special Issue:319A

31. Wyman RM. Current complications of diagnostic and therapeutic cardiac catheterization. J Am Coll Cardiol 1988;12:1400.

32. Muller DWM, Shamir KJ, Ellis SG, et al. Peripheral vascular complications after conventional and complex percutaneous coronary interventional procedures. Am J Cardiol 1992;69:63-68.

33. Schaub F, Theiss W. Heinz M, et al. New aspects in ultrasound-guided compression repair of post-catheterization femoral artery injuries. Circulation 1994;90:1861-5.

34. Hessel SJ, Adams DF, Abrams HL. Complications of angiography. Radiology 1981;138:273-281.

35. Rappaport S, Sniderman KW, Morse SS. Pseudoaneurysm: A complication of faulty technique in femoral artery puncture. Radiology 1985;529-530.

36. Moote JJ, Hilborn MD, Harris KA, et al. Postarteriographic

femoral pseudoaneurysms: treatment with ultrasound-guided compression. Annals of Vascular Surgery 1994;8:325-31.

37. Cox GS, Young JR, Gray BR, et al. Ultrasound-guided compression repair of postcatheterization pseudoaneurysms: results of treatment in one hundred cases. J Vascular Surg 1994;19:683-6.

38. Humphries AW, et al. Evaluation of the natural history and result of treatment involving the lower extremities: In Fundamentals of Vascular Grafting. McGraw-Hill, New York 1973.

39. Raithel D. Surgical treatment of acute embolization and acute arterial thrombosis. J Cardiovas Surgery. Barcelona, 1973.

40. Johnson LW, Lozner EC, Johnson S, et al. Coronary arteriography 1984-1987: A report of the registry of the Society for Cardiac Angiography and Interventions. Cathet Cardiovasc Diagn 1989;17:5-10.

41. Rooke TW. Vascular complications of interventional procedures. Radiology 1981;138:273-281.

42. Lauk EK. A survey of complications of percutaneous retrograde arteriography. Radiology 1963;81:257-263.

43. Bourassa MA, Noble J. Complication rate of coronary arteriography. Circulation. 1976;53:106-114.

44. Guss SB, Zin LM, Garrison HB, et al. Coronary occlusion during coronary angiography. Circulation 1975;52:1063-1068.

45. Feit A, Kahn R, Chowdry I, et al. Coronary artery dissection secondary to coronary arteriography: case report and review. Cathet Cardiovas Diagn 1984;10:177-181.

46. Morise AP, Hardin NJ, Bovili EG, et al. Coronary artery dissection secondary to coronary arteriography: presentation of three cases. Cathet Cardiovasc Diagn 1981;7:283-296.

47. Connors JP, Thanavaro S, Shaw RC, et al. Urgent myocardial revascularization for dissection of the left main coronary artery. J Thorac Cardiovasc Surgery 1982;84:349-352.

48. Shires TG. Principles of Surgery. Fourth Edition. McGraw-Hill, New York, 1984:240-241.

49. Boylis SM, Lausing EH, Gilas NW. Traumatic retroperitoneal hematoma. Am J Surgery 1962;103:477.

50. Caravajial JA. A thrombolism. Arch Intern Med 1967;119:539.

51. Gore J, Collins WDP. Review of the literature and a report of 16 additional cases. Am J Clin Pathol 1960;33:416.

52. Haimovici H. Vascular Emergencies. Appleton Century Crofts. 1982.

53. Colt HG, Begg RJ, Saporito JJ, et al. Cholesterol emboli after cardiac catheterization. Medicine 1988;57:389-400.

54. Gaines DA. Cholesterol embolization: A lethal complication of vascular catheterization. Lancet 1988;1:168.

55. Grines CL, Glazier S, Bakalyar D, et al. Predictors of bleeding complications following coronary angioplasty. Circulation 1991;(Suppl II);84:II-591.

56. Brown KJ, Morcher JH, Whitman GR, et al. The incidence and analysis of bleeding and vascular complications following percutaneous coronary interventional procedures. Circulation 1994;88:I-196.

57. Hillgrass WB, Brott BC, Narins CR, et al. Predictors of blood loss and bleeding complications after angioplasty. J Am Coll Cardiol 1994;March, Special Issue:69A.

58. Mansour KA, Moscucce M, Kent C, et al. Vascular complications following directional coronary atherectomy or Palmaz-Schatz stenting. J Am Coll Cardiol 1994;23:136A.

59. Oweida SW, Roubin GS, Smith RB, et al. Postcatheterization vascular complication associated with percutaneous transluminal coronary angioplasty. J Vasc Surgery 1990;12:310-315.

60. Muller D, Shamir KJ, Ellis SG, et al. Peripheral vascular complications after conventional and complex percutaneous coronary interventional procedures. Am J Cardiol 1992;69:63-68.

61. Popma JJ, Satler LF, Pichard AD, et al. Vascular complications after balloon and new device angioplasty. Circulation 1993;88:1569-1578.

62. Schweiger MJ, Wiseman A, Wolfe MW, et al. Bleeding complications of coronary angioplasty: a prospective multicenter study. Circulation 1994;90:I-621.

63. Friedman HZ, Cragg DR, Glazier SM, et al. Randomized prospective evaluation of prolonged versus abbreviated intravenous heparin therapy after coronary angioplasty. J Am Coll Cardiol 1994;24:1214-1219.

64. Carere RG, Webb JG, Dodek A. Collagen plug closure of femoral arterial punctures. Are complications excessive? Circulation 1994;90:I-621.

65. Webb JG, Carere RA, Dodek AA. Collagen plug hemostatic closure of femoral arterial puncture sites following implantation of intracoronary stents. Cathet Cardiovasc Diag 1993;30:314-6.

66. Silber S, Bjorvik A, Rosch A. Advantages of sealing arterial puncture sites after PTCA with a single collagen plug: a randomized prospective trial. J Am Coll Cardiol 1995;February, Special Issue:262A.

67. Camenzind E, Grossholz M, Urban P, et al. Mechanical compression (Femostop) alone versus combined collagen application (Vasoseal) and Femostop for arterial puncture site closure after coronary stent implantation: a randomized trial. J Am Coll Cardiol 1994;Special Issue:355A.

68. Vetter JW, Hinohara T, Ribeiro EE, et al. Percutaneous vascular surgery: suture mediated percutaneous closure of femoral artery access site following coronary intervention. J Am Coll Cardiol 1995;March, Special Issue:901-21.

69. Clark C, Popma JJ, Bucher TA, et al, A randomized study of the Femostop compression device to prevent vascular complications after coronary angioplasty. J Am Coll Cardiol 1994;March, Special Issue:106A.

70. Sridhar K, Porter K, Gupta B, et al. Reduction in peripheral vascular complications after coronary stenting by the use of a pneumatic vascular compression device. Circulation 1994;90:I-621.

71. Simon AW. Use of mechanical pressure device for hemostasis following cardiac catheterization. Am J Crit Care 1994;3:62-4.

72. Christensen BV, Iacarella CL. Manion RV, et al. Sandbags do not prevent complications after catheterization. Circulation 1994;90:I-205.

73. Reyes MP. Pyrogenic reactions after inadvertent infusion of endotoxin during cardiac catheterization. Ann Inter Med 1980;93:32.

74. McCready RA, Siderys H, Pittman JN, et al. Septic

complications after cardiac catheterization and percutaneous transluminal coronary angioplasty. J Vasc Surg 1991;14:170-4.

75. Brummitt CF, Kravitz GR, Granrud GA, Herzog CA. Femoral endarteritis due to *Staphylococcus aureus* complicating percutaneous transluminal coronary angioplasty. Am J Med 1988;86:822.

76. Frazee BW, Flaherty JP. Septic endarteritis of the femoral artery following angioplasty. Review of Infectious Diseases 1991;13:620-3.

77. Braunwald E, Swan HJC (eds). Cooperative Study on Cardiac Catheterization.

78. Adams DF, Fraser DB, Abrams HL. The complications of coronary arteriography. Circulation 1973;48:609.

79. Kennedy JW, et al. Complications associated with cardiac catheterization and angiography. Cathet Cardiovasc Diagn 1982;8-5.

80. Califf RM. Risks and complications of thrombolytic therapy. Clinical Challenges in Acute Myocardial Infarction. 1989;1:3-6.

81. Grines CL, Schreiber TL, Savas V, et al. A randomized trial of low osmolar ionic versus nonionic contrast media in patients with myocardial infarction or unstable angina undergoing PTCA. J Am Coll Cardiol 1996;27:1381-6.

82. Chatterjee T, Do-Dai D, Kaufmann U, et al. Ultrasound-guided compression repair for treatment of femoral artery pseudoaneurysm. Cathet & Cardiovasc Diagn 1996;38:335.

83. Samore MH, Wessolossky MA, Lewis SM, et al. Frequency, risk factors, and outcome for bacteremia after percutaneous transluminal coronary angioplasty. Am J Cardiol 1997;79:873-877.

84. Weaver WD, Goldberg S, Feldman RL, et al. Non-ionic contrast during high risk PTCA is associated with subsequent ischemic events. Circulation 1996;94:I-369.

85. Kodali UR, Kaplan BM, Shoukfeh MM, et al. Cholesterol embolization - Is a particular guiding catheter at increased risk? Circulation 1996;94:I-369.

86. Schaub F, Theiss W, Busch R, et al. Management of 219 consecutive cases of postcatheterization pseudoaneurysm. J Am Coll Cardiol 1997;30:670-5.

87. Porter GA. Experimental contrast-associated nephropathy and its clinical implications. Am J Cardiol 1990;66:18F-22F.

88. Myers GE, Crick W, King SW, Mumma M, Friedberg HD, Jamieson DM, Bloom F. Latex versus iodinated contrast media anaphylaxis in the cardiac cath lab. Cathet Cardiovasc Diagn 1995;35:228-231.

89. Rudnick MR, Goldfarb S, Wexler L, Ludbrook PA, Elkan MJ, Halpern F, Hill JA, Winniford M, Cohen MB, VanFossen DB, for the Iohexol Cooperative Study. Nephrotoxicity of ionic and nonionic contrast media in patients: A randomized trial. Kidney Int 1995;47:254-261.

90. Stevens MA, McCullough PA, Tobin KJ, Speck JP, Westveer DC, Allen DA, Timmis GC, O'Neill, WW. A Prospective randomized trial of prevention measures in patients at high risk for contrast nephropathy. J Am Coll Cardiol 1999;33:403-411.

91. Cigarroa RG, Lange RA, Williams RH, Hillis LD. Dosing of contrast material to prevent contrast nephropathy in patients with renal disease. Am J Med 1989;86:649-652.

92. Solomon R, Werner C, Mann D, D'Ella J, Silva P. Effects of saline, mannitol, and furosemide on acute decreases in renal function induced by radiocontrast agents. N Engl J Med 1994;331:1416-1420.

93. Altmann DB, Zwas D, Spatz A, Bergman G, Spokojny A, Riva S, Sanborn TA. Use of the contrast volume to estimated creatinine clearance ratio to predict renal failure after angiography. J Interven Cardiol 1997;10:113-119.

94. Schrader R, Esch I, Ensslen R, Fach WA, Merle H, Scherer D, Sievert H, Spies HF, Zeplin HE. A randomized trial comparing the impact of a nonionic (Iomeprol) versus an ionic (Ioxaglate) low osmolar contrast medium on abrupt vessel closure and ischemic complications after coronary angioplasty. J Am Coll Cardiol 1999;33:395-402.

95. Malekianpour M, Bonan R, Lesperance J, Gosselin G, Hudon G, Doucet S, Laurier J, Duval D. Comparison of ionic and nonionic low osmolar contrast media in relation to thrombotic complications of angioplasty in patients with unstable angina. Am Heart J 1998;135:1067-1075.

96. Greinacher A, Michels I, Kiefel V, Eckhardt C. A rapid and sensitive test for diagnosing heparin-associated thrombocytopenia. Thromb and Haemost 1991;66:734-736.

97. Eichler P, Budde U, Haas S, Kroll H, Loreth RM, Meyer O, Pachmann U, Potzsch B, Schabel A, Albrecht D, Greinacher A. First workshop for detection of heparin-induced antibodies: validation of the heparin-induced platelet-activation test (HIPA) in comparison with a pf4/heparin ELISA. Thromb Haemost 1999;81:625-629.

98. Moore JA, Burket MW, Puri S, Armos P, Lachant N, Skeel R. Ancrod infusion for anticoagulation during and after PTCA in a patient with heparin-induced thrombocytopenia. Cathet Cardiovasc Diagn 1994;32:286-287.

99. Cines DB, Kaywin P, Bina M, Tomaski A, Schreiber AD. Heparin-associated thrombocytopenia. N Engl J Med 1980;303:788-795.

100. Cines DB, Tomaski A, Tannenbaum S. Immune endothelial-cell injury in heparin-associated thrombocytopenia. N Engl J Med 1987;316:581-689.

101. Brieger DB, Mak KH, Marchant KK, Topol EJ. Heparin-induced thrombocytopenia. J Am Coll Cardiol 1998;31:1449-1459.

102. Lewis BE, Ferguson JJ, Grassman ED, et al. Successful coronary interventions performed with argatroban anticoagulation in patients with heparin-induced thrombocytopenia and thrombosis syndrome. J Invas Cardiol 1996;8:410-417.

103. Berkowitz SD, Sane DC, Sigmon KN, et al. For the Evaluation of c7E3 for the Prevention of Ischemic Complications (EPIC) Study Group. J Am Coll Cardiol 1998;32:311-319.

104. Kereiakes DJ, Essell JH, Abbottsmith CW, et al. Abciximab-associated profound thrombocytopenia: Therapy with immunoglobulin and platelet transfusion. Am J Cardiol 1996;78:1161-1163.

105. Slaughter PMP, Chetty R, Flintoft VF, et al. A single center randomized trial assessing use of a vascular hemostasis device versus conventional manual compression following PTCA: what are the potential resource savings? J Invas Cardiol 1998;10:3C-8C.

106. Shrake KL, Zuck VP. Developing effective physican partnerships: the VasoSeal® experience. J Invas Cardiol 1998;10:9C-12C.

107. Foran JPM, Patel D, Brookes J, et al. Early mobilization after percutaneous cardiac catheterization using collagen plug (VasoSeal) hemostasis. J Invas Cardiol 1998;10:13C-19C.

108. Silber S, Bjorvik A, Muhling H, Rosch A. Usefulness of collagen plugging with VasoSeal® after PTCA as compared to manual compression with identical sheath dwell times. Cathet Cardiovasc Diagn 1998;43:421-427.

109. Camenzind E, Grossholz M, Urban P, et al. Collagen application versus manual compression: a prospective randomized trial for arterial puncture site closure after coronary angioplasty. J Am Coll Cardiol 1994;24:655-662.

110. Silber S. Hemostasis success rates and local complications with collagen after femoral access for cardiac catheterization: Analysis of 6007 published patients. Am Heart J 1998;135:152-156.

111. Carere RG, Webb JG, Miyagishima R, et al. Groin complications associated with collagen plug closure of femoral arterial puncture sites in anticoagulated patients. Cathet Cardiovasc Diagn 1998;43:124-129.

112. Silber S. Rapid hemostasis of arterial puncture sites with collagen in patients undergoing diagnostic and interventional cardiac catheterization. Clinic Cardiol 1997;20:981-992.

113. Kussmaul WG, Buchbinder M, Whitlow PL, et al. Femoral artery hemostasis using an implantable device (Angio-Seal™) after coronary angioplasty. Cathet Cardiovasc Diagn 1996;37:362-365.

114. Fry SM. Review of the Angio-Seal™ hemostatic puncture closure device. J Invas Cardiol 1998;10:111-120.

115. Seidelin PH, Adelman AG. Mobilization within thirty minutes of elective diagnostic coronary angiography: A feasibility study using a hemostatic femoral puncture closure device. J Interven Cardiol 1997;10:409-415.

116. Ward SR, Casale P, Raymond R, et al. Efficacy and safety of a hemostatic puncture closure device with early ambulation after coronary angiography. Am J Cardiol 1998;81:569-572.

117. Cremonesi A, Castriota F, Tarantino F, et al. Femoral artery hemostasis using the Angio-Seal™ system after coronary and vascular percutaneous angioplasty and stenting. J Invas Cardiol 1998;10:464-469.

118. Carere RG, Webb JG, Ahmed T, Dodek AA. Initial experience using Prostar™: A new device for percutaneous suture-mediated closure of arterial puncture sites. Cathet Cardiovasc Diagn 1996;37:367-372.

119. Muramatsu T, Tsukahara R, Akimoto N, et al. Efficacy of percutaneous vascular hemostasis system Prostar: comparison to manual compression. J Interven Cardiol 1997;10:4427-434.

120. Nordrehaug JE, Chronos NAF, Priestley KA, et al. Randomized evaluation of an inflatable femoral artery compression device after cardiac catheterization. J Interven Cardiol 1996;9:381-387.

121. Muller DW, Shamir KJ, Ellis SG, Topol EJ. Peripheral vascular complications after conventional and complex percutaneous coronary interventional procedures. Am J Cardiol 1992 Jan 1;69(1):63-8.

122. Kalinowski EA, Trerotola SO. Postcatheterization retroperitoneal hematoma due to spontaneous lumbar arterial hemorrhage. Cardiovasc Intervent Radiol 1998 Jul-Aug;21(4):337-9.

123. Kent KC, Moscucci M, Mansour KA, DiMattia S, Gallagher S, Kuntz R, Skillman JJ. Retroperitoneal hematoma after cardiac catheterization: prevalence, risk factors, and optimal management. J Vasc Surg 1994 Dec;20(6):905-10; discussion 910-3.

124. Omoigui NA, Califf RM, Pieper K, Keeler G, O'Hanesian MA, Berdan LG, Mark DB, Talley JD, Topol EJ. Peripheral vascular complications in the Coronary Angioplasty Versus Excisional Atherectomy Trial (CAVEAT-I). J Am Coll Cardiol 1995 Oct;26(4):922-30.

125. Kennedy AM, Grocott M, Schwartz MS, Modarres H, Scott M, Schon F. Median nerve injury: an underrecognized complication of brachial artery cardiac catheterization? J Neurol Neurosurg Psychiatry 1997 Oct;63(4):542-6.

126. Steffenino G, Dellavalle A, Ribichini F, Russo P, Conte L, Dutto S, Giachello G, Lice G, Tomatis M, Uslenghi E. Ambulation three hours after elective cardiac catheterization through the femoral artery. Heart 1996 May;75(5):477-80.

127. Metz D, Chapoutot L, Brasselet C, Jolly D. Randomized evaluation of four versus five French catheters for transfemoral coronary angiography. Clin Cardiol 1999 Jan;22(1):29-32.

128. de Belder AJ, Smith RE, Wainwright RJ, Thomas MR. Transradial artery coronary angiography and intervention in patients with severe peripheral vascular disease. Clin Radiol 1997 Feb;52(2):115-8.

129. Mann T, Cubeddu G, Brown J, Schneider JE, Arrowood M, Newman WN, Zellinger MJ, Rose GC. Stenting in acute coronary syndromes: a comparison of radial versus femoral access sites. J Am Coll Cardiol 1998 Sep;32(3):572-6.

130. Kiemeneij F, Laarman GJ, Odekerken D, Slagboom T, van der Wieken R. A randomized comparison of percutaneous transluminal coronary angioplasty by the radial, brachial and femoral approaches: the ACCESS study. J Am Coll Cardiol 1997 May;29(6):1269-75.

131. Kiemeneij F, Laarman GJ, Odekerken D, Slagboom T, van der Wieken R. Outpatient coronary stent implantation. J Am Coll Cardiol 1997 Feb;29(2):323-7.

132. Lotan C, Hasin Y, Mosseri M, Rozenman Y, Admon D, Nassar H, Gotsman MS. Transradial approach for coronary angiography and angioplasty. Am J Cardiol 1995 Jul 15;76(3):164-7.

133. Hildick-Smith DJ, Ludman PF, Lowe MD, Stephens NG, Harcombe AA, Walsh JT, Stone DL, Shapiro LM, Schofield PM, Petch MC. Comparison of radial versus brachial approaches for diagnostic coronary angiography when the femoral approach is contraindicated. Am J Cardiol 1998 Mar 15;81(6):770-2.

134. Brachmann J, Ansah M, Kosinski EJ, Schuler G. Improved clinical effectiveness with a collagen vascular hemostasis device for shortened immobilization time following diagnostic angiography and percutaneous transluminal coronary angioplasty. Am J Cardiol 1998 Jun 15;81(12):1502-5.

135. Waksman R, King SB 3rd, Douglas JS, Shen Y, Ewing H, Mueller L, Ghazzal ZM, Weintraub WS. Predictors of groin

complications after balloon and new-device coronary intervention. Am J Cardiol 1995 May 1;75(14):886-9.

136. Pracyk JB, Wall TC, Langabaugh JP, et al. A randomized trial of vascular hemostasis techniques to reduce femoral vascular complications after coronary intervention. Am J Cardiol 1998 Apr 15;81(8):970-6.

137. Fitzgerald J, Andrew H, Conway B, et al. Outpatient angiography: a prospective study of 3 French catheters in unselected patients. Br J Radiol 1998 May;71(845):484-6.

138. Haviv YS, Nahir M, Pikarski A, et al. A late retroperitoneal hematoma mimicking acute appendicitis—an unusual complication of coronary angioplasty. Eur J Med Res 1996 Nov 25;1(12):591-2.

139. Heintzen MP, Strauer BE. Peripheral arterial complications after heart catheterization. Herz 1998 Feb;23(1):4-20.

140. Johnson LW, Esente P, Giambartolomei A, et al. Peripheral vascular complications of coronary angioplasty by the femoral and brachial techniques. Cathet Cardiovasc Diagn 1994 Mar;31(3):165-72.

141. Davis C, VanRiiper S, Longstreet J, et al. Vascular complications of coronary interventions. Heart Lung 1997 Mar-Apr;26(2):118-27.

142. Grier D, Hartnell, G. Percutaneous femoral artery puncture: practice and anatomy. Br J Radiol 1990Aug;63:602-4.

143. Sridhar K, Fischman D, Goldberg S, Zalewski A, Walinsky P, Porter D, Fenton S, Gupta B, Rake R, Gebhardt S, Savage M. Peripheral vascular complications after intracoronary stent placement: prevention by use of a pneumatic vascular compression device. Cathet Cardiovasc Diagn 1996 Nov;39(3):224-9.

144. Ricci MA, Trevisani GT, Pilcher DB. Vascular complications of cardiac catheterization. Am J Surg 1994 Apr;167:375-8.

145. Shrake KL, et al. A cost analysis of complications associated with arterial closure following diagnostic and therapeutic cardiac catheterization. J Cardiovasc Manag 1998 Nov-Dec;9(6):26-33.

146. Nasser TK, Mohler ER, Wilensky RL, Hathaway DR. Peripheral vascular complications following coronary interventional procedures. Clin Cardiol 1995 1995 Nov;18(11):609-14.

147. Pan M, Medina A, Suarex de Lezo J, Romero M, Hernandez E, Segura J, Melian F, Wanguemert F, Landin M, Benitez F, Amat M. Obliteration of femoral pseudoaneurysm complicating coronary intervention by direct puncture and permanent or removable coil insertion. Am J Cardiol 1997 Sep 15;80(6):786-8.

148. Dangas G, Mehran R, Duvvuri S, Ambrose JA, Sharma SK. Use of a pneumatic compression system (FemoStop) as a treatment option for femoral artery pseudoaneurysms after percutaneous cardiac procedures. Cathet Cardiovasc Diagn 1996 Oct;39(2):138-42.

149. Lennox A, Griffin M, Nicolaides A, Mansfield A. Regarding percutaneous ultrasound guided thrombin injection: a new method for treating postcatheterization femoral pseudoaneurysms." J Vasc Surg 1998 Dec;28(6):1120-1.

150. Liau CS, Ho FM, Chen MF, Lee YT. Treatment of iatrogenic femoral artery pseudoaneurysm with percutaneous thrombin injection. J Vasc Surg 1997 Jul;26(1):18-23.

151. Kang SS, Labropouls N, Mansour MA, Baker WH.

Percutaneous ultrasound guided thrombin injection: a new method for treating postcatheterization femoral pseudoaneurysms. J Vasc Surg 1998 Jun;27(6):1032-8.

152. Bapat VN, Agrawal NB, Tendolkar AG. Femoral nerve compression: a rare presentation of femoral artery pseudoaneurysm following cardiac catheterization. Indian Heart J 1996 Nov-Dec;48(6):715-6.

153. Kazmers A, Meeker C, Nofz K, et al. Nonoperative therapy for postcatheterization femoral artery pseudoaneurysms. Am Surg 1997 Feb;63(2):199-204.

154. Nagai S, Abe S, Sato T, et al. Ultrasonic assessment of vascular complications in coronary angiography and angioplasty after transradial approach. Am J Cardiol 1999 Jan 15;82(2):180-6.

155. Saklayen MG, Gupta S, Suryaprasad A, Azmeh W. Incidence of atheroembolic renal failure after coronary angiography. A prospective study. Angiology 1997 Jul;48(7):609-13.

156. Karalis DG, Quinn V, Victor MF, Ross JJ, Polansky M, Spratt KA, Chandrasekaran K. Risk of catheter-related emboli in patients with atherosclerotic debris in the thoracic aorta. Am Heart J 1996 Jun;131(6):1149-55.

157. Finkelhor RS, Youssefi ME, Lamont WE, Bahler RC. Embolic risk based on aortic atherosclerotic morphologic features and aortic spontaneous echocardiographic contrast. Am Heart J 2000 Jun;137(6):1088-93.

158. Keeley EC, Grines CL. Scraping of aortic debris by coronary guiding catheters: a prospective evaluation of 1,000 cases. J Am Coll Cardiol 1998 Dec;32(7):1861-5.

159. Shmuely H, Zoldan J, Sagie A, et al. Acute stroke after coronary angiography associated with protruding mobile thoracic aortic atheromas. Neurology 1997 Dec;49(6):1689-91.

160. Roye GD, Breazeale EE, Byrnes JP, et al. Management of catheter emboli. South Med J 1966 Jul;89(7):714-7.

161. Gagliardi JM, Batt M, Avril G, et al. Neurologic complications of axillary and brachial catheter arteriography in atherosclerotic patients: predictive factors. Ann Vasc Surg 1990 Nov;4(6):546-9.

162. de Swart H, Dijkman L, Hofstra L, et al. A new hemostatic puncture closure device for the immediate sealing of arterial puncture sites. Am J Cardiol 1993; 72(5):445-9.

163. Saito S, Ikei H, Hosokawa G, et al. Influence of the ratio between radial artery inner diameter and sheath outer diameter on radial artery flow after transradial coronary intervention. Catheter Cardiovasc Interv 1999 Feb;46(2):173-8.

164. Cheng TO. Influence of learning curve on the success of transradial coronary angioplasty. 1998 Oct;45(2):215-6.

165. Heuser RR. Outpatient coronary angiography: indications, safety, and complication rates. Herz 1998 Feb:23(1):21-6.

166. Kussmaul WG, Buchbinder M, Aker U, et al. Rapid arterial hemostasis and decreased access site complications after cardiac catheterization and angioplasty: results of a randomized trial of a novel hemostasis device. J Am Coll Cardiol 1995;25(7):1685-92

167. Sharma S, King T, Dangas G, et al. Early and safe ambulation after cardiac procedures using a vascular closure device (Perclose) in high-risk patients. Am J Cardiol 1998 Oct;82(7A):108S.

168. Aker UT, Kensey KR, Heuser RR, et al. Immediate arterial hemostasis after cardiac catheterization: initial experience with a new puncture closure device. Cath Cardiovasc Diagn 1994; 31(3):228-32.

169. Gerckens U, Cattelaens N, Muller R, et al. Percutaneous suture of femoral artery access sites after diagnostic heart catheterization and or coronary intervention. Safety and effectiveness of a new arterial suture technique. Herz 1998 Feb;23(1):27-34.

170. Morice MC, Lefevre T. Immediate post PTCA percutaneous suture of femoral arteries with the Perclose Device: results of high volume users. JACC 1998 Feb;31-2, suppl. A:1033-104 101A.

171. Baim D, Pinkerton C, Schatz R, et al. Acute results of the STAND II percutaneous vascular surgical device trial. Circulation 1997 Oct;96-98(2468):1-443.

172. Schwarten D, Pinkerton C, Vetter J, et al. Acute results of the STAND I percutaneous vascular surgical device trial. Circulation 1997 Oct;96-98(761):1-137.

173. Lowrie M. Hemostasis after arterial puncture: a randomized trial assessment of the Kensey Nash hemostatic puncture closure device (HPCD) vs. manual pressure. Am J Crit Care 1994; 3(3):244.

174. Sticherling C, Berkefeld J, Auch-Schwelk W, et al. Transient bilateral cortical blindness after coronary angiography [letter]. Lancet 1998 Feb 21; 351(9102):570.

175. ter Woorst FJ, Berry LL, de Swart HJ, et al. A rare complication of coronary arteriography. Cath & Cardiovasc Diagn. 1998 Apr;43(4):455-6.

176. Farah B, Prendergast B, Garbarz E, et al. Antegrade transseptal coronary angiography: an alternative technique in severe vascular disease. Cath & Cardiovasc Diagn. 1998 Apr;43(4):444-6.

177. Leker RR, Pollak A, Abramsky O, Ben-Hur T. Abundance of left hemispheric embolic strokes complicating coronary angiography and PTCA [letter]. 1999 Jan;66(1):116-7.

178. Shmuely H, Zoldan J, Sagie A, Maimon S, Pitlik S. Acute stroke after coronary angiography associated with protruding mobile thoracic aortic atheromas. Neuro 1997 Dec;49(6):1689-91.

179. Carere RG, Webb JG, Miyagishima R, Djurdev O, Ahmed T, Dodek A. Groin complications associated with collagen plug closure of femoral arterial puncture sites in anticoagulated patients. Cathet & Cardiovasc Diagn 1998 Feb;43(2):124-129.

180. Fine MJ, Kapoor W, Falanga V. Cholesterol crystal embolization: a review of 221 cases in the English literature. J Vasc Diseases 1987 Oct:769-84.

181. Botti M, Williamson B, Steen K, McTaggart J, Reid E. The effect of pressure bandaging on complications and comfort in patients undergoing coronary angiography: a multicenter randomized trial. Heart & Lung 1998 Nov-Dec;27(6):360-73.

182. Birnbaum Y, Fishbein MC, Kass R, Samuels B, Luo H, Siegel RJ. Dissection of the ascending aorta induced by coronary angiography. Am J Cardiol 1997 Aug 15;80(4):537.

183. Kipshidze N, Ferguson JJ III, Macris MP, et al. Percutaneous application of fibrin sealant to achieve hemostasis following arterial catheterization. J Invas Cardiol 1998 April;10:133-141.

184. Gershony G, Brock JM, Powell JS. Novel vascular sealing device for closure of percutaneous vascular access sites. Cathet Cardiovasc Diagn 1998;45:82

185. Personal communication: Ramee S, White C, Jenkins S, Collins T, Oschner Clinic, New Orleans.

186. Waigand J, Uhlich F, Gross CM, et al. Percutaneous treatment of pseudoaneurysms and arteriovenous fistulas after invasive vascular procedures. Cathet. Cardiovasc. Intervent. 1999;47:157-164.

187. Eggebrecht H, Oldenburg O, Dirsch O, et al. Potential embolization by atherosclerotic debris dislodged from aortic wall during cardiac catheterization: Histologic and clinical findings in 7,621 patients. Cathet Cardiovasc Intervent 2000;49:389-394.

188. McClure M, Berkowitz S, Sparapani R, et al. Clinical significance of thrombocytopenia during a non-ST-elevation acute coronary syndrome. The platelet glycoprotein IIb/IIIa in unstable angina: receptor suppression using integrilin therapy (PURSUIT) trial experience. Circulation 1999;99:2892-2900.

189. Vahdat B, Canavy I, Fourcade L, et al. Fatal cerebral hemorrhage and severe thrombocytopenia during abciximab treatment. Cathet Cardiovasc Intervent. 2000;49:177-180.

190. Sane D, Damaraju L, Topol E, et al. Occurrence and clinical significance of pseudothrombocytopenia during abciximab therapy. J Am Coll Cardiol 2000;36:75-83.

191. Gare M, Haviv Y, Ben-Yehuda A, et al. The renal effect of low-dose dopamine in high-risk patients undergoing coronary angiography. J Am Coll Cardiol 1999;34:1682-8.

192. Rihal C, Sutton-Tyrrell, K, Guo P, et al. Increased incidence of periprocedural complications among patients with peripheral vascular disease undergoing myocardial revascularization in the Bypass Angioplasty Revascularization Investigation. Circulation 1999;100:171-177.

193. Greinacher A, Janssens U, Berg G, et al. Lepirudin (recombinant hirudin) for parenteral anticoagulation in patients with heparin-induced thrombocytopenia. Circulation 1999;100:587-593.

194. Steinhubl S, Tan W, Foody J, et al. Incidence and clinical course of thrombotic thrombocytopenic purpura due to ticlopidine following coronary stenting. JAMA 1999;281:806-810.

195. Chatterjee T, Do DD, Mahler F, et al. A prospective, randomized evaluation of nonsurgical closure of femoral pseudoaneurysm by compression device with or without ultrasound guidance. Cathet. Cardiovasc. Intervent. 1999;47:304-309.

196. Brophy D, Sheiman R, Amatulle P, et al. Iatrogenic femoral pseudoaneurysms: Thrombin injection after failed US-guided compression. Radiology 2000;214:278-282.

197. Thalhammer C, Kirchherr A, Uhlich F, et al. Postcatheterization pseudoaneurysms and arteriovenous fistulas: Repair with percutaneous implantation of endovascular covered stents. Radiology 2000;214:127-131.

198. Tepel M, Van Der Giet M, Schwarzfeld C, et al. Prevention of radiographic-contrast-agent-induced reductions in renal function by acetylcysteine. N Engl J Med 2000;343:180-4.

199. Nygren A, Ulfendahl HR, Hansell P, et al. Effects of intravenous contrast media on cortical and medullary blood

flow in the rat kidney. Invest Radiol 1988;23:753-61.

200. Kien N, Moore P, Jaffe R, et al. Blood flow distribution during controlled hypotension induced by fenoldopam in anesthetized dogs. Anesth Analog 1990;70:5203.

201. Bakris GL, Lass NA, Glock D. Renal hemodynamics in radiocontrast medium-induced renal dysfunction: A role for dopamine-1 receptors. Kidney Int 1999;56:206-10.

202. Hunter D. Fenoldopam: A dopamine type-1 receptor agonist in the prevention of renal injury associated with the administration of intravenous contrast. J Vasc Interv Radiol 2000;11:396-8.

203. Tumlin J, Mathur V. Prophylactic efficacy of fenoldopam in radiocontrast nephropathy (RCN): A randomized, double-blind, placebo-controlled trial. J Vasc Interv Radiol 2000;11:175.

204. Maydoon H. Use of fenoldopam to prevent radiocontrast nephropathy (RCN) in high risk patients. J Vasc Interv Radiol 2000;11:175-176.

205. Mahaffey K, Harrington R, Simoons M, et al. Stroke in patients with acute coronary syndromes. Incidence and outcomes in the platelet glycoprotein IIb/IIIa in unstable angina: receptor suppression using integrilin therapy (PURSUIT) trial. Circulation 1999;99:2371-2377.

206. Lanzino G, Fessler R, Wakhloo A, et al. Successful intracranial thrombolysis for cerebral thromboembolic complications resulting from cardiovascular diagnostic and interventional procedures. J Invas Cardiol 1999;11:439-443.

207. Madan M, Berkowitz S. Understanding thrombocytopenia and antigenicity with glycoprotein IIb/IIIa inhibitors. Am Heart J 1999;138:S317-S326.

208. Blankenship J. Bleeding complications of glycoprotein IIb/IIIa receptor inhibitors. Am Heart J 1999;138:S287-S296.

209. Juran N. Minimizing bleeding complications of percutaneous coronary intervention and glycoprotein IIb/IIIa antiplatelet therapy. Am Heart J 1999;138:S297-S306.

210. Cantor W, Leblanc K, Garvey B, et al. Combined use of Orgaran and Reopro during coronary angioplasty in patients unable to receive heparin. Cathet Cardiovasc Intervent 1999;46:352-355.

211. Wilentz J, Mishkel G, McDermott D, et al. Outpatient coronary stenting using the femoral approach with vascular sealing. J Invas Cardiol 1999;11:709-717.

212. Chamberlin J, Lardi A, McKeever L, et al. Use of vascular sealing devices (VasoSeal and Perclose) versus assisted manual compression (Femostop) in transcatheter coronary interventions requiring abciximab (ReoPro). Cathet Cardiovasc Intervent 1999;47:143-147.

213. Goyen M, Manz S, Kroger K, et al. Interventional therapy of vascular complications caused by the hemostatic puncture closure device Angio-Seal. Cathet Cardiovasc Intervent 2000;49:142-147.

214. Carere R, Webb J, Buller C, et al. Suture closure of femoral arterial puncture sites after coronary angioplasty followed by same-day discharge. Am Heart J 2000;139:52-8.

215. Warren B, Warren S, Miller S. Predictors of complications and learning curve using the Angio-Seal™ closure device following interventional and diagnostic catheterization. Cathet Cardiovasc Intervent 1999;48:162-166.

216. Shrake K. Comparison of major complication rates associated with four methods of arterial closure. Am J Cardiol 2000;85:1024-25.

217. Gerckens U, Cattelaens N, Lampe EG, et al. Management of arterial puncture site after catheterization procedures: Evaluating a suture-mediated closure device. Am J Cardiol 1999;83:1658-1663.

218. Silber S, Gershony G, Schon B, et al. A novel vascular sealing device for closure of percutaneous arterial access sites. Am J Cardiol 1999;83:1248-1252.

219. Muller CE, Buerkle G, Buettner HJ et al. Prevention of contrast-media associated nephropathy: Randomized comparison of two hydration regimens in 1620 patients undergoing elective or emergent PTCA. Circulation 2000;102:II-643.

220. Feldman, T. Percutaneous suture closure for management of large french size arterial and venous puncture. J Interven Cardiol 2000:13:237-241.

221. Cura FA, Kapadia SR, L'Allier P, et al. Safety of femoral closure devices after percutaneous coronary interventions in the era of glycoprotein IIb/IIIa platelet blockade. Am J Cardiol 2000;86:780-782.

222. Mooney MR, Ellis SG, Gershony G, et al. Immediate sealing of arterial puncture sites after cardiac catheterization and coronary interventions: Initial U.S. feasibility trial using the Duet vascular closure device. Cathet Cardiovasc Intervent 2000;50:96-102.

223. Coto H. Thrombocytopenia complications associated with coronary therapeutic drugs. Platelet receptor glycoprotein IIb/IIIa inhibition with eptifibatide in a patient with thrombocytopenia after treatment with abciximab.

224. Elmi F, Peacock T, Schiavone J. Thrombocytopenia complications associated with coronary therapeutic drugs. Isolated profound thrombocytopenia associated with clopidogrel. J Invas Cardiol 2000;12:532-535.

225. Zidar JP, Batchelor W, Berger PB, et al. Does the low-molecular-weight enoxaparin reduce stent thrombosis in high-risk stent patients? Results from ATLAST trial. Enoxaparin plus antiplatelet therapy vs. antiplatelet therapy alone in patients at increased risk of stent thrombosis. Circulation 1999;100:I-380

IV

Interventional Devices

26

CORONARY STENTS

Robert D. Safian, M.D.
James Zidar, M.D., James Hermiller, M.D.
Adam B. Greenbaum, M.D., Sheldon Goldberg, M.D.

In 1964, Dotter and Judkins proposed the concept of implanting intravascular stents to support the arterial wall following coronary angioplasty.[1] Since that time, stents have become the most important mechanical technique for percutaneous revascularization. In 1994, fewer than 1% of 270,000 PCTAs utilized stents; in 2001, more than 900,000 stents will be implanted in 700,000 interventions in the United States alone. All stents share common goals of enlarging the vascular lumen, covering dissections, decreasing early ischemic complications, and preventing late restenosis. However, stents differ in their fundamental designs and have undergone enormous change since their introduction 10 years ago.[3]

STENT DESIGNS (Tables 26.1, 26.2)

A. SELF-EXPANDING STENTS

1. **Magic Wallstent™ (Figure 26.1).** The prototype of the self-expanding stent is the Wallstent (Boston Scientific Scimed), which consists of an interwoven mesh of 18-20 stainless steel wire filaments.[4] A specially designed stent delivery system permits release of the stent within the target lesion, followed by continued expansion of the stent until an equilibrium is achieved between the elastic constraint of the vessel wall and the dilating force of the stent. Stents should be selected to achieve diameters 20% larger than the diameter of the adjacent reference segment. European trials of the original prototype were interrupted over the high incidence of acute and subacute stent thrombosis.[5] A second-generation Wallstent had less metal surface area with a platinum inner core and a cobalt-based alloy outer core to enhance its radiopacity. The new "magic" delivery system replaced the original pressurized-membrane to facilitate delivery and ease deployment. The Wallstent has had favorable results in native coronaries and saphenous vein bypass grafts, and the new Magic Wallstent was approved by the FDA in 1999.[6-8] The Magic Wallstent may be particularly useful for long segments of diffuse disease, tapering vessels, and saphenous vein bypass grafts; stent shortening after deployment must be anticipated.

2. **Radius™ Stent (Figure 26.2).** The first self-expanding stent approved in the United States was the Radius™ stent (Boston Scientific Scimed), a multi-segmented, flexible, slotted-tube structure made of nitinol™ (nickel and titanium), employing thermal memory as the mechanism of self-expansion.[9] Similar to the Wallstent, the stent is sized 20% larger than the maximum reference vessel diameter, and deployment is accomplished by retracting a constraining sheath. Compared to the Wallstent, the radius stent has less radiopacity, but shortens <5% after deployment. Observational and randomized studies document higher technical and procedural success and equivalent angiographic

and clinical outcomes compared with first-generation balloon expandable stents,[10,11] confirming its flexibility and ease of insertion.

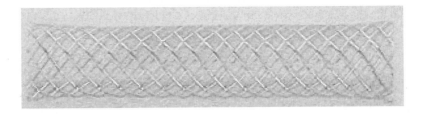

Figure 26.1. Magic Wallstent™

Courtesy of Boston Scientific Scimed

B. BALLOON-EXPANDABLE STENTS. The variety of balloon-expandable stents far exceeds that of self-expanding stents, and their structural designs are classified as coil, slotted-tubes, and hybrid.

1. Coil Stents

  a. Gianturco-Roubin® Stent. Although no longer in use today, the first coronary stent approved by the FDA was the Gianturco-Roubin Flex-Stent (Cook, Inc., Bloomington, IN), formed by wrapping a single strand of stainless steel filament around a balloon catheter.[12] By contemporary standards, the stent was bulky and difficult to deliver. A low-profile GR-II® with flat-wire stent construction and a single longitudinal strut added radial strength and enhanced deliverability and was approved in the United States in 1996 for acute or threatened closure.[13,14,15,16] The GR-II stent was associated with more recoil than other balloon-expandable designs, which necessitated slight oversizing, sometimes leading to dissection.[17,18] The GR-II is no longer available.

  b. Wiktor® Stent. The Wiktor stent (Medtronic Arterial Vascular Engineering, Inc., Santa Rosa, CA) consisted of a single strand of tantalum wire wrapped around an angioplasty balloon in a U-shaped configuration.[19] The Wiktor Rival was FDA-approved in 1997,[20,21,22] but after the merger between Medtronic and AVE, production was discontinued in favor of the other designs (see below).

2. Slotted-tube Stents

  a. Palmaz-Schatz (PS)™ **and Crown**™ **Stents.** The original Palmaz-Schatz (PS) stent (Cordis, Johnson and Johnson, Inc., Warren, NJ) consisted of two laser-cut, stainless steel segments each measuring 7 mm in length, connected by a 1 mm bridge ("articulation") for flexibility.[23] In the US, the stent was pre-mounted on a balloon covered by a 5F protective sheath, enabling delivery of the articulated stent with high degrees of success and reliability. This stent was highly resistant to elastic recoil, provided an excellent scaffold to support the arterial wall, and was implanted in over one million patients worldwide. The PS stent was the first device to reduce restenosis rates, and it was the gold-standard to which all other coronary stents were initially compared.[24,25] A heparin-coated PS stent with a spiral articulation virtually eliminated subacute stent thrombosis, but is no longer available. Non-articulated biliary and iliac versions are still used in saphenous vein grafts, large native vessels,[26] and peripheral circulation. The Crown™ stent (better flexibility by virtue of laser-cut sinusoidal slots, rather than straight slots) and the Minicrown™ stent (fewer circumferential rows and reduced strut thickness for vessels 2.25-3.25 mm in diameter) have been replaced by the BX-velocity stent (see below).

b.   BX-Velocity™ Stent (Figure 26.3). The BX-Velocity™ stent (Cordis/Johnson & Johnson, Inc.) has replaced the older Crown stent, and is a closed-cell design allowing independent modulation of radial strength and flexibility. The unique FlexSegment connectors between struts enhances flexibility, conformability, and sidebranch access. In contrast to other third generation balloon expandable stents which increase in diameter by 10% between nominal and rated burst pressures of the stent-deployment balloon, the BX-velocity stent will increase in diameter by exactly 0.25 mm. A heparin-coated version is also available.

c.   Multi-Link,™ Duet,™ and Tristar™ Stents. The Multi-Link™ stent (Guidant, Santa Clara, CA) was a second-generation balloon-expandable tubular stent consisting of a stainless-steel cylinder with laser-etched overlapping loops and bridges.[27] The version in the United States had a protective delivery sheath. As with all slotted tube stents, advantages included its strength and scaffolding, but with enhanced flexibility compared to the PS™ and Crown designs.[28-32] Disadvantages included poor radiopacity and a compliant delivery balloon. In contrast, the Multi-Link Duet™ stent had greater strut thickness (0.055"), resulting in added radial strength and better radiopacity, and a corrugated ring pattern connected by alternating 3-2-3 links. The Duet stent was mounted on a low-profile, high-pressure (16 atm) stent delivery balloon,[33] but concerns about secure nesting of the stent and balloon overhang led to development of a newer delivery balloon on the Multi-Link Tristar™ stent. Although the Tristar and Duet stents were identical, the Tristar delivery balloon incorporated S.T.E.P.™ technology (Short Transitional Edge Protection), to reduce balloon overhang and potential edge dissections. Other features of the Tristar delivery system included a special stent crimping process (GRIP™) to ensure stent retention, and a trifold "propeller" balloon to facilitate even inflation pressure and uniform stent expansion.

d.   Multi-Link TETRA™ and Multi-Link ULTRA™ Stents (Figures 26.4, 26.5). The Multi-Link TETRA™ stent utilizes Variable Thickness Strut (VTS™) stent technology, which allows for excellent scaffolding (3-3-3 link design), conformability, and radiopacity. The thickness of the stent ranges from 0.0049-inch regions that provide good radiopacity, to 0.0036-inch regions where flexibility is required. The Multi-Link TETRA™ also incorporates S.T.E.P.™ Balloon technology (first seen on the Tristar™ stent) to reduce balloon overhang and potential edge dissections, and advanced GRIP™ technology to provide excellent stent retention and allow an unexpanded stent to be retracted into a 5F guiding catheter. The Multi-Link

ULTRA™ stent is designed for larger native coronary arteries and vein grafts (vessel diameter 3.5-5.0 mm), and the corrugated rings are connected by 3-3-3 links, which enhance surface coverage. The trifold balloon and GRIP technology are employed in the delivery system to facilitate ideal stent deployment.

e. **NIR® Elite and NIROYAL™ Elite Stents (Figure 26.6).** The NIR® stent (Boston Scientific Scimed) is a modular, cellular, stainless steel stent designed for flexibility and radial strength by allowing each cell to elongate and expand individually.[34,35,36,37] The NIR stent family is designed with a transformable geometry, which allows greater flexibility during delivery and enhanced radial support after deployment. NIR stents are available with (NIROYAL™ Elite) and without (NIR® Elite) gold plating, which markedly enhances stent radiopacity, and is extremely useful when precise stent placement is required. NIR® and NIROYAL™ Elite stents offer elastomeric restraining sleeves ("sox"), which cover 0.75 mm of each stent end, providing seamless edge protection and ensuring reliable stent delivery without embolization.

f. **BeStent™2 (Figure 26.7).** The BeStent™2 (Medtronic AVE) is a laser-cut stent with gold markers at each end to facilitate ideal positioning. Balloon expansion of the stent results in rotation of non-stress junctions and orthogonal "locking," resulting in excellent radial strength without stent shortening.

C. MODULAR STENTS

1. **MicroStent II, GFX, and GFX-2 Stents.** The MicroStent-II™ and GFX™ stents (Medtronic AVE) utilized a balloon-expandable, sinusoidal-ring design, composed of elements fused in a helical pattern, creating flexibility with radial strength after deployment.[38,39] At the time these stents were released, they offered unique deliverability which was unmatched by other stent designs. Element length was reduced from 3 mm (MicroStent-II) to 2 mm (GFX stent) for improved flexibility and scaffolding. The GFX-2 stent combined the flexibility, good radial strength, and radiopacity of the GFX stent with a low-profile and high-pressure delivery system.

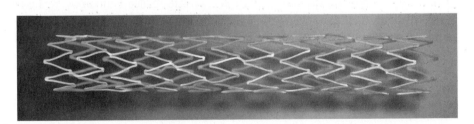

Figure 26.2. Radius™ Stent

Courtesy of Boston Scientific Scimed

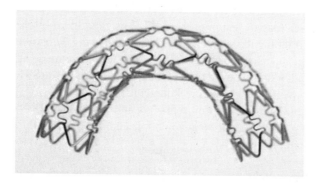

Figure 26.3. BX-Velocity Stent

Courtesy of Cordis/J & J

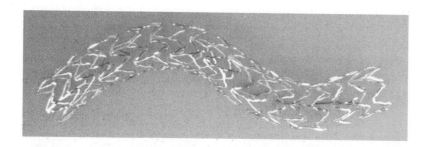

Figure 26.4. Multi-Link TETRA™ Stent

Courtesy of Guidant

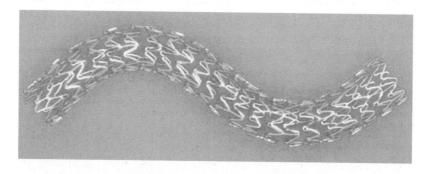

Figure 26.5. Multi-Link ULTRA™ Stent

Courtesy of Guidant

2. **S670, S660, and S7 Stents (Medtronic AVE) (Figures 26.8, 26.9).** To further improve flexibility and scaffolding, the "open" design of the GFX-2 was modified by the design of the S670 stent, which included shortening the segments to 1.5 mm and using 7 crowns. Further shortening of the segments to 1.0 mm and using 10 crowns was accomplished in the S7 stent, which is pending FDA approval in the United States. In keeping with its early designs, the S7 has excellent deliverability, with tissue support (cell area) exceeding slotted tube stents. The S660 stent is designed for smaller vessels (2.2-2.9 mm), and has 1.5 mm segments and 6 crowns. All Medtronic AVE stents offer Secure Technology for excellent stent retention and Discrete Technology to minimize excess balloon working length.

D. **OTHER STENTS (Table 26.2).** Several stents are currently used outside the United States, and some are under investigation in the United States. The BioDivYsio™ stent (Biocompatibles, Ltd., Surrey, UK) is a balloon-expandable, stainless steel tube coated with a phosphorylcholine (PC) polymer, which may reduce thrombogenicity and offer the potential for drug-attachment and delivery.[43,44] The BioDivYsio stent is available in added support, open cell, and small vessel designs; markers on the delivery system facilitate placement. FDA-approval of the BioDivYsio stent is imminent. The JOSTENT® (JOMED GmbH, Helsingborg, Sweden) is a balloon-expandable slotted tubular stent that is designed specifically for radial strength, flexibility, sidebranch preservation (JOSTENT Sidebranch), and bifurcations (JOSTENT Bifurcation) (Figure 26.10). The JOSTENT Coronary Stent Graft (PTFE sandwiched between two JOSTENTS) is under evaluation for treatment of perforations, aneurysms, and degenerated vein grafts; preliminary studies suggest no additional thrombogenicity.[45,46] Many other stent designs are described in Table 26.2.

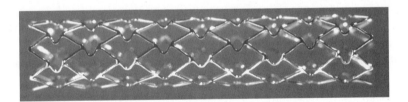

Figure 26.6. NIR® Elite and NIROYAL™ Elite Stents

The NIROYAL™ Elite stent is gold-plated. Courtesy of Boston Scientific Scimed

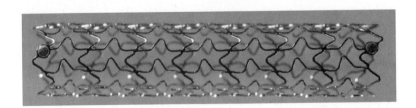

Figure 26.7. BeStent™2

Courtesy of Medtronic AVE

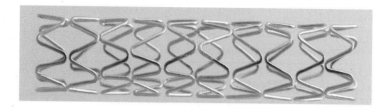

Figure 26.8. S660 Stent

Courtesy of Medtronic AVE

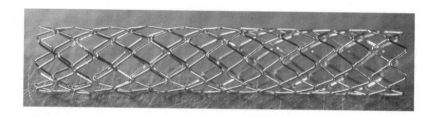

Figure 26.9. S670 Stent

Courtesy of Medtronic AVE

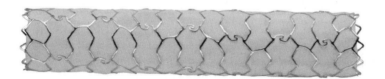

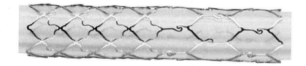
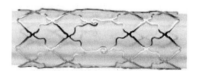

Figure 26.10. JOSTENTS

Coronary Stent Graft (top), Bifurcation stent (bottom left), and Sidebranch stent (bottom right). Courtesy of JOMED

Table 26.1. Intracoronary Stents: Technical Features

	NIR®/NIROYAL™ Elite (BSC)++	Radius™ (BSC)	Wallstent™* (BSC)	BX-Velocity™ (Cordis/J & J)
Expansion	Balloon	Self	Self	Balloon
Material	Stainless steel Gold-plated (NIROYAL)	Nitinol	Platinum/cobalt	Stainless steel
Configuration	Closed cell, transformable geometry	Multisegmented slotted tube, square struts	Woven wire mesh, round wires	Curved sections and interconnected N-links
Strut thickness (mm/inch)	0.1 / 0.004	0.11 / 0.0045	0.08 / 0.003	0.14 / 0.0055
Metal surface area (%)	12 - 16	20	14	15-20
Shortening (%)	< 5	< 5	15-20	< 1.5 mm
Recoil (%)	< 0.5	0	0	0
Delivery sheath	No	Yes	Yes	No
Delivery profile (mm)	1.1 - 1.2	1.42	1.53	1-1.2
Minimum guide ID (in)	0.064	0.066	0.064	0.067
Length (mm)	9,12,15,18,25,31	14,20,31	17-48	8,13,18,23,28,33
Expanded diameter (mm)	2.5-4.0	3.0-4.0‡	3.5-6.0†	2.25-5.0
Deployment pressure (atm)	8	NA	NA	10-16
Rated burst pressure (atm)	16	NA	NA	16

AVE = Arterial Vascular Engineering; BSC = Boston Scientific Scimed; J & J = Johnson & Johnson
* "Less-shortening" Magic Wallstent, second-generation prototype
† For vessels 3.0-5.5 mm in diameter
‡ For vessels 2.75-4.25 mm in diameter
++ Manufactured by Medinol; distributed by Boston Scientific Scimed
NA = not available

Table 26.1. Intracoronary Stents: Technical Features

MultiLink TETRA™ (Guidant)	MultiLink ULTRA™ (Guidant)	BeStent™2 (Medtronic AVE)	S660™ (Medtronic AVE)	S670™ (Medtronic AVE)
S.T.E.P™ Balloon	Balloon	Balloon	Balloon	Balloon
Stainless steel	Stainless steel	Stainless steel	Stainless steel	Stainless steel
Slotted tube, multiple corrugated rings connected with multiple links	Slotted tube, multiple corrugated rings connected with multiple links	Laser-cut tubular stent system with Discrete Technology	Sinusoidal rings, elliptorectangular elements	Sinusoidal ring elements, elliptorectangular struts
VTS™ Technology 0.09-0.12 / 0.036-0.0049	0.13 / 0.005	0.085 / 0.033	0.13 x 0.15 / 0.005	0.13 x 0.15 / 0.005 x 0.006
14	19	12 - 17	~ 20	17 - 23
2.7	2.7	~ 0$^+$	~ 1.5	3.5
< 2	1.7	< 2.2	~ 2	1.5
No	No	No	No	No
1.0-1.2	1.4-1.42	~ 1.0	1.0	1.1
0.056	0.066-0.075	0.064	0.064	0.064
8,13,18,23,28,33,38	13,18,28,38	9,12,15,18,24,30	9,12,15,18,24	9,12,15,18,24,30
2.5-4.0 Post-expansion 4.5	3.5-5.0 Post-expansion 5.5	3.0-4.5 (USA)	2.5	3.0-4.0
8 (nominal)	9 (nominal)	8	8	8
16	14	16 (3.0, 3.5 mm) 15 (4.0 mm)	16	16 15 (4.0 mm)

AVE = Arterial Vascular Engineering; BSC = Boston Scientific Scimed; J & J = Johnson & Johnson
* "Less-shortening" Magic Wallstent, second-generation prototype
† For vessels 3.0-5.5 mm in diameter
‡ For vessels 2.75-4.25 mm in diameter
++ Manufactured by Medinol; distributed by Boston Scientific Scimed
NA = not available

Table 26.2. Other Coronary Stent Designs

Stent	Company	Design	Comment
AccuFlex	Navius	Twin backbone radial bands	Locking design eliminates recoil; radial strength with flexibility
Actone	PAS	Slotted tube	Nitinol stent with single articulation
Angiostent	AngioDynamics	Single wire contained coil	Radial strength with sidebranch preservation
Bard XT	Bard	Interconnected modules	Zig-zag modules on a flexible spine allow differential expansion in tapering vessels
BioDiamond	Plasmachem	Laser-cut stainless steel slotted-tube	Coated with diamond-like carbon to reduce release of cytotoxic heavy metal ions
BioDivYsio	Biocompatibles	Laser-cut stainless steel slotted-tube	Thromboresistant phosphorylcholine coating; drug-delivery capabilities
C-1	Medex	Laser-cut stainless steel hybrid	Modular, multicellular design
Carbostent	Sorin Biomedica	Hybrid, stainless steel tube	Biocompatible Carbofilm™ coating; complex multicellular architecture results in 0% shortening
Cardiocoil	Medtronic InStent	Single wire open coil	Self-expanding Nitinol restrained on delivery catheter by sutures and a release wire; excellent recrossing
Coroflex	B. Braun Melsurgen	Laser-cut stainless steel slotted-tube	Low profile, excellent flexibility
Enforcer	CardioVascular	Uniform cellular mesh	Stainless steel mesh stent
Freedom	Global Therapeutics	Single wire, fish scale pattern	Unique design allows optimal vessel alignment; available in lengths up to 60mm
Genius	EuroCor	Stainless steel slotted-tube	Multicellular modular ring design; low profile; flexible with good radial strength
Igaki-Tamai[785]	Igaki Medical	Poly-L-lactic acid monopolymer	Biodegradable self-expanding stent
InFlow	InFlow Dynamics	Laser-cut stainless steel slotted-tube	Homogeneous gold coating, potentially resulting in more intimal proliferation; excellent visibility
IRIS	Uni-Cath	Laser-cut stainless steel slotted-tube	Alternating "C" with diagonal struts; radial strength with deliverability
JOSTENT	Jomed	Laser-cut stainless steel slotted-tube	Sidebranch, bifurcation, and PTFE-coated stent graft versions
LP	IVT Europe	Chemically-etched stainless steel slotted-tube	Unique trapezoid strut design; flexible with good radial strength
M Saint-Come	Saint Come	Laser-cut stainless steel slotted-tube	Excellent radial strength
MAC	amg GmbH	Laser-cut stainless steel slotted-tube	Low crossing profile (< 1 mm) with good radial strength
Med-X	Med-Xcor	Laser-cut stainless steel	Zig-zag rings and rectangular struts
MSM-BSM	MiroScience Medical	Laser-cut stainless steel	Implantation of surface tantalum to eliminate heavy metal release

Table 26.2. Other Coronary Stent Designs

Stent	Company	Design	Comment
Nexus	Ocaam International	Laser-cut stainless steel tube	Multiple cells and V-connections
Omega	amg GmbH	Laser-cut stainless steel slotted-tube	Low crossing profile with good radial strength
Paragon	Vascular Therapies	Slotted-tube	Balloon-expandable Nitinol™; radial strength with deliverability
Parallel-Serial Jang	In VentCa Technologies	Slotted-tube	Interlocking rhomboidal strut pattern is easily reformatted for specific performance characteristics
PURA	Devon Medical	Laser-cut stainless steel slotted-tube	Y-shaped geometry; extremely low-profile, flexible stent for a variety of lesions
QuaDS	Quanam Medical	Balloon-expandable stent	"Sleeve" covering stent may have drug delivery capability
R-stent	Orbus	Laser-cut stainless steel tube	Dual helical spiral configuration with exceptional performance; compatible with 5F guides; excellent sidebranch access
Seaquence	Nycomed Amersham	Stainless steel tube	Circumferential cells and links between segments provide flexibility and radial strength
Stent Tech	Stent Tech	Laser-cut stainless steel tube	S-articulations enhance flexibility
TENAX	Biotronik	Laser-cut stainless steel slotted-tube	Antithrombogenic amorphous silicon carbide coating
Terumo	Terumo	Stainless steel tube	Mono-linked diamond cell structure enhance conformability and radial strength
V-Flex	Cook	Laser-cut stainless steel slotted-tube	Crown units linked by alternating "V" bridge; radial strength with conformability

STENT CHARACTERISTICS (Tables 26.3-26.5)

Each stent and delivery system has characteristics which offer certain advantages and disadvantages. These design features may be concordant (such as better flexibility and deliverability) or discordant (better scaffolding but worse sidebranch access). It is crucial to understand the characteristics of each product.[668]

A. BIOCOMPATIBILITY. This refers to the ability of the stent material to resist thrombosis and corrosion. Of all the stent materials currently used, those made of stainless steel seem to be the most susceptible to thrombosis. The tendency for thrombosis is minimized by using highly polished, ultra-pure grades of stainless steel (316L stainless steel), by minimizing the metal surface area of the stent, and by using thromboresistant coatings (heparin, gold, phosphorylcholine).[43,637] Pre-clinical experimental studies suggested that stents made of tantalum or nitinol were somewhat less thrombogenic than stainless steel stents, but this potential difference is not clinically evident.[47,48,49] All patients receiving stents require medications to prevent thrombosis (see "Adjunctive Therapy" below).[50,51]

B. **CONFORMABILITY.** This term is often used interchangeably with flexibility, but actually refers to the degree to which an expanded stent can bend around its longitudinal axis after deployment. Some stents conform nicely to the shape of tortuous vessels (S670, Multi-Link TETRA, Wallstent), while others may straighten the vessel after deployment (NIR Elite). In the past, flexible stents were more conformable but had less radial strength. Today, newer stents are designed both for flexibility during delivery and radial strength after deployment. Longitudinal straightening of vessels after stent deployment (due to loss of stent conformability) was suggested as a predictor of late ischemic events,[761] although extending this observation to differences in in-vitro conformability between different stent designs may not be possible.

C. **DELIVERABILITY.** The ability to deliver a stent to the desired location depends on multiple factors, including flexibility, flaring, integrity of the delivery system, and trackability. Trackability refers to the ease of travel over the guidewire and is affected by shaft coating, stiffness, distal tapering, and profile. Most current stent designs deliver without difficulty; from a performance standpoint, differences in deliverability are difficult to discern.

D. **FLEXIBILITY.** This refers to the degree to which an unexpanded stent can bend around its longitudinal axis. Flexibility is an extremely important consideration because of the tortuosity of the coronary arterial circulation and the angulated shape of many guiding catheters. Historically, balloon-expandable stents were less flexible than self-expanding stents, and slotted-tube designs were less flexible than coil designs. However, design and manufacturing changes have allowed development of flexible balloon-expandable stents, while retaining many of the scaffolding features of older slotted-tube designs. Although coaxial guiding catheter alignment is important for proper stent deployment, the routine use of extra-support guidewires and large-lumen guiding catheters ($\geq$ 8F) is no longer necessary. Nevertheless, in-vitro studies have identified differences in flexibility between stent designs, but most of the differences are attributable to the delivery balloon rather than the stent.[757] However, the relationship between flexibility and in-vivo performance is uncertain, and statistical differences in flexibility may not be clinically relevant.

E. **RADIAL STRENGTH.** This characteristic is a measure of a stent's ability to resist recoil of the arterial wall. Stent design and strut thickness are key determinants of radial strength, which may adversely impact flexibility and conformability. Greater radial strength may be beneficial for ostial lesions, where elastic forces are high. For rigid lesions, balloon-expandable stents provide better expansion than self-expanding stents. In-vitro studies have reported significant differences in passive and stress-induced elastic recoil, varying from less than 2% recoil to 18% recoil depending on stent design. In general, coil stents demonstrated the most recoil, followed by hybrid stents and slotted tubular stents.[758,759] However, differences in recoil with newer stent designs were less apparent, and although marked differences in recoil may correlate with late outcome[762]—such as differences in restenosis between the Palmaz-Schatz and GR-II stents—subtle differences in in-vitro recoil may not be clinically important.[760-30] "Locking" stent designs (e.g., BeStent-2, Navius stent) appear to have the most radial strength without sacrificing flexibility.[758,759]

F. SCAFFOLDING. This refers to the ability of a stent to completely cover a lesion (radial and longitudinal coverage), and is dependent on radial strength and stent surface area, which varies from 7-20% (Table 26.1). Inadequate scaffolding may result in plaque protrusion through the stent struts into the lumen, facilitating stent thrombosis and restenosis.[52] However, excessive scaffolding may reduce sidebranch access, flexibility, deliverability, and conformability. Higher metal surface area may also facilitate thrombus formation (and partially explain the high rates of stent thrombosis with the original Wallstent).[53]

G. SIDEBRANCH ACCESS AND PRESERVATION. These characteristics are related to metal surface area and stent design. In general, as metal surface area increases, access to sidebranches decreases. However, for a given metal surface area, subtle differences in architecture can improve access, such as flattened or elliptical struts and rounded cell designs.

H. VISIBILITY of a stent by fluoroscopy is dependent on the stent material, design, strut thickness, and X-ray imaging equipment. Visibility is particularly important during overlapping or ostial stent placement. Historically, the radiopacity of older tantalum stents (e.g., Wiktor, Crossflex stents) was superior to older stainless steel stents (Palmaz-Schatz, Gianturco-Roubin). However, most contemporary stainless steel stents have good radiopacity, which can be enhanced by gold plating (NIROYAL Elite) or markers (BeStent).

I. IMPLICATIONS OF DIFFERENT STENT DESIGNS. Although stent characteristics can affect procedural success, it is very difficult to discern important clinical differences between contemporary stent designs. Experimental studies have identified a relationship between stent design, post-deployment luminal geometry, and subsequent intimal hyperplasia,[750] but such a relationship was not demonstrated in several randomized clinical trials. However, one randomized trial reported significant differences in 1-year outcome between the Palmaz-Schatz stent and four other second generation stents,[784] suggesting that the relationship between stent design and restenosis has not been resolved.[786] Some concern was raised about gold plating of stents when an early gold-coated stent was associated with more restenosis than its stainless steel counterpart;[783] however, techniques used for gold plating are highly variable, and the findings reported in this study may not be broadly applicable to other gold-coated stents.

Table 26.3. Intracoronary Stents: Characteristics of Commonly Used Designs

Characteristic	NIROYAL Elite (BSC)	Radius (BSC)	Wallstent (BSC)	BX-Velocity (Cordis/J & J)	MultiLink TETRA (Guidant)	MultiLink ULTRA (Guidant)	BeStent-2 (Medtronic AVE)	S670 (Medtronic AVE)
Flexibility (pre-deployment)	+++	+++	+++	++++	++++	+++	+++	++++
Deliverability	++++	+++	+++	++++	++++	+++	++++	++++
Conformability (post deployment)	+++	++++	++++	++++	+++	+++	++++	++++
Radial strength	++++	++	++	++++	+++	++++	+++	++++
Scaffolding	++++	++	+++	++++	+++	++++	+++	+++
Sidebranch access	++	+++	++	++++	++	++	++++	++++
Visibility	++++	++	++++	+++	+++	+++	++++	+++
Diversity (sizes and lengths)	+++	++	+++	++++	+++	+++	++	++++
MRI Safety	Yes	Yes	Yes	Yes	Yes	Yes	Yes	Yes
Monorail available	Yes	No	Yes*	Yes*	Yes	Yes	Yes	Yes

Abbreviations: AVE = Arterial Vascular Engineering; BSC = Boston Scientific Scimed
* Outside USA

Table 26.4. Stent Characteristics

Characteristic	Definition	Determinants
Biocompatibility	Resistance to corrosion, thrombosis	Material, coatings, metal surface area
Conformability	Degree to which an expanded stent can bend around its longitudinal axis	Material, stent design
Deliverability	Ability to deliver stent to target lesion	Longitudinal flexibility, crossing profile, trackability, nesting
Expansion ratio	Degree of stent expansion when fully deployed (opposite of recoil)	Stent design, strut thickness, metal surface area, stent recoil
Flaring	Separation of the stent strut from the delivery balloon during insertion around bends	Stent design (bigger problem with open or coil designs)
Flexibility	Degree to which an unexpanded stent can bend around its longitudinal axis	Material, stent design
Metal surface area	Percent of surface area covered by metal after stent deployment	Stent design, strut thickness
Nesting	Security of stent attachment to delivery system	Stent design, profile
Radial strength	Resistance to vessel recoil	Stent design, strut thickness
Radiopacity	Ability to identify stent during fluoroscopy	Strut thickness, material (nitinol, steel)
Scaffolding	Ability of stent to completely cover and support the vessel	Material, stent design, strut thickness, metal surface area, radial strength
Shortening	Decrease in stent length when fully deployed	Stent design
Trackability	Ease of movement over guidewire	Profile, shaft coating, stiffness, distal tapering

Table 26.5. Comparison of Commonly Used Stents

Stent	Advantages	Disadvantages
Balloon-Expandable Stents		
BeStent-2	Superb overall performance	
BX-Velocity	Superb overall performance	Moderate radiopacity
MultiLink ULTRA	Well-suited for large vessels and vein grafts	Not as trackable or flexible as stents designed for smaller vessels
MultiLink TETRA	Superb overall performance	Moderate radiopacity
NIR/NIROYAL Elite	Superb overall performance	Sidebranch access
S660	Superb overall performance for small vessels	Not designed for vessels ≥ 3 mm
S670	Superb overall performance	Moderate radiopacity
Self-Expanding Stents		
Radius	Flexibility, protective sheath, deliverability, low profile, does not shorten	Variable precision in placement, radiopacity
Wallstent	Flexibility, protective sheath, radiopacity, conformability	Shortens by 15-20%

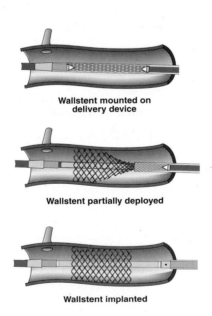

Wallstent mounted on
delivery device

Wallstent partially deployed

Wallstent implanted

Figure 26.11. Wallstent Deployment Technique

TECHNIQUE OF STENT PLACEMENT

A. SELF-EXPANDING STENTS. To facilitate Wallstent placement and removal of the delivery catheter, target lesions in native vessels should be predilated using a balloon matched to the vessel diameter. After predilatation, the angioplasty balloon is exchanged for the stent delivery system and the stent is deployed by retracting the constraining sheath (Figure 26.11). The selected stent should be 0.5-1.0 mm larger than the adjacent normal reference segment; greater degrees of stent oversizing may reduce stent-shortening.[54] If necessary, the inner surface of the stent may be smoothed by further balloon inflations using balloon/artery ratio ~ 1.0; balloon oversizing is not recommended due to the risk of dissection or perforation. The technique for implanting the Radius stent is similar, but stent shortening does not occur. In degenerated vein grafts at risk for distal embolization, direct stenting without predilatation is reasonable; gentle balloon inflations (inflation pressure 2-4 ATM) can be used if necessary after stent deployment. In contrast to balloon-expandable stents, which do not expand further after high-pressure deployment, the Wallstent and Radius stent continue to expand even after high-pressure adjunctive PTCA.[662]

B. BALLOON-EXPANDABLE STENTS. All coronary balloon-expandable stents in the United States are pre-mounted on a delivery balloon, whereas many "bare-mounted" stents are available outside the United States. With recent improvements in stent profile and securement ("nesting") to the delivery balloon, the need for a protective sheath has been virtually eliminated. By most manufacturers' guidelines, pretreatment with a conventional angioplasty balloon or other device is recommended prior to stent insertion. Besides facilitating stent insertion, predilatation can confirm that the balloon (and therefore the stent) can be fully inflated. The inability to fully release a rigid stenosis with a high-pressure balloon or Rotablator is a contraindication to stenting. Many operators employ "direct stenting" without predilatation; theoretical advantages include less dissection and lower cost (see below). Numerous studies suggest reasonable safety and efficacy,[55] but in the presence of extreme tortuosity or calcification, predilatation is strongly recommended to avoid premature stent delivery, stent embolization, and suboptimal lumen enlargement. In situations where a stent cannot be delivered because of proximal vessel tortuosity, techniques to improve success include the use of guiding catheters that enhance coaxial alignment and optimize backup support, heavy-duty or extra-support guidewires to facilitate stent advancement, and the Wiggle-wire (Guidant) to deflect the tip and facilitate delivery of the stent delivery balloon (Table 26.6). The 0.014-inch Platinum-Plus™ guidewire (Meditech, Watertown, MA) and the 0.014-inch Ironman™ wire (Guidant) provide the most straightening force and support, and are particularly useful for difficult procedures (although pseudolesions are common). With newer stent designs, successful delivery is often readily achieved without extra-support guidewires.

Ideal placement of the stent should be confirmed by contrast injections prior to stent delivery. The stent delivery system should be advanced across the lesion, and the stent deployed at the recommended inflation pressure for 15-30 seconds. Adjunctive angioplasty is recommended using high-pressure noncompliant balloons matched to the normal reference diameter (balloon/artery ratio = 1.0-1.1) at 12-18 atm.[56] Older delivery balloons have been replaced by higher-rated, less compliant delivery balloons, which can be used for post-dilatation.[57] Intravascular ultrasound may be useful for identifying the reference vessel diameter and for confirming ideal stent deployment.[60,61] In some cases, multiple stents may be required to cover long lesions or dissections. In general, it is desirable to place the most distal stent first, although in some cases (e.g., aorto-ostial lesions) it may be necessary to place the proximal stent first.

C. **RADIAL OR BRACHIAL ARTERY TECHNIQUE.** Most operators use the femoral artery approach for stent implantation. With lower profile and more flexible delivery systems, several centers use the percutaneous brachial or radial artery approach with 6F guiding catheters.[649,650] Advantages of these techniques are primarily related to patient comfort, reduction in bleeding and vascular complications, and shorter hospital stay (Chapter 2).[62-65]

D. **IMPACT OF STENT DEPLOYMENT TECHNIQUE ON OUTCOME.** The relationship between stent implantation pressure and outcome is controversial. IVUS studies suggested better stent dimensions using higher inflation pressures,[755] while some reports indicated more vessel injury and higher restenosis rates when inflation pressures exceeded 15 ATM (or with balloon:artery ratios > 1.1).[751,752,754] In contrast, one randomized trial reported no relationship between inflation pressure (15-20 ATM vs. 8-13 ATM) and either stent thrombosis, ischemic complications at 30 days, angiographic restenosis at 6 months, or event-free survival at 1 year.[756]

E. **DIRECT STENT TECHNIQUE.** Because of reliable delivery of second and third generation stent designs, many operators now perform direct stenting without predilatation. Probable advantages of direct stenting include less procedural time, fluoroscopy time, contrast volume, and cost. Theoretical advantages include less balloon-induced injury and lower restenosis (Table 26.7). For vein grafts, direct stenting (particularly with self-expanding stents) is often performed to reduce the risk of distal embolization and no-reflow. Disadvantages of direct stenting include failure to deliver the stent to the target lesion (which could lead to stent embolization during retrieval), and inability to fully expand the stent in an unsuspected rigid lesion. Virtually all failures of direct stenting are treated by subsequent successful stenting after predilatation or Rotablator. Reports in relatively small numbers of patients suggest that direct stenting is successful in > 90% with a low (< 2%) incidence of stent embolization (Table 26.8). In the PREDICT trial, 400 patients were randomized to direct stenting vs. conventional stenting with predilatation (Table 26.9). Despite the fact that lesions were highly selected (*de novo* focal lesion ≤ 15 mm in length, no calcification, reference vessel 3-4 mm, no tortuosity), direct stenting failed in 8%. However, all failures were readily managed by subsequent predilatation, and final procedural success was similar for both groups. Differences in procedural time and contrast volume favored direct stenting, although the incremental benefit was small: 2.7 minutes in total procedural time, 1.2 minutes in fluoroscopy time, and 15cc of radiographic contrast. There were no differences in hospital or late MACE. Results in the randomized SWIBAP trial were similar (Table 26.8).[866]

Table 26.6. Troubleshooting with Stents

Problem	Solution
Moderate disease proximal to target lesion	• Place stent in target lesion then reassess proximal disease • Dilate proximal disease; if dissection occurs, stent
Inadvertent unstented proximal disease	• Insert another tandem stent (1 mm overlap)
Inadvertent unstented distal disease	• Post-dilate stent with high-pressure balloon • Optimize guide and wire support • Insert another tandem stent (1 mm overlap)
Undilatable target lesion	• Rotational atherectomy followed by high-pressure balloon
Delivery system will not cross lesion	• Predilate with larger balloon • Rotational atherectomy • Improve guide support, alignment • Extra-support guidewire or Wiggle-wire • "Buddy" wire† • More flexible wires may be helpful with newer stent designs • Alternate stent or shorter stent
Proximal vessel tortuosity	• Strong guide support with excellent coaxial alignment • Extra-support guidewire or Wiggle-wire • "Buddy" wire† • More flexible wires may be helpful with newer stent designs
Angulated lesion	• Strong guide support with excellent coaxial alignment • Extra-support guidewire • More flexible wires may be helpful with newer stent designs • Shorter, overlapping stents
Ostial lesion	• Predilate with noncompliant full-size balloon • Consider debulking with rotational atherectomy prior to stenting • Avoid "aggressive" guiding catheters
Tapering vessel	• Deploy stent at low pressure • Retract balloon into confines of stent then fully deploy • Post-dilate proximal half of stent with short, high-pressure balloon
Sidebranch occlusion	• Post-dilate stent with high-pressure balloon • Dilate sidebranch; use fixed-wire or over-the-wire balloon after wiring through stent strut into branch • If angioplasty result is suboptimal, deploy second stent into sidebranch with overlap into initial stent ("T" or "Y" stent)
In-stent result is suboptimal	• Consider IVUS to guide therapy • Repeat PTCA with larger balloon or higher pressure • Overlapping stent (stent "sandwich") for protruding plaque
Loss of guidewire after stent deployment	• Recross stent with large "J" tip on floppy wire • Prolapse "J" wire across stented segment • Pass undeployed balloon or IVUS catheter completely through stent to ensure proper wire position • Post-dilate stent

Table 26.6. Troubleshooting with Stents

Problem	Solution
Balloon rupture during stent deployment	• Gently retract delivery balloon (may need to advance first) • If unable to retract, rapid inflation with full-strength contrast with manual inflation or power injector may deploy stent • Use low-profile, high-pressure balloon to further expand stent
Balloon rupture during post-stent PTCA	• Use noncompliant balloon
Difficulty removing delivery balloon	• Neutral pressure • Advance and rotate slightly prior to retraction • Reinflate, then deflate • "Buddy" wire and advance second, low-profile balloon into stent next to delivery balloon; remove both together
Removing undeployed stent	• If stent is beyond guiding catheter, align catheter and gently retract into guide; then remove • Consider disengaging guide from ostium prior to retraction • If unable to retract into guide (especially true with 6F guides), remove guide and delivery system en bloc; "buddy" wire may help support and maintain wire position during removal of guide • If unable to remove from artery, deploy in proximal vessel
Undeployed stent slipped off delivery balloon	• Attempt to retrieve with snare • If unable to snare in coronary, advance undersized, low-profile balloon within stent; inflate to 1 atm and attempt to remove or deploy stent in site
PTCA balloon will not cross stent after deployment	• See comments for proximal vessel tortuosity • Use balloon deflection technique[††]

† Buddy wire approach: Use double extra-support or heavy-duty wires to straighten the vessel; once the stent delivery system is in position across the target lesion, remove the buddy wire; do not deploy the stent until the buddy wire has been removed

†† Leave balloon in place and pass another buddy wire and balloon up to stent; use first balloon to "deflect second balloon into stent

Based on available data, we believe that highly complex lesions (such as calcified, ostial, and angulated lesions or total occlusions) are best treated by conventional stenting after pretreatment with PTCA or Rotablator. If direct stenting is considered, the greatest chance for success will be achieved by careful case selection, ideal guiding catheter alignment and support, and use of low-profile third generation stents. We do not recommend direct stenting of native coronary arteries with self-expanding stents due to the risk of suboptimal lumen enlargement. Issues surrounding the use of direct stent technique have more to do with convenience than safety or late outcome.

Table 26.7. Comparison of Direct Stenting to Conventional Stenting with Predilatation

Technique	Advantages	Disadvantages
Direct stent	• Less procedural time, radiation exposure, contrast volume, cost • Theoretical benefit of less balloon injury and lower restenosis • Theoretical benefit of less distal embolization in vein grafts	• Not well-suited for complex anatomy • Rigid lesion maybe more difficult to treat after stent deployment • Potential stent embolization if stent will not cross target lesion
Stent after predilatation	• Ensures that lesion will "yield" prior to stent deployment • Well-suited for complex anatomy (calcification, angulation, ostial or total occlusion)	• More procedural time, radiation exposure, contrast volume, cost

Table 26.8. Direct Stenting Without Predilatation

Study	Technique	N	ACC/AHA (%)	Success (%)	Comments
Bedossa[686] (2001)	DS PTCA/S	197 199	- -	97.5 99	Randomized trial. Less procedural time and contrast with DS; no difference in MACE or TLR at 30 days
Chan[763] (2000)	DS	158	A/B (88)	98.1	Less fluoroscopy and procedural time than PTCA/S
Wilson[764] (2000)	DS PTCA/S	777 3176	A/B (40) A/B (52)	96.3 96.4	No difference in in-hospital MACE or 1-yr EFS; DS had less contrast and fluoroscopy and fewer dissections
Bedossa[767] (2000)	DS	106	A/B$_1$ (100)	94	Complex lesions were excluded
Ormiston[768] (2000)	DS PTCA/S	39 42	A/B$_1$ (85) A/B$_1$ (93)	92 100	DS had lower cost and less procedural time; no difference in contrast volume, fluoroscopy time, or outcome
Herz[769] (2000)	DS PTCA/S	221 161	- -	89 98	All failures after DS underwent successful stenting after PTCA; less cost after DS
Hernandez[771] (2000)	DS	50	A/B$_1$ (90)	100	38% did not have optimal stenting by IVUS
SWIBAP[868] (2000)	DS PTCA/S	192 197	- -	97.5 99	Prospective randomized trial. DS had less procedural time and contrast, but no difference in fluoroscopy time or MACE
Danzi[765] (1999)	DS PTCA/S	61 61	A/B$_1$ (49) A/B$_1$ (49)	97 100	No difference in hospital or late MACE; DS had less contrast and procedural time
SWOP[766] (1999)	DS	240	A/B$_1$ (65)	93	All failures underwent successful stenting after PTCA or Rotablator
Briguori[770] (1999)	DS	123	A/B$_1$ (84)	96	DS had less procedural time, radiation exposure, contrast, and cost
Hamon[772] (1999)	DS	122	A/B (40)	96	Stent embolization after failed DS (1.6%)

Abbreviations: ACC/AHA = lesion type per AHA/ACC classification system; DS = direct stenting without predilatation; EFS = event-free survival; IVUS = intravascular ultrasound; MACE = major adverse cardiac events; PTCA/S = predilatation with PTCA followed by stenting; SWIBAP = Stenting Without Balloon Predilatation; SWOP = Stenting Without Predilatation; - = not reported

Table 26.9. Results of PREDICT: Predilatation vs. Direct Stenting In Coronary Treatment[891]

	Direct Stent	Predilatation
Baseline QCA		
MLD (mm)	0.94	0.90
DS (%)	68	69
Success* (%)		
1° technical	96.6	92
2° technical	99.5	99
Procedural	93.9	92.5
Procedural technique		
Total time (min)	33.2	35.9
Fluoroscopy time (min)	9.2	10.4
Contrast volume (cc)	154	169
Balloons used (n)	0.6	1.3
MACE at 6 months (%)	18.7	19.4

Abbreviations: MLD = minimum lumen diameter; DS = diameter stenosis; MACE = major adverse cardiac events (death, MI, repeat revascularization)

* 1° technical success = successful stent delivery and deployment without adjunctive intervention
   2° technical success = successful stent delivery and deployment with and without adjunctive intervention
   Procedural success = technical success and no in-hospital MACE

INDICATIONS FOR STENTING (Table 26.10)

Since their approval in 1994 for "bail-out" indications, stents have been extensively evaluated in a large range of clinical and angiographic settings. The ACC Expert Consensus Document on Coronary Artery Stents, while conservative, provides an objective overview of published data and current indications for stents.[66] Indications are broadly classified as "definite" (FDA-approved based on compelling observational data and randomized clinical trials); "probable" (observational data continues to mount but randomized data are lacking); and "possible" (stents are commonly employed, but controversy persists). Definite indications for stenting include treatment for abrupt and threatened closure, and elective use in *de novo* and restenotic lesions in native coronary arteries and vein grafts. Contraindications are relative and continue to diminish. Nevertheless, it is important to recognize that the routine, clinical application of stents goes well beyond published data from randomized trials. Furthermore, results from randomized trials cannot necessarily be extrapolated to widespread current clinical practice; for example, compared to lesion types included in STRESS and BENESTENT, restenosis rates may be 4-fold higher when stents are used in certain long and complex lesions.[666]

A. REVERSAL OF ABRUPT OR THREATENED VESSEL CLOSURE (Table 26.11). The incidence of acute closure after PTCA was 4-12%.[67-70] Older methods to reverse acute closure (repeat balloon inflations, vasodilators, and thrombolytic agents) reduced the need for emergency surgery, but were associated with substantial morbidity in 40% and in-hospital mortality in 5% of patients.[70,71] In TASC II and in several smaller series, stenting was more effective than prolonged balloon inflations for failed PTCA in reducing emergency CABG and recurrent ischemic events at 6 months (Table 26.12).[67-72] Given these results and numerous other studies demonstrating success rates > 95%,[72-75] stents have essentially replaced all other techniques for reversing acute closure. Nearly every stent approved in the United States has been successfully applied to patients with abrupt or threatened closure.[76-88,89-98] Older studies reported substantial patient morbidity after bail-out stenting, including stent thrombosis (0-32%), myocardial infarction (2-16%), emergency bypass surgery (0-16.5%), and death (0-10%).[89-98] However, most of these data were reported prior to routine use of antiplatelet regimens, high-pressure adjunctive PTCA, and the common practice of stenting high-risk dissections *before* the vessel becomes occluded (Table 26.13).

B. ELECTIVE STENT PLACEMENT. In general, stents offer the best opportunity for immediate enlargement of the vascular lumen, particularly in large vessels. It has now been clearly established that in STRESS/BENESTENT lesions (*de novo,* length < 15 mm, native vessel in > 3 mm), stenting can be performed with high success (> 95%), low complication rates (< 5%), and less restenosis compared to PTCA alone (Tables 26.14-26.17). [99-116] The favorable impact of stenting on restenosis relates to its ability to achieve superior lumen enlargement and minimize elastic recoil and negative remodeling.[117,118]

Table 26.10. Indications for Stenting*

Definite
　Acute and threatened closure
　Focal, *de novo* lesions in native vessels ≥ 3 mm
　Chronic total occlusion
　LAD stenosis
　Saphenous vein graft (focal or tubular lesions)
　Restenotic lesions

Probable
　Aorto-ostial lesions

Possible
　Long lesions/diffuse disease
　Saphenous vein graft (degenerated)
　Bifurcation lesions
　Vessels < 3 mm
　Left main disease (unprotected)
　In-stent stenosis
　Perforation/pseudoaneurysm (covered stents)

Contraindications (relative)
　Excessive thrombus
　Undilatable lesion
　Poor distal run-off

Abbreviations: LAD = left anterior descending coronary artery
* Compared to other methods of percutaneous revascularization

The excellent results of stenting have led to its use in 50-80% of all interventional procedures. However, it is estimated that more than 80% of lesions currently treated by stents would have been excluded from the STRESS and BENESTENT studies,[801] including vessels < 3 mm, lesions > 20 mm in length, bifurcation or ostial lesions, chronic total occlusions, and unprotected left main stenoses. Stent deployment in such complex lesions is associated with more late revascularization than in simple lesions.[153,154] In fact, while two studies of over 80,000 patients suggested clear superiority of stents compared to PTCA with respect to in-hospital ischemic complications, there was no difference in late revascularization.[802,803] Another large population-based study of nearly 10,000 patients reported a significant decline in late MACE from 1994-1997 (which coincided with increasing utilization of stents),[804] but the 21% reduction in late events (from 28.8% to 22.8%) was relatively modest compared to the dramatic increase in stent utilization (from 14.2% to 58.7%).[809]

1. **Native Coronary Arteries.** Three multicenter, randomized trials confirmed that stenting resulted in better lumen enlargement, higher procedural success, lower restenosis rates, fewer repeat procedures, and better event-free survival compared to PTCA alone (Tables 26.14, 26.17).[115,116,119] Newer, more flexible stent designs have demonstrated equivalence to the Palmaz-Schatz stent during long-term follow-up and are preferred in current interventional practice (Table 26.18).[644] In the WIN trial (Wallstent In Native vessels), 586 patients were randomized to PTCA or Wallstent. Clinical and angiographic results were similar at 6 months, but 37% of PTCA patients crossed over to stenting because of suboptimal results (Table 26.16). Numerous industry-sponsored registries and observational studies have also been reported (Tables 26.19, 26.20).

2. **Saphenous Vein Bypass Grafts (Chapter 17).** Stent placement is now the treatment of choice for focal or tubular lesions in nondegenerated vein grafts. Numerous observational studies reported successful stent delivery in 95-100% of lesions, with a low incidence of stent thrombosis (0-3%), emergency CABG (0-2.8%), myocardial infarction (0-4%), death (0-2%), and restenosis (17-35%) (Table 26.21). In the largest multicenter prospective randomized trial of PTCA and stents in vein grafts (SAVED), Palmaz-Schatz stents were associated with higher procedural success (92% vs. 69%, p < 0.001), superior lumen enlargement (immediately and at 6 months), less restenosis (37% vs. 46%, p = 0.02) and less MACE at 6 months (27% vs. 42%, p = 0.03) (Table 26.12).[126] Wallstents has also been evaluated in saphenous vein grafts (Tables 26.15, 26.22). In WINS, 268 patients with saphenous vein graft lesions were randomized to the Wallstent or Palmaz-Schatz stent; in-hospital and 6-month outcomes were similar. A nonrandomized registry of Wallstents in large vein grafts (vessel diameter 4.1-5.5 mm) demonstrated angiographic restenosis in 28%, target lesion revascularization in 8%, and major adverse cardiac events or stroke at 6 months in 27%. In contrast to PTCA, stenting of vein grafts does not appear to be influenced by graft age.[122] However, late morbidity is worse than after stenting in native coronary arteries; 2-year event-free survival after vein graft stenting was only 55%, due primarily to unfavorable clinical characteristics and progressive disease at non-stented sites.[125-127] The PercuSurge GuardWire reduced ischemic complications by 50-60% following vein graft intervention in the SAFER trial; other distal protection devices are currently under investigation (Chapters 9, 17). The ideal intervention for degenerated vein grafts is still unknown.[128,129,653]

3. **Left Anterior Descending Artery Stenoses.** Patients with proximal LAD disease have a worse prognosis than patients with other forms of single-vessel disease.[132-134] PTCA is more effective at improving symptoms, exercise performance, and quality of life than medical therapy;[135,136] however, intervention on the LAD is associated with greater risk (since the LAD can supply 50% of total myocardium)[137,138] and more restenosis than for other vessels.[139] In the only randomized comparison between elective stenting and PTCA for isolated proximal LAD stenosis, stenting was associated with fewer ischemic complications at 12 months (13% vs. 30%, p = 0.04) and less angiographic restenosis (19% vs. 40%, p = 0.02).[140] Ostial LAD lesions appear to have lower success rates than other lesions after stenting (Table 26.23).

4. **Ostial Lesions (Table 26.23) (Chapter 14).** PTCA of aorto-ostial lesions is frequently suboptimal because of the elasticity and rigidity of the aorta; final diameter stenoses > 50% are common. High procedural success rates after stenting can be achieved, but stent implantation is technically challenging because of difficulties seating the guiding catheter, obtaining adequate images to optimize stent placement, ensuring proper stent position to adequately cover the entire lesion, and preventing stent migration and embolization (Figure 26.12). For calcified aorto-ostial lesions, pretreatment with rotational atherectomy facilitates full balloon expansion before stenting. Intravascular ultrasound may be useful for aorto-ostial lesions to assess the degree and depth of calcification, to ensure adequate stent sizing, to confirm complete stent apposition and lesion coverage, and to avoid excessive stent protrusion into the aorta. In several small observational studies, stents were successfully implanted in more than 95% of ostial lesions, with restenosis rates ranging from 15% for native vessels to 62% for vein grafts.[141-143] In a small randomized study of PTCA and Wiktor stents in ostial RCA lesions, stents resulted in better lumen enlargement, but there was no difference in early or late outcome.[144] In contrast, other nonrandomized studies reported higher procedural success (96% vs. 88% vs. 77%) and less target vessel revascularization (24% vs. 47% vs. 40%) when ostial RCA lesions were treated by stenting compared to debulking devices (ELCA, DCA, Rotablator) or PTCA.[145,146] However, unprotected lesions at the origin of the LAD or left circumflex may be less suitable for stenting, since proper lesion coverage requires stenting of the distal left main, which may be a risk factor for ischemic complications.[147] In one small study, DCA of origin LAD lesions resulted in less compromise of the origin of the LCX than stenting.[931]

5. **Chronic Total Occlusions (Chapter 16).** Several observational (Table 26.24) and randomized (Table 26.12) trials demonstrated better immediate results, less restenosis, and fewer adverse clinical events (death, MI, or TLR) after stenting vs. PTCA.[148-152] Late outcomes after stenting also included a decrease in LV volume and an increase in ejection fraction.[670] In suitable total occlusions, stenting is preferable to PTCA.

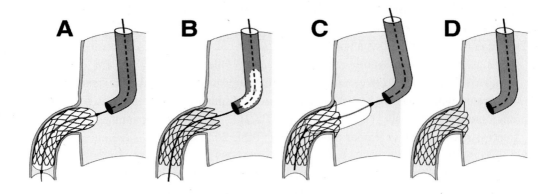

Figure 26.12. Aorto-Ostial Lesions: Stent Technique

A. Position the stent-delivery balloon so 1-2 mm of stent extends into the aorta. The guide must be retracted 1-2 cm before deploying the stent

B. Remove the delivery balloon while maintaining backward tension on the guide to prevent it from advancing into the ostium and damaging the stent

C. Perform adjunctive PTCA with a high-pressure balloon to ensure full stent expansion and apposition. Flaring the proximal end of the stent with a slightly larger balloon is useful

D. Final result

6. **Diffuse Disease and Long Lesions (Chapter 15).** Earlier observational studies of stents for diffuse disease reported subacute thrombosis in 1.2-5%.[155-166] Some studies reported similar long-term results for PTCA and stenting, but others reported better long-term results after stenting (Table 26.25).[167-169] One randomized study suggested less angiographic restenosis after stenting but no difference in clinical outcome (Table 26.12).[734] Multiple stents for long segments of disease are associated with more restenosis than single stents for focal lesions;[170-173] the risk of restenosis after stenting is approximately 1% per mm of stent. An alternative approach to use of long stents for diffuse disease is to "spot stent" more focal areas of severe disease amidst longer segments of diffuse disease;[545] the best approach is unknown.

7. **Small Vessels.** Early FDA guidelines did not recommend elective stenting in vessels < 3 mm. Nevertheless, stents have been successfully implanted in small vessels with excellent results (Table 26.26).[174-176] A post-hoc subgroup analysis in the STRESS trial suggested that the relative benefit of stents compared to PTCA was better in vessels < 3 mm than in vessels > 3 mm,[178] and a metanalysis of 1109 patients in the STRESS and BENESTENT trials suggested that the greatest benefit of stenting was in vessels 2.6-3.4-mm in diameter.[179] In contrast, a nonrandomized comparative study of stents in large and small vessels reported similar procedural success rates and in-hospital MACE, but significantly higher angiographic restenosis and TLR after small vessel stenting.[797] One criticism of these studies was that stents designed for vessels ≥ 3 mm were deployed in smaller vessels; new stent designs for vessels < 3 mm are now approved by the FDA.[180]

Pooled data from numerous observational studies indicate procedural success rates in 95% and restenosis in 35% of patients,[801] and a small randomized study showed a trend toward fewer late ischemic complications after stenting (Table 26.12).[858]

8. **Bifurcation Lesions (Chapter 10).** Experimental data showed that flow into nondiseased sidebranches was well-preserved after stent placement, and several angiographic studies suggested a low incidence of sidebranch occlusion (see below). Nevertheless, stents should be used cautiously in patients with stenoses involving sidebranches > 2.0 mm in diameter.[182] Important considerations include the likelihood of immediate and future revascularization of the sidebranch, the size of the sidebranch, and the amount of myocardium served by that branch. In general, jeopardy of acute marginal branches of the right coronary artery, small diagonal branches of the LAD, and small obtuse marginal branches of the left circumflex do not represent significant contraindications to stent placement. In some anatomically suitable vessels, there is now considerable experience with "kissing" stents, T-stents, and Culotte stents[183] (Figure 26.13; Chapter 10). These techniques are technically demanding and should be reserved for experienced stent operators (Table 26.27).[184-186] Most contemporary stent designs allow ready access to large branches. New stent designs (JOMED Sidebranch, NIRSIDE stents, and BeStent bifurcation) are undergoing clinical testing, but are not commercially available in the United States. Bifurcation lesions are perhaps the most challenging to treat with stents, even in the hands of experienced operators. The risk of sidebranch occlusion is highest when the branch ostium is diseased, and is similar to the risk of occlusion after PTCA.[672] Emerging strategies utilizing debulking techniques prior to stent deployment may result in less plaque shift and better long-term outcomes; further study is needed. When stenting a lesion immediately proximal to a bifurcation (pseudobifurcation lesion), the "skirt technique" may be useful to facilitate ideal placement.[741] This technique involves passing guidewires into each branch and hand mounting the stent on kissing balloons sized to each branch. The assembly is advanced so the tip of each balloon is in the origin of each branch, and the stent is deployed by "kissing" balloon inflations.

9. **Restenotic Lesions.** In contrast to *de novo* lesions, elective stenting of restenotic lesions resulted in procedural success > 95%, major complications rates < 3%, and re-restenosis in 25-40% (Table 26.28).[104,187,188] The prospective randomized Restenosis Stent (REST) study suggested that compared to PTCA of restenotic lesions, there was less target vessel revascularization after stenting (11.7% vs. 27%) (Table 26.12).[189,475]

10. **Lesions with Gross Thrombus (Chapter 9).** Stenting may be reasonable if thrombus can be removed prior to stent implantation.[215,221,222] Potentially useful adjuncts include TEC atherectomy,[216-218] systemic or intracoronary infusion of thrombolytics,[219] local delivery of heparin or lytics,[220] or AngioJet thrombectomy.[223] For patients who are clinically stable, a 2-5-day infusion of heparin, overnight infusion of a glycoprotein IIb/IIIa inhibitor, or a 2-3-week course of warfarin or low-molecular-weight heparin may "clean up" the vessel and permit stent implantation (Table 26.28). Older concerns about stenting thrombotic lesions have been attenuated by the excellent experience with primary stenting for acute MI.

Table 26.11. In-hospital Outcome After "Bail-Out" Stenting*

| Series | N | In-hospital Complications (%) | |
		Stent Thrombosis	D / MI /CABG
Linnemeier[852] (1998)	173	-	0.6 / 0.6 / 1.2
Steffenino[251] (1997)	150	6.6	5.3 / - / 2.7
Glatt[254] (1997)	266	2.3	4.9 / 0.8 / 1.1
Spaulding[256] (1997)	124	0.8	6.5 / 0 / 3.2
Monassier[252] (1996)	134	3	6.8 / 4.5 / 4.5
Schomig[76] (1994)	339	6.9	1.3 / 4.0 / 9
Sutton[81] (1994)	415	-	3 / 5 / 12
Agrawal[82] (1994)	240	7	-
Vrolix[85] (1994)	180	13.3	3.3 / 12 / 16.5
Garratt[86] (1994)	308	3	3.7 / 2.7 / 8.7
George[83] (1993)	518	8.7	2.2 / 5.5 / 4.3
Roubin[84] (1992)	115	7.6	1.7 / 16 / 4.2

Abbreviations: CABG = emergency coronary artery bypass surgery; D = death; MI = myocardial infarction
* Limited to studies with N $\geq$ 100

11. **Heavy Calcification (Chapter 12).** Heavy calcification is a frequent cause of failure to deliver a stent to the target lesion, and may impair full stent expansion. Virtually all experienced operators recommend rotational atherectomy in this setting prior to stenting (Table 26.28).[224]

C. **PROVISIONAL STENTING.** The role of provisional stenting, in which stenting is reserved only for suboptimal PTCA, is controversial. A post-hoc analysis of BENESTENT suggested that a "stent-like" result after PTCA (final diameter stenosis < 30%) was associated with similar outcomes compared to stents.[657] In contrast, data from the NHLBI Registry suggested that despite a final diameter stenosis < 10% after PTCA, ischemic complications at 10 years were higher than after stenting.[652] The primary motivations for provisional stenting were to decrease bleeding and vascular complications (in the era of warfarin-anticoagulation), reduce cost (use of multiple balloons for pre- and post-dilatation, increased length of hospital stay), and avoid the dilemma of treating in-stent restenosis. The principle of provisional stenting is sound, but the practice has a number of important limitations (Table 26.29). .

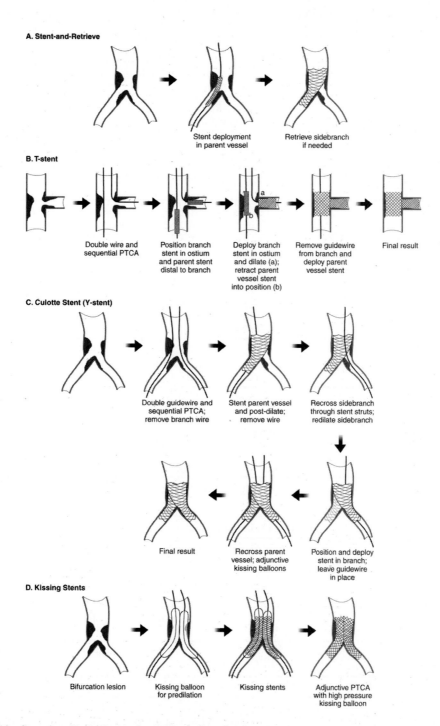

Figure 26.13. Stenting Techniques for Bifurcation Lesions

Table 26.12. Randomized Trials of Stent vs. PTCA for Specific Indications

Trial	N	Stent	Result (Stent vs. PTCA)
CHRONIC TOTAL OCCLUSION			
MAJIC[847] (1999)	220	Wiktor	Less reocclusion (2.1% vs. 9.3%, p < 0.05) and TLR (29% vs. 46%, p < 0.001) at 6 months
SARECCO[855] (1999)	110	-	Less ARS (26% vs. 62%, p = 0.01) and reocclusion (2% vs. 14%, p = 0.05) at 4 months; higher EFS at 2 years (52% vs. 26%, p = 0.05)
TOSCA[478] (1999)	410	HC-PS	Less MACE (15.8% vs. 23.1%, p = 0.08) and TVR (8.4% vs. 15.4%, p < 0.05)
STOP[549] (1999)	96	-	Less TLR at 6 months (19% vs. 39%)
Hoher[962]	85	-	Less restenosis (32% vs. 64%), less reocclusion (3% vs. 24%), and higher EFS (70% vs. 45%, p = 0.024)
GISSOC[844] (1998)	110	PS	Less ARS (32% vs. 68%, p < 0.001) and TLR (5.3% vs. 22%, p < 0.05) at 6 months
SPACTO[861] (1997)	47	Wiktor	Less ARS (32% vs. 74%, p < 0.01) and MACE (8% vs. 17%, p < 0.05) at 6 months
SICCO[477] (1996)	119	PS	Less ARS (32% vs. 74%, p < 0.001) and TLR at 6 months (22% vs. 42%, p < 0.05)
Mori[534] (1996)	43 53	Stent PTCA	Less restenosis (28% vs. 57%) and rePTCA (28% vs. 49%) at 6 months, and less MI + CABG (2.3% vs. 11%). Stenting (not PTCA) was associated with improvement in LV ejection fraction
Sato[970] (1996)	34 35	Stent PTCA	Similar reocclusion (6.3% vs. 11.4%), restenosis (36.7% vs. 34.4%), and TLR (20% vs. 25%)
SAPHENOUS VEIN GRAFTS			
BENESTENT (2000)	150	Wiktor	Less ARS (21.9% vs. 35.6%, p = 0.009), TLR (11.5% vs. 25%, p < 0.05) and MACE (19.5% vs. 36.1%, p < 0.05) at 6 months
SAVED (1997)	220	PS	Higher procedural success (92% vs. 69%) and less ARS (36% vs. 47%)
SMALL VESSELS (< 3 mm)			
RAP[687] (2001)	426	BeStent	Less restenosis (27% vs. 37%, p < 0.05) and reocclusion (1.4% vs. 2.7%, p < 0.01), but similar MACE (11% vs. 14%) at 6 months
SISCA[688] (2001)	145	BeStent	Less late MACE (2.4% vs. 9.5%%)
SISA[689] (2000)	325	BeStent	Trend toward less MACE at 6 months (22% vs. 31%)
STRESS I-II[532] (1998)	331	PS	Less ARS (33% vs. 54%) and higher EFS (78% vs. 67%)
LONG LESIONS (> 20 mm)			
Oemrawsingh[690] (2001)	100	GFX XL	IVUS-guided stenting resulted in less restenosis compared to stenting without IVUS (18% vs. 36%, p = 0.04)
ADVANCE (2000)	288	Nir	Less ARS (27% vs. 42%, p < 0.01), but no difference in EFS at 9 months (81% vs. 86%)

Table 26.12. Randomized Trials of Stent vs. PTCA for Specific Indications

Trial	N	Stent	Result (Stent vs. PTCA)
PROXIMAL LAD			
Thiele[691] (2001)	220	-	Less relief of angina and more reintervention (27% vs. 6%, p = 0.02) compared to minimally invasive bypass surgery
Versaci[473] (1997)	120	PS	Less ARS (19% vs. 40%) and better EFS (87% vs. 70%)
OTHER SETTINGS			
TASC-1[867,868] (1995)	270	PS	De novo or restenotic lesions. Less MACE at 6 months for restenotic lesions (4.8% vs. 20%), but not for de novo lesions
TASC-II[869] (1995)	43	PS	Abrupt or threatened closure. Higher procedural success (90% vs. 42%, p < 0.01)
REST[475] (1998)	383	PS	Restenotic lesions in native arteries. Less ARS (18% vs. 32%) and TVR (10% vs. 27%)

Abbreviations: ARS = angiographic restenosis; HC-PS = Heparin-coated Palmaz-Schatz; MACE = major adverse cardiac events; TLR = target lesion revascularization; CTO = chronic total occlusion; SVG = saphenous vein graft; EFS = event-free survival; TVR = target vessel revascularization; PS = Palmaz-Schatz

Acronyms: See Table 26.55, p. 587

‡ For stent trials in patients with diabetes mellitus, see Table 26.41

First, several studies confirm the insensitivity of immediate angiography for identifying "optimal PTCA";[787,788,850] IVUS, Doppler flow, pressure measurements, or delayed angiography at 30 minutes are needed (Table 26.30). Second, concerns about the cost of stents and balloons may be less important when considering the additional cost of IVUS catheters and Doppler flow or pressure measurements to assess all PTCA results. Third, most studies suggest that more than 50% of PTCA patients have suboptimal results and would require stenting anyway.[787,791,834] Finally, virtually all of the concerns about complications and cost are less compelling today because of standard antiplatelet therapy without warfarin, frequent use of direct stenting without routine post-dilation, and emerging use of vascular closure devices to reduce length of stay.

D. CONTRAINDICATIONS TO STENTING: POOR DISTAL RUNOFF. Coronary stents should not be placed in vessels which lack sufficient runoff to support flow across the stent due to the risk of stent thrombosis

Table 26.13. Principles of Bailout Stenting

Principle	Rationale	Technique
Complete coverage of dissection	Ensure laminar flow into and out of stent	Place stents distal to proximal; identify complete extent of dissection
Optimal stent sizing	Ensure complete apposition, expansion, and symmetry	Use high-pressure balloon and IVUS
Antiplatelet therapy	Reduce the risk of bleeding and stent thrombosis	Aspirin (325 mg QD) and clopidogrel (75 mg QD) for 2-4 weeks

Table 26.14. Multicenter Randomized Trials of PTCA vs. Palmaz-Schatz Stent[++]

	STRESS[471] (n = 407)		BENESTENT[472] (n = 516)	
	PTCA	Stent	PTCA	Stent
In-hospital Results (%)				
Procedural success	89.6	96.1**	91	92.7
Final diameter stenosis	35	19*	33	22*
All ischemic events	7.9	5.9	6.2	6.9
Death	1.5	0	0	0
Q-wave MI	3	2.9	0.8	1.9
non-Q-wave MI	2	1.5	2.3	1.5
CABG	4	2	3.9	3.1
PTCA	1	2	1.2	0.4
Bleeding/vascular	4	7.3	3.1	13.5*
Vessel occlusion[+]	10.2	3.4	6.2	3.5
Length of stay (days)	2.8	5.8*	3.1	8.5*
6-month Follow-up (%)				
Angiographic restenosis	42	31**	32	22*
Ischemic events	23	17	24	14
Target lesion revascularization	22	14**	27	18**
Event-free survival	72	78**	60	70**

Abbreviations: STRESS = Stent Restenosis Study; BENESTENT = Belgium Netherlands Stent Trial; CABG = emergency coronary artery bypass surgery

* $p < 0.001$
** $p < 0.005$
+   Vessel occlusion due to abrupt closure (PTCA group) or stent thrombosis (stent group)
++ Both studies utilized older warfarin-based regimens for stent patients

Table 26.15. Multicenter Wallstent Trials in North America

	WIN	WINS	WINS Registry
Description	Wallstent in Native Vessels	Wallstent in Saphenous Vein Grafts	Wallstent in Saphenous Vein Grafts
Design	Prospective, multicenter randomized trial	Prospective, multicenter randomized trial	Prospective, multicenter registry
Setting	Native coronary arteries (*de novo*, restenotic)	Saphenous vein grafts (*de novo*, restenotic)	Saphenous vein grafts (*de novo*, restenotic)
N (patients)	586	268	210
Study groups	PTCA vs. Wallstent	PS stent vs. Wallstent	Wallstent
1° Endpoint	MACE + stroke at 6 months	MACE + stroke at 6 months	MACE + stroke at 6 months
Vessel diameter	3.0-5.5 mm	3.0-4.0 mm	4.1-5.5 mm
Lesion length	≤ 22 (3-4 mm vessels) ≤ 35 (4.1-5.5 mm vessels)	≤ 22	≤ 35

Abbreviations: MACE = major adverse cardiac events (death, MI, rePTCA, CABG); PS stent = Palmaz-Schatz stent

Table 26.16. WIN Randomized Trial: Wallstent vs. PTCA in Native Vessels

	Wallstent	PTCA
N (patients)	299	287
In-hospital Results (%)		
Device success	96	60*
Procedure success	97	96
Final diameter stenosis	19	26*
Acute closure	1.7	1.9
MACE + stroke	8.0	5.9
Transfusion	4.0	1.7
Vascular complications	7.7	8.4
6-month Results (%)		
Diameter stenosis	45	46
Angiographic restenosis	38	38
Target lesion revascularization	13	15
MACE + stroke	20	20

Abbreviations: MACE = major adverse cardiac events (death, MI, rePTCA, or CABG); WIN = Wallstent In Native vessels
* $p < 0.05$

Table 26.17. Results of BENESTENT-II: PTCA vs. Heparin-coated Palmaz-Schatz Stent[829]

	PTCA (n = 413)	HCPSS (n = 414)
6-month Outcome (%)		
Death	0.5	0.2
Restenosis	31	16*
CABG	1.5	1.9
PTCA	13.7	8.0*
MACE	19.3	12.8*
1-year Outcome (%)		
Death	1.0	1.0
CABG	1.5	1.9
PTCA	15.6	9.4*
MACE	22.4	15.7*

Abbreviations: BENESTENT = Belgium-Netherlands Stent Investigation; HCPSS = Heparin-coated Palmaz-Schatz Stent; MACE = major adverse cardiac events (death, MI, PTCA, CABG)
* Statistically significant in favor of stenting

Table 26.18. Stent vs. Stent Trials

Trial	N	Stent Comparison	Outcome
BEST	650	BeStent vs. PSS	Pending
TENISS[869] (2000)	494	Tenax coated stent vs. Nir	No difference in hospital MACE or 6-month ARS (20.7% vs. 20.9%).
DISTINCT (2000)	628	BioDivYsio vs. MultiLink Duet	No difference in ARS (19.6% vs. 19.7%) or TVR at 6 months (8.0% vs. 7.1%)
MULTILINK-DUET[809] (1999)	270	MultiLink vs. MultiLink Duet	No difference in 30-day MACE or ARS at 6 months
ASCENT[692]	1040	MultiLink vs. PSS	No difference in ARS (15.6% vs. 20.5%) or TVR at 9 months (12.3% vs. 13.1%)
SMART[37]	662	MicroStent-II vs. PSS	No difference in ARS (25% vs. 23%), TLR, or MACE (16.1% vs. 14.8%) at 6 months
SCORES (1998)	1096	Radius vs. PSS	No difference in ARS or TVR at 9 months
NIRVANA[695] (1998)	849	Nir vs. PSS	No difference in ARS (20% vs. 21%) or TLR at 9 months (7.4% vs. 9.0%)
GRII[696]	755	GRII vs. PSS	More ARS (43% vs. 19%) and TLR at 12 months (26.6% vs. 14.9%) for GRII
WINS	268	Wallstent vs. PSS (SVG)	No difference (Table 26.16)
EXTRA[840] (1998)	649	Bard XT vs. PSS	No difference in ARS or MACE at 30 days

Abbreviations: ARS = angiographic restenosis; MACE = major adverse cardiac effects (death, MI, PTCA, CABG); PSS = Palmaz-Schatz stent; TLR = target lesion revascularization; TVR = target vessel revascularization
Acronyms: See Table 26.55, p. 587

Table 26.19. Observational Studies of Stents in Native Coronary Arteries

Stent Type	N	Reference #
Bard XT	355	515, 807, 511
BeStent	391	516, 519, 810
BioDivYsio	218	808
Microstent-II	2780	506, 512, 509, 510, 101, 111, 106
MultiLink	873	110, 503, 504, 507, 513, 514, 520, 872
MultiLink Duet	270	809
NIR Elite	614	508, 518, 843
NIROYAL Elite	165	808
Radius	207	805, 806, 811
Wiktor	1003	517, 103, 112, 107, 876

Acronyms: See Table 26.55, p. 587

Table 26.20. Multicenter Nonrandomized Stent Registry Studies

Study	N	Stent	Description
BeStent-2	250	BeStent 2	Pending
DISTINCT (2000)	200	BioDivYsio	BioDivYsio Stent in Coronary Artery Disease Therapy-Abrupt Closure (pending)
ESSEX[811] (2000)	103	Radius	European Scimed Stent Experience
FINESS-I[518] (1997)	255	NIR	First International Endovascular Stent Study
FINESS-2 (2000)	156	NIR	Second International Endovascular Stent Study
FREEDOM[842] (1996)	169	Freedom	The Freedom Stent for Bailout Indications
HEPACIS[845] (2000)	105	Heparinized	Heparin-coated Stents in Patients with Acute Ischemic Syndromes
HEPACOAT	200	BX-Velocity HC	Heparin-coated Bx-Velocity Stent (pending)
RECREATE[852] (1998)	173	MultiLink	Rescue of Closed Arteries Treated by Stent for Threatened Abrupt Closure
SCORES-SVG (1998)	155	Radius	Scimed Stent Comparative Restenosis Trial (SVG)
Wallstent SVG[873] (1998)	109	Wallstent	The Wallstent in Vein Graft Study
WEST-I[872] (1997)	102	MultiLink	West European Stent Trial-I
WEST-II[874] (1998)	165	MultiLink	West European Stent Trial-II (IVUS guidewire and reduced anticoagulation)
WIKTOR[875] (2000)	355	Wiktor	The Wiktor Stent Threatened or Abrupt Closure Registry

Table 26.21. Observational Studies of Stents for Saphenous Vein Grafts

Series	Stent	Lesions (N)	Success (%)	SAT (%)	Complications (%) D / MI / CABG	VSR/XF (%)	Restenosis (%)
Roffi[685] (2001)	Stent Other devices	206 72	- -	- -	- -		30-day MACE: 20.4 18.1
Leon[881] (2001)	Symbiot (PTFE-coated)	25	-	-	-	-	6.7
Ahmed[880] (2000)	PSS (diabetic) PSS (nondiabetic)	290 618	95 92	1.2 1.6	2.2 / 1.3 / 1.3 0.3 / 1.2 / 0.6	 -	1-yr EFS: 67 79
Hanekamp[871] (2000)	Wiktor PTCA	78 72	91 89	- -	9 9.7	- -	21.9 35.6
Choussat[527] (2000)	Wall++	126	-	-	3.2 / 8.7 / 0	-	44
Nishida[978] (2000)	Multiple	129	97	-	1 / 10.9 / 2	-	21
Horlitz[694] (2000)	Multiple (ostial)	30	90	3.3	0 / 3.3 / 6.6	-	38.5
Briguori[699] (2000)	PTFE Stent Stent	25 62	96 97	0 0	0 / 4 / 0 0 / 12 / 1.6	- -	31 39
Bhargava[695] (2000)	Single Multiple	649 70	99 98	0.7 0	1.3 / 17.1 / 0.9 2.8 / 30.8 / 0		23.2 20.9
Stoerger[693] (2000)	PTFE Stent	70	99	3.2	1.6 / 1.6 / -		22
Dharmadhikari[689] (2000)	PTFE Stent Stent PTCA	30 125 31	- - -	- - -	3.2 / 0 / 0 0 / 8.8 / 0 32. / 6.4 / 3.2	- - -	12-mo EFS: 73 56 48
Scavetta[555] (1999)	Multiple	92	95	3.3	3.3 / 8 / 0	2.2 / 9.8	-
Gruberg[559] (1999)	PTCA+ Stent+	182 77	96 99	0 0	1 / 11.5 / 0 0 / 12.0 / 1	6 4	25 14
Safian[617] (1999)	Wall PSS	139 130	- -	0.7 0.8	-	-	38.6 40.8
Winters[618] (1999)	TEC Stent PTCA	85 127 82	99 99 88	- - -	-	-	-
Safian[614] (1998)	PSS Wall	114 101	100 95	- -	-	-	32 13
Al-Mubarak[615] (1998)	TEC (<15mm) Wall (>15mm)	18 21	- -	0 4.7	0 / 0 / 0 0 / 0 / 0	-	-
Frimerman[892] (1997)	PSS, B	186	97.3	1.6	1.1 / 1.1 / 0/5	4.8 / 8.0	45
deJaegere[588] (1996)	PSS, Wall	62	89	3.0	3 / 3 / 5	12.9 / 9.8	30**

Table 26.21. Observational Studies of Stents for Saphenous Vein Grafts

Series	Stent	Lesions (N)	Success (%)	SAT (%)	Complications (%) D / MI / CABG	VSR/XF (%)	Restenosis (%)
Wong[127] (1995)	PSS	624	98.8	1.4	1.7 / 0.3 / 0.9	8.0 / 6.3	30
Rechavia[674] (1995)	PSS, B	29	100	0	0	3.4 / 6.8	-
Wong[700] (1995)	PSS, B	309	95.3	1.7	1.3 / 0.9 / 0.4	8.4 / 25	-
Denardo[701*] (1995)	PSS, B	300	93.3	6.7	0	16.7	-
Piana[125] (1994)	PSS, B	200	98.5	0.6	- / 0.6 / 0	8.5 / 14.0	0

Abbreviations: Success = procedural success (some studies do not distinguish between angiographic vs. clinical success); RS = restenosis; SAT = subacute thrombus; MI = in-hospital myocardial infarction (some studies do not distinguish between Q-wave vs. non-Q-wave MI); CABG = emergency coronary artery bypass surgery; VSR/XF = vascular surgery repair/blood transfusion; Wall = Wallstent; Wik = Wiktor stent; PSS = Palmaz-Schatz stent; B = biliary stent; GRS = Gianturco-Roubin stent; - = not reported

* Thrombotic vein grafts; adjunctive urokinase infusion for 20.5 hrs.

** 5-year event-free survival (no death, MI, TLR)

\+ Distal anastomotic lesions

\++ Diffusely degenerated grafts

Table 26.22. WINS Trial: Wallstent vs. Palmaz-Schatz Stent for Saphenous Vein Grafts

	WINS Randomized Trial		WINS Registry
	Wallstent	**PS Stent**	**Wallstent**
N (patients/lesions)	139/156	129/141	210/236
In-hospital Results (%)			
Procedure success	98	99	95
Final diameter stenosis	5.4	8.5	7.9
Stent thrombosis	0.7	0.8	2.4
MACE + stroke	8.6	7.8	16.7
Transfusion	5.0	3.9	6.7
Vascular complications	6.5	6.2	9.0
6-month Results (%)			
Diameter stenosis	42	46	39
Angiographic restenosis	33	33	28
Target lesion revascularization	13	12	8
MACE + stroke	28	23	27

Abbreviations: MACE = major adverse cardiac events (death, MI, rePTCA, CABG); PS = Palmaz-Schatz

Table 26.23. Observational Studies of Stents for Ostial Stenosis

Series	Device	Lesion	N	Success (%)	In-hospital MACE (%)	Other Results
Ahmed[889] (2000)	Debulk/Stent Stent	SVG	133 187	- -	- -	Similar 1-year EFS and TVR (19.4% vs. 18.2%)
Park[928] (2000)	Stent	AO LAD	111	97	4.5	ARS (26%); TLR (11.7%); 2-yr EFS (84.6%)
Mintz[929] (2000)	Stent	Ostial vs. nonostial	-	-	-	TLR higher in ostial group (17.4% vs. 12.0% p = 0.02)
Wishmeyer[930] (1999)						Diss(%) / AC(%) / 6-moTLR(%)
	PTCA	AO	73	97	-	22 4.1 22
	Debulk	AO	32	100	-	16 3.1 19
	Stent	AO	73	100	-	1.4 0 25
	PTCA	BO	98	93	-	15 2.0 16
	Debulk	BO	24	100	-	8.3 0 17
	Stent	BO	23	100	-	0 0 29
Peterson[546] (1999)	Stent	AO RCA	88	98	-	-
Asakaura[931] (1998)	PSS DCA	LAD LAD	11 13	100 100	0 0	More plaque shift after stenting than DCA
Mathur[932] (1997)	PSS GRS	BO BO	14 34	100 100	0 0	TLR (7.1% vs. 17.6%)
Kurbaan[933] (1997)	MLS, WS	AO	11	100	0	Cutting balloon before stenting
Jain[145] (1997)	PTCA ROTA/DCA ELCA/Stent	RCA RCA RCA	23 20 54	88 77 96	0 0 2	TLR: 47% 40% 24%
DeCesare[935] (1996)	PSS	LAD	23	87	0	RS (22%)
Colombo[60] (1996)	Stent	AO	35	100	0	RS (23%)
DeCesare[537] (1996)	Stent	Ostial LAD	23	100	0	RS (22%)
Rocha-Singh[143] (1995)	Stent	AO + BO	41	93	5	RS (28%)
Rechavia[141] (1995)	PSS	AO	29	100	-	RS (15%)
Wong[146] (1995)	PSS	AO SVG	104	97	2	RS (62%)

Abbreviations: AC = acute closure; AO = aorto-ostial; BO = branch-ostial; DCA = directional coronary atherectomy; EFS = event-free survival (freedom from death, MI, CABG, repeat PTCA); ELCA = excimer laser coronary angioplasty; GRS = Gianturco-Roubin stent; ILCA = infrared laser coronary angioplasty; MACE = major adverse cardiac events; MLS = MultiLink stent; PSS = Palmaz-Schatz stent; ROTA = Rotablator; RS = restenosis; TEC = transluminal extraction catheter; TLR = target lesion revascularization; WS = Wallstent; - = not reported

Table 26.24. Observational Studies of Stents for Chronic Total Occlusion[‡]

Series	Device	N	Results
Gruberg[960] (2000)	Debulk*/stent Stent alone	44 108	In-hospital MACE (2.3% vs. 6.5%); no difference in TLR (14.4% vs. 16.3%) or MACE (19.6% vs. 25.6%) at 14 months
Azuma (2000)	Debulk+/stent Stent alone	52 224	Debulk/stent with less restenosis
Anzuini[963] (1998)	Stent	89	Success (98%); in-hospital MACE (5.6%); restenosis (32%) and reocclusion (4%) at 19 months; MACE at 1 year (13%) and 3 years (28%)
Suttorp[964] (1998)	Stent	38	Restenosis (40%) and reocclusion (23%) at 6 months
Yamasaki[965] (1998)	Stent PTCA	143 75	Stents with greater patency at 3 years (88% vs. 63%)
Carere[966] (1998)	Stent OPTCA SOPTCA	194 122 74	OPTCA and stents had similar 6-month patency, TLR, and angiographic restenosis. Both were significantly better than SOPTCA
Rau[968] (1998)	Stent	143	Restenosis (22%) and reocclusion (7%) at 4.5 months
Elezi[969] (1997)	Stent (CTO) Stent (no CTO)	54 972	CTO group had more restenosis (40% vs. 26%) and reocclusion (14% vs. 3%)
Mathey[169] (1997)	Stent	143	Restenosis (28%); reocclusion (7%)
Ozaki[961] (1996)	Stent PTCA	20 66	Similar restenosis (29% vs. 45%)
Ooka[905] (1995)	Stent PTCA	47 65	Stents had less restenosis (44% vs. 68%) and reocclusion (10% vs. 35%)
Goldberg[163] (1995)	PSS	60	Restenosis (20%); 14-month EFS (77%)

Abbreviations: CTO = chronic total occlusion; MACE = major adverse cardiac events (death, MI, repeat revascularization); OPTCA = optimal PTCA; SOPTCA = suboptimal PTCA; TLR = target lesion revascularization;
* DCA, ELCA, or Rotablator prior to stenting
+ DCA or Rotablator prior to stenting
‡ See Table 26.12 for randomized trials

Table 26.25. Observational Studies of Stents for Long Lesions[‡]

Series	Stent (lesion)	N	Success (%)	MACE (%) Early	Late	ARS (%)	TLR (%)
Kornowski[936] (2000)	Stent (> 25 mm)	116	96	3.4	-	-	14.5
	Stent (< 20 mm)	1110	98	1.0	-	-	13.8
Hong[937] (2000)	Multiple ≥ (20 mm)	246	-	-	-	32	-
Ormiston[938] (2000)	MultiLink (25, 35 mm)	120	98		3	32	14
DeGregorio[939] (2000)	Spot stenting (IVUS)	101	-	3.0	22	26	20
	Long stent	143	-	3.5	36	38	32
Kobayashi[940] (1999)	Stent (≤ 20 mm)	565	96	-	-	24	-
	Stent (21-35 mm)	278	98	-	-	35	-
	Stent (> 35 mm)	247	92	-	-	47	-
Schalij[941] (1999)	Micro Stent II	119	98	5.4	10.1	-	-
Williams[942] (1999)	Wallstent	182	99	3.7	-	41	-
Nakagawa[943] (1999)	GFX ≤ 18	64	97	-	-	23.4	14.1
	GFX 24	56	96	-	-	35.7	21.4
	GFX 30	26	96	-	-	46.2	34.6
Kerr[660] (1998)	Various	34	94	-	-	18	24
Rankin[944] (1998)	Stent (< 16 mm)	-	-	-	-	-	6.3
	Stent (16-32 mm)	-	-	-	-	-	13.2
	Stent (> 32 mm)	-	-	-	-	-	17.8
Kobayashi[945] (1998)	PSS	-	92	-	-	16.5	-
	Nir 16	-	93	-	-	13.3	-
	Nir 32	-	93	-	-	51.3	-
Elezi[946] (1998)	Stent (≥ 15 mm)	371	-	-	28.3	33.7	-
	Stent (< 15 mm)	1420	-	-	21.8	25.2	-
LeBreton[947] (1998)	Nir 32	187	93	3.5	19.6	-	6
Antoniucci[948] (1998)	Freedom (> 20 mm)	27	100	0	11	38	11
Maiello[158] (1995)	PSS, GRS, Wiktor	108	93	6	-	35	-
Akira[949] (1995)	PSS	62	-	-	-	39	-
	GRS	26	-	-	-	35	-
	Wiktor	21	-	-	-	24	-

Abbreviations: ARS = angiographic restenosis; GRS = Gianturco-Roubin stent; MACE = major adverse cardiac events (death, MI, CABG, rePTCA); PSS = Palmaz-Schatz stent; SAT = subacute thrombosis; TLR = target lesion revascularization; - = not reported
‡ See Table 26.12 for randomized trials

Table 26.26. Observational Studies of Stents for Small Vessels[‡]

Series	Device	N	Success	Early MACE	Other Results
Feres[697] (2001)	Stent ($\leq$ 2.5 mm)	397	98	-	Less TVR at 9 months for largest balloon diameter > 2.5 mm vs. $\leq$ 2.5 mm (12.3% vs. 21.7%, p = 0.005)
Stankovic[698] (2001)	Stent ($\leq$ 2.8 mm) *Final balloon < 3 mm* *Final balloon = 3 mm*	124 385	- -	5.6 6.3	Study of balloon sizing after stenting vessels $\leq$ 2.8 mm. Similar late MACE, restenosis, and TLR
Germing[800] (2000)	Stent (< 3 mm) Stent (> 3 mm)	128 92	- -	- -	No difference in hospital MACE or SAT (1.6% vs. 1.1%); more late TLR in small vessels
Briguori[799] (2000)	PTCA (< 3mm) Stent (< 3 mm)	97 12	95 97	- -	No difference in hospital or late MACE; trend towards more restenosis after PTCA; SAT
Caputo[951] (2000)	XT stent PSS	178 160	- -	- -	Late MACE (18% vs. 12%); TLR (12% vs. 18%); RS (41% vs. 32%)
Al Suwaidi[952] (2000)	Stent (2.5 mm) Stent ($\geq$3.0 mm)	108 4077	97 97	- -	Late MACE (35% vs. 21%)
Mori[953] (2000)	PTCA/stent (3.0/2.5 mm) PTCA/stent (2.5/2.5 mm)	31 53	- -	- -	RS (12% vs. 53%); TLR (10% vs. 35%)
Kastrati[954] (2000)	PTCA (diabetes) Stent (diabetes)	49 51	- -	- -	No difference in death (4%), MI (4%), TLR (30% vs. 25%), or RS (44%) at 7 months
Hamasaki[955] (1999)	PTCA PSS MultiLink	199 1005 303	87 92 92	- - -	ARS (56% vs. 31% vs. 23%); TLR (40% vs. 19% vs. 13%)
Akiyama[797] (1998)	Stent ($\geq$ 3 mm) Stent (< 3 mm)	696 602	95 96	- -	No difference in hospital MACE or SAT; 1-yr EFS better for small vessels (71% vs. 63%, p < 0.01)
Shuhlen (1998)	Stent	574	-	-	SAT (2.8%); ARS (38%); 1-yr TLR (24%); 1-yr MACE (26%). Similar ARS with high/low pressure inflations
Farshid[528] (1998)	BeStent	135	99	-	SAT (0.7%); ARS (12.6%)
Michael[956] (1998)	PTCA Stent	83 54	84 93	-	TLR at 6 months (10.8% vs. 11.1%)
Elezi[529] (1998)	Stent (< 2.8 mm) Stent (2.8-3.2 mm) Stent (> 3.2 mm)	870 866 866	- - -	4.5 3.3 2.9	SAT (2.4% vs. 2.5% vs. 2.0%); ARS (39% vs. 28% vs. 20%)
Waksman[957] (1998)	PTCA Stent	148 284	95 92	- -	Late MACE (31% vs. 34%); TLR (22% vs. 27%)
Deutsch[959] (1998)	Stent ($\geq$3.0 mm) Stent (< 3.0 mm)	88 122	- -	- -	ARS: (25% vs. 34%)

Abbreviations: ARS = angiographic restenosis; DM = diabetes mellitus; GR II = Gianturco-Roubin II stent; MACE = major adverse cardiac events (death, MI, CABG, rePTCA); PSS = Palmaz-Schatz stent; RS = restenoses; SAT = subacute stent thrombosis; TLR = target lesion revascularization; - = not reported

‡ See Table 26.12 for randomized trials

Table 26.27. Observational Studies of Stents for Bifurcation Lesions

Series	N	Stent	Technique	Results
Suwaidi[921] (2000)	77 (A)	Various	Stent in one branch; PTCA in other branch	Procedural success (89.5% in group A vs. 97.4% in group B). In-hospital MACE higher with Culotte stenting vs. T-stenting (p = 0.004). No difference in MACE at 1 year
	54 (B)	Various	T-stent, Culotte stent	
Yamashita[922] (2000)	53 (A)	-	Stent in one branch; PTCA in other branch	Acute procedural success similar. Group B had lower residual stenosis (p < 0.001) and higher in-hospital MACE (p < 0.05); 6-month TVR and MACE were similar
	39 (B)	-	Stent in both branches	
de Scheerder[552] (1999)	21	V-Flex	Culotte stent	Procedural success (100%); CK elevation (10%)
Sheiban[547] (1999)	54	Various	T-stent	Procedural success (100%); ARS (45%)
Anzuini[553] (1998)	59	Wiktor	Culotte stent, T-stent, stent-and-retrieve	Procedural success 96% (similar for different techniques); more in-hospital MACE (43% vs. 17%) and higher restenosis (41% vs. 19%) using Culotte and T-stent techniques vs. stent-and-retrieve
Brunel[554] (1998)	107	-	Multiple	Angiographic success (93%); higher restenosis (57% vs. 21%) and TLR (43% vs. 8%) in double-stent techniques vs. stent-and-retrieve
Carrie[923] (1998)	54	Wiktor	Culotte stent, T-stent	Clinical success (91%); sidebranch occlusion (5.5%); ARS (25.6%)
Chevalier[924] (1998)	50	Various	Culotte stent	Clinical success (94%); non-Q-MI (6%); TLR (24%)
Lefevre[925] (1998)	161	-	Multiple	Procedural success (96%); significant learning curve suggested by lower TLR (10.9% vs. 36.7%) and less MACE (14.6% vs. 45.6%) during later experience
Pan[926] (1998)	70	-	Stent-and-retrieve, T-stent	T-stent patients had similar procedural success (91% vs. 93%) but more MACE at 15 months (39% vs. 13%)

Abbreviations: ARS = angiographic restenosis; MACE = major adverse cardiac events (death, MI, repeat revascularization); TLR = target lesion revascularization

Table 26.28. Observational Studies of Stents for Other Lesion Subsets

Series	Stent	Subset	N	Success (%)	SAT (%)	Comments
Bossi[714] (2001)	PCI	Prox LAD	224	-	-	In-hospital MACE (3.1%); follow-up at 1.6 yrs: death (2.6%); MI (1.3%); TLR (16.5%)
Singh[715] (2001)	PTCA ± Stent ROTA	Calcified	2065 447	- -	10.9 13.0	Residual stenosis < 50% (93% vs. 98%, p < 0.0001)
Kobayashi[716] (2001)	Stent	No/Mild Ca^{++} Mod. Ca^{++} Severe Ca^{++}	215 75 76	- - -	- - -	Final lumen cross-sectional area > 6.0 mm^2 (71% vs. 60% vs. 58%). Only 73% of severely calcified lesions by IVUS were calcified on angiography
Dauerman[796] (2000)	Stent PTCA	Lytic failure Lytic failure	45 63	88 78	2.2 -	Nonrandomized study of "rescue" after failed lytic therapy for acute MI; 1-yr MACE lower for stents (9.7% vs. 31%, p < 0.05)
Wong[521] (1997)	PSS GRS	Allograft	12	100	8.3	Less restenosis with stenting compared to PTCA
Jain[934] (1997)	Stent	Allograft	10	100	-	
Heublein[544] (1997)	Tenax NIR	Allograft	27		0	ARS (25%)
Colombo[525] (1996)	PSS	Restenosis	128	98	0.8	ARS (23%)
Hoffman[426] (1998)	Stent ROTA/Stent ROTA/PTCA	Calcified (> 3 mm)	103 56 147	98 98 99	-	In-hospital MACE (3.0% vs. 3.6% vs. 1.4%); TLR (21% vs. 15% vs. 28%)
Moussa[224] (1997)	Various	Calcified, complex	106	94	2.8	ARS (23%); TLR (18%); adjunctive Rotablator in all lesions
Mintz[227] (1995)	PSS	Calcified	88	100	-	Adjunctive Rotablator in all lesions
Alfonso[225] (1997)	Various	Thrombus	86	96	1.0	1-yr EFS (77%); ARS (33%)
Kaul[221] (1996)	PSS	Thrombus	12	100	0	No complications; warfarin in 58%
Menafoglio[524] (1998)	Micro	< 8 mm	-	96	-	

Abbreviations: ARS = angiographic restenosis; EFS = event-free survival; GRS = Gianturco-Roubin stent; MACE = major adverse cardiac events; PSS = Palmaz-Schatz stent; SAT = subacute thrombosis; TLR = target lesion revascularization - = not reported

Table 26.29. Comparison of Planned vs. Provisional Stenting

Strategy	Advantages	Disadvantages
Planned stenting	• Excellent immediate angiographic results • Low-risk of in-hospital MACE • Most operations rely on angiographic criteria	• Most lesions are not STRESS/BENESTENT lesions • Lack of ideal therapy for restenosis • Stenting not clearly beneficial • Higher procedural costs than PTCA • Higher risk of asymptomatic CK release
Provisional stenting	• Stenting is still feasible • Ideal PTCA result leaves open the option for future stenting • Potential cost-savings • Preserves access to sidebranches	• Angiography alone is unable to assess result • Need IVUS, FFR, or CFR

Abbreviations: CFR = coronary flow reserve; FFR = fractional flow reserve; IVUS = intravascular ultrasound; MACE = major adverse cardiac events

STENT RESTENOSIS

A. **INCIDENCE.** Quantitative angiography after stenting frequently reveals angiographic restenosis rates of 26-33% in vein grafts and 8-23% in native vessels.[76,79,81,83,99,104,105,108,127] Two large multicenter randomized trials (STRESS, BENESTENT) compared immediate and long-term results of elective Palmaz-Schatz stenting vs. PTCA in *de novo* lesions in native coronary arteries (Table 26.14);[115,116] both studies confirmed that stenting resulted in less restenosis, in addition to better lumen enlargement, higher procedural success, fewer repeat procedures, and better event-free survival. Similar findings were reported in a trial of Palmaz-Schatz stenting vs. PTCA in patients with isolated stenosis of the proximal LAD[191] and in a multicenter randomized trial in Spain.[192] Importantly, the benefits of stenting and target lesion revascularization were preserved at 1 year in BENESTENT (10% vs. 21%)[119] and at 4 years in START (12% vs. 25%).[863] In contrast to the excellent results in focal, *de novo* lesions, elective stenting of restenotic lesions resulted in more restenosis (39% vs. 14%),[189] and stent deployment in complex lesions (which would not meet inclusion criteria for the STRESS/BENESTENT trials) resulted in higher rates of late revascularization compared to simple lesions.[153,154] In contrast to other trials of PTCA vs. stent, the WIN trial failed to show a restenosis advantage for stenting (Table 26.16); however, 36% of PTCA patients crossed over to Wallstent, which obscured differences in restenosis rates based on intention-to-treat (i.e., patients who crossed over to Wallstent were analyzed as PTCA patients). Several trials demonstrated similar rates of angiographic restenosis and late revascularization among various stent designs (Tables 26.14, 26.17, 26.18).

B. **TIME COURSE FOR STENT RESTENOSIS.** The time course of stent restenosis is similar to PTCA.[193,194] However, several angiographic studies suggest that in-stent minimal lumen diameter improves between 6 months and 3 years after implantation, suggesting that 6-month angiography may underestimate the long-term benefit of stenting.[195-197] In one study, 85% of target vessel revascularization procedures were performed within 12 months, whereas 15% were performed between

1-3 years after stenting.[198] In another report, recurrent ischemia beyond 12 months after native-vessel stenting was virtually always due to progressive disease in a non-stented vessel.[199]

C. **PREDICTORS OF STENT RESTENOSIS AND EVENT-FREE SURVIVAL.** Comparisons of late outcome after stenting are hampered by different indications for stents (abrupt closure vs. elective stents), different stent designs, and different target lesions (native vessels or vein grafts). Angiographic, procedural, and IVUS predictors of stent restenosis include multiple stents, vessel diameter < 3.0 mm, restenotic lesions, ostial lesions, lesion length >10 mm, small stent lumen cross-sectional area and MLD, and large baseline plaque burden.[200-204,415,625,,646] In addition, several clinical variables have been associated with adverse late outcome, including diabetes, post-procedural non-Q-wave MI, and multivessel disease.[203,646,805]

D. **PATTERNS OF STENT RESTENOSIS.** In one report, angiographic patterns of stent restenosis included diffuse stent restenosis (33%), focal restenosis at the edges of the stent (26%), and focal in-stent restenosis involving the articulation (33%) or body of the stent (8%) (Figure 24.7).[205]

E. **TREATMENT OF STENT RESTENOSIS (Chapter 24).** Although treatment of stent restenosis is easy, safe, and highly successful from a technical standpoint, long-term outcomes have been disappointing. Potential strategies include mechanical techniques, pharmacotherapy, and intracoronary brachytherapy; of these, brachytherapy appears to hold the most promise (Table 26.31).

1. **PTCA.** Conventional PTCA is the most common technique for treatment of stent restenosis, but recurrent restenosis ranges from 30-80%, depending on the target lesion and pattern of restenosis (Figure 24.7).[654] Mechanisms of lumen enlargement with PTCA include compression and extrusion of intimal tissue.[207,664,773] IVUS is useful to exclude "pseudorestenosis," since further PTCA with larger balloons may result in better stent expansion (Chapter 31). Predictors of recurrent restenosis after PTCA included longer lesion length, diabetes, and small final MLD.[639]

2. **Debulking Techniques.** Directional atherectomy, rotational atherectomy, and ELCA have been employed with high procedural success and low complication rates. Despite initial enthusiasm for these techniques based on superior immediate angiographic results compared to PTCA,[211,212] randomized trials have not demonstrated a consistent restenosis advantage (Table 26.32); late MACE after treatment for diffuse stent restenosis was lower after Rotablator compared to PTCA in ROSTER, but not in ARTIST.

3. **Stenting.** Additional stenting within a previously deployed stent ("stent-in-a-stent" or "stent-wich") is a reliable and effective means to achieve excellent lumen enlargement and immediate angiographic results. However, the long-term consequences of this approach are unknown. A modification of this approach is the use of a PTFE-covered stent,[779] particularly for conduit vessels without significant sidebranches (such as the RCA or vein grafts); long-term results are pending.

4. **Cutting Balloon Angioplasty.** Observational studies suggest that compared to conventional PTCA, cutting balloon angioplasty increases immediate lumen dimensions when applied to coronary artery stenoses. Recently, the cutting balloon has been applied to stent restenosis,[780,781] and similar immediate angiographic results have been observed. However, experience with ELCA

Table 26.30. Adjunctive IVUS and Doppler for Stents

Study	N	Purpose	Comment
IVUS-GUIDED STENTING			
Abizaid[899] (2001)	2883	Evaluate IVUS-guided stenting vs. angiography	Observational study. IVUS with larger final lumen CSA and less TVR (12.3% vs. 15.1%, p = 0.04) and MACE (15.1% vs. 18.4%, p = 0.02) at 6 months
CRUISE[831] (2000)	1650	Evaluate IVUS-guided stenting vs. angiography	Prospective randomized trial. IVUS resulted in better lumen dimensions and less TLR at 9 months (8.5% vs. 15.3%, p < 0.05)
RESIST[853] (2000)	155	Stent deployment with and without IVUS guidance (small vessels)	Prospective randomized trial. Less TLR (27% vs. 41%, p < 0.05) but higher cost with IVUS
OSTI-1[851] (1999)	89	IVUS-guided high-pressure stent deployment	As implantation pressure increased from 12 to 18 atm, IVUS stent dimensions increased, but QCA was unable to identify these changes
START[862] (1999)	122	Evaluate IVUS-guided DCA vs. stenting	Prospective randomized trial. IVUS-guided DCA resulted in less ARS at 6 months (15.8% vs. 32.8%) and less TLR at 1 year (15% vs. 29%, p = 0.06)
MUSIC[849] (1998)	161	Evaluate aspirin alone after IVUS-guided stenting	Prospective multicenter registry. 1-month MACE (5.1%); 6-month ARS (9.7%)
WEST-II[874] (1998)	165	Evaluate aspirin alone after IVUS-guided stenting	Prospective multicenter registry. Aspirin alone was safe when using IVUS-guided optimal stenting and QCA
SIPS[857] (1997)	269	Stent deployment with and without IVUS guidance	Multicenter randomized trial. IVUS associated with less ARS (21% vs. 41%, p < 0.001), repeat PTCA (18% vs. 24%, p < 0.05), and MACE (24% vs. 33%, p = 0.09) at 6 months
AVID[826] (1996)	800	Evaluate IVUS-guided stenting vs. angiography alone	Prospective randomized trial. No difference in hospital MACE or stent thrombosis; better lumen dimensions with IVUS and lower TLR at 1 year in SVG lesions, vessels > 2.5 mm, and stenosis > 70%
APLAUSE[824] (1996)	280	Evaluate aspirin plus ticlopidine after IVUS-guided stenting	Prospective observational study. 1-year TLR: native vessels (11.8%), SVG (18.7%)
IMPRESS[846]	245	IVUS assessment of intimal proliferation after local delivery of nadroparin during stenting	Multicenter randomized trial. Local delivery of low molecular weight heparin had no impact on intimal proliferation after stenting
DOPPLER-GUIDED STENTING			
FROST[843] (2000)	251	Evaluate routine vs. provisional stenting using Doppler flow	Provisional stenting was required in 48% of PTCA patients. TLR (15% vs. 14.4%) and ARS (27.1% vs. 21.4%) were similar for provisional and routine stenting; "optimal PTCA" not evaluated
DESTINI[834] (1999)	769	Evaluate Doppler-guided optimal PTCA vs. stenting	Multicenter, prospective randomized trial. Optimal PTCA by Doppler still had higher TLR (18.1% vs. 9.2% vs. 8.4%) and clinical restenosis (26.2% vs. 12.3% vs. 14.6%) than provisional or planned stenting
DEBATE-II[833] (1998)	620	Evaluate Doppler-guided optimal PTCA vs. stenting	Multicenter, prospective randomized trial. Stent and PTCA patients with final CFR ≥ 2.5 had better outcomes than those with CFR < 2.5; MACE at 12 months was lower for stents than PTCA, regardless of CFR

Abbreviations: ARS = angiographic restenosis; CFR = coronary flow reserve; IVUS = intravascular ultrasound; MACE = major adverse cardiac events; PCI = percutaneous coronary intervention; QCA = quantitative coronary angiography; SVG = saphenous vein graft; TLR = target lesion revascularization; *Acronyms*: See Table 26.55, p. 587

Table 26.31. Treatment Strategies for Stent Restenosis

Technique	Comment
Mechanical Approaches	
PTCA	Success rates exceed 90%; restenosis rates vary from 30-80% depending on pattern of stent restenosis and nature of target lesion[207-210,641,654,664,773]
Debulking (DCA, Rotablator, ELCA)	Despite initial enthusiasm,[211,212,823] randomized trials show no benefit compared to PTCA (Table 26.17)
Stenting ("stent-wich")	Achieves the best immediate angiographic results; long-term outcomes are uncertain[774]
Cutting balloon	May facilitate immediate lumen enlargement but further study is needed
Pharmacologic Approaches (Table 26.28)	
Anti-sense DNA	No benefit (ITALICS trial)
Abciximab	No benefit (ERASER trial)
Trapidil	TRAPIST trial pending
Tranilast	Trials pending
Brachytherapy (Chapter 24)	Shows the most promise for inhibition of intimal proliferation; efficacy of beta- and gamma-radiation are established; residual issues include edge effect, delayed thrombosis, and unknown late effects

and Rotablator suggest that interventions which result in superior immediate angiographic results do not necessarily ensure better long-term results. Disadvantages of the cutting balloon include its large profile, short length, and frequent need for extra-support guidewires to access distal vessels. On the other hand, its large profile virtually eliminates any concerns about "watermelon seeding" once positioned in the target lesion.

5. **Pharmacologic Approaches.** The results of pharmacologic trials to prevent stent restenosis have been disappointing (Table 26.33). IVUS was employed to determine if anti-sense DNA (ITALICS trial) or abciximab (ERASER trial) could inhibit intimal proliferation; both studies were negative. Studies using trapidil and the anti-keloid drug tranilast are underway.[213,214]

6. **Local Drug Delivery.** Several studies are in progress to evaluate local delivery of ethanol or taxol to prevent recurrent stent restenosis.

7. **Helixcisor.** The Helixcisor (Prolifix Medical, Inc.) is a novel 4F device that rotates at 17,500 rpm and is designed specifically for stent restenosis. When used with a special 0.014-inch helical guidewire, the Helixcisor can cut and aspirate intimal tissue, achieving a large, smooth lumen. Preclinical studies are in progress.

8. **Brachytherapy**. Intracoronary brachytherapy is the most promising therapy for stent restenosis, and is discussed in detail in Chapter 24.

Table 26.32. Results of Debulking Strategies for Stent Restenosis

Series	Device	N	Comments
ROSTER[681] (2001)	ROTA PTCA	100 100	Randomized trial. ROTA had similar 30-day MACE (2% vs. 3%), but less TLR (32% vs. 45%, p = 0.04)
LARS	ELCA PTCA	160 160	Prospective multicenter randomized trial (pending)
ARTIST[682] (2000)	PTCA ROTA	146 152	Randomized trial for diffuse stent restenosis; ROTA had similar success (89% vs. 88%), but higher MACE (14.5% vs. 6.8%, p < 0.05), ARS (65% vs. 51%, p < 0.05), and TLR (48% vs. 36%) at 6 months
Mehran[704] (2000)	ELCA ROTA	158 161	Success (100%); compared to ROTA, ELCA had similar late MACE and 1-year TLR (28% vs 26%)
Koster[775] (2000)	ELCA	96	Poor outcomes at 6 months: ARS (54%); TLR (49%)
Haase[776] (1999)	ELCA	440	Success (92%); in-hospital MACE (6.4%). Non-randomized LARS trial
Lauer[703] (1999)	ELCA ROTA PTCA	78 83 124	Immediate lumen enlargement was better for ELCA and ROTA than PTCA, but at 6 months ROTA results were better than ELCA and PTCA
Mehran[706] (1999)	PTCA ELCA ROTA Stent	314 250 126 131	Immediate lumen enlargement was best for stenting, but no difference in 1-year TLR (PTCA 26.6%, ELCA 31%, ROTA 23.1%, stent 27%); device was not a predictor of TLR
Koster[707] (1998)	ELCA	90	Low incidence of complications
Haase[709] (1998)	ELCA PTCA	47 49	Randomized trial. ELCA had similar success (98%), in-hospital complications (8%), late MACE (25% vs. 30%), and ARS (52% vs. 47%)
Dauerman[710] (1998)	PTCA ROTA or DCA	40 40	Success in both groups (100%); better final diameter stenosis after debulking (18% vs. 26%, p = 0.01); TLR at 1 year was lower after debulking (28% vs. 46%, p = 0.18). Predictors of restenosis were diabetes, long lesion length, and smaller final MLD
Sharma[711] (1998)	ROTA	100	Success (100%); ARS (28%); TVR (26%). Predictors of re-restenosis were burr/artery ratio <0.6%, ostial lesion, stent for a restenotic lesion, and diffuse in-stent restenosis
Lee[712] (1998)	ROTA PTCA	36 45	Clinical restenosis was lower after ROTA (2.5% vs. 47%, p < 0.05) and angina-free survival was higher (72% vs. 49%, p = 0.02) at 6 months
Mehran[713] (1997)	ELCA PTCA	54 44	ELCA was associated with greater lumen gain and a trend toward less TLR (21% vs. 38%, p = 0.08)

Abbreviations: ARS = angiographic restenosis; ARTIST = Angioplasty vs. Rotational Atherectomy for Treatment of Diffuse In-Stent Restenosis; ELCA = excimer laser coronary angioplasty; LARS = Laser Angioplasty for Restenosed Stents; MACE = major adverse cardiac events; MLD = minimum lumen diameter ROTA = Rotablator; TLR = target lesion revascularization

Table 26.33. Randomized Trials of Pharmacologic Treatment for Stent Restenosis

Trial	Study Groups	N	Hypothesis	Comments
TRAPIST	Trapidil Placebo	(160) (160)	Trapidil will inhibit intimal hyperplasia	Pending
ERASER[819] (1999)	Abciximab (12 hrs) Abciximab (24 hrs) Placebo	79 75 71	Abciximab will inhibit intimal hyperplasia	No difference in IVUS parameters at 6 months
ITALICS[818] (1998)	Placebo Antisense-DNA*	40 45	Antisense DNA will inhibit intimal hyperplasia	No difference in angiographic restenosis or intimal volume by IVUS at 6 months

Abbreviations: TRAPIST = Trapidil on Restenosis after Stenting; ERASER = Evaluation of ReoPro and Stenting to Eliminate Restenosis; ITALICS = Investigation by the Thoraxcenter on Antisense-DNA given by Local delivery and assessed by IVUS after Coronary Stenting
* Anti C-myc RNA

SPECIAL CLINICAL SITUATIONS

Stents are the dominant platform for percutaneous revascularization.[231-236] The indications and spectrum of patient subsets now eligible for stenting have been broadly expanded.[7]

A. ACUTE MYOCARDIAL INFARCTION (Chapter 5)

1. **Rationale for Stents.** Primary PTCA for acute myocardial infarction is superior to intravenous thrombolysis, but is limited by recurrent ischemia in 10-15%, reocclusion of the infarct-related artery in 5-10% (half of which cause reinfarction), and restenosis in 37-49%.[238-240] The primary angiographic predictors of recurrent ischemia after primary PTCA— residual stenosis > 30% and residual dissection[241]—are readily treated with stents. Despite initial concerns about deploying a metal stent in a thrombosed vessel, the ability of stents to seal dissections, prevent recoil, and eliminate residual stenosis suggests that laminar flow is more important clinically than the potential prothrombotic characteristics of stents.[242-249]

2. **Stents for Failed PTCA.** Pooled results from 13 registries of bailout stenting for MI comprising more than 1000 patients suggest high procedural success (96%), infrequent stent thrombosis (3.4%), and an acceptable risk of ischemic complications (death 5.4%, reinfarction 1.2%, repeat PTCA 5.1%, and CABG 1.9%). In Stent-PAMI, 15.1% of primary PTCA patients required bailout stenting, which was associated with less restenosis (15.9% vs. 36.9%, p = 0.007) and target vessel revascularization (6.9% vs. 16.2%, p = 0.07) than successful PTCA.[262] Available studies suggest that bailout stenting during acute MI has favorable short- and long-term clinical outcomes. Anticoagulation should include aspirin and clopidogrel; although three days of heparin were utilized in Stent-PAMI, post-procedural heparin is not routinely prescribed.

3. **Primary Stenting.** In contrast to bailout stenting, primary stenting is a planned strategy of stenting the infarct-related artery regardless of PTCA success. Observational studies of primary stenting reported procedural success > 95% and low rates of recurrent ischemic events (Table 26.34), and several randomized studies of primary stenting vs. PTCA suggest less recurrent ischemia and target vessel revascularization after stenting (Table 26.35). In Stent-PAMI, stenting resulted in less target vessel revascularization (12.8 vs. 21.9%, p < 0.001), angiographic restenosis (22% vs. 33.5%, p = 0.002), and vessel reocclusion (5.1% vs. 9.3%, p = 0.039) at 6 months, but lower TIMI-3 flow rates at 30 days and higher mortality at 1 year.[278] These data suggested that primary stenting may be associated with less target vessel revascularization and recurrent ischemic events, but more distal embolization, slow flow, and mortality.[280] However, these adverse outcomes were not confirmed in CADILLAC, the largest randomized trial of primary stenting vs. PTCA to date (Tables 26.36-26.38). The CADILLAC trial and the role for GP IIb/IIIa inhibitors are discussed below.

4. **Rescue Stenting.** Lytic failures after acute MI are frequently treated by rescue angioplasty or stents.[282-285] In a small observational series, rescue stenting achieved higher procedural success and fewer ischemic complications at 1 year compared to rescue PTCA.[796]

B. **UNSTABLE ANGINA (Chapter 5).** The immediate and long term results for stent implantation in patients with stable and unstable angina are similar.[286-290,642] In more than 7000 patients with unstable angina treated with stents or PTCA, stents resulted in fewer in-hospital ischemic complications including death (1.5% vs. 2.6%, p = 0.003), recurrent angina (23.5% vs. 47.4%, p < 0.00001), Q-wave MI (0.4% vs. 1.9%, p < 0.00001), repeat PTCA (13.8% vs. 30.6%, p < 0.00001), and CABG (6.5% vs. 19.6%, p < 0.00001),[291] but no difference in mortality at 1 year.

C. **SINGLE PATENT VESSEL.** Stenting of a single patent coronary artery or bypass graft may be considered for patients who are not candidates for CABG when the target lesion is anatomically suitable for stenting and there is good distal runoff. Technical considerations include brief balloon inflations to minimize ischemia, predilatation of the lesion to ensure full balloon inflation and maximize the chance of rapid stent deployment, use of large lumen guides with sideholes to permit passive perfusion during intervention, prophylactic IABP or CPS, platelet GP IIb/IIIa inhibitors, and IVUS to ensure optimal stenting. Distal embolic protection devices may improve the safety of stenting single-remaining bypass grafts by preventing distal embolization and no-reflow (Chapter 17).

D. **UNPROTECTED LEFT MAIN (Table 26.39).** The approach to stenting patients with unprotected left main disease is similar to that of patients with a single patent vessel. In particular, prophylactic IABP may reduce the risk of intervention, especially in patients with low ejection fractions (Chapter 6). Although a variety of stents have been employed, slotted tubular stents are preferred for the left main ostium, where elastic recoil is prominent and a stent with excellent radial strength is necessary. For distal left main disease, a bifurcation stenting strategy may be employed but is technically challenging (Chapter 14). For bulky eccentric plaques, directional and rotational atherectomy have been employed prior to stenting,[293] but the utility of this approach has not been proven. Pooled data suggest high procedural success rates (> 95%) in highly selected patients and restenosis in 14-23%.[801] Late ischemic complications depend on whether stenting is emergent or elective, and the degree of LV dysfunction. For elective stenting, patients with LV ejection fractions > 40% have 6-month event-free survivals of 86%, compared to 22% for those with ejection fractions < 40%.[295] For emergency stenting, in-hospital mortality exceeds 50% and 6-month event free survival is about 40%.[294-301] Despite satisfactory results of stenting, we still recommend CABG for most patients with unprotected left main stenoses. For patients who are not candidates for CABG, stenting is reasonable, particularly for lesions not involving the bifurcation. Coronary angiography at 6-8 weeks may detect early restenosis.[295]

E. SEALING PERFORATIONS AND PSEUDOANEURYSMS. There have been several experimental[302] and clinical [303-306,630-632,645] reports of stents with vein allografts to seal perforations, pseudoaneurysms (Figure 26.14), and coronary artery fistulae.[307] This technique is technically challenging and is not appropriate for inexperienced stent operators or for patients with profound hemodynamic collapse. Autologous arterial covered stent grafts (using the radial artery) have also been described,[628,702] but PTFE-covered stents offer a more expeditious alternative for rapid bailout from acute perforations not responding to prolonged balloon inflations.[308-310] The JOMED Coronary Stent Graft is extremely well-suited for these purposes, but is not yet available in the United States. Several reports describe sealing of narrow neck aneurysms and adjacent stenoses with uncovered stents; the mechanism of sealing is probably plaque shift into the aneurysm neck (Table 26.40).[311]

F. WOMEN (Chapter 7). In the STRESS trial, women were older and had smaller vessels and more vascular complications than men, but restenosis and long-term outcomes were similar.[312-313] Other reports suggest better late results in men.[314-315] In EPISTENT, the 30-day event rate for elderly women was higher after stent/abciximab compared to PTCA/abciximab (14.4% vs 2.2%, p = 0.01).[316] In Stent-PAMI, women randomized to stenting had higher 6-month mortality (5.6% vs. 10.2%, p = 0.21), but no difference in composite adverse cardiac events (20.3% vs. 21.3%, p = 0.87);[317] these outcomes appeared to result from smaller vessel size, rather than gender per se.[316]

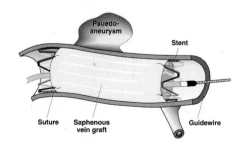

Figure 26.14. Stent-Vein Allograft for Coronary Pseudoaneurysm

G. DIABETES (Table 26.41). The presence of diabetes mellitus does not have an adverse impact on major in-hospital complications after stenting, but increases the risk for late cardiac events and target vessel revascularization (TVR), particularly in diabetics requiring insulin.[318-319] One retrospective report suggested optimal glycemic control reduced TVR in diabetics, resulting in 1-year outcomes which were indistinguishable from nondiabetics.[320] In a metanalysis of 5905 patients from three randomized stent trials, independent predictors of stent restenosis were lesion length, in-stent minimum lumen diameter, and diabetes;[321] the odds ratio for restenosis among diabetics was 1.5. The adverse long-term outcome in diabetics may result from an exaggerated neointimal response to stenting and larger pre-intervention plaque burden.[322,323] Despite higher restenosis rates compared to nondiabetics, diabetics have better immediate and late outcomes after stenting compared to PTCA.[324]

H. ELDERLY (Table 26.42). The immediate and late results of stenting are similar in younger (age < 65 years) and older patients (age > 65 years).[326]

I. MULTIVESSEL DISEASE (Chapter 3). Patients with multivessel disease are routinely treated with stents. In the prospective multicenter ARTS (Arterial Revascularization Therapy Study) trial, 1200 patients were randomized to CABG vs. stenting. At 1 year, there was no difference in total- or infarct-free survival, but stent patients required more late revascularization (Table 26.43).[825] In the smaller Argentine ERACI-II trial, stenting of high-risk patients compared to CABG resulted in less death or MI at 30 days and 1 year, but more late revascularization (4.8% vs. 16.8%, p < 0.002).[643]

J. STENTS AND MAGNETIC RESONANCE IMAGING (MRI). All currently available stents have been evaluated for safety in an MRI field. Coronary stents made of 316L stainless steels, nitinol, tantalum, and other proprietary metals are non-ferromagnetic and have never been shown to be associated with any complications during MRI. Several studies confirm that coronary stents do not move in an MRI field; waiting 4-6 weeks for endothelialization is not necessary.[655,656]

K. SUBOPTIMAL CORONARY STENTING. There are no generally accepted definitions for "suboptimal stenting," and ultrasound criteria for optimal results are more stringent and objective than angiographic criteria (see Chapter 31). Most trials of suboptimal stenting relied on angiographic criteria, including diameter stenosis > 10% after high-pressure PTCA, new or residual thrombus, NHLBI dissection grade $\geq$ D at any time during the procedure, and final TIMI flow < 3. Patients with suboptimal PTCA in the nonrandomized STARS registry had higher mortality and more non-Q-wave MI at 30 days and more clinical restenosis at 9 months than patients in the randomized cohort with "ideal" stenting.[792] Optimal management of patients with suboptimal stenting is unknown; low-molecular-weight heparin[744] and use of "rescue" glycoprotein platelet receptor antagonists have not been uniformly beneficial.

L. STENTING BEFORE NONCARDIAC SURGERY. Patients requiring urgent noncardiac surgery are sometimes referred for preoperative coronary revascularization. In one small study, urgent noncardiac surgery performed within 2 weeks of stent implantation was associated with an unacceptably high risk of perioperative death and MI due to stent thrombosis.[794] This observation suggests that failure to complete a 2-4 week course of standard antiplatelet therapy after stenting may predispose patients to serious ischemic complications after noncardiac surgery.

M. OTHER CLINICAL SITUATIONS. Stents have been successfully used for refractory coronary spasm,[327,328] spontaneous coronary dissection,[329-331] myocardial bridging,[332,333] and cardiac allograft vasculopathy.[334-336]

Table 26.34. Large Observational Studies of Stents for Acute MI

Study	N	In-hospital Outcome (%)			Comments
		Success	**SAT**	**Death**	
Mattos[829] (2000)	84 PTCA 74 Stent	72 96	- -	7.1 6.8	Acute MI due to SVG occlusion; no difference in hospital MACE
Antoniucci[795] (1999)	190	85	-	4	Late TLR (15%)
Stone[594] (1999)	236	98	6.4	0.8	Late TLR (27%)
Dirschinger[604] (1999)	100	96	-	38.9	Patients in cardiogenic shock
Mattos[610] (1999)	780 Stent 2018 PTCA	97 84	-	1.6 / 18* 2.2 / 31*	Higher procedural success with stents (p < 0.001); mortality advantage for patients with severe heart failure or stroke
Hsieh[600] (1998)	117	100	0.9	0	
Monassier[602] (1997)	269	96	3.0	5.2	French STENTIMI Registry

Abbreviations: MACE = major adverse cardiac events (death, MI, stroke); MI = myocardial infarction; NR = not reported; SVG = saphenous vein graft; TLR = target lesion revascularization
* Killip class III/IV, p = 0.02

Table 26.35. Randomized Trials of PTCA vs. Stenting for Acute MI

Trial	N	Stent	Summary (Stent vs. PTCA)	Comment
CADILLAC[190] (2000)	2082	MultiLink MultiLink-Duet	See Tables 26.37, 26.38	See Table 26.39
STENTIM-2[883] (2000)	211	Wiktor	Less ARS (23.3% vs. 39.6%, p < 0.05); no difference in procedural success, EFS, or TLR at 6 and 12 months	Stents associated with less angiographic restenosis
STOPAMI[884] (2000)	140	-	Stent + abciximab vs. t-PA; smaller infarct size (p < 0.05), better myocardial salvage (p < 0.001) and lower MACE at 6 months (8.5% vs. 23.2%, p < 0.05)	Stents plus abciximab resulted in better myocardial salvage and event-free survival than t-PA
FRESCO[885] (2000)	150	GR	Less MACE (9% vs. 28%, p < 0.01) and ARS (17% vs. 43%, p < 0.001) at 6 months	Stents associated with less MACE and restenosis
STENT-PAMI[878] (1999)	900	HCPSS	Less TIMI-3 flow (89% vs. 93%, p < 0.05); less ischemic TVR at 6 months (7.7% vs. 17%, p < 0.001) and 1 year (10.6% vs 21%, p < 0.0001); less ARS at 6 months (23% vs. 35%, p < 0.001); less MACE (17% vs. 24.8%, p < 0.01) but higher mortality at 1 year (5.8% vs. 3.0%, p = 0.054)	Stents associated with less ischemic complications but worse TIMI-3 flow and a trend toward higher mortality at 1 year
PASTA[879] (1999)	136	PSS	Similar success (99% vs. 97%); less in-hospital MACE(6% vs. 19%, p < 0.05) and 1-year MACE (22% vs. 49%, p < 0.001); less ARS at 6 months (17% vs. 37.5%, p < 0.05)	Stents associated with better in-hospital and late outcome
STAT (1999)	123	-	Stent vs. t-PA: Less recurrent MI (6.5% vs. 16.4%, p = 0.09), TVR (14.5% vs. 50.8%, p < 0.001), and MACE (24.2% vs. 57.4%, p < 0.001) at 6 months	Stents associated with less recurrent ischemia and better outcomes at 6 months
GRAMI[876] (1998)	104	GR-II	Similar procedural success; less in-hospital MACE (3.8% vs. 19.2%, p = 0.05) and better TIMI-3 flow (98% vs. 83%, p < 0.01); better EFS (82.7% vs. 65.4%, p < 0.01) but similar TLR at 1 year	Stents superior to PTCA for in-hospital complications, TIMI-flow, and late MACE
Jacksch[612] (1998)	462	Various	Less in-hospital MACE (9.9% vs. 15.6%, p < 0.001); less ARS (23% vs. 42%, p < 0.001) at 6 months	Stents associated with less in-hospital MACE and restenosis
ESCOBAR[877] (1998)	225	PSS	Less recurrent MI (1% vs. 7%, p < 0.05), TLR (4% vs. 17%, p < 0.01), and MACE (5% vs. 20%, p < 0.01) at 6 months; no mortality difference	Stents associated with better outcome at 6 months
PRISAM (1997)	300	Wiktor	Better lumen dimensions and less TLR (11% vs. 36%, p < 0.01) at 3 months	Stents associated with less TLR at 3 months

Abbreviations: ARS = angiographic restenosis; EFS = event-free survival; TLR = target lesion revascularization; MACE = major adverse cardiac events; - = not reported. *Acronyms*: See Table 26.55, p. 587

Table 26.36. CADILLAC Trial: Baseline Characteristics[190]

	PTCA	PTCA/abciximab	Stent	Stent/abciximab
N	516	529	512	525
Age (yrs)	60	61	60	59
Diabetes (%)	15.4	15.7	16.2	19.3
Prior MI (%)	13.5	15.7	11.9	12.8
Killip Class $\geq$ 2 (%)	9.7	11.1	11.4	11.3
Symptoms to PCI (hr)	3.8	3.6	3.9	3.8
MI Location (%)				
Anterior	37.4	35	38.7	34.1
Inferior	57.2	57.7	57.0	59.1
Lateral	19.2	17	16.8	16.4
Extent of CAD (%)				
1-VD	55.2	49.7	49.2	51.8
2-VD	31.2	32.4	35.5	33.3
3-VD	13.6	17.9	15.3	14.9
LVEF (%)	48	50	50	50
QCA				
Ref (mm)	3.0	2.9	2.9	3.0
Lesion length (mm)	13.2	12.1	12	13.6
Abciximab (%)	9.1	99.4	6.1	99.5

Abbreviations: CAD = coronary artery disease; LVEF = left ventricular ejection fraction; MI = myocardial infarction; PCI = percutaneous coronary intervention; QCA = quantitative coronary angiography; ref = reference vessel diameter

Table 26.37. CADILLAC Trial: In-hospital and 6-month Outcomes[190]

	PTCA (n = 516)	PTCA/abciximab (n = 529)	Stent (n = 512)	Stent/abciximab (n = 525)
Angiographic Results				
Final DS (%)	26.6	26.9	11.0*	9.8*
Final TIMI-3 (%)	94.9	96.1	93.8	96.1
Clinical Endpoints (6-month)				
MACE	19.3**	15.2**	10.9**	10.8**
Death	4.3	2.3	2.8	3.8
Reinfarction	1.6	2.1	1.2	2.3
Ischemic TVR	14.2+	12.1+	7.4	5.0

Abbreviations: DS = diameter stenosis; MACE = major adverse cardiac events (death, MI, TVR); TVR = target vessel revascularization
+   p = NS (PTCA vs. PTCA/abciximab)
*   p < 0.001 compared to PTCA
**   p = NS (PTCA vs. PTCA/abciximab; stent vs. stent/abciximab); p = 0.001 (stent vs. PTCA)

Table 26.38. CADILLAC Summary

In acute MI without shock, Multi-Link stenting resulted in marked improvement in event-free survival at 6 months compared to PTCA

In contrast to PAMI-STENT (heparin-coated Palmaz-Schatz stent), Multi-Link stenting did not result in impaired TIMI-3 flow or late survival compared to PTCA

Abciximab was associated with a trend toward better event-free survival at 6 months in PTCA patients, but had no major long-term clinical benefit in stent patients

Table 26.39. Observational Studies of Stents for Unprotected Left Main Lesions

Series	Stent	N	Success (%)	SAT (%)	Comments
Park[821] (2000)	Various	100	99	1	ARS (16%); EFS at 1.6 years (82%)
Sharma[822] (2000)	Various	72	100	0	Total survival at 9 months (83%)
Siegel[551] (1999)	Nir	24	100	0	
Kornowski[522] (1998)	Various	88	98		1-year TLR (15%)
Park[543] (1998)	Various	42	100	0	ARS (22%)
Amin[539] (1997)	Various	16	94	6.3	
Ellis[798] (1997)	Various	26	100	-	In-hospital mortality (5.9%); ARS (14.3%); 1-year survival (70.5%)
Wong[536] (1996)	PS	6	100	0	

Abbreviations: ARS = angiographic restenosis; PSS = Palmaz-Schatz; - = not reported

Table 26.40. Potential Advantages and Disadvantages of Covered Stents

Advantages	Disadvantages
Exclusion of aneurysms, pseudoaneurysms	Difficult to deliver
Seal perforations	Excludes sidebranches
Exclude thrombus	Unknown impact on restenosis
Prevent embolization	Endoleaks
Drug delivery	Infection

Table 26.41. Results of Stents for Patients with Diabetes Mellitus

Series	Group	N	Results
Abizaid[899] (2001)	Stent Diabetic Stent Nondiabetic	195 560	Elective multivessel stenting. Similar procedural success and in-hospital MACE. Diabetics with more TLR (17.7% vs. 9.1%, p = 0.004) and MACE (34.8% vs. 19.2%, p < 0.001) at 1 year
DESTINI[900] (2001)	Stent Diabetic Stent Nondiabetic	65 302	In-hospital results: no death; MI (4.6% vs. 2.3%); CABG (0% vs. 1%). 1-yr follow-up: EFS (72% vs. 79%); CABG (9.4% vs. 1.7%); rePTCA (17% vs. 17%)
CADILLAC[901] (2001)	Stent Diabetic PTCA Diabetic	184 162	Stenting vs. PTCA with and without abciximab for acute MI. Stent group had less ischemic TVR at 6 months (7.1% vs. 17.3%, p = 0.0003), but similar death, reinfarction, disabling stroke, and MACE. 6-month MACE was increased in diabetics vs. nondiabetics (17.1% vs. 12.3%, p < 0.02)
Kugelmass[682] (2001)	Stent-Male Diabetic Stent-Female Diabetic	409 314	Procedural success higher among females (92.6% vs. 87.5%, p = 0.026); no difference in hospital death or emergency CABG.
Villareal[902] (2000)	Stent Diabetic CABG Diabetic	468 762	CABG group had more in-hospital death (5.5% vs. 0.4%) and MI (5% vs. 1.5%), but less TLR (0.4% vs. 3.2%). 2-yr survival for NIDDM better with stents
Dangas[903] (2000)	Stent Nondiabetic Stent NIDDM Stent IDDM	584 121 89	Multivessel stenting. Significant difference in 1-yr MACE (nondiabetic 24.8% vs. NIDDM 37.9% vs. IDDM 48.6%, p < 0.001) and 1-yr TVR (10.7% vs. 17.9% vs. 25.7%, p = 0.01). No difference in angiographic success or in-hospital MACE
STENT-PAMI[904] (2000)	Stent Diabetic PTCA Diabetic Stent Nondiabetic PTCA Nondiabetic	72 63 377 381	Randomized trial for acute MI. Death, recurrent MI, stroke, or ischemic TVR at 1 year: nondiabetics (stent 17% vs. PTCA 25%, p = 0.005); diabetics (stent 20% vs. PTCA 30%, p = 0.21)
Ahmed (2000)	Stent Diabetic (SVG) Stent Nondiabetic (SVG)	290 608	Diabetics had higher in-hospital mortality (2.2% vs. 0.3%, p = 0.003), 1-yr TLR (16.6% vs. 12.3%, p = 0.03), and lower 1-yr EFS (68% vs. 79%, p = 0.0003). No difference in early or late outcomes between IDDM vs. NIDDM
Pereira[906] (2000)	Stent Diabetic CABG Diabetic	44 46	Randomized trial. Similar MACE at 1 year (22.7% vs. 19.5%)

Table 26.41. Results of Stents for Patients with Diabetes Mellitus

Series	Group	N	Results
Schofer[907] (2000)	Stent Nondiabetic Stent IDDM Stent NIDDM	1439 48 177	Nondiabetics with less late loss, lower loss index, and less TLR than diabetics; no difference between IDDM and NIDDM
Gaxiola[908] (2000)	Stent Diabetic Stent Nondiabetic	118 430	In-hospital outcomes: death (0.8% vs. 0.5%); MI (0.8% vs. 0.5%); CABG (1.7% vs. 0.5). Diabetics with more late TLR (26% vs 13%) and CABG (12% vs. 3%). Multiple stents and diabetes were independent predictors of TLR
Silva[909] (1999)	Stent Diabetic Stent Nondiabetic	28 76	Primary stenting for acute MI. MACE at 1 and 6 months were higher in diabetics than nondiabetics; EFS at 6 months was worse in diabetics (54% vs. 88%)
Joseph[910] (1999)	Stent Nondiabetic Stent IDDM Stent NIDDM	1910 58 214	In-hospital outcomes: death (0.8% vs. 0% vs. 0.5%); MI (1.4% vs. 0% vs. 0.5%); CABG (0.1% vs. 0% vs. 0%). Greater 1-yr survival in NIDDM vs. IDDM (97% vs. 90.7%), but similar TLR (10.5% vs. 8.2%)
Gencbay[911] (1999)	Stent Nondiabetic Stent NIDDM	96 96	Similar angiographic restenosis at 6 months (18% vs. 17%)
Alonso[912] (1999)	Stent Nondiabetic Stent Diabetic	849 134	MACE at 28 months was higher in diabetics (54% vs. 33%)
Bhaskaran[913] (1999)	Stent Diabetic PTCA Diabetic	188 570	Stent group had higher acute success (99.5% vs. 96%), higher 1-yr EFS (91% vs. 78%), and less TLR (8% vs. 16.3%)
Lansky[914] (1999)	Stent Nondiabetic Stent NIDDM Stent IDDM	386 76 102	Similar in-hospital outcomes. 1-yr TLR was highest in IDDM (27%) compared to NIDDM (10.4%) and non-diabetics (13.4%)
Carrozza[915] (1998)	Stent Diabetic Stent Nondiabetic	- -	Diabetics had more late loss, late loss index, angiographic restenosis (31% vs. 24%), and TLR (15% vs. 10%)
STRESS[916] (1997)	Stent Diabetic PTCA Diabetic	47 45	Stent group had higher acute success (100% vs. 82%), less restenosis (24% vs. 60%), and less TLR (13% vs. 31%)
Abizaid[917] (1998)	Stent Nondiabetic Stent NIDDM Stent IDDM	706 151 97	In-hospital complication rates were similar. TLR was higher in diabetics on insulin (28%) compared to those on oral therapy (18%) or nondiabetics (16%)
Elezi[918] (1997)	Stent Diabetic Stent Nondiabetic	190 991	More angiographic restenosis in diabetics (40% vs. 24%)
Yokoi[919] (1997)	Stent Diabetic Stent Nondiabetic	263 668	Acute clinical success was similar (96%), but diabetics had more restenosis (29% vs. 22%)
Van Belle[920] (1997)	Stent Diabetic Stent Nondiabetic	56 244	Similar angiographic restenosis (26%), late loss (0.78 mm), and late vessel occlusion (2%)

Abbreviations: EFS = event-free survival; IDDM = insulin-dependent diabetes mellitus; MACE = major adverse cardiac events; MI = myocardial infarction; NIDDM = non-insulin-dependent diabetes mellitus; TLR = target lesion revascularization

Table 26.42. Results of Stents in the Elderly

Series	Age	N	Success[†] (%)	Complications (%) D / Q-MI / CABG	Other Results
Trabattoni[683] (2001)	> 75 51-75 31-50	130 200 150	91 95 96	3.8 / - / 0.7 1.0 / - / 0 0 / - / 0	No difference in late MACE or restenosis between groups
Baklanov[684] (2001)	> 80	197	93	2 / - /	Stroke (2%). High-risk octogenarians: acute MI or unstable angina (65%); prior MI (66%); 3-vessel disease (48%)
Kobayashi[892] (2001)	< 70 70-79 ≥ 80	476 251 94	- 	0.2 / 0.5 / 0.2 0.4 / 0.4 / 0 0 / 0 / 0	No difference in 30-day CABG (~ 0.1%), mortality (~ 0.5%), or MACE (~ 1.5%). Vascular complications were higher in patients ≥ 80 years (1.0% vs. 1.6% vs. 4.3%, p = 0.05)
Alfonso[893] (1999)	≥ 65 < 65	378 601	93 95	4.7 / 4.2 / 0 1.3 / 3.4 / 0.3	More in-hospital death and MACE (6.8% vs. 3.4%) in the elderly.
Bage[894] (1998)	> 70	87	-	4.6 / 0 / 0	EFS at 8.6 months (84%)
DeGregorio[895] (1998)	< 75 > 75	2551 137	- -	0.1 / 1.7 / 1.4 2.2 / 2.9 / 3.7	1-yr survival (91%); 1-yr EFS (54%); elderly with lower EF, more multivessel disease, and more unstable angina
Chauhan[622] (1998)	< 80 ≥ 80	5624 265	99 99	0.2 / 0.8 / - 0.8 / 1.1 / -	TLR (12.6% vs. 11.7%); more vascular and bleeding complications in the very elderly
Gaxiola[620] (1998)	< 75 ≥ 75	280 282	97 94	0.7 / 0.7 / 0.7 3.7 / 2.4 / 1.2	EFS at 6 months (81% vs. 77%)
Moschi[623] (1998)	> 80	50	94	-	More non-Q-wave MI in the very elderly
Shawl[624] (1998)	> 80	34	100	-	1-month mortality (18%)
Nasser[621] (1997)	< 65 65-74 ≥ 75	252 258 35	97 97 97	1.0 / 0.5 / 4.0 0 / 6.5 / 4.3 0 / 0 / 0	EFS at 9 months (90% vs. 89% vs. 90%)
Lefevre[619] (1996)	≥75	245	-	-	1-month follow-up: death (3%); MI (1.6%); subacute closure (1.6%); vascular complications (2.1%)
Yokoi[896] (1995)	65-69 70-74 ≥ 75	131 126 74	96 94 86	0.8 / 0.8 / 0 1.6 / 1.6 / 2.4 4.1 / 1.4 / 1.4	EFS at 6-12 months (81% vs. 84% vs. 75%)
Fishman[897] (1995)	< 70 ≥ 70	388 116	96 91	0.8 3.5	DCA plus stents
Elliott[898] (1994)	> 70	29	86	13.8	Vascular complications (45%)

Abbreviations: CABG = emergency coronary artery bypass grafting; D = in-hospital death; DCA = directional coronary atherectomy; EF = ejection fraction; EFS = event-free survival (without death, MI, CABG, re-PTCA); MACE = major adverse cardiac events; MI= in-hospital Q-wave myocardial infarction; PSS = Palmaz Schatz stent; - = not reported
† Device + adjunctive PTCA as needed

Table 26.43. Randomized Trials of Multivessel Stenting vs. CABG[827]

	CABG	Stent	p-Value
ERACI-II[643]*			
No.	225	225	-
30-day MACE	12.3	3.6	0.002
Death	5.7	0.9	< 0.013
Q-wave MI	5.7	0.9	< 0.013
18-month Follow-up			
Death	7.5	3.1	< 0.017
MI	6.6	2.3	< 0.017
TLR	4.8	16.8	< 0.002
ARTS[825]**			
No.	600	600	-
1-yr death, MI, or stroke	8.8	9.5	0.69
1-yr MACE	12.2	27.3	0.001

Abbreviations: ARTS = Arterial Revascularization Therapy Study; ERACI = Argentine Randomized Study: Coronary Angioplasty vs. Coronary Bypass Surgery in Multivessel Disease; MACE = major adverse clinical events (death, MI, TLR, or stroke); MI = myocardial infarction; TLR = target lesion revascularization

* Inclusion criteria: Class III-IV angina or no/minimal angina with $\geq$ 2 myocardial perfusion defects; > 70% stenosis in at least one major artery and > 50% stenosis in other vessels

** Inclusion criteria: Objective evidence of ischemia with multivessel disease amenable to CABG and stenting

---

ADJUNCTIVE THERAPY

Adjunctive therapy is essential for all stent patients. Pharmacologic adjuncts are used to ensure adequate platelet inhibition, and mechanical adjuncts are used to ensure optimal stent implantation.

A. ADJUNCTIVE PHARMACOTHERAPY (Tables 26.44-26.48; Chapter 34)

    1. Intensive Anticoagulation Regimen. The original (and still FDA-approved) post-stent anticoagulation regimen included aspirin, dipyridamole, dextran, and continuous intravenous heparin followed by oral warfarin. The high incidence of bleeding and vascular complications (transfusion or surgical repair in 25%), prolonged hospital stay (5-7 days), and high costs (patient charges were 80-100% higher than PTCA) offset many of the benefits of stenting. Subsequently, experimental studies reported a 2-fold increase in platelet deposition after aspirin plus warfarin compared to aspirin plus ticlopidine,[337] suggesting that warfarin-based regimens predisposed to stent thrombosis. Clinical studies also demonstrated exaggerated platelet aggregation following warfarin.[338,339] These important observations led to a search for alternative medical regimens after stenting, which coincided with the routine application of high-pressure adjunctive PTCA after stent deployment.

2. **Oral Antiplatelet Therapy.** In an effort to decrease bleeding and vascular complications, length of stay, and cost, post-procedure anticoagulation was abandoned in favor of intensive antiplatelet therapy.[340-360] The majority of these regimens used "optimal stenting" (post-stent angioplasty with high-pressure balloons inflated to 14-20 ATM), and consisted of intraprocedural heparin and post-procedural antiplatelet agents. Dipyridamole, dextran, prolonged heparin, and warfarin were omitted from these regimens. Numerous observational studies comprising thousands of patients treated with aspirin alone (Table 26.47), aspirin plus ticlopidine (Table 26.45), aspirin plus clopidogrel (Table 26.46), and ticlopidine vs. clopidogrel (Table 26.44) suggested the superiority of combination antiplatelet therapy over aspirin alone or aspirin plus warfarin. Randomized trials have unequivocally confirmed the superiority of the aspirin plus ticlopidine compared to aspirin plus warfarin after uncomplicated stenting (Tables 26.49, 26.50):[361-365] In STARS, there was a 5-fold reduction in stent thrombosis; in ISAR, there was a 7-10-fold reduction in stent thrombosis, ischemic complications and bleeding; and in FANTASTIC,[626] there was a 77% reduction in hospital ischemic complications and a 40% reduction in vascular complications. A recent metanalysis of these trials indicated a 33% reduction in major adverse cardiac events at 30 days—equivalent to 25 fewer events per 1000 patients treated—and a 47% reduction in bleeding complications in favor of aspirin plus ticlopidine (Table 26.50).[743] Because of the relatively slow onset of action of ticlopidine, pretreatment is beneficial; the incidence of non-Q-wave MI was 28%, 14% and 5% (p = 0.002) for patients receiving ticlopidine < 1 day, 1-2 days, and ≥ 3 days prior to stenting, respectively.[366] Hematologic side effects (TTP, neutropenia) have limited the utility of ticlopidine, which has been replaced by clopidogrel (300 mg oral loading dose followed by 75 mg/day for 4 weeks). Many observational and randomized studies of clopidogrel vs. ticlopidine suggested that clopidogrel had a better safety profile, earlier onset of action, better tolerability (lower incidence of diarrhea and rash), and equivalent efficacy.[367-370] Randomized trials of aspirin alone vs. aspirin plus warfarin indicated fewer ischemic complications but more bleeding and vascular complications with warfarin[742,743] (Table 26.49). Overall, these data suggest that combination antiplatelet therapy with aspirin plus clopidogrel is preferable to aspirin alone, aspirin plus ticlopidine, or aspirin plus warfarin in patients with optimal or suboptimal stenting.

3. **Low-Molecular-Weight Heparin (LMWH) (Tables 26.48; Chapter 34).** Enoxaparin has been used with aspirin and ticlopidine to reduce the risk of acute ischemic events following stenting in high-risk patients (suboptimal results, multiple stents, residual dissection, small vessels, persistent thrombus). In ATLAST, this regimen was not superior to antiplatelet therapy alone, and patients receiving enoxaparin had more bleeding complications. Preliminary reports suggest substituting enoxaparin for unfractionated heparin during routine stent implantation is feasible,[372] and in the ENTICES trial, the combination of enoxaparin plus aspirin and ticlopidine was associated with fewer bleeding and vascular complications than aspirin plus warfarin (5% vs. 16%, p < 0.05), but there was no difference in ischemic complications at 30 days.[371]

4. **Intravenous GP IIb/IIIa Inhibitors (Table 26.52; Chapter 34).** Early randomized studies of platelet GP IIb/IIIa antagonists reported less need for and improved outcome after bailout

stenting.[144-147] Patients with complex or suboptimal stent deployment (> 2 contiguous stents, combination stent designs, incomplete expansion, or uncovered dissection) are commonly treated with platelet GP IIb/IIIa antagonists, although randomized data are not available.[144] The impact of IIb/IIIa blockers in elective stenting has been favorable (Table 26.51). EPISTENT reported a 57% reduction in major ischemic complications at 30 days (5.3% vs. 10.8%, p < 0.01)[383] and a 58% reduction in mortality at 1 year (1.0% vs. 2.4%, p = 0.037).[830] Diabetics treated with abciximab had a 49% reduction in ischemic complications (13.0% vs. 25.2%, p = 0.005) and a 56% reduction in TVR at 6 months (8.1% vs 16.6%, p < 0.02).[837] In ESPRIT, eptifibatide reduced ischemic complications at 48 hours (6.6% vs. 10.5%, p = 0.0015) and at 30 days (6.8% vs. 10.5%, p = 0.0034)[841] in patients undergoing elective native vessel stenting.[839] Results at 6 months demonstrated persistent benefit for eptifibatide on the combined endpoint of death, MI, or TVR (14.2% vs. 18.3%, p = 0.0083), although the rate of late revascularization among diabetics appeared to increase (14.9% vs. 10.2%).[830] In TARGET, stent patients randomized to tirofiban had worse 30-day MACE than those treated with abciximab (7.6% vs. 6.0%, p < 0.05), driven completely by differences in MI (6.9% vs. 5.4%); abciximab showed the greatest reduction in 30-day MACE for patients with acute coronary syndromes (6.3% vs. 9.3%), whereas patients without acute coronary syndromes had similar outcomes (tirofiban 4.5% vs. abciximab 5.6%).[732] These data offer compelling evidence supporting routine use of abciximab (or possibly eptifibatide) during elective stenting. The optimal choice between abciximab and eptifibatide is unknown: Abciximab is more expensive, but has demonstrated 50-55% reductions in ischemic endpoints (including mortality) at 1 year in diabetics and nondiabetics; eptifibatide has shown a 35% reduction for a combined ischemic endpoint at 6 months, with a lesser effect among diabetics. (One-year data from ESPRIT are not yet available.) Ultimately a direct head-to-head comparison of abciximab vs. eptifibatide may be required. The efficacy and safety of oral platelet GP IIb/IIIa antagonists in stent patients is uncertain;[381,382] studies thus far have failed to show benefit.

In contrast to the established benefit of GP IIb/IIIa blockers during stenting in patients with non-ST-elevation acute coronary syndromes (non-Q-wave MI and unstable angina), benefits in patients with acute MI and ST-segment elevation are not as clear (Tables 26.37, 26.51; Chapters 5, 34). Some studies suggested benefit (Munich Trial, ADMIRAL, ISAR-2), while the largest randomized trial did not (CADILLAC). Since CADILLAC demonstrated modest benefit for abciximab in patients treated with primary PTCA for acute MI, it seems reasonable to initiate therapy with abciximab when the operator makes the decision to perform primary intervention. If PTCA alone is utilized, abciximab should be continued; if stents are implanted, the abciximab infusion may or may not be continued.

5. **Thrombolytic Therapy.** Intracoronary urokinase (250,000-500,000 U bolus over 5-15 minutes or continuous infusion of 50,000-200,000 U/hr for 8-24 hours) was used as an adjunct to recanalize vessels with stent thrombosis[383] or in degenerated vein grafts,[344] but is no longer on the market (Chapter 17). Lytic therapy is not recommended for intraluminal haziness, and in the era of potent platelet inhibitors, thrombolytic agents are rarely necessary.

6. **Vasodilators.** Many interventional cardiologists empirically treat stent patients with long-acting nitrates and calcium antagonists, beginning 24 hours prior to stent placement and continuing for several weeks after discharge. This regimen seems reasonable to prevent vasospasm in arterial segments adjacent to the stent, but its value has not been rigorously tested.

7. **Antibiotics.** Routine antibiotic therapy in patients receiving intravascular stents was abandoned many years ago. Although only four endovascular stent infections have been reported,[435,436,384,733] it is reasonable to prescribe prophylactic antibiotics for patients who require dental procedures, endoscopy, or other invasive procedures within 3 months of stent placement (until endothelialization is complete).[385]

8. **Other Medications.** Cilostazol, a potent antiplatelet agent which is FDA-approved for patients with lower extremity claudication, may be an effective alternative to ticlopidine and clopidogrel,[745,746] but is contraindicated in patients with a history of congestive heart failure. In experimental and preliminary clinical studies, cilostazol reduced in-stent restenosis. Large-scale clinical trials are planned (Table 26.49).[156] There are no data to support the use of corticosteroids, colchicine, or other antiproliferative drugs.

9. **Local Drug Delivery.** Local delivery of various drugs is under evaluation for preventing stent thrombosis and restenosis.[647] Further study is needed.

B. **ADJUNCTIVE MECHANICAL METHODS (Table 26.30)**
   1. **Intravascular Ultrasound (IVUS) (Chapter 31)**
      a. **Use of IVUS.** Potential uses for IVUS include assessment of lesion severity, accurate measurement of reference vessel dimensions and lesion length for stent sizing, assessment of extent and distribution of calcium to guide debulking, and assessment of parameters for optimal stent implantation (Table 31.11). IVUS is particularly useful for evaluating the cause of angiographic "haziness" after stenting, which may be due to nonobstructive plaque or occult dissection.[157] IVUS is also essential for recognizing pseudorestenosis resulting from inadequate expansion or misplacement of the stent,[158] and for determining the cause of stent thrombosis. Automatic pullback and dynamic 3-D reconstruction may further enhance image analysis.[159,160] It is important to recognize that most studies of IVUS for assessment of stent results have been performed in patients with balloon-expandable stents; criteria for optimizing results after balloon-expandable stents may not apply to self-expanding stents.[627] Three multicenter randomized trials (TRAPIST, ERASER, ITALICS) utilized IVUS to evaluate the efficacy of different pharmacologic agents (trapidil, abciximab, antisense DNA) for preventing stent restenosis (Table 26.33).[640] Given the low incidence of subacute stent thrombosis, it is difficult to prove that IVUS decreases acute complications.[402]

      b. **Impact of IVUS on Stent Results (Table 26.30).** Although IVUS may add cost and time,[391] the routine use of high-pressure PTCA does not ensure optimal stent implantation.[392,393] IVUS studies have shown that up to 60% of stents implanted with "optimal" technique have inadequate expansion.[394,395,665,813] In the POST registry (Predictors and Outcomes of Stent Thrombosis), 95% of patients with subacute thrombosis had at least one IVUS abnormality (malapposition 64%, underexpansion 53%, plaque protrusion 27%, thrombus 23%, edge dissection 23%), whereas angiography identified an abnormality in only 39%.[174] IVUS can improve stent dimensions and apposition not discernible by angiography,[397-400] although the discrepancy between IVUS and quantitative angiography decreases with progressively higher inflation pressures.[171,672] The AVID (Angiography Versus Intravascular Ultrasound-Directed) trial reported that 29% of patients with high-pressure stent deployment failed to satisfy IVUS criteria for "optimal stenting" because of malapposition, malexpansion, and unrecognized edge dissection.[402] Further IVUS-guided intervention resulted in substantial increases in lumen diameter and cross sectional area.[402,403] AVID also reported less target lesion revascularization in patients undergoing IVUS-guided stenting, which was particularly important in vessels < 3 mm or > 4.5 mm, in females and diabetics, and in long and ostial lesions (Chapter 31).[886-890] In CRUISE, a nonrandomized substudy of the STARS trial,[406] IVUS patients had significantly larger minimum lumen diameters and stent cross-sectional areas, and lower target vessel revascularization at 6 months (14.8% vs 8.9%, p = 0.04) (Table 26.30).[177] Numerous studies have focused on IVUS criteria for optimal stenting and for predicting stent restenosis.[178-180,625] Proposed criterion for optimal stent expansion include minimum stent cross-sectional area > 90% of the distal reference lumen area, and minimum stent cross-sectional area > 55% of the reference vessel cross-sectional area.[408,814] A minimum in-stent cross-sectional area > 9 mm^2 was associated with target vessel revascularization in < 5%, but can only be achieved in large vessels;[181] a minimum stent area > 55% of the reference vessel cross-sectional area is associated with low restenosis rates even in smaller vessels.[410] A new IVUS imaging guidewire and on-line 3-dimensional reconstruction may have useful applications for stent implantation.[389,390,403]

2. **Debulking with Atherectomy or ELCA (Table 26.51).** The rationale for debulking before stenting is based on several observations: First, despite high pressure deployment, lumen areas after stenting are only 57% of maximum (due to balloon underexpansion and stent recoil).[412] Second, post-dilatation using larger balloons (balloon/artery ratios > 1.2) could increase minimum in-stent areas, but also increases the risk of ischemic complications.[183] Third, multiple studies suggest that residual plaque area is an independent predictor of stent restenosis.[184-187] Finally, lesion calcification (particularly superficial calcification) is an independent predictor of suboptimal stent expansion.[422-424] Based on these data, debulking with atherectomy has been used to improve stent expansion and potentially reduce restenosis.[669,816] The SOLD (Stenting after Optimal Lesion Debulking) pilot registry[418-420] reported angiographic restenosis in only 11% and TVR in 7% after aggressive DCA and stenting, although non-Q-wave MI occurred in 9.9%. Other observational studies reported similar favorable results.[421] Randomized studies and technical improvements in DCA catheters are needed before directional atherectomy is routinely employed. In a study of matched lesions in vessels ≥ 3 mm, rotational atherectomy and stenting resulted in better lumen gain and less TVR

(12.2% vs 31.6%, p < 0.05) compared to stenting alone.[425] Like DCA, there was a relatively high rate of non-Q-wave MI following Rotablator, particularly with an aggressive burr strategy.[420,426] However, aggressive debulking of heavily calcified lesions prior to stenting may decrease the risk of restenosis compared to less aggressive debulking.[815] Both TEC[427-431] and ELCA[427] have been used in high-risk vein grafts as adjuncts to stenting.

3. **Doppler Flow.** Stenting may normalize coronary flow reserve after otherwise "successful" PTCA, suggesting that Doppler techniques may be used to identify suboptimal lumen enlargement after "successful" stenting.[421-434,817]

4. **Angioscopy.** IVUS is far superior to angioscopy in assessing stent size, geometry, and optimal implantation.

Table 26.44. Observational Studies Comparing Anticoagulation Regimens After Stenting

| Series | Regimen | N | In-hospital Complications (%) | |
			SAT	D / MI / CABG
Moussa[864]	A, T	1390	1.5	0.9 / 1.8 / 0.4
(1999)	A, C	281	1.4	1.0 / 0.7 / 0.7
Mishkel[865]	A, T	361	0	1.4
(1999)	A, C	514	0.6	2.1
Chauhan[717]	A, T	40	0	0 / 5.0 / 0
(1997)	A, C	42	2.4	0 / 4.8 / 0
Hall[576]	A, T	123	0.8	0 / 0.8 / 0
(1996)	A	103	2.9	2.9 / 3.9 / 0

Abbreviations: A = aspirin; C = clopidogrel; CABG = emergency coronary bypass surgery; D = death; MI = myocardial infarction; SAT = subacute thrombosis; T = ticlopidine

Table 26.45. Observational Studies of Aspirin/Ticlopidine After Stenting

Series	Regimen	N	In-hospital Complications (%)	
			SAT	D / MI / CABG
Berger[571] (1999)	A, T (2 weeks)	827	0.4	0.6 / 0.5 / -
Wang[589] (1999)	A, T	1192	-	1.1 / 1.0 / -
Wilson[590] (1999)	A, T	1914	0.7	-
Fischman (1999)	A, T	240	-	0.8 / 3.7 / 4.1
Berger[572] (1998)	A, T	234	0	0 / 0 / 0
Elsner[579] (1998)	T	263	-	0.8 / 1.9 / -
Meketic[570] (1997)	A, T	124	0.8	0.8 / 0.8 / 0.8
Barragan[580] (1997)	T	1051	0.95	0.2 / 0.6 / 0.1
Lawerence[573] (1996)	A, T	322	0	0 / 3 / 0
Antoniucci[718] (1997)	A, T	134	0.7	1.0 / 7.0 / 1.0
Nakamura[719] (1997)	A, T	137	2.9	0 / 3.2 / 0.8
Morice[721] (1996)	A, T	260	1.2	- / 1.9 / 0.4
Goods[722] (1996)	A, T	296	0.7	0.3 / - / 0.7
Elias[724] (1996)	A, T	182	1.0	1 / - / 0
Hall[99] (1995)	A or T	411	1.0	0.3 / 1.0 / 0.5
Barragan[343] (1995)	A, T	208	0.5	1.0 / 1.0 / 0.5
Morice[358] (1995)	A, T	1156	1.6	0.3 / 2.7 / 0.3

Abbreviations: A = aspirin; CABG = emergency coronary bypass surgery; D = death; MI = myocardial infarction; SAT = subacute thrombosis; T = ticlopidine; - = not reported

Table 26.46. Observational Studies of Aspirin/Clopidogrel After Stenting

Series	Regimen	N	In-hospital Complications (%)	
			SAT	D / MI / CABG
Kolansky[747] (2000)	A, C	253	0.8	0.8 / 0 / 0
Jauhar[748] (1999)	A, C	250	0.8	0.4 / 4.0 / 0
Mishkel[582] (1999)	A, C	345	0.9	0.6 / 0.4 / 0.3
L'Allier[584] (1999)	A, C	232	-	0.5 / 0 / 0
Berger[585] (1999)	A, C	345	-	0.9 / 1.4 / 0.3

Abbreviations: A = aspirin; C = clopidogrel; CABG = emergency coronary bypass surgery; D = death; MI = myocardial infarction; SAT = subacute thrombosis; - = not reported

Table 26.47. Observational Studies of Aspirin Alone After Stenting

Series	Regimen	N	In-hospital Complications (%)	
			SAT	D / MI / CABG
Sankardas[575] (1996)	A	243	0.9	0 / 0.9 / 0
Columbo[350] (1995)	A or T	359	0.9	1.1 / 3.9 / 3.9
Hall[99] (1995)	A or T	411	1.0	0.3 / 1.0 / 0.5

Abbreviations: A = aspirin; CABG = emergency coronary bypass surgery; D = death; MI = myocardial infarction; SAT = subacute thrombosis; T = ticlopidine

Table 26.48. Observational Studies of Subcutaneous Heparin After Stenting

Series	Regimen	N	In-hospital Complications (%)	
			SAT	D / MI / CABG
Lefevre[720] (1996)	A, T, LMWH	245	2.0	3 / 1.6 / 0
Elias[724] (1996)	A, T, LMWH	240	3.6	1.2 / - / 1.2
Morice[100] (1995)	A, T, LMWH	1250	1.7	0.7 / 0.6 / 0.4
Morice[340] (1995)	A, T, LMWH	397	1.5	1.0 / 0.3 / 1.0
Morice[341] (1995)	A, T, LMWH	246	1.2	0.4 / 0 / 0.8
Cavalho[725] (1994)	A, T, LMWH	87	1.1	0 / 0 / 0
Barragan[359] (1994)	T, UFH	238	3.8	1.6 / 1.2 / 0
Elias[728] (1994)	A, T, LMWH	79	1.3	0 / 0 / 0
Aubry[730] (1994)	A, T, LMWH	643	2.5	3.7 / 3.7 / 1.3

Abbreviations: A = aspirin; CABG = emergency coronary bypass surgery; D = death; LMWH = low-molecular-weight heparin; MI = myocardial infarction; SAT = subacute thrombosis; UFH = subcutaneous unfractionated heparin; T = ticlopidine

Table 26.49. Randomized Trials of Adjunctive Antiplatelet Therapy During Coronary Stenting

Trial	N	Primary Endpoint	Agents	Result
CLASSICS[818] (2000)	-	Bleeding, neutropenia, thrombocytopenia, or drug discontinuation	ASA/ticlopidine vs. ASA/clopidogrel	No difference between ticlopidine and clopidogrel (9.1% vs. 4.6%); loading dose of clopidogrel (300 mg) was well tolerated and had fewer adverse events than clopidogrel without loading dose (2.9 vs. 6.3%)
TOPPS[870] (2000)	1016	MACE (30 d)	ASA/ticlopidine vs. ASA/clopidogrel	Clopidogrel was better tolerated than ticlopidine and had similar clinical efficacy
ATLAST[744] (1999)	1121	MACE (30 d)	Enoxaparin (1 mo. post-stenting)	Study stopped because of low event rates (placebo 2.7% vs. enoxaparin 1.8%, p = NS); more bleeding with enoxaparin
Yoon[746] (1999)	296	MACE, SAT (30 d)	ASA/ticlopidine vs. ASA/cilostazol	No differences in SAT, MACE, or bleeding complications
Park[745] (1999)	490	MACE, (30 d)	ASA/ticlopidine vs. ASA/cilostazol	No differences in SAT, MACE, or bleeding complications
CVT[832] (1999)	1327	MACE (30 d)	ASA/ticlopidine vs. ASA/clopidogrel	Nonrandomized case-control study; clopidogrel is an acceptable substitute for ticlopidine: no difference in MACE (0.8% vs. 1.6%) or SAT (0.2% vs. 0.7%)
Machraoui[742] (1999)	164	MACE (21 d)	ASA alone vs. ASA/warfarin (no IVUS)	More ischemic complications with ASA alone but more bleeding with warfarin
ENTICES[371] (1998)	122	MACE (30 d) 2°: MACE (6 mo)	ASA, ticlopidine, enoxaparin vs. ASA/warfarin	Ticlopidine/enoxaparin had fewer bleeding complications (5% vs. 16%, p < 0.05) and less MACE at 30 days (5% vs. 20%, p = 0.01) and 6 months (14% vs. 27%, p = 0.07)
MATTIS[848] (1998)	350	MACE (30 d)	ASA/ticlopidine vs. ASA/warfarin	Less MACE (10% vs. 19%, p = 0.07) and bleeding (3% vs. 12%, p < 0.05) with ticlopidine
SALTS[854] (1998)	99	Death, SAT, thrombocytopenia, neutropenia (30 d)	ASA/ticlopidine for 30 d vs. 10 d	Ticlopidine for 10 days was not associated with more adverse events
FANTASTIC[626] (1998)	485	Bleeding (6 wks) MACE (6 wks)	ASA/ticlopidine vs. ASA/warfarin	Less bleeding with antiplatelet therapy (13.5% vs. 21%, p < 0.05) and no difference in MACE
STARS[481] (1998)	1650	SAT (30 d)	ASA/warfarin vs. ASA/ticlopidine vs. ASA alone	Lowest SAT in ASA/ticlopidine (0.6%), compared to ASA/warfarin (2.4%) or aspirin alone (3.6%) (p < 0.001)
ISAR[480] (1996)	517	MACE (30 d) 2°: MACE (6 mo), ARS (6 mo), SAT (30 d)	ASA/warfarin vs. ASA/ticlopidine	Less MACE (2% vs. 12.6%, p < 0.01) and SAT (0% vs. 11.5%, p < 0.001) at 30 days with anti-platelet therapy; no difference in ARS

Abbreviations: ARS = angiographic restenosis; MACE = major adverse cardiac events; MI = myocardial infarction; TVR = target vessel revascularization

Acronyms: See Table 26.55, p. 587

Table 26.50. Metanalysis of Randomized Trials of Aspirin/Ticlopidine vs. Aspirin/Warfarin After Coronary Stenting[743]

Study	N	30-day MACE (%)	
		Ticlopidine	Warfarin
ISAR	517	1.6	6.2
FANTASTIC	473	5.8	10.0
STARS	1097	0.6	2.4
Total	**2087**	**2.0**	**3.0***

Abbreviations: MACE = major adverse cardiac events. *Acronyms:* FANTASTIC = Full Anticoagulation Versus Aspirin and Ticlopidine; ISAR = Intracoronary Stenting and Antithrombotic Regimen; STARS = Stent Anti-Thrombotic Regimen Study

* $p < 0.001$. Ticlopidine resulted in 25 fewer adverse cardiac events per 1000 patients treated at 30 days, and a 47% reduction in bleeding complications

Table 26.51. Debulking Strategies Prior to Stenting

Study	Device	N	Comments
AMIGO	DCA	750	Prospective multicenter randomized trial; MultiLink stent with and without DCA; results pending
Kiesz[823] (1998)	DCA	60	ADAPTS study (prospective, observational); in-hospital MACE (5%); 6-month ARS (13%) and TLR (10%)
EDRES[836] (1998)	ROTA/stent Stent	75 75	Small prospective randomized trial; debulking with Rotablator did not improve final stent diameter, but did reduce 6-month ARS (27% vs. 34%, $p < 0.05$)
SOLD[860] (1998)	DCA	90	Prospective registry; aggressive DCA before stenting resulted in excellent acute and mid-term outcome (ARS 11%, TLR 7% at 6 months)

Abbreviations: AMIGO = Atherectomy before MultiLink Improves Lumen Gain Outcome; ADAPTS = Acute Directional Atherectomy Prior To Stenting; EDRES = Effect of Debulking on Restenosis; SOLD = Stenting after Optimal Lesion Debulking. *Acronyms*: See Table 26.55, p. 587

Table 26.52. Randomized Trials of GP IIb/IIIa Inhibitors During Stenting

Trial	N	1° Endpoint	Design	Results
CADILLAC[190] (2000)	2082	MACE (6 mo)	(PTCA vs. stent) ± abciximab for acute MI	See Table 26.38
ESPRIT[830] (2000)	2066	MACE (48 hrs) 2°: MACE (30 d)	Placebo vs. eptifibatide for 18-24 hours prior to elective stenting	Eptifibatide pretreatment was associated with less MACE at 48 hours (6.6% vs. 10.5%, p < 0.01), 30 days (10.4% vs. 6.8%, p < 0.01), 6 months
TARGET[732] (2000)	4812	MACE (30 d)	Tirofiban vs. abciximab during coronary stenting	Less MACE (6.0% vs. 7.6%, p < 0.05) for abciximab, driven completely by differences in MI (5.4% vs. 6.9%); patients with ACS had the most benefit (MACE 6.3% vs. 9.3%). Similar MACE for patients without ACS (4.5% vs. 5.6%)
EPISTENT[838] (1999)	2399	MACE (30 d) 2°: MACE (6 mo)	PTCA/abciximab vs. stent/abciximab vs. stent	Lowest MACE for stent/abciximab (5.3%) compared to PTCA/abciximab (6.9%) or stent alone (10.8%) (p < 0.01); benefits persisted at 6 months. Less restenosis in diabetics treated with stent/abciximab
ISAR-2[611] (2000)	401	MACE (30 d)	Stent ± abciximab for acute MI	Less MACE with abciximab (4.5 vs. 9.5%, p < 0.05); no difference in recurrent MI or mortality
ADMIRAL[970] (2000)	299	MACE (30 d)	Stent ± for acute MI	Less MACE with abciximab (10.7% vs. 20%, p < 0.03)
EPISTENT-DIABETES[839] (1999)	491	MACE (6 mo)	PTCA/abciximab vs. stent/abciximab vs. stent	Stent/abciximab was superior to stent alone with respect to MACE (13% vs. 25.2%, p < 0.01) and TVR (8.1% vs. 16.6%, p < 0.05), but similar to PTCA/abciximab
Munich Trial[591] (1998)	200	MACE (in-hospital)	Stent ± abciximab for acute MI	Less MACE with abciximab (2.0% vs. 9.2%, p < 0.05). Benefits not present at 30 days (p = 0.16)

Abbreviations: MACE = major adverse cardiac events.
Acronyms: See Table 26.55, p. 587

STENT COMPLICATIONS

A. STENT THROMBOSIS

1. **Incidence.** Chest pain in the days following stenting is more common than after PTCA (41.2% vs. 12.1%, p < 0.001).[435] Except for patients with acute ECG changes or known suboptimal stent deployment, the vast majority of these patients do not require repeat angiography. When evaluating chest pain after stenting, the best clinical predictors of stent thrombosis include ST-segment elevation and persistent chest pain.[206] Acute stent thrombosis (i.e., before the patient leaves the cath

lab) is rare (< 1%) and virtually always associated with readily identifiable causes such as incomplete stent expansion or uncovered dissection. Unsuspected intramural hematoma, detectable only by IVUS, can also cause lumen compromise and stent thrombosis.[437] The median time to stent thrombosis was 3-5 days after stenting with aspirin/warfarin regimens and 12 hours after stenting with aspirin/ticlopidine;[749] stent thrombosis was rare after 2 weeks.[208] Randomized trials of various stent designs suggest no difference in stent thrombosis. Predictors of stent thrombosis include multiple stents, pre-intervention thrombus, suboptimal stent expansion, smaller vessels, residual dissection, slow flow, and bailout rather than elective indication.[439-441] By IVUS, the strongest predictors of stent thrombosis are residual plaque burden in the stented segment (odds ratio 15.7) and small stent cross-sectional area (odds ratio 6.8).[661] The risk of stent thrombosis is less in saphenous vein grafts than in native vessels, probably because of differences in vessel caliber.[442]

2. **Prevention.** The optimal medical regimen for preventing stent thrombosis has been the subject of intense investigation. Because of the tendency of intravascular metals to form blood clots, original guidelines for medical management focused on the use of aggressive anticoagulation regimens to prevent stent thrombosis. In the early Wallstent experience in Europe, stent thrombosis occurred in 20-25% of lesions despite the use of aspirin, dipyridamole, heparin, urokinase, dextran, and warfarin. In contrast, when the medical regimen was changed from aspirin alone to aspirin, dipyridamole, and warfarin, the incidence of stent thrombosis after Palmaz-Schatz stenting of chronic total occlusions decreased from 16% to 2%. Nevertheless, these aggressive anticoagulation regimens were associated with a high incidence of bleeding and vascular complications, prolonged hospital stays, and increased cost, which offset the expected benefits of stenting. Largely due to the pioneering work of Colombo and colleagues, stent thrombosis is now viewed as a mechanical problem that can be prevented by optimal stent implantation without the need for aggressive anticoagulation. "Optimal stenting" requires meticulous technique to ensure complete coverage of the lesion, complete apposition of the stent to the vessel wall, full stent expansion, and stent symmetry. Adjunctive angioplasty after stent implantation using high-pressure balloons inflated to at 12-14 ATM is a key component of "optimal stenting," and IVUS may be valuable to confirm optimal technique. Data from numerous trials confirm the superiority of antiplatelet therapy without warfarin (Table 26.49).[361-363] Using this approach, the incidence of stent thrombosis is 1%.

3. **Treatment and Outcome.** Clinical manifestations of stent thrombosis are similar to abrupt closure after other devices and usually include chest pain and ST-segment elevation. Thrombosis of a previously occluded vessel, however, may be clinically silent. In most cases, emergency angiography and revascularization are recommended. Potential remedial causes should be sought and corrected, including inadequate stent apposition, improper stent sizing, and failure to adequately cover distal disease or dissection. Rarely, stent thrombosis may be secondary to protrusion of intimal flaps through stent struts, which is managed by overlapping stents.[213] Most cases of stent thrombosis can be successfully managed by repeat PTCA or stenting, with or without antecedent thrombectomy (AngioJet). When crossing the stented segment with a guidewire, it is important to put a large J-curve on the wire tip to prevent the wire from passing between the stent

and the vessel wall. If this occurs and goes unrecognized—excessive resistance to balloon advancement is an important clue—subsequent balloon inflations can separate the stent from the vessel wall and lead to stent compression, stent embolization, and further thrombus formation.[444] IVUS is an extremely useful adjunct for evaluating identifying the cause of stent thrombosis and optimizing treatment. The role of intravenous platelet GP IIb/IIIa antagonists is unproven but not unreasonable.[445,446] Thrombolytic therapy (intracoronary bolus, prolonged intracoronary infusion, or local delivery directly into the stented segment) is rarely needed.[447] Patients who are successfully revascularized should be treated with soluble aspirin (325 mg QD-BID) and clopidogrel (75 mg QD). Data from ATLAST do not suggest additional benefit for low-molecular-weight heparin. For refractory stent thrombosis, CABG is usually advised. Stent thrombosis remains an uncommon but important complication of stenting due to the high incidence of ischemic complications (death 7-19%, MI 57-85%, emergency CABG 30-44%).[667]

B. ISCHEMIC COMPLICATIONS. Ischemic complications arise as a consequence of failed PTCA or stent thrombosis. When stents are used to reverse out-of-lab abrupt closure, significant patient morbidity should be anticipated, including nonfatal myocardial infarction (2-26%), emergency CABG (0-16%), and death (0-10%). Independent predictors of ischemic complications included delayed use of stents for abrupt closure, sidebranch occlusion, need for multiple stents, and incomplete coverage of dissection.[448]

C. BLEEDING AND VASCULAR INJURY. Warfarin anticoagulation after stenting was associated with bleeding and vascular complications in up to 15% of stent patients, compared to only 3.5% of patients treated with antiplatelet therapy after optimal stent technique.[219] Risk factors for vascular complications included age > 70 years, female gender, multiple procedures during the same hospitalization, and use of warfarin.[220,221] To minimize bleeding and vascular complications, sheaths should be removed immediately after the procedure (when ACT ≤170 seconds). Compared to overnight heparin and sheath removal the following morning, immediate sheath removal resulted in a 2-3-fold reduction in bleeding and vascular complications.[222] In patients given platelet GP IIb/IIIa inhibitors, weight-adjusted heparin and early sheath removal minimize groin complications (Chapters 25, 34).[148]

D. FAILED STENT DELIVERY AND STENT EMBOLIZATION. In older series of patients undergoing stenting with first generation balloon-expandable stents, failed coronary stent deployment occurred in 8-15% of patients.[453,736] In contemporary practice, stent embolization occurs in less than 1% of cases.[456,457] Management usually involves stent deployment at the site of embolization,[228] since retrieval with a wire snare is a feasible but technically difficult.[459-461,633,634,735] Maintaining wire position within the stent is essential.[739] In cases in which the stent cannot be retrieved from the coronary artery, crushing the stent against the vessel wall and deploying a second stent over the first has been successful.[462-464,736] Rupture of the deployment balloon may occur during stent placement: one report described use of a power injector to momentarily inflate the stent balloon, allowing successful stent expansion.[465] Coronary stents embolized into the lower extremity are at low risk for complications. Safe retention and retrieval of a dislodged stent has also been reported using the PercuSurge GuardWire.[738]

E. **SIDEBRANCH OCCLUSION.** Experimental and clinical studies have shown that flow into sidebranches is usually preserved after stenting, and stenting sometimes results in reappearance of sidebranches that are initially occluded after PTCA.[237] The management of sidebranch occlusion is more straightforward with contemporary stents, since guidewires and balloons can readily be passed through the struts of most stents. In general, low-profile balloons work best, but a fixed wire-balloon may be required. Atherectomy (rotational or directional) may be useful for preventing sidebranch occlusion prior to stenting, and in EPISTENT, abciximab reduced the risk of sidebranch occlusion after stenting (stent/abciximab 2.4% vs. stent 4.5%).[378]

F. **PERFORATION.** Coronary perforation occurs more often after laser and atherectomy than after PTCA or stenting. Our own stent experience suggests several potential mechanisms for coronary artery perforation after stenting, including use of oversized balloons (balloon/artery ratio > 1.2) during or after stent deployment; high-pressure balloon inflations outside the stent; stenting of vessels with significant tapering; stenting of contained perforations after other devices; recrossing lesions with antecedent severe dissections or abrupt closure; and stenting total occlusions when there has been unrecognized subintimal passage of the guidewire. Prompt action can be lifesaving: Severe perforation requires prolonged (20-30 minute) balloon inflations, discontinuation and reversal of heparin with protamine, platelet transfusion if abciximab has been given, and prompt pericardiocentesis if tamponade leads to hemodynamic instability (Chapter 22). The availability of PTFE stent grafts in the near future should allow rapid repair of perforations that otherwise would require emergency bypass surgery.[308-310]

G. **STENT INFECTION.** Transient bacteremia during coronary intervention is rare; coronary stent infection has been reported in 4 patients[384,435,436,733] and is usually fatal. Strict aseptic technique is recommended during stent implantation, and endocarditis prophylaxis is reasonable during the first 3 months after stent implantation if a patient requires an invasive procedure which is likely to be associated with transient bacteremia.

SUMMARY OF RANDOMIZED STENT TRIALS

In the last few years, several randomized stent trials have been completed, including trials of stent vs. PTCA, pharmacologic agents, and stent vs. stent. In all, these trials demonstrate:

- Superiority of stents compared to PTCA for patients with angina pectoris and single focal *de novo* lesions in native coronary arteries
- Superiority of stents compared to PTCA for higher risk populations including isolated proximal LAD lesions, focal *de novo* lesions in vein grafts, restenotic lesions in native coronary arteries, vessels 2.5-3.0 mm in diameter, and chronic total occlusions
- Controversy about the relative benefits of stents compared to PTCA for acute MI
- Superiority of antiplatelet regimens (aspirin plus ticlopidine or clopidogrel) compared to older antithrombotic regimens (aspirin, dipyridamole, dextran, heparin, warfarin)
- Greater benefit for abciximab as an adjunct to stents for unstable angina and non-Q-wave MI compared to Q-wave MI
- Benefit for IIb/IIIa inhibitors in elective stenting, especially for higher risk patients
- Equivalence of most balloon-expandable stents

FUTURE DIRECTIONS IN STENTING

In the last 10 years there has been tremendous proliferation of metallic stent designs. In the future, new biodegradable and nonbiodegradable polymer stents may become available, combining the benefits of current metallic stents (scaffolding) with local delivery of antithrombotic, antiplatelet, or antiproliferative agents (Tables 26.53, 26.54).[637,651,659]

Table 26.53. Drugs Used on Polymer-Coated Stents[782]

Drug	Description
Heparin	Used with biocompatible polymer coating; less platelet adhesion and thrombosis in animal models. No known impact on restenosis. Used in BENESTENT-II trial; heparin-coated BX-Velocity stent is available
Methotrexate	No known impact on stent thrombosis or restenosis
Corticosteroids	May attenuate inflammatory reaction in animal models; variable impact on restenosis
Angiopeptin	No known impact on restenosis
Argatroban	Inhibits platelet deposition in animal models
Nitric oxide donors	May inhibit thrombosis and intimal proliferation
Glycoprotein IIb/IIIa receptor antagonists	Tirofiban, abciximab may have antithrombotic effects
Paclitaxel	Shows promise for reducing intimal hyperplasia; taxol-coated stents are being evaluated in Europe

Table 26.54. Stent Coatings to Reduce Complications

Coating	Description
Cell coatings	Endothelial-cell coating of stent struts to reduce thrombogenicity and intimal reaction (stent "passivation"); genetically modified cells can deliver t-PA
Fibrin biopolymer	Animal models show less stent thrombosis and restenosis
Metallic coatings	Silicon carbide inhibits stent thrombosis in humans; experimental models suggest benefit of copper and platinum coatings
Biocompatible polymers	Such polymers "insulate" the vessel wall from the metal stent and can serve as reservoirs for local drug delivery. Polymers may or may not be biodegradable

Table 26.55. Acronyms of Stent Trials

APPLAUSE	Antiplatelet Treatment After Intravascular Ultrasound Guided Optimal Stent Expansion
ASCENT	ACS Multi-Link Stent Trial
AVID	Angiography vs. Intravascular Ultrasound Directed Coronary Stent Placement
BEST	BeStent Trial
CADILLAC	Controlled Abciximab and Device Investigation to Lower Late Angioplasty Complications
CLASSICS	Clopidogrel Aspirin Stent International Cooperative Study
CRUISE	Can Routine Ultrasound Influence Stent Expansion
CVT	Clopidogrel vs. Ticlopidine after Intracoronary Stent Placement
DEBATE-II	Doppler Endpoint Balloon Angioplasty Trial Europe-II
DESTINI	Doppler Endpoint Stenting International Investigation Coronary Flow Reserve
DISTINCT	BioDivYsio Stent in Randomized Control Trial
ENTICES	Enoxaparin and Ticlopidine after Elective Stenting
EPISTENT	Evaluation of Platelet IIb/IIIa Inhibitor for Stenting
ESCOBAR	European Stenting Compared to Conventional Balloon Angioplasty Randomized Trial
ESPRIT	Enhanced Suppression of the Platelet IIb/IIIa Receptor with Integrilin Therapy
EXTRA	Evaluation of the XT Stent for Restenosis in Native Arteries
FANTASTIC	Full Anticoagulation Versus Aspirin and Ticlopidine
FRESCO	Florence Randomized Elective Stenting in Acute Coronary Occlusions
FROST	French Randomized Optimal Stenting Trial
GRAMI	GR-II Stent in Acute MI
IMPRESS	IVUS Makes Possible Reliable Assessment of Neointima After Stenting
ISAR	Intracoronary Stenting and Antithrombotic Regimen
MATTIS	Multicenter Aspirin and Ticlopidine Trial after Intracoronary Stenting
MUSIC	Multicenter Ultrasound Stenting in Coronary Arteries
NIRVANA	Nir Vascular Advanced North American Trail
OSTI-I	Optimal Stent Implantation Trial-1
PAMI-Stent	PAMI Heparin-Coated Stent Randomized Trial
PASTA	Primary Angioplasty and Stent Implantation in Acute MI
PRISAM	Primary Stenting for Acute MI
RESIST	Restenosis After IVUS Stenting
SALTS	Strategic Alternatives with Ticlopidine in Stenting Study
SCORES	Scimed Stent Comparative Restenosis Trial
SIPS	Strategy of IVUS-guided PTCA and Stenting
SMART	Study of AVE-Microstent Ability to Limit Restenosis Trial
STARS	Stent Anti-Thrombotic Regimen Study
START	Stent vs. Directional Atherectomy Randomized Trial
STAT	Stenting vs. Thrombolysis in Acute MI Trial
STENTIM-2	Stent in Acute MI-2
STOPAMI	Stent vs. Thrombolysis for Occluded Coronary Stenosis in Patients with Acute MI
TENISS	Tenax versus Nir Stent Study
TOPPS	Ticlid or Plavix Post Stent
WEST-II	West European Stent Trial-II

* * * * *

REFERENCES

1. Dotter CT, Judkins MR. Transluminal treatment of arteriosclerotic obstructions. Circulation 1964;30:654.

2. Topol EJ. Coronary artery stents—gauging, gorging, and gouging [editorial; comment]. New Engl J Med 1998;339(23):1702-4,

3. Eeckhout E, Kappenberger L, Goy JJ. Stents for intracoronary placement: Current status and future directions. J Am Coll Cardiol 1996;27:757-65.

4. Sigwart U, Puel J, Mirkovitch V, et al. Intravascular stents to prevent occlusion and restenosis after transluminal angioplasty. N Engl J Med 1987;316:701.

5. Serruys PW, Strauss BH, Beatt KJ, et al. Angiographic follow up after placement of a self-expanding coronary artery stent. N Engl J Med 1991;324:13.

6. Ozaki Y, Keane D, Ruygrok P, et al. Six-month clinical and angiographic outcome of the new, less shortening Wallstent in native coronary arteries. Circulation 1996;93(12):2114-20.

7. Gambhir DS, Dusha R, Trehan V, et al. Immediate and six-month outcome of self-expanding Wallstent for long lesions in native coronary arteries. Indian Heart Journal 1997; 49(1):53-9.

8. Pinheiro LF, Pimentel Filho W, de Oliveira WAS, et al. Anatomic reconstruction of native coronary arteries and vein graft with less shortening wallstent. [Portuguese] Arquivos Brasileiros de Cardiologia. 1997;68(5):321-6,

9. Cragg A, Lund G, Rysavy J, et al. Nonsurgical placement of arterial endoprostheses: A new technique using nitinol wire. Radiology 1983;147(1):261-3.

10. van der Giessen WJ, Grollier G, Hoorntje JC, et al. The ESSEX study: First clinical experience with the self-expanding, nitinol radius stent. European Heart Journal 1997;18:Abstr P1014

11. Wilson SH, Han RO, Schwartz RS, Goldberg S, Angiographic outcomes in self-expanding and balloon-expandable stents: Importance of procedural technique in determining late patency. Supplement to Circulation. Vol. 98, No 17, 829A.

12. Macander PJ, Agrawal SK, Roubin GS. The Gianturco-Roubin balloon-expandable intracoronary flexible coil stent. J Interven Cardiol 1991;3:85.

13. Leon MB, Fry ETA, O'Shaughnessy D, et al. Preliminary multicenter experiences with the new GR-II stent for abrupt and threatened closure syndrome. Supplement to Circulation. Vol. 94, No 8, I-207.

14. Multicenter GR-II™ Investigator Group, Leon MB. A multicenter randomized trial comparing the second-generation Gianturco-Roubin (GR II™) and the Palmaz-Schatz coronary stents. Supplement to JACC 1997;29:170A.

15. O'Shaughnessy CD, Popma JJ, Dean LS, et al. The new Gianturco-Roubin coronary stent is an improved therapy for abrupt and threatened closure syndrome. Supplement to JACC 1997;29:416A.

16. Zidar JP, O'Shaughnessy CD, Dean LS, et al, for the GR II™ Clinical Investigators: Elective second generation stenting in small diameter vessels: A multicentre trial (abstract). Eur Heart J 1997;18(suppl):156.

17. Grégoire J, Smith D, et al. Effect of stent design and configuration on collapse resistance to external circumferential pressure. Supplement to JACC 1997;29:414A.

18. Dean LS, O'Shaughnessy CD, Moore PB, et al, on behalf of the GR II™ Clinical Investigators: Elective stenting of *de novo* lesions: Randomized, multicentre trial comparing two stent designs (abstract). Eur Heart J 1997;18(suppl):349.

19. Buchwald A, Unterberg C, Werner G, et al. Initial clinical results with the Wiktor stent: A new balloon-expandable coronary stent. Clin Cardiol 1991;14:374.

20. Eeckhout E, Goy JJ, Stauffer JC, et al. Comparison of the Wallstent, Palmaz-Schatz stent, and Wiktor stent late after intracoronary stenting. Am J Cardiol. 1994;74(6):609-12,

21. Tierstein PS, Massullo V, Jani S, et al. Catheter-based radial therapy to inhibit restenosis after coronary stenting. N Engl J Med 1997;336:1697-1703.

22. White CJ, Ramee SR, Collins TF. Elective placement of the Wiktor stent after coronary angioplasty. Am J Cardiol. 1994;74(3):274-6.

23. Schatz RA. A view of vascular stents. Circulation 1989;79:445.

24. Fischman DL, Leon MB, Baim DS, Schatz RA, et al. A randomized comparison of coronary stent placement and balloon angioplasty in the treatment of coronary artery disease. N Engl J Med 1994;331:496-501.

25. Serruys P, de Jaegere P, Kiemeneij F, et al. A comparison of balloon-expandable stent implantation with balloon angioplasty in patients with coronary artery disease. N Engl J Med 1994;331:489-495.

26. Serruys P, Emanuelsson H, van der Giessen W, et al. Heparin-coated Palmaz-Schatz Stents in human coronary arteries. Early outcome of the Benestent-II pilot study. Circulation 1996;93:412-422.

27. Waigand J, Uhlich F, Gulba DC, et al. Intracoronary stenting with the Multi-Link stent: Single centre experience (abstract). Circulation 1996;94 (suppl I):I-506.

28. Carrozza JP, Yock PG, Linnemeier TJ, et al. Serial expansion of the ACS Multi-Link stent after 8, 12, and 16 atmospheres: A QCA and IVUS pilot study (abstract). Circulation 1996;94 (suppl I):I-509.

29. Chevalier B, Royal T, Glatt B, et al. Early clinical experience with the Multi-Link coronary stent (abstract). Circulation 1996;94 (suppl I):I-1198.

30. Dawkins KD, Emanuelsson HU, van der Giessen WJ, et al. Preliminary results of a European multicentre feasibility and safety registry on an innovative stent: The "W.E.S.T." Study (abstract). Circulation 1995;92 (suppl I):I-280.

31. van der Giessen W, Emanuelsson H, Dawkins K, et al. Six-month clinical outcome and angiographic follow up of the WEST study (abstract). Eur Heart J 1996;17 (suppl):990.

32. Hermiller JB, Baim DS, Linnemeier TJ et al. Clinical results with the ACS Multi-Link stent in the US pilot phase (abstract). Circulation 1996;94 (suppl I):I-505.

33. Kereiakes DJ, Midei M, Hermiller J, et al. Procedural and late outcomes following Multi-Link Duet™ coronary stent deployment;final report for the US registry. Supplement to JACC 1999, 33:2, 95A.

34. Almagor Y, Feld S, Kiemeneij F, et al, for the FINESS Trial Investigators: First International New Intravascular Rigid-flex Endovascular Stent study (FINESS): Clinical and angiographic results after elective and urgent stent implantation. J Am Coll Cardiol 1997;30:847-854.

35. Almagor Y, Feld S, Kiemeneij F, et al. First International New Intravascular Rigid-flex Endovascular Stent Study: Angiographic results and six-month clinical follow up. Eur

Heart J 1997;18 (suppl):156.

36. Zheng H, Corcos T, Pentousis D, et al. Preliminary experience with the NIR coronary stent (abstract). Am J Cardiol 1997;80 :35S.

37. Baim DS, Cutlip DE, Lansky AJ, et al. Results of the NIRVANA equivalency trial comparing the Nir Primo stent to the Palmaz-Schatz stent. Circulation suppl 98:661A.

38. Webb GG, Popma JJ, Lansky AJ, et al. Early and late assessment of the Micro Stent PL coronary stent for restenosis and suboptimal balloon angioplasty. Am Heart J 1997;133:369-374.

39. Kiemeneij F, Laarman, GJ, Odekerken D, et al. Safety and efficacy of AVE GFX stent implantation via 6 French guiding catheters: Results of a pilot study (abstract). Am J Cardiol 1997; 80 (suppl 7A):29S.

40. Rothman MT, Serruys PW, Horntje JCA, et al, on behalf of the EASI Investigators: EASI study: 6-months results of a multicentre evaluation of a short-wave tantalum coil stent (abstract). Eur Heart J 1997;18 (suppl):152.

41. Ozaki Y, Keane D, Noboyoshi M, et al. Coronary lumen at 6-months follow up of a new radio-opaque Cordis tantalum stent using quantitative angiography and intracoronary ultrasound. Am J Cardiol 1995;76:1135-1143.

42. Penn IM, Barbeau G, Brown RIG, et al. Initial human implants with a flexible radio-opaque tantalum stent (abstract). J Am Coll Cardiol 1995;25:288A.

43. Chronos NAF, Robinson KA, Kelly AB, et al. Thromboresistant phosphorylcholine coatings for coronary stents (abstract). Circulation 1995;92 (suppl I):I-685.

44. Bonan R, Paiement P, Tanguay JF, et al. Recoil evaluation of a new stent with phosphorylcholine coating in porcine coronary arteries (abstract). Eur J Cardiol 1997;18 (suppl):153.

45. Gerckens U, Muller R, Cattelaens N, Rowold S, Grube E. Coronary stent graft JoStent reverses conventional stent design in complex coronary lesions. JACC (suppl) 1999;33:36A.

46. Morice M-C, Kumar R, Lefevre T, et al. The French registry of coronary stent grafts;acute and long-term results. JACC (suppl)1999;33:36A.

47. Buchwald AB, Stevens J, Zilz R, et al. Influence of increased wave density of coil stents on the proliferative response in a minipig coronary stent-angioplasty model (abstract). Euro Heart J 1997;18 (suppl):152.

48. Baier R. Initial events and interaction of blood with a foreign surface. J Biomed Mater Res 1969;3:191-206.

49. De Palma VE, Baier R. Investigation of three surface properties of several metals and their relation to blood biocompatibility. J Biomed Mater Res 1972;6:37-75.

50. Leon MB, Baim DS, Popma JJ, et al. A clinical trial comparing three antithrombotic drug regimens after coronary artery stenting. Stent anticoagulation restenosis study investigators. N Engl J Med 1998;339:1665-1671.

51. Karrilon GJ, Morice M-C, Benveniste E, et al. Intracoronary stent implantation without ultrasound guidance and with replacement of conventional anticoagulation by antiplatelet therapy. Thirty-day clinical outcome of the French multicenter registry. Circulation 1996;94:1519-1527.

52. den Heijer P, van Dijk R, Twisk SP, Lie K. Early stent occlusion is not always caused by thrombosis. Cathet Cardiovasc Diagn. 1993;29:136-140.

53. Serruys PW, Strauss BH, Beatt KJ, et al. Angiographic follow up after placement of a self-expanding coronary artery stent. N Engl J Med 1991 324:13.

54. Ozaki Y, Keane D, Ruygrok P, van der Giessen W, de Feyter P. Six-month clinical and angiographic follow up of the new less shortening Wallstent in native coronary arteries. Circulation 1995;92:I-79.

55. Herz I, Assaly A, Solodky A, et al. Primary stenting without pre-dilatation "Stent Alone". Is it possible? Am J Cardiol 1997;80:31S.

56. Colombo A, Hall P, Martini G. Ultrasound-guided coronary stenting without anticoagulation. In Current Review of Interventional Cardiology, Second Edition. Topol EJ, Serruys PW (eds). Current Medicine, Philadelphia, PA. 1995, pg. 115.

57. Mudra H, Regar E, Wener F, Rothman M. A focal high-pressure dilatation of Palmaz-Schatz stents can safely achieve maximal stent expansion using a single balloon catheter approach. First results from the MUSCAT Trial. Circulation 1995;92:I-280.

58. Waksman R, Shen Y, Ghazzal Z, et al. Optimal balloon inflation pressures for stent deployment and correlates of stent thrombosis and in-stent restenosis. Circulation 1996;94,I-258.

59. Savage MP, Fischman DL, Douglas JS, et al. The dark side of high-pressure stent deployment. J Am Coll Cardiol 1997;29 (Suppl. A):368A.

60. Colombo A, Itoh A, Maiello L, et al. Coronary stent implantation in aorto-ostial lesions: Immediate and follow-up results. J Am Coll Cardiology 1996;27:253A.

61. Kiemeneij F, Laarman G, Slagboom T. Mode of deployment of coronary Palmaz-Schatz stents after implantation with the stent delivery system: An intravascular ultrasound study. Am Heart J 1995;129:638-644.

62. Kiemeneij F, Laarman GJ, Slagboom T, Stella P. Transradial Palmaz-Schatz coronary stenting on an outpatient basis: Results of a prospective pilot study. J Inv Cardiol 1995;7:5A-11A.

63. Kiemeneij F, Laarman GJ. Transradial artery Palmaz-Schatz coronary stent implantation: Results of a single center feasibility study. Am Heart J 1995;130:14-21.

64. Kiemeneij F, Laarman GJ, Slagboom T. Percutaneous transradial coronary Palmaz-Schatz stent implantation, guided by intravascular ultrasound. Cathet Cardiovasc Diagn. 1995;34:133-136.

65. Kiemeneij F, Laarman G, Slagboom T, van der Wieken R. Transradial coronary stenting in outpatients. Circulation 1995;92:I-535.

66. Holmes DR, Hirschfeld J, Faxon D, et al. ACC expert consensus document on coronary artery stents. JACC 32:1471-1482.

67. Penn I, Ricci D, Brown R, et al. Randomized study of stenting versus prolonged balloon dilatation in failed angioplasty (PTCA): Preliminary data from the Trial of Angioplasty and Stents in Canada (T.A.S.C.II). Circulation 1993;88:I-601.

68. Ricci D, Buller C, O'Neill B, et al. Coronary stent vs. prolonged perfusion balloon for failed coronary angioplasty. A randomized trial. Circulation 1994;90:I-651.

69. Ray S, Penn I, Ricci D, et al. Mechanism of benefit of stenting in failed PTCA. Final results from the Trial of Angioplasty and Stents in Canada (TASC II). J Am Coll Cardiol 1995;25:156A.

70. Ricci D, Ray S, Buller C, et al. Six-month follow up of patients randomized to prolonged inflation or stent for abrupt occlusion during PTCA-clinical and angiographic data: TASC II. Circulation 1995;92:I-475.

71. Meckel C, Kjelsberg M, Ahmed W, et al. Bailout stenting for

abrupt closure during coronary angioplasty. Circulation 1995;92:I-688.

72. Hui N, Brass N, Klinke P. Effect of coronary stents on PTCA practice in a hospital without cardiac surgery. Circulation 1995;92:I-409.

73. Goy JJ, Eeckhout E, Stauffer JC, Vogt P, Kappenberger L. Emergency endoluminal stenting for abrupt vessel closure following coronary angioplasty: A randomized comparison of the Wiktor and Palmaz-Schatz stents. Cathet Cardiovasc Diagn. 1995;34:128-132.

74. Urban P, Chatelain P, Brzostek T, et al. Bailout coronary stenting with 6F guiding catheters for failed balloon angioplasty. Am Heart J 1995;129:1078-83.

75. Metz D, Urban P, Camenzind E, et al. Improving results of bailout coronary stenting after failed balloon angioplasty. Cathet Cardiovasc Diagn. 1994;32:117-124

76. Schomig A, Kastrati A, Mudra H, et al. Four-year experience with Palmaz-Schatz stenting in coronary angioplasty complicated by dissection with threatened or present vessel closure. Circulation 1994;90:2716-2724.

77. Kiemeneij F, Laarman G, van der Wieken R, Suwarganda J. Emergency coronary stenting with the Palmaz-Schatz stent for failed transluminal coronary angioplasty: Results of a learning phase. Am Heart J 1993;126:23-31.

78. Reifart N, Haase J, Preusler W, et al. Randomized trial comparing two devices: The Palmaz-Schatz stent and the Strecker stent in bailout situations. J Interven Cardiol 1994;7:539-547.

79. Hermann H, Buchbinder M, Cleman M, et al. Emergent use of balloon-expandable coronary artery stenting for failed percutaneous coronary angioplasty. Circulation 1992;86:812-819.

80. Chan C, Tan A, Koh T, Koh P. Intracoronary stenting in the treatment of acute or threatened closure in angiographically small coronary arteries (<3.0 mm) complicating percutaneous transluminal coronary angioplasty. Am J Cardiol 1995;75:23-25.

81. Sutton J, Ellis S, Roubin G, et al. Major clinical events after coronary stenting. The multicenter registry of acute and elective Gianturco-Roubin stent placement. Circulation 1994;89:1126-1137.

82. Agrawal S, Ho D, Liu M, et al. Predictors of thrombotic complications after placement of the flexible coil stent. Am J Cardiol 1994;73:1216-1219.

83. George B, Voorhees W, Roubin G, et al. Multicenter investigation of coronary stenting to treat acute or treated closure after percutaneous transluminal coronary angioplasty: Clinical and angiographic outcomes. J Am Coll Cardiol 1993;22:135-143.

84. Roubin G, Cannon A, Agrawal S, et al. Intracoronary stenting for acute and threatened closure complicating percutaneous transluminal coronary angioplasty. Circulation 1992;85:916-927.

85. Vrolix MC, Rutsch W, Piessens J, et al. Bailout stenting with Medtronic Wiktor: Results from the European stent study group. J Interven Cardiol 1994;7:549-555.

86. Garratt K, White C, Buchbinder M, et al. Wiktor stent placement for unsuccessful coronary angioplasty. Circulation 1994;90:I-279.

87. Ozaki Y, Keane D, Ruygrok P, et al. Acute clinical and angiographic results with the new AVE micro coronary stent in bailout management. Am J Cardiol 1995;76:112-116.

88. Metz D, Urban P, Hoang V, et al. Predicting ischemic complications after bailout stenting following failed coronary angioplasty. Am J Cardiol 1994;74:271-274.

89. Carrozza J, George C, Curry C. Palmaz-Schatz stenting for non-elective indications: Report from the new approaches to coronary intervention (NACI) Registry. Circulation 1995;92:I-86.

90. Hermiller J, Fry E, Peters T, et al. Multiple Gianturco-Roubin stent for long dissections causing acute and threatened coronary artery closure. J Am Coll Cardiol 1994;23:73A.

91. Recreate ref Linnemeier

92. Sankardas M, Garrahy J, McEniery PT. Sequential implantation of dissimilar tandem stents for long dissections complicating percutaneous transluminal coronary angioplasty. Cathet Cardiovasc Diagn. 1995;34:155-158.

93. Agrawal S, Liu M, Hearn J, et al. Can preemptive stenting improve the outcome of acute closure? J Am Coll Cardiol 1993;21:291A.

94. Lincoff M, Topol E, Chapekis A, et al. Intracoronary stenting compared with conventional therapy for abrupt vessel closure complicating coronary angioplasty: A matched case-control study. J Am Coll Cardiol 1993;21:866-875.

95. Stauffer JC, Eeckhout E, Goy JJ, et al. Major dissection during coronary angioplasty: Outcome using prolonged balloon inflation versus coronary stenting. J Invas Cardiol 1995;7:221-227.

96. Garratt K, Voorhees W, Bell M, et al. Complications related to intracoronary stents placed for moderate and severe dissections: Cook FlexStent Registry report. J Am Coll Cardiol 1994;23:102A.

97. Pilon C, Foley JB, Penn I, Brown R. A costing study of coronary stenting in failed angioplasty. J Am Coll Cardiol 1994;23:73A.

98. Gaspard P, Didier B, Lienhart Y, et al. Emergency temporary stenting should be preferred to permanent stenting for abrupt closure during coronary angioplasty. J Am Coll Cardiol 1994;23:103A.

99. Hall P, Nakamura S, Maiello L, et al. Clinical and angiographic outcome after Palmaz-Schatz stent implantation guided by intravascular ultrasound. J Inv Cardiol 1995;7:12A-22A.

100. Morice M-C. Advances in post stenting medication protocol. J Inv Cardiol 1995;7:32A-35A.

101. Colombo A, Maiello L, Nakamura S, et al. Preliminary experience of coronary stenting with the MicroStent. J Am Coll Cardiol 1995;25:239A.

102. Hamasaki N, Nosaka H, Nobuyoshi M. Initial experience of Cordis stent implantation. J Am Coll Cardiol 1995;25:239A.

103. Karouny E, Khalife K, Monassier J-P, et al. Clinical experience with Medtronic Wiktor stent implantation: A report from the French Multicenter Registry. J Am Coll Cardiol 1995;25:239A.

104. Savage M, Fischmann D, Schatz R, et al. Long-term angiographic and clinical outcome after implantation of a balloon-expandable stent in the native coronary circulation. J Am Coll Cardiol 1994;24:1207-1212.

105. Popma J, Colombo A, Chuang YC, et al. Late angiographic outcome after ultrasound-guided stent deployment in native coronary arteries using adjunct high-pressure balloon dilatation. Circulation 1994;90:I-612.

106. Webb J, Abel J, Allard M, Carere R, Evans E, Dodek A. AVE MicroStent: Initial human experience. Circulation 1994;90:I-612.

107. de Jaegere P, Serruys P, Bertrand M, et al. Angiographic

predictors of recurrence of restenosis after Wiktor stent implantation in native coronary arteries. Am J Cardiol 1993;72:165-9.

108. Carrozza J, Kuntz R, Levine M, et al. Angiographic and clinical outcome of intracoronary stenting: Immediate and long-term results from a large single-center experience. J Am Coll Cardiol 1992;20:328-337.

109. Strauss B, Serruys P, Bertrand M, et al. Quantitative angiographic follow up of the coronary Wallstent in native vessels and bypass grafts (European experience--March 1986 to March 1990). Am J Cardiol 1992;69:475-481.

110. Dawkins K, Emanuelson H, Wine VdG, et al. Preliminary results of a European multicenter feasibility and safety registry of an innovative stent: The WEST Study. Circulation 1995;92:I-280.

111. Chevalier B, Royer T, Glatt B, et al. Preliminary experience of coronary stenting with the MicroStent. Circulation 1995;92:I-409.

112. Goy J, Eeckhout G, Stauffer J-C, Vogt P. Stenting of the right coronary artery for de novo stenoses. A comparison of the Wiktor and the Palmaz-Schatz stents. Circulation 1995;92:I-536.

113. Levine M, Leonard B, Burke J, et al. Clinical and angiographic results of balloon-expandable intracoronary stents in right coronary artery stenoses. J Am Coll Cardiol 1990;16:332-339.

114. Fischman D, Savage M, Zalewski A. Overview of the Palmaz-Schatz stent. J Interven Cardiol 1991;3:75.

115. Fischman DL, Leon MB, Baim DS, et al. A randomized comparison of coronary stent placement and balloon angioplasty in the treatment of coronary artery disease. Stent Restenosis Study investigators. N Engl J Med 1994;331:496-501.

116. Serruys PW, de Jaegere P, Kiemeneij F, et al. A comparison of balloon-expandable stent implantation with balloon angioplasty in patients with coronary artery disease. BENESTENT Study Group. N Engl J Med 1994;331:489-95.

117. Fernandez-Ortiz A, Goicolea J, Perez-Vizcaynio M, et al. Is coronary stent recoil different for Gianturco-Roubin and Palmaz-Schatz stent? Circulation 1995;92:I-94.

118. Kimura T, Yokoi H, Nakagawa Y, et al. Three-year follow up after implantation of metallic coronary artery stents. N Engl J Med 1996;334:561-66.

119. Macaya C, Serruys PW, Ruygrok P, et al. Continued benefit of coronary stenting versus balloon angioplasty: one-year clinical follow up of BENESTENT trial. BENESTENT Study Group. J Am Coll Cardiol 1996;27:255-61.

120. Serruys PW, et al. BENESTENT-II Trial: subgroup analysis of patients assigned either to angiographic and clinical follow or clinical follow up alone. Circulation 1997;3650A-00.

121. Leon MB, Tierstein PS, Lansky AJ, et al. Intracoronary gamma radiation to reduce in-stent restenosis: The multi-center GAMMA I randomized clinical trial. JACC 1999;33:19A.

122. Wong SC, Chuang YC, Hong MK, et al. Stent placement is safe and effective in the treatment of older (>4 years) saphenous vein graft lesions. JACC 1995;25:79A.

123. Sketch MH, Jr., Wong SC, Chuang YC, et al. JJIS Stent Investigators. Progressive deterioration in late (2-year) clinical outcomes after stent implantation in saphenous vein grafts: The multicenter JJIS experience. JACC 1995;25:79A.

124. Wong SC, Popma JJ, Pichard A Kent, K. Comparison of clinical and angiographic outcomes after saphenous vein graft angioplasty using coronary versus 'biliary' tubular slotted stents. Circulation 1995;91:339-50.

125. Piana RN, Moscucci M, Cohen DJ, et al. Palmaz-Schatz stenting for treatment of focal vein graft stenosis: Immediate results and long-term outcome. J Am Coll Cardiol 1994;23:1296-1304.

126. Savage MP, Douglas JS, Fischman DL, et al. Stent placement compared with balloon angioplasty for obstructed coronary bypass grafts. Saphenous Vein *De Novo* Trial Investigators. N Engl J Med 1997;337:740-7.

127. Wong SC, Baim DS, Schatz RA, et al. Immediate results and late outcomes after stent implantation in saphenous vein graft lesions: The multicenter US Palmaz-Schatz stent experience. The Palmaz-Schatz Stent Study Group. J Am Coll Cardiol 1995;26:704-12.

128. Kaplan BM, Safian RD, Grines CL, Goldstein JA, et al. Usefulness of adjunctive angioscopy and extraction atherectomy before stent implantation in high-risk aortocoronary saphenous vein grafts. Am J Cardiol 1995;76:822-824.

129. Denardo SJ, Morris NB, Rocha-Singh KJ, Curtis GP, et al. Safety and efficacy of extended urokinase infusion plus stent deployment for treatment of obstructed, older saphenous vein grafts. Am J Cardiol 1995;76:776-780.

130. Hadjimiltiades S, Gourassas PJ, Louridas G, Tsifodimos D. Stenting the distal anastomotic site of the left internal mammary artery graft: A case report. Catheterization & Cardiovascular Diagnosis 1994;32(2):157-61.

131. de la Torre JM, Riesco F, Zueco J, Figueroa A, Colman T. Primary stenting without predilatation, "stent alone," at the origin of a left internal mammary artery graft equivalent to a left main coronary artery. Journal of Invasive Cardiology 1998;10(9):555-7.

132. Califf RM, Tomabechi Y, Lee KL, et al. Outcome in one-vessel coronary artery disease. Circulation 1983;67(2):283-90.

133. Brooks N, Cattell M, Jennings K, et al. Isolated disease of left anterior descending coronary artery. Angiocardiographic and clinical study of 218 patients. British Heart Journal 1982;47(1):71-7.

134. Klein LW, Weintraub WAS, Agarwal JB, et al. Prognostic significance of severe narrowing of the proximal portion of the left anterior descending coronary artery. AJC 1986;58(1):42-6.

135. Parisi AF, Folland ED, Hartigan P. A comparison of angioplasty with medical therapy in the treatment of single-vessel coronary artery disease. Veterans' Affairs ACME Investigators. N Engl J Med 1992;326(1):10-6.

136. Strauss WE, Fortin T, Hartigan P, Folland ED, Parisi AF. A comparison of quality of life scores in patients with angina pectoris after angioplasty compared with after medical therapy. Outcomes of a randomized clinical trial. Veterans' Affairs Study of Angioplasty compared to Medical Therapy Investigators. Circulation 1995;92(7):1710-9.

137. Mahmarian JJ, Pratt CM, Boyce PTM, Verani MS. The variable extent of jeopardized myocardium in patients with single-vessel coronary artery disease: Quantification by thallium-201 single photon emission computed tomography. JACC 1991;17(2):355-62.

138. Kalbfleisch H, Hort W. Quantitative study on the size of coronary artery supplying areas postmortem. American Heart Journal 1977;94(2):183-8.

139. Bailey SR, Keisz RS, Linnemeier TJ, Cooper-Reade GM, Roberts DK, St. Gore FG, Stone G. Stent implantation in

small vessels using ultrasound-guided implantation: Comparison of late outcome of LAD and non-LAD lesions. JACC 1999;33:68A.

140. Versaci F, Gaspardone A, Phil M, et al. A comparison of coronary artery stenting with angioplasty for isolated stenosis of the proximal left anterior descending coronary artery. N Engl J Med 1997;336:817-22.

141. Rechavia E, Litvack F, Macko G, Eigler N. Stent implantation of saphenous vein graft aorto-ostial lesions in patients with unstable ischemic syndromes: Immediate angiographic results and long-term clinical outcome. J Am Coll Cardiol 1995;25:866-870.

142. Zampieri P, Colombo A, Almagor Y, Mairello L, Finci L. Results of coronary stenting of ostial lesions. Am J Cardiol 1994;73:901-903.

143. Rocha-Singh K, Morris N, Wong C, et al. Coronary stenting for treatment of ostial stenosis of native coronary arteries or aortocoronary saphenous venous grafts. Am J Cardiol 1995;75:26-29.

144. Eeckhout E, Stauffer J-C, Vogt P, Debbas N, Kappenberger L, Goy J-J. A comparison of intracoronary stenting with conventional balloon angioplasty for the treatment of new onset stenoses of the right coronary artery. J Am Coll Cardiol 1995;25:196A.

145. Jain SP, Liu MW, Dean LS, et al. Comparison of balloon angioplasty versus debulking devices versus stenting in right coronary ostial lesions. Am J Cardiol 1997;79:1334-1338.

146. Wong SC, Popma J, Hong M, et al. Procedural results and long-term clinical outcomes in aorto-ostial saphenous vein graft lesions after new device angioplasty. J Am Coll Cardiol 1995;25:394A.

147. Schuhlen H, Hadamitzky M, Walter H, et al. Major benefit from antiplatelet therapy for patients at high risk for adverse cardiac events after coronary Palmaz-Schatz stent placement. Circulation 1997;95:2015-2021.

148. Mori M, Kurogane H, Hayashi T, et al. Comparison of results of intracoronary implantation of the Palmaz-Schatz stent with conventional balloon angioplasty in chronic total coronary lateral occlusion. American Journal of Cardiology 1996;78(9):985-9.

149. Sirnes PA, Golf S, Myreng Y, et al. Stenting in Chronic Coronary Occlusion (SICCO): A randomized, controlled trial of adding stent implantation after successful angioplasty. JACC 1996;28(6):1444-51.

150. Rubartelli P, Giommi L, Vassanelli C, et al. Stent implantation versus balloon angioplasty in chronic coronary occlusions: Results from the GISSOC trial. Gruppo Italiano di Studio sullo Stent nelle Occlusioni Coronariche. JACC 1998;32(1):90-6.

151. Sirnes PA, Golf S, Myreng Y, et al. Sustained benefit of stenting chronic coronary occlusion: Long-term clinical follow up of the Stenting in Chronic Coronary Occlusion (SICCO) study. JACC 1998;32(2):305-10.

152. Title LM, Buller CE, Catellier D, et al. Efficacy of stenting versus balloon angioplasty in small-diameter (<3mm) total coronary occlusions: A Total Occlusion Study of Canada substudy. Circulation Supp 1998;17;I-639,3362.

153. Tilli FV, Aliabadi D, Kinn JW, et al. Real life stenting: A comparison of target vessel revascularization in BENESTENT-STRESS lesions to non BENESTENT-STRESS lesions. Circulation 1996;94,I-333.

154. Bell MR, Wood DL, Berger PB, et al. Intracoronary stents for high-risk patients: Early clinical outcome and economic

analysis. Circulation 1996;94,I-333.

155. Medina A, Melian F, deLezo J, et al. Effectiveness of coronary stenting for the treatment of chronic total occlusion in angina pectoris. Am J Cardiol 1994;73:1222-1224.

156. Hsu Y-S, Tamai H, Ueda K, et al. Clinical efficacy of coronary stenting in chronic total occlusions. Circulation 1994;90:I-613.

157. Ooka M, Suzuki T, Kosokawa H, et al. Stenting vs. non-stenting after revascularization of chronic total occlusion. Circulation 1994;90:I-613.

158. Maiello L, Hall P, Nakamura S, et al. Results of stent implantation for diffuse coronary disease assisted by ultravascular ultrasound. J Am Coll Cardiol 1995;25:156A.

159. Reimers B, Di Mario C, Nierop P, et al. Long-term restenosis after multiple stent implantation. A quantitative angiographic study. Circulation 1995;92:I-327.

160. Shaknovich A, Moses J, Undemir C, et al. Procedural and short-term clinical outcomes of multiple Palmaz-Schatz stents (PSS) in very long lesions/dissections. Circulation 1995;92:I-535.

161. Akira I, Hall P, Maiello L, et al. Coronary stenting of long lesions (greater than 20 mm)-A matched comparison of different stents. Circulation 1995;92:I-688.

162. Ooka M, Suzuki T, Yokoya K, et al. Stenting after revascularization of chronic total occlusion. Circulation 1995;92:I-94.

163. Goldberg SL, Colombo A, Maiello L, Borrione M, et al. Intracoronary stent insertion after balloon angioplasty of chronic total occlusion. J Am Coll Cardiol 1995;26:713-719.

164. Yokoi H, Nobuyoshi M, Nosaka H, et al. Coronary stenting for long lesions (lesion length >20 mm) in native coronary arteries: Comparison of three different types of stent. Circulation 1996;94,I-685.

165. Nienaber CA, Fratz S, Lund GK, et al. Primary stent placement or balloon angioplasty for chronic coronary occlusions: A matched pair analysis in 100 patients. Circulation 1996;94,I-686.

166. Elezi S, Schuhlen H, Hausleiter J, et al. Six-month angiographic follow up after stenting of total coronary occlusions. J Am Coll Cardiol 1997;29 (Suppl. A):16A.

167. Sato Y, Kimura T, Nosaka H, Nobuyoshi M. Randomized comparison of balloon angioplasty (BA) versus coronary stent implantation (CS) for total occlusion (TO): Preliminary result. Circulation 1995;92:I-475.

168. Sievert H, Rohde S, Schulze R, et al. Stent implantation after successful balloon angioplasty of a chronic coronary occlusion - a randomized trial. J Am Coll Cardiol 1997;29 (Suppl. A):15A.

169. Mathey DG, Seidensticker A, Rau T, et al. Chronic coronary artery occlusion: Reduction of restenosis- and reocclusion-rates by stent treatment. J Am Coll Cardiol 1997;29 (Suppl. A):396A.

170. Gaxiola E, Vlietstra RE, Browne KF, et al. Six-month follow up of patients with multiple stents in a single coronary artery. J Am Coll Cardiol 1997;29 (Suppl. A):276A.

171. Hamasaki N, Nosaka H, Kimura T, et al. Influence of lesion length on late angiographic outcome and restenotic process after successful stent implantation. J Am Coll Cardiol 1997;29 (Suppl. A):239A.

172. Aliabadi D, Bower TR, Tilli FV, et al. Multiple stents increases target vessel revascularization rates. J Am Coll Cardiol 1997;29 (Suppl. A):276A.

173. Moussa I, Di Mario C, Moses J, et al. Single versus multiple

Palmaz-Schatz stent implantation: Immediate and follow-up results. J Am Coll Cardiol 1997;29 (Suppl. A):276A.

174. Teirstein P, Schatz R, Russo R, Guarneri E, Stevens M. Coronary stenting of small-diameter vessels: Is it safe? Circulation 1995;92:I-281.

175. Hall P, Colombo A, Itoh A, et al. Gianturco-Roubin stent implantation in small vessels without anticoagulation. Circulation 1995;92:I-795.

176. Koning R, Cribier A, Chan C, et al. Palmaz-Schatz coronary stenting for de novo lesions in small coronary arteries: Clinical and quantitative angiographic results of a prospective pilot study. Circulation 1996;94,I-685.

177. Rechavia E, Litvack F, Macko G, Eigler NL. Influence of expanded balloon diameter on Palmaz-Schatz stent recoil. Cathet Cardiovasc Diagn 1995;36:11-16.

178. Wong SC, Hirschfeld J, Teirstein P, Schatz R, Shaknovich A, Nobuyoshi M. Differential impact of stent versus PTCA on restenosis in large (> or less 3 mm) vessels in the Stent Restenosis Trial. J Am Coll Cardiol 1995;25:375A.

179. Azar AJ, Detre K, Goldberg S, Kiemeneij F, et al. A meta-analysis on the clinical and angiographic outcomes of stents vs. PTCA in the different coronary vessel sizes in the BENESTENT-I and STRESS ½ trials. Circulation 1995;92:I-475.

180. Greenbaum AB, Popma JJ, O'Shaughnessy CD, Mann JT, Hoff JG, Cox DA, Gardner LH, Parhizgar A, Zidar JP. Bailout stenting in small vessels: Preliminary in-hospital results of the ULTRA acute or threatened closure registry. JACC 1999;33:68A.

181. Guarneri E, Sklar M, Russo R, Claire D, Schatz R, Teirstein P. Escape from stent jail: An in-vitro model. Circulation 1995;92:I-688.

182. Caputo RP, Chafizedeh ER, Stoler RC, et al. "Stent jail"— A minimum security prison. Am J Cardiol 1996 (in-press).

183. Carrie D, Elbaz M, Mebarkia M, et al. "T"-shaped stent placement: A technique for the treatment of coronary bifurcation lesions. J Am Coll Cardiol 1997;29 (Suppl. A):16A.

184. Colombo A, Gaglione A, Nakamura S. "Kissing" stents for bifurcational coronary lesion. Cathet Cardiovas Diag. 1993;30:327-330.

185. Zampieri P, Colombo A, Almagor Y, et al. Results of coronary stenting of ostial lesions. Am J Cardiol 1994;73:901-903.

186. Colombo A, Maiello L, Itoh A, Hall P, et al. Coronary stenting of bifurcation lesions: Immediate and follow-up results. J Am Coll Cardiology 1996;27:277A.

187. Colombo A, Ferraro M, Itoh A, et al. Results of coronary stenting for restenosis. J Am Coll Cardiol 1996;28:830.

188. Penn I, Ricci D, Almond DG, et al. Stenting results in increased early complications and fewer late reinterventions: Final clinical data from the Trial of Angioplasty and Stents in Canada (TASC) I. Circulation 1995;92:I-475.

189. Erbel R, Hande M, Hopp HW, et al. REstenosis STent (REST) study: Randomized trial comparing stenting and balloon angioplasty for treatment of restenosis after balloon angioplasty. J Am Coll Cardiology 1996;27:139A.

190. Stone GW. Oral presentation, TCT 2000, Washington, D.C.

191. Versaci F, Gaspardone A, Phil M, et al. A comparison of coronary artery stenting with angioplasty for isolated stenosis of the proximal left anterior descending coronary artery. N Engl J Med 1997;336:817-22.

192. Masotti M, Serra A, Fernandez-Aviles F, et al. Stent trials and registries. Circulation 1996;94,I-685.

193. Kastrati A, Schomig A, Dietz R, Neumann F-J. Time course of restenosis during the first year after emergency coronary stenting. Circulation 1993;87:1498-1505.

194. Kimura T, Nosaka H, Yokoi H, et al. Serial angiographic follow up after Palmaz-Schatz stent implantation: Comparison with conventional balloon angioplasty. J Am Coll Cardiol 1993;21:1557-1163.

195. Kimura T, Yokoi H, Tamura T, Nakagawa et al. Three years follow-up after implantation of metallic coronary artery stents. N Engl J Med 1996;334:561-6.

196. Hermiller J, Fry E, Peters T, et al. Late lesion regression within the Gianturco-Roubin Flex stent. J Am Coll Cardiol 1995;25:375A.

197. Hermiller J, Fry E, Peters T, et al. Late coronary artery stenosis regression within the Gianturco-Roubin intracoronary stent. Am J Cardiol 1996;77:247-51.

198. Klugherz BD, DeAngelo DL, Kim BK, et al. Three-year clinical follow up after Palmaz-Schatz stenting. J Am Coll Cardiol 1996;27:1185-91.

199. Laham RJ, Carrozza JP, Berger JP, et al. Long-term (4-6 year) outcome of Palmaz-Schatz stenting: Paucity of late clinical stent-related problems. J Am Coll Cardiol 1996;28:820-6.

200. Matthew V, Hasdai D, Holmes DR. Clinical outcome of patients undergoing endoluminal coronary artery reconstruction with three or more stents. J Am Coll Cardiol 1997;30:676-81.

201. Kobayashi, et al. The relationship between length of stented segment and outcome (abstract). J Am Coll Cardiol 1998;31:366A.

202. Baim D, Levine M, Leon M, et al. Management of restenosis within the Palmaz-Schatz coronary stent (the US multicenter experience). Am J Cardiol 1993;71:364-366.

203. Laham R, Carrozza J, Berger C, et al. Long-term (4-6 year) outcome of Palmaz-Schatz coronary stenting. Circulation 1995;92:I-281.

204. Kastrati A, Schuhlen H, Hausleiter J, et al. Restenosis after coronary stent placement and randomization to a 4-week combined antiplatelet or anticoagulant therapy. Circulation 1997;96:462-467.

205. Yokol H, Kimura T, Nobuyoshi M. Palmaz-Schatz coronary stent restenosis: Pattern and management. J Am Coll Cardiol 1994;23:117A.

206. Ikari Y, Hara K, Tamura T, et al. Luminal loss and site of restenosis after Palmaz-Schatz coronary stent implantation. Am J Cardiol 1995;76:117-120.

207. Gordon P, Gibson M, Cohen D, et al. Mechanisms of restenosis and redilation within coronary stents-quantitative angiographic assessment. J Am Coll Cardiol 1993;21:1166-1174.

208. Macander P, Roubin G, Agrawal S, et al. Balloon angioplasty for treatment of in-stent restenosis: Feasibility, safety, and efficacy. Cathet Cardiovasc Diagn. 1994;32:125-131.

209. Reimers B, Moussa I, Akiyama T, et al. Long-term clinical follow up after successful repeat percutaneous intervention for stent restenosis. J Am Coll Cardiol 1997;30:186-92.

210. Sridhar K, Teefy PJ, Almond DG, et al. Long-term clinical outcomes of patients with in-stent restenosis. Circulation 1996;94,I-454.

211. Sharma SK, et al. Rotation atherectomy achieves a higher acute luminal gain vs. PTCA in the treatment of diffuse in-stent restenosis: Insights from the randomized ROSTER trial. JACC (suppl) 1999;33(2)49A.

212. Pathan A, Butte A, Harrell L, et al. Directional coronary atherectomy is superior to PTCA for the treatment of Palmaz-Schatz stent restenosis. J Am Coll Cardiol 1997;29 (Suppl. A):68A.

213. Tamai H, Katou K, Hayakawa H, et al. The impact of Tranilast on restenosis following coronary angioplasty: The second Tranilast restenosis following angioplasty trial (TREAT-2). Circulation 1996;94,I-620.

214. Hsu Y-S, Tamai H, Ueda K, et al. Efficacy of Tranilast on restenosis after coronary stenting. Circulation 1996;94,I-620.

215. Kaul U, Agarwal R, Mathur A, Wasir HS. Intracoronary stent placement in thrombus containing vein graft lesions. J Inv Cardiol 1995;7:248-250.

216. Kaplan BM, Safian RD, Grines CL, Goldstein JA, et al. Usefulness of adjunctive angioscopy and extraction atherectomy before stent implantation in high-risk aortocoronary saphenous vein grafts. Am J Cardiol 1995;76:822-824.

217. Annex BH, Ajluni SC, Larkin TJ, et al. Angioscopic guided interventions in a saphenous vein bypass graft. Cathet Cardiovasc Diagn 1994;31:330-333.

218. Hong MK, Pichard A, Kent KM, et al. Assessing a strategy of standalone extraction atherectomy followed by staged stent placement in degenerated saphenous vein graft lesions. J Am Coll Cardiol 1995;25:394A.

219. Denardo SJ, Morris NB, Rocha-Singh KJ, et al. Safety and efficacy of extended urokinase infusion plus stent deployment for treatment of obstructed, older saphenous vein grafts. Am J Cardiol 1995;76:776-780.

220. Glazier J, Kiernan F, Bauer H, et al. Treatment of thrombotic saphenous vein graft stenoses/occlusions with local urokinase delivery with the dispatch catheter - initial results. Circulation 1995;92:I-671.

221. Kaul U, Agarwal R, Jain P, Wasir H. Safety and efficacy of intracoronary stenting for thrombus-containing lesions. Am J Cardiol 1996;77:425-7.

222. Alfonso F, Rodriguez P, Phillips P, et al. Clinical and angiographic implications of coronary stenting in thrombus-containing lesions. J Am Coll Cardiol 1997;29:725-33.

223. Cohen DJ, Cosgrove R, Berezin R, Popma JJ, Leon MB, Kuntz RE, Ramee S. Cost-effectiveness of rheolytic thrombectomy for thrombus-containing coronary lesions: Results from the VEGAS 2 trial. J Am Coll Cardiol 1999;33:47A.

224. Moussa I, Di Mario C, Moses J, et al. Coronary stenting after rotational atherectomy in calcified and complex lesions. Circulation 1997;96:128-136.

225. Alfonso F, Rodriguez P, Phillips P, et al. Clinical and angiographic implications of coronary stenting in thrombus-containing lesions. J Am Coll Cardiol 1997;29:725-33.

226. Kaul U, Agarwal R, Jain P, Wasir H. Safety and efficacy of intracoronary stenting for thrombus-containing lesions. Am J Cardiol 1996;77:425-7.

227. Mintz G, Dussaillant G, Wong SC, et al. Rotational atherectomy followed by adjunct stents: The preferred therapy for calcified lesions in large vessels? Circulation 1995;92:I-329.

228. Teirstein P, Schatz R, Russo R, Guarneri E, Stevens M. Coronary stenting of small diameter vessels: Is it safe? Circulation 1995;92:I-281.

229. Hall P, Colombo A, Itoh A, et al. Gianturco-Roubin stent implantation in small vessels without anticoagulation. Circulation 1995;92:I-795.

230. Colombo A, Maiello L, Nakamura S, et al. Preliminary experience of coronary stenting with the MicroStent. J Am Coll Cardiol 1995;25:239A.

231. Leon MB, Wong SC. Intracoronary stents: A breakthrough technology or just another small step? Circulation 1994;89:1323-1327.

232. Oesterle SN, Whitbourn R, Fitzgerald PJ, et al. The stent decade: 1987 to 1997. Am Heart J 1998;136:578-599.

233. Colombo A. Coronary stenting: Current state of the art. J Interven Cardiol 1997;10:137-144.

234. Sigwart U. Ten years of stenting: What next? J Interven Cardiol 1997;10:195-205.

235. Ruygrok PN, Serruys PW. Intracoronary stenting: From concept to custom. Circulation 1996;94:882-890.

236. Fry ETA, Hermiller JB, Pinkerton CA. New intracoronary stent designs: form follows function versus function follows form. Current Opinion in Cardiol 1998;13:232-239.

237. Holmes DR Jr, Bell MR, Holmes DR. et al. Interventional cardiology and intracoronary stents-a changing practice: Approved vs. non-approved indications. Cathet Cardiovasc Diagn 1997;40:133-138.

238. Grines CL, Browne KR, Marco J. et al. A comparison of primary angioplasty with thrombolytic therapy for acute myocardial infarction. N Eng J Med 1993;328:673-679.

239. Weaver WD, Grines J, Betriu A et al. Comparison of primary coronary angioplasty and intravenous thrombolytic therapy for acute myocardial infarction. JAMA 1997;278:2093-2098.

240. The Global Use of Strategies to Open Occluded Coronary Arteries in Acute Coronary Syndromes (GUSTO-IIb) Angioplasty Substudy Investigators. A clinical trial comparing primary coronary angioplasty with tissue plasminogen activator for acute myocardial infarction. N Eng J Med 1997;336:1621-1628.

241. Benzuly KH, O'Neill WW, Brodie B et al. Predictors of maintained infarct artery patency after primary angioplasty in high risk patients in PAMI-2. J Am Coll Cardiol 1996;27:279A.

242. Walton AS, Oesterle SN, Yeung AC. Coronary artery stenting for acute closure complicating primary angioplasty for acute myocardial infarction. Cathet Cardiovasc Diagn. 1995;34:142-146.

243. Ahmad T, Webb JG, Carere RR, Dodek A. Coronary stenting for acute myocardial infarction. Am J Cardiol 1995;76:77-80.

244. Wong PH, Wong CM. Intracoronary stenting in acute myocardial infarction. Cathet Cardiovasc Diagn. 1994;33:39-45.

245. Benzuly KH, Goldstein JA, Almany SL, et al. Feasibility of stenting in acute myocardial infarction. Circulation 1995;92:I-616.

246. Iyer S, Bilodeau L, Cannon A, et al. Stenting the infarct related artery within 15 days of the acute event: Immediate and long term outcome using the Flexible Metallic Coil stent. J Am Coll Cardiol 1993;21:291A.

247. Capers Q, Thomas C, Weintraub W, King S, Douglas J, Scott N. Emergent stent placement: Worse out come in the patients with a recent myocardial infarction. J Am Coll Cardiol 1994;23:71A.

248. Levy G, De Boisgelin X, Volpiliere R, Gallay P, Bouvagnet P. Intracoronary stenting in direct angioplasty: Is it dangerous? Circulation 1995;92:I-139.

249. Saito S, Kim K, Hosokawa G, Hatano K, Tanaka S. Primary Palmaz-Schatz implantation without coumadine in acute myocardial infarction. Circulation 1995;92:I-796.

250. Stone GW. Stenting in acute myocardial infarction: Observational studies and randomized trials – 1998. J Inv Cardiol 1998;10(suppl A):16A-26A.

251. Steffenino G, Chierchia S, Fontanelli A, et al. Use of stents during emergency coronary angioplasty in patients with high-risk acute myocardial infarction: In-hospital results from the Italian multicenter registry (RAI). Eur Heart J 1997;18:272

252. Monassier J, Elias J, Raynaud J, et al. STENTIM I: The French registry of stenting in acute myocardial infarction. J Am Coll Cardiol 1996;27:279A.

253. Steinhubl SR, Moliterno DJ, Teirstein PS, et al. Stenting for acute myocardial infarction: The early United States experience. J Am Coll Cardiol 1996;27:279A.

254. Glatt B, Stratiev V, Guyton B, et al. Two years experience of primary stenting in unselected acute myocardial infarction: One month follow-up. Eur Heart J 1997;18:274.

255. Neuman FJ, Walter H, Richardt G, et al. Coronary Palmaz-Schatz stent implantation in acute myocardial infarction. Heart 1996;75:1592-1595.

256. Spaulding C, Cador R, Benhamda K, et al. One-week and six-month angiographic controls of stent implantation after occlusive and nonocclusive dissection during primary balloon angioplasty for acute myocardial infarction. Am J Cardiol 1997;79:1592-1595.

257. Repetto S, Onofri M, Castiglioni B, et al. Stenting of the infarct related artery during complicated angioplasty in acute myocardial infaarction. J Invas Cardiol 1996;8:177-183.

258. Horstkotte D, Piper C, Anderson D, et al. Stent implantation in acute myocardial infarction: Results of a pilot study with 80 consecutive patients. Eur Heart J 1996;17:297.

259. Hans-Jurgen R, Thomas V, Jurgen T, et al. Short and long-term results of stent implantation within 12 hours after failed PTCA in acute myocardial infarction. Circulation 1996;94:I-577.

260. Himbert D, Juliard JM, Benamer H, et al. Hospital outcomes after bail-out coronary stenting in patients with acute myocardial infarction Eur Heart J 1997;18:125.

261. Setiha ME, El Gamal M, Koolen J, et al. Coronary stenting for failed angioplasty in acute myocardial infarction. Cathet Cardiovasc Diagn 1996;39:149-154.

262. Stone GW, Morice MC, Cox D, et al. Outcomes of bail-out Stenting after failed primary angioplasty in acute myocardial infarction – analysis from the PAMI stent trial. J Am Coll Cardiol 1999;33:361A.

263. Stone GW, Brodie BR, Griffin JJ, et al. A prospective multicenter study of the safety and feasibility of primary stenting in acute myocardial infarction: In-hospital and 30 day results of the PAMI stent pilot trial. J Am Coll Cardiol 1998;31:23-30.

264. Ahmad T, Webb JG, Carere R, Dodek A. Coronary stenting for acute myocardial infarction. Am J Cardiol 1995;76:77-80.

265. Delcan JL, Garcia E, Soriano J, et al. Primary coronary stenting in acute myocardial infarction. J Am Coll Cardiol 1996;28:74-81.

266. Valeix BH, Labrunie PJ, Massiani PF. Systematic coronary stenting in the first eight hours of acute myocardial infarction. Circulation 1996;94:I-577.

267. Turi ZG, McGinnity JG, Fischman D, et al. Retrospective comparative study of primary intracoronary stenting versus balloon angioplasty for acute myocardial infarction. Cathet Cardiovasc Diagn 1997;40:235-239.

268. Saito S, Hosokawa G, Kim K, et al. Primary stent implantation in acute myocardial infarction. J Am Coll Cardiol 1996;28:74-81.

269. Gibson CM. Primary angioplasty compared with thrombolysis: New issues in the era of glycoprotein IIb/IIIa inhibition and intracoronary stenting. Ann Intern Med 1999;130:842-846.

270. Surapranata H, vsn't Hof AWJ, Hoorntje JCA, et al. Randomized comparison of coronary stenting with balloon angioplasty in selected patients with acute myocardial infarction. Circulation 1998;97:2505-2505.

271. Saito S, Hosokawa G, Suzuki S, et al. Primary stent implantation is superior to balloon angioplasty in acute myocardial infarction – The results of the Japanese PASTA (Primary Angioplasty versus Stent Implantation in Acute Myocardial Infarction) trial. J Am Coll Cardiol 1997;29:390A.

272. Rodriguez A, Bernardi V, Fernandez M, et al. In-hospital and late results of coronary stents versus conventional balloon angioplasty in acute myocardial infarction (GRAMI trial). Am J Cardiol 1998;81:1286-1291

273. Antoniucci D, Santoro GM, Bolognese L, et al. Elective stenting in acute myocardial infarction: Preliminary results of the Florence Randomized Elective Stenting in Acute Coronary Occlusion (FRESCO) study. J Am Coll Cardiol 1997;29:456A.

274. Maillard L, Marial H, Monassier JP, et al. STENTIM 2. Six months angiographic results. Elective Wiktor stent implantation in acute myocardial infarction compared with balloon angioplasty. Circulation 1998;98:I-21.

275. Stone GW. Predictors of six month event-free survival after mechanical reperfusion in acute myocardial infarction – The PAMI stent randomized trial. Circulation 1999;33:379A.

276. Scheller B, Hennen B, Severin-Kneib S, et al. Follow up of the PSAAMI study population (Primary Stenting vs. Angioplasty in Acute Myocardial Infarction). J Am Coll Cardiol 199;33:29A.

277. Stone G. Primary stenting in acute myocardial infarction. Circulation 1998;97:2482-2485.

278. Stone GW, Morice MC, Lansky A, et al. Routine stent implantation reduces restenosis after primary angioplasty in acute myocardial infarction – results from the PAMI stent randomized trial. J Am Coll Cardiol 1999;33:361A.

279. Lansky A, Stone GW, Mehran R, et al. Impact of baseline TIMI flow on outcomes after primary stenting versus primary PTCA in acute myocardial infarction. Results from PAMI stent. J Am Coll Cardiol 1999;33:368A.

280. Escobar J, Marchant E, Fajuri A. Stenting could decrease coronary blood flow during primary angioplasty in acute myocardial infarction. J Am Coll Cardiol 1999;33:368A.

281. Neuman FJ, Blasini R, Schmitt C, et al. Effect of glycoprotein IIb/IIIa receptor blockade on recovery of coronary flow and left ventricular function after the placement of coronary-artery stents in acute myocardial infarction. Circulation 1998;98:2695-2701.

282. Murdock D, Logemann T, Hoffmann M, et al. Coronary artery stenting for suboptimal PTCA: Results in acute myocardial infarction in patients treated with abciximab: Early and six-month outcome. Cathet Cardiovasc Diagn 1997;42:173-179.

283. Schultz RD, Heuser R, Hatler C, et al. Use of c7E3 FAB in conjunction with primary coronary stenting for acute myocardial infarction complicated by cardiogenic shock. Cath Cardiovasc Diagn 1996;39:143-146.

284. Silva JA, Nunez E, Krishnamoorthy V, et al. Cardiogenic shock complicating acute myocardial infarction: A comparison of primary angioplasty versus primary stenting in

in-hospital outcomes. J Am Coll Cardiol 1999;33:368A.

285. Dirschinger J, Pache J, Kastrati A, et al. Clinical outcomes after rescue stenting in patients with acute myocardial infarction. J Am Coll Cardiol 1999;33:368A.

286. Malosky S, Hirshfeld J, Herrmann H. Comparison of results of intracoronary stenting in patients with unstable vs. stable angina. Cathet Cardiovasc Diagn 1994;31:95-101.

287. Robinson NMK, Thomas MR, Wainwright RJ, Jewitt DE. Is unstable angina a contraindication to intracoronary stent insertion? J Invas Cardiol 1996;8:351-356.

288. Marzocchi A, Piovaccari G, Marrozzini C, et al. Results of coronary stenting for unstable versus stable angina pectoris. Am J Cardiol 1997;79:1314-1318.

289. Shimada K, Kawarabyashi T, Ryuushi K, et al. Efficacy and safety of early coronary stenting for unstable angina. Cath Cardiovasc Diagn 1998;43:381-385.

290. Chauhan A, Ricci DR, Buller C, et al. Multiple coronary stenting in unstable angina: Early and late clinical outcomes. Cath Cardiovasc Diagn 1998;43:11-16.

291. Singh M, Holmes DR, Garratt KN, et al. Stents versus conventional PTCA in unstable angina. J Am Coll Cardiol 1999;33:29A.

292. Singh M, Holmes DR, Garratt KN, et al. Changing outcome of percutaneous intervention in patients with unstable angina. J Am Coll Cardiol 1999;33:31A.

293. Park SJ, Park SW, Lee CW, et al. Long-term outcome of unprotected left main coronary in patients with normal left ventricular function: Is debulking atherectomy prior to stenting beneficial? J Am Coll Cardiol 1999;33:15A.

294. Laham RJ, Carrozza JP, Baim DS. Treatment of unprotected left main stenoses with Palmaz-Schatz stenting. Cath Cardiovasc Diagn 1996;37:77-80.

295. Ellis S, Tamai H, Nobuyoshi M, et al. Contemporary percutaneous treatment of unprotected left main coronary stenoses: Initial results from a multicenter registry analysis 1994-1996. Circulation 1997;96:3867-3872.

296. Chauhan A, Zubaid M, Ricci D, et al. Left main intervention revisited: Early and late outcome of PTCA and stenting. Cathet Cardiovasc Diagn 1999;41:21-29.

297. Park SJ, Park SW, Hong MK, et al. Stenting of unprotected left main coronary artery stenoses: Immediate and late outcomes. J Am Coll Cardiol 1998;31:37-42.

298. Kornowski R, Klustein M, Satler L, et al. Impact of stents on clinical outcomes in percutaneous left main coronary artery revascularization. Am J Cardiol 1998;82:32-37.

299. Amin F, Kelly P, Kurbaan A, et al. Stenting for unprotected and protected left main stem disease: A comparison of short- and long-term outcome. J Interven Cardiol 1997;10:401-407.

300. Lopez JJ, Ho KKL, Stoler R, et al. Percutaneous treatment of protected and unprotected left main coronary stenoses with new devices: Immediate angiographic results and intermediate-term follow-up. J Am Coll Cardiol 1997;29:345-52.

301. Wong P, Wong V, Tse K, et al. A prospective study of elective stenting in unprotected left main coronary disease. Cathet Cardiovasc Diagn 1999;46:153-159.

302. Stefanadis C, Toutouzas K, Vlachopoulos C, et al. Stents wrapped in autologous vein: An experimental study. J Am Coll Cardiol 1996;28:1039-1046.

303. Stefanadis C, Tsiamis E, Vlachopoulos C, et al. Arterial autologous graft-stent for treatment of coronary artery disease: A new technique. Cathet Cardiovasc Diagn 40:302-307, 1997.

304. Colon PJ, Ramee S, Mulingtapang R, et al. Percutaneous

305. Stefanadis C, Tsiamis E, Vlachopoulos C, et al. Autologous vein graft-coated stents for the treatment of thrombus-containing coronary artery lesions. Cathet Cardiovasc Diagn 1997;40:217-222.

306. Araujo JO, Akstein C, Moraes PC, et al. Coronary aneurysm treated with vein on stent. J Inv Cardiol 1999;11:79-82.

307. Saijo Y, Izutsu K, Sonobe T, et al. Successful closure of coronary-bronchial artery fistula with vein graft-coated stent. Cathet Cardiovasc Diagn 1999;46:214-217.

308. Heuser RR, Woodfield S, Lopez A. Obliteration of a coronary artery aneurysm with a PTFE-covered stent: Endoluminal graft for coronary disease revisited. Cathet Cardiovasc Intervent 1999;46:113-116.

309. Ramsdale DR, Mushahwar SS, Morris JL. Repair of coronary artery perforation after rotastenting by implantation of the Jostent covered stent. Cathet Cardiovasc Diagn 1998;45:310-313.

310. De Gregorio J, Corvaja N, Adamian M, et al. Experience with the PTFE covered stent in percutaneous coronary interventional procedures: Indications and outcomes. J Am Coll Cardiol 1999;33:96A

311. Gruberg L, Grenadier E, Beyar R. Percutaneous closure of a coronary artery aneurysm with a bare stent. J Inv Cardiol 1999;11:141-143.

312. Fenton S, Fischman D, Savage M, Rake R, Goldberg S. Influence of gender on outcome after elective coronary stent implantation. Circulation 1995;92:I-86.

313. Nasser TK, Fry ETA, Peters TF, et al. Coronary stenting in women: Clinical outcomes are equivalent to men. J Am Coll Cardiol 1997;29 (Suppl. A):71A.

314. Mehran R, Bucher TA, Lansky AJ, et al. Coronary stenting in women: Early in-hospital and long-term clinical outcomes. J Am Coll Cardiol 1997;29 (Suppl. A):454A

315. Weintraub W, Thompson TD, Ghazzi Z, et al. Does gender influence outcome of coronary stenting. Circulation 1997;98:I-78.

316. Foody J, Balog C, Cho L, et al. Older women benefit from balloon PTCA rather that stenting when combined with IIb/IIIa anti-platelet therapy: A gender specific treatment interaction from EPISTENT. J Am Coll Cardiol 1999;1006-41:12A.

317. Stone GW, Marcovitz P, Lansky AJ, et al. Differential effects of stenting and angioplasty in women versus men undergoing a primary mechanical reperfusion strategy in acute myocardial infarction – The PAMI stent randomized trial. J Am Coll Cardiol 1999;33:357A.

318. Abizaid A, Mehran R, Bucher TA, et al. Does diabetes influence clinical recurrence after coronary stent implantation? J Am Coll Cardiol 1997;29 (Suppl. A):188A.

319. Elezi S, Schuhlen H, Wehinger A, et al. Stent placement in diabetic versus non-diabetic patients. Six-month angiographic follow-up. J Am Coll Cardiol 1997;29 (Suppl. A):188A.

320. Al-Rashddan IR, Rankin JM, Elliott TG, et al. Glycemic control and major adverse cardiac events after PTCA in patients with diabetes. J Am Coll Cardiol 1990;33:97A.

321. Carrozza JP, Ho KL, Neimann D, et al. Diabetes mellitus is associated with adverse 6-month angiographic and clinical outcome following coronary stenting. Circulation 1998;98:I-79.

322. Moussa I, Moses J, Wang X, et al. Why do the coronary vessels in diabetics appear to be angiographically small. J Am

Coll Cardiol 1999;1159-55:78A

323. Kornowski R, Mintz GS, Kent KM, et al. Increased restenosis in diabetes mellitus after coronary interventions is due to exaggerated intimal hyperplasia: A serial intravascular ultrasound study. Circulation 1997;95:1366-1369.

324. Bhaskaran A, Siegel R, Barker B, et al. Stenting during coronary intervention improves procedural and long-term clinical outcomes in diabetics. J Am Coll Cardiol 1999;33:97A.

325. Lefèvre T, Morice MC, Eltchaninoff H et al. One-month results of coronary stenting in patients > 75 years of age. Am J Cardiol 1998;82:17-21.

326. Nasser T, Fry ETA, Annan K, et al. Comparison of six-month outcome of coronary artery stenting in patients <65, 65-75, and >75 years of age. Am J Cardiol 1997;80:998-1001.

327. Nakamura T, Keizou F, Uchiyama H, et al. Stent placement for recurrent vasospastic angina resistant to medical treatment. Cathet Cardiovasc Diagn 1997;42:440-443.

328. Clark DA. The fight against coronary spasm - one more weapon. Cathet Cardiovasc Diagn 1997;42:444.

329. Vale PR, Baron D. Coronary artery stenting for spontaneous coronary artery dissection: A case report and review of the literature. Cathet Cardiovasc Diagn 1998;45:280-286.

330. Klutstein MW, Tzivoni D, Bitran D. Treatment of spontaneous coronary artery dissection: Report of three cases. Cathet Cardiovasc Diagn 1997;40:372-376.

331. Leclerc KM, Mascette AM, Schachter DT et al. Spontaneous coronary artery dissection in a young woman treated with extensive coronary stenting. J Inv Cardiol 1999;4:237-240.

332. Klues HG, Schwarz ER, vom Dahl J et al. Disturbed intracoronary hemodynamics in myocardial bridging. Circulation 1997;96:2905-2913.

333. Smith SC, Taber MT, Robiolio PA, et al. Acute mycardial infarction caused by a myocardial bridge treated with intracoronary stenting. Cathet Cardiovasc Diagn 1997;42:209-212.

334. Heublein B, Pethig K, Maas C, et al. Coronary artery stenting in cardiac allograft vascular disease. Am Heart 1997;134:930-938.

335. Topaz O, Cowley MJ, Pramod K, et al. Percutaneous revasculariztion modalities in heart transplant recipients. Cathet Cardiovasc Diagn 1999;46:227-237.

336. Wong PMT, Piamsomboon C, Mathur A, et al. Efficacy of coronary stenting in the management of cardiac allograft vasculopathy. Am J Cardiol 1998:239-240

337. Tanguay JF, Crowley JJ, Kruse K, et al. Antiplatelet versus warfarin therapy: Platelet, neutrophil, and thrombus deposition for intracoronary stents in a porcine model. J Interven Cardiol 1997;10:349-356.

338. Neumann FJ, Gawaz M, Dickfeld T, et al. Antiplatelet effect of ticlopidine after coronary stenting. J Am Coll Cardiol 1997;29:1515-9.

339. Gawaz M, Neumann FJ, Ott I, et al. Platelet activation and coronary stent implantation. Effect of antithrombotic therapy. Circulation 1996;94:279-285.

340. Morice M-C, Bourdonnec C, Lefevre T, et al. Coronary stenting without coumadin. Phase III. Circulation 1994;90:I-125.

341. Morice M, Zemour G, Benveniste E, et al. Intracoronary stenting without coumadin: One month results of a French multicenter study. Cathet Cardiovasc Diagn. 1995;35:1-7.

342. Lablanche J-M, Grollier G, Danchin N, et al. Full antiplatelet therapy without anticoagulation after coronary stenting. J Am

Coll Cardiol 1995;25:181A.

343. Barragan P, Silverstri M, Sainsous J, et al. Prevention of subacute occlusion after coronary stenting with ticlopidine regimen without intravascular ultrasound guided stenting. J Am Coll Cardiol 1995;25:182A.

344. Colombo A, Nakamura S, Hall P, Maiello L, Ferraro M, Martini G. A prospective study of Gianturco-Roubin coronary stent implantation without anticoagulation. J Am Coll Cardiol 1995;25:50A.

345. Wong C, Popma J, Chuang Y, et al. Economic impact of reduced anticoagulation after saphenous vein graft stent placement. J Am Coll Cardiol 1995;25:80A.

346. Buszman P, Clague J, Gibbs S, et al. Improved post stent management: High gain at low risk. J Am Coll Cardiol 1995;25:182A.

347. Fajadet J, Jordon C, Carvalho H, et al. Percutaneous transradial coronary stenting without coumadin can reduce vascular access complications and hospital stay. J Am Coll Cardiol 1995;25:182A.

348. Blasini R, Mudra H, Schuhlen H, et al. Intravascular ultrasound guided optimized emergency coronary Palmaz-Schatz stent placement without post procedural systemic anticoagulation. J Am Coll Cardiol 1995;25:197A.

349. Colombo A, Nakamura S, Hall P, Maiello L, Finci L, Martini G. A prospective study of Wiktor coronary stent implantation without anticoagulation. J Am Coll Cardiol 1995;25:239A.

350. Colombo A, Hall P, Nakamura S, et al. Intracoronary stenting without anticoagulation accomplished with intravascular ultrasound guidance. Circulation 1995;91:1676-1688.

351. Mehan V, Saizmann C, Kaufmann U, Meier B. Coronary stenting without anticoagulation. Cathet Cardiovasc Diagn. 1995;34:137-140

352. Reifart N, Haase J, Vandormael M, et al. Gianturco-Roubin Stent Acute Closure Evaluation (GRACE): Thirty-day outcomes compared to drug regimen. Circulation 1995;92:I-409.

353. Lablanche J-M, Grollier G, Bonnet J-L, et al. Ticlopidine Aspirin Stent Evaluation (TASTE);A French multicenter study. Circulation 1995;92:I-476.

354. Russo R, Schatz R, Morris N, Stevens M, Teirstein P. Ultrasound-guided coronary stent placement without warfarin anticoagulation: Six-month clinical follow-up. Circulation 1995;92:I-543.

355. Haase H, Reifart N, Baier T, et al. Bail-out stenting (Palmaz-Schatz) without anticoagulation. Circulation 1995;92:I-795.

356. Goods C, Al-Shaibi K, Iyer S, et al. Flexible coil coronary stenting without anticoagulation or intravascular ultrasound: A prospective observational study. Circulation 1995;92:I-795.

357. Belli G, Whitlow P, Gross L, et al. Intracoronary stenting without oral anticoagulation: The Cleveland Clinic Registry. Circulation 1995;92:I-796.

358. Morice M, Breton C, Bunouf P, et al. Coronary stenting without anticoagulant, without intravascular ultrasound. Results of the French Registry. Circulation 1995;92:I-796..

359. Barragan P, Sainsous J, Silestri M, et al. Ticlopidine and subcutaneous heparin as an alternative regimen following coronary stenting. Cathet Cardiovasc Diagn. 1994;32:133-138.

360. Morice M-C. Advances in post stenting medication protocol. J Inv Cardiol 1995;7:32A-35A.

361. Leon MB, Baim DS, Popma JJ, et al. A clinical trial comparing three antithrombotic-drug regimens after coronary-artery stenting. N Engl J Med 1998;339:1665-71.

362. Schömig A, Neuman FJ, Kastrati, et al. A randomized comparison of antiplatelet and anticoagulant therapy after the placement of coronary-artery stents. N Engl J Med 1996;334:1084-9.

363. Bertrand ME, Legrand V, Boland J, et al. Randomized multicenter comparison of conventional anticoagulation versus antiplatelet therapy in unplanned and elective coronary stenting. The full anticoagulation versus aspirin and ticlopidine (FANTASTIC) study. Circulation 1998;98:1597-1603.

364. Urban P, Macaya C, Rupprecht HJ, et al. randomized evaluation of anticoagulation versus antiplatelet therapy after coronary stent implantation in high-risk patients. The multicenter aspirin and ticlopidine trial after intracoronary stenting (MATTIS). Circulation 1998;98:2126-2132.

365. Hall P, Nakamura S, Maiello L, et al. A randomized comparison of combined ticlopidine and aspirin therapy versus aspirin therapy alone after successful intravascular ultrasound-guided stent implantation. Circulation 1996;93:215-222.

366. Steinhubl SR, Lauer MS, Mukherjee DP, et al. The duration of pretreatment with ticlopidine prior to stenting is associated with the risk of procedure-related non-Q-wave myocardial infarctions. J Am Coll Cardiol 1998;32:1366-70.

367. Moussa I, Oetgen M, Roubin G, et al. Effectiveness of clopidogrel and aspirin versus ticlopidine and aspirin in preventing stent thrombosis after coronary stent implantation. Circulation 1999;99:2364-2366.

368. L'Allier P, Aronow H, Yadav J, et al. Is clopidogrel a safe and effective adjunctive anti-platelet therapy for coronary artery stenting? J Am Coll Cardiol 1999;33:40A.

369. Berger PB, Bellot V, Melby S, et al. Clopidogrel versus ticlopidine for coronary stents. J Am Coll Cardiol 1999;33:34A.

370. Mishkel GJ, Lucore CL, Ligon RW, et al. Clopidogrel for the prevention of stent thrombosis. J Am Coll Cardiol 1999;33:34A.

371. Zidar J. Low-molecular-weight heparins in coronary stenting (The ENTICES trial) Am J Cardiol 1998;82:29L-32L.

372. Rabah MM, Premmereur J, Graham M, et al. Comparison of an intravenous bolus of enoxaparin versus unfractionated heparin in elective coronary angioplasty. J Am Coll Cardiol 1999;33:14A.

373. Colombo A, Hall P, Nakamura S, et al. Preliminary experience using protamine to reverse heparin immediately following a successful coronary stent implantation. J Am Coll Cardiol 1995;25:182A.

374. Kereiakes DJ. Preferential benefit of platelet glycoprotein IIb/IIIa receptor blockade: Specific considerations by device and disease state. Am J Cardiol 1998;81(7A):49E-54E.

375. Zidar JP, Kruse KR, Thel MC, et al. Integrilin for emergency coronary artery stenting. J Am Coll Cardiol 1996;27:138A.

376. Kereiakas DJ, Lincoff AM, Miller DP, et al. Abciximab therapy and unplanned coronary stent deployment: favorable effects on stent use, clinical outcomes, and bleeding complications. Circulation 1998;97:857-864.

377. Kereiakas DJ, Lincoff AM, Simoons ML, et al. Complementarity of stenting and abciximab for percutaneous coronary intervention. J Am Coll Cardiol 1998;31:54A.

378. The EPISTENT Investigators. Randomized placebo-controlled and balloon-angioplasty-controlled trial to assess safety of coronary stenting with use of platelet glycoprotein-IIb-IIIa blockade. Lancet 1998;352:87-92.

379. Cura FA, L'Allier PL, Sapp S, et al. Comparison of the protection against restenosis afforded by stenting and abciximab. J Am Coll Cardiol 1999;33:11A.

380. L'Allier PL, Cura FA, Sapp S, et al. EPISTENT: A large scale randomized trial of primary versus provisional coronary stenting with background platelet glycoprotein IIb/IIIa blockade. J Am Coll Cardiol 1999;33:32A.

381. Vorchheimer DA, Fuster V. Oral platelet glycoprotein IIb/IIIa receptor antagonists: The present challenge is safety. Circulation 1998;97:312-314.

382. Theroux P. Oral inhibitors of platelet membrane receptor glycoprotein IIb/IIIa in clinical cardiology: issues and opportunities. Am Heart J. 1998;135:S107-S112.

383. Denardo SJ, Morris NB, Rocha-Singh KJ, Curtis GP, et al. Safety and efficacy of extended urokinase infusion plus stent deployment for treatment of obstructed, older saphenous vein grafts. Am J Cardiol 1995;76:776-780.

384. Leroy O, Martin E, Prat A, et al. Fatal infection of coronary stent implantation. Cathet Cardiovasc Diagn 1996;39:168-170.

385. Roubin GS. Stent infection: A timely reminder. Cathet Cardiovasc Diagn 1996;39:171.

386. Yoon Y, Lee D, Pyun W, et al. Comparison of cilostazol and ticlopidine after coronary artery stenting: Immediate and long-term results. J Am Coll Cardiol 1999;33:40A.

387. Ziada KM, Tuzcu EM, De Franco AC, et al. Intravascular ultrasound assessment of the prevalence and causes of angiographic "haziness" following high-pressure coronary stenting. Am J Cardiol 1997;80:116-121.

388. Hermiller JB, Fry ETA, Peters TF, et al. Update on management of in-stent restenosis. J Interven Cardiol 1998;11[Suppl]S51-S56.

389. Birgelen C, Kutryk MJB, Serruys PW. Three-dimensional intravascular ultrasound analysis of coronary stent deployment and in-stent neointimal volume: current clinical practice and concepts of TRAPIST, ERASER, and ITALICS. J Invas Cardiol 1998;10-17-26.

390. Prati F, Di Mario C, Gill R, et al. Usefulness of on-line three-dimensional reconstruction of intracoronary ultrasound for guidance of stent deployment. Am J Cariol 1996;77:455-461.

391. Mudra H, Klauss V, Blasini R, Kroetz M. Ultrasound guidance of Palmaz-Schatz intracoronary stenting with a combined intravascular ultrasound balloon catheter. Circulation 1994;90:1252-1261.

392. Gorge G, Haude M, Ge J, et al. Intravascular ultrasound after low and high inflation pressure coronary artery stent implantation. J Am Coll Cardiol 1995;26:725-730.

393. Golderberg SL, Hall P, Nakamura S, et al. Is there a benefit from intravascular ultrasound when high-pressure stent expansion is routinely performed prior to ultrasound imaging? J Am Coll Cardiology 1996;27:306A.

394. Gil R, Prati F, Ligthart J, von Birgelen C, van Camp G, Serruys P. Is quantitative angiography a substitute for intracoronary ultrasound in guidance of stent deployment? Circulation 1995;92:I-327.

395. Fitzgerald P. Lesion composition impacts size and symmetry of stent expansion: Initial report from the STRUT registry. J Am Coll Cardiol 1995;25:49A.

396. Caputo R, Lopez J, Ho K, et al. Intravascular ultrasound analysis of routine high pressure balloon post-dilatation after Palmaz-Schatz stent deployment. J Am Coll Cardiol 1995;25:49A.

397. Wong SC, Popma J, Mintz G, et al. Preliminary results from

the Reduced Anticoagulation in Saphenous Vein Graft Stent (RAVES) Trial. Circulation 1994;90:I-125.

398. Popma J, Colombo A, Mintz G, Wong SC, Pichard A. The impact of intravascular ultrasound (IVUS) on post-stent deployment balloon dilatation. J Am Coll Cardiol 1995;25:49A.

399. Jain S, Liu M, Iyer S, Parks M, Babu R, Yadav S. Do high-pressure balloon inflations improve acute gain within flexible metallic coil stents? An intravascular ultrasound assessment. J Am Coll Cardiol 1995;25:49A.

400. Mudra H, Klauss V, Blasini R, et al. Intracoronary ultrasound guidance of stent deployment leads to an increase of luminal gain not discernible by angiography. J Am Coll Cardiol 1994;23:71A.

401. Nunez B, Foster-Smith K, Berger P, Melby S, Garratt K, Higano S. Benefit of intravascular ultrasound guided high pressure inflations in patients with a "perfect" angiographic result: The Mayo Clinic Experience. Circulation 1995;92:I-545.

402. Blasini R, Neumann FJ, Schmitt C, et al. Comparison of angiography and intravascular ultrasound for the assessment of lumen size after coronary stent placement: impact of dilation pressures. Cathet Cardiovasc Diagn 1997;42:113-119.

403. Russo RJ, Nicosia A, Teirstein PS, et al. Angiography versus intravascular ultrasound-directed stent placement. J Am Coll Cardiol 1997;29:60A.

404. Carrozza JP, Hosley DJ, Cohen DS, et al. In-vivo assessment of balloon expansion and stent recoil in normal porcine coronary arteries: on-line measurement using an imaging guidewire. J Am Coll Cardiol 1998;31:493A.

405. Hall P, Nakamura S, Maiello L, Blengino S, Martini G, Colombo A. Factors associated with procedural complications during high pressure optimized Palmaz-Schatz intracoronary stent implantation. Circulation 1994;90:I-612.

406. Uren NG, Schwarzacher SP, Metz JA, et al. Intravascular ultrasound prediction of stent thrombosis: Insights from the POST registry. J Am Coll Cardiol 1997;29:60A.

407. Hayase M, Oshima A, Zidar JP, et al. Comparison of ultrasound vs. angiographic guidance for stenting in the CRUISE study. Circulation 1997;96:I-222.

408. Fitzgerald PJ, Hayase M, Mintz GS et al. CRUISE: Can routine intravascular ultrasound influence stent expansion? Analysis of outcomes. J Am Coll Cardiol 1998;31:396-A.

409. Schiele F, Seronde MF, Gupta S, et al. Optimal intravascular ultrasound criteria for stent deployment: Comparison of different ultrasound criteria on the 6 months restenosis rate. J Am Coll Cardiol 1999;33:101A.

410. Hong MK, Mintz G, Hong MK, et al. Intravascular ultrasound predictors of target lesion revascularization after stenting of protected left main coronary artery stenoses. Am J Cardiol 1999;83:175-179.

411. Moussa I, Moses J, Di Mario C, et al. Does the specific intravascular ultrasound criterion used to optimize stent expansion have an impact on the probability of stent restenosis? Am J Cardiol 1999;83:1012-1017.

412. Moussa I, Di Mario C Moses J, et al. The predictive value of different intravascular ultrasound criteria for restenosis after coronary stenting. J Am Coll Cardiol 1997;29:60A.

413. Bermejo J, Botas J, García E, et al. Mechanisms of residual lumen stenosis after high-pressure stent implantation. Circulation 1998;98:112-118.

414. Carrozza, JP, Hermiller JB, Linnemeier et al. Quantitative coronary angiographic and intravascular ultrasound assessment of a new nonarticulated stent: Report from the advanced cardiovascular systems multilink stent pilot study. J Am Coll Cardiol 1998;31:50-6.

415. Hoffmann R, Mintz GS, Roxana M, et al. Intravascular ultrasound predictors of angiographic restenosis in lesions treated with Palmaz-Schatz stents. J Am Coll Cardiol 1998;31:43-9.

416. Hoffmann R, Mintz GS, Kent KM, et al. Serial intravascular ultrasound predictors of restenosis at the margins of Palmaz-Schatz stents. Am J Cardiol 1997;79:951-953.

417. Prati F, Di Mario C, Parma A, et al. The amount of residual plaque burden after coronary stent implantation is associated with the development of late in-stent neointimal proliferation. An intravascular ultrasound study. J Am Coll Cardiol 1999;33:60A.

418. Dangas G, Mintz GS, Mehran R, et al. Pre-intervention arterial remodeling: A new risk factor for restenosis after non-stent coronary interventions. J Am Coll Cardiol 1999;33:86A.

419. Moussa I, Moses JW, Strain JE, et al. Angiographic and clinical outcome of patients undergoing "stenting after optimal lesion debulking": The "SOLD" pilot study. Circulation 1997;96:I-81.

420. Moussa I, Moses J, Strain J et al. Angiographic and clinical outcome of patients undergoing stenting after optimal lesion debulking: The "SOLD" pilot study. Circulation 1997;98:I-443.

421. Moussa I, Colombo A. Influence of debulking strategies before coronary stenting. Indian Heart J 1998;50(Suppl I) 79-88.

422. Bramucci E, Angoli L, Angelica P, et al. Adjunctive stent implantation following directional coronary atherectomy in patients with coronary artery disease. J Am Coll Cardiol 1998;32:1855-60.

423. Albrecht D, Kaspers S, Füssl R, et al. Coronary plaque morphology affects stent deployment: Assessment by intracoronary ultrasound. Cathet Cardiovasc Diagn 1996;38:229-235.

424. Marsico F, De Servi S, Kubica J, et al. Influence of plaque composition on luminal gain after balloon angioplasty, directional atherectomy, and coronary stenting. Am Heart J 1995;130:971-5.

425. Nicosia A, Russ PS, Teirstein PJ, et al. Factors associated with inadequate stent expansion IVUS analysis of 225 patients enrolled in the AVID study. J Am Coll Cardiol 1997;29:59A.

426. Hoffman R, Mintz G, Kent KM, et al. Comparative early and nine-month results of rotational atherectomy, stents, and the combination of both for calcified lesions in large coronary arteries. Am J Cardiol 1998;81:552-557.

427. Moussa I, Di Mario C, Moses J, et al. Coronary stenting following rotational atherectomy in calcified and complex lesions: angiographic and clinical follow-up results. Circulation 1997;96:128-13.

428. Hong MK, Wong SC, Popma JJ, et al. Favorable results of debulking followed by immediate adjunct stent therapy for high risk saphenous vein graft lesions. J Am Coll Cardiology 1996;27:179A.

429. Annex BH, Ajluni SC, Larkin TJ, et al. Angioscopic guided interventions in a saphenous vein bypass graft. Cathet Cardiovasc Diagn 1994;31:330-333.

430. Hong MK, Pichard A, Kent KM, et al. Assessing a strategy of stand-alone extraction atherectomy followed by staged stent placement in degenerated saphenous vein graft lesions. J Am Coll Cardiol 1995;25:394A.

431. Annex BH, Ajluni SC, Larkin TJ, et al. Angioscopic guided

interventions in a saphenous vein bypass graft. Cathet Cardiovasc Diagn 1994;31:330-333.

432. Hong MK, Pichard A, Kent KM, et al. Assessing a strategy of stand-alone extraction atherectomy followed by staged stent placement in degenerated saphenous vein graft lesions. J Am Coll Cardiol 1995;25:394A.

433. Kern M, Aguirre F, Thomas D, Bach R, Caracciolo E. Impact of lumen narrowing of coronary flow after angioplasty and stent: Intravascular ultrasound Doppler and imaging data in support of physiological-guided coronary angioplasty. Circulation 1995;92:I-263.

434. Verna E, Gil R, Di Mario C, et al. Does coronary stenting following balloon angioplasty improve distal coronary flow reserve? Circulation 1995;92:I-536.

435. Haude M, Baumgart D, Caspari G, Erbel R. Does adjunct coronary stenting in comparison to balloon angioplasty have an impact of Doppler flow velocity parameters? Circulation 1995;92:I-547.

436. Jeremias A, Kutscher S, Haude M, et al. Nonischemic chest pain induced by coronary interventions: A prospective study comparing coronary angioplasty and stent implantation. Circulation 1998;98:2656-2658.

437. Hearne S, Amsterdam PB, Baker WA, et al. Diagnosing coronary arterial stent thrombosis and arterial closure. Am J Cardiol 1998;82:666-667.

438. Abizaid A, Hoffman RH, Walsh CL, et al. Intramural coronary artery hematomas: Intravascular ultrasound and angiographic findings. Circulation 1997;96:I-153.

439. Wilson SH, Rihal CS, Bell MR, et al. Timing of coronary stent thrombosis in patients treated with ticlopidine and aspirin. Am J Cardiol 1999;83:1006-1011.

440. Mak KH, Belli G, Ellis SG, et al. Subacute stent thrombosis: Evolving issues and current concepts. J Am Coll Cardiol 1996;27:494-503.

441. Moussa I, Di Mario C, Reimers B, et al. Subacute stent thrombosis in the era of intravascular ultrasound-guided coronary stenting without anticoagulation: Frequency, predictors and clinical outcome. J Am Coll Cardiol 1997;29:6-12.

442. Werner GS, Gastmann O, Ferrari M, et al. Risk factors for acute and subacute stent thrombosis after high-pressure stent implantation: A study by intracoronary ultrasound. Am Heart J 1998;135:300-9.

443. Fischman DL, Savage MP, Goldberg S, et al. The varying behavior of stent thrombosis in native coronary arteries versus aorto-coronary saphenous vein bypass grafts. J Invas Cardiol 1997;9:407-409.

444. Ponde CK, Aroney CN, McEniery PT, et al. Plaque prolapse between the struts of the intracoronary Palmaz-Schatz stent: Report of two cases with a novel treatment of this unusual problem. Cathet Cardiovasc Diagn 1997;40:353-357.

445. Safian RD, Freed M. Stent: Subacute thrombosis. J Invas Cardiol 1997;9:609-611.

446. Henry P, Boughalem K, Rinaldi JP, et al. Use of anti-GP IIb-IIIa in acute thrombosis after intracoronary stent implantation. Cathet Cardiovasc Diagn 1998;43:105-107.

447. Casserly IP, Hasadai D, Berger PB, et al. Usefulness of abciximab for treatment of early coronary artery stent thrombosis. Am J Cardiol 1998;82:981-984.

448. Mitchel J, McKay R. Treatment of acute stent thrombosis with local urokinase therapy using catheter-based, drug delivery systems: A case report. Cathet Cardiovasc Diagn. 1995;34:149-154.

449. Metz D, Urban P, Hoang V, Camenzind E, Chatelain P, Meier B. Predicting ischemic complications after bailout stenting following failed coronary angioplasty. Am J Cardiol 1994;74:271-274.

450. Morice M-C. Advances in post stenting medication protocol. J Inv Cardiol 1995;7:32A-35A.

451. Mansour K, Moscucci M, Kent C, et al. Vascular complications following directional coronary atherectomy or Palmaz-Schatz stenting. J Am Coll Cardiol 1994;23:136A.

452. Dean L, Voorhees W, Sutor C, Roubin G. Female gender: A risk factor for complications following intracoronary stenting? A Cook multicenter registry report. Circulation 1994;90:I-620.

453. Moscucci M, Mansour K, Kuntz R, et al. Vascular complications of Palmaz-Schatz stenting: Predictors, management and outcome. J Am Coll Cardiol 1994;23:134A.

454. Cantor WJ, Lazzam C, Cohen EA, et al. Failed coronary stent deployment. Am Heart J 1998;136:1088-95.

455. Lohavanichbutr K, Webb JG, Carere RG, et al. Mechanisms, management and outcome of failure of delivery of coronary stents. Am J Cardiol 1999;83:779-781.

456. Buller CE. Failed stent delivery: Importance for modern interventional cardiology. Am Heart J 1998;136:945-7.

457. Cishek MB, Laslett L, Gershony G. Balloon catheter retrieval of dislodged coronary artery stents: A novel technique. Cathet Cardiovasc Diagn 1995;34:350-352.

458. Rozenman Y, Burstein M, Hasin Y, Gotsman M. Retrieval of occluding unexpanded palamaz-Schatz stent from a saphenous aorto-coronary vein graft. Cathet Cardiovasc Diagn. 1995;34:159-161.

459. McGinnity JG, Glazier JJ, Spears JR, et al. Successful redeployment of an unexpanded coronary stent. Cathet Cardiovasc Diagn 1998;44:52-56.

460. Pan M, Medina A, Romero M, et al. Peripheral stent recovery after failed intracoronary delivery. Cathet Cardiovasc Diagn 1992;27:230-233.

461. Elsner M, Peifer A, Kasper W. Intracoronary loss of balloon-mounted stents: Successful retrieval with a 2 mm-"microsnare"-device. Cathet Cardiovasc Diagn 1996;39:271-276.

462. Farshid A, Pitney MR. Intracoronary embolization and retrieval of radio-opaque ring marker on the ACS multi-link stent sheath. Cathet Cardiovasc Diagn 1998;43:306-307.

463. Miketíc S, Carlsson J, Tebbe U. Treatment of a "lost" unexpanded intracoronary stent in a patient with unstable angina. Am J Cardiol 1995;76:1317-1318.

464. Chu TNT, Ling FS. Successful management of Palmaz-Schatz stents deformed by inadvertent angioplasty outside the stents. Cathet Cardiovsc Diagn 1997;41:435-439.

465. Eeckhout E, Vogt P. Stent by stent crush: Procedural outcome and angiographic follow-up. Cathet Cardiovasc Diagn 1998, 45:54-56.

466. Keelan ET, Nunez BD, Berger PB. Management of balloon rupture during rigid stent deployment. Cathet Cardiovasc Diagn 1995;35:211-215.

467. Iniguez A, Macaya C, Alfonso F, Goicolea J. Early angiographic changes of side branches arising from a Palmaz-Schatz stented coronary segment: Results and clinical implications. J Am Coll Cardiol 1994;23:911-915.

468. Mazur W, Grinstead C, Hakim A, et al. Fate of side branches after intracoronary implantation of the Gianturco-Roubin flex-stent for acute or threatened closure after percutaneous transluminal coronary angioplasty. Am J Cardiol 1994;74:1207-1210.

469. Kinoshita T, Kobayashi Y, Nameki M, et al. Difference in security of stent jail among Palmaz-Schatz stent, NIR stent, and multi-link stent: Effect of balloon inflation through stent struts. J Am Coll Cardiol 1999;33;84A.

470. Colombo A, Hall P, Nakamura S, et al. Intracoronary stenting without anticoagulation accomplished with intravascular ultrasound guidance. Circulation 1995;91:1676-1688.

471. Fischman D, Leon M, Baim d, et al. A randomized comparison of coronary-stent placement and balloon angioplasty in the treatment of coronary disease. N Engl J Med 1994;331:496-501.

472. Serruys P, De Jaegere P, Kiemeneji F, et al. A comparison of balloon expandable-stent implantation with balloon angioplasty in patients with coronary artery disease. N Engl J Med 1994;331:489-495.

473. Versaci F, Gaspardone A, Tomai F, et al. A comparison of coronary-artery stenting with angioplasty for isolated stenosis of the proximal left anterior descending coronary artery. N Engl J Med 1997;336:817-22.

474. Savage MP, Douglas JS, Fischman DL, et al. Stent placement compared with balloon angioplasty for obstructed coronary bypass gafts. N Engl J Med 1997;337:740-7.

475. Erbel R, Haude M, Hopp HW, et al. Coronary-artery stenting compared with balloon angioplasty for restenosis after initial balloon angioplasty. N Engl J Med 1998;339:1672-8.

476. Savage MP, Fischman DL, Rake R, et al. Efficacy of coronary stenting versus balloon angioplasty in small coronary arteries. J Am Coll Cardiol 1997;31:307-311.

477. SICCO trial. J Am Coll Cardiol 1996;28:144-51.

478. Buller CE,Vladimir D, Carere RG, et al. Primary stenting versus balloon angioplasty in occluded coronary arteries. Circulation 1999;100:236-242.

479. Stone GW, Brodie BR, Griffin JJ, et al. Prospective, multicenter study of the safety and feasibility of primary stenting in acute myocardial infarction: In-hospital and 30-day results of the PAMI Stent Trial. J Am Coll Cardiol 1998;31:23-30.

480. Schomig A, Neumann F, Kastrati A, et al. A randomized comparison of antiplatelet and anticoagulant therapy after the placement of coronary-artery stents. N Engl J Med 1996;334:1084-9.

481. Leon MB, Baim DS, Popma JJ, et al. A clinical trial comparing three antithrombotic-drug regimens after coronary-artery stenting. N Engl J Med 1998;339:1665-71.

482. EPISTENT Investigators. Evaluation of platelet IIb/IIIa inhibitor for stenting. Randomized placebo-controlled and balloon-angioplasty-controlled trial to assess safety of coronary stenting with use of platelet glycoprotein-IIb/IIIa blockade. Lancet 1998 Jul 11;352(9122):87-92.

483. Antoniucci D, Valenti R, Santoro GM et al. Preliminary experience with stent-supported coronary angioplasty in long narrowings using the long Freedom Force stent: Acute and six month clinical and angiographic results in a series of 27 consecutive patients. Cathet Cardiovasc Diagn 1998;43: 163-167.

484. Chalij MJ, Savalle LH, Tresukosol D, et al. Micro stent I, initial results, and six months follow-up by quantitative coronary angiography. Cathet Cardiovasc Diagn 1998;43: 19-27.

485. Ozaki Y, Keane D, Ruygrok P, et al. Six-month clinical and angiographic outcome of the new, less shortening wallstent in native coronary arteries. Circulation 1996;93: 2114-2120.

486. Nakano Y, Nakagawa Y, Yokoi H, et al. Initial follow-up results of the ACS multi-link stent: A single center experience. Cathet Cardiovasc Diagn 1998;45: 368-374.

487. Hamasaki N, Nosada H, Kimura T, et al. Initial experience with the Cordis stent: Analysis of serial angiographic follow-up. Cathet Cardiovasc Diagn 1997;42: 166-172.

488. Park SJ, Park SW, Lee CW, et al. Immediate results and late clinical outcomes after new crossflex coronary stent implantation. Am J Cardiol 1999;83: 502-506.

489. Kornowski R, Mehran R, Hong MK, et al. Procedural results and late clinical outcomes after placement of three or more stents in single coronary lesions. Circulation 1998;97: 1355-1361.

490. Alonso JJ, Fernandez-Aviles F, Duran JM, et al. Influence of diabetes mellitus on the initial and long-term outcome of patients treated with coronary stenting. J Am Coll Cardiol 1999;33 (2 Suppl A): 98A.

491. Lansky AJ, Mehran R, Popma JJ,et al. Insulin treatment of diabetic women predicts a worse outcome after intracoronary stenting. Clinical results of 564 consecutive patients. J Am Coll Cardiol 1999;33 (2 Suppl A) 97A-98A.

492. Fernandez-Aviles F, Alonso JJ, Duran JM, et al. Long-term prognosis of patients with unstable angina undergoing coronary stenting. J Am Coll Cardiol 1999;33 (2 Suppl A): 391A-392A.

493. Rutherford BD, Jones PG, Vacek JL, et al. Multiple vessel stenting compared to multiple vessel angioplasty: In-hospital outcome and long-term follow-up. J Am Coll Cardiol 1999;33 (2 Suppl A): 13A.

494. Tsuchikane E, Kobayashi T, Nakamura T, et al. One year clinical follow-up results of stent versus atherectomy randomized trial. JACC 1999;33 (2 Suppl A): 15A.

495. Bhargava B, Kornowski R, Hong M, et al. Procedural results and late clinical outcomes following multiple saphenous vein graft stenting.

496. Bhaskaran A, Siegel R, Barker B, et al. Stenting during coronary intervention improves procedural and long-term clinical outcomes in diabetics. JACC 1999;33 (2 Suppl A): 97A.

497. Herzog CA, Ma JZ, Collins AJ. Comparative survival of dialysis patients in the United States after coronary artery bypass surgery, coronary angioplasty, and coronary stenting. Circulation 1998;98 (Suppl I): I-78.

498. Bartorelli AL, Montorsi P, Fabbiocchi F, et al. Does coronary stenting eliminate gender difference in percutaneous revascularization outcome? Circulation 1998;98 (Suppl I): I-77.

499. Carrozza JP, Ho KKL, Neimann D, Kuntz RE, Cutlip DE. Diabetes mellitus is associated with adverse 6-month angiographic and clinical outcome following coronary stenting. Circulation 1998;98 (Suppl I): I-79.

500. Alonso JJ, Duran JM, Gimeno F, et al. Five-year follow-up after coronary stenting: Survival, event-free survival and freedom from new revascularization. Circulation 1998;98 (Suppl I): I-287.

501. Karam C, Aoun A, Cortina R, et al. Nine-year outcome of Palmaz-Schatz intracoronary stenting in 107 patients. Circulation 1998;98 (Suppl I): I-287.

502. Farshid A, Friend CA, Allan RM, et al. Favourable acute and six-month follow-up results after coronary stenting using the small BeStent in 2.5-3.0 mm arteries. Circulation 1998;98 (Suppl I): I-639.

503. Emanuelsson H, Serruys PW, van der Giessen WJ, et al. Clinical and angiographic results with the Multi-Link

coronary stent system B the West European Stent Trial (WEST). J Invas Cardiol 1997;9: 561-568.

504. Carrozza JP Jr., Hermiller JB Jr., Linnemeier TJ, et al. Quantitative coronary angiographic and intravascular ultrasound assessment of a new nonarticulated stent: Report from the Advanced Cardiovascular Systems MultiLink Stent Pilot Study. J Am Coll Cardiol 1998;31: 50-6.

505. Watson PS, Ponde CK, Aroney CN, Cameron J, et al. Angiographic follow-up and clinical experience with the flexible tantalum Cordis stent. Cathet Cardiovasc Diagn 1998;43: 168-173.

506. Oemrawsingh PV, Tuinenburg JC, Schalij MJ, et al. Clinical and angiographic outcome of MicroStent II implantation in native coronary arteries. Am J Cardiol 1998;81: 152-7.

507. Ruygrok P, Barron G, Ormiston J, et al. Introduction of the Multilink stent into routine angioplasty practice: early angiographic and clinical outcome. Cathet Cardiovasc Diagn 1998;43: 147-52.

508. Zheng H, Corcos T, Favereau X, et al. Preliminary experience with the NIR coronary stent. Cathet Cardiovasc Diagn 1998;43: 153-8.

509. Rozenman Y, Lotan C, Mosseri M, et al. Experience with the AVE micro stent in native coronary arteries. Am J Cardiol 1996 Sept 15;78: 685-7.

510. Tresukosol D, Schalij MJ, Savalle LH, et al. Micro Stent, Quantitative coronary angiography, and procedural results.. Cathet Cardiovasc Diagn 1996;38: 135-43.

511. Pentousis D, Guerin Y, Favereau X, et al. Preliminary clinical experience with the Bard XT coronary stent. Am Heart J 1998;136: 786-90.

512. Pomerantsev EV, Colombo A, de la Fuenta L, et al. Microstent to GFX: Experience in 2,325 patients. J Interven Cardiol 1998;11:101-6.

513. Hamaski N, Nakano Y, Nosaka H, et al. Initial experience with the ACS Multilink stent: Serial angiographic follow-up and comparison with the Palmaz-Schatz stent in matched lesions. J Invas Cardiol 1998;10: 76-82.

514. Serruys PW, van der Giessen W, Garcia E, et al. Clinical and angiographic results with the Multi-link stent implanted under intravascular ultrasound guidance (WEST-2 study). J Invas Cardiol 1998;10 (Suppl B): 20B-27B.

515. Ravat H, Cannon A. Early experience with the Bard XT stent. Cathet Cardiovasc Diagn 1998;45: 462-70.

516. Beyar R, Roguin A, Hamburger J, et al. Multicenter pilot study of a serpentine balloon-expandable stent (beStent): acute angiographic and clinical results. J Interven Cardiol 1997;10: 277-86.

517. Carrie D, Puel J, Khalife K, et al. Clinical experience with Wiktor stent implantation: a report from the French multicentric registry. J Interven Cardiol 1996;9: 279-286.

518. Almagor Y, Feld S, Kiemeneij F, et al. First international new intravascular rigid-flex endovascular stent study (FINESS): clincal and angiographic results after elective and urger stent implantation. J Am Coll Cardiol 1997;30: 847-54.

519. Roguin A, Grenadier E, Peled B, et al. Acute and 30-day results of the serpentine balloon expandable stent implanation in simple and complex coronary arterial narrowings. Am J Cardiol 1997;80: 1155-62.

520. Pentousis D, Guerin Y, Funck F, et al. Direct stent implantation without predilatation using the Multilink stent. Am J Cardiol 1998;82: 1437-40.

521. Wong PMT, Piamsombom C, Mathur A, et al. Efficacy of coronary stenting in the management of cardiac allograft vasculopathy. Am J Cardiol 1998 Jul 15;82: 239-41.

522. Kornowski R, Klutstein M, Satler LF, et al. Impact of stents on clincal outcomes in percutaneous left main coronary artery revascularization. Am J Cardiol 1998;82: 32-37.

523. Pubartelli P, Niccoli L, Verna E, et al. Stent implantation versus balloon angiplasty in chronic coronary occlusions: results from the GISSOC trial. J Am Coll Cardiol 1998;32: 90-6.

524. Menafoglio A, Eeckhout E, Debbas N, et al. Randomized comparison of Micro Stent I with Palmaz-Schatz placement for the elective treatment of short coronary stenoses. Cathet Cardiovasc Diagn 1998;43: 403-7.

525. Colombo A, Ferraro M, Itoh A, et al. Results of coronary stenting for restenosis. J Am Coll Cardiol 1996;28: 830-6.

526. Zidar JP, O'Shaughnessy CD, Dean LS, et al. Elective GR II stenting in small vessels: multicenter results. J Am Coll Cardiol 1998;(??): 274A.

527. Nishida T, Colombo A, Briguori C, et al. Contemporary percutaneous treatment of saphenous vein graft stenosis: Immediate and late outcomes. J Invas Cardiol 2000;12:505-512.

528. Farshid A, Friend CA, Allan RM, et al. Favourable acute and six month follow-up results after coronary stenting using the small BeStent in 2.5 B 3.0 arteries. Circulation 1998;98 (Suppl I): I-639.

529. Elezi S, Kastrati A, Neumann FJ, et al. Vessel size and long-term outcome after coronary stent placement. Circulation 1998;98: 1875-80.

530. Lau KW, He Q, Ding ZP, Johan A. Safety and efficacy of angiography-guided stent placement in small native coronary arteries of <3.0mm in diameter. Clin Cardiol 1997;20: 711-6.

531. Koning R, Chan C, Eltchaninoff H, et al. Primary stenting of de novo lesions in small coronary arteries: A prospective, pilot study. Cathet Cardiovasc Diagn 1998;45: 235-8.

532. Savage MP, Fischman DL, Rake R, et al. Efficacy of coronary stenting versus balloon angioplasty in small coronary arteries. J Am Coll Cardiol 1998;31: 307-11.

533. Hamasaki N, Nosaka H, Kimura T, et al. Stenting for small vessel using new generation flexible stent B comparison of balloon angioplasty and Palmaz-Schatz stent. J Am Coll Cardiol 1999;2 (Suppl A): 32A.

534. Mori M, Kurogane H, Hayashi T, et al. Comparison of results of intracoronary implantation of the Palmaz-Schatz stent with conventional balloon angioplasty in chronic total coronary arterial occlusion. Am J Cardiol 1996;78: 985-9.

535. Phillips PS, Segovia J, Alfonso F, et al. Advantage of stents in the most proximal left anterior descending coronary artery. Am Heart J 1998;135: 719-25.

536. Wong P, Wong CM, Ko P, Fong PC. Elective stenting of unprotected left main coronary disease. Cathet Cardiovasc Diagn 1996;39: 347-54.

537. DeCesare NB, Bartorelli AL, Galli S, et al. Treatment of ostial lesions of the left anterior descending coronary artery with Palmaz-Schatz coronary stent. Am Heart J 1996;132: 716-20.

538. Itoh A, Hall P, Maiello L, et al. Implantation of the peripheral Wallstent for diffuse lesions in coronary arteries and vein grafts. Cathet Cardiovasc Diagn 1996;37: 322-30.

539. Amin FR, Kelly PA, Kurbaan AS, et al. Stenting for unprotected and protected left main stem disease: A comparison of short- and long-term outcome. J Interven Cardiol 1997;10:401-7.

540. Moussa I, DiMario C, Moses J, et al. Comparison of angiographic and clinical outcomes of coronary stenting of

chronic total occlusion versus subtotal occlusions. Am J Cardiol 1998;81:1-6.

541. Keane D, Azar AJ, de Jaegere P, et al. Clinical and angiographic outcome of elective stent implantation in small coronary vessels: An analysis of the BENESTENT trial. Semin Intervent Cardiol 1996;1:255-62.

542. Lau KW, He Q, Bing ZP, Johan A. Safety and efficacy of angiography-guided stent placement in small native coronary arteries of <3.0mm in diameter. Clin Cardiol 1997;20: 711-16.

543. Park SJ, Park SW, Hong MK, et al. Stenting of unprotected left main coronary artery stenoses: Immediate and late outcomes. J Am Coll Cardiol 1998;31:37-42.

544. Heublein B, Pethig K, Maab C, et al. Coronary artery stenting in cardiac allograft vascular disease. Am Heart J 1997;134: 930-8.

545. DeGregorio J, Kobayashi N, Adamaian M, et al. A matched comparison between spot stenting and traditional stenting for the treatment of long lesions. J Am Coll Cardiol 1999;33 (2 Suppl A):33A.

546. Peterson M, Carter A, Mehran R, et al. Can debulking prior to stenting be justified as standard treatment for right coronary artery ostial lesions? J Am Coll Cardiol 1999;33 (2 Suppl A):27A.

547. Sheiban I, Albiero R, Marsico F, et al. Immediate and long term results AT stenting in bifurcational coronary lesions. J Am Coll Cardiol 1999;33 (2 Suppl A): 91A.

548. Coussement P, Dens J, Desmet W, Piessens J, Bijnens B, De Scheerder I. Side branch evaluation after stent implantation. J Am Coll Cardiol 1999;33 (2 Suppl A): 74A.

549. Lotan C, Krakover R, Tugeman Y, et al. The STOP study B: A randomized multicenter Israeli study for stents in total occlusion and restenosis prevention. J Am Coll Cardiol 1999;33 (2 Suppl A):28A.

550. Tamura T, Kimura T, Nosaka H,et al. Stent treatment for unprotected left main coronary artery stenosis: long-term follow-up result. J Am Coll Cardiol 1999;33 (2 Suppl A): 33A.

551. Siegel R, Bhaskaran A, Underwood P, et al. Stenting of left main coronary artery: A viable alternative in patients with prohibitive surgical risk. J Am Coll Cardiol 1999;33 (2 Suppl A):52A.

552. de Scheerder I, Dens J, Desmet W, et al. Treatment of bifurcation lesions using a new tubular stent. J Am Coll Cardiol 1999;33 (2 Suppl A):97A.

553. Anzuini A, Rosanio S, Legrand V, et al. Implantation of the Wiktor stent in coronary bifurcation lesions: Immediate and follow-up results. Circulation 1998;98 (Suppl I): I-638.

554. Brunel P, Commeau P, Koning R, et al. Assessment of coronary bifurcation lesions treated with stent implantation on the parent vessel and with balloon or stent on the sidebranch. Circulation 1998;98 (Suppl I): I-639.

555. Scavetta K, Oh C, Caldron R, et al. Results of saphenous vein graft stent implantation: Single center results from use of oversized balloon catheters. Angiography 1999;50:891-899.

556. Tamai H, Tsuchigane E, Suzuki T, et al. Circulation 1998;98 (Suppl I): I-639.

557. DeGregorio J, Kobayashi Y, Albiero R, et al. Long term results of IVUS guided PTCA and spot stenting in long lesions and small vessels. Circulation 1998;98 (Suppl I): I-90.

558. Shizuta S, Kimura T, Nosaka H,et al. Serial angiographic follow-up after stent implantation for chronic total occulusion. Circulation 1998;98 (Suppl I): I-284.

559. Gruberg L, Hong MK, Mehran R, et al. In-hospital and long-term results of stent deployment compared with balloon angioplasty for treatment of narrowing at the saphenous vein graft distal anastomosis site. Am J Cardiol 1999;84:1381-1384.

560. Clague JR, Vasudeva A, Ward DE, Pumphrey CW, Redwood DR. The AVE micro coronary stent as a bailout device. J Invas Cardiol 1997;9:339-43.

561. Murdock DK, Logemann T, Hoffmann MT,et al. Coronary artery stenting for suboptimal PTCA results in acute myocardial infarction in patients treated with abciximab: early and six-month outcome. Cathet Cardiovasc Diagn 1997;42:173-9.

562. Lau KW, Gao W, Ding ZP, Kowk V. Single bailout stenting for threatened coronary closure complicating balloon angioplasty: Acute and mid-term outcome. Coronary Artery Disease 1996;7:327-33.

563. Chauhan A, Zubaid M, Buller CE, et al. Comparison of bailout versus elective stenting: Time to reassess our benchmarks of outcome. Cathet Cardiovasc Diagn 1997;41: 40-7.

564. Witkowski A, Chmielak Z, Dabrowski M, et al. High-pressure bail-out coronary stenting without anticoagulation: Early outcome and follow-up results. J Invas Cardiol 1998;10: 83-88.

565. Ortiz-Fernandez A, Goicolea J, Perez-Vizcayna MJ, et al. Six-month follow-up of successful stenting for acute dissection after coronary angioplasty: Comparison between slotted tube (Palmaz-Schatz) and flexible coil (Gianturco-Roubin) stent designs. J Interven Cardiol 1998;11:41-7.

566. Bertrand OF, Legrand V, Bilodeau L, et al. Emergency coronary stenting with Wiktor stent B: Immediate and late results. J Invas Cardiol 1997;9:2-9.

567. Himbert D, Juliard JM, Benamer H, et al. Hospital outcome after bailout coronary stenting in patients with acute myocardial infarction. Cathet Cardiovasc Diagn 1998;44: 371-77.

568. Eeckhout E, Stauffer JC, Vogt P, et al. Placement of multiple and different stent types for very long dissections during coronary angioplasty. Cathet Cardiovasc Diagn 1996;39:302-8.

569. Machraoui A, Germing A, von Dryander S, et al. High pressure coronary stenting: Efficacy and safety of aspirin versus coumadin plus aspirin. J Invas Cardiol 1997;9: 171-6.

570. Miketic S, Carlsson J, Tebbe U. Safety and efficacy of angiographic guided elective Palmaz-Schatz stent implantation without coumadin: comparison of stent implantation and angioplasty. J Inteven Cardiol 1997;10: 265-70.

571. Berger PB, Bell MR, Hasdai D, et al. Safety and efficacy of ticlopidine for only 2 weeks after successful intracoronary stent placement. Circulation 1999;99: 248-53.

572. Berger PB, Bell MR, Grill DE, et al. Frequency of adverse clinical events in the 12 months following successful intracoronary stent placement in patients treated with aspirin and ticlopidine (without warfarin). Am J Cardiol 1998;81: 713-18.

573. Lawrence ME, Burtt DM, Shaftel PA, et al. Intracoronary stent placement without coumadin or intravascular ultrasound. J Invas Cardiol 1996;8: 428-32.

574. Albiero R, Hall P, Itoh A, et al. Results of a consecutive series of patients receiving only antiplatelet therapy after optimized stent implantation. Comparison of aspirin alone versus combined ticlopidine and aspirin therapy. Circulation

1997;95: 1145-56.

575. Sankardas MA, McEniery T, Aroney CN, Bett JHN. Elective implantation of intracoronary stents without intravascular ultrasound guidance or subsequent warfarin. Cathet Cardiovasc Diagn 1996;37: 355-59.

576. Hall P, Nakamura S, Maiello L, et al. A randomized comparison of combined ticlopidine and aspirin therapy versus aspirin therapy alone after successful intravascular ultrasound-guided stent implantation. Circulation 1996;93: 215-222.

577. Karrillon GJ, Morice MC, Benveniste E, et al. Intracoronary stent implantation without ultrasound guidance and with replacement of conventional anticoagulation by antiplatelet therapy: 30-day clinical outcome of the French Multicenter Registry. Circulation 1996;94: 1519-27.

578. Goods CM, Al-Shaibi KF, Liu MW, et al. Comparison of aspirin alone versus aspirin plus ticlopidine after coronary artery stenting. Am J Cardiol 1996;78: 1042-44.

579. Elsner M, Peifer A, Drexler M, et al. Clinical outcome at six months of coronary stenting followed by ticlopidine monotherapy. Am J Cardiol 1998;81: 147-51.

580. Barragan P, Sainsous J, Silverstri M, et al. Coronary artery stenting withough anticoagulation, aspirin, ultrasound guidance, or high balloon pressure: prospective study of 1, 051 consecutive patients. Cathet Cardiovasc Diagn 1997;42: 367-73.

581. Park SW, Lee HJ, Lee CW, et al. A randomized comparison of cilostazol versus ticlopidine therapy after elective coronary stent placement. J Am Coll Cardiol 1999;33 (2 Suppl A): 255A.

582. Mishkel GJ, Lucore CL, Ligon RW, Trokey J. Clopidogrel for the prevention of stent thrombosis. J Am Coll Cardiol 1999;33 (2 Suppl A): 34A.

583. Yoon Y, Lee DH, Pyun WB, et al. Comparison of cilostazol and ticlopidine after coronary artery stenting: immediate and long-term results. J Am Coll Cardiol 1999;33 (2 Suppl A): 40A.

584. L'Allier PL, Aronow HD, Yadav JS, et al. Is clopidogrel a safe and effective adjunctive anti-platelet therapy for coronary artery stenting? J Am Coll Cardiol 1999;33 (2 Suppl A): 40A.

585. Berger PV, Bellot V, Melby S, et al. Clopidogrel versus ticlopidine for coronary stents.

586. Rabah MM, Premmereur J, Graham M, et al. Comparison of an intravenous bolus of enoxaparin versus unfractionated heparin in elective coronary angioplasty. J Am Coll Cardiol 1999;33 (2 Suppl A): 14A.

587. Rau T, Schluter M, Schofer J, . Restenosis after stent implantation: Impact of preintervention ticlopidine and the duration of postintervention iticlopidine treatment. J Am Coll Cardiol 1999;33 (2 Suppl A): 72A.

588. deJaegere PP, van Domburg RT, de Feyter PJ, et al. Long-term clinical outcome after stent implantation in saphenous vein grafts. J Am Coll Cardiol 1996;28:89-96.

589. Wang X, Oetgen M, Maida R, et al. The effectiveness of the combination of plavix and aspirin versus ticlid and aspirin after coronary stent implantation. J Am Coll Cardiol 1999;33 (2 Suppl A): 13A.

590. Wilson SH, Rihal CS, Bell MR, et al. Timing of coronary stent thrombosis in patients treated with ticlopidine and aspirin. J Am Coll Cardiol 1999;33 (2 Suppl A): 91A.

591. Neumann FJ, Blasini R, Schmitt C, et al. Effect of glycoprotein IIb/IIIa receptor blockade on recovery of coronary flow and left ventricular function after the placement of

coronary-artery stents in acute myocardial infarction. Circularion 1998;98:2695-701.

592. Webb JG, Carere RG, Hilton JD, et al. Usefulness of coronary stenting for cardiogenic shock. Am J Cardiol 1997;79: 81-84.

593. Rodriguez A, Bernardi V, Fernandez M, et al. In-hospital and late results of coronary stents versus conventional balloon angioplasty in acute myocardial infarction (GRAMI trial). Am J Cardiol 1998;81: 1286-91.

594. Stone GW, Brodie BR, Griffin JJ, et al. Prospective, multicenter study of the safety and feasibility of primary stenting in acute myocardial infarction: In-hospital and 30-day results of the PAMI stent pilot trial. J Am Coll Cardiol 1998;31: 23-30.

595. Mahdi NA, Lopez J, Leon M, et al. Comparison of primary coronary stenting to primary balloon angioplasty with stent bailout for the treatment of patients with acute myocardial infarction. Am J Cardiol 1998;81: 957-63.

596. Saito S, Hosokawa G, Kim K, et al. Primary stent implantation without coumadin in acute myocardial infarction. J Am Coll Cardiol 1996;28: 74-81.

597. LeMay MR, Labinaz M, Beanlands RSB, et al. Usefulness of intracoronary stenting in acute myocardial infarction. Am J Cardiol 1996;78: 148-52.

598. Antoniucci D, Valenti R, Buonamici P, et al. Direct angioplasty and stenting of the infarct-related artery in acute myocardial infarction. Am J Cardiol 1996 Sept 1;78: 568-71.

599. Garcia-Cantu E, Spaulding C, Corcos T, et al. Stent implantation in acute myocardial infarction. Am J Cardiol 1996;77: 451-54.

600. Hsieh IC, Change HJ, Chern MS, et al. Late coronary artery stenting in patients with acute myocardial infarction. Am Heart J 1998;136: 606-12.

601. Rodriguez AE, Fernandez M, Santaera O, et al. Coronary stenting in patients undergoing percutaneous transluminal coronary angioplasty during acute myocardial infarction. Am J Cardiol 1996;77: 685-9.

602. Monassier JP, Hamon M, Elias J, et al. Early versus late coronary stenting following acute myocardial infarction: results of the STENTIM I study (French registry of stenting in acute myocardial infarction. Cathet Cardiovasc Diagn 1997;42: 243-8.

603. Silva JA, Nunez E, Vivekananthan K, et al. Cardiogenic shock complicating acute myocardial infarction: A comparison of primary angioplasty versus primary stenting in in-hospital outcomes. J Am Coll Cardiol 1999;33 (2 Suppl A): 368A.

604. Dirschinger J, Kastrati A, Schuhlen H, et al. Coronary stent placement in patients with acute myocardial infarction complicated by cardiogenic shock. One-year clinical follow-up. J Am Coll Cardiol 1999;33 (2 Suppl A): 28A-29A.

605. Stone GW, Marcovitz P, Lansky AJ, et al. Differential effects of stenting and angioplasty in women versus men undergoing a primary mechanical reperfusion strategy in acute myocardial infarction B: The PAMI stent randomized trial. J Am Coll Cardiol 1999;33 (2 Suppl A): 357A.

606. Cox DA, Stone GW, Grines CL, et al. Do proximal LAD lesions in acute myocardial infarction benefit from stenting? The PAMI stent randomized trial. J Am Coll Cardiol 1999;33 (2 Suppl A): 353A.

607. L'Allier PL, Cura FA, Sapp S, et al. EPISTENT: Large scale randomized trial of primary versus provisional coronary stenting with background platelet glycoprotein IIb/IIa blockade. J Am Coll Cardiol 1999;33 (2 Suppl A): 32A.

608. Scheller B, Hennen B, Severin-Kneib S, et al. Follow-up of the

PSAAMI study population (Primary Stenting vs. Angioplasty in Acute Myocardial Infarction). J Am Coll Cardiol 1999;33 (2 Suppl A): 29A.

609. Garg M, Chowdhry S, Vacek JL. Influence of initial thrombolytic therapy on outcomes of stent placement in angioplasty for acute myocardial infarction. J Am Coll Cardiol 1999;33 (2 Suppl A): 374A.

610. Mattos L, Sousa A, Neto CC, Labrunie A, Alves CR, Carvalho H, Saad J. Primary stenting versus PTCA on acute myocardial infarction: In hospital results from the Brazilian Interventional Registry. J Am Coll Cardiol 1999;33 (2 Suppl A): 29A-30A.

611. Neumann FJ, Kastrati A, Schmitt C, Blasini R, Hadamitzky M, Mehilli J, Gawaz M, Schleef M, Seyfarth M, Dirschinger J, Schömig A. Effect of glycoprotein IIb/IIIa receptor blockade with abciximab on clinical and angiographic restenosis rate after the placement of coronary stents following acute myocardial infarction. J Am Coll Cardiol 2000;35:915-21.

612. Jacksch R, Niehues R, Knobloch W, Schiele T. PTCA vs. stenting in acute myocardial infarction (AMI). Circulation 1998;98 (Suppl I): I-307.

613. Hong MK, Mehran R, Satler LF, et al. Long-term clinical results and predictors after successful stent implantation in saphenous vein grafts. Circulation 1998;98 (Suppl I): I-286.

614. Safian RD, Kaplan B, Schreiber T, et al. Interim results of the Wallstent endoprothesis in saphenous vein graft trial (WINS). Circulation 1998;98 (Suppl I): I-662.

615. Al-Mubarak NA, Liu MW, Al-Saif SM, et al. Combined transluminal extraction atherectomy (TEC) and wallstents for treatment of saphenous vein graft disease.Circulation 1998;98 (Suppl I): I-717.

616. Holmes Jr. DR, Berger PB, Williams DO, et al. Contemporary vein graft intervention: A report from the NHLBI dynamic registry. J Am Coll Cardiol 1999;33 (2 Suppl A): 50A.

617. Safian RD, Kaplan B Schreiber T, et al. Final results of the randomized wallstent endoprosthesis in saphenous vein graft trial. J Am Coll Cardiol 1999;33 (2 Suppl A): 37A.

618. Winters KJ, Taniuchi M, Smith SC, et al. Myocardial infarctions after saphenous vein graft revascularization: Comparison of angioplasty, stenting, and transluminal extraction catheter atherectomy. J Am Coll Cardiol 1999;33 (2 Suppl A): 51A.

619. Lefevre T, Morice MC, Labrunie B, et al. Coronary stenting in elderly patients. Results from the stent without coumadin French registry. J Am Coll Cardiol 1996;27:252A.

620. Gaxiola E, Vlietstra RE, Browne KF, et al. Is the outcome of coronary stenting worse in elderly patients? J Interven Cardiol 1998;11:37-40.

621. Nasser TK, Fry ETA, et al. Coronary stenting in women: Clinical outcomes are equivalent to men. J Am Coll Cardiol 1997;29(Suppl. A):71A.

622. Chauhan MS, Schmidt JM, Cutlip DE. Outcome of stenting in the aged. Circulation 1998;98 (Suppl I): I-78.

623. Moschi G, Antoniucci D, Valkenti R, et al. Unconditional primary PTCA in the elderly. Results in patients aged 80 years or above. Circulation 1998;98 (Suppl I): I-153.

624. Shawl FA, Lapetine FL, Kadra WY, et al. Stent supported carotid angioplasty (SSCA) has more favorable outcome in octogenarians (Oct) compared to non-octogenarians (non-Oct). Circulation 1998;98 (Suppl I): I-304.

625. Kasoka S, Tobis, JM, Akiyama T, Reimers B, et al. Angiographic and intravascular ultrasound predictors of in-stent restenosis. J Am Coll Cardiol 1998;32:1630-1635.

626. Bratrand ME, Legrand V, Boland J, Fleck E, et al.

Randomized multicenter comparison of conventional anticoagulation versus antiplatelet therapy in unplanned and elective coronary stenting. The Full Anticoagulation versus Aspirin and Ticlopidine (FANTASTIC) study. Circulation 1998;98:1597-1603.

627. von Birgelen C, Gil Robert, Ruygrok P, Prati F, et al. Optimized expansion of the Wallstent compared with the Palmaz-Schatz stent: On-lone observations with two- and three-dimensional intracoronary ultrasound after angiographic guidance. Am Heart J 1996;131:1067-1075.

628. Stefanadis C, Tsiamis E, Vlachopoulos C, Toutouzas K, et al. Arterial autologous graft-stent for treatment of coronary artery disease: A new technique. Cathet Cardiovasc Diagn 1997;40:302-307.

629. Elsner M, Peifer A, Kasper W. Intracoronary loss of balloon-mounted stents: Successful retrieval with a 2 mm-"microsnare" device. Cathet Cardiovasc Diagn 1996;39:271-276.

630. Kaplan BM, Stewart RE, Sakwa MP, O'Neill WW. Repair of a coronary pseudoaneurysm with percutaneous placement of a saphenous vein allograft attached to a biliary stent. Cathet Cardiovasc Diagn 1996;37:208-212.

631. Stefanadis C, Toutouzas K, Vlachopoulos C, Tsiamis E, et al. Autologous vein graft-coated stent for treatment of coronary artery disease. Cathet Cardiovasc Diagn 1996;38:159-170.

632. Colombo A, Itoh A, Di Mario C, Maiello L, et al. Successful closure of a coronary vessel rupture with a vein graft stent: Case report. Cathet Cardiovasc Diagn 1996;38:172-174.

633. Kobayashi Y, Nongi H, Miyazaki S, et al. Successful retrieval of unexpanded Palmaz-Schatz stent from left main coronary artery. Cathet Cardiovasc Diagn 1996;38:402-404.

634. Eisenhauer AC, Piemonte TC, Gossman DE, Ahmed ML. Extraction of fully deployed coronary stents. Cathet Cardiovasc Diagn. 1996;38:393-401.

635. Leroy O, Martin E, Prat A, et al. Fatal infection of coronary stent implantation. Cathet Cardiovasc Diagn 1996;39:168-170.

636. Gunther HU, Strupp G, Volmar J, et al. Coronary stent-implantation: Infection and myocardial abscess with lethal outcome. Z Kardiol 1993;82:521-525.

637. Bertrand OF, Siehia R, Mongrain R, Rodes J, et al. Biocompatibility aspects of new stent technology. J Am Coll Cardiol 1998;32:562-567.

638. Blasini R, Neumann FJ, Schmitt C, et al. Restenosis rate after intravascular ultrasound-guided coronary stent implantation. Cathet Cardiovasc Diagn 1998;44:380-386.

639. Dauerman HL, Baim DS, Cutlip DE, Sparano AM, et al. Mechanical debulking versus balloon angioplasty for the treatment of diffuse in-stent restenosis. Am J Cardiol 1998;82:277-284.

640. Von Birgelen C, Kutryk MJB, Serruys PW. Three-dimensional intravascular ultrasound analysis of coronary stent deployment and in-stent neointimal volume: Current clinical practice and the concepts of TRAPIST, ERASER, and ITALICS. J Invas Cardiol 1998;10:17-26.

641. Bauters C, Banos JL, van Belle E, Mcfadden EP, et al. Six-month angiographic outcome after successful repeat percutaneous intervention for in-stent restenosis. Circulation 1998;97:318-321.

642. Chauhan A, Vu E, Ricci DR, Bullr CE, et al. Multiple coronary stenting in unstable angina: Early and late clinical outcomes. Cathet Cardiovasc Diagn 1998;43:11-16.

643. Rodriguez A, Bernardi V, Navia J, et al. Argentine

randomized study: coronary angioplasty with stenting versus coronary bypass surgery in patients with multiple-vessel disease (ERACCI II): 30-day and one-year follow-up results. J Am Coll Cardiol 2001;37:51-8.

644. Foley DP, Serruys PW. Provisional stenting—stent-like balloon angioplasty: evidence to define the continuing role of balloon angioplasty for percutaneous coronary revascularization. Semin Intevent Cardiol 1996;1:269-273.

645. Wong SC, Kent KM, Mintz GS, Pichard AD, et al. Percutaneous transcatheter repair of a coronary aneurysm using a composite autologous cephalic vein-coated Palmaz-Schatz biliary stent. Am J Cardiol 1995;76:990-991.

646. Kastrati A, Schomig A, Elezi S, Schuhlen H, et al. Predictive factors of restenosis after coronary stent placement. J Am Coll Cardiol 1997;30:1428-1436.

647. Bartorelli AL, DeCesare N, Kaplan AV, Fabbiocchi F, et al. Local heparin delivery prior to coronary stent implantation: Acute and six-month clinical and angiographic results. Cathet Cardiovasc Diagn 1997;42:313-320.

648. Nakamura T, Furukawa K, Uchiyama H, et al. Stent placement for recurrent vasospastic angina resistant to medical treatment. Carthet Cardiovasc Diagn 1997;42:440-443.

649. Schneider JE, Mann T, Cubeddu G, Arrowood ME. Transradial coronary stenting: A United States experience. J Invas Cardiol 1997;9:569-574.

650. Nolan J, Batin P, Welsh C, Lindsay S, et al. Feasibility and applicability of coronary stent implantation with the direct brachial approach: Results of a single-center study. Am Heart J 1997;134:939-944.

651. Labinaz M, Zidar JP, Stack RS, Phillips HR. Biodegradable stents: The future of interventional cardiology? J Interven Cardiol 1995;8(4):395-404.

652. Holmes DR, Kip KE, Yeh W, Kelsey SF, et al. Long-term analysis of conventional coronary balloon angioplasty and an initial "stent-like" result. The NHLBI PTCA Registry. J Am Col Cardiol 1998;32:590-595.

653. Braden GA, Xenopoulos NP, Young T, et al. Transluminal extraction catheter atherectomy followed by immediate stenting in treatment of saphenous vein grafts. J Am Coll Cardiol 1997;30:657-663.

654. Eltchaninoff H, Koning R, Tron C, et al. Balloon angioplasty for the treatment of coronary in-stent restenosis: Immediate results and 6-month angiographic recurrent restenosis rate. J Am Coll Cardiol 1998;32:980-984.

655. Jost C, Kumar V. Are current cardiovascular stents MRI safe? J Invas Cardiol 1998;10:477-479.

656. Scott NA, Pottigren NI. Absence of movement of coronary stent after placement in a magnetic resonance imaging field. Am J Cardiol 1996;73:900-901.

657. Rodriguez A, Ayala F, Bernardi V, Santaera O, et al. Optimal coronary balloon angioplasty with provisional stenting versus primary stent (OCBAS). Immediate and long-term follow-up results. J Am Coll Cardiol 1998;32:1351-1357.

658. Sharma SK, Duvvuri S, Dangas G, Kini A, et al. Rotational atherectomy for in-stent restenosis: Acute and long-term results of the first 100 cases. J Am Coll Cardiol 1998;32:1358-1365.

659. Aggarwal RK, Ireland DC, Azrin MA, et al. Antithrombotic potential of polymer-coated stents eluting platelet glycoprotein IIb/IIIa receptor antibody. Circulation 1996;94:3311-3317.

660. Kerr AJ, Stewart RAH, Low CJS, et al. Long stenting in native coronary arteries: Relation between vessel size and outcome. Cathet Cardiovasc Diagn 1998;44:170-174.

661. Werner GS, Gastmann O, Ferrari M, Schuenemann S, et al. Risk factors for acute and subacute stent thrombosis after high-pressure stent implantation: A study by intracoronary ultrasound. Am Heart J 1998;135:300-309.

662. von Birgelen C, Airiian SG, de Feyter P, Foley DP, et al. Coronary Wallstents show significant late, postprocedural expansion despite implantation with adjunct high-pressure balloon inflations. Am J Cardiol 1998;82:129-134.

663. Lee SG, Lee CW, Cheong SS, Hong MK, et al. Immediate and long-term outcomes of rotational atherectomy versus balloon angioplast alone for treatment of diffuse in-stent restenosis. Am J Cardiol 1998;82:140-143.

664. Shiran A, Mintz GS, Waksman R, Mehran R, et al. Early lumen loss after treatment of in-stent restenosis. An intravascular ultrasound study. Circulation 1998;98:200-203.

665. Bermejo J, Botas J, Garcia E, Elizaga J, et al. Mechanisms of residual lumen stenosis after high-pressure stent implantation. A quantitative coronary angioplasty and intravascular ultrasound study. Circulation 1998;98:112-118.

666. Antoniucci D, Valenti R, Santoro G, Bolognese L, et al. Restenosis after coronary stenting in current clinical practice. Am Heart J 1998;135-510-518.

667. Hasdai D, Garratt KN, Holmes DR, et al. Coronary angioplasty and intracoronary thrombolysis are of limited efficacy in resolving early intracoronary stent thrombosis. J Am Coll Cardiol 1996;28:361-367.

668. Nguyen T, Dave V, Jia S, Fang C, et al. Practical clinical evaluation of stents. J Interven Cardiol 1998;11[Suppl]:S101-S110.

669. Bramucci E, Angoli L. Merlini A, Barberis P, et al. Adjunctive stent implantation following directional coronary atherectomy in patients with coronary artery disease. J Am Coll Cardiol 1998;32:1855-1860.

670. Van Belle E, Blouard P, McFadden EP, et al. Effects of stenting of recent or chronic coronary occlusions on late vessel patency and left ventricular function. Am J Cardiol 1997;80:1150-1154.

671. Aliabadi D, Tilli FV, Bowers TR, Benzuly KH, et al. Incidence and angiographic predictors of side branch occlusion following high-pressure intracoronary stenting. Am J Cardiol 1997;80:994-997.

672. Blasini R, Neumann FJ, Schmitt C, et al. Comparison of angiography and intravascular ultrasound for the assessment of lumen size after coronary stent placement: Impact of dilation pressures. Cathet Cardiovasc Diagn 1997;42:113-119.

673. Mehran R, Mintz GS, Satler LF, Pichard AD, et al. Treatment of in-stent restenosis with excimer laser coronary angioplasty. Mechanisms and results compared with PTCA alone. Circulation 1997;96:2183-2189.

674. Rechavia E, Litvack F, Macko G, Eigler N. Stent implantation of saphenous vein graft aorto-ostial lesions in patients with unstable ischemic syndromes: Immediate angiographic results and long-term clinical outcome. J Am Coll Cardiol 1995;25:866-870.

675. Fenton S, Fischman D, Savage M, et al. Long-term angiographic and clinical outcome after implantation of balloon-expandable stents in aortocoronary saphenous vein grafts. Am J Cardiol 1994;74:1187-1191.

676. Leon MB, Wong SC, Pichard A. Balloon expandable stent implantation in saphenous vein grafts. In Hermann HC, Hirschfeld JW (Eds). Clinical Use of the Palmaz-Schatz Intracoronary Stent. Futura Publishing Company Inc.

1993;111-121.

677. Fortuna R, Heuser R, Garratt K, Schwartz R, M B. Intracoronary stent: experience in the first 101 vein graft patients. J Am Coll Cardiol 1993;26:I-308.

678. Pomerantz R, Kuntz R, Carrozza J, et al. Acute and long-term outcome of narrowed saphenous venous grafts treated by endoluminal stenting and directional atherectomy. Am J Cardiol 1992;70:161-167.

679. Strauss B, Serruys P, Bertrand M, et al. Quantitative angiographic follow-up of the coronary Wallstent in native vessels and bypass grafts (European experience--March 1986 to March 1990). Am J Cardiol 1992;69:475-481.

680. de Scheerder I, Strauss B, de Feyter P, et al. Stenting of venous bypass grafts: A new treatment modality for patients who are poor candidates for reintervention. Am Heart J 1992;123:1046-1054.

681. Sharma SK, Kini AS, King T, et al. Multivariate predictors of target lesion revascularization in the randomized trial of PTCA versus rotablator for diffuse in-stent restenosis (ROSTER). J Am Coll Cardiol 2001;37(2):56A.

682. Kugelmass AD, Mehta S, Simon AW, et al. Gender differences in outocmes among diabetic patients undergoing percutaneous coronary interventions. J Am Coll Cardiol 2001;37(2):65A.

683. Trabattoni D, Montorsi P, Loaldi A, et al. How is the outcome of coronary stenting in the elderly compared to younger patients? J Am Coll Cardiol 2001;37(2):160A.

684. Baklanov DV, Marcu CB, Chawarski MC, et al. Coronary stenting is safe and effective in a high risk octogenarian patient cohort. J Am Coll Cardiol 2001;37(2):1101-57A

685. Roffi, Marco Chan A, Chew DP, et al. Stents and glycoprotein IIb/IIIa inhibitors do not improve 30-day outcome in bypass graft percutaneous interventions: A retrospective registry-based analysis. J Am Coll Cardiol 2001;37(2):76A.

686. Bedossa M, Commeau P, Brunnel P, et al. Direct coronary stenting without balloon predilation: Immediate and 6 month results of a multicenter prospective randomized trial. J Am Coll Cardiol 2001;37(2):11A

687. Garcia E, Gomez-Recio M, Moreno Raul, et al. Stent reduces restenosis in small vessels. Results of the RAP study. J Am Coll Cardiol 2001;37(2):32-4A

688. Moer R, Myreng Y, Albertsson P, et al. Stenting in small coronary arteries (SISCA): A randomized comparison of heparin coated bestent and balloon angioplasty. J Am Coll Cardiol 2001;37(2):836-2A

689. Dharmadhidari A Di Mario C, Tzifos V, et al. Comparison of procedural and one-year outcome with only balloon angioplasty, covered stents and non-covered stents in saphenous vein grafts. J Am Coll Cardiol 2000;35:26A.

690. Oemrawsingh PV, Schalij M, van der Wall EE, et al. Guidance of long stent implantation by intravascular ultrasound has a significantly better outcome compared to implantation guided by angiography alone: Final results of a randomized study (the TULIP study). J Am Coll cardiol 2001;37(2)1089-23A

691. Thiele H, Diegeler A, Lauer B, et al. Minimal invasive bypass surgery versus stentimplantation is isolated proximal high lesions of the LAD in more than 200 patients. J Am Coll Cardiol 2001;37(A)883-2A

692. Baim DS, et al. ACS Multi-link StENT Trial. The Manual of Interventional Trials 2000.

693. Stoerger H, Haase J, Hofmann M, Schwarz F. Implantation of coronary PTFE-grafts in degenerated saphenous vein grafts: Acute and intermediate term results. Circulation 2000;102:II-642.

694. Horlitz M, Amin FR, Sigwart U, Clague JR. Coronary stenting of aorto-ostial saphenous vein graft lesions. J Intervent Cardiol 2000;13:303-8.

695. Bhargava B, Kornowski R, Mehran R, et al. Procedural results and intermediate clinical outcomes after multiple saphenous vein graft stenting. J Am Coll Cardiol 2000;35:389-97.

696. Lansky AJ, Popma JJ, Hanzol, GS, et al. Predictors of late clinical outcome after gianturco-Roubin II stent use. Final results of the GR II randomized clinical trial. Circulation 1998;98:I-662.

697. Feres F, Costa MA, Staico R, et al. Is stent oversizing the best strategy to treat small vessels? J Am Coll Cardiol 2001;37(2):1070-11

698. Stankovic GR, Nishida T, Corvaja N, et al. Effect of balloon oversizing in stenting small vessels. J Am Coll Cardiol 2001;37(2):1256-28A

699. Briguari C, DeGregorio J, Nishida T, et al. Polytetrafluoroethylene-covered stent for the treatment of narrowings in aortocoronary saphenous vein grafts. Am J Cardiol 2000;86:343-346.

700. Wong SC, Popma J, Pichard A, Kent K. Comparison of clinical and angiographic outcomes after saphenous vein grafts angioplasty using coronary versus "biliary" tubular slotted stents. Circulation 1995;91:339-350.

701. Denardo SJ, Morris NB, Rocha-Singh, KJ, et al. Safety and efficacy of extended urokinase infusion plus stent deployment for treatment of obstructed, older saphenous vein grafts. Am J Cardiol 1995;76:776-780.

702. Stefanadis C, Toutouzas K, Tsiamis E, et al. Implantation of stents covered by autologous arterial grafts in human coronary arteries: A new technique. J Invas Cardiol 2000;12:7-12.

703. Lauer B, Schmidt E, Ambrosch H, et al. Optimal treatment of in-stent-retenosis: Excimer laser-angioplasty, rotational atherectomy or conventional angioplasty? J Am Coll Cardiol 1999;33(Suppl A):I-62A.

704. Mehran R, Dangas G, Mintz GS, et al. Excimer laser vs. rotational atherectomy for the treatment of diffuse in-stent restenosis: acute and long-term results. J Am Coll Cardiol 1999;33(Suppl A):I-62A.

705. Siegel R, Bhaskran A, Underwood P, et al. Excimer laser coronary angioplasty in in-stent restenosis: acute and long-term clinical outcomes. J Am Coll Cardiol 1999;33(Suppl A):I-63A.

706. Mehran R, Dangas G, Mintz GS, et al. In-stent restenosis: "The Great Equalizer" - disappointing clinical outcomes with ALL interventional strategies. J Am Coll Cardiol 1999;33(Suppl A):I-63A.

707. Koster R, Hamm CW, et al. Treatment of in-stent coronary restenosis by excimer laser angioplasty. Am J Cardiol 1998;80(11):1424-1428.

708. Margolis J, Beyarano J, Draz P, et al. Laser approach for coronary artery or vein raft in stent restenosis. Eur Heart J 1997;18:497.

709. Hasse J, Reifart N, Schwart F, et al. Is excimer laser angioplasty superior to balloon dilatation for the treatment of in-stent restenosis? Results of prospective single center study. J Am Coll Cardiol 1998;31(Suppl C):400C.

710. Dauerman HL, Baim DS, Cutlip DE, Sparano AM, et al. Mechanical debulking versus balloon angioplasty for the

treatment of diffuse in-stent restenosis. Am J Cardiol 1998;82:277-284.

711. Sharma SK, Duvvuri S, Dangas G, Kini A, et al. Rotational atherectomy for in-stent restenosis: Acute and long-term results of the first 100 cases. J Am Coll Cardiol 1998;32:1358-1365.

712. Lee SG, Lee CW, Cheong SS, Hong MK, et al. Immediate and long-term outcomes of rotational atherectomy versus balloon angioplasty alone for treatment of diffuse in-stent restenosis. Am J Cardiol 1998;82:140-143.

713. Mehran R, Mintz GS, Satler LF, Pichard AD, et al. Treatment of in-stent restenosis with excimer laser coronary.

714. Bossi I, Klersy C, Jordan C, et al. Isolated proximal left anterior descending coronary artery stenosis: Long-term clinical outcome after percutaneous interventions. J Am Coll Cardiol 2001;37(2)1073-38A.

715. Singh M, Mathew V, Lennon RJ, et al. Comparison of rotational atherectomy versus PTCA with or without stenting in calcified lesions: In-hospital and 6-month outcome. J Am Coll Cardiol 2001;37(2):1070-14A

716. Kobayashi Y, Mehran R, Dangas G, et al. Effect of coronary plaque calcification on the final lumen dimensions after stenting without rotational atherectomy: An intravascular ultrasound study. J Am Coll Cardiol 2001;37(2):1070-18A.

717. Chauhan A, Zubaid M, Buller CE, et al. Reduced anticoagulation with antiplatelet therapy alone is safe and effective after "bail-out" stenting for failed angioplasty. J Invas Cardiol 1997;9:398-406.

718. Antoniucci D, Valenti R, Santor GM, et al. Bailout coronary stenting without anticoagulation or intravascular ultrasound guidance: Acute and six-month angiographic results in a series of 120 consecutive patients. Cathet Cardiovasc Diagn. 1997;41:14-19.

719. Nakamura S, Hall P, Gaglion A, et al. High pressure assisted coronary stent implantation accomplished without intravascular ultrasound guidance and subsqent anticoagulation. J Am Coll Cardiol 1997;29:21-7.

720. Lefevre T, Morice M, Labrunie B, et al. Coronary stenting in elderly patients. Results from the Stent Without Coumadin French Registry. J Am Coll Cardiology 1996;27:252A.

721. Morice MC, Valelx B, Marco J, et al. Preliminary results of the MUST trial, major clinical events during the first month. J Am Coll Cardiology 1996;27:137A.

722. Goods CM, Al-Shaibi KF, Dean LS, et al. Is ticlopidine a necessary component of antiplatelet regimens following coronary artery stenting. J Am Coll Cardiology 1996;27:137A.

723. Marco J, Fajadt J, Brunel P, et al. First use of the second-generation Gianturco-Roubin stent without coumadin. Am J Cardiol 1996 (in-press).

724. Elias J, Monassier JP, Carrie D, et al. Final results of phases II, III, IV and V of Medtronic Wiktor stent implantation without coumadin. J Am Coll Cardiology 1996;27:15A.

725. Carvalho H, Fajadet J, Jordan C, et al. A lower rate of complications after Gianturco-Roubin coronary stenting using a new antiplatelet and anticoagulant protocol . Circulation 1994;90:I-125.

726. Jordan C, Carvalho H, Fajadet J, et al. Reduction of acute thrombosis rate after coronary stenting using a new anticoagulant protocol. Circulation 1994;90:I-125.

727. Colombo A, Nakamura S, Hall P, et al. A prospective study of Wiktor Coronary stent implantation treated only with antiplatelet therapy. Circulation 1994;90:I-124.

728. Elias J, Monassier JP, Puel J, et al. Medtronic Wiktor stent implantation without coumadin: Hospital outcome. Circulation 1994;90:I-124.

729. Hall P, Colombo A, Nakamura S, et al. A prospective study of Gianturco-Roubin coronary stent implantation without subsequent anticoagulation. Circulation 1994;90:I-124.

730. Aubry P, Royer T, Spaulding C, et al. Coronary stenting without coumadin: Phase II and III, the bail-out group. Circulation 1994;90:I-124.

731. Blengino S, Maiello L, Hall P, et al. Randomized trial of coronary stent implantation without anticoagulation: aspirin vs. ticlopidine. Circulation 1994;90:I-124.

732. Topol EJ, Oral presentation, American Heart Association meeting, New Orleans, 2000.

733. Dieter, RS. Coronary artery stent infection. Clin Cardiol 2000;23:808-810.

734. Serruys PW. Presented at the XXII European Society of Cardiology, 2000.

735. Bogart DB. Dislodged stent: A simple retrieval technique. Cathet Cardiovasc Intervent 1999;47:323-324.

736. Lohavanichbutr K, Webb JG, Carere RG, et al. Mechanisms, management, and outcome of failure of delivery of coronary stents. Am J Cardiol 1999;83:779-781.

737. Akhtar S, Johnson KB, Dalton R, et al. Balloon rupture during stent implantation: A novel technique of salvage with a new manual power injector. Cathet Cardiovasc Intervent 1999;48:74-77.

738. Webb JG, Solankhi N, Carere RG. Facilitation of stent retention and retrieval with an emboli containment device. Cathet Cardiovasc Intervent 2000;50:215-217.

739. Satler LF, Mintz G. Patience in the pursuit of perfection. Cathet Cardiol Intervent 2000;50:218-220.

740. Abernethy WB III, Choo JK, Oesterle SN, Jang IK. Balloon deflection technique: A method to facilitate entry of a balloon catheter into a deployed stent. Cathet Cardiovasc Intervent 2000;51:312-313.

741. Kobayashi Y, Colombo A, Adamian M, et al. The skirt technique: A stenting technique to treat a lesion immediately proximal to the bifurcation (pseudobifurcation). Cathet Cardiovasc Intervent 2000;51:347-351.

742. Machraoui A, Germing A, von Dryander S, et al. Comparison of the efficacy and safety of aspirin alone with coumadin plus aspirin after provisional coronary stenting: Final and follow-up results of a randomized study. Am Heart J 1999;138:663-9.

743. Tcheng JE, Kong DF. Vale, warfarin: A stentorian farewell. Am Heart J 1999;138:602-5.

744. Zidar JP, Batchelor W, Berger PB, et al. Does the low-molecular-weight enoxaparin reduce stent thrombosis in high-risk stent patients? Results from ATLAST trial. Enoxaparin plus antiplatelet therapy vs. antiplatelet therapy alone in patients at increased risk of stent thrombosis. Circulation 1999;100:I-380.

745. Park SW, Lee CW, Kim HS, et al. Comparison of cilostazol versus ticlopidine therapy after stent implantation. Am J Cardiol 1999;84:511-514.

746. Yoon Y, Shim WH, Lee DH, et al. Usefulness of cilostazol versus ticlopidine in coronary artery stenting. Am J Cardiol 1999;84:1375-1380.

747. Kolansky DM, Klugherz BD, Curran SC, et al. Combination therapy with clopidogrel and aspirin after coronary stenting. Cathet Cardiovasc Intervent 2000;50:276-279.

748. Jauhar R, Bergman G, Savino S, et al. Effectiveness of aspirin and clopidogrel combination therapy in coronary stenting.

Am J Cardiol 1999;84:726-728.

749. Wilson SH, Rihal CS, Bell MR, et al. Timing of coronary stent thrombosis in patients treated with ticlopidine and aspirin. Am J Cardiol 1999;83:1006-1011.

750. Garasic JM, Edelman ER, Squire JC, et al. Stent and artery geometry determine intimal thickening independent of arterial injury. Circulation 2000;101:812-818.

751. Lee DP, Lo ST Suzuki T, et al. Optimizing clinical outcomes with intracoronary stenting: The importance of minimizing vessel injury. Stent 2000;3:2-6.

752. Fujise K, Yhip PA, Anderson V, et al. Balloon to artery ratio, not inflation pressure, correlates with adequate stent deployment: Size is more important than pressure. J Intervent Cardiol 2000;13:223-229.

753. Leosco D, Fineschi M, Pierli C, et al. Intracoronary serotonin release after high-pressure coronary stenting. Am J Cardiol 1999;84;1317-1322.

754. Hoffmann R, Mintz GS, Mehran R, et al. Tissue proliferation within and surrounding Palmaz-Schatz stents is dependent on the aggressiveness of stent implantation technique. Am J Cardiol 1999;83:1170-1174.

755. Stone GW, St. Goar FG, Hodgson JM, et al. Analysis of the relation between stent implantation pressure and expansion. Am J Cardiol 1999;83:1397-1400.

756. Dirschinger J, Kastrati A, Neumann FJ, et al. Influence of balloon pressure during stent placement in native coronary arteries on early and late angiographic and clinical outcome. A randomized evaluation of high-pressure inflation. Circulation. 1999;100:918-923.

757. Ormiston JA, Dixon SR, Webster MWI, et al. Stent longitudinal flexibility: A comparison of 13 stent designs before and after balloon expansion. Cathet Cardiovasc Intervent 2000;50:120-124.

758. Barragan P, Rieu R, Garitey V, et al. Elastic recoil of coronary stents: A comparative analysis. Cathet Cardiovasc Intervent 2000;50:112-119.

759. Yamamoto Y, Brown DL, Ischinger TA, et al. Effect of stent design on reduction of elastic recoil: A comparison via quantitative intravascular ultrasound. Cathet Cardiovasc Intervent 1999;47:251-257.

760. Costa MA, Sabate M, Kay IP, et al. Three-dimensional intravascular ultrasonic volumetric quantification of stent recoil and neointimal formation of two new generation tubular stents. Am J Cardiol 2000;85:135-139.

761. Gyongyosi M, Yang P, Khorsand A, et al. Longitudinal straightening effect of stents is an additional predictor for major adverse cardiac events. J Am Coll Cardiol 2000;35:1580-9.

762. Hong MK, Pard SW, Lee CW, et al. Intravascular ultrasound comparison of chronic recoil among different stent designs. Am J Cardiol 1999;84:1247-1250.

763. Chan AW, Carere RG, Solankhi N, et al. Coronary stenting without predilatation in broad spectrum of clinical and angiographic situations. J Invas Cardiol 2000;12:75-79.

764. Wilson SH, Berger PB, Mathew V, et al. Immediate and late outcomes after direct stent implantation without balloon predilation. J Am Coll Cardiol 2000;35:937-43.

765. Danzi GB, Capuano C, Fiocca L, et al. Stent implantation without predilation in patients with a single, noncalcified coronary artery lesion. Am J Cardiol 1999;84:1250-1254.

766. Herz I, Assali A, Solodky A, et al. Effectiveness of coronary stent deployment without predilation. Am J Cardiol 1999;84:89-91.

767. Bedossa M, Commeau P, Leclercq C, et al. Direct coronary stenting in noncomplex and noncalcified lesions: Immediate and mid-term results of a prospective registry. J Intervent Cardiol 2000;13:231-235.

768. Ormiston JA, Webster MWI, Ruygrok PN, et al. A randomized study of direct coronary stent delivery compared with stenting after predilatation: The NIR future trial. Cathet Cardiovasc Intervent 2000;50:377-381.

769. Herz I, Assali A, Solodky A, et al. Coronary stenting without predilatation (SWOP): Applicable technique in everyday practice. Cathet Cardiovasc Intervent 2000;49:384-388.

770. Briguori C, Sheiban I, De Gregorio J, et al. Direct coronary stenting without predilation. J Am Coll Cardiol 1999;34:1910-5.

771. Hernandez JM, Gomez I, Rodriguez-Entem F, et al. Evaluation of direct stent implantation without predilatation by intravascular ultrasound. Am J Cardiol 2000;85:1028-1030.

772. Hamon M, Richardeau Y, Lecluse E, et al. Direct coronary stenting without balloon predilation in acute coronary syndromes. Am Heart J 1999;138:55-9.

773. Schiele F, Vuillemenot A, Meneveau N, et al. Effects of increasing balloon pressure on mechanism and results of balloon angioplasty for treatment of restenosis after Palmaz-Schatz stent implantation: An angiographic and intravascular ultrasound study. Cathet Cardiovasc Intervent 1999;46:314-312.

774. Antoniucci D, Valenti R, Moschi G, et al. Stenting for in-stent restenosis. Cathet Cardiovasc Intervent 2000;49:376-381.

775. Koster R, Kahler J, Terres W, et al. Six-month clinical and angiographic outcome after successful excimer laser angioplasty for in-stent restenosis. J Am Coll Cardiol 2000;36:69-74.

776. Haase J, Storger H, Hoffmann M, Schwarz F. Excimer laser angioplasty with adjunctive balloon dilation versus balloon dilation alone for the treatment of in-stent restenosis: Results of a randomized single-center study. J Intervent Cardiol 1999;12:513-518.

777. Koster R, Hamm CW, Seabra-Gomes R, et al. Laser angioplasty of restenosed coronary stents: Results of a multicenter surveillance trial. Am Coll Cardiol 1999;34:25-32.

778. Radke PW, Klues HG, Haager PK, et al. Mechanisms of acute lumen gain and recurrent restenosis after rotational atherectomy of diffuse in-stent restenosis. J Am Coll Cardiol.1999;34:33-9.

779. Baldus S, Reimers J, Koster R, et al. Recurrent coronary in-stent restenosis: Potential of membrane-covered stents. J Intervent Cardiol 2000;13:167-172.

780. Albiero R, Nishida T, Karvouni E, et al. Cutting balloon angioplasty for the treatment of in-stent restenosis. Cathet Cardiovasc Intervent 2000;50:452-459.

781. Kurbaan AS, Foale RA, Sigwart U, et al. Cutting balloon angioplasty for in-stent restenosis. Cathet Cardiovasc Intervent 2000;50:480-483.

782. Swanson N, Gershlick A. The stent as a local delivery device. Stent 1999;2:66-73.

783. Kastrati A, Schomig A, Dirschinger J, et al. Increased risk of restenosis after placement of gold-coated stents. Results of a randomized trial comparing gold-coated with uncoated steel stents in patient with coronary artery disease. Circulation 2000;101:2478-2483.

784. Kastrati A, Dirschinger J, Boekstegers P, et al. Influence of stent design on 1-year outcome after coronary stent placement: A randomized comparison of five stent types in 1147 unselected patients. Cathet Cardiovasc Intervent 2000;50:290-297.

785. Tamai H, Igaki K, Kyo E, et al. Initial and 5-month results of biodegradable poly-*l*-lactic acid coronary stents in humans. Circulation 2000;102:399-404.

786. Escaned J, Goicolea J, Alfonso F, et al. Propensity and mechanisms of restenosis in different coronary stent designs. J Am Coll Cardiol 1999;34:1490-7.

787. Cantor WJ, Peterson ED, Popma JJ, et al. Provisional stenting strategies: Systematic overview and implications for clinical decision-making. J Am Coll Cardiol 2000;36:1142-51.

788. Dangas G, Ambrose JA, Rehmann D, et al. Balloon optimization versus stent study (BOSS): Provisional stenting and early recoil after balloon angioplasty. Am J Cardiol 2000;85:957-961.

789. Muhlestein JB, Maycock CA. Routine stenting or provisional stenting: Which is better? A look at presently existing data. J Intervent Cardiol 1999;12:389-394.

790. Abizaid A, Pichard AD, Mintz GS, et al. Acute and long-term results of an intravascular ultrasound-guided percutaneous transluminal coronary angioplasty/provisional stent implantation strategy. Am J Cardiol 1999;84:1298-1303.

791. van Liebergen RAM, Piek JJ, Koch KT, et al. Hyperemic coronary flow after optimized intravascular ultrasound-guided balloon angioplasty and stent implantation. J Am Coll Cardiol 1999;34:1899-906.

792. Cutlip DE, Leon MB, Ho KKL, et al. Acute and nine-month clinical outcomes after "suboptimal" coronary stenting. Results from the Stent Anti-thrombotic Regimen Study (STARS) registry. J Am Coll Cardiol 1999;34:698-706.

793. Gaspardone A, Tomai F, Versaci F, et al. Coronary artery stent placement in patients with variant angina refractory to medical treatment. Am J Cardiol 1999;84:96-89.

794. Kaluza GL, Joseph J, Lee JR, et al. Catastrophic outcomes of noncardiac surgery soon after coronary stenting. J Am Coll Cardiol 2000;35:1288-94.

795. Antoniucci D, Valenti R, Santoro GM, et al. Primary coronary infarct artery stenting in acute myocardial infarction. Am J Cardiol 1999;84:505-510.

796. Dauerman HL, Prpic R, Andreou C, et al. Angiographic and clinical outcomes after rescue coronary stenting. Cathet Cardiovasc Intervent 2000;50:269-275.

797. Akiyama T, Moussa I, Reimers B, et al. Angiographic and clinical outcome following coronary stenting of small vessels: A comparison with coronary stenting of large vessels. J Am Coll Cardiol 1998;32:1610-8.

798. Ellis SG, Tamai G, Nobuyoshi M, et al. Contemporary percutaneous treatment of unprotected left vein coronary stenosis: Initial results from a multicenter registry analysis 1994-1996. Circulation 1997;96:3867-3872.

799. Briguori C, Nishida T, Adamian M, et al. Coronary stenting versus balloon angioplasty in small coronary artery with complex lesions. Cathet Cardiovasc Intervent 2000;50:390-397.

800. Germing A, Von Dryander S, Machraoui A, et al. Coronary artery stenting in vessels with reference diameter < 3 mm. J Intervent Cardiol 2000;13:309-314.

801. Wong P, Lau KW, Lim YL, Oesterle SN. Stent placement for non-STRESS/BENESTENT lesions: A critical review. Cathet Cardiovasc Intervent 2000;51:223-233.

802. Heuser R, Houser F, Culler SD, et al. A retrospective study of 6671 patients comparing coronary stenting and balloon angioplasty. J Invas Cardiol 2000;12:354-362.

803. Ritchie JL, Maynard C, Every NR, Chapko MK. Coronary artery stent outcomes in a Medicare population: Less emergency bypass surgery and lower mortality rates in patients with stents. Am Heart J 1999;138:437-40.

804. Rankin JM, Spinelli JJ, Carere RG, et al. Improved clinical outcome after widespread use of coronary-artery stenting in Canada. N Engl J Med 1999;341:1957-65.

805. Mathew V, Grill DE, Scott CG, et al. Baseline clinical and angiographic variables associated with long-term outcome after successful intracoronary stent implantation. Am J Cardiol 1999;84:789-794.

806. Hirayama A, Kodama K, Adachi T, et al. Angiographic and clinical outcome of a new self-expanding intracoronary stent (RADIUS): Results from multicenter experience in Japan. Cathet Cardiovasc Intervent 2000;49:401-407.

807. Bueno RRL, Guerios EE, Tarastchuk JC, et al. Angiographic results and late clinical follow-up after Bard-XT intracoronary stent implantation. J Invas Cardiol 2000;11:661-666.

808. Cremonesi A, Benit E, Carlier M, et al. Multicenter registry to evaluate the efficacy of the NIROYAL™ stent in De Novo or restenotic coronary stenosis. J Invas Cardiol 2000;12:225-232.

809. Kereiakes DJ, Midei M, Hermiller J, et al. Procedural and late outcomes following MULTI-LINK DUET coronary stent deployment. Am J Cardiol 1999;84:1385-1390.

810. Lau WK, Ding ZP, Johan A, Hung JS. Mid-term clinical and angiographic follow-up outcome after placement of a new balloon expandable stent in native coronary arteries. Cathet Cardiovasc Intervent 2000;49:348-351.

811. Kay IP, Sabate M, Van Langenhove G, et al. The ESSEX (European Scimed Stent Experience) study. Cathet Cardiovasc Intervent 2000;50:419-425.

812. Galli M, Bartorelli A, Bedogni F, et al. Italian Biodiv Ysio open registry (Biodiv Ysio PC-coated stent): Study of clinical outcomes of the implant of a PC-coated coronary stent. J Invas Cardiol 2000;12:452-458.

813. Choi JW, Vardi GM, Meyers SN, et al. Role of intracoronary ultrasound after high-pressure stent implantation. Am Heart J 2000;139:643-8.

814. Moussa I, Moses J, Di Mario C, et al. Does the specific intravascular ultrasound criterion used to optimize stent expansion have an impact on the probability of stent restenosis? Am J Cardiol 1999;83:1012-1017.

815. Kobayashi Y, De Gregorio J, Kobayashi N, et al. Lower restenosis rate with stenting following aggressive versus less aggressive rotational atherectomy. Cathet Cardiovasc Intervent 1999;46:406-414.

816. Moussa I, Di Mario C, Colombo A. Plaque removal prior to stent implantation in native coronary arteries: Why? When? and How? J Invas Cardiol 1999;11:36-41.

817. Hanekamp CEE, Koolen JJ, Pijls NHJ, et al. Comparison of quantitative coronary angiography, intravascular ultrasound, and coronary pressure measurement to assess optimum stent deployment. Circulation 1999;99:1015-1021.

818. Mehran R, et al. The Manual of Interventional Trials, TCT 2000.

819. The ERASER Investigators. Acute platelet inhibition with abciximab does not reduce in-stent restenosis (ERASER Study). Circulation 1999;100: 799-806.

820. Vom Dahl J, Dietz U, Silber S, et al. Angioplasty versus

rotational atherectomy for treatment of diffuse in-stent restenosis: Clinical and angiographic results from a randomized multicenter trial (ARTIST Study). J Am Coll Cardiol 2000;7a: 79-1.

821. Park S-J, Park S-W, Lee C W, et al. Stenting for unprotected left main coronary stenosis: Acute and long-term results of the first 100 cases. J Am Coll Cardiol 2000;61a: 1008-167.

822. Sharma S K, Kini A, Reich D, et al. Intervention of unprotected left main stenosis in high risk patients: Acute and long term results. JACC 2000;62a: 1008-168.

823. Kiesz RS, Rozek MM, Mego DM, et al. Acute directional coronary atherectomy prior to stenting in complex coronary lesions: ADAPTS Study. Cathet Cardiovasc Diagn. 1998;45: 105-112.

824. Hong M K, Wong S C, Pichard A D, et al. Long-term results of patients enrolled in the anti-platelet treatment after intravascular ultrasound guided optimal stent expansion (APLAUSE). Circulation 1996;94: I686

825. Serruys PW, et al. Arterial revascularisation therapy study: The ARTS study, a randomised trial of bypass-surgery versus stenting in multivessel coronary disease. Circulation 2000;I498: 2620.

826. Russo R J, Teirstein P S. Angiography versus intravascular ultrasound-directed stent placement, AVID STUDY. Circulation 1996;94: I263 (1536).

827. Serruys PW, Van Hout B, Bonnier H, et al. Randomised comparison of implantation of heparin-coated stents with balloon angioplasty in selected patients with coronary artery disease. Lancet 1998;352: 674-81.

828. Koning RA. In-hospital results and six-month clinical and angiographic follow-up of coronary stenting in small coronary arteries: Final results of the BEstent in SMall ARTeries (BESMART)Study. J Am Coll Cardiol 2000;36: 314-5.

829. Mattos L, Sousa A, Neto CC, et al. Primary stenting versus balloon PTCA for the treatment of acute vein graft occlusion in myocardial infarction: In-hospital results from the Brazilian coronary interventional registry (CENIC). J Am Coll Cardiol 2000;39a.

830. The ESPRIT investigators. Lancet 2000;256:2037-44.

831. Fitzgerald PJ, Oshima A, Hayase M, et al. Final results of the Can Routine Ultrasound Influence Stent Expansion (CRUISE) study. Circulation 2000;102: 523-30.

832. Berger P, Bell MR, Rihal CS, et al. Clopidogrel versus ticlopidine after intracoronary stent placement. J Am Coll Cardiol 1999;34: 1891-4.

833. De Bruyne B, et al. Debate II: A randomized study to evaluate provisional stenting after guided balloon angioplasty. Circulation 1998;I498: 2622

834. DiMario C, The DESTINI-CFR Study Group. Doppler and QCA guided aggressive PTCA has the same target lesion revascularization of stent implantation. 6-Month results of the DESTINI study. Am Coll Cardiol 1999;47a: 810-2

835. Mehran R, et al. The Manual of Interventional Trials. TCT 2000

836. The EDRES trial. Circulation 1998;98:98:(Supp. I);I-709.

837. Marso SP, Lincoff AM, Ellis SG, et al. Optimizing the percutaneous interventional outcomes for patients with diabetes, Results of the EPISTENT (Evaluation of Platelet IIb/IIIa Inhibitor for STENTING trial diabetic) substudy. Circulation 1999;100: 2477-84.

838. Topol EJ, Mark DB, Lincoff AM, Cohen E, Burton J, Kleiman N, Talley D, Sapp S, Booth J, Cabot CF, Anderson KM, Califf RM. Outcomes at 1 year and economic implications of platelet glycoprotein IIb/IIIa blockade in patients undergoing coronary stenting: results from a multicentre randomised trial. EPISTENT Investigators. Evaluation of platelet IIb/IIIa inhibitor for stenting. Lancet 1999;354(9195):2019-24.

839. Marso SP, Lincoff AM, Ellis SG, Bhatt DL, Tanguay JF, Kleiman NS, Hammoud T, Booth JE, Sapp SK, Topol EJ. Optimizing the percutaneous interventional outcomes for patients with diabetes mellitus: results of the EPISTENT (Evaluation of platelet IIb/IIIa inhibitor for stenting trial) diabetic substudy. Circulation 1999;100(25):2477-84.

840. Carruzza J P, et al;Final acute, 30-day, and 6-month clinical and angiographic outcome from the multicenter randomized EXTRA trial comparing the operator-mounted XT and Palmaz-Schatz coronary stents. Circulation 1998;I661: 3474

841. Mehran R, et al. The Manual of Interventional Trials. TCT 2000

842. DeScheerder I K, Wang K, Kerdsinchai P, et al. Clinical and angiographic experience with coronary stenting using freedom stent. J Invas Cardiol 1996;8: 418-27.

843. Lafont A, Dubois-Rande JL, Steg PG,et al. The French randomized optimal stenting trial: A prospective evaluation of provisional stenting guided by coronary velocity reserve and quantitative coronary angiography FROST. J Am Coll Cardiol 2000;36: 404-9.

844. Rubartelli P, Niccoli L, Verna E, et al. Stent implantation versus balloon angioplasty in chronic coronary occlusions: Results from the GISSOC trial. J Am Coll Cardiol1998;32: 90-96.

845. Mehran R. et al. The Manual of Interventional Trials. TCT 2000.

846. Schiele F, et al. Intravascular Ultrasound Makes Possible Reliable ASSessment of Neo Intima After Stenting. J Am Coll Cardiol 1999;33:Abstract 1188-94.

847. Tamai H, Tsuchikane E, et al. Mayo-Japan investigation for chronic total occlusions (MAJIC). Circulation 1999;I436.

848. Urban P, Macaya C, Rupprecht HJ, et al. Randomized evaluation of anticoagulation versus antiplatelet therapy after coronary implantation in high-risk patients: The Multicenter Aspirin and Ticlopidine Trial after Intracoronary Stenting (MATTIS). Circulation 1998; 98: 2126-32.

849. De Jaegere P, Mudra H, Figulla H, et al. Intravascular ultrasound-guided optimized stent deployment. Immediate and clinical and angiographic results from the multicenter ultrasound stenting in coronaries study, Eur Heart J 1998;19: 1214 – 23.

850. Rodriguez A, Ayala F, Bernardi V, et al. Optimal coronary balloon angioplasty with provisional stenting versus primary stent (OCBAS). J Am Coll Cardiol 1998;32: 1351 – 57.

851. Stone GW, St Goar FG, Hodgson JM, et al. Analysis of the relation between stent implantation pressure and expansion, optimal stent implantation (OSTI) investigators. Am J Cardiol 1999;83: 1397 – 400.

852. Linnemeier T J, Cannon L A, et al. Preliminary acute results of the RECREATE Trial – an evaluation of the ACS multilink stent in the treatment of abrupt or threatened abrupt closure. Circulation 1998;I854: 4481.

853. Schiele F, Meneveau N, Seronde M F, et al;Medical costs over 18 months after stent implantation with versus without intravascular ultrasound guidance. results of the randomized "REStenosis After Intravascular Ultrasound STenting" (RESIST) Study. J Am Coll Cardiol 2000;3a.

854. Szto G Y, Linnemeier T J, Lewis S J, et al. Safety of 10 days of ticlopidine after coronary stenting-a randomized

comparison with 30 days: strategic alternatives with ticlopidine in stenting study (SALTS). J Am Coll Cardiol 998;352a.

855. Sievert H, Rohde S, Utech A, et al. Stent or angioplasty after recanalization of chronic coronary occlusions? (The SARECCO Trial). Am J Cardiol 1999;84: 386-90.

856. Mehran R, et al. The Manual of Interventional Trials. TCT 2000.

857. Frey A W, Roskamm H, Hodgson J M, et al. IVUS– guided stenting: Does acute angiography predict long term outcome? Insights from the strategy of IVUS-guided PTCA and stenting, SIPS Trial. Circulation 1997;I222.

858. Doucet S, Schalig M J, Hilton D, et al. The SISA study: A randomized comparison of balloon angioplasty and stent to prevent restenosis in small arteries. J Am Coll Cardiol 2000;8a.

859. Heuser R, Kuntz R, Lansky A, et al. A comparison of the long AVE Micro Stent II and the Palmaz-Schatz stent: A SMART Trial Registry. J Am Coll Cardiol 1998;31:80a.

860. Moussa I, Moses J, Di Mario C, et al. Stenting after optimal lesion debulking (SOLD) registry. Angiographic and clinical outcome. Circulation 1998;16: 1604-9.

861. Hoher M, Grebe O, Woehrle J, et al. Wiktor stent implantation in chronic total occlusions reduces restenosis rate-initial results of the SPACTO trial. Circulation 1997;I268.

862. Tsuchikane E, Sumitsuji S, Awata N, et al. Final results of the Stent versus directional coronary Atherectomy Randomized Trial (START). J Am Coll Cardiol 1999;34: 1050 –7.

863. Betriu A, Masotti M, Serra A, et al. Randomized comparison of coronary stent implantation and balloon angioplasty in the treatment of de novo coronary artery lesions (START):A four-year follow-up. J Am Coll Cardiol1999;34: 1498-1506.

864. Moussa I, Oetgen M, Roubin G, et al. Effectiveness of clopidogrel and aspirin versus ticlopidine and aspirin in preventing stent thrombosis after coronary stent implantation. Circulation 1999;99: 2364 – 6.

865. Mishkel GJ, Aguirre FV, Ligon RW, et al. Clopidogrel as adjunctive antiplatelet therapy during coronary stenting. J Am Coll Cardiol 1999;34: 1884 – 90.

866. Mehran R, et al. The Manual of Interventional Trial. TCT 2000.

867. TASC-I trial. J Am Coll Cardiol 1995;156A.

868. TASC-I trial. Circulation 1995;92:I-475.

869. TASC-II trial. J Am Coll Cardiol 1995;156A.

870. Mehran R, et al. The Manual of Interventional Trials. TCT 2000.

871. Choussat R, Black AJR, Bossi I, et al. Long-term clinical outcome after endoluminal reconstruction of diffusely degenerated saphenous vein grafts with less-shortening Wallstents. J Am Coll Cardiol 2000;36:387-94.

872. Emanuelsson H, Serruys PW, Van Der Giessen WJ, et al. Clinical and angiographic results with the multi-link coronary stent system – the West European Stent Trial (WEST). J Invas Cardiol 1997;9: 561 – 8.

873. The Wallstent SVG Study. J Am Coll Cardiol 1998;30:216A.

874. Serruys PW, Van der Giessen W, Garcia E, et al. Clinical and angiographic results with the multi-link stent implanted under intravascular ultrasound guidance (WEST-2 study). J Inv Cardiol 1998;10: 20b-27b.

875. Wiktor study. Am J Cardiol 199;84:644-649.

876. Rodriquez A, Bernardi V, Fernandez M, et al. Hospital and late results of coronary stents versus conventional balloon angioplasty in acute myocardial infarction (GRAMI Trial). Am J Cardiol 1998;81: 1286-91.

877. Suryapranata H, Van't Hof AW, Hoorntje J, et al. Randomized comparison of coronary stenting with balloon angioplasty in selected patients with acute myocardial infarction. Circulation 1998;97:2502-05.

878. Grines C L, Cox D A, Stone G W, et al. Coronary angioplasty with or without stent implantation for acute myocardial infarction. N Engl J Med 1999;341:1949-56.

879. Saito S, Howokawa G, Tanaka S, et al. Primary stent implantation is superior to balloon angioplasty in acute myocardial infarction: Final results the primary angioplasty versus stent implantation in acute myocardial infarction (PASTA) Trial. Cathet Cardiovasc Intervent. 1999;48: 262-8.

880. Hanekamp CEE, Koolen JJ, Den Heyer P, et al. A randomized comparison between balloon angioplasty and elective stent implantation in venous bypass grafts;the Venestent study. J Am Coll Cardiol 2000;35:9A.

881. Ahmed JM, Hong MK, Mehron R, et al. Influence of diabetes mellitus on early and late clinical outcomes in saphenous vein graft stenting. J Am Coll Cardiol 2000;36:1186-93.

882. Leon, M Strumpf R, Buchbinder M, et al. Preliminary findings using a PTEE-coated stent in patients with saphenous vein graft disease. J Am Coll. Cardiol 2001;1038(15):2A.

883. Maillard L, Hamon M, Khalife K, et al. A comparison of systematic stenting and conventional balloon angioplasty during primary percutaneous transluminal coronary angioplasty for acute myocardial infarction. J Am Coll Cardiol 2000;35:1729 –36.

884. Schoming A, Kastrati A, Dirschinger J, et al. Coronary stenting plus platelet glycoprotein IIb/IIIa blockade compared with tissue plasminogen activator in acute myocardial infarction. Stent versus thrombolysis occluded coronary arteries in patients with acute myocardial infarction study investigators. N Engl J Med. 2000;43:385-91.

885. Antoniucci D, Santoro G M, Bolognese L, et al. A clinical trial comparing primary stenting of the infarct-related artery with optimal primary angioplasty of acute myocardial infarction. Results from the Florence Randomized Elective Stenting in Acute Coronary Occlusions (FRESCO) trial. J Am Coll Cardiol 1998;31: 1234 – 9.

886. Kastrati A, Elezi S, Dirschinger J, Hadamitzky M, Neumann FJ, Schomig A. Influence of lesion length on restenosis after coronary stent placement. Am J Cardiol 1999;83(12):1617-22.

887. Sheifer SE, Canos MR, Weinfurt KP, Arora UK, Mendelsohn FO, Gersh BJ, et al. Sex differences in coronary artery size assessed by intravascular ultrasound. Am Heart J 2000;139(4):649-53.

888. de Feyter PJ, Kay P, Disco C, Serruys PW. Reference chart derived from post-stent-implantation intravascular ultrasound predictors of 6-month expected restenosis on quantitative coronary angiography. Circulation 1999;100(17):1777-83.

889. Ahmed JM, Hong MK, Mehran R, et al. Comparison of debulking followed by stenting versus stenting alone for saphenous vein graft aortoostial lesions: immediate and one-year clinical outcomes. J Am Coll Cardiol 2000;35(6):1560-8.

890. Hong MK, Park SW, Mintz GS, et al. Intravascular ultrasonic predictors of angiographic restenosis after long coronary stenting. Am J Cardiol 2000;85(4):441-5.

891. Baim DS. PREDICT: A prospective multicenter randomized trial of stent implantation with vs. without predilatation. Presented at TCT 2000.

892. Frimerman A, Rechavia E, Eigler N, et al. Long-term follow-up of a high risk cohort after stent implantation in saphenous

vein grafts. J Am Coll Cardiol 1997;30:1277-1283.

893. Alfonso F, Azcona L, Perez-Vizcayna MJ, et al. Initial results and long-term clinical and angiographic implications of coronary stenting in elderly patients. J Am Coll Cardiol 1999;149:1483-87.

894. Bage MD, Bauman WB, Gupta R, et al. Coronary stenting in the elderly: Longitudinal results in a wide spectrum of patients treated with a new and more practical approach. Cathet Cardiovasc Diagn 1998;44:397-404.

895. De Gregorio J, Kobayashi Y, Albiero R, et al. Coronary artery stenting in the elderly: Short-term outcome and long-term angiographic and clinical follow-up. J Am Coll Cardiol 1998;32:577-583.

896. Yokoi H, Kimur T, Sawada Y, Nosaka H, et al. Efficacy and safety of Palmaz-Schatz stent in elderly (> 75 years old) patients: Early and follow-up results. J Am Coll Cardiol 1995;February Special Issue:47A.

897. Fishman RF, Kuntz RE, Carrozza JP, et al. Acute and long-term results of coronary atherectomy in women and the elderly. Circulation (in-press).

898. Elliot JM, MacIsaac AI, Lefkovits J, et al. New coronary devices in the elderly: Comparison with angioplasty. Circulation 1994;90:4:I

899. Abizaid A, Dangas G, Mehran R, et al. One-year results after multivessel stenting in diabetic vs. non-diabetic patients. J Am Coll Cardiol 2001;37(2):68A.

900. Moussa I, Colombo A, DiMario C, et al. Long-term outcome of patients with versus without diabetes mellitus in the DESTINI Trial. J Am Coll Cardiol 2001;37(2):65A.

901. Stuckey T, Grines CL, Cox D, et al. Does stenting and glycoprotein IIb/IiIa receptor blockade improve the prognosis of diabetics undergoing primary angioplasty in acute myocardial infarction? The CADILLAC trial. J Am Coll Cardiol 2001;37(2):342A.

902. Villareal RP, Lee V, Elayda M, Wilson JM. Survival after coronary artery bypass surgery or coronary stenting in patients with diabetes mellitus. Circulation 2000;102:II549.

903. Dangas G, Kobayashi Y, D'Agate D, et al. Long term results after multivessel stenting in diabetic patients. Circulation 2000;102:II-194.

904. Mattos L, Grines C, Sousa JE, et al. One year follow-up after primary coronary interventions for acute myocardial infarction in diabetic patients: STENT-PAMI trial results. J Am Coll Cardiol 2000;35:72A.

905. Ooka M, Suzuki T, Yokoya K, Hayase M, et al. Stenting after revascularization of chronic total occlusion. Circulation 1995;92:I-94.

906. Pereira CF, Bernardi V, Martinez J, et al. Diabetic patients with multivessel disease treated with percutaneous coronary revascularization had similar outcome than those treated with surgery;one year follow up results from two Argentine randomized studies (ERACI-ERACI II). J Am Coll Cardiol 2000;35:3A.

907. Schofer J, Schluter M, Rau, et al. Influence of treatment modality on angiographic outcome after coronary stenting in diabetic patients: a controlled study. J Am Coll Cardiol 2000;35:1554-9.

908. Gaxiola E, Vliestra RE, Brenner AS, et al. Diabetes and multiple stents independently double the risk of short-term revascularization. J Interven Cardiol 2000;13:87-91.

909. Silva JA, Ramee SR, White CJ, et al. Primary stenting in acute myocardial infarction: Influence of diabetes mellitus in angiographic results and clinical outcome. Am Heart J 1999;138:446-55.

910. Joseph T, Fajadet J, Jordan C. et al. Coronary stenting in deabetics: immediate and mid-term clinical outcome. Cathet Cardiovasc Intervent 1999;47:279-284.

911. Gencbay M, Degertekin M, Dinar I, Turan, F. Coronary stent implantation in patients with non-insulin dependent diabetes mellitus. J Am Coll Cardiol 1999;33[suppl A]:98A.

912. Alonso JJ, Fernandez-Aviles F, Duran JM, et al. Influence of diabetes mellitus on the initial and long-term outcome of patients treated with coronary stenting. J Am Coll Cardiol 1999;33[suppl A]:98A.

913. Bhaskaran A, Siegel R, Barker B, et al. Stenting during coronary intervention improves procedural and long-term clinical outcomes in diabetics. J Am Coll Cardiol 1999;33[suppl A]:97A.

914. Lansky AJ, Mehran R, Popma JJ, et al. Insulin treatment of diabetic women predicts a worse outcome after intracoronary stenting. Clinical results of 564 consecutive patients. J Am Coll Cardiol 1999;33[suppl A]:97A.

915. Carrozza JP, Neimann D, Kuntz RE, Cutlip D. Diabetes mellitus is associated with adverse 6-month angiographic and clinical outcome following coronary stenting. Circulation 1998;98[suppl I]:I-79.

916. Savage MP, Fischman DL, et al. Coronary intervention in the diabetic patient: Improved outcome following stent implantation versus balloon angioplasty. J Am Coll Cardiol 1997;29(Suppl. A):188A.

917. Abizaid A, Kornowski R, Mintz GS, et al. The influence of diabetes mellitus on acute and late clinical outcomes following coronary stent implantation. J Am Coll Cardiol 1998;32:584-9.

918. Elezi S, Schuhlen H, et al. Stent placement in diabetic versus non-diabetic patients. Six-month angiographic follow-up. J Am Coll Cardiol 1997;29(Suppl. A):188A.

919. Yokoi H, Nosaka H, et al. Coronary stenting in the diabetic patients: Early and follow-up results. J Am Coll Cardiol 1997;29(Suppl. A):455A.

920. Van Belle E, Bauters C, Hubert E, et al. Restenosis rates in diabetic patients. A comparison of coronary stenting with balloon angioplasty in native coronary vessels. Circulation 1997;96:1454-60.

921. Suwaidi JA, Berger PB, Rihal CS, et al. Immediate and long-term outcome of intracoronary stent implantation for true bifurcation lesions. J Am Coll Cardiol 2000;35:929-36.

922. Yamashita R, Nishida T, Adamian MG, et al. Bifurcation lesions: Two stents versus one stent—immediate and follow-up results. J Am Coll Cardiol 2000;35:1145-51.

923. Carrie D, Elbaz M, Dambrin G, et al. Coronary stenting of bifurcation lesions using "T" or "reserve Y" configuration with Wiktor stent. Am J Cardiol 1998;82:1418-1421.

924. Chevalier B, Glatt B, Royer T, Guyon P. Placement of coronary stents in bifurcation lesions by the "culotte" technique. Am J Cardiol 1998;82:943-949.

925. Lefevre T, Louvard Y, Morice MC, et al. Stenting of bifurcation lesions: Seven-month follow-up of a prospective study. Circulation 1998;98(suppl I):I-638.

926. Pan M, de Lezo JS, Romero M, et al. Simple and complex stent strategies for bifurcated coronary lesions. Circulation 1998;98(suppl I):I-638.

927. Stefanadis C, Toutouzas K, Tsiamis E, et al. Stents covered by autologous venous grafts: Feasibility and immediate and long-term results. Am Heart J 2000;139:437-45.

928. Park SJ, Lee CW, Hong MK, et al. Stent placement for ostial

left anterior descending coronary artery stenosis: Acute and long-term (2-year) results. Cathet Cardiovasc Intervent 2000;49:267-271.

929. Mintz GS, Mehran R, Jackson M, et al. Diabetes and ostial lesion location have an additive effect on target lesion revascularization after stent implantation. J Am Coll Cardiol 2000;35:17A.

930. Wischmeyer JB, Huber KC, Johnson WJ, et al. Procedural outcomes of aorto-ostial vs. coronary ostial lesions. J Am Coll Cardiol 1999;33:82A.

931. Asakaura Y, Takagi S, Ishikawa S, et al. Favorable strategy for the ostial lesion of the left anterior descending coronary artery: Influence on narrowing of circumflex coronary artery. Cathet Cardiovasc Diagn. 1998;43:95-100.

932. Mathur A, Liu MW, Goods CM, et al. Results of elective stenting of branch ostial lesions. Am J Cardiol 1997;79:472-474.

933. Kurbaan AS, Kelly PA, Sigwart U. Cutting balloon angioplasty and stenting for aorto-ostial lesions. Heart 1997;77:350-352.

934. Jain SP, Zhang S, et al. Is coronary stenting a better option in palliative treatment of cardiac allograft vasculopathy? J Am Coll Cardiol 1997;29(Suppl. A):28A.

935. DeCesare NB, Bartorelli AL, Galli S, et al. Treatment of ostial lesions of the left anterior descending coronary artery with Palmaz-Schatz coronary stent. Am Heart J 1996;132:716-720.

936. Kornowski R, Mehran R, Lansky AJ, Fuchs S. Procedural results and late clinical outcomes following percutaneous interventions using long (≥ 25 mm) stents. J Am Coll Cardiol 1998;33(Suppl A):69A.

937. Hong MK, Park SW, Mintz GS, et al. Intravascular ultrasonic predictors of angiographic restenosis after long coronary stenting. Am J Cardiol 2000;85:441-445.

938. Ormiston J, Ruygrok PN, Webster M, et al. Stenting of long coronary lesions: a prospective 6-month quantitative angiographic study (STELLA trial). J Am Coll Cardiol 2000;35:62A.

939. De Gregorio J, Moussa I, Kobayashi Y, et al. The use of IVUS-guided PTCA and spot stenting in the treatment of long lesions: A comparison to traditional stenting. J Am Coll Cardiol 2000;35:62A.

940. Kobayashi Y, DeGregorio J, Reimers B, et al. The length of the stented segment is an independent predictor of restenosis. J Am Coll Cardiol 1999;33(Suppl A):366A.

941. Schalij MJ, Udayachalerm W, Oemrawsingh P, et al. Stenting of long coronary artery lesions: Initial angiographic results and 6-month clinical outcome of the Micro Stent II-XL. Cathet Cardiovasc Intervent 1999;48:105-112.

942. Williams IL, Thomas MR, Robinson NMK, et al. Angiographic and clinical restenosis following the use of long coronary wallstents. Cathet Cardiovasc Intervent 1999;48:287-293.

943. Nakagawa Y, Yufu K, Tamura T, Tokoi H, et al. Stenting for long lesions with long GFX stent. J Am Coll Cardiol 1999;33(Suppl I):69A.

944. Rankin JM, Lohavanichbutr K, Carere RG, et al. Low rate of repeat revascularization despite stenting long segments. Circulation 1998;98(suppl I):I-285.

945. Kobayashi Y, DeGregorio J, Reimers B, et al. Immediate and follow-up results following implantation of the long and short NIR stent: Comparison with the Palmaz-Schatz stent. J Am Coll Cardiol 1998;33(Suppl A):312A.

946. Elezi S, Kastrati A, Wehinger A, Walter H, et al. Stent placement in long (≥ 15 mm) coronary lesions. J Am Coll Cardiol 1998;33(Suppl A:31(Suppl A):273A.

947. Le Breton H, Bedossa M, Commeau P, et al. Clinical and angiographic results of stenting for long coronary arterial atherosclerotic lesions. Am J Cardiol 1998;82:1539-1542.

948. Antoniucci D, Valenti R, Santoro GM, et al. Preliminary experience with stent-supported coronary angioplasty in long narrowings using the long Freedom Force stent: Acute and six-month clinical and angiographic results in a series of 27 consecutive patients. Cathet Cardiovasc Diagn 1998;43:163-167.

949. Akira I, Hall P, Maiello L, Blengino S, et al. Coronary stenting of long lesions (greater than 20 mm) — a matched comparison of different stents. Circulation 1995;92:I-688.

950. Schalij MJ, Doucet S, Hilton D., et al. The SISA study: A randomized comparison of balloon angioplasty and stent to prevent restenosis in small arteries: 6 Month angiographic and 12 month clinical outcome. Circulation 2000;102:II-663.

951. Caputo RP, Giambartolomei A, Simons A, et al. Small vessel stenting-Comparison of modular vs. slotted tube design. Six month results from the EXTRA trial. J Am Coll Cardiol 2000;35:56A

952. Al Suwaidi J, Garratt KN, Rihal CS, et al. Immediate and one-year outcome of coronary stent implantation in small coronary vessels using 2.5 mm stents. J Am Coll Cardiol 2000;35:63A.

953. Mori F, Tsurumi Y, Nakamura A, et al. Stenting in small coronary vessels (<2.5mm): Impact of stent over-dilatation following initial stent deployment. Circulation 2000;102:II-641.

954. Kastrati A, Mehilli J, Dirschinger J, et al. Is stenting superior to PTCA for lesions in small coronary vessels in diabetic patients? Results from the ISAR-SMART randomized trial. Circulation 2000:102:II-387.

955. Hamasaki N, Nosaka H, Kimura T, et al. Stenting for small vessels using new generation flexible stent: Comparison of balloon angioplasty and Palmaz-Schatz stent. J Am Coll Cardiol 1999;33(Suppl I):32A.

956. Michael L, Buller CE, Catellier D, et al. Efficacy of stenting vs. balloon angioplasty in small diameter (<3 mm) total coronary occlusions: A total occlusion study of Canada substudy. Circulation 1998;98(Suppl I):I-639.

957. Waksman R, Mehran R, Saucedo JF, et al. Balloons PTCA is equivalent to stents in patients with small coronaries: A comparative retrospective matching study. J Am Coll Cardiol 1999;33(Suppl I):273A.

958. Schunkert H, Harrell L. Small coronary vessels: A suitable target for percutaneous revascularization in the new device era? J Am Coll Cardiol 1999;33(Suppl I):275A.

959. Deutsch E, Martin JL, Fischman DL, et al. The late benefit of coronary stenting in small vessels is reduced in diabetic patients. J Am Coll Cardiol 1999;33(Suppl I):275A

960. Gruberg L, Mehran R, Dangas G, et al. Effect of plaque debulking and stenting on short- and long-term outcomes after revascularization of chronic total occlusions. J Am Coll Cardiiol 2000;35:151-6.

961. Ozaki Y, Violaris AG, Hamburger J, et al. Short- and long-term clinical and quantitative angiographic results with the new, less shortening Wallstent for vessel reconstruction in chronic total occlusion: A quantitative angiographic study. J Am Coll Cardiol 1996;28:354-360.

962. Hoher M, Wohrle J, Grebe OC, et al. A randomized trial of elective stenting after balloon recanalization of chronic total occlusions. J Am Coll Cardiol 1999;34:722-9.

963. Anzuini A, Rosanio S, Legrand V, et al. Wiktor stent for treatment of chronic total coronary artery occlusions: Short- and long-term clinical and angiographic results from a large multicenter experience. J Am Coll Cardiol 1998;31:281-288.Suttorp MJ, Mast EG, Plokker HWT, et al. Primary coronary stenting after successful balloon angioplasty of chronic total occlusions: A single-center experience. Am Heart J 1998;135:318-322.

964. Yamasaki K, Nakamura T, Yung-Sheng H, et al. Three-year angiographic follow-up of coronary stenting in patients with chronic total occlusion. Circulation 1998;98:I-283-I-284.

965. Carere RG, Barbeau G, Dzavik V, et al. Do superior balloon angioplasty resutls provided stent-like outcomes in coronary occlusions. Circulation 1998;98:I-284.

966. Title LM, Buller Ce, Catellier D, et al. Efficacy of stenting vs. balloon angiopaslty in small diameter (< 3 mm) total coronary occlusions: A total occlusion study of Canada substudy. Circulation 1998;98:I-639.

967. Rau T, Schofer J, Schulter M, et al. Stenting of nonacute total coronary occlusions: Predictors of late angiographic outcome. J Am Coll Cardiol 1998;31:275-280.

968. Elezi S, Schuhlen H, et al. Six-month angiographic follow-up after stenting of chronic total coronary occlusions. J Am Coll Cardiol 1997;29(Suppl. A):16A.

969. Barragan P, Beauregard C. Montalescot G, Wittenberg O, Ecollan P, Elhadad S, Villain P, Boulenc JM, Maillard L, Pinton P. Abciximab associated with primary angioplasty and stenting in acute myocardial infarction: The Admiral Study, 6-month results. Circulation 2000;102(18):II-663 (Abstract).

970. Sato Y, Nosaka H, Kimura T, et al. Randomized comparison of balloon angioplasty versus coronary stent implantation for total occlusion. J Am Coll Cardiol 1996;27:152A.

27 ROTABLATOR ATHERECTOMY

Mark Reisman, M.D.
Robert D. Safian, M.D.

A. DESCRIPTION. The Rotablator system (Boston Scientific Scimed) (Figures 27.1, 27.2) consists of a reusable console that controls the rotational speed of an olive-shaped, nickel-plated, brass burr, which is coated on its leading edge with 20-30 micron diamond chips and is bonded to a flexible drive shaft. The drive shaft is enclosed in a 4.3 F flexible Teflon sheath, which protects the arterial wall from the rotating drive shaft and serves as a conduit for saline flush solution, which cools and irrigates the system. The speed of burr rotation is regulated by a compressed-air or nitrogen-driven turbine, which is controlled by the console and activated by a foot pedal; rotational speed is monitored by a fiberoptic tachometer (Figure 27.3). The are several specialized 0.009-inch stainless steel Rotablator guidewires (floppy and extra-support) with transitional zones that taper distally allowing for improved tracking and variable bias within the artery. To perform atherectomy, the Rotablator guidewire is steered into the target vessel so that the platinum tip is distal to the lesion (the burr will not advance over the large diameter tip). Alternatively, a conventional flexible PTCA guidewire may be used to cross the target lesion, after which time a balloon or transfer catheter can be used to exchange for the Rotablator wire. The burr is then advanced over the guidewire until it lies just proximal to the stenosis. Thereafter, the saline flush is infused, rotation is initiated, and using a control knob on the top of the advancer, the rotating burr (140,000-160,000 RPM depending on burr size) is gently advanced through the lesion.

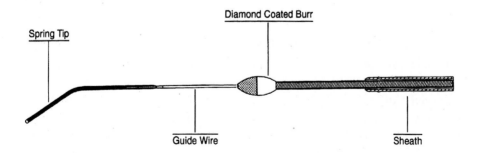

Figure 27.1. The Rotablator Burr

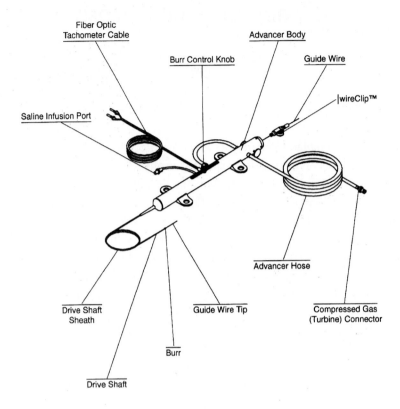

Figure 27.2. The Rotablator Setup

B. **PHYSICAL PRINCIPLES AND DESIGN CHARACTERISTICS.** The two physical principles that enable the Rotablator system to preferentially ablate atherosclerotic plaque are differential cutting and orthogonal displacement of friction:

1. **Differential Cutting** is defined as the ability of a device to selectively cut one material while maintaining the integrity of another, based on differences in substrate composition. In the case of high-speed rotational atherectomy, this results in pulverization of inelastic material such as fibrotic atheromatous plaque and lipid-rich tissue; in contrast, nondiseased vessel segments, which retain their viscoelastic properties, are deflected away from the advancing burr and spared from ablation.

2. **Orthogonal Displacement of Friction** explains the easy passage of the burr through tortuous and diseased segments of the coronary vasculature. At rotational speeds ≥ 60,000 RPM, the longitudinal friction vector is virtually eliminated, resulting in reduced surface drag and unimpeded advancement and withdrawal of the burr.

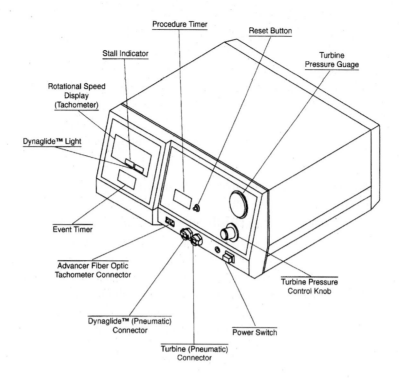

Figure 27.3. The Rotablator Control Panel

C. IMPACT OF HIGH-SPEED ROTATIONAL ABLATION

1. **Effect on the Vessel Wall.** Histological[1] and IVUS [2,3] studies have demonstrated that fibrotic, calcified, and soft plaque are removed after Rotablator, leaving a smooth internal surface devoid of endothelium without medial injury. The segments proximal and distal to the treatment site show no change in diameter at follow-up angiography 3 and 6 months after atherectomy, suggesting that Rotablator does not accelerate atherosclerosis.[4]

2. **Microparticulate Debris.** The size of microparticulate debris generated during atherectomy is determined by the size of the diamond chips and by the speed and pressure of the advancing burr. Larger particles are generated at slow (< 75,000 RPM)[5] burr speeds and heat is generated by forceful advancement of the burr, characterized by a fall in RPM > 5000.[54] Conversely, smaller particles and a lower particulate burden are generated at speeds > 140,000 RPM and during gentle advancement of the burr, although rotational speeds of 180,000 RPM seem to be associated with more frequent platelet aggregation and larger platelet aggregates. Experimental studies reported that 77% of the particles generated by the Rotablator were < 5 microns and 88% were < 12 microns,[5] and that particulate concentrations 10-30 times greater than those observed in human

Rotablator studies were needed to reduce coronary blood flow.[6] Most particles pass harmlessly through the circulation and are cleared by the liver, lungs, and spleen.[7] While some studies using positron emission tomography (PET)[8] and simultaneous transesophageal echocardiography[9] found no effect on hemodynamic performance, global LV function, or regional wall motion, other studies demonstrated transient (30-40 minutes) myocardial stunning.[10] Studies with the Doppler wire demonstrated persistent abnormality in coronary flow reserve even after successful adjunctive PTCA,[65] but these abnormalities were corrected by stenting, suggesting that Doppler flow impairment after Rotablator is due to inadequate lumen enlargement, not distal embolization.

3. **Efficiency of Ablation.** Quantitative angiographic analyses suggest that Rotablator atherectomy achieves a lumen that is 90% of the selected burr size;[13] lumen dimensions may increase even further over the following 24 hours,[14] possibly due to release of elastic recoil and/or vasospasm. Intravascular ultrasound (IVUS) studies show that the primary mechanism of lumen enlargement after the Rotablator is plaque ablation,[15] characterized by a decrease in plaque plus media area (plaque removal), an increase in lumen diameter, no change in external elastic membrane area (no arterial expansion), and a decrease in the arc of target lesion calcium. In contrast, adjunctive PTCA was shown to enlarge the lumen primarily through arterial expansion (an increase in external elastic membrane in 80% of lesions) and not by plaque removal (no change in plaque plus media area). Typical IVUS findings after Rotablator atherectomy included an intimal-luminal interface that was distinct and circular, and lumen dimensions that were frequently larger than the final burr diameter.[16]

4. **Costs.** Limited data are available concerning cost-effectiveness.[17,18] In a randomized trial of PTCA, Rotablator atherectomy, and excimer laser angioplasty, the incremental cost of Rotablator over PTCA was 23%; however, this was accompanied by an increase in procedural success (93% vs. 83% for PTCA) and a decrease in length of stay (3.5 days vs. 4.2 days for PTCA).

D.   ROTABLATOR PROCEDURE

1. **Preprocedural Assessment.** The approach to Rotablator is similar to PTCA, although several factors are worth special emphasis. For target lesions in a dominant RCA, dominant circumflex, or ostial LAD, or when using a 2.5 mm burr, the development of heart block may warrant prophylactic insertion of a temporary pacemaker. Bradycardia usually occurs immediately upon burr activation and typically reverses 5-60 seconds after ablation is terminated. The mechanism of bradycardia is unknown, but may be due to microcavitation, microparticulate embolization, vasospasm, guidewire vibration, or an unknown reflex. Continuous monitoring of pulmonary artery pressure is strongly recommended when Rotablator atherectomy is used in patients with severe LV dysfunction[53] or when the target vessel supplies a large myocardial territory. In select high-risk cases (e.g., a single patent vessel), prophylactic insertion of an IABP is recommended to prevent hemodynamic instability should transient myocardial dysfunction occur.

2. **Adjunctive Medication.** As for all interventions, aspirin (325 mg/d beginning at least 1 day prior to atherectomy) is mandatory. Adequate hydration and calcium channel blockers are also recommended prior to the case and may reduce the frequency of vasospasm, which can occur in up to 15% of patients. During the procedure, heparin (10,000 units IV bolus with supplements as needed) is used to maintain the ACT > 350 seconds throughout the case. If IIb/IIIa inhibitors are used, standard ACT guidelines should be followed. Although severe vasospasm is uncommon, intracoronary nitroglycerin should be readily available; a common technique is to administer a 100-150 mcg bolus after each ablation run. Intracoronary verapamil or diltiazem (injected through a balloon or transport catheter into the distal vessel) may be helpful in reversing slow-flow or no-reflow (Chapter 21). Finally, some operators prepare a "cocktail" of nitroglycerin, verapamil and heparin in the flush solution, to provide continuous delivery of coronary vasodilators during Rotablation and possibly reduce the incidence of no-reflow.[19,55,56] Rotaglide lubricant is used by some operators to reduce friction between the drive coil and guidewire. Platelet IIb/IIIa inhibitors are associated with a 50% reduction in CPK elevation[62] and less burr-induced platelet aggregation,[63,64] and are routinely utilized in many institutions.

3. **Rotablator Technique**
   a. **Guide Catheter Selection and Guidewire Placement.** A critical step in the procedure is selection of a guide catheter that ensures coaxial alignment. Since ablation occurs along the path of the guidewire, tangential orientation of the guidewire (guidewire bias) may direct the burr into the arterial wall, resulting in suboptimal debulking and increasing the risk of dissection or perforation.[20] The internal diameter of the guiding catheter must be 0.004 inches larger than the burr; the 1.25 mm, 1.50 mm, 1.75 mm, 2.0 mm, and 2.15 mm burrs can be advanced through a giant-lumen 8F guide (ID $\geq$ 0.089-inch); 2.25 mm burrs through a 9F guide (ID > 0.093-inch); 2.38 mm burrs through a giant-lumen 9F guide (ID $\geq$ 0.098-inch); and 2.50 mm burrs through a 10F guiding catheter (ID $\geq$ 0.102-inch).

   b. **Burr Selection and Placement.** A two-burr approach, beginning with a burr-to-artery ratio of 0.5-0.6 and ending with a burr-to-artery ratio of 0.75-0.8, is often recommended to minimize the microparticulate burden and allow the operator to assess the progress of the procedure. Initiating treatment with a burr-to-artery ratio < 0.5 is usually reserved for total occlusions, lesions on severe bends, or lesions greater than 30 mm in length. After the burr is tested outside the body, it is advanced to a position just proximal to the target lesion (i.e., the "platform segment"). The burr must have unimpeded rotation in the platform segment; if the burr is activated while in contact with the arterial wall, the risk of vessel injury is greatly increased. Free flow of contrast around the burr will confirm adequate positioning. Prior to activating the burr, all forward tension should be neutralized by gentle retraction on the drive shaft itself; no resistance should be felt when the advancer knob is loosened and "jiggled." If tension remains in the drive shaft, activation of the device will cause the burr to lurch forward, possibly resulting in dissection. Once tension is released, the burr is activated in the platform segment and the platform speed (RPM proximal to lesion) is adjusted according to the burr size. Traditional guidelines recommend a platform speed of 160,000 RPM for burrs > 2 mm and 180,000 RPM for burrs ≤ 2 mm. However, some operators favor lower speeds to reduce platelet aggregation and other complications.[63,65]

c. **Ablation Technique.** The most important principle of Rotablator technique is the use of *RPM surveillance* to guide slow and careful advancement of the burr through the lesion. Aggressive burr advancement, indicated by excessive deceleration (rotational speed falls > 5,000 RPM below the platform speed), increases the risk of vessel trauma and ischemic complications caused by heat and the formation of large particles. Intermittent contrast injections should be performed to provide visual assessment of burr advancement; these injections identify the borders of the lesion, the orientation of the device in tortuous segments, the burr-to-artery relationship, and may induce reactive hyperemia. If egress of contrast is not observed, the burr is withdrawn slightly to re-establish antegrade flow and allow clearance of particles. The optimal duration of ablation is based on lesion morphology, distal runoff, and hemodynamic and clinical parameters. In general, each run lasts 15-30 seconds, with time between runs (30 seconds to 2 minutes depending on patient's response) sufficient to allow particle clearance and the administration of vasodilators. When ECG changes, significant chest discomfort, or hemodynamic compromise occur, the interval between ablations should be increased until the patient is clinically stable. Several ablation runs are usually required to completely treat the lesion. The burr is removed when there is no tactile resistance or drop in RPM during burr advancement. Meticulous attention to technical details can produce excellent results with few complications, even in very complex lesions.[56]

d. **Adjunctive Treatment.** Since most burrs are small in relation to the target vessel, adjunctive PTCA is required to achieve definitive lumen enlargement in over 90% of lesions. In general, most of the lumen enlargement occurs after PTCA.[70] There is still controversy about the ideal Rotablator and adjunctive angioplasty strategy. Some operators use a lesion modification strategy employing smaller burrs (burr/artery ratio ≤ 0.6) to gently alter lesion compliance, followed by conventional PTCA (balloon/artery ratio ~ 1.0). In contrast, others use a more aggressive debulking strategy (burr/artery ratio > 0.7) with slightly oversized balloons (balloon/artery ratio ~1.1) at low pressure. Although preliminary data from two large multicenter randomized trials failed to demonstrate a clinical or angiographic advantage for use of aggressive debulking techniques prior to PTCA (Table 27.1),[60,62,82] heavily calcified lesions may require greater debulking to achieve satisfactory results.[69] Rotablator atherectomy followed by directional atherectomy has been applied synergistically to calcified lesions in large diameter vessels. In one report,[21] the Rotablator appeared to render calcified plaque more susceptible to directional atherectomy. In another study using IVUS, adjunctive DCA after Rotablator achieved lumen enlargement which was superior to adjunctive PTCA.[57] Many patients are now being treated with Rotablator and stents (Rotastent) in complex lesions (calcified lesions, long lesions, diffuse disease) (Table 27.2). Compared to adjunctive PTCA, adjunctive stenting resulted in a larger lumen and smaller final stenosis.[22] An IVUS study of

Rotablator followed by PTCA, DCA, or stent for calcified lesions in vessels > 3 mm found that Rotablator/stent resulted in the largest lumen and lowest residual stenosis.[52,64] The SPORT trial (Stenting Post Rotablator Treatment) is a multicenter randomized trial comparing Rotastent vs. PTCA-stent in large calcified lesions; observational data suggested less restenosis after Rotastent.[66] Finally, IVUS has been used to assess the extent and distribution of lesion calcium and guide interventional strategy. The preferred treatment of superficial calcium is the Rotablator, whereas lesions with deep calcium (without superficial calcium) can be treated by PTCA, DCA, or stenting (Chapter 12). Although Rotablator seems to facilitate final stent expansion in calcified lesions, an aggressive debulking strategy (final burr ≥ 2.25 mm or final burr/artery ratio > 0.8) was associated with more in-hospital MI (Q-wave and non-Q-wave) and less restenosis (31% vs. 50%, $p < 0.05$).[71]

    e. Postprocedure Management. Postprocedure management is similar to that of conventional PTCA.

E. RESULTS. Older Rotablator data were based on earlier techniques; important modifications in technique (especially avoidance of excessive burr deceleration) may have had significant beneficial impact on immediate and long-term results.

   1. Success. In a multicenter registry of 2976 patients (3717 lesions), procedural success was achieved in 94.5%.[24] In 90% of cases, adjunctive angioplasty was needed to obtain a residual stenosis < 30%. Procedural success was greater in restenotic lesions than de novo lesions, but was not predicted by patient age, gender, multivessel disease, or unstable angina.

Table 27.1. STRATAS Trial: **Impact of Rotablator Technique on Heavily Calcified Lesions**

	Routine Debulking* (n = 246)	Aggressive Debulking** (n = 248)
In-hospital Results		
Reference vessel (mm)	2.5	2.5
Baseline diameter stenosis (%)	66	67
Final diameter stenosis (%)	26	27
9-month Outcome (%)		
Diameter stenosis	50	54
Angiographic restenosis	52	57
Target lesion revascularization	29	34

STRATAS = Study To Determine Rotablator And Transluminal Angioplasty Strategy
*   Burr-to-artery ratio 0.6-0.8 with adjunctive PTCA
** Burr-to-artery ratio 0.7-0.9 with no- or low-pressure (1 atm) PTCA

Table 27.2. Results of Rotastenting

Series	Description	N	Procedural Success (%)	Restenosis (%)	Comments
Braden[113] (2001)	CTO	139	-	20	
EDRES[114] (2000)	Rotastent Stent	75 75	- -	27 34	Debulking with Rotablator did not improve final stent diameter, but reduced restenosis at 6 months
Kini[63] (2000)	CTO	200	99	-	
Motwani[96] (2000)	Ostial	119	98	18	
SPORT[66] (2000)	Rotastent Stent	328 342	84 89	- -	No difference in in-hospital MACE (17% vs. 13.7%) or reintervention (11.6% vs. 9.9%)
Kobayashi[73] (1999)	Aggressive debulking Routine debulking	56 106	89 95	31 50	Increased risk of Q-wave MI with aggressive debulking
Hoffman[95] (1998)	Calcified (> 3 mm vessel)	56	98	15	
Wang[84] (1998)	-	178	-	41	
Moussa[75] (1997)	Complex	106	93	23	

Abbreviations: CTO = chronic total occlusion; MACE = major adverse cardiac events; - = not reported
Acronyms: EDRES = The Effects of Debulking on Restenosis; SPORT = Stenting Post Rotational Atherectomy Trial
+ Target lesion revascularization

Results from other studies are similar (Table 27.3). An angiographic study revealed further lumen enlargement 24 hours post-Rotablator, suggesting release of elastic recoil and/or vasospasm.[14,69]

2. **Complications.** In the multicenter registry and other observational studies (Table 27.4), clinical complications rates were similar to those reported for PTCA, including death in 1.0%, Q-wave MI in 1.2%, and emergency CABG in 2.5%.[24] Elevated CK-MB more than 2 times normal—the most conservative definition of non-Q-wave MI—occurred in 6-8% of patients; there is growing concern that patient experiencing these "minor" elevations in CK-MB may have a poorer long-term prognosis.[25] As shown in Table 27.5, angiographic complications included dissection (10-13%), abrupt closure (1.8-11.2%), slow-flow (1.2-7.6%), perforation (0-1.5%), and severe spasm (1.6-6.6%); differences in complication rates between series are likely the result of different definitions, the growth in operator experience, and evolving technique. Due to the slightly larger sheath size ($\geq$8F), significant bleeding (need for transfusion, decrease in hemoglobin > 3 gm/dL, or hematoma > 4 cm) occurred in 1.0-7.7%,

while groin complications requiring surgery occurred in 2-3% of patients. In high-risk patients undergoing Rotablator, prophylactic insertion of an IABP may reduce the incidence of hypotension and non-Q-wave MI.[53] In the Dilatation vs. Ablation Restenosis Trial (DART), dissection and bailout stenting were more frequent after PTCA (14% vs. 6%, p < 0.05), but no-reflow was more frequent after Rotablator (8% vs. 0.5%, p < 0.01). Sidebranch occlusion is more common in the presence of ostial side branch disease and during treatment of stent restenosis.[92]

Table 27.3. Rotablator Atherectomy: Procedural Success and Restenosis

Series	N	Results (%)			
		Success[†]	PTCA	Final Stenosis	Restenosis
Kini[91] (1999)	1000	94-98	96	14-24	-
Bersin[93] (1999)	126	90	100	27	-
Levin[67] (1998)	240	94	100	19	18
Zimarino[70] (1997)	70	-	100	18	-
Reisman[61] (1997)	3153	96	-	-	-
Stertzer[56] (1995)	656	94.5	65	-	-
MacIsaac[35] (1995)	2161	95.2	74	22	-
Safian[26] (1994)	116	91	77	30	51
Ellis[34*] (1994)	400	94.7	-	27	-
Warth[32*] (1994)	874	93.4	42	-	38
Barrione[29] (1993)	166	91.7	100	24	-
Guerin[30] (1993)	67	94	100	-	-

Abbreviations: - = not reported
† Residual stenosis < 50% without death, Q-wave MI, or emergency bypass surgery
†† PTCA = adjunctive PTCA
* Subset of multicenter registry

Table 27.4. Rotablator Atherectomy: In-hospital Complications

Series	N	Complications (%)				
		Death	CABG	Q-MI	non-Q-MI	Other
Mehran[90] (2000)	161	0.7	0	0	8.0	Stent restenosis
Kini[91] (1999)	1000	≤1.7	≤ 1.7	≤ 2.3	≤ 1.7	
Bersin[93] (1999)	126	3.2	1.0	-	8.5	
Radke[72] (1999)	45	0	0	0	0	
Kobayashi[73] (1999)	162	1.8 0	1.8 2.8	8.9 1.9	11.0 1.9	Aggressive technique Routine technique
Braden[79] (1999)	139	2.0	1.6	0	7.5	
Kiesz[76] (1999)	111	0	0	0	4.5	
Levin[67] (1998)	240	1.1	2.2	2.8	-	Vascular (1.9%)
Sharma[74] (1998)	100	0	0	0	2.0	
Buttner[81] (1998)	32	0	0	0	-	
Safian[89] (1998)	222	0 0	0 0.7	1.6 2.2	2.5 0	Burr/artery > 0.7 Burr/artery < 0.7
Bass[82] (1998)	104	0 8.7	0 2.0	1.9 0	24.5 17.6	Aggressive technique Routine technique
Reisman[61] (1997)	200 2953	3.0 1.0	2.5 2.5	0.5 1.2	6.0 6.1	After 1994 Before 1994
Moussa[75] (1997)	75	1.3	4.0	1.3	6.7	
Erbel[86] (1997)	502	0.4 1.2	2.0 1.2	2.0 1.6	-	Rotablator PTCA
Goldberg[85] (1997)	153	2.2	-	-	-	
Reisman[87] (1997)	442	-	-	-	-	MACE (1.3%)

Table 27.4. Rotablator Atherectomy: In-hospital Complications

Series	N	Complications (%)				
		Death	CABG	Q-MI	non-Q-MI	Other
Stertzer[56] (1995)	656	0.5	1.4	3.4	-	
MacIsaac[35] (1995)	2161	0.8	2.0	0.7	8.8	
Ellis[34]* (1994)	316	0.3	0.9	2.2	5.7	
Vandormeal[27] (1994)	215	-	-	-	-	MACE (2.3%)
Warth[32]* (1994)	743	0.8	1.7	0.9	3.8	Vascular (2.2%); arrhythmia (1.9%)
Safian[26] (1993)	104	1	1.9	4.8	2.9	Bleeding (7.7%); vascular (2.9%); arrhythmia (1.8%)
Barrione[29] (1993)	166	1.8	0	0.6	8.4	
Guerin[30] (1993)	61	0	1.6	1.6	6.6	Arrhythmia (6.6%)
Gilmore[31] (1993)	108	0.9	2.8	0.9	2.8	
Stertzer[33]* (1993)	302	0	1.0	2.6	-	

Abbreviations: CABG = emergency coronary bypass grafting; Q-MI = Q-wave myocardial infarction; non-Q-MI = non-Q-wave myocardial infarction; MACE = major adverse cardiac events; - = not reported
† Need for transfusion, drop in hemoglobin ≥ 3 gm/dL, or hematoma > 4 cm
* Subset of multicenter registry

3. **Restenosis.** Restenosis rates are comparable to balloon angioplasty and have ranged from 39% in the multicenter registry to 62% in the randomized ERBAC trial (Table 27.6).[27] A study of restenosis by lesion length and calcium showed that restenosis was twice as likely in long lesions and noncalcified lesions.[36] Restenosis rates were lowest (6.3%) for short calcified lesions and highest (37.2%) for noncalcified lesions > 20 mm in length.[36] In DART, a randomized trial of PTCA vs. Rotablator + PTCA for type A and B$_1$ lesions in vessels ≤ 3.0 mm, there was no difference in late revascularization (22% for PTCA vs. 18% after Rotablator) or angiographic restenosis (48% for PTCA vs. 52% for Rotablator). Two other trials showed no restenosis advantage for aggressive debulking compared to more conservative debulking strategies.[62,68]

Table 27.5. Rotablator Atherectomy: Angiographic Complications

Series	N	Complications (%)					
		Acute Closure	Slow Flow	Perforation	Dissection	Sidebranch Occlusion	Severe Spasm
Kini[91] (1999)	1000	≤ 4.0	≤ 9.0	≤ 1.0	≤ 5.0	≤ 5.0	< 7.0
Bersin[93] (1999)	126	4.0	-	1.0	6.1	2.8	-
Kobayashi[73] (1999)	162	1.8	-	2.7	-	-	-
Levin[67] (1998)	240	5.1	-	1.7	-	-	-
Sharma[74] (1998)	100	-	3	-	7	-	-
Bass[82] (1998)	104	-	11.3[#] 3.9[##]	-	2.0 0	-	-
Reisman[61] (1997)	200[+] 2953[++]	3.4 4.1	- -	0.4 0.6	- -	- -	-
Moussa[75] (1997)	75	2.8	-	-	-	-	-
Reisman[87] (1997)	442	-	8.0* 0.5**	1.8 0.4	8.0 16.0	-	-
Stertzer[56] (1995)	656	2.7	1.8	0.6	10.4	1.7	5.3
MacIsaac[35] (1995)	2161	3.6	-	0.7	13	-	-
Ellis[34] (1994)	400	5.5	7.6	1.5	-	-	-
Warth[32*] (1994)	874	3.1	1.2	0.5	10.5	0.1	1.6
Safian[26] (1993)	116	11.2	6.1	0	-	1.8	-
Barrione[29] (1993)	166	1.8	-	-	-	-	-

Abbreviations: - = not reported
*   Rotablator alone
**   PTCA alone
#   Aggressive technique
Routine technique
+   After 1994
++   Before 1994

Table 27.6. ERBAC Trial[27]

	PTCA (n = 210)	ELCA (n = 195)	Rotablator (n = 215)	p-Value
B₂/C lesions (%)	72	78	85	-
Final DS (%)	36	32	31	< 0.05
In-hospital MACE (%)	4.8	6.2	2.3	< 0.05
6-month Outcome (%)				
Death	3.1	0	2.6	NS
QMI	3.8	0.7	3.2	NS
TLR	35	46	46	< 0.05
ARS	54	60	62	NS

Abbreviations: B₂/C = ACC/AHA classification type B₂ or C; DS = diameter stenosis; ERBAC = Excimer Rotablator Balloon Angioplasty Comparison; MACE = major adverse cardiac events; QMI = Q-wave myocardial infarction; TLR = target lesion revascularization; ARS = angiographic restenosis

4. **Impact of Plaque Composition on Results (Table 27.7)**
   a. **Calcification.** Procedural success and major complications are similar among calcified and noncalcified lesions treated with the Rotablator.[35,37] Reports differ with respect to restenosis: The multicenter registry reported no difference,[35] while another report found less restenosis among calcified lesions. In large, calcified vessels treated by stenting, initial debulking with Rotablator was superior to pretreatment with PTCA alone with respect to final diameter stenosis (4.2% vs. 13.1%, p < 0.0001) and late revascularization (12.2% vs. 24.5%, p < 0.05).[64]

   b. **Soft Plaque.** Intravascular ultrasound has shown that Rotablator is capable of ablating soft plaque.[38]

5. **Impact of Lesion Morphology on Results (Table 27.7)**
   a. **Complex Lesions.** The ERBAC trial compared Rotablator atherectomy, PTCA, and excimer laser angioplasty in type B and C lesions.[27] Despite its use in more B₂ and C lesions compared to PTCA (85% vs. 72%), Rotablator had higher success (91% vs. 80%), lower residual stenosis (27% vs. 35%), and fewer ischemic complications (1.5% vs. 7.0%). Restenosis rates at 6 months were high in all groups (PTCA 51.4% vs. Rotablator 62%; p = NS).

   b. **Long Lesions.** In the multicenter registry, there was no difference in procedural success or restenosis for lesions 1-10 mm, 11-15 mm, and 15-25 mm in length.[39] In a retrospective study[40] of lesions 10-20 mm in length, procedural success and major complications were higher after Rotablator than after PTCA (success: 95% vs. 91%; complications: 1.4% vs. 0.5%);

success was also higher after the Rotablator in lesions > 20 mm (84% vs. 76% for PTCA), but there was a high (10%) incidence of major complications in both groups.

c. **Ostial Lesions.** Treatment of ostial lesions by the Rotablator has been analyzed in several reports.[41-44] The largest of these studies reported success in 97%, dissection in 17%, spasm in 2.8%, CABG in 1.9%, and angiographic restenosis in 32%.[42]

d. **Chronic Total Occlusions.** Among 145 chronic total occlusions in the multicenter registry, Rotablator success was achieved in 91%.[45] In-hospital death and non-Q-wave MI occurred in 1.4% and 4.3%, respectively. Restenosis was observed in 62.5%, although angiographic follow-up was recorded in only 49% of patients. Multivariate predictors of success and restenosis were vessel diameter and diabetes, respectively.

e. **Undilatable Lesions.** The Rotablator is particularly useful for management of fibrocalcific lesions resistant to PTCA,[46-49] with procedural success in 90% of such lesions.[47]

f. **Restenotic Lesions.** Comparison of de novo and restenotic lesions from the multicenter Registry revealed a higher initial success rate in restenotic lesions with no difference in restenosis (38%) at follow-up.[50]

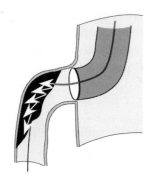 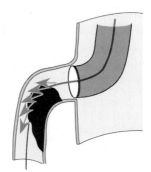

Lesion on Outer Curve:
Device directed into lesion

Lesion on Inner Curve:
Device deflected into disease-free wall

Figure 27.4. Angulated Lesions: Impact of Lesion Location

Angulated lesions with plaque situated along the outer curve may sometimes be considered for ELCA, TEC, or Rotablator. In contrast, when plaque is situated along the inner curve, these devices may deflect away from the plaque and into the disease-free wall, increasing the risk of dissection or perforation.

Table 27.7. Rotablator Procedural Success by Lesion Morphology

Series	N	Adjunctive Treatment	Procedural Success (%)	Other
CHRONIC TOTAL OCCLUSION				
Kini[63] (2000)	200	PTCA, Stent	99.5	
Braden[79] (1999)	139	PTCA, Stent	-	RS (20%)
Levin[68] (1996)	15	PTCA	100	
Omoigui[45] (1995)	145	PTCA	91	-
COMPLEX LESION MORPHOLOGY				
Kiesz[76] (1999)	146	PTCA	98.1	RS (28%)
Bass[82] (1998)	104	PTCA	82	
Levin[67] (1998)	240	PTCA	94	
Moussa[75] (1997)	106	Stent	93	RS (23%)
Erbel[86] (1997)	502	None PTCA	74* 77**	RS (36% vs. 29%)
Vandormael[27] (1994)	215	PTCA	91	
OSTIAL LESIONS				
Motwani[96] (2000)	119	PTCA, Stent	98	RS (18%)
Koller[41] (1994)	29	PTCA	93	RS (39%)
Zimarino[43] (1994)	69	PTCA	92	
Cowley[97] (1995)	109	PTCA	93	RS (52%)
Ellis[98] (1994)	68	-	91	
Commeau[99] (1994)	142	PTCA	95	
Popma[42] (1993)	105	PTCA	97	

Table 27.7. Rotablator Procedural Success by Lesion Morphology

Series	N	Adjunctive Treatment	Procedural Success (%)	Other
CALCIFIED LESIONS				
Singh[100] (2001)	447 2065	PTCA ± Stent PTCA ± Stent (no ROTA)	- -	FDS < 50% (98% vs. 93%, p < 0.0001); no difference in in-hospital MACE
Kiesz[101] (1999)	101	-	98	Non-Q-MI (4.5%); RS (28%); TLR (19%)
Hoffman[95] (1998)	147 103 56	PTCA Stent (no ROTA) Stent	98 98 98	TLR (28% vs. 21% vs. 15%)
Moussa[102] (1997)	106	Stent	94	TLR (18%)
Dussaillant[103] (1996)	83 120 235	Stent DCA PTCA	- - -	FDS (12% vs. 16% vs. 24%)
MacIsaac[35] (1995)	1078 1083 (noncalcified)	PTCA PTCA	94 95	-
Mintz[104] (1995)	88	Stent	-	No subacute thrombosis
Warth[105] (1995)	107 346 (noncalcified)	PTCA PTCA	97 95	MACE (1.9% vs. 2.6%)
Altmann[37] (1993)	No/mild calcium Moderate calcium Heavy calcium	PTCA PTCA PTCA	96 96 92	Total no. lesions = 670
LONG LESIONS				
Ellis[106] (1994)	286 (0-4 mm) 27 (9-12 mm) 6 (13-16 mm)	-	-	In-hospital MACE (4.2% vs. 18.5% vs. 50%)
Warth[107] (1994)	588 (≤ 10 mm) 195 (11-25 mm)	-	-	In-hospital MACE (0.2% vs 2.1%)
Reisman[39] (1993)	953 (< 10 mm) 180 (11-15 mm) 143 (15-25 mm)	PTCA PTCA PTCA	95 97 92	-
Favereau[40] (1992)	215 73	PTCA PTCA	95 84	-

Table 27.7. Rotablator Procedural Success by Lesion Morphology

Series	N	Adjunctive Treatment	Procedural Success (%)	Other
UNDILATABLE LESIONS				
Reisman[46] (1993)	34	PTCA	97	-
Brogan[47] (1993)	41	PTCA	90	-
Sievert[49] (1993)	32	PTCA	97	-
Rosenblum[48] (1992)	40	PTCA	97	-
OTHER LESION MORPHOLOGIES				
Schiele[88] (1998)	9	PTCA (IVUS)	100	Small vessels
Bass[50] (1992)	428	PTCA	97	Restenotic lesions
Chevalier[51] (1994)	123	PTCA	86	Angulated lesions

Abbreviations: FDS = final diameter stenosis; IVUS = intravascular ultrasound; MACE = major adverse cardiac events; RS = restenosis; TLR = target lesion revascularization
*   Rotablator alone
** PTCA alone

g.   **Angulated Lesions.** Compared to Rotablator atherectomy of nonangulated lesions, lesion angulation > 45 degrees resulted in lower procedural success (86% vs. 94%), more death (2.7% vs. 0.3%), and a higher incidence in total ischemic events (5.4% vs 1.3%).[51] When performing Rotablator in angulated lesions, it is important to begin with small burrs, use a maximum burr-to-artery ratio of 0.6-0.7, and use adjunctive PTCA or stenting rather than larger burrs. Lesions on the outer curve are better suited for the Rotablator than inner curve lesions (Chapter 11) (Figure 27.4).

h.   **Stent Restenosis.** In contemporary practice, rotational atherectomy is often used for treatment of stent restenosis (Table 27.8); plaque displacement by IVUS was shown to be better after Rotablator than after ELCA.[72] The ROSTER (Rotablator for Stent Restenosis) trial, a single center randomized trial of 100 lesions, demonstrated less clinical restenosis after rotational atherectomy plus PTCA than PTCA alone (20% vs. 38%, p < 0.04) for vessels 2.7-3.5 mm in diameter.[64] Another report indicated less repeat revascularization after Rotablator plus PTCA compared to PTCA alone, but the difference was not statistically significant (28% vs. 46%, p = 0.18).[83] ELCA and Rotablator seemed to be equally effective in debulking stent restenosis, although non-Q-MI and in-hospital MACE were more common after ELCA. Despite these favorable observations, a prospective multicenter randomized trial of Rotablator plus PTCA vs. PTCA alone for diffuse stent restenosis (ARTIST) demonstrated worse clinical and angiographic results (final diameter stenosis, angiographic restenosis, TLR) after Rotablator, despite better initial results (Table 27.9).[80]

  i.   **Bifurcation Lesions.** The incidence of sidebranch occlusion after Rotablator was 7.5% in one study; persistent sidebranch occlusion >24 hours was unusual.[58] Rotational atherectomy with stenting may reduce the frequency of sidebranch occlusion compared to PTCA followed by stenting (6% vs 20%, p < 0.02).[74]

Table 27.8. Studies of Rotational Atherectomy for Stent Restenosis

Series	Device	N	Adjunctive Treatment	Procedural Success (%)	Other Results
ROSTER[112] (2001)	ROTA PTCA	100 100	PTCA, Stent Stent (31%)	- -	Single center randomized trial. 30-day MACE (2% vs. 3%); TLR (32% vs. 45%, p = 0.04)
Mehran[109] (2000)	ROTA ELCA	158 161	PTCA, Stent	100 100	Similar 1-yr TLR (28% vs. 26%) and late MACE
vom Dahl[78,94] (2000)	ROTA	298	PTCA, Stent	88	ARS (65%)
Lauer[110] (1999)	ROTA ELCA PTCA	83 78 124	PTCA, Stent		Immediate lumen enlargement better for ROTA and ELCA; at 6 months ROTA results best
Mehran[111] (1999)	ROTA PTCA ELCA STENT	126 314 250 131	PTCA, Stent	-	Immediate lumen enlargement best for stenting, but no difference in 1-yr TLR
Radke[72] (1999)	ROTA	45	PTCA	100	ARS (45%)
Lee[108] (1998)	ROTA PTCA	36 45	PTCA, Stent		ROTA had less CRS (2.5% vs. 47%, p < 0.05) and better angina-free survival at 6 months (72% vs. 49%, p = 0.02)
Sharma[74] (1998)	ROTA	100	PTCA	100	CRS (28%)
Buttner[81] (1998)	ROTA	32	PTCA	100	ARS (56%)
Silber[77] (1998)	ROTA	52	PTCA		ARS (56%)

Abbreviations: ARS = angiographic restenosis; CRS = clinical restenosis; MACE = major adverse cardiac events; ROSTER = Rotablator for Stent Restenosis; TLR = target lesion revascularization

Table 27.9. The ARTIST Trial: Rotablator vs. PTCA for In-Stent Restenosis[80]

	PTCA (n = 146)	Rotablator (n = 152)	p-Value
Baseline QCA			
Reference vessel (mm)	2.8	2.8	NS
MLD (mm)	0.7	0.7	NS
Diameter stenosis (%)	77	74	NS
Lesion length (mm)	17	17	NS
Final QCA			
MLD (mm)	2.1	2.3	< 0.05
Diameter stenosis (%)	25	17	< 0.05
Burr/artery ratio	-	0.8	-
Balloon/artery ratio	1.2	1.3	NS
6-month Outcome			
Diameter stenosis (%)	56	64	0.005
Late loss index	0.5	0.7	-
Angiographic restenosis (%)	51.2	64.8	0.04
TLR (%)	36.2	47.8	0.06
Total occlusion (%)	1.4	6.6	0.04

Abbreviations: QCA = quantitative coronary angiography; MLD = minimal lumen diameter; TLR = target lesion revascularization; ARTIST = Angioplasty vs. Rotational Atherectomy for Treatment of Diffuse In-stent Restenosis

j. **Other Lesions.** Rotational atherectomy is not recommended in the body of saphenous vein grafts due to the risk of distal embolization. In contrast, rotational atherectomy may be used for rigid lesions at the aorto-ostial junction or at the distal anastomosis, and for stent restenosis within the body of a vein graft.

G. **SUMMARY.** Rotational atherectomy has expanded the applications for percutaneous techniques, particularly for revascularization of rigid, calcified lesions that cannot be treated by other methods.

* * * * *

REFERENCES

1. Fourrier JL, Stankowiak C, Lablanche JM, et al. Histopathology after rotational angioplasty of peripheral arteries in human beings. J Am Coll Cardiol 1988;11:109A.

2. Kovach J, Mintz G, Pichard A, Kent K, et al. Sequential intravascular ultrasound characterization of the mechanisms of rotational atherectomy and adjunct balloon angioplasty. J Am Coll Cardiol 1993;22:1024-32.

3. Mintz G, Potkin B, Keren G, Satler L, et al. Intravascular ultrasound evaluation of the effect of rotational atherectomy in obstructive atherosclerotic coronary artery disease. Circulation 1992; 86:1383-1393.

4. Cowley M, Buchbinder M, Warth D, Dorros G, et al. Effect of coronary rotational atherectomy abrasion on vessel segments adjacent to treated lesions . J Am Coll Cardiol 1992;19:333A.

5. Prevosti LG, Cook JA, Unger EF, Sheffield CD, et al. Particulate debris from rotational atherectomy: size distribution and physiologic effect. Circulation 1988;78:II-83.

6. Friedman HZ, Elliott MA, Gottlieb GJ, O'Neill WW. Mechanical rotational atherectomy: The effects of microparticle embolization on myocardial blood flow and function. J Interv Cardiol 1989;2:77-83.

7. Hansen DD, Auth DC, Hall M, Ritchie JL. Rotational endarterectomy in normal canine coronary arteries: preliminary report. J Am Coll Cardiol 1988; 11:1073-77.

8. Sherman C, Brunken R, Chan A, et al. Myocardial perfusion and segmental wall motion after coronary rotational atherectomy. Circulation 1992;86:I-652.

9. Pavlides G, Hauser A, Grines C, et al. Clinical, hemodynamic, electrocardiographic, and mechanical events during nonocclusive coronary atherectomy and comparison to balloon angioplasty. Am J Cardiol 1992;70:841-845.

10. Williams MJA, Dow CJ, Newell JB, et al. Prevalence and timing of regional myocardial dysfunction after rotational coronary atherectomy: J Am Coll Cardiol 1996;28:861-9.

11. Huggins GS, Williams MJA, Yang J, et al. Transient wall motion abnormalities following rotational atherectomy are reflective of myocardial stunning more than myocardial infarction. J Am Coll Cardiol 1995;25:96A.

12. Nunez BD, Keelan ET, Lerman A, et al. Coronary hemodynamics after rotational atherectomy. J Am Coll Cardiol 1995;25:95A.

13. Safian R, Freed M, Lichtenberg A, et al. Are residual stenoses after excimer laser angioplasty and coronary atherectomy due to inefficient or small devices? Comparison with balloon angioplasty. J Am Coll Cardiol 1993;22:628-1634.

14. Reisman M, Buchbinder M, Bass T, et al. Improvement in coronary dimensions at early 24-hour follow-up after coronary rotational ablation: Implications for restenosis. Circulation 1992;86:I-332.

15. Kovach JA, Mintz GS, et al. Sequential intravascular ultrasound characterization of the mechanisms of rotational atherectomy and adjunct balloon angioplasty. J Am Coll Cardiol 1993;22:1024-32.

16. Mintz GS, Douek P, et al. Target lesion calcification in coronary artery disease: An intravascular ultrasound study. J Am Coll Cardiol 1992;20:1149-55.

17. Nino C, Free M, Blankenship L, et al. Procedural cost and benefits of new interventional devices. Am J Cardiol 1994;74:1165-1166.

18. Vandormael M, Reifart N, Preusler W, et al. In-hospital costs comparison of excimer laser angioplasty, rotational atherectomy (Rotablator) and balloon angioplasty for complex coronary lesions: A randomized trial (ERBAC). J Am Coll Cardiol 1994;89:223A.

19. Cohen BM, Weber VJ, Blum RR, et al. Cocktail alternation of rotational ablation flow effects (CARAFE) study pilot. Cathet Cardiovasc Diag 996;Suppl 3:69-72.

20. Reisman M, Harms V. Guidewire bias: A potential source of complications with rotational atherectomy. Cathet Cardiovasc Diagn 1996;3:64-68.

21. Mintz GS, Pichard AD, et al. Transcatheter device synergy: preliminary experience with adjunct directional coronary atherectomy following high-speed rotational atherectomy or excimer laser angioplasty in the treatment of coronary artery disease. Cathet Cardiovasc Diagn 1993;28:37-44.

22. Mintz GS, Dussaillsnt GR, Wong SC, et al. Rotational atherectomy followed by adjunct stents: The preferred therapy for calcified large vessels? Circulation 1995;92:I-329.

23. Mintz GS, Pichard AD, et al. Impact of preintervention intravascular ultrasound imaging on transcatheter treatment strategies in coronary artery disease. Am J Cardiol 1994;73:423-430.

24. MacIsaac A, Whitlow P, Cowley M, Buchbinder M. Angiographic predictors of outcome of coronary rotational atherectomy from the completed multicenter registry. J Am Coll Cardiol 1994;23:353A.

25. Redwood SR, Popma JJ, Kent KM, Pichard AD, et al. "Minor" CPK-MB elevations are associated with increased mortality following new-device angioplasty in native coronary arteries. Circulation 1995;92:I-544.

26. Safian RD, Niazi KA, et al. Detailed angiographic analysis of high-speed mechanical rotational atherectomy in human coronary arteries. Circulation 1993;88:961-8.

27. Reifart N, Vandormael M, et al. Randomized comparison of angioplasty of complex coronary lesions at a single center: Excimer laser, rotational atherectomy, and balloon angioplasty comparison (ERBAC) Study. Circulation 1997;96:91-98.

28. Dietz UR, Erbel R, et al. Angiographic and histologic findings in high frequency rotational ablation in coronary arteries in vitro. Zeitschrift fur Kardiologie 1991;80:222-9.

29. Barrione M, Hall P, et al. Treatment of simple and complex coronary stenosis using rotational ablation followed by low pressure balloon angioplasty. Cathet Cardiovasc Diagn 1993;30:131-7.

30. Guerin Y, Rahal S, et al. Coronary angioplasty combining rotational atherectomy and balloon dilatation. Results in 67 complex stenoses. Arch Mal du Coeur 1993;86:1535-41.

31. Gilmore PS, Bass TA, et al. Single site experience with high-speed coronary rotational atherectomy. Clin Cardiol 1993;16:311-6.

32. Warth DC, Leon MB, et al. Rotational atherectomy multicenter registry: Acute results, complications and 6-month angiographic follow-up in 709 patients. J Am Coll Cardiol 1994;24:641-8.

33. Stertzer SH, Rosenblum J, et al. Coronary rotational ablation: initial experience in 302 procedures. J Am Coll Cardiol 1993;21:287-95.

34. Ellis SG, Popma JJ, et al. Relation of clinical presentation, stenosis morphology, and operator technique to the procedural results of rotational atherectomy and rotational atherectomy facilitated angioplasty. Circulation 1994;89:882-92.

35. MacIsaac AI, Bass TA, Buchbinder M, et al. High speed rotational atherectomy: Outcome in calcified and noncalcified coronary artery lesions. J Am Coll Cardiol 1995;26:531-6.

36. Leguizamon JH, Chambre DF, Torresani EM, et al. High speed coronary rotational atherectomy: Are angiographic factors predictive of failure, major complications or restenosis? J Am Coll Cardiol 1995;25:95A.

37. Altmann D, Popma J, Kent K, et al. Rotational atherectomy effectively treats calcified lesions. J Am Coll Cardiol 1993;21:443A.

38. Dussaillant GR, Mintz GS, Pichard AD, et al. Effect of rotational atherectomy in noncalcified atherosclerotic plaque: A volumetric intravascular ultrasound study. J Am Coll Cardiol 1996;28(4):856-860.

39. Reisman M, Cohen B, Warth D, Fenner J, et al. Outcome of long lesions treated with high speed rotational ablation. J Am Coll Cardiol 1993;21:443A.

40. Favereaux X, Chevalier B, Commeau P, et al. Is rotational atherectomy more effective than balloon angioplasty for the treatment of long coronary lesions? SCA & I Meeting Abstracts, 92.

41. Koller PT, Freed M, Grines CL, O'Neill WW. Success, complications, and restenosis following rotational and transluminal extraction atherectomy of ostial stenoses. Cathet and Cardiovas Diagn 1994;31:255-260.

42. Popma J, Brogan W, Pichard A, et al. Rotational coronary atherectomy of ostial stenoses. Am J Cardiol 1993;71:436-438.

43. Zimarino M, Corcos T, Favereau X, et al. Rotational coronary atherectomy with adjunctive balloon angioplasty for the treatment of ostial lesions. Cathet Cardiovas Diagn 1994;33:22-27.

44. Sabri MN, Cowley MJ, DiSciascio G, DeBottis D, et al. Immediate results of interventional devices for coronary ostial narrowing with angina pectoris. Am J Cardiol 1994;73:122-125.

45. Omoigui N, Booth J, Reisman M, et al. Rotational atherectomy in chronic total occlusions. J Am Coll Cardiol 1995;25:97A.

46. Reisman M, Devlin P, Melikian J, et al. Undilatable noncompliant lesions treated with the Rotablator: outcome and angiographic follow-up. Circulation 1993;88: I-547.

47. Brogan W, Popma J, Pichard A, Satler L, et al. Rotational coronary atherectomy after unsuccessful coronary balloon angioplasty. Am J Cardiol 1993;71:794-798.

48. Rosenblum J, Stertzer S, Shaw R, et al. Rotational ablation of balloon angioplasty failures. J Invas Cardiol 1992;4:312-317.

49. Sievert H, Tonndorf S, Utech A, Schulze R. High frequency rotational angioplasty (rotablation) after unsuccessful balloon dilatation Z Cardiol 1993;82:411- 414.

50. Bass T, Gilmore P, Buchbinder M, et al. Coronary rotational atherectomy (PTCA) in patients with prior coronary revascularization: a registry report. Circulation 1992;86:I-653.

51. Chevalier B, Commeau P, Favereau X, et al. Limitations of rotational atherectomy in angulated coronary lesions. J Am Coll Cardiol 1994;23:285A.

52. Dussaillant GR, Mintz GS, Pichard AD, et al. The optimal strategy for treating calcified lesions in large vessels: Comparison of intravascular ultrasound results of rotational atherectomy + adjunctive PTCA, DCA, or stents. J Am Coll Cardiol 1996;27:153A.

53. O'Murchu B, Foreman RD, Shaw RE, et al. Role of intraaortic balloon pump counterpulsation in high risk coronary rotational atherectomy. J Am Coll Cardiol 1995;26:1270-5.

54. Reisman M, DeVore LJ, Ferguson M, et al. Analysis of heat generation during high-speed rotational ablation: Technical implications. J Am Coll Cardiol 1996;27:292A.

55. Coletti RH, Haik BJ, Wiedermann JG, et al. Marked reduction in slow-reflow after rotational atherectomy through the use of a novel flushing solution. TCT Meeting 1996;Washington DC

56. Stertzer SH, Pomerantsev EV, Fitzgerald PJ, et al. Effects of technique modification on immediate results of high speed rotational atherectomy in 710 procedures on 656 patients. Cathet Cardiovasc Diagn 1995;304-310.

57. Dusaillant GR, Mintz GS, Pichard AD, et al. Mechanisms and immediate and long-term results of adjunct directional coronary atherectomy after rotational atherectomy. J Am Coll Cardiol 1996;27:1390-1397.

58. Walton AS, Pomerantsev EV, Oesterle SN, et al. Outcome of narrowing related sidebranches after high-speed rotational atherectomy. Am J Cardiol 1996;77:370-3.

59. Stertzer SH, Pomerantsev EV, Fitzgerald PS, et al. Effects of technique modification on immediate results of high-speed rotational atherectomy in 710 procedures in 656 patients. Cathet Cardiovasc Diagn 1995;36:304-10.

60. Bass TA, Whitlow PL, et al. Acute complications related to coronary rotational atherectomy strategy: A report from the STRATAS trial. J Am Coll Cardiol 1996;29(Suppl. A):68A.

61. Reisman M, Harms V, et al. Comparison of early and recent results with rotational atherectomy. J Am Coll Cardiol 1997;29:353-7.

62. Safian RD, Feldman T, Muller DWM, et al. Coronary Angioplasty and Rotablator Atherectomy Trial (CARAT): Immediate and late results of a prospective multicenter randomized trial. Cathet Cardiovasc Interv 2001 (in press).

63. Kini A, Reich D, Bertea T, et al. Rotational atherectomy for chronic total coronary occlusions: acute results and predictors of target vessel revascularization. J Am Coll Cardiol 2000; 35 (Suppl A):87A.

64. Hoffmann R, Mintz GS, Kent KM, et al. Comparative early and nine-month results of rotational atherectomy, stents, and the combination of both for calcified lesions in large coronary arteries. Am J Cardiol 1998;81:552-557.

65. Bowers TE, Stewart RE, O'Neill WW, Reddy VM, Safian RD. Effect of Rotablator atherectomy and adjunctive balloon angioplasty on coronary blood flow. Circulation 1997;95:1157-1164.

66. Buchbinder M, Fortuna R, Sharma SK, et al. Debulking prior

to stenting improves acute outcomes: early results from the SPORT trial. J Am Coll Cardiol 2000;35(Suppl A):8A.

67. Levin TN, Holloway S, Feldman T. Acute and late clinical outcome after rotational atherectomy for complex coronary disease. Cathet Cardiovasc Diagn 1998;45:122-130.

68. Levin TN, Carroll J, Feldman T. High-speed rotational atherectomy for chronic total coronary occlusions. Cathet Cardiovasc Diagn 1996;3:34-39.

69. Reisman M, Buchbinder M, Harms V, et al. Quantitative angiography of coronary artery dimensions 24 hours after rotational atherectomy. Am J Cardiol 1998;81:1427-1432.

70. Zimarino M, Corcos T, Favereau X, et al. Rotational coronary atherectomy with adjunctive balloon angioplasty: Evaluation of lumen enlargement by quantitative angiographic anlaysis. Am Heart J 1997;133:203-209.

71. Kobayashi Y, DeGregorio J, Kobayashi N, Akiyama T, et al. Lower restenosis rate with stenting following aggressive versus less aggressive rotational atherectomy. Cathet Cardiovasc Intervent 1999;46:406-414.

72. Radke PW, Klues HG, Haager PK, et al. Mechanisms of acute lumen gain and recurrent restenosis after rotational atherectomy to diffuse in-stent restneosis. J Am Coll Cardiol 1999;34:33-39.

73. Kobayashi Y, DeGrgorio J, Kobayashi N, et al. Lower restenosis rate with stenting following aggressive versus less aggressive rotational atherectomy. Cathet Cardiovasc Intervent 1999;46;406-414.

74. Sharma SK, Duvvuri S, Dangas G, et al. Rotational atherectomy for in-stent restenosis: Acute and long-term results of the first 100 cases. J Am Coll Cardiol 1998;32:1358-1365.

75. Moussa I, Moses JM, Reimers B, et al. Coronary stenting after rotational atherectomy in calcified and complex lesions. Circulation 1997;96:128-136.

76. Kiesz RS, Rozek MM, Ebersole DG, et al. Novel approach to rotational atherectomy results in low restenosis rates in long, calcified lesions: Long-term results of the San Antonio Rotablator Study (SARS). Cathet Cardiovasc Intervent 1999;48:48-53.

77. Silber S, Seidel N, Muehlinh H, et al. Rotablation is not the cure for diffuse in-stent restenosis. Circulation 1998;98:511.

78. vom Dahl J, Klues HG, Radke P, et al. Long-term outcome and predictors of recurrent restenosis after percutaneous transluminal rotational atherectomy for treatment of diffuse in-stent restenosis. J Am Coll Cardiol 1999;33(Suppl A):27A.

79. Braden GA, Young TM, Love WM, et al. Rotational atherectomy of chronic total coronary occlusion is associated with very low clinical rates; the treatment of choice. J Am Coll Cardiol 1999;33(Suppl A):48A.

80. Vom Dahl J, Silber S, Niccoli SE, et al. Angioplasty versus rotational atherectomy for treatment of diffuse in-stent restenosis: clinical and angiographic results from a randomized multicenter trial (ARTIST Study). J Am Coll Cardiol 2000;35(Suppl A):7A.

81. Buttner HJ, Muller C, Hodgson J, et al. Rotational atherectomy with adjunctive low-pressure balloon dilatation in diffuse in-stent restenosis: Immediate and follow-up results. J Am Coll Cardiol 1998;31:141A.

82. Bass TA, Williams DO, Ho KKL, et al. Is an aggressive

Rotablator strategy preferable to a standard Rotablator strategy in patients with heavily calcified coronary lesions? A report from the STRATAS Trial. J Am Coll Cardiol 1998;31:378A.

83. Dauerman HL, Baim DS, Sparano AM, et al. Balloon angioplasty versus debulking for treatment of diffuse in-stent restenosis. J Am Coll Cardiol 1998;31:455A.

84. Wang X, Mossa I, Colombo A. Coronary stenting after rotational atherectomy versus coronary stenting alone: An angiographic comparison. J Am Coll Cardiol 1998;31:456A.

85. Goldberg SL, Shawl F, Buchbinder M, et al. Rotational atherectomy for in-stent restenosis: The BARASTER Registry. Circulation 1997;96:80A.

86. Erbel R, Dill T, Weber PW, et al. A randomized study of high-speed rotational atherectomy and percutaneous transluminal coronary angioplasty in patients with complex coronary stenoses (COBRA Study). Circulation 1997;96:80A.

87. Reisman M, Buchbinder M, Sharma SK, et al. A multicenter randomized trial of rotational atherectomy vs PTCA: DART. Circulation 1997;96:I467A.

88. Schiele F, Meneveau N, Vuillemenot A, et al. Treatment of in-stent restenosis with high speed rotational atherectomy and IVUS guidance in small < 3.0 mm vessels. Cathet Cardiovasc Diagn 1998;44:77-82.

89. Safian RD, Feldman, Muller DWM, et al. Coronary angioplasty and Rotablator for atherectomy trial (CARAT): Immediate and late results of a prospective multicenter randomized trial. J Am Coll Cardiol 1998;31:378A.

90. Mehran R, Dangas G, Mintz GS, et al. Treatment of in-stent restenosis with excimer laser coronary angioplasty versus rotational atherectomy. Circulation 2000;101:2484-2489.

91. Kini A, Marmur JD, Duvvuri S, et al. Rotational atherectomy: improved procedural outcome with evolution of technique and equipment. Single center results of first 1000 patients. Cathet Cardiovasc Intervent 1999;46:305-311.

92. Cho G-Y, Lee CW, Hong M-K, et al. Side-branch occlusion after rotational atherectomy of in-stent restenosis: incidence, predictors and clinical significance. Cathet Cardiovasc Intervent 2000;50:406-416.

93. Bersin RM, Cedarholm JC, Kowalchuk GJ, et al. Long-term clinical follow-up of patients treated with the coronary rotablator: single center experience. Cathet Cardiovasc Intervent 1999;46:399-405.

94. vom Dahl J, Radke PW, Haager PK, et al. Clinical and angiographic predictors of recurrent restenosis after percutaneous transluminal rotational atherectomy for treatment of diffuse in-stent restenosis. Am J Cardiol 1999;83:862-867.

95. Hoffmann R, Mintz GS, Kent KM, Pichard AD, Satler LF, et al. Comparative early and nine-month results of rotational atherectomy, stents, and the combination of both for calcified lesions in large coronary arteries. Am J Cardiol 1998;81:552-557.

96. Motwani JG, Raymond RE, Franco I, et al. Effectiveness of rotational atherectomy of right coronary artery ostial stenosis. Am J Cardiol 2000;85:563-567.

97. Cowley CA, Patterson PE, Kipperman RM, Chuang YC, Pacera JH, Popma JJ. Multicenter rotational coronary atherectomy registry experience in coronary artery ostial stenoses. TCT Course (Washington DC), February, 1995.

98. Ellis S, Popma J, et al. Relation of clinical presentation, stenosis morphology, and operator technique to the procedural results of rotational atherectomy-facilitated angioplasty. Circulation 1994;89:882-892.

99. Commeau P, Zimarino M, Lancelin B, et al. Rotational coronary atherectomy for the treatment of aorto-ostial and branch-ostial lesions. Circulation 1994;90:I-213.

100. Singh M, Mathew V, Lennon R, et al. Comparison of rotational atherectomy vs. PTCA with or without stenting in calcified lesions. J Am Coll Cardiol 2001; 37 (2); 10A.

101. Kiesz SR, Rozek MM, Ebersole DG, et al. Novel approach to rotational atherectomey results in low restenosis rates in long, calcified lesions: Long-term results of the San Antonio Rotablator Study (SARS). Cathet Cardiovasc Intervent 1999;48:48-53.

102. Moussa I, Di Mario C, Moses J, Reimers B, et al. Coronary stenting after rotational atherectomy in calcified and complex lesions. Angiographic and clinical follow-up results. Circulation 1997;96:128-136.

103. Dussaillant GR, Mintz GS, Pichard AD, et al. The optimal strategy for treating calcified lesions in large vessels: Comparison of intravascular ultrasound results of rotational atherectomy + adjunctive PTCA, DCA, or stents. J Am Coll Cardiol 1996;27:153A.

104. Kiesz SR, Rozek MM, Ebersole DG, et al. Novel approach to rotational atherectomey results in low restenosis rates in long, calcified lesions: Long-term results of the San Antonio Rotablator Study (SARS). Cathet Cardiovasc Intervent 1999;48:48-53.

105. Warth D, Leon M, et al. Rotational atherectomy multicenter registry: Acute results, complications and 6-month angiographic follow-up in 709 patients. J Am Coll Cardiol 1994;24:641-648.

106. Ellis, S., J. Popma, et al. Relation of clinical presentation, stenosis morphology, and operator technique to the procedural results of rotational atherectomy-facilitated angioplasty. Circulation 1994;89:882-892. Warth D, Leon MB, O'Neill W, Zacca N, Polissar NL, Buchbinder M. Rotational atherectomy multicenter registry: Acute results, complications and 6-month angiographic follow-up in 709 patients. J Am Coll Cardiol 1994;24: 641-648.

107. Lee SG, Lee CW, Cheong SS, Hong MK, et al. Immediate and long-term outcomes of rotational atherectomy versus balloon angioplasty alone for treatment of diffuse in-stent restenosis. Am J Cardiol 1998;82:140-143.

108. Mehran R, Dangas G, Mintz GS, et al. Excimer laser vs. rotational atherectomy for the treatment of diffuse in-stent restenosis: acute and long-term results. J Am Coll Cardiol 1999;33(Suppl A):I-62A.

109. Lauer B, Schmidt E, Ambrosch H, et al. Optimal treatment of in-stent-retenosis: excimer laser-angioplasty, rotational atherectomy or conventional angioplasty? J Am Coll Cardiol 1999;33(Suppl A):I-62A.

110. Mehran R, Dangas G, Mintz GS, et al. In-stent restenosis: "The Great Equalizer" - disappointing clinical outcomes with ALL interventional strategies. J Am Coll Cardiol 1999;33(Suppl A):I-63A.

111. Sharma SK, Kini AS, Sterling FD, et al. Multivariate predictors of target lesion revascularization in the randomized trial of PTCA versus Rotablator for diffuse in-stent restenosis (ROSTER). J Am Coll Cardiol 2001;37(2):55A.

112. Braden GA, Kutcher MA, Ranking KM, et al. Debulking using rotational atherectomy of chronic total coronary occlusion leads to high initial success and very low restenosis rates. J Am Coll Cardiol 2001;37(2)46A.

113. Dunn, et al. Circulation 1998;98:I-709.

28 DIRECTIONAL CORONARY ATHERECTOMY

Robert D. Safian, M.D.

A. DESCRIPTION. Directional coronary atherectomy (DCA) (Guidant Corporation, Santa Clara, CA) is a percutaneous, over-the-wire cutting and retrieval system (Figure 28.1). The prototype of the directional atherectomy catheter is the Simpson Coronary AtheroCath™, which consists of a metal housing with an affixed balloon, a nosecone collection chamber, and a hollow torque tube that accommodates a 0.014" guidewire. A cup-shaped cutter inside the housing is attached to a flexible drive shaft, and is activated by a hand-held battery-operated motor drive unit (Figure 28.2). The AtheroCath is advanced into the lesion over a 0.014" wire with the cutting window oriented toward the atheroma. The balloon is inflated, pushing the plaque into the cutting window and holding the housing in place. The motor drive is activated, and then a lever on the motor drive unit allows the operator to slowly advance the cutter through the lesion as it rotates at 2000 RPM. Excised atheroma is stored in the distal nosecone collection chamber. The balloon is deflated, the AtheroCath rotated and reoriented, and the process repeated until the desired angiographic result is achieved.

B. DCA EQUIPMENT. The Simpson Coronary AtheroCath was approved by the FDA in 1990.

  1. Guiding Catheters (Figure 28.3, Table 28.1). The entire line of 11F guiding catheters has been replaced by 9.5F and 10F guiding catheters with enhanced torque response. Rather than the typical primary and secondary curves of conventional left Judkins catheters, DCA guiding catheters for

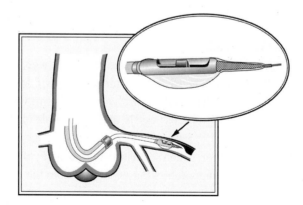

Figure 28.1. Directional Coronary Atherectomy (DCA)

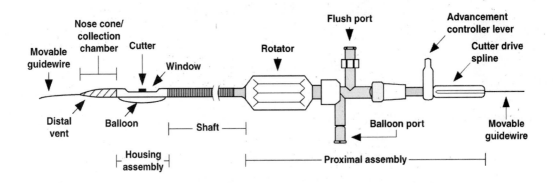

Figure 28.2. Directional Coronary Atherectomy: AtheroCath Components

the left coronary artery have gentle C-curves (called JCL guides), which permit easy cornering of the AtheroCath through the guiding catheter. Standard sizes for the left coronary artery include JCL3.5, JCL4.0, JCL4.5, and JCL5.0, depending on the diameter of the aortic root. For the right coronary artery, the JCR4.0 is available in standard-length and short-tip (S) designs. The JCR4S is the recommended for the RCA. Additional guides for the RCA include the JCR4IF (for inferior takeoff), the Hockey Stick (for horizontal, anterior, or superior takeoff), and the JCRGRF (for superior takeoff or Shepherd Crook origin). For bypass grafts, available guiding catheters include the JCRGRF (for anterior grafts with gentle upward takeoff), the JCLGRF (for anterior grafts with marked superior takeoff), and the Multipurpose guide (for grafts with vertical takeoff). The manufacturer has developed an 8F guiding catheter to be used with its next generation AtheroCath (ID = 0.091").

2. **AtheroCath Designs (Table 28.2)**
    - **SCA-EX.** Enhanced torque and an improved nosecone design were the key modifications of this second generation AtheroCath. The EX has a 9 mm cutting window and is available in 6F, 7F, and 7F Graft sizes. The EX is also available with a short (5 mm) window, which may be better suited for very focal lesions and tortuous vessels, and is available in all sizes except the 7F Graft.

    - **SCA-GTO.** This third generation AtheroCath is available in 5F, 6F, and 7F sizes. The GTO has a redesigned shaft with better support and torque control than the EX (Figure 28.4).

    - **Bantam.** The Bantam is available in 5F, 6F, and 7F sizes, and has a smaller shaft for use in 9F guiding catheters. The smaller shaft has a spiral inflation lumen and does not torque as well as the GTO device.

Table 28.1. Guiding Catheter Selection for DCA

Vessel	Configuration	Guiding Catheter
LCA	Normal	JCL4.0
	Narrow aortic root or superior origin	JCL3.5
	Wide aortic root or posterior origin	JCL4.5, JCL5.0
RCA	Normal	JCR4S, JCR4
	Anterior origin	Hockey stick
	Horizontal origin	Hockey stick
	Superior origin or Shepherd Crook	Hockey stick, JCRGRF
	Inferior origin	JCR4.IF, JCR4S
Vein Grafts to LCA	Normal	JCR4, JCR4S, Hockey stick
	Superior origin	Hockey stick, JCRGRF, JCLGRF
Vein Grafts to RCA	Normal	Multipurpose, JCR4IF
	Horizontal origin	JCR4, Hockey stick

Abbreviations: LCA = left coronary artery; RCA = right coronary artery; IF = inferior; JCL = JC left; JCR = JC right; S = short tip; JCRGRF = modified right graft; JCLGRF = modified left graft

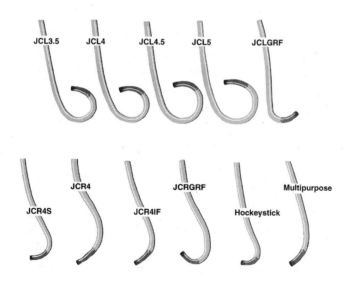

Figure 28.3. Directional Coronary Atherectomy Guiding Catheters

Table 28.2. AtheroCaths for Directional Coronary Atherectomy

Type	Balloon Material	Housing Length (mm) Rigid/Window	Sizes
SCA-EX	PET	17 / 9	5F, 6F, 7F, 7FG
SCA-EX short	PET	12 / 5	5F, 6F, 7F
AtheroCath GTO	PET	16 / 9	5F, 6F, 7F
Bantam	PET	17 / 9	5F, 6F, 7F
Flexi-Cut	PEBAX	12 / 9	6F housing (3 balloon sizes)

Abbreviations: SCA = Simpson Coronary AtheroCath; GTO = greater torque output; PET = polyethylene terephthalate (Dacron); F = French size; G = graft cutter

- **Flexi-Cut™.** This new atherectomy device has been designed to enhance performance, ease-of-use, and clinical utility. Compared to other designs, the Flexi-Cut has a smaller shaft for compatibility with 8F (minimum ID = 0.087") guiding catheters, a shorter rigid length for enhanced flexibility, and a Titanium Nitride-coated cutter for more effective cutting of soft and hard plaque.

3. **Ancillary Equipment.** Other ancillary equipment for DCA includes a large-bore rotating hemostatic valve (internal diameter > 0.094-inch), the motor drive unit (MDU), and 0.014-inch guidewires. Guiding catheters may be advanced into the central circulation using either a 7F tapered introducer and a 0.035" guidewire, or a 0.063" guidewire without the introducer. The MDU has a locking mechanism to prevent cutter movement while the device is advanced through the target vessel.

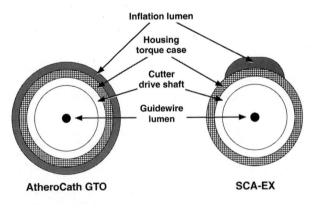

Figure 28.4. Directional Coronary Atherectomy: Construction

Comparison of the GTO and SCA-EX devices.

Table 28.3. Recommendations for DCA Based on Operator Experience and Lesion Morphology

Morphology	Level 1: Requires 0 to 5 cases	Level 2: Requires > 5 cases	Level 3: Requires > 20 cases	Level 4: Not recommended
Vessel	Proximal & mid LAD	Ostial LAD	Distal LAD, RCA, non-degenerated SVG, LCX, protected LM	Degenerated SVG, unprotected LM
Angulation of takeoff	Shallow	Shallow	Moderate	Severe
Tortuosity (proximal or distal to lesion)	None	Mild	Moderate	Severe
Lesion length	≤ 10mm	≤ 10mm	11-20 mm	-
Vessel diameter	≥ 3.0 mm	≥ 3.0 mm	≥ 2.5 mm	< 2.5 mm
Vessel dissection	Absent	Absent	Focal flap, not angulated	Severe flap, angulated, long or spiral dissection
Lesion morphology	Eccentric, concentric	Ulcerated	Thrombus	Heavily calcified
Lesion type	Restenosis	De novo	All	Friable, grumous
Calcification	None	Mild	Moderate	Heavy, especially in tortuous vessels

Abbreviations: LAD = left anterior descending coronary artery; RCA = right coronary artery; SVG = saphenous vein graft; LCX = left circumflex coronary artery; LM = left main coronary artery

C. **DCA TECHNIQUE.** Most interventional cardiologists do not have much experience with directional atherectomy. General guidelines for lesion selection are based on operator experience (Table 28.3).

1. **Preparation of the AtheroCath.** Unlike the SCA-EX, which required a single negative aspiration prep, preparation of the GTO requires a *triple* negative aspiration prep, each lasting 30-45 seconds. The balloon should then be inflated to 2-3 ATM for a few seconds, and then deflated completely. This technique ensures elimination of air and permits adequate visualization of the balloon during inflation. The Flexi-Cut™ device requires a double negative aspiration prep.

2. **Guiding Catheter Manipulation.** Because of the caliber and rigidity of the AtheroCath, proper guiding catheter position is crucial. The most important feature is coaxial alignment of the tip of the guide with the vessel ostium (Table 28.1); guiding catheter maneuvers such as over-rotation and deep-seating increase the risk of vessel injury and should be avoided.

3. **AtheroCath Deployment.** To properly position the AtheroCath, it is important to gently rotate and advance the device into the lesion; forward advancement without rotation will increase resistance and can result in proximal vessel dissection or failure to cross the lesion. In contrast to PTCA, the AtheroCath should never be "jack-hammered" across a lesion; if the device does not cross, ensure coaxial alignment of the guiding catheter, exchange for a heavier-duty guidewire, and use more device rotation (to "screw" it across the lesion); changing to a smaller or short-cutter device or predilating the lesion with a 2.0 mm balloon will also improve crossing rates. To avoid perforation, the window should be oriented towards angiographically-apparent plaque before initiating the cutting sequence. Periodic contrast injections should be performed every 6-8 cuts to assess progress. Free mobility of the distal guidewire should be maintained at all times. Loss of wire mobility after several cuts suggests that the nosecone collection chamber is full; forceful removal of the device at this point greatly increases the risk of guidewire fracture. If free mobility cannot be achieved, the guidewire and AtheroCath should be removed together as a single unit.

4. **Adjunctive Medical Therapy.** Adjunctive medical therapy for DCA is similar to PTCA, including preprocedural aspirin (325 mg/d starting at least 1 day prior to DCA) and intraprocedural heparin. Long acting nitrates and/or calcium antagonists are administered at the discretion of the operator to minimize vasospasm. If a satisfactory angiographic result is obtained, heparin is discontinued at the end of the case and the vascular sheaths are removed 4-6 hours later. In EPIC, bolus plus infusion of abciximab was shown to decrease the incidence of major complications and possibly restenosis (Chapter 34).[1] Abciximab resulted in a 71% reduction in non-Q-wave MI (15.4% to 4.5%) in DCA patients.[137] In EPILOG, abciximab was associated with a 57% reduction in major ischemic complication (20% to 8.7%) in DCA patients.[138] Weight-adjusted heparin (70 U/kg bolus) is recommended if abciximab is used.

5. **Adjunctive Devices.** PTCA, Rotablator, and ELCA have been used to facilitate subsequent passage of the AtheroCath when it fails to cross the lesion;[2,3] this is more common in aorto-ostial, angulated and calcified lesions, and in tortuous vessels. Intravascular ultrasound may be particularly useful to assess the depth and extent of calcification; for superficial calcification, Rotablator is the device of choice, but for deep calcification, DCA alone or DCA followed by PTCA may be considered.

6. **Optimal Atherectomy.** The goal of optimal atherectomy is to create a large lumen diameter without complications. For initial DCA passes, begin with an AtheroCath according to the practical guidelines in Table 28.4. Initial cuts should be directed toward angiographically-apparent plaque (as guided by multiple orthogonal views). Initial balloon inflation pressures of 10-20 psi are used, and the AtheroCath is usually removed and emptied after 6-8 cuts. If repeat angiography demonstrates a residual stenosis > 15%, additional atherectomy is performed using higher inflation pressures (20-40 psi). If a residual stenosis > 15% is still evident, the decision to perform DCA with a larger cutter (vs. PTCA or stenting) depends on the cutter-to-artery ratio. If upsizing complies with the sizing guidelines in Table 28.4, DCA is performed; if the next size cutter is too

large for the target vessel, PTCA or stenting is performed. PTCA should be performed using a balloon-to-artery ratio of 1.0-1.2 and inflation pressures of 4-6 atm. In one report, adjunctive stenting resulted in superior immediate lumen enlargement compared to PTCA.[10] Although some data suggest that intravascular ultrasound can be used to achieve larger lumen diameters,[4-7] other data suggest that comparable lumen enlargement can be achieved using angiography alone.[8,9] The "ideal" residual stenosis is unknown; one study suggested a reduction in late cardiac events when the final diameter stenosis was 10-20%, with no incremental benefit for residual stenoses < 10%.[11] Most operators attempt to achieve a residual stenosis < 20%.

D. MECHANISM OF LUMEN ENLARGEMENT. Although DCA can excise tissue and plaque, the amount of tissue removal (usually 6-45 mg) may not fully account for the magnitude of luminal enlargement. IVUS studies suggest that tissue removal accounts for about 50-75% of the luminal improvement after DCA,[15-18,134] the rest being due to angioplasty effects.

E. PROCEDURAL RESULTS. The results of DCA have been reported in numerous single and multicenter observational studies (Tables 28.5, 28.6, 28.7, 28.8) and in several large, multicenter, prospective, randomized trials (Tables 28.9, 28.10, 28.11).

   1. Immediate Angiographic Results. As shown in Tables 28.5 and 28.6, observational studies report DCA success in 83-99%, final diameter stenoses of 5-29%, and major complications in 1.5-10% of patients. In the three largest randomized studies comparing DCA and PTCA in native vessels (CAVEAT-I, CCAT) and vein grafts (CAVEAT-II), DCA resulted in better immediate lumen enlargement, higher procedural success, and similar major complications rates (Table 28.9).

Table 28.4. Recommendations for DCA Sizing

AtheroCath Size (F)	Vessel Diameter (mm)*	Vessel Diameter (mm), Practical **
5F	2.5-2.9	≤ 2.5
6F	3.0-3.4	2.5-3.0
7F	3.5-3.9	3.0-3.5
7FG	≥ 4.0	3.5-4.0

Abbreviations: F = French size; G = graft cutter
*   These guidelines are based on the product label; recommended by the FDA
** These guidelines are not approved by the FDA, but may allow for more "optimal atherectomy"

Table 28.5. Immediate Results and Clinical Complications After DCA

Series	N (pts)	Final DS (%)	Success (%)	MACE (%)	Comments
Haberbasch[144] (2000)	50	20	96	2.0	DCA for stent restenosis
START[127,130,143] (1999)	122	13	100	0	TLR (15%)
ABACAS[110,111,114,116] (1999)	225	15	95	0.9	TLR (15%)
OARS[112] (1998)	199	7	97	2.5	1-yr TLR (18%)
Grewal[108] (1997)	187	-	91	3	2-yr TLR (18%); clinical restenosis (16%)
NACI[109] (1997)	1196	19	88	3	TLR (23%); death (0.6%); MI (1.5%); CABG (2.8%)
Fortuna[19] (1995)	310	16	95	5	VSR (1.3%); TLR (28%)
Umans[20] (1994)	150	29	90	10	Worse 2-yr EFS with unstable angina
Popma[21] (1993)	306	14	95	2.6	nQMI (5.6%); CRS (28%)
Cowley[22] (1993)	300	-	95	4.6	
Baim[23] (1993)	873	-	92	4.9	DCA Registry: ARS (42%); nQMI (5%); VSR (1.1%)
Feld[24] (1993)	116	8	99	4	nQMI (6%); dissection (13%)
Fishmann[37] (1992)	190	7	97	3	nQMI (7.4%); ARS (32%); 1-yr EFS (74%)
Popma[25] (1992)	1020	-	83	-	Death (0.2%); MI (1.7%); CABG (2.5%)
Garratt[26] (1992)	158	-	91	7	ARS (58%)
Ellis[27] (1991)	378	-	88	6.3	
Hinohara[28] (1991)	339	15	94	3.4	Success: noncalcified (78%); calcified (52%)
Safian[12] (1990)	67	5	88	1.5	VSR (3%); nQMI (4.5%)

Abbreviations: ARS = angiographic restenosis; CRS = clinical restenosis; EFS = event-free survival; MACE = major in-hospital complications (death, Q-wave myocardial infarction, emergency coronary artery bypass surgery); nQMI = non-Q-wave myocardial infarction; TLR = target lesion revascularization; VSR = vascular surgical repair;- = not reported;

Table 28.6. Immediate Results and Clinical Complications After DCA in Vein Grafts

Series	N	Success (%)	MACE** (%)
Stephan[146] (1997)	57	86	0
NACI[109] (1997)	209	86	2.2
Cowley[31] (1993)	363	86	2.5*
Garratt[26] (1992)	26	96	4.2
Pomerantz[32] (1992)	35	94	0
DiScasio[32a] (1992)	96	97	1.4
Ghazzal[33] (1992)	286	87	2.1
Selmon[34] (1991)	87	91	2.6

*   U.S. DCA Registry: vascular repair (3.5%); non-Q-wave MI (3%); restenosis (38% de novo lesions, 75% restenotic lesions)

** In-hospital major adverse cardiac events (death, MI, emergency bypass surgery)

Although adjunctive PTCA after DCA was initially discouraged, PTCA may actually improve DCA outcome and can often result in residual stenoses <10%.[4,5,8,9] In lesions with 3 or more complex characteristics, the success rate of atherectomy decreased from 97% to 84%, but increased to nearly 90% after adjunctive PTCA.[28] In another study, adjunctive PTCA converted "suboptimal" DCA to "optimal" DCA, and improved late outcome.[56] Four prospective trials of optimal atherectomy have been completed (Table 28.10, 28.11, 28.12), and all confirm the safety of optimal DCA. Together, these studies suggest better immediate and late lumen enlargement and less angiographic restenosis after optimal DCA (compared to DCA or PTCA alone), but no difference in late TLR. Surprisingly, in the START trial, aggressive DCA resulted in superior angiographic and clinical outcomes compared to primary stenting.[143]

2. **Angiographic Complications (Table 28.7).** In general, the overall incidence of angiographic complications after DCA is similar to PTCA.[12,19-58]

    a. **Dissection and Abrupt Closure.** Nonocclusive dissection and severe dissection leading to abrupt closure occur in 20%[29] and 0-7% of cases, respectively (Tables 28.7, 28.9). In CAVEAT-II and CCAT, the incidence of abrupt closure after DCA and PTCA were similar (Table 28.9). In CAVEAT-I, abrupt closure was more common after DCA (8% vs. 3.8%, p = 0.005) and occurred at a site *other* than the target lesion in 42% (presumably from guide catheter or nosecone trauma).[98]　Finally, reports from the NACI Registry [85] and OARS [100] indicated abrupt closure rates of only 1.3% and 1%, respectively. Whereas the principal mechanism of abrupt closure after PTCA is dissection, vessel thrombosis is more often the cause after DCA.[25] Dissection may be caused by the guiding catheter (particularly for the RCA), the guidewire, and the atherectomy device itself (from the cutting mechanism, integrated balloon, or nosecone). Guiding catheter-induced injury can be reduced by avoiding over-rotation and deep-seating.

b.　**Thrombosis.** Local thrombosis was felt to complicate approximately 2% of DCA procedures and account for $\geq$50% of acute closures after DCA.[25,57] However, given the poor predictive accuracy of angiography for thrombus, it is possible that many filling defects attributed to thrombus were due to dissection. Treatment includes PTCA and stenting, or CABG for refractory cases (Chapter 9).

c.　**Distal Embolization and No-Reflow.** Distal embolization causing abrupt cutoff of the target vessel beyond the original target lesion has been reported in 0-13.4% of DCA procedures (Tables 28.7, 28.9). This type of macroembolization is usually due to dislodgement of thrombus or friable plaque from the target vessel, or less often, from release or incomplete capture of tissue stored in the nosecone collection chamber. Distal embolization occurs more often after DCA in vein grafts than in native vessels, probably due to the frequent presence of loose friable atherothrombotic debris in vein grafts. Platelet receptor antagonists are effective for preventing distal embolization and CPK elevation after DCA, and should be strongly considered prior to intervention (Chapter 34). Like distal embolization, no-reflow is more frequent after DCA (and other percutaneous interventions) in vein grafts and in lesions with thrombus. Intracoronary calcium antagonists are the most effective form of therapy, whereas nitrates, thrombolytic agents, and CABG are usually ineffective in restoring flow (Chapter 21).

d.　**Vasospasm.** Severe epicardial vasospasm is an infrequent (< 2%) complication of DCA,[55,99] probably because most patients are routinely pretreated with parenteral nitrates. Spasm may occur at the site of the original lesion, but more commonly occurs distal to the lesion, probably from nosecone vibration. Spasm responds readily to intracoronary nitroglycerin or gentle, low-pressure balloon inflations (Chapter 19).

e.　**Perforation.** Coronary artery perforation is an important complication because of its associated morbidity and mortality (Chapter 22). The incidence of perforation after DCA is < 1% (Tables 28.7, 28.11), which is probably lower than other devices that ablate or remove plaque (TEC, ROTA, ELCA), but higher than the 0.2% incidence after PTCA. Some perforations occurred when DCA was used to excise dissection flaps. In contemporary practice, stents are routinely used to seal dissections; DCA should not be considered.

Table 28.7. Angiographic Complications After DCA

Series	N	Vessel	Complications (%)			
			Acute Closure	DE or No-reflow	Branch Occlusion	Perforation
OARS[112] (1998)	213	N	2.0	1.4	3.0	1.0
NACI[109] (1997)	1329	N, SVG	1.1	1.4	0.8	1.0
Stephan[36] (1995)	160	N, SVG	4.0	4.0	-	-
Fortuna[19] (1995)	396	N, SVG	3.6	-	-	-
Umans[20] (1994)	150	N	1.3	0	0.7	0
Popma[21] (1993)	306	N, SVG	2.3	1.3	0.7	0.3
Cowley[22] (1993)	318	SVG	1.9	7.2	0.3	0.6
Baim[23] (1993)	1032	N, SVG	3.9	1.8	3.8	0.6
Pomerantz[32] (1992)	35	SVG	0	2.9	0	0
Fishman[37] (1992)	225	N, SVG	3.2	0	3.7	0.5
Popma[25] (1992)	1140	N, SVG	4.2	-	-	0.6
Garratt[26] (1992)	165	N, SVG	-	2.0	1.0	-
Hinohara[28] (1991)	382	N, SVG	3.7	2.1	2.6	0.8
Rowe[29] (1990)	91	N	2.2	-	7.7	-
Safian[12] (1990)	76	N, SVG	1.5	1.5	1.5	0
Kaufmann[30] (1989)	50	N, SVG	4.0	4.0	2	0

Abbreviations: N = native vessel; NACI = New Approaches to Coronary Intervention; OARS = Optimal Atherectomy Restenosis Study; SVG = saphenous vein graft; DE = distal embolization; - = not reported

f. Sidebranch Occlusion. The incidence of significant sidebranch occlusion after DCA is 0.7-7.7% (Table 28.7). However, among true bifurcation lesions, sidebranch narrowing or occlusion may occur in up to 37%. Fortunately, most cases can be managed by PTCA; for suitable vessels (diameter ≥ 3mm without severe lesion angulation), DCA can be used to salvage the sidebranch. [61] Risk factors for sidebranch occlusion are similar to PTCA and include origin of the sidebranch from the target lesion and baseline narrowing of the sidebranch origin.[67] In a CAVEAT substudy, DCA of bifurcations was associated with higher procedural success, more abrupt closure, and less angiographic restenosis than PTCA.[133]

3. **Clinical Complications (Tables 28.5, 28.6, 28.8, 28.9, 28.11).** Abrupt closure is the most common cause of clinical complications after DCA (and other devices). In one report, abrupt closure was associated with a 16-fold increase in mortality and a 23-fold increase in MI. [25]

a. **Major Clinical Complications.** The incidence of death, MI, or emergency CABG after DCA is 0-10% and similar to other devices. In one report prior to the use of stents, indications for emergency CABG included obstructive complications at the target lesion (57%), perforation (9%), guiding catheter injury (13%), device-related complications (8%), and complications related to adjunctive PTCA (11%).[57] Many of these complications would now be eliminated by stents.

b. **Non-Q-Wave MI.** In most observational studies of DCA, the reported incidence of non-Q-wave MI is 3-12.5% (Tables 28.5, 28.8, 28.9). In CAVEAT-I, but not in CCAT or CAVEAT-II, there was a higher incidence of non-Q-wave MI after DCA compared to PTCA. Risk factors for CK-MB elevation include high-risk patients, de novo lesions, and complex lesion morphology.[63-65] Platelet receptor antagonists administered prior to DCA can reduce the incidence of non-Q-wave MI.[66]

c. **Vascular Injury (Tables 28.5, 28.6, 28.8).** The incidence of vascular injury requiring blood transfusion or vascular repair is approximately 1-5%. The incidence of any peripheral vascular complication in CAVEAT-I was 6.6% and was similar between PTCA and DCA groups.[68] Steps to minimize vascular complications are described in Chapter 25.

4. **Restenosis and Late Outcome.** Several observational studies have reported restenosis rates of 25-58% after DCA (Tables 28.5, 28.6), but comparisons between studies are hindered by incomplete follow-up, different definitions, and different patient populations and target lesions. Three large multicenter randomized trials failed to demonstrate differences in restenosis between DCA and PTCA in native vessels (CAVEAT-I, CCAT) or in saphenous vein grafts (CAVEAT-II) (Table 28.9).[53-55] A comparative study of PTCA and DCA using matched lesions with similar baseline and immediate post-intervention results reported greater late loss of lumen diameter after DCA than PTCA (2.0 vs. 1.8 mm, p = 0.001); these data support the use of optimal atherectomy to

Table 28.8. Results of DCA for Special Situations

Series	N	Success (%)	MACE (%)	Comments
OSTIAL LESIONS				
Jain[119] (1997)	26 (PTCA) 26 (DCA) 58 (Stent)	77 88 96	- - -	TLR (47% vs. 40% vs. 24%)
Stephen[36] (1995)	160	87	0	nQMI (9%); restenosis: de novo lesions (48%), in restenotic lesions (61%), restenotic SVG lesions (93%)
CAVEAT[148] (1995)	41 (LAD)	86	7	ARS (48%)
Popma[149] (1993)	81	98	-	EFS at 3 months (66%)
Popma[46] (1991)	7 (RCA)	86	0	Final DS (14%); ARS (14%)
ECCENTRIC LESIONS				
Popma[149] (1993)	71 (concentric) 235 (eccentric)	96 94		
Hinohara[150] (1991)	116 (concentric) 122 (mild-mod eccentric) 85 (severe eccentric)	92 86 95	- - -	In-hospital CABG (1.7% vs. 3.3% vs. 2.4%)
BIFURCATION LESIONS				
Dauerman[104] (1998)	40	97	2.5	Adjunctive Rotablator (15%)
Brenner[147] (1996)	34	-	9	SBO (15%)
CAVEAT[133] (1995)	DCA PTCA	88 74	- -	ARS (50% vs. 61%); AC (6.9% vs. 2.6%)
Lewis[47] (1994)	30	97	0	nQMI (67%); SBO (37%)
SUBOPTIMAL PTCA				
Bergelson[38] (1994)	16	100	0	Final DS (17%); restenosis at 9 months (17%)
Harris[39] (1994)	16	63	0	Final DS (41%; 21% if DCA successful)
McCluskey[40] (1993)	103	91	14.0	Perforation (1%)
Movsowitz[41] (1993)	40	80	0	Procedural success: for severe dissection (38%); for focal dissection, elastic recoil, or thrombus (88-100%)
Hofling[42] (1992)	40	92	0	

Table 28.8. Results of DCA for Special Situations

Series	N	Success (%)	MACE (%)	Comments
MYOCARDIAL INFARCTION				
Dangas[142] (1998)	DCA PTCA	96 92	0 9	AC (2% vs. 9%)
Kurisu[140] (1997)	32	97	death (0)	AC (3%); ARS (41%); TLR (34%)
Saito[118] (1996)	21	86	death (0)	3-month ARS (47%)
Baldwin[51] (1993)	11	91	death (0)	Adjunctive PTCA (73%); urokinase (45%); AC (18%)
CALCIFIED LESIONS				
Popma[149] (1993)	306 (all lesions) 60 (calcified)	95 94	- -	1-yr EFS (72% vs. 80%)
Hinohara[151] (1991)	105 (Type A) 70 (calcified)	98 87	0 5.7	
Ellis[152] (1991)	47	-	-	Relative risk of failure (1.98)
OTHER SUBSETS				
Mahdi[121] (1998)	46 (ISR)	100	0	10-mo TLR (28.3%); 12-mo EFS (65%)
Garratt[132] (1996)	57 (calcified) - (angulated) 87 (thrombotic) 47 (tortuosity) 57 (bifurcation)	85 84 88 88 86	15.8 12.6 5.8 7.6 4.4	Final DS (51%) Distal embolization (1.4%) SBO (2.2%)
Laster[49] (1994)	25 (left main, protected)	88	0	nQMI (4.5%); CRS (16%); EFS at 2 years (89%)
Emmi[52] (1993)	58 (thrombotic)	76	15.4	More CABG compared to lesions without clot (p = 0.03); no difference in success or final outcome
Mooney[48] (1993)	88 (> 10 mm)	97	0	AC (4.6%); final DS (18%)
Dick[50] (1991)	7 (total occlusion)	86	0	Final DS (32%); duration of occlusion 5-10 days
Hinohara[56] (1991)	10 (total occlusion)	90	0	

Abbreviations: AC = acute closure; ARS = angiographic restenosis; CABG = coronary artery bypass surgery; CRS = clinical restenosis; DS = diameter stenosis; EFS = event-free survival; MACE = In-hospital major adverse cardiac events (death, MI rePTCA, or CABG); nQMI = non-Q-wave myocardial infarction; QMI = Q-wave myocardial infarction; SBO = sidebranch occlusion; - = not reported

compensate for the greater late loss.[70] Using "optimal" atherectomy technique, angiographic restenosis may be lower after DCA than PTCA, but there is no benefit in reducing late target lesion revascularization. The major mechanism of restenosis after DCA is controversial. Some studies suggest that vascular remodeling accounts for most of the late loss of lumen diameter after DCA,[72,73,103,139,141] but other IVUS studies suggest that intimal proliferation is the major mechanism of restenosis.[74] Tranilast shows promise in reducing restenosis.[75] In the EUROCARE trial, carvedilol failed to reduce restenosis after DCA.[128] In one report of DCA vs. stenting in native coronary arteries, DCA resulted in higher residual stenosis and more angiographic restenosis and late revascularization.[136] This contrasts with the START trial, which demonstrated a lower rate of restenosis with aggressive DCA compared to primary stenting (15.8% vs. 32.8%, $p = 0.032$).

5. **Correlates of Outcome**
   a. **Angiographic Results.** Lesion morphologies associated with lower procedural success include lesion calcification, lesion length > 10 mm, lesion angulation, proximal tortuosity, and thrombus. As the number of unfavorable Type B or C characteristics increases, DCA success decrease (B_1 success = 88%, B_2 success = 75%; C = 75%).[27] Of all lesion morphologies, heavy calcification is the most powerful predictor of procedural failure; in one report, DCA was successful in only 52% of calcified lesions.[76] However, after initial Rotablator atherectomy, adjunctive DCA results in better lumen enlargement than adjunctive PTCA.[101]

   b. **Complications.** The development of angiographic complications was associated with operator experience (relative risk 6.6), treatment of a de novo lesion (relative risk 2.2), and lesion angulation (relative risk 2.7).[27]

   c. **Restenosis.** Several observational studies reported different predictors of restenosis, most likely due to differences in patient population, lesion morphology, and definitions of restenosis. In these studies, risk factors for restenosis included target lesion in a vein graft or the LAD, hypertension, lesion length $\geq$10 mm, vessel diameter < 3 mm, use of a 6F device, final lumen diameter < 3 mm, cholesterol > 200 mg/dl, and diabetes. [21,37,77,78] In CAVEAT, the most important determinant of 6-month lumen diameter was the final lumen diameter after intervention; less important determinants included reference vessel diameter, a history of diabetes, and target lesion in the proximal LAD.[53] In CCAT, the only predictor of 6-month restenosis was the presence of unstable angina before intervention.[54] The amount of residual plaque burden also seems to be an important predictor of restenosis.[124,117]

Table 28.9. Results of Randomized Trials of PTCA vs. DCA

Outcome	CAVEAT-I[53]		CCAT[54]		CAVEAT-II[55]	
	PTCA (n = 500)	DCA (n = 512)	PTCA (n = 136)	DCA (n = 138)	PTCA (n = 156)	DCA (n = 149)
In-hospital (%)						
Final DS	36	29	33	25**	38	32**
Success	76	82*	88	94+	79	89*
Abrupt closure	3	7	5.1	4.3	2.6	4.7
Death, QMI, CABG	4.4	5	4.4	2.1	5.7	4.7
Any MI	8	19**	3.7	4.3	11.5	17.4
Distal embolization	-	-	-	-	5.1	13.4*
Follow-up (6 months) (%)						
Final DS ≥ 50%	57	50	4.3	46	46	51
TLR	37.2	36.5	26.4	28.3	26	19
EFS	63	60	71	71	56	60

Abbreviations: CAVEAT = Coronary Angioplasty Versus Excisional Atherectomy Trial (I = native vessels; II = saphenous vein grafts); CCAT = Canadian Coronary Atherectomy Trial (LAD only); DS = diameter stenosis; QMI = Q-wave myocardial infarction; CABG = emergency coronary artery bypass surgery; TLR = target lesion revascularization; EFS = event-free survival; n = number of patients; - = not reported
* p < 0.05
+ p = 0.06
** p < 0.01

F. SPECIAL CONSIDERATIONS

1. **Deep Tissue Resection.** Deep wall components (media and adventitia) can be identified in up to 2/3 of DCA specimens.[12,79] Although immediate post-procedure lumen diameter is an important determinant of restenosis and is the central theme of the "bigger-is-better" hypothesis,[80] there is concern among some interventionalists that achieving large lumen diameters by partial excision of plaque and deep vessel wall components may increase the risk of perforation, restenosis, and aneurysm formation.[81] Although perforation is slightly more frequent after DCA than PTCA, there does not appear to be any relationship between retrieval of deep wall components and perforation. The controversy surrounding restenosis[81,82] appears to have been resolved by a report from the CAVEAT I and II investigators, who found that deep wall resection did *not* increase the risk of restenosis.[102] Finally, no relationship was observed between deep tissue resection and the late development of coronary aneurysms.[83]

Table 28.10. Multicenter Trials of DCA in Native Coronary Arteries

	CAVEAT-I[53]	CCAT[54]	OARS[4]	BOAT[8]
No. Patients	1012	548	200	1000
Year[1]	1993	1993	1995	1995
# Cases/Operator[2]	50	-	> 200	> 200
Qualify[3]	No	No	Yes	Yes
AtheroCath[4]	Suryln, EX	Surlyn, EX	EX, GTO	EX, GTO
PTCA[5]	No	No	Yes	Yes
IVUS[6]	No	No	Yes	No
Goal (final DS %)[7]	< 50	< 50	< 15	< 15

Abbreviations: CAVEAT-I = Coronary Angioplasty Versus Excisional Atherectomy Trial (native vessels); CCAT = Canadian Coronary Atherectomy Trial (LAD); OARS = Optimal Atherectomy Restenosis Study; BOAT = Balloon vs. Optimal Atherectomy Trial; - = not reported
1. Year of primary publication
2. Co-investigators had to perform a minimum number of DCA cases
3. Co-investigators had to submit angiograms to Core Lab to document their ability to achieve good results
4. Type of AtheroCaths used during study period
5. Use of adjunctive PTCA: No = not permitted; Yes = permitted
6. Routine use of IVUS
7. Co-investigators attempted to achieve a predefined target diameter stenosis

2. **Unstable Angina.** The use of DCA for patients with unstable ischemic syndromes is controversial. In many early observational studies, high procedural success and low complication rates were achieved, despite inclusion of many patients with unstable angina. However, other reports indicate that 2-year event-free survival may be lower in patients with unstable angina (54% vs. 69% for stable angina, $p < 0.02$).[20,84]

3. **Acute MI.** The results of DCA in patients with recent MI are less favorable than in patients without previous infarction, primarily due to a higher incidence of dissection (7.1% vs. 2.8%, $p < 0.05$) and abrupt closure (4.7% vs. 1.2%, $p < 0.05$).[85] Other studies reported more angiographic[85] and major ischemic complications after recent MI (9.7% vs. 2.6%, $p < 0.01$) despite overall procedural success rates of 92-97%. DCA is rarely considered as primary treatment for acute MI because of the high success rates of PTCA with and without stenting.

4. **Elderly.** While there may be a higher incidence of major complications (4.2-10.9%), procedural failure (3.3-13.8%), and need for blood transfusion (3.3-17%) in the elderly, final diameter stenosis (18-22%), abrupt closure (0.8-4.9%), perforation (0-0.8%), and stroke (0-2.4%) appear to be unrelated to age.[88]

Table 28.11. Optimal Atherectomy Trials

		BOAT	BOAT[113]		ABACAS[114]		START[143]
	OARS[4,5,67,112]	PILOT[8,9]	PTCA	DCA	DCA	DCA + PTCA	DCA + PTCA
No. lesions	218	192	497	492	106	108	60
Procedure success (%)	97	96	87**	93	94	94	100
Adjunctive PTCA (%)	89	67	100	81	0	100	23
Final DS (%)	8	10	28**	15	15	11	13
Complications (%) Death	0	0.5	0.4	0	0	0	0
nQMI/QMI	11/1.5	17/1.6	- / 1.2	6/2	0.9/0.9	0.9	3.3
CABG	1.0	1.0	2.0	1.0	0	0	0
Perforation	0.5	0.5	-	1.4	-	0.9	0
Angiographic restenosis	30.3	-	40	31*	20	24	16
Target lesion revascularization	-	-	18	15	15	21	15
Event-free survival	-	-	75	79	-	-	-

Abbreviations: ABACAS = Adjunctive Balloon Angioplasty After Coronary Atherectomy Study; BOAT = Balloon versus Optimal Atherectomy Trial; CABG = emergency coronary artery bypass surgery; DS = diameter stenosis; nQMI = non-Q-wave myocardial infarction; OARS = Optimal Atherectomy Restenosis Study; - = not reported
* $p < 0.05$
** $p < 0.01$

5.   **Debulking Prior to Stenting (Table 28.13).** Several IVUS studies suggest that residual plaque burden is an important determinant of restenosis after percutaneous intervention.[124,117] To reduce plaque burden, mechanical debulking with DCA or Rotablator has been employed as an adjunct to stenting. Observational studies suggest that DCA/stenting is associated with less restenosis than stenting alone.[105-17,131,145] Further studies are pending.

G.   LESION-SPECIFIC APPLICATIONS

1.   **Ostial Lesions (Table 28.8).** Percutaneous intervention on ostial lesions is frequently limited by lesion rigidity and elastic recoil, leading to suboptimal results. For noncalcified ostial lesions in vessels ≥3 mm, DCA is associated with procedural success in 87% and major complications in <1% of patients.[36,46] Although immediate angiographic results in highly selected lesions are excellent, DCA of ostial lesions is limited by a high incidence of restenosis (48% in de novo lesions, 61% in restenotic lesions, and 93% in restenotic vein graft lesions).[36] One study of ostial LAD lesions treated by DCA vs. Palmaz-Schatz stenting suggested similar lumen enlargement, but more compromise of the ostium of the LCX after stenting.[122]

Table 28.12. Comparative Results of "Conventional" vs. "Optimal" Atherectomy Techniques

	Conventional DCA		Optimal DCA		
	CAVEAT-1[53]	CCAT[54]	OARS[112]	BOAT[113]	START[143]
Reference Vessel (mm)	2.8	3.13	3.28	3.25	3.29
Final DS (%)	29	26	7	15	13
7F AtheroCath (%)	46	29	95	95	100
# Cuts (mean)	11	-	19	19.5	22
Adjunctive PTCA (%)	3	8	87	82	23
Procedure Success (%)	88	94	98	93	100
Angiographic Restenosis (%)	49.6	46	29	31	16
TLR (%)	37.0	22.6	17.8	15.3	150

Abbreviations: DS = diameter stenosis; TLR = target lesion revascularization; CAVEAT = Coronary Angioplasty Versus Excisional Atherectomy Trial; CCAT = Canadian Coronary Atherectomy Trial; OARS = Optimal Atherectomy Restenosis Study; BOAT = Balloon versus Optimal Atherectomy Trial; - = not reported

2. **Bifurcation Lesions (Table 28.8).** Percutaneous intervention on bifurcation lesions is often complicated by "shifting plaque," leading to "snow-plow" injury, sidebranch occlusion, and suboptimal results. As with PTCA, the risk of sidebranch occlusion with DCA is greatest when the sidebranch originates from the target lesion and when the origin of the branch is stenotic. The approach to atherectomy of bifurcations includes DCA of the main vessel followed by sequential PTCA or DCA of the branch, depending on vessel size, calcification, and angulation. In some cases, a double guidewire technique can be used; nitinol guidewires are resistant to injury after DCA and can be used to protect sidebranches during atherectomy of the main vessel.[45] In highly selected cases, procedural success has been reported in 97-100% with major complications in 0-3% (Figure 28.5).[43,44,47] In these studies, transient sidebranch occlusion occurred in 37% but was successfully retrieved in most patients by PTCA or DCA; final diameter stenosis was 6-12% in the main vessel and 0-17% in the branch. In CAVEAT-I, DCA of bifurcation lesions was associated with higher success (88% vs. 74%, p < 0.001), more ischemic complications (9.5% vs. 3.7%, p < 0.01), and less restenosis (50% vs. 61%, p < 0.001) compared to PTCA.[90]

3. **Thrombus-Containing Lesions.** DCA should not be used in vessels that contain a large clot burden due to the risk of acute closure. In one study, the presence of thrombus was associated with a higher incidence of emergency CABG, but no difference in success or other complications compared to lesions without thrombus.[52] In another series, the presence of a "complex, probable thrombus-containing" lesion was actually predictive of *higher DCA success*,[27] although vessels with a large clot burden were generally not treated by DCA. However, DCA is rarely considered for

Table 28.13. Debulking with DCA Prior to Stenting

	SOLD Registry[106]		Bramucci[105]		Hopp[145]
	PTCA + Stent	DCA + Stent	PTCA + Stent	DCA + Stent	DCA + Stent
No. Lesions	75	75	94	94	167
Lesion Length (mm)	12.5	11.9	11.3	11.9	-
Diameter Stenosis (%)					76
Baseline	74	74	76	76	
Final	4	0.3*	11	5	5
MLD (mm)					
Baseline	0.85	0.85	0.80	0.79	1.0
Final	3.15	3.48**	2.0	2.26	3.6
Acute Gain (mm)	2.30	2.63**	2.2	2.43*	2.6
Late Loss (mm)	1.02	0.91	1.04	0.82	0.5
Loss Index	0.46	0.33*	0.54	0.31**	0.19
Restenosis Rate (%)	21	11*	30	7**	10.8

Abbreviations: acute gain = post-procedure MLD minus pre-procedure MLD; DS = diameter stenosis; late loss = post-procedure MLD minus follow-up MLD; loss index = late loss/acute gain; MLD = minimal luminal diameter
* $p < 0.05$
** $p < 0.01$

most thrombus-containing lesions because of the success of other mechanical techniques (TEC, AngioJet), adjunctive platelet receptor antagonists, and the frequent use of stents.

4. **Saphenous Vein Grafts.** For focal lesions in nondegenerated vein grafts, numerous observational studies report procedural success in 86-96% and major complications in 0-7% (Table 28.6). Although one study reported angiographic restenosis in 25%,[32] another reported restenosis in 57%, including 38% for de novo lesions and 75% for restenotic lesions.[31] In CAVEAT-II, DCA resulted in better lumen enlargement and higher procedural success, but no difference in angiographic restenosis, target lesion revascularization, or event-free survival compared to PTCA (Table 28.9).[55] In most centers, stents have replaced DCA for vein graft intervention, although DCA may be useful for debulking rigid ostial vein graft lesions prior to stenting.

5. **Left Main Disease.** Stenoses in the left main coronary artery are well-suited for DCA because of their proximal location and large vessel caliber.[49,120,125] In one study of protected left main lesions, procedural success was 88% and emergency CABG was required in 4.5%.[49] Nevertheless, most operators prefer stents.

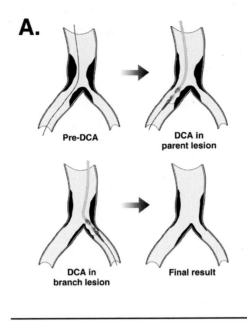

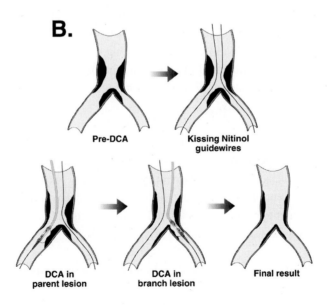

Figure 28.5. Bifurcation Lesions: DCA Techniques

A. Sequential guidewires and sequential DCA
B. Kissing nitinol guidewires and sequential DCA

6. **Suboptimal PTCA (Table 28.8).** DCA may be applied to lesions after suboptimal PTCA due to elastic recoil. In highly selected focal lesions in large vessels, DCA success ranged from 63-92%, with death, Q-wave MI, and emergency CABG reported in 0-2%, 0-6.3%, and 0-12.5% of patients, respectively.[38-42,56] Because of the risk of perforation and the reliability and effectiveness of stents, DCA should not be used to treat dissections (Chapter 20).

7. **Restenotic Lesions.** In a recent study of 1087 patients with restenotic lesions, procedural success was 94-96% for conventional PTCA, DCA, and Palmaz-Schatz stenting. Although DCA and stents resulted in significantly better immediate lumen enlargement compared to PTCA, the incidence of major in-hospital complications, 6-month cardiac events (clinical restenosis), and 3-year event-free survival were similar for all 3 devices.[91] For restenotic ostial lesions, recurrent restenosis after DCA was 61% in native vessels and 93% in vein grafts. [35]

8. **Stent Restenosis.** Although DCA has been used to treat stent restenosis,[89,129,144] there are no data to suggest superiority over conventional PTCA. In fact, there have been several instances of partial excision of stent struts and coils. Histologic studies of DCA for stent restenosis confirm a high incidence of intimal hyperplasia, virtually identical to that observed after restenosis following other interventions.

H. **TISSUE ANALYSIS.** The application of DCA to patients with peripheral vascular and coronary artery disease provided the opportunity for sampling of atherosclerotic vascular tissue from living patients. The availability of such tissue has led to several interesting observations, which may have important implications for further understanding and treatment of atherosclerosis:

1. De novo lesions frequently consist of fibrosis, necrotic debris, foam cells, cholesterol, and calcium, typical findings of atherosclerosis.

2. In 20-40% of de novo lesions, intimal proliferation is evident and is indistinguishable from similar cellular proliferation in restenotic lesions.[92,94] Thus, intimal proliferation is not specific for restenosis, but is a nonspecific response to injury. Such injury may be due to spontaneous events (plaque rupture), interventional devices, or other causes. Intimal hyperplasia in de novo lesions was associated with younger age and lesions in the LAD, and was not associated with higher rates of restenosis than de novo lesions without intimal hyperplasia.

3. Immunohistochemical studies confirm that proliferative tissue consists primarily of smooth muscle cells.

4. There is a higher prevalence of mural thrombus, plaque hemorrhage, and inflammation in unstable compared to stable angina (22% vs. 2% in one study; 44% vs. 17% in another); this is lower than the prevalence of thrombus in angiographic studies, but similar to necropsy studies.[92,93,95,96,135]

5. Human tissue factor, a crucial activator of blood coagulation and intimal proliferation, is detectable

in 43% of patients with unstable coronary syndromes and only 12% of patients with stable coronary syndromes. [97]

6. Increased plasminogen activator inhibitor levels have been detected in DCA specimens from patients with non-insulin dependent diabetes compared to those without diabetes, suggesting a potential factor predisposing to vessel thrombosis.[123]

* * * * *

REFERENCES

1. Topol E, Califf R, Weisman H, et al. Randomized trial of coronary intervention with antibody against platelet IIb/IIIa integrine for reduction of clinical restenosis: results at six months. Lancet 1994;343:881-886.

2. Mintz GS, Pichard AD, Kent KM, et al. Transcatheter device synergy: Preliminary experience with adjunct directional coronary atherectomy following high-speed rotational atherectomy or excimer laser angioplasty in the treatment of coronary artery disease. Cathet Cardiovasc Diagn 1993;Suppl 1:37-44.

3. Dussaillant GR, Griffin J, Weaver TK, Deible RA, Pichard AD. Transcatheter device synergy: Intravascular ultrasound assessment of rotational atherectomy followed by adjunct directional coronary atherectomy in the treatment of calcified coronary artery disease. Circulation 1995;92:I-329.

4. Leon M, Kuntz R, Popma J, et al. Acute angiographic, intravascular ultrasound and clinical results of directional atherectomy in the optimal atherectomy restenosis study. J Am Coll Cardiol 1995;25:137A.

5. Simonton CA, Leon MB, Kuntz RE, et al. Acute and late clinical and angiographic results of directional atherectomy in the optimal atherectomy restenosis study (OARS). Circulation 1995;92:I-545.

6. Doi T, Tamai H, Ueda K, et al. Impact of intracoronary ultrasound-guided directional atherectomy on restenosis. Circulation 1995;92:I-545.

7. Bauman RP, Yock PG, Fitzgerald PJ, Annex BH, et al. "Reference Cut" method of intracoronary ultrasound guided directional coronary atherectomy: Initial and six month results. Circulation 1995;92:I-546.

8. Baim D, Kuntz R, Popma J, Leon M. Results of directional atherectomy in the "Pilot" phase of BOAT. Circulation 1994;90:I-214.

9. Baim DS, Kuntz RE, Sharma SK, Fortuna R, et al. Acute results of the randomized phase of the balloon versus optimal atherectomy trial (BOAT). Circulation 1995;92:I-544.

10. Mintz GS, Pichard AD, Dussaillant GR, et al. Acute results of adjunct stents following directional coronary atherectomy. Circulation 1995;92:I-326.

11. Waksman R, Weintraub WS, Ghazzal ZMB, et al. Directional coronary atherectomy (DCA): Is much bigger much better? Circulation 1995;92:I-329.

12. Safian R, Gelbfish J, Erny R, et al. Coronary atherectomy. Clinical, angiographic, and histological findings and observations regarding potential mechanisms. Circulation 1990;82:69-79.

13. Baim D, Kuntz R. Directional coronary atherectomy: How much lumen enlargement is optional? Am J Cardiol 1993;72:65E-70E.

14. Penny W, Schmidt D, Safian R, Erny R, Baim D. Insights into the Mechanism of Luminal Improvement After Directional Coronary Atherectomy. Am J Cardiol 1991;67:435-437.

15. Matar F, Mintz G, Farb A, Douek P. The contribution of tissue removal to lumen improvement after directional coronary atherectomy. Am J Cardiol 1994;74:647-650.

16. Tenaglia AN, Buller CE, Kisslo KB, Stack RS. Mechanisms of balloon angioplasty and directional coronary atherectomy as assessed by intracoronary ultrasound. J Am Coll Cardiol 1992;20:685-691.

17. Braden G, Herrington D, Downes T, et al. Qualitative and quantitative contrasts in the mechanisms of lumen enlargement by coronary balloon angioplasty and directional coronary atherectomy. J Am Coll Cardiol 1994;23:40-48.

18. Umans V, Baptisla J, di Mario C, et al. Angiographic, ultrasound, and angioscopic assessment of the coronary artery wall and lumen area configuration after directional atherectomy: The mechanism revisited. Am Heart J 1995;130:217-227.

19. Fortuna R, Walston D, Hansell H, Schulz G. Directional coronary atherectomy: Experience in 310 patients. J Invas Cardiol 1995;7:57-64.

20. Umans V, de Feyter P, Deckers J, et al. Acute and long-term outcome of directional coronary atherectomy for stable and unstable angina. Am J Cardiol 1993;74:641-646.

21. Popma J, Mintz G, Satler L, et al. Clinical and angiographic outcome after directional coronary atherectomy: A qualitative and quantitative analysis using coronary arteriography and intravascular ultrasound. Am J Cardiol 1993;72:55E-64E.

22. Cowley M, DiSciascio G. Experience with directional coronary atherectomy since pre-market approval. Am J Cardiol 1993;72:12E-20E.

23. Baim D, Tomoaki H, Holmes D, et al. Results of directional coronary atherectomy during multicenter preapproval testing. Am J Cardiol 1993;72:6E-11E.

24. Feld H, Schulhoff N, Lichstein E, et al. Coronary atherectomy versus angioplasty: The CAVA study. Am Heart J 1993;126:31-38.

25. Popma J, Topol E, Hinohara T, et al. Abrupt vessel closure after directional coronary atherectomy. J Am Coll Cardiol 1992;19:1372-1379.

26. Garratt K, Holmes D, Bell M, et al. Results of directional atherectomy of primary atheromatous and restenosis lesions in coronary arteries and saphenous vein grafts. Am J Cardiol 1992;70:449-454.

27. Ellis S, DeCesare N, Pinkerton C, Whitlow P. Relation of stenosis morphology and clinical presentation to the procedural results of directional coronary atherectomy. Circulation 1991;84:644-653.

28. Hinohara T, Rowe MH, Robertson GC, et al. Effect of lesion characteristics on outcome of directional coronary atherectomy. J Am Coll Cardiol 1991;17:1112-20.

29. Rowe MH, Hinohara T, White NW, Robertson GC. Comparison of dissection rates and angiographic results following directional coronary atherectomy and coronary angioplasty. Am J Cardiol 1990;66:49-53.

30. Kaufmann UP, Garratt KN, Vlietstra RE, Menke KK. Coronary atherectomy: First 50 patients at the Mayo Clinic. Mayo Clin Proc 1989;64:747-752.

31. Cowley M, Whitlow P, Baim D, Hinohara T, et al. Directional coronary atherectomy of saphenous vein graft narrowings: Multicenter investigational experience. Am J Cardiol 1993;72:30E-34E.

32. Pomerantz R, Kuntz R, Carrozza J, et al. Acute and long-term outcome of narrowed saphenous venous grafts treated by endoluminal stenting and directional atherectomy. Am J Cardiol 1992;70:161-167.

32a. DiScasio G, Cowley MJ, Vetrovec GW, Goudreau E, et al. Directional coronary atherectomy of saphenous vein graft lesions unfavorable for balloon angioplasty: Results of a single center experience. Cathet Cardiovasc Diagn 1992;26:75.

33. Ghazzal ZMB, Douglas JS, Holmes DR, et al. Directional atherectomy of saphenous vein grafts: Recent multicenter experience. J Am Coll Cardiol 1991;17:219A.

34. Selmon MR, Hinohara T, Robertson GC, Rowe MH, et al. Directional coronary atherectomy for saphenous vein graft stenoses. J Am Coll Cardiol 1991;17:23A.

35. Kaufmann U, Garratt K, Vlietstra R, Holmes D. Transluminal atherectomy of saphenous vein aortocoronary bypass grafts. Am J Cardiol 1990;65:1430-1433.

36. Stephan W, Bates E, Garratt K, Hinohara T, Muller D. Directional atherectomy of coronary and saphenous vein graft ostial stenoses. Am J Cardiol 1995;75:1015-1018.

37. Fishman R, Kuntz R, Carrozza J, et al. Long-term results of directional coronary atherectomy: Predictors of restenosis. J Am Coll Cardiol 1992;20:1101-1110.

38. Bergelson B, Fishman R, Tomaso C, et al. Acute and long-term outcome of failed percutaneous transluminal coronary angioplasty treated by directional coronary atherectomy. Am J Cardiol 1994;73:1224-1226.

39. Harris W, Berger P, Holmes D, Garratt K. "Rescue" directional coronary atherectomy after unsuccessful percutaneous transluminal coronary angioplasty. Mayo Clin Proc 1994;69:717-722.

40. McCluskey E, Cowley M, Whitlow P. Multicenter clinical experience with rescue atherectomy for failed angioplasty.

Am J Cardiol 1993;72:42E-46E.

41. Movsowitz H, Emmi R, Manginas A, et al. Directional coronary atherectomy for failed balloon angioplasty: Outcome depends on the underlying pathology. Circulation 1993;88:I-601.

42. Hofling B, Gonschior P, Simpson L, Bauriedel G. Efficacy of directional coronary atherectomy in cases unsuitable for percutaneous transluminal coronary angioplasty (PTCA) and after unsuccessful PTCA. Am Heart J 1992;124:341-348.

43. Mansour M, Fishman RF, Kuntz RE, Carrozza JP. Feasibility of directional atherectomy for the treatment of bifurcation lesions. Cor Art Dis 1992;3:761-765.

44. Eisenhauer AC, Clugston RA, Ruiz CE. Sequential directional atherectomy of coronary bifurcation lesions. Cathet Cardiovasc Diagn 1993;Suppl 1:54-60.

45. Grossman ED, Leya FS, Lewis BE, Johnson SA, et al. Examination of common PTCA guide wires used for side branch protection during directional coronary atherectomy of bifurcation lesions performed in vivo and in vitro. Cathet Cardiovasc Diagn 1993;1:48-53.

46. Popma JJ, Dick RJL, Haudenschild CC, Topol EJ, Ellis S. Atherectomy of right coronary ostial stenoses: Initial and long-term results, technical features and histologic findings. Am J Cardiol 1991;67:431-433.

47. Lewis B, Leya F, Johnson S, et al. Acute procedural results in the treatment of 30 coronary artery bifurcation lesions with a double-wire atherectomy technique for side-branch protection. Am Heart J 1994;127:1600-1607.

48. Mooney M, Mooney-Fishman J, Madison J, Nahhan A, Van Tassel R. Directional atherectomy for long lesions: Improved results. Cathet Cardiovasc Diagn 1993;1:26-30.

49. Laster S, Rutherford B, McConahay D, Giorgi L, Johnson W. Directional atherectomy of left main stenoses. Cathet Cardiovasc Diagn 1994;33:317-322.

50. Dick RJL, Haudenschild CC, Popma JJ, Ellis SG. Directional atherectomy for total coronary occlusions. Cor Art Dis 1991;2:189-199.

51. Baldwin TF, Lash RE, Whitfeld SS, Toalson WB. Directional coronary atherectomy in acute myocardial infarction. J Inv Cardiol 1993;5:288-294.

52. Emmi R, Movsoqitz H, Manginas A, et al. Directional coronary atherectomy in lesions with coexisting thrombus. Circulation 1993;88:3204.

53. Topol E, Leya F, Pinkerton C, et al. A comparison of directional atherectomy with coronary angioplasty in patients with coronary artery disease. N Engl J Med 1993;329:221-227.

54. Adelman A, Cohen E, Kimball B, et al. A comparison of directional atherectomy with balloon angioplasty for lesions of the left anterior descending coronary artery. N Engl J Med 1993;329:228-233.

55. Holmes D, Topol E, Califf R, et al. A multicenter, randomized trial of coronary angioplasty versus directional atherectomy for patients with saphenous vein bypass graft lesions. Circulation 1995;91:1966-1974.

56. Gordon P, Kugelmass A, Cohen D, et al. Balloon postdilation can safely improve the results of successful (but suboptimal) directional coronary atherectomy. Am J Cardiol 1993;72:71E-79E.

57. Carrozza J, Baim J. Complications of directional coronary atherectomy: Incidence, causes, and management. Am J Cardiol 1993;72:47E-54E.

58. Carrozza JP, Baim DS, Safian RD, et al. Risks and complications of coronary atherectomy. In: Atherectomy, eds. Holmes DR, Garratt KN; Blackwell Scientific Publication, 1992, p.132-148.

59. Van Suylen RJ, Serruys PW, Simpson JB, et al. Delayed rupture of right coronary artery after directional atherectomy for bail-out. Am Heart J 1991;121:914-917.

60. Selmon MR, Robertson GC, Simpson JB, et al. Retrieval of media and adventitia by directional coronary atherectomy and angiographic correlation. Circulation 1990;82:III-624.

61. Safian R, Schreiber T, Baim D. Specific indications for directional coronary atherectomy: Origin left anterior descending coronary artery and bifurcating lesions. Am J Cardiol 1993;72:35E-41E.

62. Campos-Esteve M, Laird J, Kufs W, Wortham CD. Side-branch occlusion with directional coronary atherectomy: Incidence and risk factors. Am Heart J 1994;128:686-690.

63. Hinohara T, Vetter JW, Robertson GC, Selmon MR, et al. CK MB elevation following directional coronary atherectomy. Circulation 1995;92:I-544.

64. Tauke JT, Kong TW, Meyers SN, et al. Prognostic value of creatinine kinase elevation following elective coronary artery interventions. J Am Coll Cardiol 1995;25:269A.

65. Kugelmass AD, Cohen DJ, Moscucci M, et al. Elevation of the creatine kinase myocardial isoform following otherwise successful directional coronary atherectomy and stenting. Am J Cardiol 1994;74:748-754.

66. Lefkovits J, Blankenship JC, Anderson K, et al. Increased risk of non-Q MI after directional atherectomy is platelet dependent: Evidence from the EPIC trial. J Am Coll Cardiol 1996;28:849.

67. Cutlip DE, Ho KKL, Senerchia C, Baim DS, et al. Classification of myocardial infarction after directional coronary atherectomy and relation to clinical outcome: Results of the OARS trial. Circulation 1995;92:I-616.

68. Omoigui N, Califf R, Pieper K, et al. Peripheral vascular complications in the coronary angioplasty versus excisional atherectomy trial (CAVEAT-I). J Am Coll Cardiol 1995;26:922-930.

69. Elliott J, Berdan L, Holmes D, et al. One-year follow-up in the coronary angioplasty versus excisional atherectomy trial (CAVEAT I). Circulation 1995;91:2158-2166.

70. Umans V, Keane D, Foley D, Boersma E, et al. Optimal use of directional coronary atherectomy is required to ensure long-term angiographic benefit: A study with matched procedural outcome after atherectomy and angioplasty. J Am Coll Cardiol 1994;24:1652-1659.

71. Morris D, Weintraub W, Liberman H, Douglas J, King S. A case matched comparison of directional atherectomy to balloon angioplasty. Circulation 1993;88:3232.

72. Mintz GS, Fitzgerald PJ, Kuntz RE, Simonton CA, et al. Lesion site and reference segment remodeling after directional coronary atherectomy: An analysis from the optimal atherectomy restenosis study. Circulation 1995;92:I-93.

73. Mintz GS, Kent KM, Satler LF, Wong SC, Hong MK, Griffin J, Pichard AD. Dimorphic mechanisms of restenosis after

74. Mitsuo K, Degawa T, Nakamura S, Ui K, et al. Serial intravascular ultrasound evaluation of the mechanism of restenosis after directional coronary atherectomy. Circulation 1995;92:I-149.

75. Kosuga K, Tamai H, Ueda K, Hsu YS, et al. Efficacy of tranilast on restenosis after directional coronary atherectomy (DCA). Circulation 1995;92:I-346.

76. Popma JJ, DeCesare NB, Ellis SG, Holmes DR. Clinical, angiographic and procedural correlates of quantitative coronary dimensions after directional coronary atherectomy. J Am Coll Cardiol 1991;18:1183-1189.

77. Umans V, Robert A, Foley D, et al. Clinical, histological and quantitative angiographic predictors of restenosis after directional coronary atherectomy: A multivariate analysis of the renarrowing process and late outcome. J Am Coll Cardiol 1994;23:49-58.

78. Hinohara T, Robertson G, Selmon M, et al. Restenosis after directional coronary atherectomy. J Am Coll Cardiol 1992;20:623-632.

79. Garratt KN, Kaufmann UP, Edwards WD, Vlietstra RE. Safety of percutaneous coronary atherectomy with deep arterial resection. Am J Cardiol 1989;64:538-542.

80. Kuntz RE, Gibson MC, Nobuyoshi M, Baim DS. Generalized model of restenosis after conventional balloon angioplasty, stenting and directional atherectomy. J Am Coll Cardiol 1993;21:15-25.

81. Garratt K, Holmes D, Bell M, et al. Restenosis after directional coronary atherectomy: Differences between primary atheromatous and restenosis lesions and the influence of subintimal resection. J Am Coll Cardiol 1990;16:1665-1671.

82. Kuntz R, Hinohara T, Safian R, et al. Restenosis after directional coronary atherectomy. Effects of luminal diameter and deep wall excision. Circulation 1992;86:1394-1399.

83. Bell M, Garratt K, Bresnahan J, Edwards W, Holmes D. Relation of deep arterial resection and coronary artery aneurysms after directional coronary atherectomy. J Am Coll Cardiol 1992;20:1474-1481.

84. Abdelmeguid A, Ellis S, Sapp S, Simpfendrofer C. Directional coronary atherectomy in unstable angina. J Am Coll Cardiol 1994;24:46-54.

85. Ghazzal Z, Hinohara T, Scott N, et al. Directional coronary atherectomy in patients with recent myocardial infarction. A NACI Registry Report. J Am Coll Cardiol 1993;21:32A.

86. Robertson G, Hinohara T, Vetter J, et al. Directional coronary atherectomy for patients with recent myocardial infarction. J Am Coll Cardiol 1994;23:219A.

87. Poelnitz AV, Backa D, Bauriedel G, Nerlich A. Coronary directional atherectomy: Rescue for failed balloon angioplasty and treatment of complicated lesions. J Interven Cardiol 1991;4:5-11.

88. Movsowitz H, Manginas A, Emmi R, et al. Directional coronary atherectomy can be successfully performed in the elderly. Am J Cardiol 1994;31:261-263.

89. Strauss B, Umans V, van Suylen R-J, et al. Directional atherectomy for treatment of restenosis within coronary stents: Clinical, angiographic and histologic results. J Am Coll

Cardiol 1992;20:1465-1473.

90. Lewis B, Leya F, Johnson S, et al. Outcome of angioplasty (PTCA) and atherectomy (DCA) for bifurcation and non-bifurcation lesions in CAVEAT. Circulation 1993;88:I-601.

91. Waksman R, Weintraub WS, Ziyad MB, et al. Balloon angioplasty, Palmaz-Schatz stent, and directional coronary atherectomy for restenotic lesions: Retrospective comparison in a single center. J Am Coll Cardiol 1995;25;330A.

92. Escaned J, van Suylen R, MacLeod D, et al. Histologic characteristics of tissue excised during directional coronary atherectomy in stable and unstable angina pectoris. Am J Cardiol 1993;71:1442-1447.

93. Rosenschein U, Ellis S, Haudenschild C, et al. Comparison of histopathologic coronary lesions obtained from directional atherectomy in stable angina versus acute coronary syndromes. Am J Cardiol 1994;73:508-510.

94. Miller M, Kuntz R, Friedrich S, et al. Frequency and consequences of intimal hyperplasia in specimens retrieved by directional atherectomy of native primary coronary artery stenoses and subsequent restenoses. Am J Cardiol 1993;71:652-657.

95. DiSciascio G, Cowley M, Goudreau E, et al. Histopathologic correlates of unstable ischemic syndromes in patients undergoing directional coronary atherectomy: In vivo evidence of thrombosis, ulceration, and inflammation. Am Heart J 1994;128:419-26.

96. Arbustini E, De Servi S, Bramucci E, et al. Comparison of coronary lesions obtained by directional coronary atherectomy in unstable angina, stable angina, and restenosis after either atherectomy or angioplasty. Am J Cardiol 1995;75:675-682.

97. Annex B, Denning S, Channon K, et al. Differential expression of tissue factor protein in directional atherectomy specimens from patients with stable and unstable coronary syndromes. Circulation 1995;91:619-622.

98. Holmes DR, Simpson JB, Berdan LG, et al. Abrupt closure: The CAVEAT I Experience. J Am Coll Cardiol 1995;26:1494-500.

99. Mehta S, Popma J, Margolis JR, et al. Complications with new angioplasty devices. Are these device specific? J Am Coll Cardiol 1996;27:168A.

100. Popma JJ, Baim DS, Kuntz RE, Mintz GS, et al. Early and late quantitative angiographic outcomes in the Optimal Atherectomy Restenosis Study (OARS). J Am Coll Cardiol 1996;27:91A.

101. Dusaillant GR, Mintz GS, Pichard AD, et al. Mechanisms and immediate and long-term results of adjunct directional coronary atherectomy after rotational atherectomy. J Am Coll Cardiol 1996;27:1390-1397.

102. Holmes DR, Garratt KN, Isner JM, et al. Effect of subintimal resection on initial outcome and restenosis for native coronary lesions and saphenous vein graft disease treated by directional coronary atherectomy: A report from the CAVEAT I and II investigators. J Am Coll Cardiol 1996;28:645-651.

103. deVrey EA, Mintz GS, von Birgelen, et al. Serial volumetric (three dimensional) intravascular ultrasound analysis of restenosis after directional coronary atherectomy. J Am Coll Cardiol 1998;32:1874-1980.

104. Dauerman HL, Higgin PJ, Sparano AM, et al. Mechanical debulking versus balloon angioplasty for the treatment of true bifurcational lesions. J Am Coll Cardiol 1998;32:1845-1852.

105. Bramucci E, Angoli L, Angelica P, et al. Adjunctive stent implantation following directional coronary atherectomy in patients with coronary artery disease. J Am Coll Cardiol 1998;32:1855-1860.

106. Moussa I, Moses J, Di Mario C, et al. Stenting after optimal lesion debulking (SOLD) registry: Angiographic and clinical outcome. Circulation. 1998;98:1604-1609.

107. Kiesz RS, Rozek MM, Mego DM, et al. Acute directional coronary atherectomy prior to stenting in complex coronary lesions. Cathet Cardiovasc Diagn 1998;45:105-112.

108. Grewal KS, Jorgensen MB, Diesto JT, et al. Long-term clinical follow-up after directional coronary atherectomy. Am J Cardiol 1997;79:553-558.

109. Waksman R, Popma JJ, Kenneard ED, et al. Directional coronary atherectomy (DCA): A report from the New Approaches to Coronary Intervention (NACI) Registry. Am J Cardiol 1997;80(10A):50K-59K.

110. Hosokawa H, Suzuki T, Ueno K, et al. Clinical and angiographic follow-up of Adjunctive Balloon Angioplasty following Coronary Atherectomy Study (ABACAS). Circulation 1996;94:I-318.

111. Suzuki T, Kato O, Fujita T, et al. Initial and long-term results of the Adjunctive Balloon Angioplasty following Coronary Atherectomy Study (ABACAS). J Am Coll Cardiol 1997;29:68A.

112. Simonton CA, Leon MB, Baim DS, et al. 'Optimal' Directional Coronary Atherectomy: Final results of the Optimal Atherectomy Restenosis Study (OARS). Circulation 1998;97:332-339.

113. Baim DS, Cutlip DE, Sharma SK, et al. Final results of the Balloon vs Optimal Atherectomy Trial (BOAT). Circulation 1998;97:322-331.

114. Suzuki T, Hosokawa H, Katoh, O, et al. Effects of adjunctive balloon angioplasty after intravascular ultrasound-guided optimal directional coronary atherectomy: the result of the Adjunctive Balloon Angioplasty After Coronary Atherectomy Study (ABACUS). J Am Coll Cardiol 1999;34:1028-35.

115. de Very E, Mintz GS, Kimura T, et al. Arterial remodelling after directional coronary atherectomy: A volumetric analysis from the Serial Ultrasound Restenosis. J Am Coll Cardiol 1997;29:280A.

116. Sumitsuji S, Suzuki T, Katoh O, et al. Restenosis mechanism after aggressive directional coronary atherectomy assessed by intravascular ultrasound in Adjunctive Balloon Angioplasty following Coronary Atherectomy Study (ABACAS). J Am Coll Cardiol 1997;29:457A.

117. Honda Y, Tsuchikane E, Aizawa T, et al. Impact of vessel wall injury on vascular response after directional coronary atherectomy: A serial intravascular ultrasound study. Circulation. 1997;96:I-583.

118. Saito S, Kim K, Hosokawa G, et al. Short and long-term clinical effects of primary directional coronary atherectomy for acute myocardial infarction. Cathet Cardiovasc Diagn 1996;39:157-165.

119. Jain Sp, Liu MW, Dean LS, et al. Comparison of balloon angioplasty versus debulking devices versus stenting in right coronary ostial lesions. Am J Cardiol 1997;79:1334-1338.

120. Ellis SG, De Cesare NB, Pinkerton CA, et al. Relation of

stenosis morphology and clinical presentation to the procedural results of directional coronary atherectomy. Circulation 1991;84:644-653.

121. Mahdi NA, Pathan AZ, Harrell L, et la. Directional coronary atherectomy for the treatment of Palmaz-Schatz in-stent restenosis. Am J Cardiol 1998;82:1345-1351.

122. Asakaura Y, Takagi S, Ishikawa S, et al. Favorable strategy for the ostial lesion of the left anterior descending coronary artery: Influence on narrowing of circumflex coronary artery. Cathet Cardiovasc Diagn. 1998;43:95-100.

123. Sobel BE, Woodcock-Mitchell J, Schneider DJ, et al. Increased plasminogen activator inhibitor Type 1 in coronary atherectomy specimens from Type II diabetic compared with non-diabetic patients: A potential factor predisposing to thrombosis and its persistence. Criculation 1998;97:2213-2221.

124. Prati F, DiMario C, Reimers B, et al. In-stent neointimal proliferation correlates with amount and distribution of residual plaque outside the stent: An intravascular ultrasound study. Circulation 1999;99:1011-1014.

125. Park SJ, Park SW, Lee CW, et al. Long-term outcome of unprotected left main coronary stenting in patients with normal left ventricular function: Is debulking atherectomy prior to stenting beneficial? J Am Coll Cardiol;33 (Suppl A):15A

126. Tanaka S, Ueda K, Hsu YS, et al. Directional coronary atherectomy in ostial lesion of left anterior descending artery —comparison with stenting. Circulation 1996;94:I258.

127. Tsuchikane E, Kobayashi T, Nakamura T, et al. One year clinical follow-up results of Stent verses Atherectomy Randomized Trial. J Am Coll Cardiol 1999;33:15A.

128. Serruys PW, Foley DP, Hofling B, et al. Carvedilol for prevention of restenosis after directional coronary atherectomy. Final results of the European Carvediol Atherectomy Restenosis (EUROCARE) Trial. Circulation 2000;101:1512-1518.

129. Dauerman HL, Baim DS, Sparano AM, et al. Balloon angioplasty versus debulking for treatment of diffuse in-stent restenosis. J Am Coll Cardiol 1998;31:455A.

130. Tsuchikane E, Sumitsuji S, Nakamura T, et al. Impact of superficial calcification of coronary plaque on lumen dilation: Comparison of stenting and atherectomy from acute results of Stent vs. Directional Coronary Atherectomy Randomized Trial (START). Circulation 1997;67:I81.

131. Kobayashi Y, Moussa I, Akiyama T, et al. Low restenosis rate in lesions of the left anterior descending coronary artery with stenting following directional coronary atherectomy. Cathet Cardiovasc Diagn 1998;45:131-138.

132. Garratt KN, Bell MR, Holmes DR Jr. Directional atherectomy of complex coronary disease: Lesion specific outcomes and treatment strategies. J Interven Cardiol 1996;9:135-144.

133. Lewis BR, Leya FS, Johnson SA, Grassman ED, et al. Assessment of outcome of bifurcation lesions and non-bifurcation lesions treated in the CAVEAT Trial. J Invas Cardiol 1995;7:251-258.

134. Weissman NJ, Palacios IF, Nidorf SM, et al. Three-dimensional intravascular ultrasound assessment of plaque volume after successful atherectomy. Am Heart J 1995;130:413-419.

135. Haft JI, Christou CP, Goldstein JE, et al. Correlation of atherectomy specimen histology with coronary arteriographic lesions morphology appearance in patients with stable and unstable angina. Am Heart J 1995;130:420-424.

136. Umans VA, Melkert R, Foley DP, et al. Clinical and angiographic comparison of matched patients with successful directional coronary atherectomy or stent implantation for primary coronary artery lesions. J Am Coll Cardiol 1996;28:637-644.

137. Lefkovitz J, Blankenship JC, Anderson KM, et al. Increased risk of non-Q-wave myocardial infarction after directional atherectomy is platelet dependent: Evidence from the EPIC trial. J Am Coll Cardiol 1996;28:849-855.

138. Ghaffari S, Kereiakes DJ, Lincoff M, et al. Platelet glycoprotein IIb/IIIa Receptor blockade with abciximab reduces ischemic complications in patients undergoing directional coronary atherectomy. Am J Cardiol 1998;82:7-12.

139. Lansky AJ, Mintz GS, Popma JJ, et al. Remodeling after directional coronary atherectomy (with and without adjunctive percutaneous transluminal coronary angioplasty): A serial angiographic and intravascular ultrasound analysis from the Optimal Atherectomy Restenosis Study. J Am Coll Cardiol 1998;32:329-337.

140. Kurisu S, Sato H, Tateishi H, et al. Directional coronary atherectomy for the treatment of acute myocardial infarction. Am Heart J 1997;134:345-350.

141. Kimura T, Kaburagi S, Tamura T, et al. Remodeling of human coronary arteries undergoing coronary angioplasty or atherectomy. Circulation 1997;96:475-483.

142. Dangas G, Mehran R, Duvvuri S, et al. Directional coronary atherectomy in acute myocardial infarction. Cardiology 1998;90:63-66.

143. Tsuchikane E, Sumitsuji S, Awata N, et al. Final results of the stent versus directional coronary atherectomy randomized trial (START). J Am Coll Cardiol 1999;34:1050-7.

144. Haberbasch W, Wolfgang W, Waldecker B, et al. Directional coronary athererectomy of in-stent restenosis: a two center experience. J Interven Cardiol 2000;13:93-100.

145. Hopp HW, Baer Fm, Ozbek C, et al. A synergistic approach to optimal stenting. J Am Coll Cardiol 2000;36:1853-9.

146. Stephan W, Bates E, Garratt K, Hinohara T, Muller D. Directional atherectomy of coronary and saphenous vein graft ostial stenoses. Am J Cardiol 1995;75:1015-1018.

147. Brenner SJ, Leya FS, Apperson-hanse C, et al. A comparison of debulking versus dilatation of bifurcation coronary arterial narrowings (from the CAVEAT I Trial). Am J Cardiol 1996;78:1039-1041.

148. Boehrer JD, Ellis SG, Pieper K, et al. Directional atherectomy versus balloon angioplasty for coronary ostial and nonostial left anterior descending coronary artery lesions: Results from a randomized multicenter trial. J Am Coll Cardiol 1995;25:1380-6.

149. Popma JJ, Mintz GS, Satler LF, et al. Clinical and angiographic outcome after directional coronary atherectomy. A qualitative and quantitative analysis using coronary arteriography and intravascular ultrasound. Am J Cardiol 1993;72:55E-64E.

150. Hinohara T, Vetter JW, Selmon MR, et al. Directional

coronary atherectomy is effective treatment for extremely eccentric lesions. Circulation 1991;84:II-520.

151. Hinohara T, Rowe MH, Robertson GC, et al. Effect of lesion characteristics on outcome of directional coronary atherectomy. Circulation 1991;17:1112-1120.

152. Ellis SG, De Cesare NB, Pinkerton CA, et al. Relation of stenosis morphology and clinical presentation to the procedural results of directional coronary atherectomy. Circulation 1991;84:644-653.

29 TRANSLUMINAL EXTRACTION ATHERECTOMY

Robert D. Safian, M.D.

A. DESCRIPTION. The Transluminal Extraction Catheter (TEC) (InterVentional Technologies, Inc., San Diego, CA) is a percutaneous over-the-wire cutting and aspiration system that consists of a conical cutting head with two stainless steel blades attached to the distal end of a flexible hollow torque-tube (Figure 29.1). The proximal end of the catheter attaches to a battery-powered hand-held motor drive unit and to a vacuum bottle for aspiration of excised atheroma, thrombus, and debris (Figure 29.2). A trigger on the bottom of the motor drive unit activates cutting blade rotation and aspiration, and a lever on top of the unit allows advancement/retraction of the cutter. During atherectomy, warmed (37°C) Lactated Ringers solution is infused under pressure to create a slurry of blood and tissue which facilitates aspiration. A special 0.014-inch stainless steel guide wire allows coaxial passage of the catheter and has a radiopaque floppy tip with a terminal 0.021" ball to prevent wire tip entrapment or advancement of the cutting blades beyond the guidewire (Figure 29.3). A large-bore rotating hemostatic valve contains a side arm for contrast injections and infusion of pressurized flush solution.

B. EQUIPMENT
   1. Cutters (Table 29.1). TEC cutters for coronary application are available in sizes from 5.5-7.5F (1.8-2.5 mm). The conical cutter head—fabricated from a cylindrical base of proprietary stainless

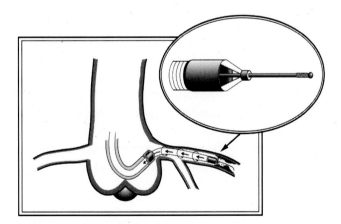

Figure 29.1. Transluminal Extraction Atherectomy (TEC)

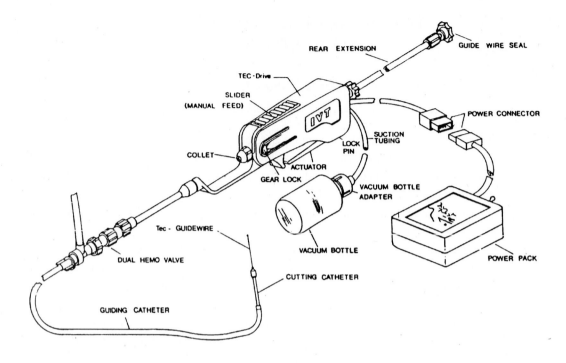

Figure 29.2. The TEC Assembly

steel—is bonded to the distal end of the catheter and contains microtome-sharp cutting edges that rotate at 750 rpm when the motor-drive is activated. The shaft of the cutter consists of a hollow inner-core through which excised material is aspirated and evacuated.

2. **Guiding Catheters (Table 29.2).** Special 90 cm 10F tungsten-braided, soft-tip guiding catheters are available in the following sizes and tip configurations: JR 4.0; JL 3.5, 4.0, 5.0; modified Amplatz; hockey stick; multipurpose; and right bypass graft. Guides from other manufacturers can be used if necessary. For TEC cutters $\leq 6.5F$ (2.2mm), 9F guiding catheters may be used; the 8F giant lumen (ID = 0.086 inches) guide can only accommodate the 5.5F cutter. Pressure damping and poor contrast opacification are common when using guiding catheters < 10F.

C. TECHNIQUE
1. **Guiding Catheter Manipulation.** The TEC guiding catheters are stiffer than conventional angioplasty guides; overrotation and deep seating greatly increase the risk of vessel injury and should be avoided. During advancement of the TEC guide to the aortic root, blood loss can be minimized by tracking the guide over a 0.063-inch guidewire, or alternatively, over a 0.035-inch guidewire and a 6F multipurpose catheter.

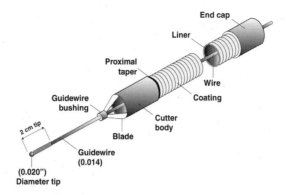

Figure 29.3. The TEC Cutter and Guidewire

2. **Hemostatic Valve.** A special rotating hemostatic valve (RHV) connects the TEC motor-drive handle to the guiding catheter. To minimize the risk of air embolism, it is extremely important to aspirate blood from the guiding catheter (once attached to the RHV), and to thoroughly flush all air out of the RHV.

3. **Guidewires.** Because the stiff 300-cm stainless-steel TEC guidewire is less steerable than conventional PTCA guidewires, a conventional guidewire should be used to cross the target lesion. Once in position, the PTCA guidewire can be exchanged for the TEC guidewire using any suitable transport catheter that will accommodate the 0.021-inch ball (the Scimed Ultrafuse-X catheter works nicely for this purpose). It is important to advance the floppy, radiopaque portion of the wire well beyond the lesion to ensure that atherectomy is performed along the stiff, radiolucent segment. Due to the stiffness of the TEC guidewire, pseudolesions are common, but generally resolve after removal of the guidewire.

Table 29.1. Cutters for TEC Atherectomy

Cutter Size (F)	Cutter Diameter (mm)	Vessel Diameter* (mm)	Guide ID** (inch)
5.5	1.8	2.5	0.088
6.0	2.0	2.75	0.088
6.5	2.17	3.0	0.090
7.0	2.33	3.25	0.096
7.5	2.5	3.5	0.103

*   Minimum vessel diameter to be used with TEC cutters
** Minimum guide catheter internal diameter

4. **Cutter Deployment.** We prefer to undersize the cutter by at least 1mm in relation to the distal reference segment (i.e., cutter-to-artery ratio of 0.5-0.7). In diffusely diseased vessels, angulated lesions, or vessels < 3 mm, our bias is to avoid TEC. Several important technical principles deserve emphasis:

- The TEC cutter must be activated proximal to the lesion. Activation within the lesion increases the risk of distal embolization and dissection and should be avoided.

- Be sure to advance the cutter slowly (10 mm/30 seconds) through the lesion to achieve a continuous stream of blood entering the vacuum bottle. Never advance a rotating cutter in the absence of flow into the vacuum bottle due to the risk of dissection and distal embolization. If blood does not flow into the vacuum bottle, determine if the vacuum has been lost; if so, change bottles. Adequate removal of thrombus and atheroma from most lesions usually requires filling of 5-10 vacuum bottles.

- Do not activate the cutter in the guiding catheter or in a bend.

- The pressurized flush should be turned on while cutting, and turned off between cutter passes. Some experienced operators feel that the pressurized flush may potentiate distal embolization, but routine TEC without flush has not been systematically evaluated.

Table 29.2. Guiding Catheters for TEC Atherectomy

Target Vessel	Configuration	Guiding Catheter
RCA	Normal	JR 4
	Anterior origin	Modified Amplatz, Hockey Stick
	Horizontal origin	Hockey Stick
	Superior origin; Shepherd Cook	Hockey Stick, RBG
	Inferior origin	JR 4, Multipurpose
LCA	Normal	JL 4.0
	Narrow root or superior origin	JL 3.5
	Wide root or posterior origin	JL 5.0
SVG to LCA	Normal	JR 4
	Superior origin	Modified Amplatz, Hockey Stick
		Modified Amplatz, RBG
SVG to RCA	Normal	Modified Amplatz, Multipurpose, RBG
	Horizontal origin	JR 4, Hockey Stick, Modified Amplatz

Abbreviations: JR = right Judkins; JL = left Judkins; RBG = right bypass graft; RCA = right coronary artery; LCA = left coronary artery; SVG = saphenous vein graft

- After completing 2-5 slow passes through the lesion, the TEC cutter should be retracted and the lesion reassessed by angiography. If a filling defect persists and there is no dissection, a larger TEC cutter may be used. If there is significant residual stenosis but no residual filling defect, adjunctive PTCA or stenting is recommended.

5. **Adjunctive Medical Treatment.** Medications are the same as those for PTCA. All patients should receive aspirin (325 mg/d at least 1 day prior to the procedure), heparin (to achieve and maintain an ACT $\geq$+9 300 seconds during the case), and intracoronary nitroglycerin (100-200 mcg just prior to cutting to attenuate spasm). In addition, intracoronary verapamil (100 mcg/min up to 1-1.5 mg) is useful for no-reflow. Abciximab has been used for intraluminal thrombus and high-risk intervention.[27]

6. **Adjunctive Intervention.** If a suboptimal result is obtained, the TEC cutter may be exchanged for a larger cutter, PTCA balloon, or stent; the rotating hemostatic valve, 0.014-inch TEC guidewire, and guiding catheter are compatible with all coronary and biliary stents.

D. **MECHANISM OF ACTION.** Angioscopy studies demonstrated partial or complete thrombus removal in 75-100% of thrombotic lesions after TEC.[1,2] Dissection was noted in virtually all cases by angioscopy[1,2] and in 36% of cases by IVUS.[4] Although gross examination of aspirated material sometimes demonstrates yellowish debris, histologic studies have failed to reveal evidence for tissue removal. It is likely that a "Dotter" effect contributes to angiographic improvement after TEC.[5]

E. **RESULTS**
1. **Native Coronary Arteries (Table 29.3).** TEC is rarely used in the native coronary circulation, but may be useful in large vessels with large thrombus burden.
   a. **Immediate Results.** Procedural success in native coronary arteries was achieved in 84-94%,[6,7] although adjunctive PTCA was required in 79-84% of lesions to enlarge lumen dimensions (72%), salvage technical failures (1%), or manage TEC-induced vessel occlusion (11%).[7] In one study, quantitative angiography revealed a residual diameter stenosis of 61% after TEC and 36% after adjunctive PTCA. The extent of elastic recoil after TEC was approximately 30%, similar to conventional PTCA.[8]

   b. **Clinical Complications.** Major in-hospital complications after TEC include death (1.4-2.3%), emergency CABG (2.6-3.4%), and Q-wave MI (0.6-3.4%).[6,7]

   c. **Angiographic Complications.** Prior to the availability of stents, angiographic complications included dissection (39% after TEC; 6.6% after adjunctive PTCA), abrupt closure (8-11%), coronary artery perforation (0.7-2.2%), distal embolization (0.5-1.6%), and sidebranch occlusion (2.7%).[6,7]

   d. **Follow-up.** Angiographic restenosis (> 50% stenosis) was reported in 56-61% of native vessels treated by TEC,[6,7] and was not affected by the use of adjunctive PTCA. Clinical restenosis (the need for target vessel revascularization, MI, or death) occurred in 29% of patients.[7] Because of the high incidence of dissection, suboptimal lumen enlargement, and restenosis, contemporary practice usually involves the use of TEC as an adjunct to stenting.

2. **Saphenous Vein Grafts (Table 29.4).** TEC appears to have a greater niche as an adjunct to vein graft interventions than native vessel interventions.

   a. **Immediate Results.** For vein graft lesions treated with TEC, procedural success rates were 82-92%;[4,6,10-12] adjunctive PTCA was required in 74-95% of lesions. In the multicenter TEC registry, procedural success was 90% in thrombotic lesions, 97% in ulcerated lesions, and 97% in grafts > 3 years old.[6]

   b. **Clinical Complications.** Prior to stents, major clinical complications after vein graft TEC included death (0-10.3%), MI (0.7-3.7%), and CABG (0.2%).[4,6,10-12]

   c. **Angiographic Complications.** Serious angiographic complications after vein graft TEC are similar to conventional PTCA, including distal embolization (2-17%), no-reflow (8.8%), and abrupt closure (2-5%). No-reflow usually responds to intragraft verapamil (100-300 mcg),[13-15] and prophylactic intragraft verapamil prior to intervention is reasonable but unproven. In one report, distal embolization was more likely to occur in grafts with one or more intraluminal filling defects, and in older grafts.[16] In a NACI Registry report, distal embolization was associated with a higher incidence of in-hospital mortality and myocardial infarction; multivariate predictors of distal embolization included noncardiac disease, stand-alone TEC, thrombus, and large vessel size.[17] To minimize the risk of distal embolization and no-reflow, some operators recommend TEC followed by staged (1-2 months later) rather than immediate stent implantation; in one report, this approach resulted in less distal embolization,[18,19] although 15% of grafts occluded before stenting.[18] In our practice, stenting is often deferred for 2-3 weeks after TEC to minimize the risk of interim graft occlusion. During this period, we empirically treat with aspirin, clopidogrel, and subcutaneous heparin (5,000-10,000 units BID) or enoxaparin (30-60 mg BID).

   d. **Follow-up.** Angiographic restenosis has been reported in 64-69% of vein graft lesions treated with TEC,[6,10] with a 29% incidence of late total occlusion in one report.[10]

Table 29.3. In-hospital Results of TEC Atherectomy in Native Coronary Arteries

	IVT[6] (1995)	Safian[7] (1994)
No. lesions	783	181
Adjunctive PTCA (%)	79	84
Success (%)	94	84
Complications (%)		
MI	0.6	3.4
Death	1.4	2.3
Acute closure	8.0	11.0
Distal embolization	1.6	0.5
No-reflow	0	0

F. SPECIAL CONSIDERATIONS. TEC atherectomy may have special utility in several situations:

    1. Acute Ischemic Syndromes. TEC has been employed for primary revascularization for acute MI, rescue after failed thrombolysis, post-infarct MI angina, and unstable angina associated with a thrombotic lesion. In a study of 110 patients with acute ischemic syndromes, overall procedural success was 94%; in-hospital complications included death in 4.3% (only 1.4% of patients not presenting in cardiogenic shock), CABG in 2.9%, repeat PTCA in 5.7%, and blood transfusion in 20%.[20] At 6 months, vessel patency was 90% and angiographic restenosis was 68%. A multicenter randomized trial comparing TEC vs. PTCA in thrombus-containing lesions (TOPIT) reported less CK elevation after TEC (Table 29.5).[24]

    2. Thrombus. Angiographic thrombus increases the risk of an adverse outcome in virtually all studies of percutaneous interventional devices. However, in the initial TEC registry, procedural success was equally high with and without thrombus, offering hope that TEC's ability to excise and aspirate thrombus would fill an important void in the interventional arena (Table 29.6). Some of these hopes were attenuated when studies of TEC in thrombotic vein grafts reported lower procedural success, and more angiographic and clinical complications.[4,21] Nevertheless, TEC is currently employed as a bailout technique after failed PTCA in the setting of acute MI,[22] and to pretreat thrombotic lesions prior to stenting.[2] Although thrombus increases the risk of TEC (and other devices) compared to lesions without thrombus, the TOPIT trial suggested superiority of TEC over PTCA for patients with acute coronary syndromes in whom thrombus is likely to be present.

Table 29.4. In-hospital Results of TEC Atherectomy in Saphenous Vein Grafts

	Bejarano[26] (1997)	Meany[11] (1995)	Twidale[12] (1994)	Safian[10] (1994)	Popma[4] (1992)
No. lesions	106	650	88	158	29
Adjunctive PTCA (%)	100	74	95	91	86
Success (%)	87	89	86	84	82
Complications (%)					
MI	6.6	0.7	3.4	2.0	3.7
Death	2.0	3.2	0	2.0	10.3
Acute closure	4.7	2.0	5.0	5.0	-
Distal embolization	11.8	2.0	4.5	11.9	17
No-reflow	-	-	-	8.8	-

Abbreviations: - = not reported

3. **Saphenous Vein Bypass Grafts.** Angioscopy revealed that TEC effectively removed thrombus and friable debris from degenerated vein grafts, albeit at an increased risk of no-reflow and distal embolization compared to interventions in native coronary arteries.[23] Patients in whom filling defects persist or transient no-reflow occurs after TEC are at increased risk for no-reflow and distal embolization after adjunctive PTCA or stenting. An angioscopic-guided study demonstrated the effectiveness of TEC followed by stenting for thrombotic and degenerated saphenous vein grafts:[2] Partial and complete thrombus extraction was evident in 100% and 65%, respectively, and all 32 high-risk lesions were successfully treated without Q-wave MI, need for emergency CABG, or death. Debulking high-risk vein grafts with TEC prior to stenting results in high procedural success and low complication rates, although late cardiac events are frequent.[25] In one small study of 17 patients, abciximab prior to TEC was associated with less distal embolization and no-reflow compared to TEC without abciximab.[27] TEC has not yet been compared to distal embolic protection devices, but the imminent release of such devices may obviate the need for TEC in many vein graft interventions.

4. **Ostial Lesions.** Older studies suggested that a combined strategy of TEC followed by PTCA results in an incremental increase in lumen diameter of 22% compared to PTCA alone.[8] In the TEC registry, high procedural success (94%) and low complications (similar to other lesions subtypes) were achieved,[6] but TEC is virtually never used as an atherectomy device for ostial lesions.

Table 29.5. TOPIT Trial: TEC or PTCA in Thrombus-Containing Lesions[28]

	TEC	PTCA	p-Value
No. lesions	131	134	-
Success (%)	98	97	NS
Ischemic complications* (%)	4.5	11.2	0.06
CK elevation (%)	4.5	15.4	0.03
Final DS (%)	27	26	NS
Dissection (%)	38	29	0.04
Distal embolization (%)	2	4	NS
No-reflow (%)	5	8	NS
Perforation (%)	0	0.7	NS
Final TIMI flow < 3 (%)	2	3	NS

Abbreviations: CK = creatine kinase; DS = diameter stenosis; NS = not statistically significant; TOPIT = Transluminal Extraction Atherectomy Or PTCA In Thrombus-Containing Lesions
* Death, MI, abrupt closure, rePTCA, CABG

5. **Contraindications.** Certain lesions are unsuitable for TEC, including moderate-to-heavily calcified lesions, severely angled stenoses, highly eccentric lesions, bifurcation lesions, and lesions in vessels < 2.5 mm. TEC is absolutely contraindicated in the setting of dissection caused by another device due to the risk of extending the dissection and perforating the vessel. Since it is often difficult to distinguish dissection from thrombus by angiography alone, adjunctive imaging techniques such as angioscopy and intravascular ultrasound can be used to guide subsequent use of TEC (for thrombus) or stents (for dissection).

G. **FUTURE DIRECTIONS.** Current TEC cutters are hampered by their small size (≤ 2.5 mm) and limited ability to aspirate. Larger cutters with improved cutting and aspiration are under development. An expandable cutter may allow the use of larger cutters without larger guiding catheters, and adjustments in cutter angles and sharpness may create smoother cuts and decrease complications. Further studies are needed to define the role of TEC as an adjunct to stents (particularly in vein graft intervention), to establish the relative benefits of TEC versus potent platelet receptor antagonists, and to compare TEC to other mechanical techniques for removal of thrombus (AngioJet, Hydrolyzer), disruption of thrombus (ultrasound thrombolysis, local drug delivery), or prevention of distal embolization (distal embolic protection devices).

Table 29.6. Impact of TEC on Thrombus in Vein Grafts

Series	N	Outcome
Misumi[29] (1996)	163	Less distal embolization after TEC than PTCA (3.9% vs. 16.7%, p < 0.01)
Meany[11] (1995)	183	Angiographic success of TEC not affected by thrombus
Dooris[21] (1995)	59	Thrombus decreased clinical success (69% vs. 88%) and increased angiographic and clinical complications (no-reflow and Q-wave MI) after TEC
Al-Shaibi[19] (1995)	124	TEC with less CK elevation compared to PTCA

* * * * *

REFERENCES

1. Annex BH, Larkin TJ, O'Neill WW, Safian RS. Evaluation of thrombus removal by transluminal extraction coronary atherectomy by percutaneous coronary angioscopy. Amer J Cardiol 1994;74:606-9.
2. Kaplan BM, Safian RS, Grines CL, Goldstein JA, et al. Usefulness of adjunctive angioscopy and extraction atherectomy before stent implantation in high risk narrowings in aorto-coronary artery saphenous vein grafts. Amer J Cardiol 1995;76:822-824.
3. Moses JW, Lieberman SM, Knopf WD, et al. Mechanism of transluminal extraction catheter (TEC) atherectomy in degenerative saphenous vein grafts (SVG): An Angioscopic Observational Study. J Am Coll Cardiol 1993;21:442A.
4. Popma JJ, Leon MB, Mintz GS, et al. Results of coronary angioplasty using the transluminal extraction catheter. Am J Cardiol 1992;70:1526-1532.
5. Pizzulli L, Kohler U, Manz M, Luderitz B. Mechanical dilatation rather than plaque removal as major mechanism of transluminal extraction atherectomy. J Intervent Cardiol 1993;6:31-39.
6. IVT Coronary TEC Atherectomy Clinical Database. 1995.
7. Safian RS, May MA, Lichtenberg A, et al. Detailed clinical and angiographic analysis of complex lesions in native coronary arteries. J Am Coll Cardiol 1995;25:848-854.
8. Safian RD, Freed M, Reddy V, et al. Do excimer laser and rotational atherectomy facilitate balloon angioplasty? Implications for lesion-specific coronary intervention. J Am Coll Cardiol (in-press)
9. Ishizaka N, Ikari Y, Hara K, Saeki F, et al. Angiographic follow-up of patients after transluminal extraction atherectomy. Am Heart J 1994; 128(4): 691-696.
10. Safian RS, Grines CL, May MA, et al. Clinical and angiographic results of transluminal extraction coronary atherectomy in saphenous vein bypass grafts. Circulation

1994; 89(1): 302-312.
11. Meany TB, Leon MB, Kramer BL, et al. Transluminal extraction catheter for the treatment of diseased saphenous vein grafts: A multicenter experience. Cathet Cardio Diagn 1995; 34: 112-120.
12. Twidale N, Barth III, CW, Kipperman RM, et al. Acute results and long-term outcome of transluminal catheter atherectomy for saphenous vein graft stenoses. Cath and Cardio Diagn 1994; 31: 187-91.
13. Kaplan BM, Benzuly KH, Bowers TR, et al. Prospective study of intracoronary Verapamil and nitroglycerin for the treatment of no-reflow after interventions on degenerated saphenous vein grafts. Circ 1995; 92:I-330.
14. Piana RN, Paik GY, Moscucci M, Cohen DJ, et al. Incidence and treatment of "no-reflow" after percutaneous coronary intervention. Circulation 1994; 89(6): 2514-2518.
15. Pomerantz RM, Kuntz RE, Diver DJ, Safian RD, Baim DS. Intracoronary verapamil for the treatment of distal microvascular coronary artery spasm following PTCA. Cathet Cardio Diagn 1991; 24: 283-285.
16. Hong MK, Popma JJ, Pichard AD, Kent KM, et al. Clinical significance of distal embolization after transluminal extraction atherectomy in diffusely diseased saphenous vein grafts. Am Heart J 1994; 127(6): 1496-1503.
17. Moses JW, Yeh W, Popma JJ, Sketch Jr. MH, NACI Investigators. Predictors of distal embolization with the TEC catheter: A NACI Registry report. Circ 1995;92:I-329.
18. Hong MH, Pichard AD, Kent KM, et al. Assessing a strategy of stand-alone extraction atherectomy followed by staged stent placement in degenerated saphenous vein graft lesions. J Amer Coll Cardiol 1995;27:394A.
19. Al-Shaibi KF, Goods CM, Jain SP, et al. Does transluminal extraction atherectomy reduce distal embolization in saphenous vein grafts? Circ 1995; 92:I-329.

20. Kaplan BM, Larkin T, Safian RD, O'Neill WW, Kramer B, Hoffmann M, Schreiber T, Grines CL. Prospective study of extraction atherectomy in patients with acute myocardial infarction. Am J Cardiol 1996;77:383-388.

21. Dooris M, Hoffman M, Glazier S, et al. Comparative results of transluminal extraction coronary atherectomy in saphenous vein graft lesions with and without thrombus. J Am Coll Cardiol 1995; 25: 1700-1705.

22. Kaplan BM, O'Neill WW, Grines CL, et al. Rescue extraction atherectomy after failed primary angioplasty in right coronary artery infarction. Am J Cardiol (in-press)

23. Tilli FV, Kaplan BM, Safian RD, Grines CL, O'Neill WW. Angioscopic plaque friability: a new risk factor for procedural complications following saphenous vein graft interventions. J Am Coll Cardiol (in-press).

24. Schreiber, TL, Kaplan B, Gregory ML, et al. Transluminal extraction atherectomy vs. Balloon angioplasty in acute ischemic syndromes (TOPIT): Hospital outcome and six-month status. J Am Coll Cardiol 1997;29(Suppl. A):132A.

25. Braden G, Xenopoulos N, Young T, et al. Transluminal extraction catheter atherectomy followed by immediate stenting in treatment of saphenous vein grafts. J Am Coll Cardiol 1997;30:657-63.

26. Bejarano J, Margolis J, Kramer B. Extraction atherectomy for recently occluded saphenous vein grafts: A retrospective study. J Invas Cardiol 1997;9:263-269.

27. Sullebarger JT, Dalton RD, Nasser A, Matar FA. Adjunctive abciximab improves outcomes during recanalization of totally occluded saphenous vein grafts using transluminal extraction atherectomy. Cathet Cardiovasc Intervent 1999;46:107-110.

28. Kaplan B. Personal communication; 2000.

29. Misumi K, Matthews RV, Sun GW, Mayeda G, Burstein S, Shook TL. Reduced distal embolization with tranlsuminal extraction atherectomy compared to balloon angioplasty for saphenous vein graft disease. Cathet Cardiovasc Diagn 1996;39:246-251.

EXCIMER LASER CORONARY ANGIOPLASTY

30

On Topaz, M.D.
Robert D. Safian, M.D.

A. BACKGROUND

1. **Laser Description.** Lasers produce intense electromagnetic energy[1,2] and may have several important cardiovascular applications (Table 30.1). The coherent laser beam is delivered via optical fibers arranged in a circular array inside a coronary catheter. Excimer lasers (XeCl) are pulsed-wave devices operating at ultraviolet wavelengths (308nm). The CVX-300 (Spectranetics, Colorado Springs, CO) is the only FDA-approved system for coronary artery revascularization and pacemaker lead extraction. The CO_2 and holmium:YAG lasers are approved for surgical and percutaneous transmyocardial revascularization (TMR).

2. **Laser Effects on Plaque.** Absorption of laser energy in a biological tissue results in photomechanical, photochemical, and photothermal effects, leading to vaporization of plaque[3-5] (Table 30.2). Laser debulking of atherosclerotic plaque invariably produce gas bubbles[6] and acoustic effects, which can cause dissection, acute closure, and coronary artery perforation. These complications can be minimized by appropriate lasing techniques,[7-9] as described below.

Table 30.1. Cardiovascular Lasers

Laser Medium	Mode	Wavelength (nm)	Penetration Depth (μm)	Comments
Argon	Continuous wave	520	400	A weak, early generation laser
CO2	Continuous wave/ pulsed wave	10600	15	Approved for TMR
Dye	Pulsed wave	480-577	330	Investigational; potential for thrombolysis
Erbium: YAG	Pulsed wave	2940	1300	Investigational; potential for calcified lesions
Holmium: YAG	Pulsed wave	2090	500	Approved for TMR
Neodymium: YAG	Continuous wave/ pulsed wave	1064	1000	Used for multiple medical purposes
Xenon-chloride (excimer)	Pulsed wave	308	35	FDA-approved for coronary interventions and pacemaker lead extraction

Table 30.2. Laser-Tissue Interactions

Laser Effect	Tissue Effect
Gas bubble formation	Perforation, dissection, acute closure
Acoustic shock waves	Dissection
Thermal (heat)	Spasm, charring, fibrosis
Absorbtion of laser energy	Thrombolysis

B. RECOMMENDATIONS FOR CASE SELECTION. Common indications and contraindications to ELCA are described in Table 30.3. Baseline left ventricular dysfunction is not a contraindication to ELCA, and since severe bradycardia or heart block is rare, prophylactic temporary pacemakers are not required.[10]

C. TECHNICAL DETAILS

1. **Equipment Selection.** Coaxial guiding catheter alignment is imperative for successful delivery of the laser to the target lesion. The rapid-exchange concentric and eccentric coronary laser catheters (Vitesse E) are available in diameters of 1.4-2.0 mm and 1.7/2.0 mm, respectively (Tables 30.4, 30.5). New concentric catheters with optimally spaced fibers (Vitesse C_{os}) have improved spacing of optic fibers[11] and a larger exit angle, resulting in a 40-60% increase in ablation area compared to other catheters. Importantly, initial catheter selection depends on baseline stenosis severity, not the normal vessel reference diameter; the greater the stenosis, the smaller the initial catheter size. Eccentric and concentric lesions can be adequately recanalized with concentric catheters, but greater plaque ablation can be achieved by 4-quadrant ablation with eccentric catheters. Eccentric catheters require careful manipulation and are frequently used for debulking stent restenosis.[12] Laser safety is important; the patient and all catheterization personnel must wear special protective goggles whenever the laser is enabled.

2. **Lasing Technique.** The most important aspect of laser angioplasty is use of the *heparinized flush technique* to eliminate contrast from the lasing field and minimize acoustic injury.[13,14] Using heparinized saline or dextrose, all contrast must be cleared from the manifold, Y connector, tubing, and guide catheter prior to lasing. Immediately before lasing, 5-10 ml of heparinized flush is rapidly injected through the guide catheter. As the operator initiates lasing (using 5 seconds "trains"), an assistant injects flush at a rate of 2-3 ml/second using a 20-30 ml syringe. Transient Q-T prolongation can be minimized by using heparinized dextrose instead of saline. Angiography can be repeated at any time, but contrast *must* be flushed from the system prior to further lasing.

Table 30.3. Excimer Laser Coronary Angioplasty: Indications and Contraindications

Lesion-Specific Indications	Contraindications
Debulking prior to stent deployment	Lesions not traversable by a guidewire
Stent restenosis	Unprotected left main stenoses
Total occlusion crossed by a guide wire	Coronary artery perforation or dissection
Saphenous vein grafts (ostial or focal lesions)	Lesion angulation > 45°
Thrombotic lesions	Extreme tortuosity of proximal target vessel
Long lesions	Degenerated saphenous vein grafts
Nondilatable lesions	
Focal lesions in heart transplant patients	

It is important to advance the laser catheter *very slowly* (0.2-0.5 mm/sec) during laser emission, since the depth of penetration is only 35-50 microns.[11] Any attempt to hasten the procedure by rapid advancement of the laser will result in "dottering" rather than plaque ablation. We recommend 2-3 trains of laser emission (total 250-375 pulses), followed by retraction of the laser catheter into the guide catheter, injection of intracoronary nitroglycerin, and repeat angiography. The laser catheter can be then readvanced, or a larger laser catheter can be used, if necessary. Such "pulse and retreat" lasing[15] minimizes acoustic injury. Lasing during retraction of the laser catheter is not recommended since the laser catheter may not be in contact with the target lesion. Energy fluence is usually set at 45 mJ/mm^2 (25 Hz), but higher energy (60 mJ/mm^2; 40 Hz) may be required for thrombotic or resistant lesions. If these energy levels are not successful, lasing should be abandoned. The composition of the target lesion affects the required energy level; restenosis lesions, known to consist largely of smooth muscle cells, require more laser pulses than de novo lesions, which contain thrombi, cholesterol plaque, and fibrosis.[16] Incorporation of safe lasing techniques results in virtual elimination of perforation, acute closure, severe dissection, and refractory spasm.[17-19] A "wireless" lasing technique for lesions resistant to guidewire crossing has recently been described for selected patients with aorto-ostial total occlusions.[20]

D. RESULTS

1. **Observational Studies.** Two large observational studies of excimer laser angioplasty were reported prior to the routine use of stents (Table 30.6): The Spectranetics Laser Registry[19] and the AIS Registry.[21] Clinical success, defined as ≤50% stenosis and no major complications, was achieved in 90% of patients. The incidence of complications tended to decrease with greater operator experience, but the benefits of routine saline infusion and slow catheter advancement were not appreciated when these studies were performed. The Holmium:YAG Laser Multicenter Study[22] was completed in 1997 (Table 30.7), and suggested that the mid-infrared laser could be successfully and safely applied to complex lesions, particularly in patients with acute ischemic syndromes. Limitations of these older lasers were cost, the need for adjunctive balloon angioplasty or stenting to achieve definitive lumen enlargement, and lack of benefit on restenosis.

Table 30.4. Comparison of Tissue Penetration and Ablation Area with Vitesse Laser Catheters

Catheter Type	Penetration Rate (μm/pulse)	p-Value	Ablated Area (mm²)	p-Value
2.0mm Vitesse C	7 ± 2.3	0.0009	1.5	0.01
2.0mm Vitesse C_{OS}	3 ± 0.3		2.7	
1.7mm Vitesse C	7 ± 1.2	0.0005	1.1	0.0003
1.7mm Vitesse C_{OS}	2 ± 0.7		1.7	
1.4mm Vitesse C	10 ± 2.3	0.0001	0.9	0.0006
1.4mm Vitesse C_{OS}	4 ± 2.3		1.3	

Abbreviations: Vitesse C = standard concentric laser catheter (Spectranetics, Colorado Springs, CO); Vitesse C_{OS} = new, optimally-spaced laser catheter (Spectranetics, Colorado Springs, CO)

2. **Randomized Trials.** Several randomized studies have been completed. In ERBAC (Excimer Laser, Rotational Atherectomy, Balloon Angioplasty Comparison), 620 patients with *de novo* type B or C lesions were randomized to conventional balloon angioplasty, rotational atherectomy, or excimer laser angioplasty (Table 30.8).[23,24] Despite better initial lumen enlargement, neither excimer laser nor Rotablator was superior to PTCA in terms of late restenosis or target lesion revascularization. The AMRO (Amsterdam-Rotterdam) Trial randomized 308 patients with long lesions to excimer laser or balloon angioplasty (Table 30.9);[25] no benefit was observed for ELCA. The laser arm did not incorporate the saline infusion or slow catheter advancement technique in either ERBAC or AMRO. The LAVA (Laser Angioplasty Versus Angioplasty) study was a prospective, randomized multicenter study comparing the holmium:YAG laser with PTCA,[26] but was prematurely terminated because of insufficient enrollment. In-hospital success rates and final diameter stenosis were similar with balloon angioplasty and laser.

E. LESION AND PATIENT APPLICATIONS

1. **Thrombotic Lesions.** The presence of intracoronary thrombus is known to increase the risk of PTCA.[27,28] In the early 1990's, many operators refrained from using lasers in patients with intracoronary thrombus because of concerns about distal embolization.[29] Since then, many of these concerns have been allayed due to refinements in catheter technology[11,30,31] and routine use of heparinized-flush techniques.[14,17] In-vitro studies of excimer laser and thrombus demonstrated significant suppression of platelet aggregation,[32-35] and recent clinical experience demonstrated considerable success in patients with thrombotic lesions[36,37] (Figure 30.1) (Table 30.10). The potential of laser energy to augment the effect of t-PA on thrombus and to reverse the resistance of old thrombus to t-PA has been recently recognized.[38]

Table 30.5. Characteristics of Excimer Laser Coronary and EPS Catheters (Spectranetics)

	Working Length (cm)	Minimum Guide Catheter, ID (inch)	Maximum Guidewire (inch)	Proximal Shaft Size (inch/Fr)	Distal Shaft Size (inch/Fr)	Number of Fibers	Fiber Core (microns)	Total Optical Area (mm²)	Repetition Range (Hertz)	Fluence Range (mJ/mm²)	Output at 45 Fluence (mJ)
Coronary Catheters											
1.4mm Vitesse C	135	0.072	0.014	.052/4.0	.055/4.2	108	61	0.32	25-40	30-60	13.1
1.7mm Vitesse C	135	0.080	0.018	.055/4.2	.063/4.8	140	61	0.40	25-40	30-60	18.9
2.0mm Vitesse C	135	0.088	0.018	.069/5.3	.076/5.8	250	61	0.73	25-40	30-60	32.0
1.4mm Vitesse C_{OS}	135	0.072	0.014	.052/4.0	.055/4.2	108	61	0.32	25-40	30-60	13.1
1.7mm Vitesse C_{OS}	135	0.080	0.018	.055/4.2	.063/4.8	140	61	0.40	25-40	30-60	18.9
2.0mm Vitesse C_{OS}	135	0.088	0.018	.069/5.3	.076/5.8	250	61	0.73	25-40	30-60	32.0
1.7mm Vitesse E	135	0.080	0.014	.057/4.4	.063/4.8	185	50	0.36	25-40	30-60	16.7
2.0mm Vitesse E	135	0.088	0.018	.066/5.0	.076/5.8	290	50	0.57	25-40	30-60	24.8
0.9mm Extreme	135	0.060	0.014	.046/3.5	.037/2.8	65	50	0.13	25-40	30-60	5.9
0.9mm Vitesse	135	0.060	0.014	.044/3.5	.037/2.8	65	50	0.13	25-40	30-60	5.9
Prima FX Laserwire*	135	0.060	NA	.018/1.4	.018/1.4	12	45	0.02	25-80	30-80	0.9
Prima SX Laserwire*	135	0.060	NA	.018/1.4	.018/1.4	12	45	0.02	25-80	30-80	0.9
Peripheral Catheters											
2.0mm Extreme‡	135	0.090	0.018	.074/5.6	.076/5.8	240	61	0.70	25-40	30-60	32.0
2.2mm Extreme‡	120	0.090	0.035	.089/6.8	.089/6.8	104	100	0.82	25-40	30-60	36.5
2.5mm Extreme‡	100	0.090	0.035	.099/7.6	.099/7.6	95	130	1.26	25-40	30-50	55.9
2.0mm Extreme OS^2*	135	0.090	0.035	.074/6.6	.076/5.8	150	61	0.44	25-40	30-60	18.9
2.2mm Extreme OS^2*	120	0.090	0.035	.084/6.4	.089/6.8	104	100	0.82	25-40	30-60	36.5
2.5mm Extreme OS^2*	100	0.090	0.035	.095/7.3	.099/7.6	95	130	1.28	25-40	30-50	55.9
Lead Removal Catheters											
12 French Laser Sheath	40	NA	0.098	.163/12.4+	.163/12.4+	82	100	0.64	25-40	30-60	32.0
14 French Laser Sheath	40	NA	0.111	.190/14.5+	.190/14.5+	101	100	0.79	25-40	30-60	32.0
16 French Laser Sheath	40	NA	0.150	.220/16.8+	.220/16.8+	118	100	0.91	25-40	30-60	36.5

* Not approved for USA distribution

‡ Investigational use

+ = maximum

NA = not applicable

Table 30.6. Observational Studies of ELCA

	Spectranetics Registry[19]	AIS Registry[21]
No. Patients	2432	3000
Device Success (%)	86	84
Clinical Success (%)*	89	90
MACE (%)		
Death	0	0.5
QMI	1.0	2.1
CABG	3.0	3.8
nQMI	2.5	2.3
Angiographic Complications (%)		
Dissection	5.5	13
Acute closure	5.0	6.5
Perforation	0.5	0.6
Angiographic Restenosis (%)	-	58**

Abbreviations: MACE = major adverse cardiac events; QMI = Q-wave myocardial infarction; nQMI = non-Q-wave myocardial infarction
* Lesion-specific success: ostial (86%), long (86%), calcified (83%), SVG (96%), total occlusion (84%)
**Pre-stent area

2. **Stent Restenosis.** Treatment of stent restenosis with laser energy has recently received considerable attention. Immediate procedural success rates exceed 92%, and complication rates are low (Chapter 26).[39-43]

3. **Heart Transplant Recipients.** Severe allograft coronary artery disease is the main cause of death in heart transplant recipients.[44] Percutaneous revascularization has been attempted with PTCA, directional atherectomy, and rotational atherectomy, with variable success.[45] Laser angioplasty (excimer and holmium:YAG) has recently been reported to be safe in complex, focal, atherosclerotic lesions in heart transplant recipients.[46-48]

4. **Saphenous Vein Grafts.** ELCA (with adjunctive stenting) can be successfully applied to aorto-ostial lesions and focal, thrombotic lesions in vein grafts with success rates > 90%.[49-51] In contrast to other devices, the presence of a saphenous vein graft lesion has been reported as a predictor for procedural success after ELCA.[37] However, diffusely degenerated grafts should not be treated by laser angioplasty.[52]

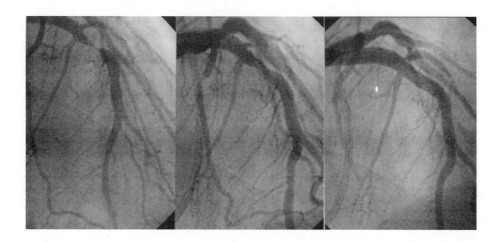

Figure 30.1. Excimer Laser for Unstable Angina

ELCA of a patient with unstable angina and anterior ischemia.
Left panel: Target lesion in the LAD
Middle panel: Post-lasing result with a 2.0 mm excimer laser (45mJ/mm^2; 25 Hz; 500 pulses)
Right panel: Final result

Table 30.7. Mid-Infrared Laser Multicenter Study[22]

No. Patients	1862
Device Success (%)	87
Procedural Success (%)	93
MACE (%)	
Death	0.8
QMI	1.2
CABG	2.5
Angiographic Complications (%)	
Perforation	2.2
Dissection	5.8
Spasm	12.0
Angiographic Restenosis (%)	54

Abbreviations: MACE = major adverse cardiac events; CABG = coronary artery bypass grafting; QMI = Q-wave myocardial infarction

Table 30.8. ERBAC Trial[24]

	PTCA (n = 210)	ELCA (n = 195)	Rotablator (n = 215)	p-Value
Type B₂/C lesions (%)	72	78	85	-
Final DS (%)	36	32	31	< 0.05
In-hospital MACE (%)	4.8	6.2	2.3	< 0.05
6-month Outcome (%)				
Death	3.1	0	2.6	NS
QMI	3.8	0.7	3.2	NS
TLR	35	46	46	< 0.05
ARS	54	60	62	NS

Abbreviations: ARS = angiographic restenosis; DS = diameter stenosis; ERBAC = Excimer Laser Rotablator Balloon Angioplasty Comparison; MACE = major adverse cardiac events; TLR = target lesion revascularization; Type B₂/C = ACC/AHA classification type B₂ or C; QMI = Q-wave myocardial infarction

5. **Total Occlusions.** The 0.018-inch excimer laser guidewire contains 12 optical fibers, a lubricious coating, and a 3-cm radiopaque tip. The laserwire can traverse about 50% of total occlusions that are refractory to other PTCA guidewires,[53] but severe dissection (7.5%) and extravascular protrusion (24%) are important limitations. The laserwire has not gained widespread acceptance because of prolonged fluoroscopy time, large contrast volumes, and the risk of tamponade. Most operators prefer to use the over-the-wire laser once the occlusion has been crossed with a guidewire.

6. **Peripheral Vascular Disease.** A variety of laser sources have been used for lower extremity arterial revascularization,[56] but more favorable experience has been reported with the excimer laser.[57,58] Biamino and colleagues [59] have utilized a "step-by-step" laser method in long occlusions that cannot be traversed with conventional guidewires. The "step-by-step" method involves advancement of the laser catheter and guidewire as a unit through the occlusion; as the laser catheter engages the obstruction, the guidewire is advanced a few millimeters into the occlusion, and the laser is activated to debulk the obstruction.

F. **LASER-INDUCED COMPLICATIONS.** The most severe complications of laser intervention include perforation, dissection, and acute closure.[60-63] The frequency of coronary artery perforation has declined with increasing operator experience, although the risk of perforation may be higher in women, bifurcation lesions, and with oversized laser catheters.[63,64] Dissection, acute closure, thrombosis, and distal embolization are rarely encountered when the saline infusion technique is employed.[64,65] Operator judgement and careful debulking can significantly reduce laser-induced complications.[57,]

Table 30.9. Dutch AMRO Study: Comparison of ELCA and PTCA[25,53,54]

	PTCA (n = 157)	ELCA (n = 151)
Angiographic Success (%)	79	80
Angiographic Complications (%)		
Dissection	55	47
Spasm	1	4
Perforation	1	3
Transient occlusion	0.7	7*
Clinical Events at 6 Months (%)		
Death	0	0
Myocardial infarction	5.7	4.6
Coronary artery bypass surgery	10.8	10.6
Repeat PTCA	18.5	21.2
Overall clinical events	29.9	33
Restenosis (stenosis > 50%)	41.3	51.6

AMRO = Amsterdam Rotterdam Trial
* $p = 0.005$

Table 30.10. ELCA in Thrombotic Lesions[36]

	Unstable Angina (n = 33)	Acute MI (n = 26)
Thrombus Area Pre-Laser (mm^2)	38 ± 16	123 ±354
Thrombus Area Post-Laser (mm^2)	1 ± 2	5 ± 7
Thrombus Reduction by Laser (%)	97	96

* * * * *

REFERENCES

1. Topaz O. Coronary laser angioplasty. In Topol EJ (ed): Textbook of Interventional Cardiology, ed 2. Philadelphia, WB Saunders, 1995, pp 235-255.

2. Milonni PW, Eberly JH. Introduction to laser operation. In: Milonni PW, Eberly JH (eds) Lasers. New York, John Wiley & Sons, 1988;pp 1-19.

3. Cross FW, Bowker TJ. The excimer laser-tissue interactions and early clinical results, In: Abela GS (ed) Lasers in Cardiovascular Medicine and Surgery: Fundamentals and Techniques. Boston, Kluwer Academic Publishers, 1990 pp 45-48.

4. Thomsen S. Pathologic analysis of photothermal and photochemical effects of laser-tissue interactions. Photochem Photobiol 1991; 53:825-826.

5. Topaz O. Plaque removal and thrombus dissolution with pulsed-wave lasers' photoacoustic energy: biotissue interactions and their clinical manifestations. Cardiology 1996;87:384-391.

6. van Leeuwen TG, van Erven I, Meertens JH, et al. Intraluminal vapor bubble induced by excimer laser pulse causes microsecond arterial dilation and invagination leading to extensive wall damage in the rabbit. Circulation 1993;87:1258-1263.

7. Hasse K, Hanke H, Baumbach A, et al. Occurrence, extent and implication of pressure waves during excimer laser ablation of normal arterial wall and atherosclerotic plaque. Lasers Surg Med 1993;13:263-270.

8. Tomaru T, Geschwind HJ, Bourssignac G. Characteristics of shock waves induced by pulsed lasers and their effect on arterial tissue: comparison of excimer, pulsed-dye and holmium:YAG lasers. Am Heart J 1992;123:896-904.

9. Abela GS. Abrupt closure after pulsed laser angioplasty: spasm or a "mille Feuilles" effect? J Intervent Cardiol 1992;5:259-262.

10. Topaz O, Rozenbaum EA, Luxenberg MG, Schumacher A. Laser assisted coronary angioplasty in patients with severely depressed left ventricular function: quantitative coronary angioplasty and clinical results. J Intervent Cardiol 1995;8:661-669.

11. Topaz O, Lippincott R, Bellendir J, Taylor K, Reiser C. Optimally spaced excimer laser coronary catheters: performance analysis. J Clin Laser Med Surg 2001 (in press).

12. Mehran R, Mintz GS, Satler LF, Pichard AD, Kent KM, Bucher TA, Popma JJ, Leon MB. Treatment of in-stent restenosis with excimer laser coronary angioplasty. Circulation 1997;96:2183-2189.

13. Ginsburg R. Laser Angioplasty Technique. In Ginsburg R, Geschwind HJ (eds). Primer on Laser Angioplasty, 2nd edition, Mount Kisco, NY, Futura 1992; pp. 269-274.

14. Tcheng JE. Saline infusion in excimer laser coronary angioplasty. Semin Intervent Cardiol 1996;1:135-141.

15. Topaz O. A new, safer lasing technique for laser-facilitated coronary angioplasty. J Intervent Cardiol 1993;6:297-306.

16. Topaz O, McIvor M, deMarchena E. Solid-state, pulsed-wave, mid-infrared coronary laser angioplasty in de novo versus restenosis lesions. Observations from a multicenter study. J Clin Laser Med Surg 1995;13:319-323.

17. Deckelbaum LI, Natarajan MK, Bittl JA, et al. Effect of intracoronary saline infusion on dissection during excimer laser coronary angioplasty: a randomized trial. J Am Coll Cardiol 1995;26:1264-1269.

18. Tcheng JE, Wells LD, Phillips HR, et al. Development of a new technique for reducing pressure pulse generation during 308nm excimer laser coronary angioplasty. Cath Cardiovasc Diagn 1995;34:15-22.

19. Bittl JA. Clinical results with excimer laser coronary angioplasty. Semin Intervent Cardiol 1996;1:129-134.

20. Perin EC, Leite-Sarmento R, Silva GV, et al. "Wireless" laser recanalization of chronic total coronary occlusions. J Invas Cardiol 2001 (In press).

21. Litvack F, Eigler N, Margolis J, et al. Percutaneous excimer laser coronary angioplasty: results in the first consecutive 3000 patients. J Am Coll Cardiol 1994;23:323-330.

22. Topaz O, McIvor M, Stone GW, et al. An analysis of acute results, complications and effect of lesion characteristics on outcome with the solid-state, pulsed-wave, mid-infrared laser angioplasty system: Final multicenter registry report. Laser Surg Med 1998;22:228-229.

23. Reifart N, Vandormael M, et al. Randomized comparison of angioplasty of complex coronary lesions at a single center. Circulation 1997;96:91-98.

24. Vandormael M, Reifart N, Preusler W, et al. Six months follow-up results following excimer laser angioplasty, rotational atherectomy and balloon angioplasty for complex lesions: ERBAC study. Circulation 1994;90:I-213A.

25. Appleman YEA, Pick JJ, Strikwerda S, et al. Randomized trial of excimer laser versus balloon angioplasty for treatment of obstructive coronary artery disease. Lancet 1996;347:79-84.

26. Stone GW, deMarchena E, Dageforde D, et al. A prospective, randomized, multi-center comparison of laser facilitated balloon angioplasty versus balloon angioplasty in patients with obstructive coronary artery disease. J Am Coll Cardiol 1997; 30:1714-1721.

27. Vetrovec GW, Cowley MJ, Overton H, et al. Intracoronary thrombus in syndromes of unstable myocardial ischemia. Am Heart J 1981;102:1202-1208.

28. White CJ, Ramee SR, Collins TJ, et al. Coronary thrombi increase PTCA risk. Circulation 1996; 93:253-258.

29. Estella P, Ryan TJ, Lanzberg JS, et al. Excimer laser assisted coronary angioplasty in lesions containing thrombus. J Am Coll Cardiol 1993;21:1550-1556.

30. Gijsbers GHM, Hamburger JN, Serruys PW. Homogeneous light distributing to reduce vessel trauma during the excimer laser angioplasty. Semin Intervent Cardiol 1996;1:143-148.

31. Taylor K, Reiser C. Large eccentric laser angioplasty catheter. In Proceeding of lasers in surgery: advanced characterization, therapeutics and systems. SPIE 1997;2970:34-41.

32. Gregory KW. Laser Thrombolysis. In Topol EJ (ed). Textbook of Interventional Cardiology, 2nd edition, WB Saunders, Philadelphia. 1993; pp 892-903.

33. Bonn D. Laser thrombolysis: safe and rapid removal of clots? Lancet 2000;355:1976.

34. Topaz O, Minisi AJ, Bernardo NL, McPherson RA, Martin E, Carr SL, Carr ME. Effect of excimer laser emission on platelet aggregation: the stunned platelets phenomenon. Submitted for publication.

35. Topaz O, Bernardo N, McQueen R, Desai P, Janin Y, Lansky AJ, Carr ME. Excimer laser angioplasty in acute coronary syndromes. Cath Cardiovasc Intervent 2000;50:154.

36. Topaz O, Bernardo NL, McQueen R, Desai P, Janin Y, Lansky AJ, Carr ME. Effectiveness of excimer laser coronary angioplasty in acute myocardial infarction or in unstable angina pectoris. Am J Cardiol 2001 (in press).

37. Bittl JA, Sanborn TA, Tcheng JE, Siegel RM, Ellis SG. Clinical success, complication and restenosis rates with excimer laser coronary angioplasty. Am J Cardiol 1992;70:1533-1539.

38. Topaz O, Morris C, Minisi AJ, Mohanty PK, Carr ME. Enhancement of t-PA induced fibrinolysis with laser energy: in-vitro observations. Lasers Med Sci 1999;14:123-128.

39. Topaz O, Vetrovec GW. The stenotic stent: mechanisms and revascularization options. Cath Cardiovasc Diagn 1996; 37:293-299.

40. Topaz O, Vetrovec GW. Rescue revascularization of tandem occluded intracoronary stents: technique and equipment. Cath Cardiovasc Diagn 1996;39:185-190.

41. Koster R, Hamm CW, Seabra-Gomes R, et al. Treatment of in-stent coronary restenosis by excimer laser angioplasty. Am J Cardiol 1998;80:1424-1428.

42. Koster R, Hamm CW, Seabra-Gomes R, et al. Laser angioplasty of restenosed coronary stents: results of a multicenter surveillance trial. J Am Coll Cardiol 1999;34:25-32.

43. Dahm JB, Kuon E. High-energy eccentric excimer laser angioplasty for debulking diffuse in-stent restenosis lead to better acute and 6-month follow-up results. J Invas Cardiology 2000;12:335-342.

44. Hosenpud JD, Shipley GD, Wagner CR. Cardiac allograft vasculopathy: currentconcepts, recent developments and future directions. J Heart Lung Transplant 1992;11:9-23.

45. Topaz O, Ebersole D, Dahn J, et al. Excimer laser revascularization: current indications, applications and technniques. Lasers Med Science 2001.

46. Topaz O, Cowley MJ, Mohanty PK, Vetrovec GW. Percutaneous revascularization modalities for heart transplant recipients. Cath Cardiovasc Intervent 1999;46:227-237.

47. Topaz O, Janin Y, Bernardo N, Bailey NT, Mohanty PK. Coronary revascularization in heart transplant recipients by excimer laser angioplasty. Laser Surg Med 2000;26:425-431.

48. Topaz O, Bailey NT, Mohanty PK. Application of solid-state, pulsed-wave, mid-infrared laser for percutaneous revascularization in heart transplant recipients. J Heart Lung Transp 1998;17:505-510.

49. Bittl JA, Sanborn TA, Yardley DE, et al. Predictors of outcome of percutaneous excimer laser coronary angioplasty of saphenous vein bypass lesions. Am J Cardiol 1994;74:144-148.

50. Tcheng JE, Bittl JA, Sanborn TA, et al. Treatment of aorto-ostial disease with percutaneous excimer laser coronary angioplasty (abstract). Circulation 1992; 86{Suppl I):512A.

51. Eigler NI, Weinstock B, Douglas JS Jr, et al. Excimer laser coronary angioplasty of aorto-ostial stenoses: results of the Excimer Laser Coronary Angioplasty Registry in the first 200 patients. Circulation 1993;88:2049-2057.

52. Topaz O, Bernardo NL, Desai P, Janin Y. Acute thrombotic-ischemic syndromes - the usefulness of TEC. Cath Cardiovasc Interventions 1999;48:406-420.

53. Foley DP, Appelman YE, Piek JJ on behalf of the AMRO group. Comparison of angiographic restenosis propensity of excimer laser coronary angioplasty (ELCA) and balloon angioplasty (BA) in the Amsterdam Rotterdam (AMRO) Trial. Circulation 1995;92:I-477.

54. Koolen J, Appelman Y, Strikwerda S, et al. I.nitial and long-term results of excimer laser coronary angioplasty versus balloon angioplasty in functional and total coronary occlusions. Eur Heart Journal 1994:832.

55. Hamburger JN, deFeyter PJ, Serruys PW. The laser guidewire experience: "crossing the Rubicon". Semin Intervent Cardiol 1996; 1:163-171.

56. Barbeau GR, Seeger TJ, Jablowski S, et al. Peripheral artery recanalization in humans using balloon and laser angioplasty. Clin Cardiol 1996;19:232-238.

57. Topaz O. Whose fault is it? Notes on "true" versus "pseudo" laser failure. Editorial. Cath Cardiovasc Diagn. 1995;36:1-4.

58. Isner JM, Rosenfield K. Redefining the treatment of peripheral artery disease: role of percutaneous revascularization. Circulation 1993;84:1534-1557.

59. Biamino GC, Ragg JC, Struk B, Schweiger U, Bottcher H. Long occlusions of the superficial femoral artery: success rate and 1 year follow-up after excimer laser assisted angioplasty. Eur Heart J 1994;15(Suppl):147 (915).

60. Topaz O. Laser. In Textbook of Interventional Cardiology, Topol EJ (ed). 3rd edition, WB Saunders, Philadelphia 1988, pp 615-633.

61. deMarchena E, Larrain G, Posada JD. Holmium laser assisted coronary angioplasty in acute ischemic syndromes. Clin Cardiol 1996; 19:315-319.

62. Topaz O, Rosenbaum EA, Schumacher A, Luxenberg MG. Solid-state, mid-infrared laser facilitated coronary angioplasty: clinical and quantitative angiographic results in 112 patients. Laser Surg Med 1996;19:260-272.

63. Holmes DR Jr, Reeder GS, Chazzal ZMB, et al. Coronary perforation after excimer laser angioplasty: The excimer laser coronary angioplasty registry experience. J Am Coll Cardiol 1994;23:330-335.

64. Baumbach A, Bittl JA, Fleck E, et al. Acute complications of excimer laser coronary angioplasty: A detailed analysis of multicenter results. J Am Coll Cardiol 1994;23:1305-1313.

65. Bittl JA, Brinker JA, Sanborn TA, et al. The changing profile of patient selection, procedural techniques, and outcomes in excimer laser coronary angioplasty. J Intervent Cardiol 1995;8:653-660.

INTRAVASCULAR ULTRASOUND

31

Anthony C. De Franco, MD, Robert D. Safian, MD,
Khaled M. Ziada, MD, E. Murat Tuzcu, MD,
Steven E. Nissen, MD

The incremental value of intravascular ultrasound (IVUS) compared to contrast angiography is due to its tomographic perspective and its ability to directly image atheroma and the vessel wall. Angiography depicts cross-sectional coronary anatomy as a planar silhouette of the lumen, whereas direct imaging by IVUS allows measurement of atheroma size, distribution, and composition. Although angiography remains the principal method to assess the extent of coronary atherosclerosis and to guide percutaneous coronary intervention, intravascular ultrasound has become a vital adjunctive imaging modality.

A.   RATIONALE FOR INTRAVASCULAR ULTRASOUND

1.   **Limitations of Angiography in Assessing Lesion and Disease Severity**. Contrast angiography has several limitations (Table 31.1).[1-9] Visual estimates of stenosis severity have significant intra- and interobserver variability,[3-5] and angiography significantly underestimates the extent of atherosclerosis detected by autopsy.[6-9] Several factors account for the inaccuracy of coronary angiography. First, angiography is a two-dimensional imaging modality, depicting complex coronary cross-sectional anatomy as a planar silhouette of a contrast-filled lumen. Necropsy and IVUS studies demonstrate that coronary lesions are often highly complex and eccentric, leading to both under- and overestimation of stenosis severity by angiography (Figure 31.1).[1,10,11] Second, visual and computer-assisted techniques to assess stenosis severity rely on comparisons to the adjacent "normal" reference segment. However, necropsy and IVUS examinations confirm that angiography frequently underestimates true disease severity,[1,2,12] since the "normal" segment is often diffusely diseased. Third, angiography is limited by the resolution of fluoroscopic imaging, motion artifacts, and inability to visualize structures smaller than 0.2 mm such as intracoronary thrombi or calcification.[13] Fourth, percutaneous interventional techniques increase the complexity and irregularity of luminal shape, exaggerating luminal eccentricity by fracturing the atheroma.[10,12,14,15]   Consequently, extensive plaque fracture frequently results in a "hazy" appearance, which typically overestimates the true vessel cross-section dimension (Figure 31.2).[12] Finally, angiography cannot assess the atheroma within the arterial wall (Figure 31.3). Vascular "remodeling" due to outward displacement of the vessel wall permits accumulation of atheroma without encroaching on the lumen.[16] Since lumen reduction does not occur until the plaque occupies more than 40% of the total vessel cross-sectional area, such lesions are frequently missed by angiography, yet are potential substrates for acute coronary syndromes due to ulceration and thrombosis.[17]

Table 31.1. Comparison of Imaging and Hemodynamic Techniques

Characteristic	Digital Angiography	Angioscopy	IVUS	Doppler FloWire	Pressure Wire
Vessel lumen detail	+	++++	++	-	-
Vessel wall detail	-	-	++++	-	-
Plaque composition	-	++	+++	-	-
Vessel dimensions	++	-	++++	-	-
Identify disease in "normal" vessel	+	++	++++	-	-
Detect diffuse disease	+	++	++++	-	-
Evaluate "haziness"	±	+++	+++	+	+
Arterial remodeling	±	-	++++	-	-
Borderline lesions - morphology	+	-	++++	-	-
Borderline lesions - physiology	-	-	+	++++	++++
Suboptimal results	+	++	+++	+++	++++
Clot vs. dissection	±	++++	+++	-	-
Predict complications	+	unknown	possible	+++	possible
Continuous record (trend)	-	-	-	+++	-
Predict restenosis	+	-	++	++	unknown
Microvascular disease	-	-	-	+++	-
Cause of ischemia	-	+++	+	-	-

Abbreviations: IVUS = intravascular ultrasound
- = no value
± = limited value
+ thru ++++ = increasing value

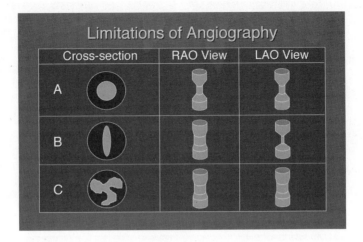

Figure 31.1. Schematic Demonstrating the Limitations of Angiography

Panel A: When the reference segment is normal and the lesion is simple and concentric, orthogonal angiographic views provide a relatively accurate assessment of lumen morphology and size. Panel B: A severe slit-like stenosis may be underestimated (RAO view) or overestimated (LAO view), depending on the angiographic projection. Panel C: Angiography cannot accurately represent complex luminal shapes; in this situation, multiple orthogonal projections will not lead to an accurate assessment of lumen diameter or lesion morophology.

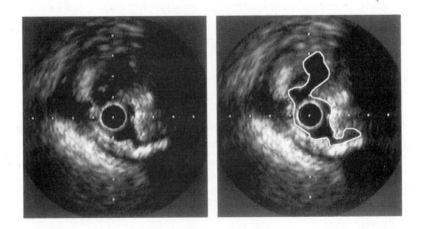

Figure 31.2. Complex Lumen Morphology After PTCA

Intraluminal haziness is commonly observed after PTCA, but IVUS frequently demonstrates complex lumen morphology and high grade residual stenosis (the intimal edge is outlined on the right).

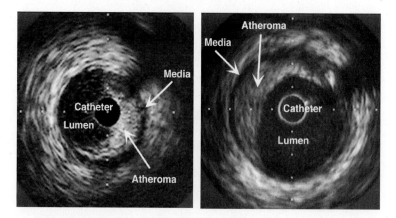

Figure 31.3. Arterial Remodeling and Occult Atherosclerosis

Angiography failed to demonstrate the atherosclerotic lesions in either vessel. Despite the presence of moderate atheroma by IVUS, the lesion appeared circular and normal by angiography.

2. **Advantages of Ultrasound (Table 31.2).** Intravascular ultrasound has several important advantages over contrast angiography. First, IVUS allows precise quantitation of disease severity.[11,19,20] Second, the tomographic orientation enables visualization of the entire circumference of the vessel wall, rather than a two-dimensional silhouette of the lumen. Third, IVUS allows characterization of plaque composition, distribution, and length, which has important implications for device selection and assessment of results. Finally, ultrasound allows the cardiologist to assess disease in vessels that are typically difficult to image by conventional angiography, including diffusely diseased segments, lesions at bifurcation sites, ostial stenoses, and highly eccentric plaques.[12] Although vessel foreshortening and overlapping structures often preclude accurate quantitative angiography, IVUS is unaffected by these factors.

Table 31.2. Advantages of IVUS

Precise Quantitative Measurements
 Lumen diameter
 Reference vessel diameter
 Cross-sectional area (CSA)
 Lesion length (automatic pulllback)

Characterization of Plaque
 Arterial remodeling (positive, negative)
 Plaque stability
 Plaque distribution (eccentric, concentric)
 Plaque composition (soft, fibrous, calcified, mixed; depth of calcium [deep, superficial])
 Dissection (length, severity of lumen compromise)

B. ULTRASOUND EQUIPMENT AND TECHNIQUE

1. **Ultrasound Catheters (Table 31.3).** All intracoronary ultrasound systems consist of two major components: a catheter incorporating a miniaturized transducer, and a console containing the electronics necessary to reconstruct the image. Since the transducer is close to the arterial wall, high frequencies (20-45 MHz) are necessary to enhance resolution (axial resolution is approximately 100 microns). The determinants of lateral resolution are more complex, but lateral resolution (for a 30 MHz device) is approximately 250 microns. Currently, there are two different types of ultrasound transducers—mechanical devices and multi-element electronic arrays—each with their own imaging and handling characteristics. Mechanical transducers (such as those manufactured by Boston Scientific Scimed) employ a drive cable that rotates a single piezoelectric transducer mounted near the distal catheter tip. For mechanical ultrasound systems, a rotation rate of 1800 rpm is used, yielding 30 images per second. In contrast, fully electronic ultrasound systems (such as those manufactured by EndoSonics Corporation) have an annular array of 64 piezoelectric elements which are activated sequentially to generate a tomographic image. The electronic signals are processed by several ultra-miniaturized integrated circuits near the catheter tip and require only two conductive wires (rather than a drive cable) within the catheter. Intracoronary ultrasound catheters currently available in the United States have an outer diameter of 2.9-3.5 French (diameter of 0.96-1.17 mm). The smallest catheters can be placed through a large lumen 6F guide, although 7 and 8F guides are sometimes preferable (as described below). Most ultrasound catheters are monorail designs to facilitate rapid exchange. Multi-element designs generally have greater flexibility, but mechanical transducers have traditionally provided better image quality. These differences have narrowed in recent years. The ultrasound console includes the computer processor, which reconstructs the image, and an integrated videotape recording system on Super-VHS tape. Digital image recording technology has recently been introduced to IVUS imaging, and at least one commercially available system permits digital recording of a 60-second pullback. This system can display the acquired "loop" at variable playback rates, provides digital freeze-frames, and permits archival of the imagine sequence to CD-ROM.

2. **Examination Technique.** Intracoronary ultrasound is performed using standard interventional techniques.[21] Intravenous heparin (to maintain the ACT > 200-250 sec) is recommended prior to imaging, although there are no controlled studies proving its necessity. Most practitioners employ a 6 or 7F guiding catheter and a flexible 0.014-inch angioplasty guidewire. A stable guiding catheter position with good support is desirable, since current ultrasound catheters have less trackability and a larger profile than PTCA catheters. We recommend intracoronary nitroglycerin (100-200 mcg) prior to each imaging run to prevent coronary spasm and to achieve maximal vasodilation. Once the lesion has been crossed by a guidewire, the imaging catheter is carefully advanced so the transducer is distal to the target lesion. The automatic pullback device is activated to retract the catheter at a constant speed (usually 0.5 mm/sec) while recording images on videotape. There are three major reasons for routine use of automatic pullback devices: First, by starting every IVUS study at a designated landmark (such as a prominent branch), the entire imaging sequence can be reviewed from the same location.

Table 31.3. Intravascular Ultrasound Systems

System	Guiding Catheter	Frequency (MHz)	Main Uses	Scanner Console Required
Atlantis SR™*	6F	40	Coronary	Scimed ClearView™ or Galaxy™
Ultracross™ 3.2*	7F	30	Coronary	Scimed ClearView™ or Galaxy™
Ultracross™ 2.9	7F	30	Tortuous anatomy, total occlusions, etc. No guidewire artifact	Scimed ClearView™ or Galaxy™
Sonicath™ 3.2*	8F	20	Renal and iliacs	Scimed ClearView™ or Galaxy™
Sonicath Ultra™ 9+	9F	9	Aorta	Scimed ClearView™ or Galaxy™
Sonicath Ultra™ 6	8F	12.5 and 20	Aorta, renal and iliacs	Scimed ClearView™ or Galaxy™
Ultra ICE™ 9 F+	9F	9	Intracardiac echo (ICE), radiofrequency ablation	Scimed ClearView™ or Galaxy™
JOMED Avanar F/X	5F	20 phased array	Coronary and peripheral applications; rapid exchange monorail	InVision™ or InVision™ Gold
JOMED Vision 0.018 PV	6F	20 phased array	Coronary and peripheral applications; rapid exchange monorail	InVision™ or InVision™ Gold
JOMED Vision PV 8.2F AAA	8F	10 phased array	Aorta and peripheral arteries	InVision™ or InVision™ Gold

* Rapid-exchange, monorail designs
+ Does not require a guidewire

Second, recording during pullback eliminates uncertainty about the direction in which the catheter was moving and qualitative analysis. Most centers use a motorized pullback device to withdraw the transducer at a constant speed. Third, automatic pullback offers the only reproducible method to measure lesion length, which can assist in estimating the length of the stent necessary to cover the lesion. However, since focal lesions (particularly those at coronary ostia and bifurcations) may be missed by rapid pullback, we recommend a motorized pullback to "survey" the coronary artery, followed by a more thorough examination of sites of interest by manual interrogation. For mechanical systems, catheter designs that allow withdrawal of the transducer within an external sheath minimize catheter rotation or changes in pullback velocity. Sidebranches are useful landmarks to facilitate interpretation and comparison of imaging sequences.

C. IMAGE INTERPRETATION

1. **Normal Coronary Arterial Morphology (Figures 31.4, 31.4A).** IVUS often depicts the normal coronary artery as a trilaminar structure.[22,23] The innermost discrete layer (at the lumen/wall interface) represents the intima. When present, it appears as a delicate, echoreflective (white) band due to acoustic reflections from the internal elastic lamina.   The media is visualized as a distinct echolucent (black or dark gray) middle layer, which is bordered by a third, outer echodense media-

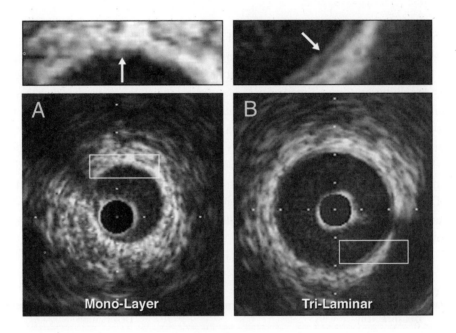

Figure 31.4. Normal Coronary Artery by Intravascular Ultrasound

Left panel: This normal vessel has a monolayer appearance because there are insufficient reflections from the internal elastic lamina to create a trilaminar appearance. Right panel: Reflections from the internal elastic lamina create a trilaminar appearance in two of four quadrants. The innermost layer (top panel) represents reflections from the internal elastic lamina. The smooth muscle cells of the media reflect ultrasound poorly and appear sonolucent (black). The bright white echoes beyond the media represent adventitia. In this example, half of the vessel appears as a monolayer. Higher magnifications are shown at the top of each panel.

adventitia interface. The characteristic trilaminar pattern is not observed in 30-50% of normal coronary arteries; the thin intimal layer reflects ultrasound poorly and often leads to signal dropout and a monolayer appearance.[20] Whether the artery is trilaminar or monolayered, the deepest layers of adventitia and peri-adventitial tissue exhibit a characteristic "onionskin" pattern. The outer border of the vessel is usually indistinct, primarily because there are no acoustic differences between the adventitia and surrounding tissues. Accordingly, total wall thickness cannot be measured reliably using ultrasound, except in vessels with a distinct outer border (such as saphenous vein bypass grafts).

2. **IVUS Measurements (Tables 31.4, 31.5, Figure 31.5).** All measurements during intravascular ultrasound are taken "leading edge to leading edge." *Intimal thickness* is defined as the distance from the intima to the external elastic membrane (adventitial leading edge). Some investigators prefer to call this the "intima-media" or "plaque plus media" thickness, because this measurement includes both media and atheroma.[24] The rationale for this convention is that the normal media is frequently indistinct because its thickness is only slightly greater than the axial resolution of the imaging system.[25,26,27] The most common IVUS measurements include the lumen cross-sectional area (Lcsa), external elastic membrane cross-sectional area (EEMcsa), maximum intimal thickness (IT-max), minimum intimal thickness (IT-min), vessel diameter, and minimum lumen diameter (MLD) (Table 31.4). Common calculations include the percent plaque burden (%PB) or the percent cross-sectional narrowing (%CSN), the intimal index, the eccentricity index, and diameter stenosis (Table 31.5).[28]

Table 31.4. Common IVUS Measurements

Measurement	Description
Intimal thickness (IT) (also called the "intima-media" or "plaque media" thickness) or "atheroma thickness" (when diseased)	Distance from the intima to the external elastic membrane (EEM)
IT-max	Maximum intimal thickness
IT-min	Minimum intimal thickness
ITcsa	Cross-sectional area of the "intima-media" or "plaque-media" space; also referred to as "atheroma area." Can be used as an absolute measure of plaque burden
Lcsa	Lumen cross-sectional area measured within the leading edge of the intima (includes transducer)
MLD	Minimum lumen diameter
EEMcsa (also called the "vessel area" or "medial-adventitial area")	Cross-sectional area measured within the external elastic membrane. It includes the plaque area (ITcsa) and lumen area (Lcsa)

3. **Artifacts and Limitations (Tables 31.6, 31.7).** IVUS artifacts may adversely affect image quality, interfere with image interpretation, and reduce the accuracy of quantitative measurements.[29] Recognition of these artifacts and understanding how to correct them is a critical part of IVUS interpretation (Figure 31.6).

   a. **Image drop-out.** Inadequate flushing of the mechanical ultrasound catheter can result in air bubbles and loss of image quality (Figure 31.6 A). This artifact is easily corrected by proper flushing.

   b. **Guidewire artifact.** With mechanical ultrasound catheters, the presence of the guidewire adjacent to the imaging transducer creates a discrete shadowing artifact, extending from the lumen into the adventitia. This shadowing generally occupies an arc < 12°, and is readily distinguished from shadowing due to vessel calcification (Figure 31.6 B). Although the guidewire artifact cannot be corrected (there is no guidewire artifact with electronic phase-array transducers), it rarely interferes with image interpretation or quantitation.

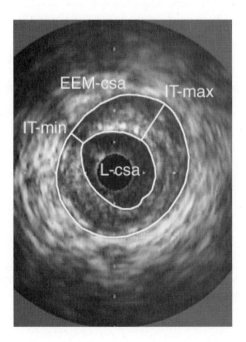

Figure 31.5. Ultrasound Measurements

Abbreviations: L-csa = lumen cross-sectional area; EEM-csa = external elastic membrane cross-sectional area (sometimes referred to as "vessel area"); IT-max = maximal intimal thickness; IT-min = minimal intimal thickness. See Tables 31.4 and 31.5 for definitions and formulas.

c.   **Ring-down artifact.** Although the diameter of most current coronary ultrasound catheters is only 1.0-1.1 mm in diameter, acoustic oscillations in the transducer result in high-amplitude signals that preclude near-field imaging. These artifacts have a characteristic appearance consisting of white circles surrounding the ultrasound catheter (Figures 31.6 C, 31.6 D). Recent catheter designs use special transducer materials, coatings, backings, and filters to suppress these artifacts. Lesion morphology and quantitative measurements may be distorted by the distending effect of the catheter, particularly in critical stenoses. There are finite limitations to further transducer miniaturization: Smaller transducers reduce the "aperture" of the device (which limits acoustic power), lateral resolution, and the signal-to-noise ratio. The resolution of small apertures may be partially enhanced by using higher frequency transducers (40-50 MHz).

d.   **Non-uniform rotational distortion (NURD).** This artifact is present only in mechanical intravascular ultrasound systems, and is due to uneven drag on the catheter drive shaft during its rotational cycle, resulting in oscillations in rotational speed. The image may exhibit circumferential "smearing" and "compression" of the contralateral vessel wall (Figure 31.6 C). NURD is most evident when the drive shaft is deformed into a small radius of curvature by

Table 31.5. Important IVUS Calculations

Variable	Unit	Significance	Formula
Plaque area (ITcsa)	mm^2	Absolute measure of plaque burden	EEMcsa - Lcsa
% PB (% CSN)	%	Relative measure of stenosis severity	([EEMcsa - Lcsa] / EEMcsa) x 100
Intimal index	none	Relative measure of plaque burden	ITcsa / EEMcsa
Eccentricity index	none	Relative measure of plaque eccentricity	([ITmax - ITmin] / ITmax) x 100
% Diameter stenosis	%	Relative measure of stenosis severity	(1 - [MLD / VD]) x 100
Minimum CSA$^+$	mm^2	Strongest predictor of TLR	

Abbreviations: CSA = cross-sectional area; CSN = cross-sectional area narrowing; EEM = external elastic membrane; IT = intimal-medial thickness; L = lumen; max = maximum; min = minimum; MLD = minimum lumen diameter; PB = plaque burden; TLR = target lesion revascularization; VD = vessel diameter
+   Stent variable. Minimum CSA is the minimum in-stent CSA

external manipulation or vessel tortuosity. Two remedial causes of NURD are excessive tightening of the hemostasis valve at the hub of the guiding catheter, and excessive slack in the catheter between the pullback sled and the guiding catheter.

e. **Blood stasis artifact.** At frequencies greater than 25 MHz, blood within the vessel lumen appears as subtle, finely textured echoes in a characteristic swirling pattern. The pattern of blood speckle varies with the velocity of blood flow. This speckle can assist the operator in confirming the communication between a dissection plane and the "true" lumen. However, when the ultrasound catheter occludes the lumen at a severe stenosis, the signal from the slowly flowing blood has increased echogenicity and a coarse texture, which can confound the distinction between lumen and atheroma distal to the target lesion (Figure 31.7).

f. **Geometric distortion.** Geometric distortion can result from imaging in an oblique plane (not perpendicular to the long axis of the vessel), resulting in an elliptical (rather than circular) cross-sectional imaging plane.[30] This phenomenon can confound quantitative measurements. It is often possible to recognize a non-orthogonal catheter position during image acquisition and manipulate the device to a more coaxial position. This artifact can be more troublesome when imaging larger vessels, such as iliac and renal arteries.

g. **Intracoronary thrombus.** The presence of intraluminal thrombi is the hallmark of an acute coronary syndrome,[31] and identification of thrombus has significant impact on therapy. The accuracy of angiography for detecting thrombus is low.[32] Unfortunately, IVUS cannot

Table 31.6. IVUS Artifacts

Image Artifacts	Description
Image drop-out	Loss of image due to air bubbles; easily corrected by flushing the catheter (mechanical transducers only)
Guidewire artifact	Discrete shadowing artifact with all mechanical transducers; rarely interferes with interpretation
Ring-down artifact	Characteristic white circles surrounding the IVUS catheter, which may impair interpretation and quantitation
Non-uniform rotational distortion (NURD)	Circumferential "smearing" and "compression" of the vessel wall when the drive shaft of mechanical transducers is deformed by vessel tortuosity, excessive tightening of the O-ring, or redundancy in the IVUS catheter outside the patient
Geometric distortion	Elliptical, rather than circular image, resulting from a tangential imaging plane; worse in larger vessels. Can interfere with quantitative measurements

reliably differentiate acute thrombus from echolucent plaque, probably due to similar echodensity. Although several small studies have attempted to define the intravascular ultrasound appearance of thrombus,[33,34] ultrasound is less accurate than angioscopy (which has sensitivity and specificity of 100%).[35] Higher frequency catheters may detect thrombus, and unprocessed ultrasound signals (backscatter) have shown some promise in differentiating thrombus from plaque.[36,37]

D. IMPACT ON UNDERSTANDING ATHEROSCLEROSIS. Ultrasound imaging is useful in studying the relationship between plaque composition and acute coronary syndromes (Table 31.2).

1. **Atheroma Distribution**. Histologically, most atheromas are eccentric.[38,39] Stenosis severity and the extent of calcification in eccentric lesions are less than in concentric lesions, suggesting that eccentric lesions represent an earlier stage of atherosclerosis.[41] Angiographic eccentricity

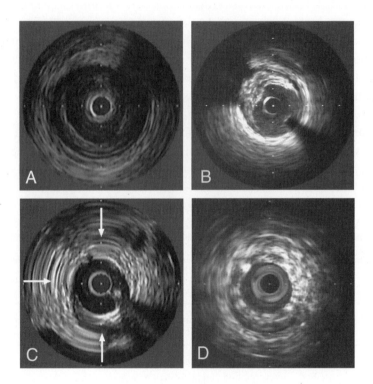

Figure 31.6. Ultrasound Artifacts

A. Image dropout due to an air bubble in the system, which can be corrected by flushing the ultrasound catheter
B. Shadowing at five o'clock is caused by a guidewire artifact, whereas shadowing at nine to eleven o'clock is caused by deep calcification
C. "Smearing" and "compression" of the image (white arrows) are due to nonuniform rotational distortion (NURD)
D. The white circles around the catheter are referred to as "ring-down" artifact

Table 31.7. Limitations of IVUS Interpretation

Limitation	Description
Evaluation of thrombus	IVUS detection of thrombus is unreliable; echolucent plaque and thrombus have similar echogenicity
Assessment of tissue histology	Tissue with similar echogenicity by IVUS may not have identical composition (e.g., thrombus and echolucent plaque)

correlates poorly with histopathologic examination[9,40] or ultrasound,[41] and many angiographically-eccentric lesions are in fact concentric by ultrasound (Figure 31.8). Atherosclerotic lesions targeted for percutaneous intervention are usually concentric, and arcs of normal arterial wall are quite uncommon.

2. **Plaque Composition (Figure 31.9).** In practice, ultrasound defines three broad classes of coronary lesions: *soft lesions,* where echogenicity of the atheroma is less than that of the adventia, *fibrous lesions,* where the atheroma is of equal density to the adventitia, and *calcific or fibrocalcific lesions,* where the atheroma is more echodense than the adventia. Overt calcification is highly likely when dense, bright echoes are accompanied by shadowing of the deeper structures. Early studies demonstrated the reliability of ultrasound in predicting plaque composition.

3. **Detection of Coronary Calcification.** Ultrasound imaging is superior to fluoroscopy and angiography in detecting coronary calcification, which is an important determinant of successful PTCA, directional atherectomy, and rotational atherectomy.[44] The degree of calcification is estimated by the angle subtended by the calcified arc of the vessel wall.[45] Detection of target lesion calcification by fluoroscopy increases when calcium exists in two or more quadrants ($\geq 180°$), extends ≥ 5 mm in length,[44] or is superficial in the arterial wall (Figures 31.10, 31.11).[46]

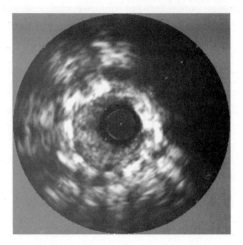

Figure 31.7. Blood Stasis Artifact

When blood velocity is low or when there is no flow in the vessel, stagnant red blood cells appear grey and can be easily confused with atheroma. This artifact may be observed when the ultrasound catheter occludes the vessel in a severe stenosis proximal to the transducer. A brisk injection of saline or contrast from the guiding catheter can restore the usual dark lumen appearance and often distinguish blood stasis from severe atheroma.

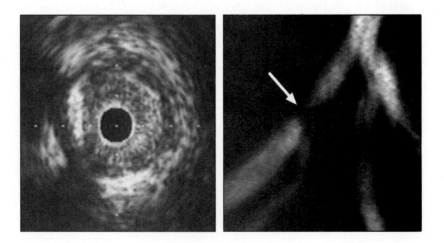

Figure 31.8. Evaluation of Atheroma Distribution

An eccentric lesion by angiography is concentric by intravascular ultrasound.

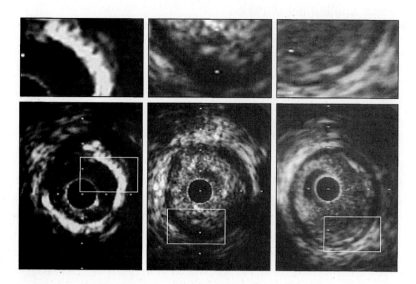

Figure 31.9. Ultrasound Characterization of Plaque Composition

Left panel: Calcified lesions are more echodense than the adventitia and have deep shadowing, since the ultrasound signals cannot penetrate these tissues. Middle panel: "Fibrous" lesions have similar echo gencity to the adventitia. Right panel: "Soft" lesions are less echogenic than the adventia. Higher magnifications are shown on the top of each panel.

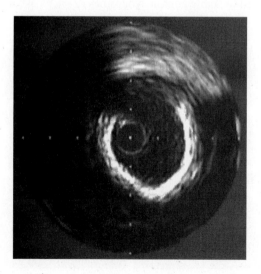

Figure 31.10. Extensive Calcification by Intravascular Ultrasound

There is a 270 degree arc of calcification from 2 o'clock to 11 o'clock, characterized by bright white echoes and dense shadowing of the ultrasound image beyond the layer of calcification.

Table 31.8. Diagnostic Applications of IVUS

Identify occult atherosclerosis in angiographically-normal vessels
Evaluation of intermediate lesions
Evaluation of lesions difficult to assess by angiography
   Indeterminate left main lesions
   Aorto-ostial lesions
   Bifurcation lesions
Determine the extent of cardiac allograft vasculopathy

4. **Unstable Plaque.** An important potential application of ultrasound is the correlation of lesion morphology with the risk of plaque rupture (Figure 31.12). Plaque rupture and acute thrombosis frequently develop in mildly diseased vessels rather than in vessels with high-grade stenoses.[17,47] Histologic examination of unstable plaques posing the highest risk of rupture usually reveals a lipid-laden core with a thin fibrous cap.[48] Although more than 70% of culprit lesions in patients with unstable angina have angiographic eccentricity or irregular ulcerated edges (Ambrose type II lesions),[49,50] angiography is unable to accurately identify "rupture-prone" atherosclerotic lesions. The size of the lipid pool and the thickness of the fibrous cap are more important than stenosis severity in predicting plaque rupture,[51] and peak circumferential stress is higher in plaques with large lipid pools and thin fibrous caps than in lesions with severe stenosis.[51] Echolucent, lipid-laden plaques correlate with acute coronary syndromes and are more frequently observed in patients with unstable compared to stable angina syndromes (74% vs. 41%, p <0.01).[14]

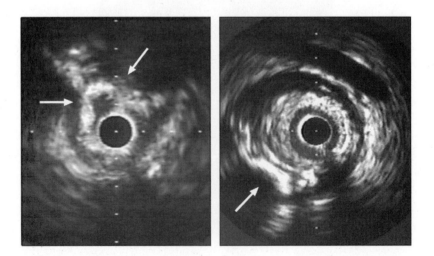

Figure 31.11. Depth of Coronary Calcification by Intravascular Ultrasound

Left panel: Superficial calcification involves two quadrants (12 to 2 o'clock and 9 to 11 o'clock [arrow]). Right panel: Deep calcification near the media-adventitial border involves one quadrant (6 to 9 o'clock, arrow).

Although coronary erosion is an important cause of acute coronary syndromes and sudden cardiac death,[52,53] ultrasound findings have not been well described.

5. **Arterial Remodeling.** Remodeling is defined as a change in vessel area due to atherosclerosis. Remodeling can be *positive* (in which vessel area increases with atheroma development) or *negative* (in which the vessel area decreases). Glagov described an increase in arterial size that appeared to accommodate the deposition of atherosclerotic plaque (Figure 31.13). In lesions with area stenosis < 30-40%, the increase in arterial size "overcompensates" for plaque deposition, leading to an increase in lumen area. With more advanced lesions (area stenosis > 40%), the degree of arterial enlargement is less, and luminal diameter becomes progressively smaller with disease progression.[16] The findings of Glagov were later confirmed *in vivo* by intracoronary ultrasound (Figures 31.3, 31.14).[54] Recently, histopathologic and ultrasound studies demonstrated negative arterial remodeling (arterial shrinkage) in *de novo* coronary lesions. At these sites, the area inside the external elastic lamina (EEMcsa) is *less* than at the corresponding reference segment.[55,56] It is important to realize that when remodeling is defined by comparing lesion-to-reference EEM areas, there is an inherent assumption that the reference EEM area represents the original vessel size at the lesion site. Since normal vessels may taper 20% over a length of 10 mm, and angiographically normal vessels may be diseased by ultrasound, quantitative angiography is not a good method for assessing remodeling. Contrast angiography frequently underestimates the severity of atherosclerosis and vessel size, which has been implicated in restenosis.[57]

E. DIAGNOSTIC APPLICATIONS OF INTRACORONARY ULTRASOUND (Table 31.8)

1. **Angiographically Normal Coronary Arteries.** In patients undergoing angiography for clinically suspected coronary artery disease, significant disease is identified in 80-90% of patients by angiography and 90-100% of patients by ultrasound (Figures 31.3, 31.14).[11,12,58,59]

2. **Indeterminate Left Main Lesions (Table 31.9).** Angiographic assessment of the severity of left main lesions is frequently difficult.[7] Often, the left main trunk is short and lacks a "normal" segment for comparison. In addition, contrast in the aortic cusp sometimes obscures the ostium, and "streaming" of contrast may result in a false impression of luminal narrowing. Furthermore, the bifurcation (or trifurcation) into branches may conceal the distal left main trunk. Finally, angiography underestimates stenosis severity, particularly in vessels with a 50-75% narrowing,[9,60-62] which is precisely the range in which left main decisions are most crucial. Accordingly, IVUS is commonly employed to quantitate left main lesions when angiographic interpretation is ambiguous (Figure 31.15).[63] The technique for examination of left main lesions is relatively simple, requiring advancement of the transducer into the circumflex or left anterior descending, followed by a slow, motorized pullback into the aorta, while the guiding catheter is slightly disengaged. Although this approach allows rapid interrogation, *manual* pullback is recommended to thoroughly investigate

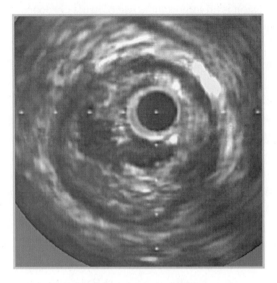

Figure 31.12. Unstable Plaque by Intravascular Ultrasound

Unstable plaque is characterized by disrupted tissue adjacent to the lumen, which could be a nidus for acute thrombosis (six o'clock). In "real time," this friable plaque was very mobile.

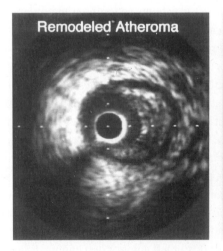 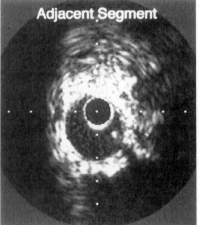

Figure 31.13. Positive Remodeling in a Coronary Artery

There is a large plaque with expansion of the adventitia (left), resulting in a lumen diameter virtually identical to an adjacent segment (right).

intermediate left main lesions. Unfortunately, there are no absolute ultrasound criteria for "critical" left main stenosis. Important considerations include the patient's symptomatic status, the presence of other lesions, and the amount of myocardium in jeopardy. Nevertheless, suggested IVUS criteria for significant left main disease are > 60% area stenosis, absolute area < 7 mm^2 in patients with symptoms, or absolute area < 6 mm^2 in asymptomatic patients. A recent study evaluated 122 patients with intermediate left main lesions (~ 42% diameter stenosis by QCA).[64] The 1-year event rate was 14% when left main revascularization was deferred based on IVUS. When patients with an event were compared to patients without an event, there were no significant differences in left ventricular function or QCA diameter stenosis, but the group with events had greater cross-sectional narrowing (70 ± 14% vs. 53 ± 18%, p = 0.0418), smaller minimum left main lumen area (6.8 ± 4.4mm^2 vs. 10.0 ± 5.3mm^2, p = 0.0127), and smaller minimum lumen diameter (2.30 ± 0.69mm vs. 2.94 ± 0.81mm, p = 0.0012). Predictors of cardiac events at one year were diabetes mellitus (OR 6.32; 95% CI 1.82-22.04, p = 0.004), any epicardial vessel with a QCA stenosis ≥50% (OR 3.80; 95% CI 1.08-13.39, p = 0.037), and left main minimum lumen diameter by IVUS (OR 1.7; 95% CI 0.05-0.59, p = 0.005). Thus, when IVUS is used to assess the severity of intermediate left main stenoses, decisions to defer revascularization must consider absolute IVUS dimensions, the presence of diabetes, and the presence of significant lesions in other major epicardial vessels.

3. **Other Intermediate Lesions (Table 31.9).** Angiography frequently underestimates stenosis severity in other vessels with 50-75% diameter stenosis (Figure 31.16).[9,60-62] Recently, several prospective studies compared IVUS, stress myocardial perfusion, and physiologic lesion assessment to evaluate intermediate lesions. In one study, a cross-sectional area < 4.0 mm^2 had a sensitivity of 88% and a specificity of 90% for identifying lesions associated with an abnormal perfusion scan, and may be more reliable than visual or QCA percent stenosis for identifying intermediate lesions which require revascularization. In another study, an absolute lumen area < 3 mm^2 demonstrated a sensitivity of 83% and a specificity of 92% in identifying hemodynamically significant lesions by fractional flow reserve (FFR). Although an absolute lumen area ≥ 4.0 mm^2 was associated with a coronary flow reserve (CFR) > 2.0 in one study,[65] another did not find a strong correlation between IVUS and CFR.[66] When intervention on intermediate lesions was deferred based on IVUS, no angiographic variables predicted subsequent events. The only independent predictors of events were diabetes mellitus, the IVUS-measured minimum lumen area, and the IVUS-determined area stenosis. Importantly, a minimum lumen area > 4.0 mm^2 identified patients with a very low risk of subsequent events. Thus, in the absence of prospective randomized data, these studies provide some guidelines for using IVUS to assess angiographically intermediate lesions in native vessels: Absolute lumen area < 4.0 mm^2 is frequently associated with myocardial ischemia (by stress perfusion imaging), and absolute lumen area < 3.0 mm^2 is associated with a physiologically significant stenosis (by CFR or FFR); strong consideration should be given to revascularizing these vessels. When in doubt, cross-sectional area stenosis > 60-70% also suggests the need for revascularization. Patients with angiographically intermediate lesions and an absolute lumen area ≥ 4.0 mm^2 can be followed clinically without intervention.

Table 31.9. IVUS Criteria for "Significant" Stenosis

Left Main Coronary Artery
   Cross-sectional area stenosis > 60%
   Lumen cross-sectional area < 7 mm^2 (symptomatic patients)
   Lumen cross-sectional area < 6 mm^2 (asymptomatic patients)
   Minimum lumen diameter < 2.3 mm

Non-Left Main Coronary Arteries
   Cross-sectional area stenosis > 60%
   Lumen cross-sectional area < 4.0 mm^2*
   Lumen cross-sectional area < 3.0 mm^2**

*   Correlates with abnormal myocardial perfusion scan (two studies)
**   Correlates with abnormal fractional flow reserve (one study only)
Note: The clinical significance of a stenosis should not be based solely on the absolute lumen cross-sectional area, but should be considered along with other factors, such as lesion length, amount of viable myocardium in jeopardy, and the results of other noninvasive functional studies. In some cases, lesions with an IVUS cross-sectional area > 4 mm^2 may produce ischemia; in other cases, lesions with a cross-sectional area < 3 mm^2 may not be associated with ischemia. These caveats emphasize the importance of integrating all available clinical, angiographic, and ultrasound data when making decisions about indeterminate lesions.

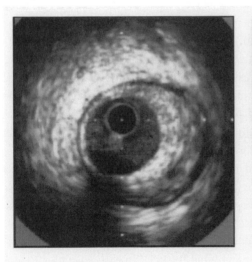 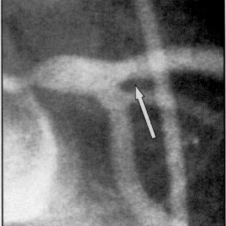

Figure 31.14. Arterial Remodeling in the Proximal LAD

Left panel: The ultrasound image demonstrates a large, eccentric atheroma extending from twelve o'clock to seven o'clock. Right panel: Angiography at this site (white arrow) suggests that the LAD is essentially normal. Comparison with the distal LAD suggests that the lesion was extensively remodeled, since the lumen is round and smooth. Multiple orthogonal projections did not reveal any abnormality.

4. **Ostial and Bifurcation Lesions.** Angiographers commonly encounter ostial and bifurcation lesions which elude accurate assessment (Figure 31.17). In these lesions, physiologic data (FFR and CFR) may be difficult to obtain and interpret. In contrast, ultrasound is relatively easy to perform, and similar criteria (absolute lumen area ≤ 4.0 mm^2, area stenosis > 60-70%) may be used to guide revascularization. When evaluating an ostial lesion, the importance of choosing a coaxial guiding catheter to prevent geometric distortion cannot be overstated, and careful manual interrogation is often necessary for accurate assessment.

5. **Cardiac Allograft Vasculopathy.** Identification of cardiac allograft atherosclerosis is important and clinically challenging, since it is a leading cause of late morbidity and mortality, and is often silent (most patients do not experience angina). Many centers perform routine IVUS at the time of annual angiography (Figure 31.18).

F. **NON-STENT INTERVENTIONAL APPLICATIONS OF ULTRASOUND (Table 31.10).** Device selection for percutaneous intervention depends on several factors, but is mostly determined by target lesion morphology and stenosis severity, which can be better characterized by ultrasound imaging than by angiography. Information from ultrasound imaging may be used to predict short- and long-term outcomes, particularly following coronary stenting.[67]

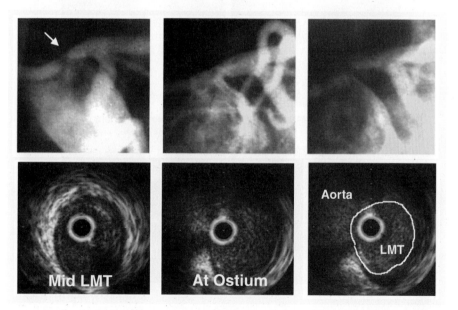

Figure 31.15. Intravascular Ultrasound Evaluation of Ambiguous Left Main Stenosis

Top panels: Initial coronary angiography suggests a critical ostial left main stenosis (white arrow), but selective angiography suggested moderate disease. Bottom panels demonstrate the IVUS findings during careful manual interrogation. Bypass surgery was cancelled since the minimal lumen diameter was > 3 mm and the cross-sectioned area was > 8 mm^2. LMT = left main trunk.

1. **Pre-Interventional Ultrasound Imaging.** Ultrasound imaging of target lesions frequently alters the approach to therapy.[67-70] During Phase I of the Guidance by Ultrasound Imaging for Decision Endpoints (GUIDE) trial, angiography and ultrasound were performed during balloon angioplasty or directional atherectomy. Operators reclassified lesion characteristics after ultrasound in 68% of lesions and the therapeutic approach was modified in 48% of patients. Ultrasound measurements revealed smaller post-procedure lumen dimensions than measured by QCA, leading to balloon upsizing.[68,69] Importantly, the incidence of angiographic dissection was not increased after ultrasound-guided balloon upsizing (37% vs. 40%, p = 0.67). In addition, the acute lumen gain achieved following angioplasty was comparable to that after stenting,[79] allowing use of "provisional" stenting for suboptimal results.[80] In another study, "acceptable" procedural results by angiography were deemed suboptimal by ultrasound in 30% of patients.[70] The impact of routine ultrasound imaging on long-term outcomes after PTCA and atherectomy remains to be determined, although restenosis is known to be dependent on final lumen dimensions.[71]

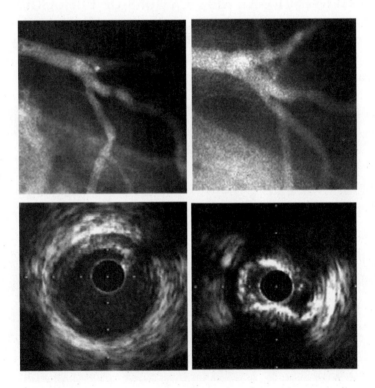

Figure 31.16. Intravascular Ultrasound Evaluation of a "Hazy" Lesion

This patient had a large reversible defect in the lateral wall during stress perfusion imaging, and angiography demonstrated a "hazy" area in a large ramus branch in one projection (top left) but not in another (top right). Ultrasound examination demonstrated mild concentric atheroma proximal to the "hazy" lesion (bottom left), and dense "napkin ring" calcification with severe lumen compromise at the lesion site (bottom right).

2. **Ultrasound Imaging and Balloon Angioplasty.** Ultrasound studies in the early 1990s demonstrated three mechanisms of lumen enlargement following PTCA, including plaque fracture/dissection (major mechanism), arterial wall stretching (particularly important in soft echolucent plaques[74,75,76]), and plaque compression/redistribution (Figures 31.2, 31.19).[10,45,72,73] Calcified lesions had a higher incidence of dissection (67% vs. 25%, p = 0.03), and there was a trend toward more restenosis in lesions without dissection.[45] Plaque compression was once suggested as the major mechanism of lumen enlargement following PTCA,[77] but recent *in vivo* ultrasound studies showed no evidence for plaque compression,[73,76] although axial redistribution of plaque may occur.[78]

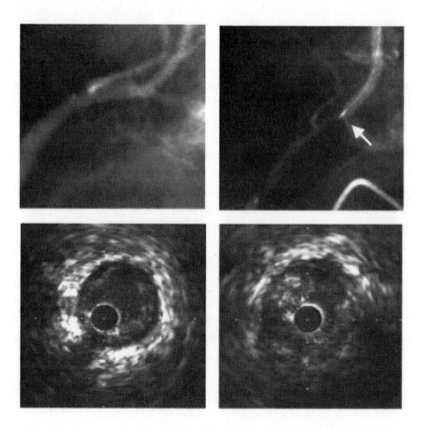

Figure 31.17. Intravascular Ultrasound Evaluation of a Borderline Ostial Lesion

This patient had a large reversible defect in the inferior wall, and angiography demonstrated moderate ostial narrowing (top panels). Intravascular ultrasound just distal to the ostium (bottom left) demonstrated mild atheroma and a large lumen. However, careful manual pullback at the aorto-ostial junction (top right, white arrow) revealed bulky atheroma and severe stenosis (bottom right).

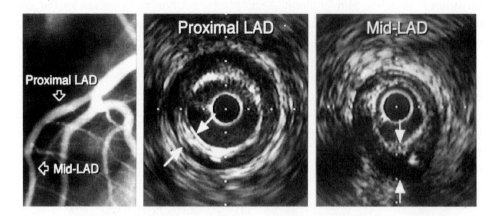

Figure 31.18. Angiographic Underestimation of Atherosclerosis in a Heart Transplant Patient

Although the angiogram is relatively normal, diffuse disease narrows the entire LAD.

3. **Ultrasound Imaging and Rotational Atherectomy.** *In vivo* ultrasound studies have confirmed the principle of differential cutting, in which normal elastic tissue is deflected away from the Rotablator burr and inelastic atheroma is abraded (Figure 31.20).[81-85] Plaque area and the arc of calcium decrease after rotational ablation, indicating that plaque pulverization is the major mechanism of lumen enlargement.[85] Vessel expansion, plaque fracture, and dissection were uncommon and did not contribute to lumen gain. Adjunctive PTCA achieved further lumen enlargement by vessel expansion (80% of lesions) and dissection (70% of lesions), but not by a change in plaque mass. Ultrasound imaging facilitates burr sizing, especially in diffusely diseased vessels where vessel size is underestimated by angiography.[85] A recent study demonstrated that late in-stent intimal proliferation directly correlates with residual plaque burden after stent implantation, suggesting that aggressive plaque removal prior to stenting may reduce restenosis;[86] the benefits of this approach await validation.

4. **Ultrasound Imaging and Directional Atherectomy.** Ultrasound imaging before and during directional atherectomy may help localize atheroma distribution, the extent of calcification, and residual plaque burden (which often exceeds 70%), thus facilitating directional atherectomy (Figure 31.21).[87,88] Although ABACAS and OARS demonstrated that aggressive IVUS-guided atherectomy was associated with low restenosis rates,[89,90] similar restenosis rates were reported in BOAT, which did not utilize routine IVUS. Since a large plaque burden prior to stenting adversely affects the final in-stent area (a major determinant of TLR and restenosis), some investigators speculate that ultrasound-guided DCA with stenting might provide better long-term outcomes than stenting alone.[86,91]

5. **Restenosis After Non-Stent Interventions.** In non-stent coronary interventions, the lumen gain observed during the first month after intervention is due to compensatory vessel enlargement, whereas late lumen loss is caused mostly by vessel shrinkage (negative remodeling) and to a lesser extent by progressive intimal hyperplasia.[93] The most important predictors of angiographic restenosis are final cross-sectional area and reference lumen area by ultrasound, and baseline diameter stenosis by QCA.[92]

G. ULTRASOUND IMAGING AND CORONARY STENTING (Table 31.10)

1. **Ultrasound Imaging Prior to Stenting.** Ultrasound imaging prior to stent deployment can provide useful information regarding the degree of ostial involvement, length of dissection, and the presence and extent of lesion calcification. These features are important since residual dissection after stenting increases the risk of stent thrombosis,[94] and in heavily calcified lesions, stenting frequently results in a small, asymmetric lumen.[95] In the Angiography Versus. Intravascular Ultrasound (AVID) trial, vessel calcification was a major determinant of suboptimal stent expansion.[96,97,98]

2. **Ultrasound to Determine the Endpoints of Stenting.** Ultrasound imaging has a pivotal role in optimizing stent results. Several studies suggest that angiography often fails to identify inadequate stent deployment (malapposition, malexpansion), which is readily evident by ultrasound (Figures 31.22, 31.23).[99-101] Angiography is unable to identify stent malapposition because contrast opacifies the entire lumen, which may be larger than the lumen occupied by the stent (Figure 31.18). Routine high-pressure inflations (15 atm) and ultrasound guidance achieve full stent expansion and complete apposition in 96% of patients.[102] High-pressure PTCA, ultrasound guidance, and reduced anticoagulation result in outstanding clinical outcomes, including subacute stent thrombosis in <1% and target vessel revascularization in 13%.[103] Following widespread acceptance of high-pressure PTCA and reduced anticoagulation regimens, the incremental benefit of routine ultrasound was debated, since excellent results were achieved with high-pressure inflations without routine ultrasound.[104,105] However, the Optimal Stent Implantation (OSTI) trial demonstrated better in-stent dimensions with IVUS than angiography alone.[106] Furthermore, minimum in-stent area was the most powerful predictor of clinical restenosis, and high-pressure inflations resulted in suboptimal stent expansion in 20-40% by IVUS (Figure 31.23).[104,105,107]

3. **Ultrasound Criteria for "Optimal" Stent Expansion (Table 31.5).** In general, criteria for optimal stent expansion relate to the degree of strut apposition to the vessel wall, in-stent minimal cross-sectional area, symmetry of the stent lumen, and adequacy of coverage of adjacent disease or dissection. Although there is no consensus on the IVUS endpoints, most operators strongly advocate complete apposition of the stent struts to the vessel and coverage of adjacent segments of disease or dissection.[97,109] Early recommendations to achieve $\geq$ 60% of the average proximal and distal reference area have been revised, so that most operators attempt to achieve $\geq$ 90% of the distal reference lumen area.[102] Other criteria for optimal expansion include $\geq$ 90% of the distal and $\geq$ 80%-90% of the average reference lumen area,[97,108] but these procedural endpoints are not achieved in most cases. In OSTI,[110] the target endpoint of > 90% of the average reference area was achieved in < 50% of patients at an inflation pressure of 15 atm, and in only 60% of patients at

Table 31.10. Interventional Application of IVUS

Precise vessel sizing for device size and length
Precise plaque characterization for device selection
Understanding mechanisms of lumen enlargement
Guiding therapy for "suboptimal" result
Predicting complications and restenosis

18 atm. Similarly, 90% of the distal reference area was achieved in < 30% of patients in AVID.[96,97] The most widely used IVUS criteria for optimal stenting is minimum in-stent CSA ≥ 55% of the reference vessel area (within the EEM), which applies to vessels of all sizes.

4. **Ultrasound and Long-term Results After Stenting.** IVUS confirms that stents improve lumen dimensions by axial redistribution of atheroma, vessel expansion, and plaque compression.[115] In contrast to non-stent interventions, restenosis after stenting is due solely to intimal hyperplasia;[93] stent recoil (at least in slotted-tubular stents) does not occur.[118] Late lumen loss is significantly greater with stents than with balloon angioplasty, but is offset by more acute lumen gain; the net gain at follow-up is significantly greater with stenting compared to PTCA or atherectomy.[119-121] Nevertheless, the impact of routine ultrasound on late target lesion revascularization remains controversial. The non-randomized CRUISE (Can Routine Ultrasound Impact Stent Expansion) substudy compared the outcome of ultrasound- and angiographically-guided stenting in 538 procedures; there was a 39% relative reduction in target vessel revascularization with ultrasound guidance.[116] In contrast, a smaller, randomized trial reported a 6.3% absolute reduction in restenosis, which was not statistically significant.[117] Possible reasons for discordant results among these trials is the use of different IVUS criteria to define "optimal" stent deployment, as well as differences in study design and patient inclusion criteria.

5. **Ultrasound Correlates of Restenosis After Stenting (Tables 31.5, 31.11).** The final in-stent area (by IVUS) is a powerful predictor of target vessel revascularization,[112,125] since a larger final area allows late intimal hyperplasia without leading to restenosis.[111,112,122-125] Ultrasound predictors of restenosis at the stent margins include smaller reference vessel and lumen size, larger plaque burden at the reference segments, and smaller final in-stent lumen area at the stent margins.[123] The amount of residual plaque outside the stent (i.e., behind the stent rather than at the stent margins) is another predictor of stent restenosis.[86] Other technical factors (stent length, high pressure, large balloon/artery ratio),[126-131] angiographic factors (final angiographic lumen diameter < 3 mm, ostial lesion location, multiple stents), and clinical factors (diabetes mellitus),[132] are also associated with stent restenosis. The risk of restenosis is inversely related to the absolute final minimum in-stent lumen area: Restenosis occurred in 8% of patients with final in-stent minimal lumen area ≥9mm^2, compared to 25% of patients with final in-stent minimal lumen area < 9 mm^2 (p < 0.0001).[111,112]

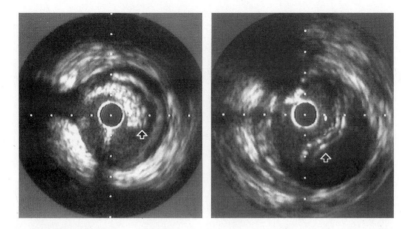

Figure 31.19. Complex Dissection After PTCA

A deep dissection (black arrow, left) is associated with a large intimal flap (black arrow, right).

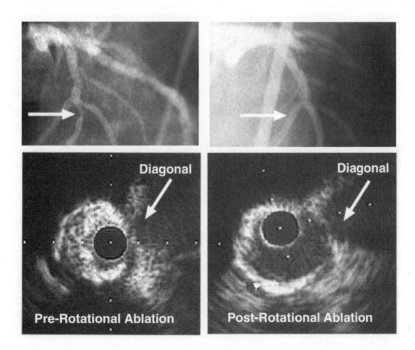

Figure 31.20. Intravascular Ultrasound of Successful Rotational Ablation of the LAD

Baseline angiography reveals severe stenosis in the mid-LAD (top left), which is densely calcified by IVUS (bottom left). After Rotoblator, angiography reveals a widely patent smooth lumen (top right) due to extensive atheroablation of fibrocalcific plaque (bottom right).

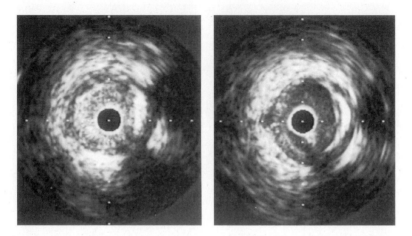

Figure 31.21. Intravascular Ultrasound Before and After DCA

Although the angiogram shows an eccentric lesion, IVUS demonstrates a concentric plaque (left). There is little residual plaque after DCA (right).

However, minimal stent lumen area ≥ 9 mm^2 was observed in only 25% of patients. Since an absolute in-stent minimum lumen cross-sectional area ≥ 9 mm^2 (optimal result) can only be achieved in the largest vessels, most operators try to achieve an in-stent minimum lumen cross-sectional area $\geq 55\%$ of the reference segment vessel area (area within the external elastic lamina), which provides the greatest predictive power of freedom from restenosis independent of vessel size and final in-stent area. Reported TLR and restenosis rates are 13% and 17% when stent area is $\geq 55\%$ of vessel area. Absolute measures of in-stent lumen area rather than stent-to-artery ratios have a stronger correlation with late restenosis and target vessel revascularization (such as a final lumen area $\geq 70\%$ of final balloon cross-sectional area),[113,114] but neither predicts stent thrombosis. A recent ultrasound analysis demonstrated that the degree of in-stent intimal hyperplasia is independent of final stent lumen size,[107] perhaps explaining higher restenosis rates in smaller vessels and poorly expanded stents.

6.   **Stent Complications Detected by IVUS.** Routine ultrasound is clearly not necessary to achieve subacute thrombosis rates < 1. However, IVUS occasionally reveals "suboptimal" results due to edge dissections, malexpansion, or malapposition even after angiographically "successful" stent placement. Routine IVUS identifies angiographically-inapparent edge dissections in approximately 11% of patients.[133] At 6 months, 75% of these dissections heal without sequelae, suggesting that small edge tears (superficial dissections confined to the intima) detected by IVUS but not by angiography may be safely observed without additional treatment. In contrast, additional treatment is recommended for edge dissections that are deep (extension into the media and/or involving more than one vessel quadrant) or long (dissection extends > 5 mm beyond the stent margin), especially when associated with malexpansion or malapposition.[94,102,113,123] Significant edge dissections

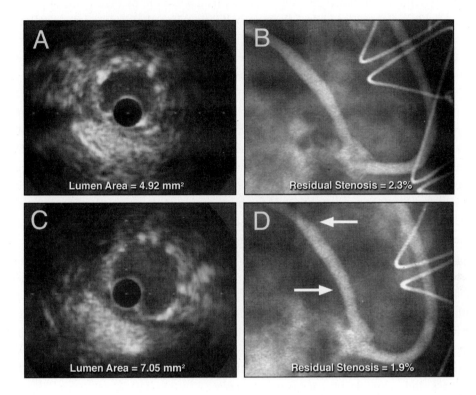

Figure 31.22. Stent Malexpansion

Despite the satisfactory angiographic result after stenting (Panel B), intravascular ultrasound demonstrates gross malexpansion at the distal stent edge (Panel A). After inflation with a larger balloon, the minimal cross-sectional lumen area increased from 4.92 mm² to 7.05 mm² (Panel C), without any detectable change by angiography (Panel D).

generally require additional stenting, whereas malapposition or malexpansion usually requires PTCA with larger and/or higher pressure balloons. The choice of a larger balloon or higher inflation pressure is often empiric.[139,140] Of course, dense, fibrocalcific plaque may not expand regardless of balloon size or pressure, so the operator must weigh the risk of vessel injury when considering high pressures (> 18 atm) and oversized balloons.[134]

7. **Stent Subsets Most Likely To Benefit From Ultrasound.** The AVID trial reported a strong correlation between IVUS and QCA at vessel diameters > 3.5 mm, but QCA tended to underestimate vessel size by more than 25% in vessels 2.5-3.25 mm in diameter. Thus, vessels measuring 2.5-2.75 mm by QCA may be 3.0 mm by IVUS. In fact, AVID reported at least 40% reduction in TVR when IVUS guidance was employed in these vessels. Since women have smaller vessels than men (even when adjusted for body mass index),[135] IVUS guidance may be useful. IVUS-guidance is also recommended in vessels > 4.5 mm, since large vessels may be predisposed to inadequate apposition or expansion using angiography alone. A large, single-center series suggested that ultrasound guidance may achieve substantial reductions in TVR in high-risk subsets such as diabetes and ostial lesions.[130,136,137] Although multiple stents are cited as a risk factor for subsequent target vessel revascularization,[128-130,138] if adequate minimum in-stent area is obtained with IVUS guidance, TVR may be similar for short (< 20 mm; TVR 10%) and long (> 20 mm; TVR 12.5%) lesions.[138] Even in patients treated with stents 20-40 mm in length, TVR was observed in < 15% if the final minimum in-stent area was > 7 mm^2. In summary, IVUS-guided stent implantation may be especially useful in vessels < 3 mm or > 4.5 mm, in females and diabetics, and in long lesions and ostial lesions.

8. **Understanding the Cause of Stent Restenosis.** Many operators advocate routine ultrasound to identify the precise mechanism of stent restenosis (Table 31.4), including inadequate initial stent implantation (larger balloons alone may lead to substantial improvement in lumen area), intimal hyperplasia (radiation therapy may be useful), or both. Stents with early restenosis (within 2 months of implantation) may have mechanical problems which could have been identified by IVUS at the time of implantation (Figures 31.24, 31.25), so-called "pseudorestenosis."[142] When these stents are interrogated by IVUS, findings often include malapposition (due to stent "slippage" at the time of deployment), malexpansion, unexpected side branch occlusion, or failure to cover the entire target lesion. Although balloon-expandable stents do not or "recoil" several months following deployment, prolapse of tissue is occasionally responsible for early recurrences (Figure 31.25). Finally, ultrasound can determine whether intimal hyperplasia has occurred entirely within the stent or in the adjacent reference segment; additional stent placement may be more effective than debulking or repeat PTCA in the latter situation.

Table 31.11. Correlates of Stent Restenosis

IVUS Variables
    Final in-stent CSA
    Reference vessel EEMcsa
    Plaque burden at the reference segment
    Residual plaque burden (behind the stent struts)

Technical Variables
    Stent length
    Final inflation pressure
    Final balloon/artery ratio
    Multiple stents

Angiographic Variables
    Final QCA lumen diameter < 3 mm
    Ostial lesion

Clinical Variables
    Diabetes mellitus

Abbreviations: CSA = cross-sectional area; EEMcsa = vessel cross-sectional area (inside the external elastic membrane); QCA = quantitative coronary angiography

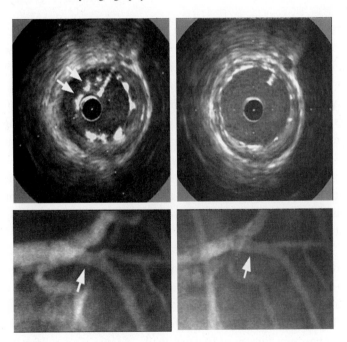

Figure 31.23. Stent Malapposition

After stent deployment in the proximal LAD, IVUS reveals malapposition of the stent (top left, white arrows), yet angiography suggests a superb result (bottom left, white arrow). After further adjunctive PTCA with a larger balloon at 16 ATM, IVUS reveals excellent apposition (top right). Angiography is unable to identify any change in vessel appearance or lumen dimensions (bottom right).

9. **Understanding the Cause of Acute Stent Thrombosis.** Although stent thrombosis occurs in less than 1-2% of cases, it is often catastrophic. Once TIMI 3 flow is restored, we recommend IVUS to identify causes of suboptimal stenting, which should be corrected as described above (Figure 31.26).

J. SAFETY OF INTRACORONARY ULTRASOUND. Intracoronary ultrasound is safe when performed by experienced operators. The most frequent complication is transient coronary spasm (5-10%), which usually responds rapidly to intracoronary nitroglycerin. Pretreatment with nitroglycerin can prevent spasm and is important to achieve maximal vasodilation to standardize vessel measurements. The incidence of spasm, dissection, or guidewire entrapment was 1.1% in patients undergoing PTCA,[143] which is 3-fold higher than during diagnostic procedures.[144,145]

K. FUTURE DEVELOPMENTS IN INTRACORONARY ULTRASOUND

1. **Guidewire-Sized Devices.** During the next several years, technological advances in intravascular imaging are anticipated, including further reduction in the size of imaging catheters to current guidewire dimensions (< 0.025 inches).[146] A guidewire ultrasound probe might improve the ease and safety of the examination and permit simultaneous imaging and revascularization.

2. **Combined Devices.** Combination devices incorporating imaging with a therapeutic device are also under development. An angioplasty balloon with an ultrasound transducer (Endosonics - Oracle™) is FDA approved, and a transducer combined with an atherectomy device is undergoing initial clinical testing.[147,148] Other IVUS catheters are under development which incorporate a tip-mounted Doppler flow probe to allow simultaneous cross-sectional area and flow velocity measurements. Finally, brachytherapy catheters (with imaging and shielding capability) and stents mounted on intravascular ultrasound catheters may become available in the future.

3. **Tissue Characterization.** Several investigators have demonstrated the feasibility of tissue characterization by analyzing tissue backscatter. Intrinsic characteristics of backscattered signals (amplitude distribution, frequency response, power spectrum of the signal) convey specific information about tissue types.[36,149-151]

4. **High Frequency Catheters.** High frequency (> 30 MHz) ultrasound catheters are in the advanced stages of development, although their incremental clinical benefit remains uncertain.[79,152-154] High frequency enables better axial and lateral resolution, but penetration is impaired compared to conventional devices. In addition, backscatter from blood cells may interfere with discrimination of the interface between lumen and vessel wall. As the demand for catheter miniaturization becomes more intense, a shorter wavelength may preserve near-field image quality.

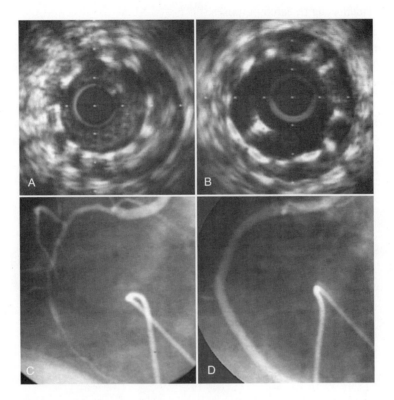

Figure 31.24. Stent Restenosis: Stent Malexpansion and Intimal Proliferation

A long dissection mandated deployment of several stents in the RCA. When the patient developed restenosis several months later, intravascular ultrasound demonstrated extensive neointimal tissue within the stent, as well as stent malexpansion (Panel A). Baseline angiography shows diffuse restenosis (Panel C). After rotational ablation and a 3.5 mm balloon at 18 ATM, IVUS demonstrates ablation of intimal tissue and better stent expansion (Panel B). The final angiographic result is excellent (Panel D).

5. **Three-Dimensional Reconstruction.** Three-dimensional (3-D) reconstruction may lead to a better understanding of the spatial relationship between structures in different tomographic cross-sections.[155-158] A prerequisite for 3D-reconstruction is the use of motorized pullback, allowing acquisition of sequential cross-sections separated by known distance.[159] However, algorithms for 3D-reconstruction assume that the catheter passes in a straight line through the center of consecutive cross-sections (leading to possible inaccuracies in tortuous vessels), and movement of the catheter in the vessel generates characteristic artifacts. Accordingly, the reconstructed images should not yet be considered faithful representations of the vessel, and should not be used for volumetric plaque determination. Simultaneous digitization of biplane fluoroscopic tracking of the

radio-opaque transducer and catheter tip may overcome some of these limitations, but is only practical for small-scale research purposes.[160-162]

6. **Guiding Intracoronary Radiation.** Intracoronary radiation is a promising technique for preventing restenosis.[157,163-168] Ultrasound is useful for vessel sizing to determine proper dose, catheter size, and treatment length.

L. **SUMMARY.** Available data support the use of IVUS in five broad clinical situations (Table 31.10). In our experience, this selective approach will result in the use of IVUS in 5% of diagnostic angiograms and in 20-30% of coronary interventions.

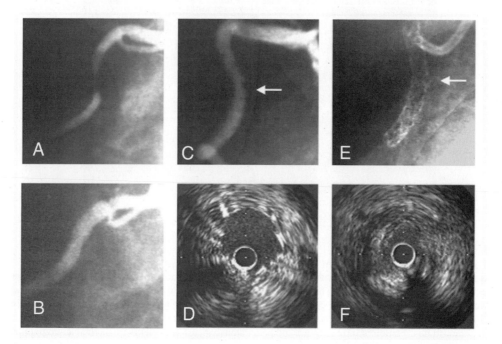

Figure 31.25. Stent Pseudorestenosis: Plaque Prolapse

A severe stenosis in a tortuous RCA (Panel A) was treated by successful PTCA and stenting (Panel B) without IVUS. Nine days later the patient developed unstable angina, and repeat angiography revealed a mild wedge-shaped defect in the middle of the stent (Panel C, white arrow). Angiographic imaging without contrast suggested excessive flaring of the stent struts (Panel E, white arrow). Careful manual pullback with IVUS showed the "gap" between the stent struts (Panel D, 7-8 o'clock) and definite tissue prolapse at the site of the lesion, which is not covered by stent struts (Panel F). Placement of a short stent across the "gap" immediately corrected this problem.

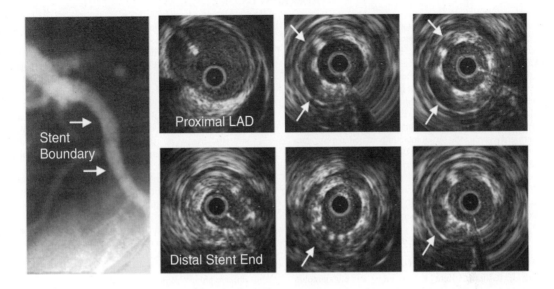

Figure 31.26. Subacute Stent Thrombosis Due to Stent Malexpansion and Malapposition

This patient underwent primary stenting of the LAD for acute MI without IVUS (left panel). Four days later, the patient developed recurrent chest pain and ST-segment elevation, and repeat angiography confirmed reocclusion and stent thrombosis. After passing a guidewire across the occlusion, IVUS demonstrated severe malexpansion (note the marked discrepancy between stent diameter and vessel diameter throughout the pullback sequence) and malapposition (note the black echolucent zones between the stent struts and the underlying wall; IVUS images with white arrows). High pressure PTCA was performed with a 4.5 mm balloon, achieving an excellent result (not shown).

* * * * *

REFERENCES

1. Roberts W, Jones A. Quantitation of coronary arterial narrowing at necropsy in sudden coronary death. Am J Cardiol 1979;44:39-44.

2. Waller BF, Orr CM, Slack JD, Pinkerton CA, Van Tassel JV, Peters T. Anatomy, histology, and pathology of coronary arteries: a review relevant to new interventional and imaging techniques--Part III. Clin-Cardiol 1992;15(8):607-15.

3. White C, Wright C, Doty D, Hiratza LF, Eastham CL, Harrison DG, et al. Does visual interpretation of the coronary arteriogram predict the physiologic importance of a coronary stenosis? N Engl J Med 1984;310:819-824.

4. Galbraith J, Murphy M, Desoyza N. Coronary angiogram interpretation: interobserver variability. JAMA 1981; 240:2053-2059.

5. Zir L, Miller S, Dinsmore R, Gilbert J, Harthorne J. Interobserver variability in coronary angiography. Circulation 1976;53:627-632.

6. Vlaodaver Z, F R, van Tassel R, Edwards J. Correlation of the antemortem coronary angiogram and the postmortem specimen. Circulation 1973;47:162-168.

7. Isner J, Kishel J, Kent K. Accuracy of angiographic determination of left main coronary arterial narrowing. Circulation 1981;63:1056-1061.

8. Grondin C, Dyrda I, Pasternac A, Campeu L, Bourassa M. Discrepancies between cineangiographic and post-mortem findings in patients with coronary artery disease and recent myocardial revascularization. Circulation 1974;49:703-709.

9. Arnett E, Isner J, Redwood C, Kent K, Baker W, Ackerstein H, et al. Coronary artery narrowing in coronary heart disase: comparison of cineangiographic and necropsy findings. Ann Intern Med 1979; 91:350-356.

10. Waller BF. "Crackers, breakers, stretchers, drillers, scrapers, shavers, burners, welders, and melters"--the future treatment of atherosclerotic coronary artery disease? A clinical-morphologic assessment. J Am Coll Cardiol. 1989;13:969-987.

11. Nissen SE, Gurley JC, Grines CL, Booth DC, McClure R, Berk M, et al. Intravascular ultrasound assessment of lumen size and wall morphology in normal subjects and patients with coronary artery disease. Circulation 1991;84(3):1087-99 issn: 0009-7322.

12. Topol E, Nissen S. Our preoccupation with coronary luminology: The dissociation between clinical and angiographic findings in ischemic heart disease. Circulation 1995;92:2333-2342.

13. Nissen SE. Radiographic Principles in Cardiac Catheterization. New York: Churchill Livingstone Inc. 1993.

14. Hodgson JM, Reddy KG, Suneja R, Nair RN, Lesnefsky EJ, Sheehan HM. Intracoronary ultrasound imaging: correlation of plaque morphology with angiography, clinical syndrome and procedural results in patients undergoing coronary angioplasty. J Am Coll Cardiol 1993;21(1):35-44.

15. Tobis JM, Mallery JA, Gessert J, Griffith J, Mahon D, Bessen M, et al. Intravascular ultrasound cross-sectional arterial imaging before and after balloon angioplasty in vitro. Circulation 1989;80(4):873-82.

16. Glagov S, Weisenberg E, Zarins C, al e. Compensatory enlargement of human atherosclerotic coronary arteries. N Engl J Med 1987;316:1371-1375.

17. Little WC, Constantinescu M, Applegate RJ, Kutcher MA, Burrows MT, Kahl FR, et al. Can coronary angiography predict the site of a subsequent myocardial infarction in patients with mild-to-moderate coronary artery disease? Circulation 1988;78:1157-1166.

18. Yamagishi M, Miyatake K, Tamai J, Nakatani S, Koyama J, Nissen SE. Intravascular ultrasound detection of atherosclerosis at the site of focal vasospasm in angiographically normal or minimally narrowed coronary segments. J Am Coll Cardiol 1994;23(2):352-7.

19. Nissen SE, Gurley JC. Application of intravascular ultrasound for detection and quantitation of coronary atherosclerosis. Int J Card Imaging 1991;6(3-4):165-77.

20. Nissen SE, Gurley JC, Booth DC, DeMaria AN. Intravascular ultrasound of the coronary arteries: current applications and future directions. Am J Cardiol 1992;69(20):18h-29h.

21. Nissen SE, Tuzcu EM, De Franco AC. Coronary Intravascular Ultrasound: Diagnostic and Interventional Applications. Philadelphia: W B Saunders 1994.

22. Fitzgerald PJ, St. Goar FG, Connolly AJ, Pinto FJ, Billingham ME, Popp RL, et al. Intravascular ultrasound imaging of coronary arteries. Is three layers the norm? Circulation 1992;86:154-8.

23. Maheswaran B, Leung CY, Gutfinger DE, Nakamura S, Russo RJ, Hiro T, et al. Intravascular ultrasound appearance of normal and mildly diseased coronary arteries: correlation with histologic specimens. Am Heart J 1995;130(5):976-86.

24. Metz JA, York PG, Fitzgerald PJ. Intravascular ultrasound: Basic interpretation. [Review] [35 refs.]. Cardiology Clinics 1997;15:1-15.

25. Lockwood GR, Ryan LK, Gotlieb AI, Lonn E, Hunt JW, Liu P, et al. In vitro high resolution intravascular imaging in muscular and elastic arteries. J Am Coll Cardiol 1992;20:153-60.

26. Yock PG, Linker DT. Intravascular ultrasound. Looking below the surface of vascular disease [comment]. Circulation 1990;81:1715-8.

27. Wong M, Edelstein J, Wollman J, Bond MG. Ultrasonic-pathological comparison of the human arterial wall. Verification of intima-media thickness. Arteriosclerosis & Thrombosis 1993;13:482-6.

28. Tuzcu EM, Hobbs RE, Rincon G, Bott Silverman C, De Franco AC, Robinson K, et al. Occult and frequent transmission of atherosclerotic coronary disease with cardiac transplantation. Insights from intravascular ultrasound. Circulation 1995;91(6):1706-13.

29. ten Hoff H, Korbijn A, Smith TH, Klinkhamer JF, Bom N. Imaging artifacts in mechanically driven ultrasound catheters. Int J Card Imaging 1989;4:195-199.

30. Di Mario C, Madretsma S, Linker D, The SH, Bom N, Serruys PW, et al. The angle of incidence of the ultrasonic beam: a critical factor for the image quality in intravascular ultrasonography. Am Heart J 1993;125(2 Pt 1):442-8.

31. Levin DC, Fallon JT. Significance of the angiographic morphology of localized coronary stenosis: histopathologic

correlations. Circulation 1982;66:316-320.

32. Ambrose JA, Winters SL, Stern A, Eng A, Teichholz LE, Gorlin R, et al. Angiographic morphology and the pathogenesis of unstable angina pectoris. J Am Coll Cardiol. 1985;5:609-616.

33. Kearney P, Erbel R, Rupprecht H, Ge J, Koch L, Voigtlander T, et al. Differences in the morphology of unstable and stable coronary lesions and theor impact on the mechanisms of angioplasty. An in vivo study with intravascular ultrasound. Eur Heart J 1995;17:721-730.

34. Bocksch W, Schartl M, Beckmann S, Dreysse S, Fleck E. Intravascular ultrasound imaging in patients with acute myocardial infarction. Eur Heart J 1995;19 Suppl J:46-52.

35. Siegel RJ, Ariani M, Fishbein MC, Chae JS, Park JC, Maurer G, et al. Histopathologic validation of angioscopy and intravascular ultrasound. Circulation 1991;84:109-17.

36. Bridal SL, Fornes P, Bruneval P, Berger G. Parametric (integrated backscatter and attenuation) images constructed using backscattered radio frequency signals (25-56 MHz) from human aortae in vitro. Ultrasound Med Biol 1997;23:215-229.

37. Hiro T, Leung CY, Karimi H, Farvid AR, Tobis JM. Angle dependence of intravascular ultrasound imaging and its feasibility in tissue characterization of human atherosclerotic tissue [In Process Citation]. Am Heart J. 1999;137:476-481.

38. Hangartner JR, Charleston AJ, Davies MJ, Thomas AC. Morphological characteristics of clinically significant coronary artery stenosis in stable angina. Br Heart J. 1986;56:501-508.

39. Schoenhagen P, Ziada KM, Kapadia SR, Crowe TD, Nissen SE, Tuzcu EM. Extent and direction of arterial remodeling in stable versus unstable coronary syndromes : an intravascular ultrasound study. Circulation 2000;101:598-603.

40. Vlodaver Z, Edwards JE. Pathology of coronary atherosclerosis. Prog Cardiovasc Dis. 1971;14:256-274.

41. Mintz GS, Popma JJ, Pichard AD, Kent KM, Satler LF, Chuang YC, et al. Limitations of angiography in the assessment of plaque distribution in coronary artery disease: a systematic study of target lesion eccentricity in 1446 lesions. Circulation 1996;93:924-31.

42. Gussenhoven EJ, Essed CE, Lancee CT, Mastik F, Frietman P, van Egmond FC, et al. Arterial wall characteristics determined by intravascular ultrasound imaging: an in vitro study. J Am Coll Cardiol 1989;14(4):947-52.

43. Potkin BN, Bartorelli AL, Gessert JM, Neville RF, Almagor Y, Roberts WC, et al. Coronary artery imaging with intravascular high-frequency ultrasound [see comments]. Circulation 1990;81(5):1575-85.

44. Mintz GS, Douek P, Pichard AD, Kent KM, Satler LF, Popma JJ, et al. Target lesion calcification in coronary artery disease: an intravascular ultrasound study. J Am Coll Cardiol 1992;20(5):1149-55.

45. Honye J, Mahon DJ, Jain A, White CJ, Ramee SR, Wallis JB, et al. Morphological effects of coronary balloon angioplasty in vivo assessed by intravascular ultrasound imaging. Circulation 1992;85(3):1012-25.

46. Tuzcu E, Berkalp B, De Franco A, Ellis S, Goormastic M, Whitlow P, et al. The dilemma of diagnosing coronary calcification: Angiography vs. intravascular ultrasound. J Am Coll Cardiol 1996;27:832-8.

47. Little WC, Downes TR, Applegate RJ. The underlying coronary lesion in myocardial infarction: implications for coronary angiography. Clin Cardiol. 1991;14:868-874.

48. Richardson PD, Davies MJ, Born GV. Influence of plaque configuration and stress distribution on fissuring of coronary atherosclerotic plaques [see comments]. Lancet 1989;2:941-944.

49. Kalbfleisch SJ, McGillem MJ, Simon SB, DeBoe SF, Pinto IM, Mancini GB. Automated quantitation of indexes of coronary lesion complexity. Comparison between patients with stable and unstable angina. Circulation 1990;82:439-447.

50. Ambrose JA, Winters SL, Arora RR, Eng A, Riccio A, Gorlin R, et al. Angiographic evolution of coronary artery morphology in unstable angina. J Am Coll Cardiol. 1986;7:472-478.

51. Loree HM, Kamm RD, Stringfellow RG, Lee RT. Effects of fibrous cap thickness on peak circumferential stress in model atherosclerotic vessels. Circulation Research 1992;71(4):850-8.

52. Virmani R, Burke AP, Farb A. Plaque rupture and plaque erosion. Thromb Haemost 1999;82(Suppl 1):1-3.

53. Arbustini E, Dal Bello B, Morbini P, Burke AP, Bocciarelli M, Specchia G, et al. Plaque erosion is a major substrate for coronary thrombosis in acute myocardial infarction. Heart 1999;82(3):269-72.

54. Hermiller J, Tenaglia A, Kisslo K, et al. In vivo validation of compensatory enlargement of atherosclerotic coronary arteries. Am J Cardiol 1993;71:665-668.

55. Pasterkamp G, Wensing PJ, Post MJ, Hillen B, Mali WP, Borst C. Paradoxical arterial wall shrinkage may contribute to luminal narrowing of human atherosclerotic femoral arteries. Circulation 1995;91(5):1444-9.

56. Mintz GS, Kent KM, Pichard AD, Satler LF, Popma JJ, Leon MB. Contribution of inadequate arterial remodeling to the development of focal coronary artery stenoses. An intravascular ultrasound study [see comments]. Circulation 1997;95(7):1791-8.

57. Kimura T, Kaburagi S, Tamura T, Yokoi H, Nakagawa Y, Hamasaki N, et al. Remodeling of human coronary arteries undergoing coronary angioplasty or atherectomy. Circulation 1997;96:475-483.

58. Erbel R, Ge J, Bockisch A, Kearney P, Gorge G, Haude M, et al. Value of intracoronary ultrasound and Doppler in the differentiation of angiographically normal coroanry arteries: a prospective study in patients with angina pectoris. Eur Heart J. 1996;17:880-889.

59. Mintz GS, Painter JA, Pichard AD, Kent KM, Satler LF, Popma JJ, et al. Atherosclerosis in angiographically "normal" coronary artery reference segments: an intravascular ultrasound study with clinical correlations. J Am Coll Cardiol 1995;25(7):1479-85.

60. Waller BF. Anatomy, histology, and pathology of the major epicardial coronary arteries relevant to echocardiographic imaging techniques. J Am Soc Echocardiogr 1989;2:232-253.

61. Isner JM, Donaldsen RF. Coronary angiographic and morphologic correlaton. In Waller BF (ed.) Cardiac Morphology. Philadelphia: Saunders 1984:571-592.

62. Marcus ML, Skorton DJ, Johnson MR, Collins SM, Harrison DG, Kerber RE. Visual estimates of percent diameter coronary stenosis: "a battered gold standard.". J Am Coll Cardiol 1988;11:882-885.

63. Hermiller JB, Buller CE, Tenaglia AN, Kisslo KB, Phillips HR, Bashore TM, et al. Unrecognized left main coronary artery disease in patients undergoing interventional procedures. Am J Cardiol 1993;71(2):173-6.

64. Abizaid AS, Mintz GS, Abizaid A, Mehran R, Lansky AJ, Pichard AD, et al. One-year follow-up after intravascular ultrasound assessment of moderate left main coronary artery disease in patients with ambiguous angiograms. J Am Coll Cardiol 1999;34(3):707-15.

65. Abizaid A, Mintz GS, Pichard AD, Kent KM, Satler LF, Walsh CL, et al. Clinical, intravascular ultrasound, and quantitative angiographic determinants of the coronary flow reserve before and after percutaneous transluminal coronary angioplasty. Am J of Cardiol 1998;82(4):423-8.

66. Moses JW, Undermir C, Strain JE, Kreps EM, Higgins JE, Gleim GW, et al. Relation between single tomographic intravascular ultrasound image parameters and intracoronary Doppler flow velocity in patients with intermediately severe coronary stenoses. Am Heart J 1998;135(6 Pt 1):988-94.

67. Mintz GS, Pichard AD, Kovach JA, Kent KM, Satler LF, Javier SP, et al. Impact of preintervention intravascular ultrasound imaging on transcatheter treatment strategies in coronary artery disease. Am J Cardiol 1994;73(7):423-30.

68. Fitzgerald PJ, Yock PG. Mechanisms and outcomes of angioplasty and atherectomy assessed by intravascular ultrasound imaging. J Clin Ultrasound 1993;21:579-588.

69. TGt i. Impact of ultrasound on device selection and endpoint assessment of interventions: phase I of the GUIDE trial [abstract]. J Am Coll Cardiol. 1993;19:1493-1499.

70. Lee DY, Eigler N, Luo H, Nishioka T, Tabak SW, Forrester JS, et al. Effect of intracoronary ultrasound imaging on clinical decision making. Am Heart J 1995;129(6):1084-93.

71. Kuntz R, Safian R, Levine M, Reis G, Diver D, Baim D. Novel approach to the analysis of restenosis after the use of three new coronary devices. J Am Coll Cardiol 1992;19:1493-1499.

72. Gil R, Di Mario C, Prati F, von Birgelen C, Ruygrok P, Roelandt JR, et al. Influence of plaque composition on mechanisms of percutaneous transluminal coronary balloon angioplasty assessed by ultrasound imaging. Am Heart J 1996;131:591-597.

73. Losordo DW, Rosenfield K, Pieczek A, Baker K, Harding M, Isner JM. How does angioplasty work? Serial analysis of human iliac arteries using intravascular ultrasound. Circulation 1992;86(6):1845-58.

74. Potkin BN, Keren G, Mintz GS, Douek PC, Pichard AD, Satler LF, et al. Arterial responses to balloon coronary angioplasty: an intravascular ultrasound study. J Am Coll Cardiol 1992;20(4):942-51.

75. Braden GA, Herrington DM, Downes TR, Kutcher MA, Little WC. Qualitative and quantitative contrasts in the mechanisms of lumen enlargement by coronary balloon angioplasty and directional coronary atherectomy. J Am Coll Cardiol. 1994;23:40-48.

76. van der Lugt A, Gussenhoven EJ, Stijnen T, van Strijen M, van Driel E, van Egmond FC, et al. Comparison of intravascular ultrasonic findings after coronary balloon angioplasty evaluated in vitro with histology. Am J Cardiol 1995;76(10):661-6.

77. Dotter CT, Judkins MP. Transluminal treatment of arteriosclerotic obstruction. Description of a new technic and a preliminary report of its application. Circulation 1964;30:654-701.

78. Mintz GS, Pichard AD, Kent KM, Satler LF, Popma JJ, Leon MB. Axial plaque redistribution as a mechanism of percutaneous transluminal coronary angioplasty. Am J Cardiol 1996;77:427-429.

79. Stone GW, Hodgson JM, St Goar FG, Frey A, Mudra H, Sheehan H, et al. Improved procedural results of coronary angioplasty with intravascular ultrasound-guided balloon sizing: the CLOUT Pilot Trial. Clinical Outcomes With Ultrasound Trial (CLOUT) Investigators. Circulation 1997;95(8):2044-52.

80. Abizaid A, Pichard AD, Mintz GS, Abizaid AS, Klutstein MW, Satler LF, et al. Acute and long-term results of an intravascular ultrasound-guided percutaneous transluminal coronary angioplasty/provisional stent implantation strategy. Am J Cardiol 1999;84(11):1298-303.

81. MacIsaac A, Bass T, Buchbinder M, Cowley M, Leon M, Warth D, et al. High speed rotational atherectomy: outcome of calcified and noncalcified coronary artery lesions. J Am Coll Cardiol 1995;26:731-6.

82. De Franco AC, Nissen SE, Tuzcu EM, Whitlow PL. Incremental value of intravascular ultrasound during rotational coronary atherectomy. Cathet Cardiovasc Diagn. 1996;Suppl:23-33.

83. Sharma SK, Duvvuri S, Dangas G, Kini A, Vidhum R, Venu K, et al. Rotational atherectomy for in-stent restenosis: acute and long-term results of the first 100 cases. J Am Coll Cardiol. 1998;32:1358-1365.

84. Schiele F, Meneveau N, Vuillemenot A, Gupta S, Bassand JP. Treatment of in-stent restenosis with high speed rotational atherectomy and IVUS guidance in small 3.0 mm vessels. Cathet Cardiovasc Diagn. 1998;44:77-82.

85. Kovach JA, Mintz GS, Pichard AD, Kent KM, Popma JJ, Satler LF, et al. Sequential intravascular ultrasound characterization of the mechanisms of rotational atherectomy and adjunct balloon angioplasty. J Am Coll Cardiol 1993;22(4):1024-32.

86. Prati F, Di Mario C, Moussa I, Reimers B, Mallus MT, Parma A, et al. In-stent neointimal proliferation correlates with the amount of residual plaque burden outside the stent: an intravascular ultrasound study. Circulation 1999;99:1011-1014.

87. Matar FA, Mintz GS, Pinnow E, Javier SP, Popma JJ, Kent KM, et al. Multivariate predictors of intravascular ultrasound end points after directional coronary atherectomy. J Am Coll Cardiol 1995;25(2):318-24.

88. Baptista J, di Mario C, Ozaki Y, Escaned J, R. G, de Feyter P, et al. Impact of plaque morphology and composition on the mechanisms of lumen enlargement using intracoronary ultrasound and quantitative angiography after balloon angioplasty. Am J Cardiol. 1996;77:115-121.

89. Simonton CA, Leon MB, Baim DS, Hinohara T, Kent KM,

Bersin RM, et al. 'Optimal' directional coronary atherectomy: final results of the Optimal Atherectomy Restenosis Study (OARS). Circulation 1998;97:332-339.

90. Suzuki T, Hosokawa H, Katoh O, Fujita T, Ueno K, Takase S, et al. Effects of adjunctive balloon angioplasty after intravascular ultrasound-guided optimal directional coronary atherectomy: the results of the Adjunctive Balloon Angioplasty After Coronary Atherectomy Study (ABACAS). J Am Coll Cardiol 1999;34(4):1028-35.

91. Moussa I, Moses J, Di Mario C, Busi G, Reimers B, Kobayashi Y, et al. Stenting after optimal lesion debulking (SOLD) registry. Angiographic and clinical outcome. Circulation 1998;98:16041-1609.

92. Mintz GS, Popma JJ, Pichard AD, Kent KM, Salter LF, Chuang YC, et al. Intravascular ultrasound predictors of restenosis after percutaneous transcatheter coronary revascularization. J Am Coll Cardiol 1996;27(7):1678-87.

93. Mintz GS, Popma JJ, Pichard AD, Kent KM, Satler LF, Wong C, et al. Arterial remodeling after coronary angioplasty: a serial intravascular ultrasound study. Circulation 1996;94:35-43.

94. Schuhlen H, Hadamitzky M, Walter H, Ulm K, Schomig A. Major benefit from antiplatelet therapy for patients at high risk for adverse cardiac events after coronary Palmaz-Schatz stent placement: analysis of a prospective risk stratification protocol in the Intracoronary Stenting and Antithrombotic Regimen (ISAR) trial. Circulation 1997;95:2011-2021.

95. Hoffmann R, Mintz GS, Popma JJ, Satler LF, Kent KM, Pichard AD, et al. Treatment of calcified coronary lesions with Palmaz-Schatz stents. An intravascular ultrasound study [see comments]. Eur Heart J. 1998;19:1224-1231.

96. Russo RJ. Ultrasound-guided stent replacement. Cardiol Clin. 1997;15:49-61.

97. Russo RJ, Nicosia A, Teirstein PS, AVID I. Angiography Versus Intravascular Ultrasound-Directed Stent Placement. J Am Coll Cardiol. 1997;29:369A.

98. Ellis SG, Savage M, Fischman D, Baim DS, Leon M, Goldberg S, et al. Restenosis after placement of Palmaz-Schatz stents in native coronary arteries. Initial results of a multicenter experience. Circulation 1992;86:1836-1844.

99. Goldberg SL, Colombo A, Nakamura S, Almagor Y, Maiello L, Tobis JM. Benefit of intracoronary ultrasound in the deployment of Palmaz-Schatz stents. J Am Coll Cardiol 1994;24(4):996-1003.

100. Kiemeneij F, Laarman G, Slagboom T. Mode of deployment of coronary Palmaz-Schatz stents after implantation with the stent delivery system: an intravascular ultrasound study. Am Heart J 1995;129(4):638-44.

101. Nakamura S, Colombo A, Gaglione A, Almagor Y, Goldberg SL, Maiello L, et al. Intracoronary ultrasound observations during stent implantation. Circulation 1994;89:2026-2034.

102. Colombo A, Hall P, Nakamura S, Almagor Y, Maiello L, Martini G, et al. Intracoronary stenting without anticoagulation accomplished with intravascular ultrasound guidance [see comments]. Circulation 1995;91(6):1676-88.

103. Gorge G, Ge J, Erbel R. Role of intravascular ultrasound in the evaluation of mechanisms of coronary interventions and restenosis. Am J Cardiol 1998;81(12A):91G-95G.

104. Goods CM, Al Shaibi KF, Yadav SS, Liu MW, Negus BH,

Iyer SS, et al. Utilization of the coronary balloon-expandable coil stent without anticoagulation or intravascular ultrasound. Circulation 1996;93(10):1803-8.

105. Karrillon GJ, Morice MC, Benveniste E, Bunouf P, Aubry P, Cattan S, et al. Intracoronary stent implantation without ultrasound guidance and with replacement of conventional anticoagulation by antiplatelet therapy. 30-day clinical outcome of the French Multicenter Registry. Circulation 1996;94:1519-1527.

106. Stone GW, St. Goar FG, Hodgson JM, Fitzgerald PJ, Alderman EL, Yock PG, et al. Analysis of the relation between stent implantation pressure and expansion. Optimal Stent Implantation (OSTI) Investigators. Am J of Cardiol 1999;83(9):1397-400, A8.

107. Hoffmann R, Mintz GS, Pichard AD, Kent KM, Satler LF, Leon MB. Intimal hyperplasia thickness at follow-up is independent of stent size: a serial intravascular ultrasound study. Am J Cardiol 1998;82(10):1168-72.

108. de Jaegere P, Mudra H, Figulla H, Almagor Y, Doucet S, Penn I, et al. Intravascular ultrasound-guided optimized stent deployment. Immediate and 6 months clinical and agiographic results from the Multicenter Ultrasound Stenting in Coronaries Study (MUSIC Study) [see comments]. Eur Heart J. 1998;19:1214-1223.

109. Goldberg SL, Hall P, Nakamura S, Maiello L, Almagor Y, Tobis J, et al. Is there a benefit from intravascular ultrasound when high pressure stent expansion is routinely performed prior to ultrasound imaging? (abstract). J Am Coll Cardiol. 1996;27:306A.

110. Stone GW, St. Goar F, Fitzgerald P, Alderman E, Yock P, Hodgson JM, et al. The Optimal Stent Implantation Trial: final core lab angiographic and ultrasound analysis (abstract). J Am Coll Cardiol. 1997;29:369A.

111. Ziada KM, Tuzcu EM, De Franco AC, Whitlow PW, Ellis SE, Nissen SE. Absolute, not relative, post-stent lumen area is a better predictor of clinical events (abstract). Circulation 1996;94:I-453.

112. Kasaoka S, Tobis JM, Akiyama T, Reimers B, Di Mario C, Wong ND, et al. Angiographic and intravascular ultrasound predictors of in-stent restenosis. J Am Coll Cardiol 1998;32(6):1630-5.

113. Ziada KM, Tuzcu EM, De Franco AC, Kim MH, Raymond RE, Franco I, et al. Intravascular ultrasound assessment of the prevalence and causes of angiographic "haziness" following high-pressure coronary stenting. Am J Cardiol 1997;80(2):116-21.

114. Moussa I, Di Mario C, Moses J, Reimers B, Blengino S, Colombo A. The predictive value of different intravascular ultrasound criteria for restenosis after coronary stenting (abstract). J Am Coll Cardiol 1997;29:60A.

115. Ahmed JM, Mintz GS, Weissman NJ, Lansky AJ, Pichard AD, Satler LF, et al. Mechanism of lumen enlargement during intracoronary stent implantation: an intravascular ultrasound study. Circulation 2000;102(1):7-10.

116. Fitzgerald PJ, Hayase M, Mintz GS, Kuntz R, Moses JW, Diver DJ, et al. CRUISE: Can Routine Intravascular Ultrasound Influence Stent Expansion? Analysis of outcomes. J Am Coll Cardiol 1998;31:396A.

117. Schiele F, Meneveau N, Vuillemenot A, Zhang DD, Gupta S,

Mercier M, et al. Impact of intravascular ultrasound guidance in stent deployment on 6-month restenosis rate: a multicenter, randomized study comparing two strategies--with and without intravascular ultrasound guidance. RESIST Study Group. REStenosis after Ivus guided STenting. J Am Coll Cardiol 1998;32(2):320-8.

118. Painter JA, Mintz GS, Wong SC, Popma JJ, Pichard AD, Kent KM, et al. Serial intravascular ultrasound studies fail to show evidence of chronic Palmaz-Schatz stent recoil. Am J Cardiol 1995;75(5):398-400.

119. Serruys P, de Jaegere P, Kiemeniej F, Magaya C, Rutsch W, Heyndrickx G, et al. A comparison of balloon-expandable-stent implantation with balloon angioplasty in patients with coronary artery disease. N Engl J Med 1994;331:489-495.

120. Serruys PW, van Hout B, Bonnier H, Legrand V, Garcia E, Macaya C, et al. Randomised comparison of implantation of heparin-coated stents with balloon angioplasty in selected patients with coronary artery disease (Benestent II) [published erratum appears in Lancet 1998 Oct 31;352(9138):1478]. Lancet 1998;352:673-681.

121. Fischman D, Leon M, Baim D, Schatz R, Savage M, Penn I, et al. A randomized comparison of coronary-stent placement and balloon angioplasty in the treatment of coronary artery disease.
N Engl J Med 1994;331:496-501.

122. Moussa I, Moses J, Di Mario C, Albiero R, De Gregorio J, Adamian M, et al. Does the specific intravascular ultrasound criterion used to optimize stent expansion have an impact on the probability of stent restenosis? Am J Cardiol 1999;83(7):1012-7.

123. Hoffmann R, Mintz GS, Kent KM, Satler LF, Pichard AD, Popma JJ, et al. Serial intravascular ultrasound predictors of restenosis at the margins of Palmaz-Schatz stents. Am J Cardiol. 1997;79:915-953.

124. Hong MK, Mintz GS, Hong MK, Pichard AD, Satler LF, Kent KM, et al. Intravascular ultrasound predictors of target lesion revascularization after stenting of protected left main coronary artery stenoses. Am J Cardiol 1999;83(2):175-9.

125. Hoffmann R, Mintz GS, Mehran R, Pichard AD, Kent KM, Satler LF, et al. Intravascular ultrasound predictors of angiographic restenosis in lesions treated with Palmaz-Schatz stents. J Am Coll Cardiol 1998;31(1):43-9.

126. Moussa I, Di Mario C, Moses J, Reimers B, Blengino S, Colombo A. Single versus multiple Palmaz-Schatz stent implantation: immediate and follow-up results. J Am Coll Cardiol (abstract) 1997;29 Suppl A:276A.

127. Aliabadi D, Bowers T, Tilli F, Spybrook M, Greenberg H, Goldstein J, et al. Multiple stents increase target vessel revascularization rates. J Am Coll Cardiol 1997;29 Suppl A:312A.

128. Kereiakes D, Linnemeier TJ, Baim DS, Kuntz R, O'Shaughnessy C, Hermiller J, et al. Usefulness of stent length in predicting in-stent restenosis (the MULTI-LINK stent trials). Am J Cardiol 2000;86(3):336-41.

129. Kasaoka S, Tobis JM, Akiyama T, Reimers B, Di Mario C, Wong ND, et al. Angiographic and intravascular ultrasound predictors of in-stent restenosis. J Am Coll Cardiol 1998;32(6):1630-5.

130. Kastrati A, Elezi S, Dirschinger J, Hadamitzky M, Neumann FJ, Schomig A. Influence of lesion length on restenosis after coronary stent placement. Am J Cardiol 1999;83(12):1617-22.

131. Hoffmann R, Mintz GS, Mehran R, Kent KM, Pichard AD, Satler LF, et al. Tissue proliferation within and surrounding Palmaz-Schatz stents is dependent on the aggressiveness of stent implantation technique. Am J Cardiol 1999;83(8):1170-4.

132. Kornowski R, Mintz GS, Kent KM, Pichard AD, Satler LF, Bucher TA, et al. Increased restenosis in diabetes mellitus after coronary interventions is due to exaggerated intimal hyperplasia. A serial intravascular ultrasound study. Circulation 1997;95(6):1366-9.

133. Sheris SJ, Canos MR, Weissman NJ. Natural history of intravascular ultrasound-detected edge dissections from coronary stent deployment. Am Heart J 2000;139(1 Pt 1):59-63.

134. Fitzgerald P. Personal communication. 2000.

135. Sheifer SE, Canos MR, Weinfurt KP, Arora UK, Mendelsohn FO, Gersh BJ, et al. Sex differences in coronary artery size assessed by intravascular ultrasound. Am Heart J 2000;139(4):649-53.

136. de Feyter PJ, Kay P, Disco C, Serruys PW. Reference chart derived from post-stent-implantation intravascular ultrasound predictors of 6-month expected restenosis on quantitative coronary angiography. Circulation 1999;100(17):1777-83.

137. Ahmed JM, Hong MK, Mehran R, Mintz GS, Lansky AJ, Pichard AD, et al. Comparison of debulking followed by stenting versus stenting alone for saphenous vein graft aortoostial lesions: immediate and one-year clinical outcomes. J Am Coll Cardiol 2000;35(6):1560-8.

138. Hong MK, Park SW, Mintz GS, Lee NH, Lee CW, Kim JJ, et al. Intravascular ultrasonic predictors of angiographic restenosis after long coronary stenting. Am J Cardiol 2000;85(4):441-5.

139. Caputo RP, Ho KL, Lopez JJ, Stoler RC, Cohen DJ, Carrozza JP. Quantitative angiographic comparison of Palmaz-Schatz stent implantation with and without intravascular ultrasound (abstract). Circulation 1995; 92:I-545.

140. Werner G, Diedrich J, Ferrari M, Buchwald A, Figulla HR. Can additional intravascular ultrasound improve the luminal area gain after high pressure stent deployment? J Am Coll Cardiol. 1996;27:225A.

141. de la Torre Hernandez JM, Gomez I, Rodriguez-Entem F, Zueco J, Figueroa A, Colman T. Evaluation of direct stent implantation without predilatation by intravascular ultrasound. Am J Cardiol 2000;85(8):1028-30, A8.

142. Mintz GS, Hoffmann R, Mehran R, Pichard AD, Kent KM, Satler LF, et al. In-stent restenosis: the Washington Hospital Center experience. Am J Cardiol 1998;81(7A):7E-13E.

143. Batkoff BW, Linker DT. Safety of intracoronary ultrasound: data from a Multicenter European Registry. Cathet Cardiovasc Diagn. 1996;38:238-241.

144. Hausmann D, Erbel R, Alibelli-Chemarin MJ, Boksch W, Caracciolo E, Cohn JM, et al. The safety of intracoronary ultrasound. A multicenter survey of 2207 examinations. Circulation 1995;91:623-630.

145. Pinto FJ, St. Goar FG, Gao SZ, Chenzbraun A, Fischell TA, Alderman, et al. Immediate and one-year safety of

intracoronary ultrasonic imaging. Evaluation with serial quantitative angiography. Circulation 1993;88:1709-1714.

146. TenHoff H, Hamm MA, Lowe GE, Koger JD. Technical aspects of ultrasound imaging guidewires. Semin Interv Cardiol. 1997;2:63-68.

147. Stone GW, St. Goar FG, Linnemeier TJ. Initial clinical experience with a novel low-profile integrated ultrasound-angioplasty catheter. Cathet Cardiovasc Diagn 1996;38:303-307.

148. Mudra H, Klauss V, Vlasini R, Kroetz M, Reiber J, Regar E, et al. Ultrasound guidance of Palmaz-Schatz intracoronary stenting with a combined intravascular ultrasound balloon catheter. Circulation 1994;90:1252-1261.

149. Hiro T, Leung CY, Karimi H, Farvid AR, Tobis JM. Angle dependence of intravascular ultrasound imaging and its feasibility in tissue characterization of human atherosclerotic tissue. Am Heart J 1999;137(3):476-81.

150. Hiro T, Leung CY, De Guzman S, Caiozzo VJ, Farvid AR, Karimi H, et al. Are soft echoes really soft? Intravascular ultrasound assessment of mechanical properties in human atherosclerotic tissue. Am Heart J 1997;133(1):1-7.

151. Barzilai B, Saffitz JE, Miller JG, Sobel BE. Quantitative ultrasonic characterization of the nature of atherosclerotic plaques in human aorta. Circ Res 1987;60:459-463.

152. Lockwood GR, Ryan LK, Foster FS. A 45 to 55 MHz needle-based ultrasound system for invasive imaging. Ultrason Imaging 1993;15:1-13.

153. Foster FS, Knapik DA, Machado JC, Ryan LK, Nissen SE. High-frequency intracoronary ultrasound imaging. Semin Interv Cardiol. 1997;2:33-41.

154. Brezinski ME, Tearney GJ, Weissman NJ, Boppart SA, Bouma BE, Hee MR, et al. Assessing atherosclerotic plaque morphology: comparison of optical coherence tomography and high frequency intravascular ultrasound. Heart 1997;77(5):397-403.

155. Bom N, Li W, van der Steen AF, Lancee CT, Cespedes EI, Slager CJ, et al. New developments in intravascular ultrasound imaging. Eur J Ultrasound 1998;7:9-14.

156. Di Mario C, von Birgelen C, Prati F, Soni B, Li W, Bruining N, et al. Three dimensional reconstruction of cross sectional intracoronary ultrasound: clinical or research tool? Br Heart J 1995;73:26-32.

157. Williams DO. Radiation vascular therapy: a novel approach to preventing restenosis. Am J Cardiol 1998;81(7A):18E-20E.

158. Prati F, Di Mario C, Gil R, von Birgelen C, Camenzind E, Montauban van Swijndregt WJ, et al. Usefulness of on-line three-dimensional reconstruction of intracoronary ultrasound for guidance of stent deployment. Am J Cardiol 1996;77:455.

159. von Birgelen C, de Vrey EA, Mintz GS, Nicosia A, Bruining N, Li W, et al. ECG-gated three-dimensional intravascular ultrasound: feasibility and reproducibility of the automated analysis of coronary lumen and atherosclerotic plaque dimensions in humans. Circulation 1997;96:2944-2952.

160. Krams R, Wentzel JJ, Oomen JA, Vinke R, Schuurbiers JC, de Feyter PJ, et al. Evaluation of endothelial shear stress and 3D geometry as factors determining the development of atherosclerosis and remodeling in human coronary arteries in vivo. Combining 3D reconstruction from angiography and IVUS (ANGUS) with computational fluid dynamics. Arterioscler Thromb Vasc Biol 1997;17:2061-2065.

161. Evans JL, Ng KH, Wiet SG, Vonesh MJ, Burns WB, Radvany MG, et al. Accurate three-dimensional reconstruction of intravascular ultrasound data. Spatially correct three-dimensional reconstructions. Circulation 1996;93:567-576.

162. Pellot C, Block I, Herment A, Sureda F. An attempt to 3D reconstruct vessel morphology from X-ray projections and intravascular ultrasounds modeling and fusion. Comput Med Imaging Graph 1996;20:141-151.

163. Kay IP, Sabate M, Van Langenhove G, Costa MA, Wardeh AJ, Gijzel AL, et al. Outcome from balloon induced coronary artery dissection after intracoronary beta radiation. Heart 2000;83(3):332-7.

164. Meerkin D, Tardif JC, Bertrand OF, Vincent J, Harel F, Bonan R. The effects of intracoronary brachytherapy on the natural history of postangioplasty dissections. J Am Coll Cardiol 2000;36(1):59-64.

165. Sabate M, Serruys PW, van der Giessen WJ, Ligthart JM, Coen VL, Kay IP, et al. Geometric vascular remodeling after balloon angioplasty and beta-radiation therapy: A three-dimensional intravascular ultrasound study. Circulation 1999;100(11):1182-8.

166. Waksman R, White RL, Chan RC, Bass BG, Geirlach L, Mintz GS, et al. Intracoronary gamma-radiation therapy after angioplasty inhibits recurrence in patients with in-stent restenosis [see comments]. Circulation 2000;101(18):2165.

167. Limpijankit T, Waksman R, Yock PG, Fitzgerald PJ. Intravascular ultrasound volumetric assessment of intimal hyperplasia in stents treated with intracoronary radiation. Am J Cardiol 1999;84(7):850-4, A8.

168. Shiran A, Mintz GS, Waksman R, Mehran R, Abizaid A, Kent KM, et al. Early lumen loss after treatment of in-stent restenosis: an intravascular ultrasound study. Circulation 1998;98(3):200-3.

32 CORONARY ANGIOSCOPY

Robert D. Safian, M.D.

Although early coronary angioscopes were limited by their large diameters and inflexibility,[1] flexible catheters with advanced fiberoptics have been designed to permit direct visualization of the luminal surface of virtually all native coronary arteries and bypass grafts. Several studies confirm the superiority of angioscopy to contrast angiography in detecting and differentiating plaque, dissection, and thrombus.[2-4,32,33] Despite the capability for accurate detection of thrombus and other intraluminal details,[5,6] angioscopy has not achieved an important role in guiding interventional therapy (Table 32.1).

A. **TECHNIQUE OF CORONARY ANGIOSCOPY.** The angioscopy system is a monorail design compatible with virtually all 8F guiding catheters and 0.014-inch guidewires. It consists of a high-intensity light source, a fiberoptic imaging bundle with over 2000 individual fibers, a video monitor for on-line imaging, and a videotape recorder for image archiving, storage, and retrieval (Figure 32.1). Despite its flexibility, advancement of the angioscope up to the lesion requires good guiding catheter support and the use of an extra-support guidewire. A blood-free field is obtained by gently inflating the occlusion cuff on the angioscope and simultaneously injecting warm heparinized saline through the irrigation port via a power injector. Special care was taken to avoid overinflation of the occlusion cuff, since the highly compliant material could expand to 6 mm in diameter and induce vessel injury. In general, cuff inflation was limited to 45-90 seconds to minimize myocardial ischemia.

B. **PROPOSED INDICATIONS FOR CORONARY ANGIOSCOPY (Table 32.2)**
   1. **Guiding Saphenous Vein Graft Interventions.** Percutaneous interventions in saphenous vein grafts are limited by a high incidence of complications and restenosis.[7] We and others frequently used angioscopy to guide therapeutic strategies based on its ability to detect intraluminal thrombus, friable plaque, and post-procedural dissection.[8,9] However, concerns about the need to identify thrombus[10-12] have been markedly attenuated by the success of stenting in vein grafts. Also, no large-scale clinical trials demonstrate a clear benefit of angioscopy in vein graft lesions. Loose friable material in vein grafts identifies a high-risk population for transient or sustained no-reflow[13,14] and can be readily identified by angioscopy, but the emerging role of distal embolic protection devices may obviate the need to identify it.

   2. **Evaluation of Suboptimal Results.** Evaluation of the "hazy" or suboptimal result after percutaneous intervention was the most valuable role for angioscopy,[15] given its ability to distinguish between thrombus, dissection, and plaque.[15,16] In practice, most operators rely on IVUS for this purpose, or more commonly use empiric stenting.

Table 32.1. Comparison of Imaging and Hemodynamic Techniques

Characteristic	Digital Angiography	Angioscopy	IVUS	Doppler FloWire	Pressure Wire
Vessel lumen detail	+	++++	++	-	-
Vessel wall detail	-	-	++++	-	-
Plaque composition	-	++	+++	-	-
Vessel dimensions	++	-	++++	-	-
Identify disease in "normal" vessel	+	++	++++	-	-
Detect diffuse disease	+	++	++++	-	-
Evaluate "haziness"	±	+++	+++	+	+
Arterial remodeling	±	-	++++	-	-
Borderline lesions - morphology	+	-	++++	-	-
Borderline lesions - physiology	-	-	+	++++	++++
Suboptimal results	+	++	+++	+++	++++
Clot vs. dissection	±	++++	+++	-	-
Predict complications	+	unknown	possible	+++	possible
Continuous record (trend)	-	-	-	+++	-
Predict restenosis	+	-	++	++	unknown
Microvascular disease	-	-	-	+++	-
Cause of ischemia	-	+++	+	-	-

Abbreviations: IVUS = intravascular ultrasound

- = no value; ± = limited value; + thru ++++ = increasing value

3. **Post-Interventional Assessment.** Angioscopic evaluation after stent placement was used to determine the adequacy of stent expansion[17] and the effects of laser angioplasty and atherectomy,[9,18,19] but has been supplanted by IVUS (Chapter 31).

4. **Assessment of Borderline Lesions.** Angioscopy was used to assess lesions of intermediate severity, particularly when associated with typical symptoms or other objective signs of ischemia. However, other modalities such as Doppler flow analysis (Chapter 33) and intravascular ultrasound (Chapter 31) are superior to angioscopy for this purpose, since they provide objective physiologic data (Doppler) or quantitative analysis (ultrasound), which cannot be derived from angioscopy.

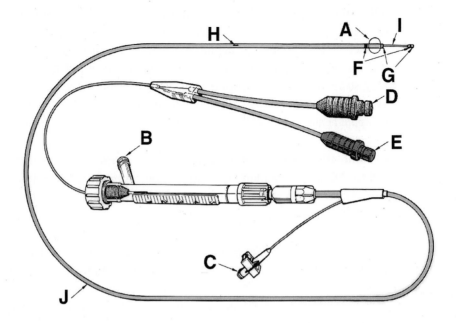

Figure 32.1 The ImageCath Coronary Angioscope

A. Balloon. B. Flush port. C. Balloon inflation port. D. Video connector. E. Light connector. F. Radiopaque markers. G. Tip of shaft and imaging core. H. Guidewire exit. I. Moveable imaging core. J. Catheter shaft.

Table 32.2. Old Indications for Angioscopy

Guiding saphenous vein bypass graft interventions

Evaluation of suboptimal results

Post-intervention assessment

Assessment of borderline lesions

Identification of "culprit" lesions

Predicting outcome after intervention

5. **Identification of Culprit Lesions.** Given the high incidence (43-80%) of thrombus in de novo unstable lesions,[20] and angioscopy's ability to detect thrombus (and the yellow lipid-rich plaques frequently associated with thrombus),[21,22] angioscopy was used to identify the "culprit" lesion in patients with multivessel disease and unstable angina.[32] Angioscopy is probably superior to IVUS for discriminating stable from unstable plaques[36] in vein grafts and in native vessels. However, most operators still rely on noninvasive functional studies or invasive techniques in which angiography is supplemented with IVUS, the pressure wire, or the Doppler FloWire.

6. **Predicting Outcome after Intervention.** Small studies suggested that plaque color, lesion ulceration, and thrombus were important predictors of outcome after intervention,[24,25,40] but the incremental value of these observations seems small in an era when stents and GP IIb/IIIa receptor antagonists are widely employed.

D. **LIMITATIONS OF ANGIOSCOPY (Table 32.3).** Angioscopy provides qualitative morphologic information, but in contrast to Doppler analysis and IVUS, it does not provide quantitative analysis of flow or lumen dimensions. Angioscopy is also suboptimal for imaging aorto-ostial lesions (due to difficulty ensuring a blood-free imaging field) and for proximal LAD or circumflex lesions (due to the need for transient occlusion of the left main coronary artery). Furthermore, blood flow from adjacent side branches may obscure the imaging field and preclude image analysis. Angioscopy catheters also lacked steerability, had a limited field of view, and lacked some sensitivity and specificity for detecting endoluminal lesions.[27] For these and other reasons, angioscopy has not been widely embraced by the interventional community.

E. **COMPLICATIONS (Table 32.4).** In general, angioscopy was a safe adjunct to other percutaneous interventions; complications were related to operator experience.[28] Coronary artery perforation due to rupture of the occlusion cuff was reported in one patient.[29] Improper technique also led to air emboli from the flush solution. Although severe angiographic complications were unusual, 9% of lesions treated with PTCA required a "touch-up" balloon inflation after angioscopy to smooth out the final result.[30] Angioscopy of degenerated vein grafts induced transient or sustained no-reflow in nearly 50% of lesions, which identified a high-risk subgroup for sustained no-reflow after further intervention.[13] Although cuff inflation lasting more than 60 seconds often induced transient myocardial ischemia, the overall incidence of major ischemic complications was less than 1%.[28]

Table 32.3. Limitations of Angioscopy

Does not provide quantitative data

Inability to reliably image aorto-ostial lesions

May lead to transient ischemia or hemodynamic instability

Not safe for imaging lesions at the origin of the LAD or LCX

Table 32.4. Complications of Angioscopy

Angiographic Complications (%)[13,20]	
Dissection *	2.8
Abrupt closure **	1.0
No-reflow***	45
Clinical Complications (%)[20]	
Death	0.1
MI	0.2
CABG	0.5
VF	1.7

Abbreviations: MI = In-hospital Q-wave myocardial infarction; CABG = emergency coronary bypass grafting;
VF = ventricular fibrillation
*   Dissection due to occlusion cuff, guidewire, or imaging bundle
**   Managed by stents or emergency CABG
*** Degenerated vein grafts

* * * * *

REFERENCES

1. Sherman TC, Litvack F, Grundfest W, et al. Coronary angioscopy in patients with unstable angina pectoris. N Eng J Med 1986;315:913-919.

2. Litvack F, Grundfest WS, Lee ME, et al. Angioscopic visualization of blood vessel interior in animals and humans. Clin Cardiol 1985;8:65-70.

3. Grundfest WS, Litvack F, Sherman T, et al. Delineation of peripheral and coronary detail by intraoperative angioscopy. Ann Surg 1985;202:394-400.

4. Sanborn TA, Rygaard JA, Westbrook BM, et al. Intraoperative angioscopy of saphenous vein and coronary arteries. J Thorac Cardiovasc Surg 1986;91:339-343.

5. King SB III. Role on new technologies in balloon angioplasty. Circulation 1991;84:2574-2579.

6. Forrester JS, Eigler N, Litvack F: Interventional cardiology: The decade ahead. Circulation 1991;84:942-944.

7. Schweiger MJ, Roccario E, Weil T. Treatment of patients following bypass surgery: a dilemma for the 1990s. Am Heart J 1992;123:268-272.

8. White CJ, Ramee SR, Collins TJ, et al. Percutaneous angioscopy of saphenous vein coronary bypass grafts. J Am Coll Cardiol 1993;21:1181-1185.

9. Annex, BH, Larkin TJ, O'Neill WW, et al. Evaluation of thrombus removal by transluminal extraction coronary atherectomy by percutaneous coronary angioscopy. Am J Cardiol 1994;74:606-609.

10. Annex BH, Ajluni SC, Larkin TJ, et al. Angioscopic-guided interventions in a saphenous vein bypass graft. Cathet Cardiovasc Diagn 1994;31:330-333.

11. Nath FC, Muller DWM, Ellis SG, et al. Thrombosis of a flexible coil coronary stent: frequency, predictors and clinical outcome. J Am Coll Cardiol 1993;21:622-627.

12. Hermann HC, Buchbinder M, Clemen MW, et al. Emergent use of balloon-expandable coronary artery stenting for failed percutaneous transluminal coronary angioplasty. Circulation 1992;86:812-819.

13. Kaplan BM, Safian RD, Grines CL, et al. Usefulness of adjunctive angioscopy and extraction atherectomy before stent implantation in high-risk aorto-coronary saphenous vein grafts. Am J Cardiol 1995;76:822-824.

14. Tilli FV, Kaplan BM, Safian RD, Grines CL, O'Neill WW. Angioscopic plaque friability: A new risk factor for procedural complications following saphenous vein graft interventions. J Am Coll Cardiol (in-press).

15. White CJ, Ramee SR, Collins TJ, et al. Percutaneous coronary angioscopy: Applications in interventional cardiology. J Interven Cardiol 1993;6:61-67.

16. Sassower MA, Abela GS, Koch JM, et al. Angioscopic evaluation of periprocedural and postprocedural abrupt closure after percutaneous coronary angioplasty. Am Heart J 1993;126:444-450.

17. Teirstein PS, Schatz RA, Rocha-Singh KJ, et al. Coronary stenting with angioscopic guidance. J Am Coll Cardiol 1992;19:223A.

18. Nakamura F, Kvasnicka J, Uchida Y, et al. Percutaneous angioscopic evaluation of luminal changes induced by excimer laser angioplasty. Am Heart J 1992;124:1467-1472.

19. Eltchaninoff H, Cribier A, Koning R, et al. Comparative angioscopic findings after rotational atherectomy and balloon angioplasty. J Am Coll Cardiol 1995;25:95A.

20. Waxman S, Mittleman MA, Manxo K, Saaower M, et al. Culprit lesion morphology in subtypes of unstable angina as assessed by angioscopy. Circulation 1995;92:I-79.

21. Waxman S, Saaower M, Mittleman MA, Nesto RW, et al. Characterization of the culprit lesion underlying thrombus: Insights from angioscopy. Circulation 1995;92:I-353.

22. Uchida Y, Nakamura F, Tomaru T, Mortia T, et al. Prediction of acute coronary syndromes by percutaneous coronary angioscopy in patients with stable angina. Am Heart J 1995;130:195-203.

23. Silva JA, Escobar A, Collins TJ, Ramee SR, White CJ. Unstable angina. A comparison of angioscopic findings between diabetic and nondiabetic patients. Circulation 1995;92:1731-1736.

24. Bauters C, Lablanche JM, McFadden E, Hamon M, Bertrand ME. Angioscopic thrombus is associated with a high risk of angiographic restenosis. Circulation 1995;92:I-401.

25. Waxman S, Sassower M, Mittleman MA, et al. Angiographic predictors of early adverse outcome after coronary angioplasty in patients with unstable angina and non-Q-wave myocardial infarction. Circulation 1996;93:2106-2113.

26. Feld S, Ganim M, Carell ES, et al. Comparison of angioplasty, intravascular ultrasound imaging and quantitative coronary angiography in predicting clinical outcome after coronary intervention in high-risk patients. J Am Coll Cardiol 1996;28:97-105.

27. Uretsky BF, Denys BG, Counihan P, et al. Accuracy of angioscopy in diagnosing endoluminal lesions. J Am Coll Cardiol;1994:23:407A.

28. Lablanche, JM, Geschwind H, Cribier A, et al. Coronary angioscopy safety survey: European multicenter experience. J Am Coll Cardiol 1995;25:154A.

29. Wolff, MR, Resar JR, Stuart RS, et al. Coronary artery rupture and pseudoaneurysm formation resulting from percutaneous coronary angioscopy. Cathet Cardiovasc Diagn 1993;28:47-50.

30. Alfonso F, Hernandez R, Goicolea J, et al. Angiographic deterioration of the previously dilated coronary segment induced by angioscopic examination. Am J Cardiol 1994;74:604-606.

31. White CJ, Ramee SR, Collins TJ, et al. Coronary thrombi increase PTCA risk: Angioscopy as a clinical tool. Circulation 1996;93:253-8.

32. Alfonso F, Segovia J, Goicolea J, et al. Angioscopic characteristics of coronary narrowing in patients with recurrent myocardial ischemia after myocardial infarction. Am J Cardiol 1997;79:1394-1396.

33. Waxman S, Mittleman MA, Zarich SW, et al. Angioscopic assessment of coronary lesions underlying thrombus. Am J Cardiol 1997;79:1106-1109.

34. Thieme T, Wernecke KD, Meyer R, et al. Angioscopic evaluation of atherosclerotic plaques: Validation by histomorphologic analysis and association with stable and unstable coronary syndromes. J Am Coll Cardiol 1996;28:1-6.

35. de Feyter PJ, Ozaki Y, Baptista J, et al. Ischemia-related lesion characteristics in patients with stable or unstable angina. A study with intracoronary angioscopy and ultrasound. Circulation 1995;92:1408-1413.

36. Silva JA, White CJ, Collins TJ, et al. Morphologic comparison of atherosclerotic lesions in native coronary arteries and saphenous vein grafts with intracoronary angioscopy in patients with unstable angina. Am Heart J 1998;136:156-163.

37. Ueda Y, Asakura M, Hirayama A, et al. Intracoronary morphology of culprit lesions after reperfusion in acute myocardial infarction: Serial angioscopic observations. J Am Coll Cardiol 1996;27:606-610.

38. Arakawa K, Mizuno K, Shibuya T, et al. Angioscopic coronary macromorphology after thrombolysis in acute myocardial infarction. Am J Cardiol 1997;79:197-202.

39. Alfronso F, Fernandez-Ortiz A, Goicolea J, et al. Angioscopic evaluation of angiographically complex coronary lesions. Am Heart J 1997;134:703-711.

40. Van Belle E, Lablanche JM, Bauters C, et al. Coronary angioscopic findings in the infarct-related vessel within 1 month of acute myocardial infarction. Natural history and the effect of thrombolysis. Circulation 1998;97:26-33.

33

INTRACORONARY DOPPLER BLOOD FLOW AND PRESSURE MEASUREMENTS

Simon Dixon, M.D.
Terry T. Bowers, M.D.
Robert D. Safian, M.D.

A. INTRODUCTION TO CORONARY FLOW RESERVE. Myocardial blood flow is regulated by changes in vascular resistance at the level of the coronary arteriole (Table 33.1). As myocardial O_2 demand increases (e.g., exercise), there is a decrease in resistance (coronary vasodilatation) and an increase in blood flow. Coronary flow reserve (CFR), defined as the ratio of hyperemic-to-resting blood flow velocity,[8] is typically > 2. In the presence of a flow-limiting epicardial stenosis, the distal microvasculature dilates to preserve resting basal blood flow;[7] however, maximal hyperemic flow is impaired and CFR is < 2. CFR and other blood flow measurements can be safely, easily, and reliably obtained in the catheterization laboratory with the use of the Endosonics FloWire, a flexible, steerable 0.014" or 0.018" guidewire with a tip-mounted piezoelectric Doppler crystal (Figure 33.1).[2-4] Doppler signals are transmitted from the tip of the FloWire to the FloMap Instrument, where they are converted into a spectral display on the monitor (Figure 33.2). Preliminary data suggest that the Doppler wire may be useful to assess the physiologic significance of a stenosis in a variety of clinical and interventional settings (see Section E, below).[8-14]

B. APPROACH TO DOPPLER BLOOD FLOW

1. **Doppler Systems (Table 33.2).** Older 3F Doppler catheters have been largely replaced by the Endosonics FloWire.

Table 33.1. Determinants of Coronary Vascular Resistance

Physiologic	Pharmacologic
Autoregulation	Norepinephrine
Increased myocardial O_2 consumption	Papaverine
Sympathetic stimulation	Dipyridamole
	Serotonin
	Vasopressin
	Nitroglycerin
	Adenosine
	EDRF (Nitric Oxide)

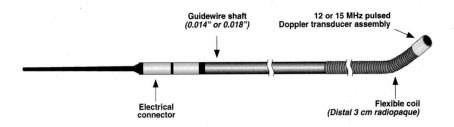

Figure 33.1. Doppler FloWire Construction

Courtesy of Endosonics, Inc.

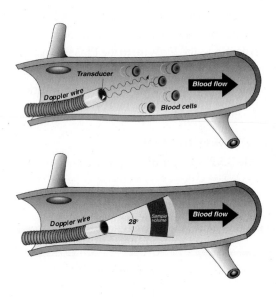

Figure 33.2. Coronary Blood Flow: Doppler Measurements

The ultrasound beam (28°) provides a large sample volume, which ensures measurement of peak flow velocity with minimal dependence on guidewire position. The sample volume is 5 mm and 4 mm from the tip of the 0.018-inch and 0.014-inch FloWire, respectively.

Table 33.2. Doppler Systems for Coronary Blood Flow Velocity Measurements

Device	Size	Crystal Position	Display	Range Gate (mm)	Doppler Signal Analysis	Frequency Shift
Numed[64,65]	3F (1.0 mm)	Side-mounted	Chart recorder	1-10	Zero-cross	20 MHZ
Millar[66]	3F (1.0 mm)	End-mounted	Chart recorder	1-10	Zero-cross	20 MHZ
FloWire[67]	0.018" 0.014"	End-mounted	On-line spectral display	5.2	Fast fourier transform	12 MHZ

2. **Coronary Blood Flow Data.** Spectral flow velocity data, along with ECG and arterial blood pressure recording, are displayed in real time on the FloMap monitor. In addition to coronary flow reserve—the parameter used to assess the functional significance of a lesion before and after intervention—other blood flow measurements can be obtained, including the beat-to-beat phasic average peak velocity (APV), diastolic-to-systolic velocity ratio (DSVR), APV trend over 1.5-90 minutes, and the proximal-to-distal translesional velocity ratio. The "normal" range of Doppler-derived flow velocity variables has been defined (Table 33.3),[3,4,16-22] but interpretation of each variable must be considered in the context of other Doppler variables, angiographic features, and clinical characteristics of the patient.[2,3] One limitation of the Doppler wire is that it measures coronary blood flow velocity rather than volumetric flow. However, if the cross-sectional area of the artery remains constant between basal and hyperemic conditions, changes in flow velocity parallel changes in volumetric flow. Administration of intracoronary nitroglycerin can be used to achieve maximum vasodilation and minimize differences in vessel dimensions between basal and hyperemic conditions, and improve the reliability of CFR measurements.[15]

a. **Coronary Flow Reserve (CFR).** CFR is defined as the ratio of hyperemic-to-baseline coronary blood flow velocity. Values > 2 are normal, while values < 2 (especially < 1.7[72]) suggest the presence of a functionally-significant epicardial obstruction. Several pharmacologic agents can be used to induce hyperemic flow (Table 33.4). In our institution, intracoronary adenosine is the preferred vasodilator because of its short duration of action, ease of use, and proven safety. CFR and relative CFR (rCFR) are the most useful Doppler measurements to assess the physiologic significance of a stenosis and the functional status of the distal microvascular bed before and after coronary intervention (Table 33.5).

b. **Blood Flow Velocity.** The instantaneous peak velocities are used to derive the average peak velocity (APV), mean velocity, and time-area relationship (integral) of diastolic and systolic velocity averaged over two cardiac cycles. The diastolic-to-systolic velocity ratio (DSVR) and APV are displayed continuously on the monitor and updated every 2 seconds.

Table 33.3. Doppler-Derived Flow Velocity Parameters

Variable	Normal Reference Range
Average Peak Velocity (APV)[3,4,16]	
Basal	$\geq$ 20 cm/sec
Hyperemic	$\geq$ 30 cm/sec
Diastolic/Systolic Mean Velocity Ratio (DSVR)[3,4,16,17]	
LAD	> 1.7
LCX	> 1.5
RCA	> 1.2*
Proximal/Distal Mean Velocity Ratio (PDR⁺)[3,4,16-18]	< 1.7
Distal Coronary Flow Reserve (CFR)[19-22]	$\geq$ 2.0
Relative Coronary Flow Reserve (rCFR)	1.0

* Normal DSVR > 1.4 in distal RCA or PDA
+ Also called Translesional Velocity Gradient (TVG)

Table 33.4. Drugs for Maximal Vasodilation

Drug	Dose	Duration
Adenosine[20,68,69]		
Intracoronary	RCA 6-10 mcg; LCA 12-20 mcg	20-45 seconds
Intravenous	100-150 mcg/kg/min	45 seconds after IV discontinued
Adenosine 5'-Triphosphate[76,77]		
Intracoronary	20-50 mcg LCA; 15-30 mcg RCA	30-60 seconds
Intravenous	140-160 mcg/kg/min	1-2 minutes after IV discontinued
Papaverine[70]		
Intracoronary	5-10 mg	45-150 seconds
Intravenous	Not recommended*	Not recommended*
Dipyridamole[71]		
Intravenous	0.56 mg/kg over 4 minutes	Peak 4-minutes; duration 20-40 minutes

Abbreviations: RCA = right coronary artery; LCA = left coronary artery
* Intravenous infusion is not recommended because of a slow systemic excretion; drug accumulation may lead to systemic hypotension.

Table 33.5. Comparison of CFR, rCFR, and FFR

	CFR	rCFR	FFR
Hemodynamic independence	No	Yes	Yes
Microvascular independence	No	Yes	Yes
Use in multivessel disease	Yes	No	Yes
Abnormal range	< 2.0	< 0.8	< 0.75

Abbreviations: CFR = coronary flow reserve; rCFR = relative coronary flow reserve; FFR = fractional flow reserve

c. **Blood Flow Patterns.** The pattern of diastolic and systolic coronary flow is important in acute myocardial infarction. Abnormal flow is characterized by the presence of rapid diastolic deceleration and early systolic flow reversal, and is associated with myocardial "no-reflow" due to severe microvascular injury.[40,93-96] Abnormal blood flow patterns are frequently seen even in patients with TIMI-3 flow after successful revascularization.

d. **Limitations of Translesional Velocity Gradients and Coronary Flow Reserve.** The application of intracoronary Doppler velocimetry demands an in-depth understanding of the limitations of the technique (Table 33.6).[2,24,25] Importantly, abnormalities of the microcirculation may falsely lower CFR and confound its interpretation. CFR may also be sensitive to changes in hemodynamic conditions, such as tachycardia (increases CFR), hypertension (decreases CFR), and increased contractility (increases CFR). Relative CFR, defined as the ratio of CFR in the distal target vessel to the CFR in the nonstenotic vessel, is a new measurement which correlates better with fractional flow reserve and percent area stenosis than CFR (Table 33.5).[81,98,99] Relative CFR is independent of hemodynamic changes and the presence of microvascular disease, but may be unreliable in the presence of 3-vessel disease. Furthermore, CFR may be less useful for assessing the functional significance of a residual stenosis in acute MI patients treated with PTCA because of the known impairment of CFR in this setting.[27,73,74] Since conditions associated with impaired microcirculation have little regional variability, normal CFR in a vessel without an epicardial stenosis reliably excludes small vessel disease as a cause of decreased CFR in a vessel with a significant epicardial stenosis. Alternatively, relative CFR and fractional flow reserve may be used.

C. **INTRODUCTION TO FRACTIONAL FLOW RESERVE.** Fractional flow reserve (FFR) is a specific index for epicardial blood flow, and represents the fraction of normal maximum flow that is achievable. FFR is defined as the ratio of maximum myocardial blood flow in the presence of a stenosis to the theoretical maximum flow if no stenosis is present. The normal value in each patient and for each coronary artery is 1.0, and unlike CFR, is independent of changes in heart rate, blood pressure, contractility, and microvascular disease[75] (Table 33.5).

D. APPROACH TO FRACTIONAL FLOW RESERVE

1. **Pressure Systems.** Pressure wires available for determination of FFR are described in Table 33.7. In contrast to the older 0.018" fiberoptic wires or the 2.2F endhole catheters, the current pressure wires have handling characteristics similar to conventional angioplasty guidewires (Figure 33.3), and are compatible with monorail balloon catheters. The Endosonics WaveWire is also extendable. After administration of intracoronary adenosine (identical to the technique used for CFR measurements), FFR is then calculated. Simultaneous measurement of FFR and CFR with a conventional pressure wire has been reported using the SmartFlow Intravascular processor.[100]

2. **Fractional Flow Reserve Data**
   a. **Calculation.** FFR is calculated as the ratio of distal mean coronary pressure during maximal hyperemia divided by the simultaneous mean aortic pressure.[82,83.] Functionally-significant lesions are identified by FFR < 0.75;[82,83,84,85] this index can be used in patients with multivessel disease and with serial lesions. Pullback pressure recordings during maximal hyperemia provide a clear demonstration of the exact location and severity of the stenosis.

   b. **Limitations.** It is important to recognize that FFR was validated as an index of stenosis severity for isolated stenoses and assumes that pharmacologically-induced microvascular vasodilatation will lead to maximum translesional flow. In the presence of a second lesion, the increase in flow may be limited, overestimating the true FFR. While the equation of FFR remains valid for determining the hemodynamic significance of both stenoses together (without intervening sidebranches), the ratio cannot be used to predict the FFR of each stenosis separately, but can be predicted by more complex equations.[91,101] Caution is required in the interpretation of FFR after myocardial infarction and in the presence of advanced microvascular disease or left ventricular hypertrophy.[92,102] Significant collateral flow may also influence FFR measurement.[101]

E. CLINICAL AND INTERVENTIONAL APPLICATIONS.

Because of the limitations of quantitative angiography,[1-11] several techniques are useful adjuncts to coronary angiography, including intravascular ultrasound (Chapter 31), Doppler blood flow measurement, and intracoronary pressure measurements. These techniques should not be viewed as competitive technologies; rather, each provides complementary information that may be extremely useful during angiography and intervention (Table 33.8). The best methods for the physiologic assessment of coronary artery disease in the catheterization laboratory are coronary flow reserve and fractional flow reserve (Table 33.9).

1. **Clinical Applications**
   a. **Syndrome X.** The "gold standard" for the diagnosis of Syndrome X (myocardial ischemia due to impaired coronary microcirculation) is the finding of abnormal CFR in the presence of angiographically "normal" epicardial arteries.[30] Since significant aortic stenosis and other causes of severe left ventricular hypertrophy can also cause angina and a low CFR,[31-33] they should be excluded before making a diagnosis of Syndrome X. The observation of abnormal CFR and normal rCFR (or FFR) suggests microvascular disease.

Table 33.6. Impact of Technical and Anatomic Factors on Doppler Data

Factor	Potential Effect
Doppler Wire Technical Considerations	
Inappropriate on-line APV tracking	APV and DSVR may be falsely low; CFR and TVG calculated from APV may be erroneous
Inappropriate ECG gating from QRS	False diastolic and systolic time intervals; erroneous DSVR
Unstable phasic Doppler signal	APV may be falsely low
Doppler probe not positioned to assess peak flow velocity	APV may be falsely low
Translesional Velocity Gradient (TVG, PDR) may be influenced by:	
Ostial lesions	No proximal value to assess lesion
Single unbranched conduits	TVG may be falsely low
Tortuous vessels	Unable to obtain reliable distal peak velocity
Diffuse distal disease	Falsely low TVG secondary to falsely elevated distal velocity
Tandem/sequential lesions	Falsely low TVG secondary to falsely elevated distal velocity (distal lesional flow acceleration)
Eccentric lesions	Falsely low TVG secondary to falsely elevated proximal velocity (acceleration at lesional flow convergence)
Coronary Flow Reserve (CFR) may be influenced by:	
Abnormal microcirculation (hypertrophy, diabetes, connective tissue disease, prior myocardial infarction, Syndrome X)	May falsely lower CFR
Sequential lesions	Distal CFR is the result of the combined physiologic effects of all lesions
Changes in vasomotor tone	May falsely lower CFR
Submaximal vasodilator dose	May falsely lower CFR
Transient increase in distal flow	May falsely lower CFR
Varying Doppler wire position between baseline and hyperemic assessment	May falsely lower CFR
Varying hemodynamic conditions	May falsely lower CFR

Abbreviations: APV = average peak velocity; DSVR = diastolic-to-systolic velocity ratio; CFR = coronary flow reserve; TVG = translesional velocity gradient; PDR = proximal-to-distal velocity ratio

Table 33.7. Pressure Wires

Name	Diameter (inch)	Sensor	Position of Sensor
Pressure Wire (Radi Medical Systems)	0.014	Electronic	3 cm from tip
Informer Wire (Boston Scientific Scimed)	0.014	Fluid-filled	3 cm from tip
WaveWire (Endosonics)	0.014	Electronic	3 cm from tip

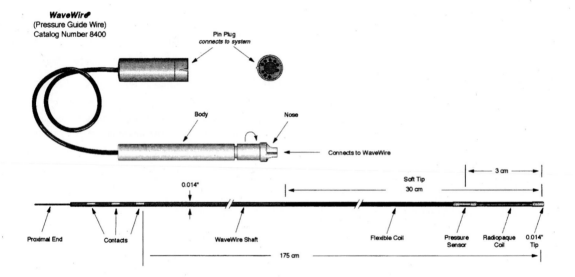

Figure 33.3. Schematic Illustration of the WaveWire

Courtesy of Endosonics.

b. **Cardiac Transplantation.** CFR may be useful in identifying rejection and diffuse coronary atherosclerosis (i.e., transplant arteriopathy) not evident angiographically, and may help guide therapeutic intervention in cardiac transplant patients.[34,78,79,103]

c. **Bypass Surgery.** Saphenous vein grafts can normalize CFR;[35,36] differences in resting phasic blood flow between internal mammary and venous conduits may have implications for long-term patency. CFR measurement in internal mammary artery grafts correlates well with graft flow determined by echocardiography, and is useful to assess graft patency.[97]

d. **Myocardial Infarction.** CFR has been used to study flow dynamics in the acute[37,38,104] and recovery[39,106] periods after myocardial infarction, and may predict recovery of microcirculatory and contractile function.[40,41,74,107-110] The coronary blood flow pattern after primary PTCA correlates with myocardial perfusion[93] and ST-segment recovery,[111] and predicts regional recovery of left ventricular function.[94,96] Preliminary data from our institution suggest abnormal coronary blood flow patterns after primary PTCA or stenting despite TIMI-3 flow, suggesting microcapillary dysfunction.

2. **Interventional Applications**
   a. **Intermediate Lesions.** CFR is reliable for assessing the physiologic significance of intermediate or borderline lesions.[8-14,18-22,72] CFR can often identify the culprit lesion in patients with multivessel coronary disease who present with unstable angina without ECG changes, and can be used to identify borderline lesions requiring intervention. Normal translesional velocity gradient and/or CFR suggest the presence of non-flow-limiting obstruction(s); intervention may be safely deferred in such lesions.[28,29,112] Translesional pressure measurement and FFR are the best techniques for the physiologic assessment of the intermediate lesion.[82-86] Identification of exact lesion location (tandem lesions) is possible with the pullback technique. FFR < 0.75 suggests a hemodynamically-significant stenosis, is associated with reversible ischemia, and supports the need for revascularization. Retrospective studies indicate that it is safe to defer intervention if FFR > 0.75;[83,87] a large randomized prospective study (DEFER) is in progress.

   b. **"Suboptimal" Results.** Coronary blood flow velocity may be used to assess the results of percutaneous intervention; normalization of APV and DSVR have been reported after successful PTCA,[3,4] DCA,[42] ELCA,[42] Rotablator,[43] and stent implantation.[44,45] In contrast, normalization of CFR after PTCA is unusual, although immediate stenting of successfully dilated lesions may normalize CFR.[45,49-51] These data suggest that in addition to further lumen enlargement, another potential use of stenting is to improve flow abnormalities after PTCA. "Suboptimal" results after intervention, characterized by intraluminal haziness, moderate residual stenosis, or non-flow-limiting dissection, may be ideal indications for Doppler flow assessment to determine the need for further intervention.[98,113] Persistent impairment of CFR after PTCA or stenting may result from a high baseline flow velocity; normalization of CFR at follow-up is associated with a decline in basal flow.[114] The Doppler Endpoint Balloon

Angioplasty Evaluation (DEBATE) study revealed that distal CFR > 2.5 and diameter stenosis < 35% predict favorable outcomes with low rates of recurrent symptoms (23% vs 47%, p = 0.005) and restenosis (16% vs 41%, p = 0.002).[52] The French Randomized Optimal Stenting Trial (FROST) applied the DEBATE criteria (CFR > 2.2 to defer stenting) and showed in a multicenter, randomized, prospective trial that Doppler-guided PTCA can reduce the need for stenting in 50% of cases without a detrimental effect on clinical or angiographic outcomes.[88] FFR values > 0.75 predict favorable clinical outcomes and lower restenosis rates after PTCA,[89] confirm optimal stent deployment, and correlate well with IVUS.[90] In patients with single vessel disease, a residual diameter stenosis < 35% and FFR ≥ 0.90 after balloon angioplasty alone predict excellent clinical outcome at two years.[115] The strategy of physiologic-guided angioplasty and stenting is being further evaluated in the DESTINI-CFR and DEBATE II studies.

c. **Complications ("Trending") (Table 33.10).** The FloMap can be placed in a trend mode to record continuous coronary blood flow velocity over time; trending is most commonly used following coronary intervention to identify angiographically-inapparent flow impairment due to dissection, vasospasm, platelet aggregation, or changes in vasomotor tone.[54-57] It is possible that post-intervention trending can be used to identify patients with unstable flow patterns who may benefit from stents or new antiplatelet agents.[59] Analysis of Doppler flow patterns confirms the utility of IABP and intracoronary nitroprusside for improving diastolic coronary blood flow.

d. **Urokinase Infusions.** Repeat angiographic studies are usually required to identify vessel patency after prolonged (8-48 hours) infusions of intracoronary urokinase for the revascularization of chronic total occlusions. In these situations, continuous monitoring with a Doppler wire may indicate restoration of distal flow, obviating the need for repeat angiography.

e. **No-Reflow.** In our laboratory, patients at risk for "no-reflow" are monitored during intervention to assess the utility of intracoronary verapamil for restoring flow. Doppler flow velocity may also be used to distinguish inapparent residual stenosis from microvascular dysfunction after primary PTCA for acute MI.[60,61]

f. **Dynamic Turbulence.** An application of the "trend" mode is measurement of dynamic flow velocity for the assessment of stenosis severity.[62] Mechanical pull-back of the Doppler guidewire from the distal to proximal artery may result in transient high velocity recordings, reflecting turbulent flow. Preliminary data suggest that turbulent blood flow may lead to underestimation of CFR in 20% of patients after PTCA.[63] Proponents of this technique believe that dynamic assessment will complement instantaneous assessment of DSVR and CFR.

Table 33.8. Comparison of Imaging and Hemodynamic Techniques

Characteristic	Digital Angiography	Angioscopy	IVUS	Doppler FloWire	Pressure Wire
Vessel lumen detail	+	++++	++	-	-
Vessel wall detail	-	-	++++	-	-
Plaque composition	-	++	+++	-	-
Vessel dimensions	++	-	++++	-	-
Identify disease in "normal" vessel	+	++	++++	-	-
Detect diffuse disease	+	++	++++	-	-
Evaluate "haziness"	±	+++	+++	+	+
Arterial remodeling	±	-	++++	-	-
Borderline lesions - morphology	+	-	++++	-	-
Borderline lesions - physiology	-	-	+	++++	++++
Suboptimal results	+	++	+++	+++	++++
Clot vs. dissection	±	++++	+++	-	-
Predict complications	+	unknown	possible	+++	possible
Continuous record (trend)	-	-	-	+++	-
Predict restenosis	+	-	++	++	unknown
Microvascular disease	-	-	-	+++	-
Cause of ischemia	-	+++	+	-	-

Abbreviations: IVUS = intravascular ultrasound
- = no value; ± = limited value; + thru ++++ = increasing value

    g. Collateral Flow. Both Doppler[116] and pressure systems may be used to assess functional collateral flow.[105] Pressure-derived fractional collateral flow correlates with ventricular recovery after acute myocardial infarction.

Table 33.9. Applications of Coronary Blood Flow Velocity

Clinical Applications	Interventional Applications
Intermediate lesions	Assess suboptimal results
Identify Syndrome X	Predict complications (trending)
Identify transplant arteriopathy	Assess no-reflow
Bypass grafts	Monitor urokinase infusions
Myocardial infarction	Dynamic turbulence

Table 33.10. Continuous Doppler-Flow Velocity Patterns (Trending)

Pattern	Cause
Abrupt flow acceleration	Transient spasm
Abrupt flow cessation	Vasovagal reaction
Abrupt flow deceleration	Abrupt closure
Cyclical flow variations	Abrupt closure/thrombus

* * * * *

REFERENCES

1. Benchimol A, Stegall HF, Gartlan JL. New method to measure phasic coronary blood velocity in man. Am Heart J 1971;81:93-101.

2. Doucette JW, Corl PD, Payne HM, et al. Validation of a Doppler guidewire for intravascular measurement of coronary artery flow velocity. Circulation 1992;85:1899-1911.

3. Segal J, Kern MJ, Scott NA, King III SB, et al. Alterations of phasic coronary artery flow velocity in humans during percutaneous coronary angioplasty. J Am Coll Cardiol 1992;20:276-286.

4. Ofili EO, Kern MJ, Labovitz AJ, St. Vrain JA, et al. Analysis of coronary blood flow velocity dynamics in angiographically normal and stenosed arteries before and after endoluminal enlargement by angioplasty. J Am Coll Cardiol 1993;21:308-316.

5. Marcus ML, Chilian WM, Kanatuka H, Dellsperger KC, et al. Understanding the coronary circulation through studies at the microvascular level. Circulation 1990;82:1-7.

6. Bone RM, Rubio R. Coronary circulation, in Berne R, Sperelakis N, (eds): Handbook of Physiology, Section 2: The Cardiovascular System, Volume 1, The Heart. Baltimore, Williams & Wilkins CO, 1979, pp 873-952.

7. Wilson RF, Laxson DD. Caveat Emptor: A clinician's guide to assessing the physiologic significance of arterial stenoses. Cathet Cardiovasc Diagn 1993;29:93-98.

8. Gould KL, Lipscomb K, Hamilton GW. Physiologic basis for assessing critical coronary stenosis. Am J Cardiol 1974;33:87-94.

9. Gould KL, Lipscomb K, Calvert J. Compensatory changes of the distal coronary vascular bed during progressive coronary constriction. Circulation 1975;51:1085-1094.

10. Kirkeeide R, Gould KL, Parsel L. Assessment of coronary stenoses by myocardial imaging during coronary vasodilation. VII. Validation of coronary flow reserve as a single integrated measure to stenosis severity accounting for all its geometric dimensions. J Am Coll Cardiol 1986;7:103-113.

11. Gould KL, Kirkeeide R, Buchi M. Coronary flow reserve as a physiologic measure of stenosis severity. Part I. Relative and absolute coronary flow reserve during changing aortic pressure. Part II. Determination from arterographic stenosis dimensions under standardized conditions. J Am Coll Cardiol 1990;15:459-474.

12. Demer L, Gould KL, Kirkeide RL. Assessing stenosis severity: Coronary flow reserve, collateral function, quantitative coronary arteriography, position imaging, and digital subtraction angiography: a review and analysis. Prog Cardiovasc Dis 1988;30:307-322.

13. Gould KL. Identifying and measuring severity of coronary artery stenosis: quantitative coronary arteriography and position emission tomography. Circulation 1988;78:237-245.

14. Wilson RF, Marcus ML, White CW. Prediction of the physiologic significance of coronary arterial lesions by quantitative lesion geometry in patients with limited coronary artery disease. Circulation 1987;75:723-732.

15. Shammas NW, Thondapu V, Gerasimou EM, et al. Effect of pretreatment with nitroglycerin on coronary flow reserve measured using bolus intracoronary adenosine. Circulation 1995;92:I-264.

16. Ofili EO, Lasovitz AJ, Kern MJ. Coronary flow velocity dynamics in normal and diseased arteries. Am J Cardiol 1993;71:3D-9D.

17. Kajiya F, Ogasawara Y, Tsujioka K, et al. Analysis of flow characteristics in post-stenotic regions of the human coronary artery during bypass graft surgery. Circulation 1987;76:1092-1100.

18. Donohue TJ, Kern MJ, Aguirre FV, et al. Assessing the hemodynamic significance of coronary artery stenosis. Analysis of translesional pressure-flow velocity relations in patients. J Am Coll Cardiol 1993;22:449-458.

19. Kern MJ, Aguirre FV, Bach RG, Caracole EA, Donohue TJ. Translesional pressure-flow velocity assessment in patients: Part I. Cathet Cardiovasc Diagn 1994;313:49-60.

20. Kern MJ, Deligonul, Tatineni S, et al. IV adenosine continuous infusion and low dose bolus administration for determination of coronary vascular reserve in patients with and without coronary artery disease. J Am Coll Cardiol 1991;18:718-729.

21. Miller DD, Donohue TJ, Younis LT, et al. Correlation of pharmacological ^{99m}Tc-Sestamibi myocardial perfusion imaging with post-stenotic coronary flow reserve in patients with angiographically intermediate coronary artery stenoses. Circulation 1994;89:2150-2160.

22. Joye JD, Schulman DS, Lesorde D, et al. Intracoronary Doppler guide wire versus stress single-photon emission computer tomographic thallium 201 imaging in assessment of intermediate coronary stenoses. J Am Coll Cardiol 1994;24:940-947.

23. Gadallah S, Thaker KB, Kawanishi D, Rashtian M, et al. Comparison of the hyperemic response to intracoronary and intravenous adenosine by intracoronary Doppler flow recording. Circulation 1995;92:I-326.

24. White CW, Wilson RF, Intracoronary Doppler Ultrasound in Nanda P (ed): Doppler Ultrasound. Philadelphia, Lea & Febiger, 1994, pp 403-412.

25. McGinn AL, White CW, Wilson RF. Interstudy variability of coronary flow reserve. Influence of heart rate, arterial pressure and ventricular preload. Circulation 1990;81:1319-1330.

26. De Bruyne B, Bartunek J, Stanislas US, et al. Feasibility and hemodynamic dependency of invasive indexes of coronary stenosis. Circulation 1995;92:I-324.

27. Claeys MJ, Vrints CJ, Bosmans JM, Cools F, et al. Coronary flow reserve measurement during coronary angioplasty in the infarct related vessel. Circulation 1995;92:I-326.

28. Kern MJ, Donohue TJ, Aguirre FV, Bach RG, et al. Clinical outcome of deferring angioplasty in patients with normal translesional pressure-flow velocity measurements. J Am Coll Cardiol 1995;25:178-187.

29. Lesser JT, Wilson RF, White CW. Physiologic assessment of coronary stenosis of intermediate severity can facilitate patient selection for coronary angioplasty. Coronary Art Dis 1990;1:697-705.

30. Cannon RO III, Camici PG, Epstein SE. Pathophysiological dilemma of Syndrome X. Circulation 1992;85:883-892.

31. Marcus ML, Doty DB, Hirratzka LF, Wright CB, Enpthan

CE. Decreased coronary reserved a mechanism of angina pectoris in patients with aortic stenosis and normal coronary arteries. N Engl J Med 1982;37:1362-1366.

32. Houghton JL, Prisant LM, Carr AA, van Dohlen TW, Frank MJ. Relationship of left ventricular mass to impairment of coronary vasodilator reserve in hypertensive heart disease. Am Heart J 1991;21:1107.

33. Cannon RO, Bonow RO, Bacharach SL, et al. Left ventricular dysfunction in patients with angina pectoris, normal epicardial coronary arteries, and abnormal vasodilator reserve. Circulation 1985;71:218-226.

34. McGinn AL, Wilson RF, Olisan MT et al. Coronary vasodilator reserve following human orthotopic cardiac transplantation. Circulation 1988;78:1200-1209.

35. Wilson RE, Wilson ML, White CW. Effects of coronary bypass surgery and angioplasty on coronary blood flow and flow reserve. Prog Cardiovasc Dis 1988;31:95-114.

36. Wilson RE, White CW. Does coronary bypass graft surgery restore normal CFR. The effect of diffuse atherosclerosis and focal obstruction lesions. Circulation 1987;76:563-571.

37. Stewart RE, Bowers TR, Ponto R, Miller DD, et al. Coronary Doppler flow velocity and PET myocardial blood flow are highly correlated and predict post-infarction perfusion in patients with TIMI-3 flow. J Am Coll Cardiol 1995;25:427A.

38. Aguirre FV, Donohue TJ, Bach RG, Caracole EA, et al. Coronary flow velocity of infarct-related arteries: Physiologic differences between complete (TIMI III) and incomplete (TIMI 0,I,II) angiographic coronary perfusion. J Am Coll Cardiol 1995;25:401A.

39. Ishihara M, Sato H, Tateishi H, et al. Time course of impaired coronary flow reserve after reperfusion in patients with acute myocardial infarction. Am J Cardiol 1996; 78: 1103-1108.

40. Wakatsuki T, Nakamura M, Tsunoda T, et al. Coronary flow velocity immediately after primary coronary stenting as a predictor of ventricular wall motion recovery in acute myocardial infarction. J Am Coll Cardiol 2000; 35: 1835-41.

41. Kim HS, Tahk SJ, Shin JH, Kim W, Cho YK, et al. Coronary flow reserve in infarct related artery and myocardial viability in patients with recent myocardial infarction. Circulation 1995;92:I-600.

42. Segal J. Applications of coronary flow velocity during angioplasty and other coronary interventional procedures. Am J Cardiol 1993;71:17D-25D.

43. Bowers TR, Stewart RE, O'Neill WW, Reddy VM, et al. Plaque pulvariation during Rotablator atherectomy: does it impair coronary flow dynamics? J Am Coll Cardiol 1995;25:96A.

44. Bach R, Kern MJ, Bell C, et al. Clinical application of coronary flow velocity for stent placement during coronary angioplasty. Am J Heart 1993;125:873-880.

45. Bowers TR, Safian RD, Stewart RE, Benzuly KH, et al. Normalization of CFR after stenting, but not after PTCA. J Am Coll Cardiol 1996 J Am Coll Cardiol 1996;27(2):19A.

46. Larman DJ, Serruys PW, Suryapranata H, et al. Inability of coronary blood flow reserve measurements to assess the efficacy of coronary angioplasty in the first 24-hours in unselected patients. Am Heart J 1991;122:631-639.

47. Wilson RF, Johnson MR, Marcus ML, Aylward PEG, et al. The effect of coronary angioplasty on coronary flow reserve.

Circulation 1988;77:873-885.

48. Kern MJ, Deligonul U, Vandormael M, Labovitz A, et al. Impaired coronary vasodilator reserve in the immediate post coronary angioplasty period: Analysis of coronary artery flow velocity indexes and regional cardiac venous efflux. J Am Coll Cardiol 1989;13:860-872.

49. Kern MJ, Aguirre FV, Donohue TJ, et al. Impact of residual lumen narrowing on coronary flow after angioplasty and stent: Intravascular ultrasound Doppler and imaging data in support of physiologically-guided coronary angioplasty. Circulation 1995;92:I-263.

50. Verna E, Gil R, Di Mario C, et al. Does coronary stenting following balloon angioplasty improve distal coronary flow reserve? Circulation 1995;92:I-536.

51. Haude M, Baumgart D, Caspari G, Erbel R. Does adjunct coronary stenting in comparison to balloon angioplasty has an impact on Doppler flow velocity parameters? Circulation 1995;92:I-547.

52. Surreys PW, di Mario C, Piek J, et al. Prognostic value of intracoronary flow velocity and diameter stenosis in assessing the short- and long-term outcomes of coronary balloon angioplasty: the DEBATE Study. Circulation 1997;96(10):3369-3377.

53. The D.E.B.A.T.E. Study Group. Doppler guide wire as a primary guide wire for PTCA. Feasibility, safety, and continuous monitoring of the results. Circulation 1995;92:I-263.

54. Eichhorn E, Grayburn PA, Willard JE, et al. Spontaneous alterations in coronary blood flow velocity before and after coronary angioplasty in patients with severe angina. J Am Coll Cardiol 1991;17:43-52.

55. Anderson HV, Kirkeeide RL, Stuart Y, et al. Coronary artery flow monitoring following coronary interventions. Am J Cardiol 1993;71:62D-69D.

56. Kern MJ, Donohue TJ, Bach RG, Aguirre FV, Bell C. Monitoring cyclical coronary blood flow alterations following coronary angioplasty for stent restenosis using a Doppler guidewire. Am Heart J 1993;125:1159-1160.

57. Kern MJ, Aguirre FV, Donohue TJ, et al. Continuous coronary flow velocity monitoring during coronary interventions: Velocity trend patterns associated with adverse events. Am Heart J 1994;128:426-34.

58. The D.E.B.A.T.E. Study Group. Cyclic flow variations after PTCA are predictive of immediate complications. Circulation 1995;92:I-725.

59. Anderson HV, Revana M, Rosales O, et al. Intravenous administration of monoclonal antibody to the platelet GP IIb/IIIa receptor to treat abrupt closure during coronary angioplasty. Am J Cardiol 1992;69:1373-1376.

60. Yaniyama Y, Iwakure K, Ito H, et al. Coronary flow velocity pattern in patients with TIMI flow grade 2: Its relation to residual coronary stenosis and microvascular dysfunction. Circulation 1995;92:I-149.

61. Nemoto T, Kimure K, Shimizu T, et al. Coronary artery flow velocity waveform in acute myocardial infarction with angiographic no-reflow. Circulation 1995;92:I-325.

62. Geschwind HJ, Melnik L, Kvasnicka J, Dupouy P. Dynamic detection of coronary stenosis by Doppler-tipped guidewire. J Am Coll Cardiol 1995;25:336A.

63. Ferrari M, Werner GS, Nargang L, Figulla HR. Turbulent flow as a cause for underestimating the coronary flow reserve. Circulation 1995;92:I-77.

64. Wilson RF, Laughlin DE, Ackell PH, Chilian WM. Transluminal subselective measurement of coronary blood flow velocity and vasodilator reserve in man. Circulation 1985;72:82-92.

65. White CW, Marcus ML, Wilson RF. Methods of measuring coronary flow in humans. Prog Cardiovasc Dis 1988;31:79-94.

66. Sibley DH, Millar HD, Hartley CJ, Whitlow PL. Subselective measurement of coronary blood flow velocity using a steerable Doppler catheter. J Am Coll Cardiol 1986;8:1332-1340.

67. Vanyi J, Bowers TR, Jarvis G, White CW. Can an intracoronary Doppler wire accurately measure changes in coronary blood flow velocity? Cathet Cardiovasc Diagn 1993;29:240-246.

68. Zijlstra F, Juilliere Y, Serruys PW, Roelandt JRTC. Value and limitations of intracoronary adenosine for the assessment of coronary flow reserve. Cathet Cardiovasc Diagn 1988;15:76-80.

69. Wilson RF, Wych K, Christensen BV, et al. Effects of adenosine on human coronary arterial circulation. Circulation 1990;82:1595-1606.

70. Wilson RF, White CW. Intracoronary papaverine: An ideal vasodilator for studies of the coronary circulation in conscious humans. Circulation 1986;73:444-452.

71. Ranhosty A, Kempthorne-Rawson J. Intravenous Dipyridamole Thallium Imaging Study Group. The safety of intravenous dipyridamole thallium myocardial perfusion imaging. Circulation 1990;81:1205-1209.

72. Heller LI, Cates C, Popma J, et al. Intracoronary doppler assessment of moderate coronary artery disease. Comparison with[201] Tl Imaging and Coronary Angiography. Circulation 1997;96:484-490.

73. Kern MJ, Puri S, Craig WR, et al. Hemodynamic rounds series II: Coronary hemodynamics for angioplasty and stenting after myocardial infarction: use of absolute, relative coronary velocity and fractional flow reserve. Cathet Cardiovasc Diagn 1998;45(2):174-182.

74. Mazur W, Bitar JN, Lechin M, et al. Coronary flow reserve may predict myocardial recovery after myocardial infarction in patients with TIMI grade 3 flow. Am Heart J 1998;136(2):335-344.

75. De Bruyne B, Bartunek J, Sys SU, et al. Simultaneous coronary pressure and flow velocity measurements in humans. Feasibility, reproducibility, and hemodynamic dependence of coronary flow velocity reserve, hyperemic flow versus pressure slope index, and fractional flow reserve. Circulation 1996;94(8):1842-1849

76. Sonoda S, Takeuchi M, Nakashima Y, Kuroiwa A. Safety and optimal dose of intracoronary adenosine 5'-triphosphate for the measurement of coronary flow reserve. Am Heart J 1998;135(4):621-627.

77. Jeremias A, Filardo SD, Whitbourn RJ, et al. Effects of intravenous and intracoronary adenosine 5'-triphosphate as compared with adenosine on coronary flow and pressure dynamics. Circulation 2000;101:318-323.

78. Wolford TL, Donohue TJ, Bach RG, et al. Heterogeneity of coronary flow reserve in the examination of multiple individual allograft coronary arteries. Circulation 1999;99(5):626-632.

79. Mazur W, Bitar JN, Young JB, et al. Progressive deterioration of coronary flow reserve after heart transplantation. Am Heart J 1998;136(3):504-509.

80. Weis M, Hartmann A, Olbrich HG, et al. Prognostic significance of coronary flow reserve on left ventricular ejection fraction in cardiac transplant recipients. Transplantation 1998;65(1):103-108.

81. Baumgart D, Haude M, Goerge G, et al. Improved assessment of coronary stenosis severity using the relative flow velocity reserve. Circulation 1998;98(1):40-46.

82. Pils NHJ, Van Gelder B, Van der Voort P, et al. Fractional flow reserve: a useful index to evaluate the influence of an epicardial coronary stenosis on myocardial blood flow. Circulation 1995;92:3183-3193.

83. Pils NHJ, De Bruyne B, Peels K, et al. Measurement of fractional flow reserve to assess the functional severity of coronary artery stenoses. N Engl J Med 1996;334:1703-1708.

84. De Bruyne B, Bartunek J, Sys SK, et al. Relation between myocardial fractional flow reserve calculated from coronary pressure measurements and exercise-induced myocardial ischemia. Circulation 1995;92:39-45.

85. Bartunek J, Marwick T, Rodriques ACT, et al. Dobutamine-induced wall motion abnormalities: correlations with myocardial fractional flow reserve and quantitative coronary angiography. J Am Coll Cardiol 1996;27:1429-1436.

86. Lederman SJ, Menegus MA, Greenberg MA. Fractional flow reserve. ACC Current Journal Review 1997;2:34-35.

87. Bech GJW, De Bruyne B, Bonnier HJRM et al. Long-term follow-up after deferral of PTCA of intermediate stenosis, on the basis of coronary pressure measurements. J Am Coll Cardiol 1998;31:841-847.

88. Lafont A, Dubois-Rande JL, Steg PG, et al. The French Randomized Optimal Stenting Trial: A prospective evaluation of provisional stenting guided by coronary velocity reserve and quantitative coronary angiography. J Am Coll Cardiol 2000;36:404-9.

89. Pils NHJ, Bech GJW, De Bruyne B, et al. Prognostic value of pressure-derived fractional flow reserve to predict restenosis after regular balloon angioplasty. Circulation 1997;96:I-649.

90. Hanekamp C, Koolen JJ, Pils NHJ, et al. Comparison of quantitative coronary angiography, intravascular ultrasound, and pressure-derived fractional flow reserve to assess optimal stent deployment. Circulation (in press).

91. Kern MJ. Coronary physiology revisited. Practical insights from the cardiac catheterization laboratory. Circulation 2000;101:1344-1351.

92. Bartunek J, Pijls NHJ, Bech GJW, et al. Fractional flow reserve: who needs the pressure wire? J Interven Cardiol 1999;12:425-430.

93. Iwakura K, Ito H, Takiuchi S, et al. Alteration in the coronary blood flow velocity pattern in patients with no reflow and reperfused acute myocardial infarction. Circulation 1996;94:1269-1275.

94. Kawamoto T, Yoshida K, Akasaka T, et al. Can coronary blood flow velocity pattern after primary percutaneous

transluminal angioplasty predict recovery of regional left ventricular function in patients with acute myocardial infarction. Circulation 1999;100:339-345.

95. Iwakura K, Ito H, Nishikawa N, et al. Early temporal changes in coronary flow velocity patterns in patients with acute myocardial infarction demonstrating the "no-reflow" phenomenon. Am J Cardiol 1999;84:415-419.

96. Akasaka T, Yoshida K, Kawamoto T, et al. Relation of phasic coronary flow velocity characteristics with TIMI perfusion grade and myocardial recovery after primary percutaneous transluminal coronary angioplasty and rescue stenting. Circulation 2000;101:2361-2367.

97. Voudris V, Athanassopoulos G, Vassilikos V, et al. Usefulness of flow reserve in the left internal mammary artery to determine graft patency to the left anterior descending coronary artery. Am J Cardiol 1999;83:1157-1163.

98. Kern MJ, Puri S, Bach RG, et al. Abnormal coronary flow velocity reserve after coronary artery stenting in patients. Role of relative coronary flow reserve to assess potential mechanisms. Circulation 1999;100:2491-2498.

99. Wieneke H, Haude M, Ge J, et al. Corrected coronary flow velocity reserve: a new concept for assessing coronary perfusion. J Am Coll Cardiol 2000;35:1713-20.

100. Gruberg L, Mintz GS, Fuchs S, et al. Simultaneous assessment of coronary flow reserve and fractional flow reserve with a novel pressure-based method. J Interven Cardiol (in press).

101. De Bruyne B, Pijls NHJ, Heyndrickx GR, et al. Pressure-derived fractional flow reserve to assess serial epicardial stenosis. Theoretical basis and animal validation. Circulation 2000;101:1840-1847.

102. Pijls NHJ, Kern MJ, Yock PG, De Bruyne B. Practice and Potential Pitfalls of Coronary Pressure Measurement. Cathet Cardiovasc Intervent 2000:49:1-16.

103. Schwarzacher SP, Uren NG, Ward MR, et al. Determinants of coronary remodeling in transplant coronary disease. A simultaneous intravascular ultrasound and Doppler flow study. Circulation 2000;101:1384-1389.

104. Kern MJ, Moore JA, Aguirre FV, et al. Determination of angiographic (TIMI grade) blood flow by intracoronary Doppler flow velocity during acute myocardial infarction. Circulation 1996;94:1545-1552.

105. Lee CW, Park SW, Cho GY, et al. Pressure-derived fractional collateral blood flow: a primary determinant of left ventricular recovery after reperfused acute myocardial infarction. J Am Coll Cardiol 2000;35:949-55.

106. Neumann FJ, Kosa I, Dickfield T, et al. Recovery of myocardial perfusion in acute myocardial infarction after successful balloon angioplasty and stent placement in the infarct-related coronary artery. J Am Coll Cardiol 1997;30:1270-1276.

107. Suryapranata H, Zijlstra F, MacLeod DC, et al. Predictive value of reactive hyperemic response on reperfusion on recovery of regional myocardial function after coronary angioplasty in acute myocardial infarction. Circulation 1994;89:1109-1117.

108. Teiger E, Garot J, Aptecar E, et al. Coronary blood flow reserve and wall motion recovery in patients undergoing angioplasty for myocardial infarction. Eur Heart J 1999;20:285-292.

109. Feldman LJ, Himbert D, Juliard JM, et al. Reperfusion syndrome: relationship of coronary blood flow reserve to left ventricular function and infarct size. J Am Coll Cardiol 2000;35:1162-9.

110. Lepper W, Hoffmann R, Kamp O, et al. Assessment of myocardial reperfusion by intravenous myocardial contrast echocardiography and coronary flow reserve after primary percutaneous transluminal coronary angioplasty in patients with acute myocardial infarction. Circulation 2000;101:2368-2374.

111. Dixon SR, O'Neill WW, Safian RD, et al. Doppler-derived phasic coronary blood flow pattern in the infarct related artery predicts ST-segment recovery after primary angioplasty. Circulation (in press).

112. Ferrari M, Schnell B, Werner GS, et al. Safety of deferring angioplasty in patients with normal coronary flow velocity reserve. J Am Coll Cardiol 1999;33:82-7.

113. Kern MJ, Dupouy P, Drury JH, et al. Role of coronary lumen enlargement in improving coronary blood flow after balloon angioplasty and stenting: a combined intravascular ultrasound doppler flow and imaging study. J Am Coll Cardiol 1997;29:1520-7.

114. van Liebergen RAM, Piek JJ, Koch KT, et al. Immediate and long-term effect of balloon angioplasty or stent implantation on the absolute and relative coronary blood flow velocity reserve. Circulation 1998;98:2133-2140.

115. Bech GJW, Pijls NHJ, De Bruyne B, et al. Usefulness of fractional flow reserve to predict clinical outcome after balloon angioplasty. Circulation 1999;99:883-888.

116. van Liebergen RAM, Piek JJ, Koch KT, et al. Quantification of collateral flow in humans: a comparison of angiographic, electrocardiographic and hemodynamic variables. J Am Coll Cardiol 1999;33:670-7.

V

Miscellaneous Topics

ADJUNCTIVE PHARMACOTHERAPY

34

James J. Ferguson, III, M.D.
Mark Freed, M.D.
Robert D. Safian, M.D.

CONSCIOUS SEDATION

Conscious sedation to ease anxiety and discomfort without compromising patient cooperation and ventilation is usually achieved by an analgesic and sedative. Popular combinations include a narcotic such as hydromorphone (Dilaudid, 0.5-1.0 mg IV) and a short-acting benzodiazepine like midazolam (Versed, 0.5-1.0 mg IV) or diazepam (Valium, 2-5 mg IV). Other useful narcotics include morphine sulfate (1-2 mg IV), fentanyl (Sublimase, 1-2 mcg/kg IV), and meperidine (Demerol, 25-50 mg IV). The major risk associated with conscious sedation is respiratory depression, particularly with fentanyl. In patients who are elderly, debilitated, chronically ill, or predisposed to hypoventilation (e.g., COPD), small initial doses should be given and sufficient time (2 or more minutes) should be allowed between additional doses to evaluate the full sedative effect. Respiratory depression caused by narcotics may be reversed with naloxone (Narcan, 0.4-2.0 mg IV up to 10 mg in 10 minutes) and respiratory depression caused by benzodiazepines may be reversed with flumazenil (Romazicon, 0.2 mg IV over 15 seconds repeated as needed every 60 seconds up to 1 mg). Demerol is contraindicated in patients who received monoamine oxidase (MAO) inhibitors within 14 days due to unpredictable and potentially fatal reactions, manifest as a narcotic-overdose like syndrome (respiratory depression, hypotension, coma) or as a neuroexcitatory syndrome (paradoxical agitation, seizures, hypertension, hyperpyrexia). Severe reactions should be treated with IV hydrocortisone (100-250 mg IV); when hypertension and hyperpyrexia are present, chlorpromazine (25 mg IV Q 6-8 hours) may be useful. Demerol should be used cautiously in patients with renal failure due to the risk of seizures from toxic accumulation of the metabolite normeperidine. Infiltration of warm xylocaine pre-heated to 37-43°C may reduce the discomfort of local anesthesia.[1,2]

PREVENTION AND TREATMENT OF CONTRAST REACTIONS

A. **PROPHYLAXIS AGAINST CONTRAST REACTIONS.** Prophylactic medical therapy is recommended for all patients with a history of urticaria, bronchospasm, or anaphylaxis after previous exposure to radiographic contrast agents. No regimen is fully protective, but premedication started 18 hours before contrast exposure reduces the risk of recurrent anaphylaxis from 40% to less than 10%.[3,4] "Standard" prophylaxis includes a corticosteroid (prednisone 40-60 mg PO, solumedrol 40-60 mg IV, hydrocortisone 100 mg IV) with or without an antihistamine (diphenhydramine 25-50 mg) given 18,

12, and 6 hours prior to the procedure; H_2 blockers are optional. Shorter periods of premedication are not reliable in preventing recurrent contrast reactions, but if emergency angiography is necessary, hydrocortisone (100 mg IV) or solumedrol (40 mg IV) should be given immediately before the procedure; low-osmolar contrast is also recommended. In patients with a previous anaphylactic reaction to contrast, it may be prudent to withhold beta-blockers on the morning of the procedure in case epinephrine is needed to treat recurrent anaphylaxis.

B. TREATMENT OF CONTRAST REACTIONS. The treatment of minor, moderate, and major contrast reactions is described in Table 34.1 and Chapter 25.

PROCEDURAL ANTICOAGULATION

Angiographic thrombus before and after intervention is a strong independent predictor of procedural failure, abrupt closure, major ischemic complications, and restenosis.[5-17] Antithrombotic and antiplatelet agents are routinely employed to decrease the risk of abrupt closure (Tables 34.2, 34.3).

Table 34.1. Contrast Reactions: Presentation, Onset, and Treatment*

Type	Presentation	Onset	Treatment
Minor	Mild urticaria, pruritus, erythema	Usually occur within minutes of exposure	Occasionally requires intervention. Treatment is supportive, including observation and cool compresses; oral diphenhydramine is sometimes useful.
Moderate	Angioedema, bronchospasm, laryngeal edema	Usually occur within minutes to hours of exposure	Usually requires intervention. Treatment includes diphenhydramine (50 mg IV), steroids (e.g., hydrocortisone 100 mg IV). Anaphylactoid reactions are also treated with epinephrine (0.1-0.5cc of a 1:1,000 dilution [0.1-0.5 mg] subcutaneously every 5-15 minutes as needed). Bronchodilator treatments (e.g., albuterol aerosol 2.5 mg nebulized mist every 1-2 hours) might be of benefit.
Severe	Anaphylaxis (cardiovascular collapse or profound hypotension)	May occur immediately with a single contrast injection	Life-threatening and requires aggressive attention. Epinephrine (1-5cc of a 1:10,000 solution [0.1-0.5 mg] via IV or endotracheal tube every 5 minutes as needed), steroids (e.g., hydrocortisone 100 mg IV or solumedrol 125 mg IV), diphenhydramine (50 mg IV), and possible intubation.

* Common side effects (chemotoxic effects) to radiographic contrast, such as nausea, vomiting, and vasovagal reactions, should not be considered "allergic" manifestations. Immediate treatment, if necessary, includes centrally-acting antiemetics (compazine 2-5 mg IV) for nausea/vomiting and atropine (0.5-1.0 mg IV) for vasovagal reactions. Pretreatment with corticosteroids is not useful for these reactions, but low-osmolar or nonionic contrast will reduce the incidence and severity of these side effects. The dose for epinephrine is the same for moderate or severe contrast reactions; the dilution, injected volume, and route of administration are different.

UNFRACTIONATED HEPARIN

Unfractionated heparin is a heterogeneous polysaccharide which binds to antithrombin to potentiate the inhibition of thrombin and factor Xa. In the cath lab, heparin effect is measured by the activated clotting time (ACT), which is the time for whole blood to form a firm, grossly-apparent clot in response to kaolin (HemoTec ACT) or diatomaceous earth (HemoChron ACT).[18,19] For the same heparin concentration, a higher ACT is obtained using the HemoChron system.[20] Intravenous heparin is virtually always employed during intervention to reduce the risk of abrupt closure.[21]

A. **PROCEDURAL HEPARIN WITHOUT GLYCOPROTEIN IIb/IIIa INHIBITORS.** There are no objective standards to identify the optimal level of anticoagulation during intervention; "therapeutic" levels have been empirically derived from the early cardiac surgery experience and from other observations.[22-36] Common practice is to maintain the HemoChron ACT at 300-350 seconds and the HemoTec ACT at 250-300 seconds, although some interventionalists prefer higher values. The average heparin dose required to achieve an ACT > 300 seconds varies with the anginal syndrome,[37,38] but a common initial weight-adjusted[39,40] dose is 100 U/kg. Lower doses of heparin (5000 U bolus) have been used in some low-risk patients,[41,42] but this practice is not recommended since the ACT level during PTCA may be inversely related to the risk of abrupt closure.[35,43] Ischemic complications after PTCA were higher in patients with a HemoTec ACT < 250 seconds compared to those with an ACT > 300 seconds.[32] The requirements for high levels of anticoagulation are not as stringent with stents, but minimum safe levels for ACT have not been established. Since the risk of bleeding increases with higher ACT levels, the ideal therapeutic ACT "window" may be relatively narrow. Patients who require larger doses of heparin to achieve a "therapeutic" ACT and the 30% of patients with elevated fibrinopeptide A levels despite "therapeutic" ACTs and high heparin levels (reflecting heparin resistance and residual thrombin activity) may have worse outcomes than other patients.[45] Unfortunately, there are no readily available bedside assays to identify these high-risk patients.

B. **PROCEDURAL HEPARIN WITH GLYCOPROTEIN IIb/IIIa INHIBITORS.** The precise recommendations for heparin administration during percutaneous intervention are somewhat ambiguous (Table 34.4, Figure 34.1). For planned abciximab, the recommended heparin bolus is 70 U/kg to achieve a target ACT of 200-250 seconds. Although the current FDA-approved labeling of eptifibatide and tirofiban includes a recommendation for a heparin dose of 100 U/kg to achieve an ACT of 300-350 seconds, most interventional cardiologists (including ourselves) recommend a heparin bolus of 70 U/kg to achieve an ACT 200-250 seconds, as with abciximab. In ESPRIT, in which patients were treated with a double bolus followed by an infusion of eptifibatide, the heparin bolus was 60 U/kg to achieve a target ACT of 200-300 seconds. For patients already receiving heparin, the guidelines are more confusing; one suggested approach is described in Figure 34.1. In our practices, the target ACT and heparin dose are identical for patients treated with abciximab, eptifibatide, or tirofiban.

C. **POSTPROCEDURAL HEPARIN.** In recent years the routine use of post-procedure heparin has declined after several studies[46-50] suggested no value for preventing ischemic events and increased risk for bleeding and vascular complications. In situations when post-procedural heparin may be recommended (e.g., patients requiring an IABP), meticulous monitoring of anticoagulation is required to prevent bleeding; bedside aPTT (Biotrack 523 Portable aPTT machine, Ciba-Corning Diagnostics, Medfield, MA) has improved the safety of heparin anticoagulation. Since rebound thrombin generation[51] and abrupt closure[52] may be temporally associated with discontinuation of prolonged heparin infusions, heparin should be tapered slowly over 6-24 hours rather than abruptly stopped.

D. **LIMITATIONS OF HEPARIN.** Heparin catalyzes the inactivation of thrombin and activated factor Xa, but must bind with antithrombin III to exert its anticoagulant effect. Heparin's antithrombotic activity is limited by its inability to inactivate clot-bound thrombin,[53] neutralization by platelet factor IV from platelet-rich thrombi, and inactivation by fibrin II monomers, which are formed by the action of thrombin on fibrinogen (Table 34.5). Accordingly, "therapeutic" concentrations of heparin may not prevent propagation of thrombus.[45,54] In addition, prolonged heparin infusions may deplete antithrombin III and potentially increase the risk of thrombosis.[55,56]

E. **ADVERSE EFFECTS.** The major adverse effect of heparin is bleeding, which is generally proportional to the heparin dose, ACT level, and use of concomitant antiplatelet and thrombolytic therapy. An infrequent but important complication of heparin therapy is heparin-induced thrombocytopenia (HIT) (Table 34.6) (Chapter 25).[57,58] Type-I HIT is due to direct (non-immune-mediated) platelet activation, results in mild thrombocytopenia, and has a benign clinical course. In contrast, Type-II HIT is due to immune-mediated platelet activation, results in moderate or severe thrombocytopenia, and is associated with serious thromboembolic complications. Platelet transfusions should not be used to treat patients with HIT due to the increased risk of thrombotic complications. An infusion of the prostacyclin analog Iloprost (Berlex laboratories) titrated to eliminate in-vitro heparin-induced platelet activation (infusion rates of 10-48 ng/kg/min) was successful in preventing recurrent HIT-2 in patients requiring cardiovascular surgery.[57,58] Anticoagulation in HIT-2 patients has also been achieved with defibrinating viper venoms like Ancrod or Reptilase, and with the heparinoid Org 10172.[58] Low-molecular-weight heparin may reduce[59,60] but not eliminate[61] the risk of HIT-1, but is absolutely contraindicated in patients with prior HIT-2. Recently, the direct-acting thrombin antagonists lepirudin (Refludan) and argatroban (Acova) have become commercially available as alternatives to heparin (see below). Heparin-induced thrombocytopenia is discussed in greater detail in Chapter 25.

Table 34.2. Antithrombotic and Antiplatelet Agents for Coronary Intervention

Antithrombotic Therapy
  Heparin (unfractionated)
  Low-molecular-weight heparin
  Direct thrombin inhibitor
        Polypeptide inhibitors (hirudin [Lepirudin], bivalirudin [Hirulog])
        Low-molecular-weight inhibitors (argatroban [Acova])
Antiplatelet Therapy
  Aspirin
  Clopidogrel
  Ticlopidine
  Dipyridamole
  Platelet GP IIb/IIIa antagonists
        Abciximab
        Eptifibatide
        Tirofiban
  Other antiplatelet agents

Table 34.3. Antithrombotic Therapy for Coronary Intervention: Effects, Indications, and Dose

Drug	Effect on Abrupt Closure	Indication and Dose
Aspirin	↓	*Elective PTCA:* 325 mg/d at least one day prior to procedure; continue indefinitely. *Urgent PTCA*: 4 chewable baby aspirins (total: 325 mg)
Dipyridamole	-	Not used
Ticlopidine	↓	*Aspirin-intolerant or allergic patient*: 250 mg PO BID starting 3-5 days prior to intervention. *Stents*: 250 mg BID x 2-4 weeks. Used less frequently now that clopidogrel is available
Clopidogrel	↓	*Aspirin-intolerant, allergic, or resistant patient*: 75 mg PO QD. *Stents:* 300 mg oral loading dose, then 75 mg PO QD x 2-4 weeks. *Radiation therapy for in-stent restenosis:* Aspirin plus clopidogrel for at least 9 months following the procedure
Heparin	↓	See Table 34.4 and Figure 34.1
LMW heparin	↓	*Alternative to unfractionated heparin for procedural anticoagulation:* Enoxaparin 1 mg/kg IV
Thrombolytics	-	*Dissolution of intracoronary thrombus:* Streptokinase (250,000 units IC) or tPA (10-20 mg IC) over 5-45 minutes
Dextran	-	Not recommended
GP IIb/IIIa inhibitors	↓	See Table 34.4 and Figure 34.1

↓ Most data suggest a decreased incidence
- No effect or unknown effect

Patient is on Heparin

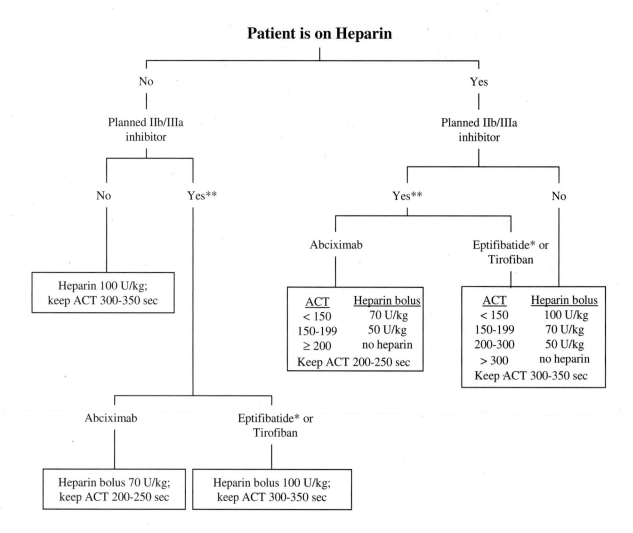

Figure 34.1. Approach to Heparin Administered During Percutaneous Intervention

*   In ESPRIT, the recommended initial heparin dose was 60 U/kg to achieve a target ACT 200-300 seconds
** In practice, many interventionalists use the same heparin and target ACT guidelines for tirofiban or eptifibatide as
     recommended for abciximab

Table 34.4. Platelet Glycoprotein IIb/IIIa Antagonists for Coronary Intervention

	Abciximab	Eptifibatide	Tirofiban
Dose for PCI	0.25 mg/kg IV bolus plus 0.125 mcg/kg/min (maximum 10 mcg/min) IV infusion for 12 hours. Low-dose heparin and early sheath removal to minimize bleeding (Table 34.24). For patients with unstable angina planning to undergo PCI within 24 hours, bolus plus infusion abciximab (PCI dose) can be started up to 24 hours prior to PCI and continued at the same rate until one hour after the procedure	**Acute coronary syndromes (PURSUIT dose):** 180 mcg/kg IV bolus plus 2.0 mcg/kg/min IV infusion. If arrive in cath lab > 4 hours after initiating therapy, no additional bolus is required. **Percutaneous intervention (ESPRIT dose):** 2 x 180 mcg/kg/min IV bolus 10 minutes apart, plus 2.0 mcg/kg/min IV infusion for 18-24 hours	10 mcg/kg IV bolus (over 3 minutes) immediately prior to PCI followed by an infusion of 0.15 mcg/kg/min for 18-24 hours. Patients with creatinine clearances < 30 cc/min should receive half the usual infusion rate
Heparin (unfractionated)	Maintain ACT at 200-250 seconds to minimize bleeding. Initial IV heparin dose based on ACT: ACT (sec) Heparin (bolus) < 150 70 U/kg 150-199 50 U/kg ≥ 200 no additional Discontinue heparin immediately after PCI	100 U/kg bolus, titrate to ACT 300-350 seconds. May also consider lower doses, as recommended for abciximab. In ESPRIT, the recommended initial heparin dose was 60 U/kg to achieve a target ACT of 200-300 seconds	100 U/kg bolus, titrate to ACT 300-350 seconds. May also consider lower doses, as recommended for abciximab
Aspirin	325 mg started at least 1 day prior to PCI and continued indefinitely; 4 chewable baby aspirin (325 mg total) for urgent intervention. For stents, add clopidogrel 300 mg oral load, then 75 mg PO daily for 2-4 weeks	See abciximab	See abciximab

Abbreviations: ACT = activated clotting time; PCI = percutaneous coronary intervention

Table 34.5. Comparison of Low-Molecular-Weight Heparins to Unfractionated Heparin

Characteristic	Unfractionated Heparin	LMW Heparins
Composition	Heterogenous mixture of polysaccharides; molecular weight 3000-30,000 Daltons	Homogenous glycosaminoglycans; molecular weight 4000-6000 Daltons
Mechanism of anticoagulation	Activates antithrombin III*; equivalent activity against factor Xa and thrombin; releases TFPI from endothelium; unable to inactivate clot-bound thrombin or FDP; inactivates fluid-phase thrombin	Less activation of antithrombin III; greater activity against factor Xa than thrombin; releases TFPI from endothelium; unable to inactivate clot-bound thrombin or FDP; weaker inactivation of fluid-phase thrombin
Pharmacokinetics	Variable binding to plasma proteins, endothelial cells, and macrophages leads to unpredictable anticoagulant effects (less available to interact with antithrombin III); half-life is short	Minimal binding to plasma proteins, endothelial cells, and macrophages leads to predictable anticoagulation; longer half-life
Laboratory monitoring	Essential because of unpredictable anticoagulant effects; use aPTT or ACT	Unnecessary except in renal failure or body weight < 50 kg or > 80 kg; use anti-factor Xa levels
Clinical uses	Prevention of venous thrombosis; treatment of venous thrombosis, unstable angina, acute MI, ischemic stroke. Routinely used during percutaneous intervention.	At least as effective as heparin for prevention of venous thrombosis in surgery and trauma patients, and for treatment of unstable angina, venous thrombosis, ischemic stroke. No definite advantage over heparin during percutaneous intervention.
Neutralization	Protamine neutralizes antithrombin activity	Protamine neutralizes antithrombin activity but only partially reverses anti-factor Xa activity.
HIT-2	Should not be used in patients with a history of HIT-2	Should not be used in patients with a history of HIT-2
Cost	Inexpensive	10-20 times more expensive than unfractionated heparin

Abbreviations: ACT = activated clotting time; aPTT = activated partial thromboplastin time; HIT = heparin-induced thrombocytopenia; TFPI = tissue factor pathway inhibitor; FDP = fibrin degradation products
* Antithrombin III is now commonly referred to as antithrombin

Table 34.6. Features of Heparin-Induced Thrombocytopenia (HIT)

	Type I HIT	Type II HIT
Incidence	10%	Rare
Mechanism	Direct platelet aggregating effect of heparin	Autoantibody (IgG or IgM) directed against platelet factor IV-heparin complex
Onset	Early (1-5 days)	Later (> 5 days); may occur sooner if prior heparin exposure
Platelet count	50,000/mm^3 - 150,000/mm^3	< 50,000/mm^3
Duration	Transient; often improves even if heparin is continued	Requires discontinuation of ALL heparin; gradual recovery in platelet count over 1-5 days in most patients
Clinical course	Benign	Recalcitrant venous and arterial thromboses and thromboembolism; may be fatal
Heparin substitute	UFH or LMWH may be continued	Argatroban (Acova) and lepirudin (Refludan) are FDA-approved

Abbreviations: UFH = unfractionated heparin; LMWH = low-molecular-weight heparin

---

LOW-MOLECULAR-WEIGHT HEPARINS

Low-molecular-weight (LMW) heparins are fragments of commercial grade heparin with potent antithrombotic properties. LMW heparins have numerous features distinct from unfractionated heparin (UFH), including a more predictable anticoagulation effect, lack of inhibition by platelet factor-4, lack of need for monitoring, and a lower risk of HIT (Table 34.7). In contrast to UFH, LMW heparins have less antithrombin activity and do not prolong the aPTT; their anticoagulant effect is mediated primarily by inhibition of Factor Xa (thrombin generation) (Table 34.5). LMW heparins have been used to prevent deep venous thrombosis and pulmonary embolism,[62] and the randomized ESSENCE [63] and TIMI-11b [64] trials demonstrated better event-free survival for enoxaparin vs. UFH in non-ST-elevation acute coronary syndromes (Table 34.8). However, studies during coronary intervention suggested little or no benefit over UFH (Table 34.9). Although ENTICES[65] and REDUCE[66] suggested a significant reduction in early ischemic events with enoxaparin or reviparin compared to UFH, these observations were not confirmed in ERA,[67] ATLAST,[68] or ENOXAPARIN[69] (Table 34.9). Likewise, some studies reported less bleeding with LMW heparin (ENTICES,[65] ATLAST[68]), while others did not (ERA,[67] ENOXAPARIN,[69] REDUCE [66]). Local delivery of enoxaparin showed a reduction in angiographic restenosis after stenting (POLONIA[70] trial), but other trials showed no difference in restenosis or late MACE between LMW heparin and UFH. LMW heparin has also been evaluated for extended therapy in high-risk post-stent patients: In ATLAST,[68] overall event rates were low, and there was no incremental benefit for enoxaparin compared to standard antiplatelet therapy. In fact, bleeding complications were more frequent after enoxaparin. More recently, observational studies of enoxaparin with (NICE-4)[71] and without (NICE-1) [72] platelet glycoprotein IIb/IIIa receptor antagonists for routine procedural anticoagulation have been completed. These studies and others[73] suggest that enoxaparin is safe and effective, and may be a reasonable alternative to UFH for procedural anticoagulation in the interventional setting. The recently completed NICE-3 study[74] demonstrated that patients with acute coronary syndromes receiving a IIb/IIIa antagonist and subcutaneous enoxaparin could safely undergo percutaneous revascularization without UFH. In ACUTE II,[75] a randomized trial of enoxaparin vs. UFH in interventional patients receiving tirofiban, safety and efficacy endpoints were similar between groups. Future data from INTERACT and CRUISE will help clarify the role of LMW heparin and IIb/IIIa antagonists in the cath lab. For now, LMW heparins are reasonable alternatives to UFH for procedural anticoagulation, but are not superior to UFH during percutaneous intervention in terms of reducing ischemic complications.

Table 34.7. Low-Molecular-Weight Heparin Preparations*

Preparation	Indications
Dalteparin (Fragmin)	Venous thrombosis, unstable angina (120 U/kg SQ BID; max. 10,000 U)
Enoxaparin (Lovenox)	Venous thrombosis, unstable angina (1 mg/kg SQ BID); PTCA (1 mg/kg IV)
Tinzaparin (Innohep)	Venous thrombosis (175 anti-Xa IU/kg SQ QD)
Ardeparin (Normiflo)	Venous thrombosis (50 U/kg SQ BID)
Danaparoid (Orgaran)**	Venous thrombosis (750 anti-Xa units SQ BID)
Nadroparin (Fraxiparin)	Not established
Reviparin (Clivarine)	Not established
Certoparin (Sandoparin)	Not established

Abbreviations: BID = twice daily; SQ = subcutaneous; QD = once daily
*   Different preparations are not interchangeable; each is classified as a distinct drug by the FDA
** Low-molecular-weight heparinoid

Table 34.8. Major Clinical Trials of Low-Molecular-Weight Heparins for Unstable Angina

Study	Drug	Setting	Endpoint	Results
FRISC[216] (n = 1506)	ASA, β-blockers for all patients; dalteparin (120 IU/kg SQ BID) vs. placebo	UA, non-Q-MI	Death, MI at 6 days	Risk reduction 68% (1.8% vs. 4.7%, p < 0.01) for dalteparin; more minor bleeding (7.9% vs. 0.3%) but similar major bleeding; less death, MI at 40 days (5.0% vs. 11%, p = 0.07)
FRIC[217] (n = 1482)	Dalteparin vs. standard heparin for 6 days	UA, non-Q-MI	Death, MI, revascularization at 45 days	No difference in outcome (14% vs. 12.9%) or bleeding (1.1% vs. 1%) for dalteparin
FRISC-Troponin[218] (n = 971)	ASA, β-blockers for all patients; dalteparin (120 mcg/kg BID for 5-7 days, or 7500 U QD for 5 weeks) vs. placebo	High-risk UA with elevated troponin-T, non-Q-MI	Death, MI at 45 days	Short- and long-term dalteparin superior to placebo
ESSENCE[63] (n = 3171)	Enoxaparin vs. standard heparin	UA, non-Q-MI	Death, MI, recurrent angina at 14 days	Enoxaparin superior to heparin (19.8% vs. 23.3%, p < 0.02); 16% relative risk reduction
TIMI-11b[63] (n = 3910)	Enoxaparin vs. standard heparin	UA, non-Q-MI	Death, MI, urgent revascularization at 8 days	Enoxaparin superior to heparin (12.4% vs. 14.5%, p = 0.048); 14% relative risk reduction
FRISC-II[219] (n = 2267)	Dalteparin in all patients for 5 days; then dalteparin vs. placebo for 3 months	UA, non-Q-MI	Death, MI at 3 months	Dalteparin superior to placebo at 1 month (3.1% vs. 5.9%), but no differences at 3 months (6.7% vs. 8%). No difference in patients treated with PCI
Gurfinkel[220] (n = 219)	Nadroparin vs. heparin vs. placebo for 5-7 days	UA	Death, MI, angina, revascularization at 7 days	Nadroparin superior to heparin
FRAXIS[221] (n = 3468)	Nadroparin (short and long duration) vs. heparin	UA, non-Q-MI	Death, MI, refractory angina at 14 days	Short- and long-term nadroparin similar to heparin
ACUTE-II[75] (n = 525)	Enoxaparin plus tirofiban vs. UFH plus tirofiban	UA	Safety and clinical outcomes	Outcomes similar with UFH and enoxaparin
NICE-3[74] (n = 616)	Enoxaparin plus IIb/IIIa antagonist (observational)	UA	Safety (non-CABG major bleeding)	Comparable safety (1.9%) and clinical efficacy
SYNERGY (n~ 8000)	Enoxaparin vs. UFH (efficacy)	UA managed invasively	Death/MI at 30 days	[Ongoing]

Abbreviations: ASA = aspirin; CABG = coronary artery bypass grafts; MI = myocardial infarction; PCI = percutaneous intervention; UA = unstable angina; UFH = unfractionated heparin
Acronyms: See Table 34.31, p. 803

Table 34.9. Major Trials of Low-Molecular-Weight Heparin for Coronary Intervention

Study	Drug	Setting	Endpoints	Results
ENTICES[65] (n = 123)	Enoxaparin (30-60 mg BID x 10d) + ASA + ticlopidine vs. ASA + dipyridamole + warfarin	Elective stent	Markers of thrombin activity and platelet activation at 10 days	No differences in markers; enoxaparin group had fewer ischemic events (5% vs. 20%, p < 0.01) and bleeding complications (16% vs. 5%, p < 0.05)
ERA[67] (n = 458)	Enoxaparin (for 1 month post-procedure)	PTCA	MACE and angiographic restenosis at 6 months	No difference in late MACE or restenosis
REDUCE[66] (n = 625)	Reviparin (procedural IV and 28 days post-procedure SQ)	PTCA	Angiographic restenosis at 6 months	Reviparin group had a 52% reduction in early ischemic events (3.9% vs. 8.2%, p < 0.05); no difference in bleeding, restenosis, or late MACE
ENOXAPARIN[69] (n = 60)	Enoxaparin (procedural only; IV)	PTCA/stent	Anticoagulation level (anti-Xa); procedural success	Similar anticoagulation effects, success, and complications
Diez[73] (n = 70)	Enoxaparin (procedural only; IV)	PTCA/stent	Procedural success	Comparable success
NICE-1[72] (n = 812)	Enoxaparin (procedural only IV without IIb/IIIa antagonists)	PTCA/stent (observational)	Safety	Low risk of bleeding and early MACE; comparable results to NICE-4
NICE-4[71] (n = 857)	Enoxaparin (procedural only IV with IIb/IIIa antagonists)	PTCA/stent (observational)	Safety	Low risk of bleeding and early MACE; comparable results to NICE-1
ATLAST[68] (n = 1121)	Enoxaparin (for 1 month post-procedure)	High-risk or suboptimal stent	Death, MI, or urgent revascularization at 30 days	Study stopped because of low event rates (placebo 2.7% vs. enoxaparin 1.8%, p = NS); more bleeding with enoxaparin
POLONIA[70] (n = 100)	Locally delivered enoxaparin via transport catheter vs. systemic UFH	Stent	Late lumen loss; loss index	Both endpoints significantly reduced
NICE-3[74] (n = 616)	Enoxaparin plus IIb/IIIa antagonist	ACS (PCI in 292 patients)	Safety (major bleeding)	Comparable bleeding (1.9% overall, 1.0% in PCI patients) and success
SYNERGY (n ~ 8000)	Enoxaparin vs. UFH (IIb/IIIa strongly encouraged)	ACS managed invasively	Death/MI	[Ongoing]

Summary: Compared to unfractionated heparin, LMW heparins have distinct advantages, including ease of administration and lack of need for intensive monitoring (primarily due to less protein binding). However, in patients undergoing percutaneous intervention, LMW heparins have not yet been shown to be superior to unfractionated heparin; cost is a clear disadvantage of LMW heparins. Further studies as adjuncts to platelet IIb/IIIa inhibitors are in progress.

Abbreviations: ACS = acute coronary syndrome; MACE = major adverse cardiac events; PCI = percutaneous coronary intervention; UFH = unfractionated heparin
Acronyms: See Table 34.31, p. 803

DIRECT THROMBIN INHIBITORS

Direct thrombin inhibitors are generally classified as polypeptide or low-molecular weight inhibitors[76] (Table 34.10). Polypeptide inhibitors such as hirudin (recombinant hirudin is lepirudin) and bivalirudin (hirulog) inactivate circulating thrombin via the active binding site and clot-bound thrombin via exosite-1. Low-molecular weight inhibitors such as argatroban also inactivate circulating thrombin via the active binding site, but do not inactivate clot-bound thrombin. Unlike heparin, direct thrombin inhibitors such as hirudin and bivalirudin do not require antithrombin for anticoagulant effect, form highly stable noncovalent complexes with circulating *and* clot-bound thrombin, and are not inhibited by platelet factor 4 (Tables 34.11, 34.12). Although a pilot study reported that bivalirudin was similar to heparin in decreasing ischemic complications after PTCA,[77] a subsequent study reported fewer ischemic and bleeding complications with bivalirudin in high-risk patients with post-infarction angina.[78] In the Hirudin European Trial versus Heparin in the Prevention of Restenosis after PTCA (HELVETICA),[79] PTCA patients with unstable angina had fewer early ischemic events after hirudin, but no difference in restenosis. A higher incidence of intracranial hemorrhage has been reported in three trials combining hirudin and thrombolytic therapy (GUSTO IIa,[80] TIMI 9A,[81] HIT-III[82]). The ongoing CACHET and REPLACE trials are evaluating the efficacy of bivalirudin (with "rescue" IIb/IIIa antagonist if necessary) vs. unfractionated heparin with routine IIb/IIIa antagonist during coronary intervention (Table 34.13). In the United States, lepirudin (Refludan, a recombinant hirudin) and argatroban (Acova, a small molecule active site inhibitor) are approved for use in patients with heparin-induced thrombocytopenia who require IV anticoagulation. In such patients, lepirudin is administered as an initial bolus of 0.4 mg/kg (maximum 44 mg) over 15-20 seconds, followed by a continuous infusion of 0.15 mg/kg/hr (maximum rate 16.5 mg/hr). Monitoring is accomplished using the same aPTT guidelines as for UFH. Bivalirudin (Angiomax) has recently been approved for procedural anticoagulation in unstable angina.

Table 34.10. Direct Thrombin Inhibitors

Polypeptide Inhibitors
      Hirudin (Lepirudin)*+
      Bivalirudin (Hirulog)

Low-Molecular-Weight Inhibitors
      <u>Noncovalent</u>
      Argatroban (Acova)+
      Napsagatran
      Inogatran
      Melogatran

      <u>Reversible-covalent</u>
      Efegatran
      Boro-arginine derivatives

*   Hirudin is derived from medicinal leech saliva. It is available by recombinant DNA technology as lepirudin (Refludan)

\+   FDA-approved for patients with HIT-2 who require anticoagulation

Table 34.11. Comparison of Unfractionated Heparin and Direct Thrombin Inhibitors*

	Unfractionated Heparin	**Direct Thrombin Inhibitors**
Effect on clot-bound thrombin, FDP	None	Inactivation
Effect on antithrombin	High-affinity interaction; inhibits thrombin and factor Xa	High affinity interaction
Effect on factor Xa bound to platelets	None	Inactivation
Binding to endothelium and plasma proteins	High; results in less heparin availability to activate antithrombin	None
Binding to PF-4	High affinity	None
Anticoagulant effects	Highly variable	Predictable
Laboratory monitoring	Essential	May be unnecessary with bivalirudin

Summary: Direct thrombin inhibitors have biologic and pharmacokinetic advantages compared to heparin. The biologic advantage reflects their ability to inactivate clot-bound thrombin via exosite 1 (polypeptide inhibitors), whereas the pharmacologic advantages produce more predictable anticoagulant effects without the need for intensive laboratory monitoring (especially bivalirudin), by less binding to endothelial and plasma proteins. Bivalirudin may block procoagulant activity associated with eptifibatide and tirofiban.

Abbreviations: FDP = fibrin degradation products; PF-4 = platelet factor-4
* Hirudin, bivalirudin

Table 34.12. Comparison of Direct Thrombin Polypeptide Inhibitors

	Hirudin	**Bivalirudin**
Source	Saliva of medicinal leech; now available by recombinant technology*	Semisynthetic
Composition	65-amino acid polypeptide	20-amino acid polypeptide
Inhibition of thrombin	Slowly reversible, highly selective	Transient, reversible
Safety margin	Narrow	Wide
Dose range	Narrow	Wide
Effect on Protein C	Inhibits activation	Promotes activation and enhances anticoagulation
Laboratory monitoring	Necessary	Probably not necessary

Summary: Compared to hirudin, bivalirudin has potential safety advantages (shorter half-life, transient reversible thrombin inhibition) and efficacy (wider dose range, promotes activation of protein C). Despite the theoretical advantages of direct thrombin inhibitors compared to heparin, clinical trials of hirudin as adjuncts to thrombolytic therapy or PTCA have not demonstrated better efficacy than heparin. Bivalirudin may be safer and more effective than hirudin; further study is needed.

* Recombinant hirudin is available as lepirudin (Refludan)

Table 34.13. Major Trials of Thrombin Antagonists for Coronary Intervention

Study	Drug	Setting	Endpoint	Results
Van den Bos[204] (n = 113)	Hirudin vs. heparin	PTCA	Safety	More reliable aPTTs with hirudin; comparable clinical outcomes
HELVETICA[79] (n = 1141)	Hirudin vs. heparin	PTCA	Death, MI, TVR, ARS at 6 months	No difference in outcome
Hirulog Pilot[77] (n = 291)	Hirulog (bivalirudin)	PTCA	Dose ranging (feasibility)	Less abrupt closure with higher doses
Hirulog Angioplasty Study[78] (n = 4098)	Hirulog vs. heparin	PTCA	Death, MI, abrupt closure, rapid clinical deterioration in hospital	Hirulog with less bleeding (3.8% vs. 9.8%, p < 0.001) and fewer events in post-MI patients (9.1% vs. 14.2%, p = 0.04), but no difference overall (11.4% vs. 12.2%, p = NS)
CACHET Pilot[205] (n = 210)	Bivalirudin (with rescue abciximab) vs. heparin/abciximab	PTCA/Stent	Clinical outcomes and bleeding	Reduction in composite events with bivalirudin
REPLACE	Bivalirudin (with rescue abciximab) vs. heparin/abciximab	PCI	Clinical outcomes	[Ongoing]

Abbreviations: ARS = angiographic restenosis; MI = myocardial infarction; TVR = target vessel revascularization; PTCA = percutaneous transluminal coronary angioplasty; PCI = percutaneous coronary intervention
Acronyms: See Table 34.31, p. 803

ANTIPLATELET THERAPY

Oral antiplatelet therapy is the cornerstone of pharmacotherapy during percutaneous coronary intervention (Table 34.14). Aspirin alone (PTCA, laser, atherectomy) and aspirin plus clopidogrel (stents) are the standard regimens in the interventional setting.

A. **ASPIRIN.** Aspirin blocks the formation of prostaglandin endoperoxides and thromboxane A2 by inhibiting prostaglandin G/H synthase and the cyclooxygenase pathway. This effect is transient in nucleated cells but is permanent for the life of anucleate platelets. Aspirin also exerts antiplatelet effects which are independent of its effects on thromboxane.[83,84] Preprocedural aspirin reduces the risk of abrupt coronary occlusion by 50-75% and is standard therapy for all coronary interventional procedures.[85,86] Other beneficial effects include prevention of coronary artery disease and stroke, improved outcome in chronic stable angina, unstable angina, and acute MI,[87-92] and maintenance of saphenous vein graft patency after coronary bypass surgery.[93] Aspirin increases the risk of bleeding complications[94,95] and has no impact on restenosis.[96]

1. **Dosage.** The optimal dose, timing, and duration of administration of aspirin are unknown, but it is customary to administer 325 mg at least one day before elective PTCA and continue it indefinitely. If urgent PTCA is required, 4 chewable baby aspirins (81 mg each) are given prior to the case. For the aspirin-allergic patient, clopidogrel (75 mg daily starting 3-5 days prior to intervention) can be substituted; dipyridamole, sulfinpyrazone, and dextran have not been studied and are not routinely recommended. Patients with acute coronary syndromes may be resistant to aspirin,[97] but the impact of higher doses has not been studied. New slow-release oral and transdermal aspirin preparations may selectively inhibit platelet aggregation without inhibiting the synthesis of prostacyclin (PGI_2), which is a potent vasodilator and platelet inhibitor. Whether these preparations offer any advantage over conventional aspirin is unknown.

2. **Limitations.** Aspirin does not prevent platelet aggregation caused by thrombin, catecholamines, ADP, serotonin, or shear-stress. These deficiencies may partially explain persistent thrombin generation and platelet activation in some patients despite "therapeutic" aspirin and heparin; unfortunately, these prothrombotic conditions are difficult to detect in routine clinical settings. Recent studies also suggest that 8-12% of patients with coronary artery disease may be unresponsive to the antiplatelet effects of aspirin;[98-100] bedside platelet function testing may soon facilitate the identification of such aspirin nonresponders.

B. **TICLOPIDINE.** Ticlopidine is a thienopyridine that blocks ADP-induced platelet activation by interfering with the signaling between the low-affinity platelet ADP receptor (P2T) and the subsequent processes of platelet activation, including activation of the platelet glycoprotein (GP) IIb/IIIa receptor.[101-103] Ticlopidine inhibits platelet aggregation in response to collagen, thrombin, and shear-stress by inhibiting ADP amplification mechanisms for platelet activation;[104] it also enhances the antiaggregatory effects of prostacyclin[105] and promotes deaggregation of thrombin-activated platelets.[106] Thienopyridines such as ticlopidine and clopidogrel are much more effective than aspirin in inhibiting shear-induced platelet activation, an important mechanism for endovascular thrombosis in coronary artery disease. In a randomized PTCA trial, ticlopidine (250 mg BID) resulted in fewer ischemic complications than aspirin plus dipyridamole (2% vs. 5%).[96] Several other trials have demonstrated superiority of aspirin plus ticlopidine vs. aspirin plus warfarin in reducing ischemic and hemorrhagic complications after stenting (STARS,[107] ISAR,[108,109] FANTASTIC, [110] MATTIS [111]) (Chapter 26). Ticlopidine has also been shown to reduce the risk of death and nonfatal MI in unstable angina,[112] prevent stroke in patients with TIAs,[113] and has been used for aspirin-allergic or intolerant patients. In patients with coronary artery disease, the combination of aspirin (50 mg/day) plus ticlopidine (250 mg twice daily) demonstrated synergistic platelet inhibition.[114]

1. **Dosage.** Ticlopidine should be administered at a dose of 250 mg PO BID for at least 3 days prior to intervention to maximize antiplatelet effect. Onset of action is 48-72 hours, and full antiplatelet effects are evident in 5-7 days. An oral loading dose of 500 mg PO BID for 48 hours may accelerate antiplatelet effects[115] and confer some benefit in emergency situations. After ticlopidine is stopped, the antiplatelet effects subside over 1-2 weeks.[106] Although ticlopidine was routinely administered for 2-4 weeks after stenting, the benefit of therapy beyond 2 weeks has been questioned.[116]

2. **Limitations.** An important side effect of ticlopidine is reversible neutropenia, which occurs in 0.5-2% of patients after 4 weeks of use;[117,118] complete blood counts are recommended every 2-4 weeks during the first few months of therapy. Sporadic cases of thrombotic thrombocytopenic purpura (TTP) have also been reported, with an estimated incidence of 0.02%; most cases occur in the third or fourth week of therapy (Chapter 25). Nausea, vomiting, and diarrhea are common and can be minimized by taking ticlopidine with food; skin rash and elevated transaminases are rare. Long-term administration of ticlopidine lowers plasma fibrinogen and increases cholesterol, but the clinical consequences of these effects are unknown.

C. **CLOPIDOGREL.** Clopidogrel is another thienopyridine derivative, analogous to ticlopidine,[119] which blocks ADP-induced platelet activation by irreversibly modifying the platelet ADP receptor. Compared to ticlopidine, clopidogrel has a longer duration of action, a faster onset of action, and is associated with fewer adverse hematologic effects.[119-122] In more than 19,000 patients randomized to clopidogrel vs. aspirin in CAPRIE,[122] there was no difference in neutropenia. In the randomized CLASSICS trial of 1020 patients undergoing elective stenting,[123] clopidogrel was better tolerated than ticlopidine without compromising clinical efficacy (Chapter 26). Clopidogrel has largely replaced ticlopidine in the United States because of its superior safety profile. The combined use of aspirin plus clopidogrel vs. aspirin alone for acute coronary syndromes was recently evaluated in the CURE (Clopidogrel in Unstable Angina to Prevent Recurrent Events) trial.[229] In this study, 12,562 patients with unstable angina or non-Q-wave MI were randomized to aspirin (75-325 mg/day) alone or aspirin plus clopidogrel (300 mg loading dose followed by 75 mg/day) for 3-12 months (average 9 months). Patients treated with IIb/IIIa inhibitors within 3 days or revascularization within 3 months were excluded from this study. As shown in Table 34.32 (below), clopidogrel resulted in a highly significant 20% relative reduction in the primary composite endpoint of cardiovascular death, MI, or stroke (9.3% vs. 11.5%, p = 0.00005). Benefits were evident within the first 30 days, and increased further beyond 30 days, demonstrating the importance of long-term therapy. Although there was a 1% absolute increase in major bleeding with clopidogrel, these cases were effectively managed by blood transfusions, and there was no increase in fatal bleeding. These compelling data suggest that patients with acute coronary syndromes should be considered for antiplatelet therapy with aspirin plus clopidogrel.

Table 34.32. Combination Antiplatelet Therapy for ACS: Results of the CURE Trial[229]

Endpoint	Aspirin (n = 6303)	Aspirin + Clopidogrel (n = 6259)	Risk Ratio	p-Value
CV death, MI, stroke (%)*	11.5	9.3	0.80	0.00005
CV death, MI, stroke, refractory ischemia (%)	19.0	16.7	0.88	0.0004
Major bleeding (%)	2.7	3.6	1.34	0.003
Minor bleeding (%)	8.6	15.3	1.78	< 0.001

Abbreviations: ACS = acute coronary syndromes; CURE = Clopidogrel in Unstable angina to prevent Recurrent Events; CV = cardiovascular; MI = myocardial infarction
* Primary endpoint

1. **Dosage.** The oral dose of clopidogrel is 75 mg daily; full antiplatelet effect is achieved in 5 days. A loading doses of 300 mg was employed in CLASSICS, CREDO, and CURE, and a 375 mg loading dose produced 60% inhibition of ADP-induced platelet aggregation in normal volunteers.[124] Higher loading doses may produce more rapid platelet inhibition. The ongoing CREDO trial will define the ideal dose and duration of clopidogrel when used with aspirin following stent implantation.

2. **Limitations.** Clopidogrel may be better tolerated than aspirin. The most frequent side effects[122] include purpura (5%), diarrhea (4%), rash (4%), and pruritus (3%). Clopidogrel is not associated with an increased risk of neutropenia, so routine hematologic monitoring is not necessary for patients on chronic therapy. A recent report[125] documented 11 cases of suspected TTP among 3 million patients exposed to clopidogrel, although the incidence of TTP is substantially lower than that associated with ticlopidine.[126] Some patients on combined aspirin and clopidogrel therapy may develop severe platelet inhibition, which could be clinically important if CABG is needed; the rapid platelet aggregation assay can be used to assess the degree of antiplatelet activity in this instance. Clopidogrel is metabolized in the liver but has little impact on hepatic enzyme induction or drug metabolism. Although clopidogrel may interfere with metabolism of fluvastatin, the significance of this interaction is unknown. Caution is recommended when clopidogrel is used in combination with nonsteroidal anti-inflammatory drugs or warfarin due to the increased risk of bleeding.

D. **DIPYRIDAMOLE.** Dipyridamole increases platelet cAMP and causes direct release of prostacyclin from the endothelium, but its antiplatelet mechanism of action is incompletely understood. Dipyridamole has a half-life of 10 days and is primarily metabolized by the liver and excreted in the bile. When used in conjunction with aspirin, dipyridamole enhances platelet survival in patients with venous and arterial thrombosis, prosthetic valves, and prosthetic grafts. In ESPS-II,[127] high-dose dipyridamole plus low-dose aspirin (50 mg/d) was superior to aspirin alone in preventing recurrent ischemic events following stroke or TIA, but acceptance of this regimen has been hampered by prior negative studies in the same clinical scenario. In PTCA patients, two studies of parenteral dipyridamole plus aspirin reported fewer ischemic complications compared to aspirin alone,[128,129] but a randomized trial of oral dipyridamole failed to demonstrate benefit.[130] At the present time, dipyridamole is not routinely recommended for coronary intervention. The usual oral dose of dipyridamole is 75 mg BID for 6 months. Side effects include exacerbation of angina, headaches, hypertension, hypotension, and tachycardia. Concurrent administration with aspirin increases the risk of GI bleeding.

E. **DEXTRAN.** Dextran is rarely used today in interventional cardiology. Despite its theoretical benefits, there is no proven benefit compared to placebo. Serious adverse effects include anaphylaxis, hypotension, and pulmonary hemorrhage.

F. **OTHER ANTIPLATELET INHIBITORS.** Other promising agents under investigation include thromboxane receptor and synthetase antagonists (Ridogrel), serotonin antagonists (Ketanserin), prostacyclin analogues (Ciprostene), intravenous ADP receptor antagonists, platelet glycoprotein Ib receptor antagonists, and other GP IIb/IIIa inhibitors.

G. **PLATELET GLYCOPROTEIN IIb/IIIa INHIBITORS (see below)**

Table 34.14. Major Trials of Oral Antiplatelet Therapy for Coronary Intervention

Study	Drug	Setting	Endpoint	Results
Ticlopidine trial[201] (n = 337)	Placebo ASA/dipyridamole Ticlopidine	PTCA	Ischemic complications; restenosis	Ischemic complications (14% vs. 4% vs. 3%); no effect on restenosis
STARS[107] (n = 1653)	ASA Warfarin + ASA Ticlopidine + ASA	Stent	Death, MI, TVR, or thrombosis at 30 days	Ischemic complications (3.6% vs. 2.8% vs. 0.5%, p = 0.001)
ISAR[109,188] (n = 517)	Warfarin + ASA Ticlopidine + ASA	High-risk stent	Cardiac death, MI, TVR at 30 days	Ischemic complications (6.2% vs. 1.6%, p < 0.01)
FANTASTIC[110] (n = 236)	Warfarin + ASA Ticlopidine + ASA	Elective and nonelective stent (Wiktor)	Bleeding; clinical events (death, MI, occlusion at 6 months)	Bleeding (21% vs. 13.5%, p = 0.03); clinical events (15.5% vs. 12.9%, p = NS)
MATTIS[111] (n = 350)	Warfarin + ASA Ticlopidine + ASA	High-risk stent	Death, MI, or TVR at 30 days	Ischemic complications (11% vs. 5.6%, p = 0.07)
Albiero[202] (n = 801)	ASA Ticlopidine + ASA	Successful optimized stent (usually with IVUS)	Stent thrombosis, major adverse clinical events	Stent thrombosis (1.9% vs. 1.9%); MACE (1.9% vs. 1.9%)
Moussa[203] (n = 1489)	ASA + ticlopidine ASA + clopidogrel (not randomized)	Stent	Clinical events; drug side effects	Clinical events (1.5% vs. 1.4%); drug side effects (10.6% vs. 0.3%, p = 0.006)
CLASSICS [123.] (n = 1020)	ASA+ ticlopidine ASA + clopidogrel ASA + clopidogrel (loaded)	Stent	1°: Safety (bleeding, neutropenia, thrombocytopenia, early drug D/C) 2°: Clinical events (death, MI, TVR at 6 months)	Safety (9.1% vs. 6.3% vs. 2.9% p = 0.005); clinical events (0.9% vs. 1.5% vs. 1.2%, p = NS)
CREDO	ASA + clopidogrel ASA + clopidogrel (loaded) Short- vs. long-term therapy	Stent	Clinical events	[Ongoing]

Abbreviations: ASA = aspirin; IVUS = intravascular ultrasound; MACE = major adverse cardiac events; MI = myocardial infarction; TVR = target vessel revascularization
Acronyms: See Table 34.31, p. 803

PLATELET GLYCOPROTEIN IIb/IIIa RECEPTOR ANTAGONISTS (Tables 34.15, 34.16)

Activation of the platelet glycoprotein (GP) IIb/IIIa receptor complex constitutes the final common pathway for platelet aggregation, and is a critical event in arterial thrombosis (Figure 40.4, Chapter 40). Potent GP IIb/IIIa receptor antagonists have been shown to improve event-free survival in a variety of interventional and non-interventional settings and are the focus of intensive investigation. Abciximab is a noncompetive antagonist (monoclonal antibody) that binds 1:1 to the GP IIb/IIIa receptor molecule to induce a conformational change that renders its fibrinogen-binding site inactive. Eptifibatide and tirofiban are competitive antagonists that reversibly inhibit the binding of fibrinogen to the GP IIb/IIIa receptor by directly interacting with its RGD binding site. From a clinical standpoint, noncompetitive inhibitors (such as abciximab) have a longer biological half-life, more cross-reactivity with other cell-surface receptors, and higher dissociation constants (more permanent binding) than competitive inhibitors, which may translate into more durable clinical efficacy (in terms of reducing ischemic complications) and less restenosis (possibly due to cross-reactivity with the vitronectin receptor). Numerous studies have evaluated these agents for acute coronary syndromes and as adjuncts for percutaneous coronary intervention (Tables 34.17-34.21). The specific agents and clinical trials are detailed below.

A. **ABCIXIMAB.** Abciximab (ReoPro, Centocor) is the Fab fragment of the chimeric monoclonal antibody 7E3. Abciximab binds to and blocks platelet GP IIb/IIIa receptors, the vitronectin receptor ($\alpha_v\beta_3$) on smooth muscle and endothelial cells, and the Mac-1 receptor on leukocytes (Table 34.22). Interaction with these receptors may confer antiplatelet, antiproliferative (i.e., restenosis), and anti-inflammatory activity, respectively. Inhibition of clot retraction, factor XIII, and PAI-I, displacement of fibrinogen, and prolongation of the ACT may confer additional anticoagulant and thrombolytic activity unique to abciximab.

1. **Abciximab Trials (Tables 34.17-34.21).** Abciximab has been studied in several large-scale, placebo-controlled randomized trials[131-139] in PTCA (EPIC, EPILOG, CAPTURE), stenting (EPISTENT), acute MI (ADMIRAL, RAPPORT, CADILLAC), and acute coronary syndromes (GUSTO-IV ACS); a comparative trial of abciximab vs. tirofiban (TARGET) has recently been completed. EPIC, EPILOG, EPISTENT, and CAPTURE all demonstrated 35-57% reductions in the primary endpoint (death, MI, TLR) favoring abciximab,[131,133-135] which was particularly evident in patients with unstable angina and acute MI. Although EPIC reported more bleeding complications with abciximab, EPILOG demonstrated that low-dose, weight-adjusted heparin (70 U/kg to achieve ACT 200-250 seconds) plus abciximab could significantly attenuate the risk of bleeding without sacrificing efficacy. Furthermore, benefits observed in high-risk PTCA patients in EPIC were extended to high and low-risk PTCA and stent patients in EPILOG and EPISTENT. Importantly, EPIC continues to demonstrate sustained benefit of abciximab at 30 days, 6 months, and 3 years.[131,132,138] EPILOG has shown persistent benefit at 1 year,[137] and EPISTENT reported sustained benefit at 6 months[135] and at 1 year (mortality: 1% vs. 2.4%).[140] Angiographic restenosis was also lower in diabetics treated with abciximab.[141] In contrast to the abciximab bolus and 12-

hour infusion utilized in EPIC, EPILOG, and EPISTENT, CAPTURE patients received an 18-24 infusion before and a 1-hour infusion after intervention; initial benefit at 30 days was not sustained at 6 months,[134] suggesting that a 12-hour infusion after intervention may be important for sustained clinical efficacy. Abciximab has also been studied as an adjunct to thrombolytic therapy for acute MI patients with ST-segment elevation (Table 34.21). In patients with acute MI undergoing primary PTCA or stenting, three trials of abciximab have reported divergent results (Table 34.18): In RAPPORT,[136] abciximab was associated with a nonsignificant 17% reduction in late MACE after primary PTCA (p = 0.07). In ADMIRAL,[142] abciximab was associated with a 47% reduction in late MACE after primary stenting (p = 0.03). In CADILLAC,[143] patients were randomized to primary PTCA vs. stenting, and abciximab vs. no abciximab. Similar to RAPPORT, the 21% reduction in late MACE after primary PTCA was not significant, and in contrast to ADMIRAL, abciximab offered no incremental benefit after primary stenting. In patients with non-ST-segment elevation acute coronary syndromes, GUSTO-IV ACS revealed no benefit for abciximab (24 or 48-hour infusion) when added to aspirin and heparin (UFH or dalteparin).[144] Finally, the TARGET trial[145] reported better results for abciximab compared to tirofiban for stent patients (death, MI, or urgent revascularization at 30 days: abciximab 6.0% vs. tirofiban 7.5%, p = 0.037), especially those presenting with an acute coronary syndrome.

2. **Dosage.** The recommended dose for abciximab for percutaneous intervention is an IV bolus of 0.25 mg/kg administered 10 minutes before intervention, followed by a continuous infusion of 0.125 mcg/kg/min (to a maximum of 10 mcg/min) for 12 hours after intervention. All patients should also receive standard aspirin therapy. The recommended heparin dose is 70 U/kg to achieve an ACT 200-250 seconds; additional heparin is not recommended after intervention. Vascular sheaths should be removed when the ACT is 150-175 seconds, and there is no need to discontinue abciximab for sheath removal. When abciximab is administered after full-dose heparinization ("rescue ReoPro"), additional heparin should be used cautiously to reduce the risk of bleeding; clear guidelines have not been established, and although some suggest partial reversal of full-dose heparin with protamine, this is not routinely recommended.

3. **Limitations (Chapter 25).** A number of safety concerns have been raised about the use of IIb/IIIa antagonists in general and about abciximab in particular. Most of these concerns are related to bleeding complications, the potential requirement for emergency CABG, severe thrombocytopenia, and potential drug interactions. Virtually all of these considerations are readily prevented and/or treated, and do not constitute significant obstacles to the use of IIb/IIIa inhibitors.

   a. **Bleeding (Table 34.23).** In most IIb/IIIa inhibitor trials,[131-133,135,136] major bleeding was defined as a drop in hemoglobin > 5 gm/dL, an absolute drop in hematocrit > 15%, or intracranial hemorrhage; minor bleeding included spontaneous gross hematuria, spontaneous hematemesis, a drop in hemoglobin > 3 gm/dL with evident blood loss, or a drop in hemoglobin > 4 gm/dL without evident blood loss. In abciximab trials utilizing standard-dose heparin to maintain high ACT levels (EPIC, EPILOG, RAPPORT), bleeding was more frequent with abciximab vs. placebo (Table 34.23); independent predictors of bleeding included acute MI, low body weight, old age, longer procedural times, repeat PTCA, and failed intervention. In contrast, trials utilizing low-dose heparin, early sheath removal, and ACT 200-250 seconds (EPILOG, CAPTURE, EPISTENT) reported no difference in major or minor bleeding for patients treated with abciximab or placebo. These studies suggest that the risk of bleeding associated with abciximab can be minimized by low-dose heparin, early sheath removal, avoidance of venous sheaths, and fastidious post-procedure groin care (Table 34.24). Importantly, patients treated with abciximab do not have a higher incidence of intracranial hemorrhage compared to placebo.

b. **Thrombocytopenia (Table 34.25).** A potential safety concern with IIb/IIIa antagonists is thrombocytopenia, which may increase bleeding complications.[146] The incidence of thrombocytopenia appears to be higher with abciximab than with eptifibatide or tirofiban. In the clinical trials, the incidence of mild thrombocytopenia ($< 100,000/mm^3$) was 2.6-5.6% and severe thrombocytopenia ($< 50,000/mm^3$) was 0.9-1.6%; platelet transfusions were administered in 1.6-5.5%. Unlike heparin-induced thrombocytopenia, abciximab-associated thrombocytopenia responds within days of discontinuing the drug, and responds promptly to platelet transfusions (Tables 34.24, 34.25). In contrast, severe thrombocytopenia after abciximab retreatment (which is 2-3 times more frequent than after first time use) may not respond promptly to platelet transfusions. Although abciximab is not FDA-approved for readministration, repeat use is common in clinical practice. One study of readministration of abciximab in 500 patients[147] reported a 3-fold higher incidence of profound thrombocytopenia than with initial administration. Although human IgG anti-chimeric antibodies (HACA) are more common after abciximab readministration,[148] a clear association between HACA and thrombocytopenia has not been identified. If readministration of abciximab is considered, early platelet counts should be obtained and abciximab should be discontinued immediately if the platelet counts fall (Chapter 25).

c. **Emergency CABG (Table 34.24).** The risk of bleeding during emergency CABG is potentiated by abciximab and heparin.[149,150] The hemostatic defect due to abciximab is largely reversible with platelet transfusions, but the benefit is not immediate or complete due to persistent platelet-bound abciximab. Transfused platelets serve as "sink" to remove excess drug from affected platelets, and it may take 3 hours to completely reverse the antiplatelet effect.[151,152] In EPIC, EPILOG, and EPISTENT, [153,154] the risk of major bleeding or blood transfusion in emergency CABG patients receiving antecedent abciximab was similar to placebo, although abciximab patients required more platelet transfusions. Key factors in reducing the risk of bleeding during emergency CABG include careful titration of heparin dose and liberal use of platelet transfusions, especially after coming off cardiopulmonary bypass.

d. **Drug Interactions.** Potential drug interactions are described in Table 34.26.

B. **EPTIFIBATIDE (Tables 34.15, 34.16)**. Eptifibatide (Integrilin; manufactured by COR Therapeutics, distributed by Shering-Plough) is a synthetic cyclic K-G-D (lysine-glycine-aspartic acid) heptapeptide and a competitive antagonist for the IIb/IIIa receptor. Unlike abciximab, eptifibatide has a short half-life (2.5 hours),[155] is very specific for the IIb/IIIa receptor, and does not cross-react with the vitronectin receptor. Platelet function returns to baseline within 4 hours after drug discontinuation.

   1. **Eptifibatide Trials.** The use of eptifibatide during coronary intervention was studied in IMPACT-II, PURSUIT, and ESPRIT (Tables 34.17-34.21). In IMPACT-II,[156] there was a nonsignificant 19% reduction in the composite primary endpoint (death, MI, revascularization, or bailout coronary stent) at 30-days in the low-dose eptifibatide group (9.2% vs. 11.4%, p = 0.063) and in the high-dose eptifibatide group (9.9% vs. 11.4%, p = 0.22). There were no differences in major bleeding or blood transfusion (Table 34.23). In PURSUIT, 10,948 patients with unstable angina or non-Q-wave MI received aspirin and intravenous heparin (initial bolus of 5000 U followed by 1000 U/hr to achieve aPTT 50-70 seconds) and were randomly assigned to eptifibatide (180 mcg/kg bolus and 2.0 mcg/kg/min infusion) or placebo.[157] A third arm using a lower dose of eptifibatide was discontinued (as specified in the original protocol) since the higher dose did not cause more bleeding complications. In a subgroup of 1,250 patients undergoing percutaneous intervention within 72 hours of randomization, eptifibatide reduced the 30-day incidence of death and MI by 31% (11.6% vs. 16.7%, p = 0.01), and the incidence of the death and MI before intervention by 69% (1.7% vs. 5.5%, p < 0.001). In ESPRIT,[158] the dose of eptifibatide was further modified to include a second bolus, 10 minutes after the first. In an elective coronary stent population, this second bolus was associated with a 37% reduction in ischemic events at 48 hours, which persisted at 30 days and at 6 months.

   2. **Dosage.** Because IMPACT II was used to support product labeling, the FDA-approved dose of eptifibatide is an IV bolus of 135 mcg/kg immediately before intervention followed by a continuous infusion of 0.5 mcg/kg/min for 12-24 hours. However, given the dosing concerns in IMPACT II and the favorable experience in PURSUIT, many physicians have adopted the higher dose employed in PURSUIT: an IV bolus of 180 mcg/kg followed by an infusion of 2 mcg/kg/min for patients with acute coronary syndromes. For therapy initiated in the cath lab (as in ESPRIT), a double bolus of eptifibatide (180 mcg/kg x 2, 10 minutes apart) is recommended, followed by an infusion of 2 mcg/kg/min.

   3. **Limitations.** Eptifibatide did not increase the risk of major bleeding complications in IMPACT II, PURSUIT, and ESPRIT. In contrast to abciximab, there may be less need to reduce the heparin dose, there is no known immune response, and the incidence of thrombocytopenia is similar to placebo. Eptifibatide should be discontinued in patients requiring emergency CABG; antiplatelet effects will resolve in 4-6 hours and platelet transfusion is ineffective. Drug clearance is longer in patients with impaired renal function.

C. **TIROFIBAN (Tables 34.15, 34.16).** Tirofiban (Aggrastat; Merck) is a synthetic, small-molecule nonpeptide competitive antagonist of the IIb/IIIa receptor. As with eptifibatide, it is rapidly reversible, highly selective, and does not cross-react with the vitronectin receptor.

1. **Tirofiban Trials**. In RESTORE,[159,160] 2,139 patients with acute coronary syndromes undergoing PTCA or DCA receiving aspirin and heparin were randomized to tirofiban (10 mcg/kg bolus and 0.15 mcg/kg/min infusion) or placebo for 36 hours. There was a 40% reduction in death, MI, and urgent revascularization (5.2% vs. 8.7%, p = 0.002) at 2 days, 30% reduction at 7 days (6.9% vs. 9.8%, p = 0.016), and 24% reduction at 30 days (8.0% vs. 10.5%, p = 0.16). The composite endpoint (death, MI, and revascularization) at 6 months was similar (24.1% with tirofiban vs. 27.1% with placebo, p = 0.11), and follow-up angiography in 417 patients showed no difference in restenosis (Tables 34.17-34.20).[160] In PRISM-PLUS,[161] patients with acute coronary syndromes were randomized to tirofiban, heparin, or tirofiban plus heparin for 48-96 hours; the tirofiban-only arm was dropped because of excess mortality at 7 days. The study was completed with 773 patients receiving tirofiban plus heparin and 797 patients receiving heparin plus placebo. The primary endpoint (death, MI, or refractory ischemia within 7 days) was significantly lower in the heparin plus tirofiban group (12.9% vs. 17.9%, p = 0.004). The composite of death and MI was also significantly lower in the heparin plus tirofiban group at 7 days, 30 days, and 6 months. The incidence of major bleeding was similar in the two groups. The recently reported TARGET trial[145] was a direct head-to-head comparison of tirofiban vs. abciximab in 4812 stent patients. Overall, tirofiban was less effective than abciximab, with a 26% relative increase in the primary endpoint of death, MI, or urgent revascularization at 30 days (7.5% vs. 6.0%, p = 0.037). In TACTICS-TIMI-18,[162] 2,220 patients with unstable angina or non-ST-elevation MI received aspirin, heparin, beta-blockers and tirofiban upon hospital admission, followed by randomization to invasive management (cath within 4 to 48 hours and revascularization where feasible) vs. conservative management (cath only for spontaneous or provokable ischemia). The primary endpoint of the trial (death, MI, or rehospitalization for ACS at 6 months) was reduced by 18% in the invasive arm (15.9% vs. 19.4%, p = 0.025); the beneficial effect was most pronounced in patients with positive troponins (14% vs. 24%).

2. **Dosage**. The dose of tirofiban used in RESTORE and TARGET was a 10 mcg/kg bolus followed by an infusion of 0.15 mcg/kg/min. In PRISM-PLUS, the dose was slightly different, a 0.4 mcg/kg/min loading infusion for 30 minutes, followed by a 0.1 mcg/kg/min maintenance infusion. In practice, physicians favor the high-dose regimen for patients undergoing coronary intervention. Therapy is usually continued for 18-24 hours after completion of the case.

3. **Limitations**. There was no increase in major bleeding complications with tirofiban in the clinical trials (Table 34.23),[159,161] and like eptifibatide, there is no known immune response and the overall incidence of thrombocytopenia is low. If patients require emergency CABG, tirofiban should be discontinued; antiplatelet effects will resolve in 6 hours, but platelet transfusion is ineffective. Clearance is longer in patients with renal failure.

D. **OTHER IIb/IIIa INHIBITORS**. Lamifiban, another intravenous GP IIb/IIIa antagonist, showed benefit for reducing ischemic complications in unstable angina patients in one study,[163] but was less efficacious in others.[164,165] Lamifiban is not currently under investigation as an adjunct to interventional procedures. Trials of oral GP IIb/IIIa antagonists have been disappointing (Tables 34.17, 34.20, 34.26). In EXCITE,[166] 7,232 patients undergoing coronary intervention were randomized to xemilofiban or placebo. The primary endpoint (death, MI and urgent intervention) was similar at 30 days and 6 months, although there appeared to be a benefit in diabetics. In OPUS-TIMI 16,[167] 10,302 patients with unstable ischemic syndromes were randomized to oral orbofiban or placebo. Enrollment was terminated because of excess 30-day mortality in the low-dose orofiban group, although patients who underwent PCI appeared to benefit from orbofiban. In SYMPHONY[168] and 2nd SYMPHONY[169] there was a trend toward higher mortality in patients with acute coronary syndromes receiving sibrafiban. The BRAVO[170] trial with lotrifiban was also terminated because of concerns about excess mortality.

E. **RECOMMENDATIONS FOR USE OF GP IIb/IIIa INHIBITORS.** GP IIb/IIIa inhibitors have been extensively studied in a variety of clinical settings (Tables 34.17, 34.28). There are compelling data to support their routine use in patients undergoing percutaneous intervention and in patients with acute coronary syndromes. Recommendations in these and other clinical setting are described in Table 34.28.

Table 34.15. Platelet Glycoprotein IIb/IIIa Receptor Antagonists

Class	Agent	Route	Type of Inhibition
Monoclonal antibody	Abciximab (ReoPro)	IV	Noncompetitive

Cyclic peptides
  RGD sequence
  KGD sequence
	
	MK-852
	Eptifibatide (Integrilin)
		IV	Competitive

Nonpeptide inhibitors	Tirofiban (Aggrastat), fradafiban, lamifiban	IV	Competitive
Oral agents	Xemilofiban, orofiban, sibrafiban, lefradafiban, lotrifiban	Oral	Competitive

Table 34.16. Comparison of Noncompetitive and Competitive Glycoprotein IIb/IIIa Inhibitors

	Noncompetitive*	Competitive**
Biological half life	Long	Short
Duration of effect	Continues after infusion	During infusion
Plasma half-life	Short	Short
GP IIb/IIIa specificity	Cross-reactivity with other receptors	Highly specific
GP IIb/IIIa binding	Permanent	Reversible

* Abciximab
** Eptifibatide, tirofiban

Table 34.17. Overview of Clinical Trials of GP IIb/IIIa Inhibitors

Trial	IIb/IIIa Inhibitor	Setting
ACUTE MI - ADJUNCT TO LYTIC THERAPY		
TAMI-8	M7E3	t-PA
IMPACT-AMI	Eptifibatide	t-PA
PARADIGM	Lamifiban	t-PA, SK, r-PA
TIMI-14A	Abciximab	t-PA, SK
SPEED	Abciximab	r-PA
GUSTO-IV MI	Abciximab	r-PA
INTRO-AMI	Eptifibatide	t-PA
ACUTE MI - ADJUNCT TO PRIMARY PTCA/STENT		
GRAPE	Abciximab	Primary PTCA
RAPPORT	Abciximab	Primary PTCA
ADMIRAL	Abciximab	Primary PTCA
CADILLAC	Abciximab	Primary stenting or PTCA
STOP-AMI	Abciximab	Stent/abciximab vs. t-PA
ISAR-2	Abciximab	Primary stenting*
PERCUTANEOUS CORONARY INTERVENTION		
EPIC	Abciximab	PTCA, DCA
EPILOG	Abciximab	PTCA, DCA
IMPACT-II	Eptifibatide	PTCA, DCA, ROTA, ELCA
RESTORE	Tirofiban	High-risk PTCA, DCA
EPISTENT	Abciximab	PTCA, PS stent
ESPRIT	Eptifibatide	Elective stent
TARGET	Tirofiban vs. abciximab	Stent (elective and ACS)
EXCITE	Xemilofiban	All percutaneous devices
ERASER	Abciximab	Stent (IVUS to assess restenosis)
UNSTABLE ANGINA/NON-ST-ELEVATION MI		
CAPTURE	Abciximab	ACS with intervention
PURSUIT	Integrilin	ACS with/without intervention
PARAGON A	Lamifiban	ACS with/without intervention
PARAGON B	Lamifiban	ACS with/without intervention
PRISM	Tirofiban	ACS: tirofiban vs. UFH
PRISM-PLUS	Tirofiban	ACS with/without intervention
GUSTO-IV ACS	Abciximab	ACS without intervention
ACUTE II	Tirofiban	ACS: LMWH vs. UFH
TACTICS (TIMI 18)	Tirofiban	ACS: conservative vs. invasive

Abbreviations: ACS = acute coronary syndromes; DCA = directional coronary atherectomy; ELCA = excimer laser coronary angioplasty; LMWH = low-molecular-weight heparin; PS = Palmaz-Schatz; r-PA = reteplase; ROTA = Rotablator; SK = streptokinase; t-PA = tissue plasminogen activator; UFH = unfractionated heparin
* Included patients with acute MI < 48 hours
Acronyms: See Table 34.31, p. 803

Table 34.18. Major Trials of IIb/IIIa Antagonists for Coronary Intervention in Acute MI

Study	Antagonist	1° Endpoint	Result	Comments
CADILLAC[143] (n = 2082)	Abciximab (PTCA vs. stent)	Death, MI, or ischemia-driven TVR at 6 months	PTCA: 19.3% PTCA/abcix: 15.2% Stent: 10.9% Stent/abcix: 10.8% (p < 0.0001)	Stenting superior to PTCA; adverse effects of stents on TIMI flow and late mortality in PAMI-STENT not observed in CADILLAC. Abciximab was associated with a trend toward better event-free survival in PTCA patients, but no benefit in stent patients
RAPPORT[136] (n = 483)	Abciximab (primary PTCA)	Death, MI, or revascularization at 6 months	Placebo: 16.1% Abciximab: 13.3% (p = 0.32)	No benefit for abciximab in primary PTCA patients
ADMIRAL[142] (n = 299)	Abciximab (stent 85%, PTCA 15%)	Death, MI, or ischemia-driven TVR at 30 days	Placebo: 20% Abciximab: 10.7% (p < 0.03)	Substantial benefit for abciximab in primary stent patients
Munich Trial[222] (n = 200)	Abciximab (primary stenting)	Hospital death, MI, revascularization	Placebo: 9.2% Abciximab: 2.0% (p < 0.05)	Abciximab group also had better regional wall motion, global LV function, and peak coronary blood flow. Short-term benefits on primary endpoint were no longer significant at 30 days (p = 0.16)
ISAR-2[180] (n = 401)	Abciximab (primary stenting)	Angiographic restenosis	No effect on restenosis	Abciximab led to reduction in 30-day MACE (5.0% vs. 10.5%). No additional benefit over time
EPIC[181] (n = 64)	Abciximab (direct or rescue PTCA)	Death, MI, or urgent revascularization at 30 days	*30-day*: Placebo 26.1% vs. abciximab+ 4.8% (p = 0.06) *6-month*: Placebo 47.8% vs. abciximab+ 4.5% (p = 0.002)	Study group represented 64 of 2099 patients in EPIC with acute MI; 42 direct PTCA, 22 rescue PTCA
GRAPE[163] (n = 60)	Abciximab (PTCA)	Infarct artery patency	TIMI-3: 18%	Abciximab before primary PTCA is safe
RESTORE[159,160] (n = 134)	Tirofiban (primary PTCA)	Death, MI, or any revascularization	56% reduction at 7 days and 22% reduction at 30 days (p = NS)	Study group represented 134 of 2141 patients in RESTORE with acute MI

Abbreviations: IVUS = intravascular ultrasound; MI = myocardial infarction; TVR = target vessel revascularization
+ Bolus plus infusion
Acronyms: See Table 34.31, p. 803

Table 34.19. Major Trials of IIb/IIIa Antagonists for Acute Coronary Syndromes

Study	Antagonist	Setting	Composite Events (30 days)	Result (Drug vs. Placebo)	RRR (%)
PURSUIT[157] (n = 10,984)	Eptifibatide	ACS	Death, MI	14.2% vs 15.7% (p = 0.04)	10
CANADIAN LAMIFIBAN STUDY[163] (n = 365)	Lamifiban	ACS	Death, MI	3.7% vs 8.1% (p = 0.07)	54
PARAGON A[164,189] (n = 2282)	Lamifiban	ACS	Death, MI	Placebo: 11.7% Low-dose lamifiban: 10.6%* High-dose lamifiban: 12.0%*	–
PARAGON B[190] (n = 5225)	Lamifiban	ACS	Death, MI, refractory ischemia	11.8% vs. 12.8%*	8
PRISM[191] (n = 3232)	Tirofiban	ACS	Death, MI, recurrent ischemia	36% risk reduction (p = 0.007) at 48 hours was not maintained at 30 days (15.9% vs. 17.1%*)	7
PRISM-PLUS[161] (n = 1915)	Tirofiban	High-risk ACS	Death, MI, recurrent ischemia	18.5% vs 22.3% (p = 0.03)	17
TACTICS[162] (n = 2220)	Tirofiban (all pts)	ACS: invasive vs. conservative	Death, MI, rehospitalization	Invasive 7.4% vs. conservative 10.5% (p < 0.001); benefit persisted at 6 months (18% risk reduction, p = 0.025)	30
CAPTURE[134] (n = 1265)	Abciximab	ACS	Death, MI, rehospitalization	11.3% vs. 15.9% (p = 0.012)	29
GUSTO-IV ACS[144] (n = 7800)	Abciximab	ACS	Death, MI	Placebo: 8.0% Abciximab (24-hr): 8.2%* Abciximab (48-hr): 9.1%*	–
ACUTE-II[75]	Tirofiban	ACS: LMWH vs. UFH	Death, MI, recurrent ischemia, ischemic CVA	Tirofiban, LMWH: 11.7 Tirofiban, UFH: 16.7	30

Abbreviations: ACS = acute coronary syndromes; LMWH = low-molecular-weight heparin; MI = myocardial infarction; PCI = percutaneous coronary intervention ; RRR = relative risk reduction; UFH = unfractionated heparin
Acronyms: See Table 34.31, p. 803
* p = NS

Table 34.20. Major Trials of IIb/IIIa Antagonists for Coronary Intervention in Acute Coronary Syndromes or Elective Indications

Study	Antagonist	1° Endpoint	Result	Comments
EPIC[131,132,138] (n = 2099)	Abciximab (high risk; PTCA or atherectomy)	Death, MI, or urgent TVR at 30 days	Placebo: 12.8% Bolus alone: 11.4% Bolus/infusion: 8.3% (p = 0.008)	Short-term benefits persisted at 6 months (RRR 23%) and 3 years (RRR 13%); first trial to show improved survival by decreasing risk of post-procedural CK elevation. Increased bleeding with abciximab
EPILOG[133,136,137] (n = 2792)	Abciximab (PCI)	Death, MI, or urgent TVR at 30 days	Placebo: 11.7% SD heparin: 5.2% LD heparin: 5.4% (p < 0.001)	Persistent benefit at 6 months (RRR 43%, p < 0.05). This study extended the benefits of abciximab to low-risk patients and proved that a reduction in heparin dose reduced bleeding complications without sacrificing efficacy
CAPTURE[134] (n = 1265)	Abciximab (PCI for refractory unstable angina)	Death, MI, or urgent TVR at 30 days	Placebo: 15.9% Abciximab: 11.3% (p = 0.012)	More major bleeding with abciximab; no difference in outcome at 6-months, suggesting the need for 12-hour drug infusion post-intervention
EPISTENT[135] (n = 2399)	Abciximab (stent)	Death, MI, or urgent TVR at 30 days	Stent alone: 10.8% PTCA/abcix: 6.9% Stent/abcix: 5.3% (p < 0.001)	No increase in bleeding; significant benefit as an adjunct to stenting; mortality benefit at 1 year
ERASER[139] (n = 225)	Abciximab (elective stent)	In-stent restenosis at 6 months (by IVUS)	Placebo: 32.4% 12-hr abcix: 37.7% 24-hr abcix: 34.2% (p = NS)	No restenosis benefit for abciximab after stenting using IVUS criteria
IMPACT-II[156] (n = 4010)	Eptifibatide (PCI)	Death, MI, or urgent TVR at 30 days	Placebo: 11.4% LD eptifib: 9.2% (p = 0.062) HD eptifib: 9.9% (p = 0.22)	No difference in bleeding; insignificant trend toward benefit with low-dose eptifibatide may have been due to inadequate drug dose
ESPRIT[158] (n = 2064)	Eptifibatide (elective stent)	Death, MI, or urgent TVR at 48 hours	Placebo: 10.4% Eptifibatide: 6.8% (p = 0.0015)	Slight increase in bleeding; modified double bolus effective in reducing short-term events in low-risk patients (RRR 35% at 30-days, p = 0.003). Long-term data not yet available
RESTORE[159,160] (n = 2141)	Tirofiban (PCI for unstable angina)	Death, MI, or any TVR at 48 hours	Placebo: 8.7 % Tirofiban: 5.4% (p = 0.005)	No difference in bleeding; used different endpoints that abciximab trials; tirofiban with persistent (but not significant) benefit at 30-days (RRR 16%)
TARGET[145] (n = 4802)	Tirofiban vs. abciximab (stent)	Death, MI, or ischemia-driven TVR at 30 days	Tirofiban: 7.6% Abciximab: 6.0% (p = 0.037)	Comparable bleeding. Tirofiban was inferior to abciximab, but may be an alternative in low-risk patients without acute coronary syndromes
EXCITE[166] (n =)	Xemilofiban (PCI)	Death, MI, or urgent TVR at 30 days	Placebo: 8.1% 10 mg: 8.1% 20 mg: 7.3% (p = NS)	Oral xemilofiban had no benefit; diabetics had slight benefit with xemilofiban

Abbreviations: HD = high-dose; IVUS = intravascular ultrasound; LD = low-dose; MI = myocardial infarction; RRR = relative risk reduction; SD = standard dose; TVR = target vessel revascularization
Acronyms: See Table 34.31, p. 803

Table. 34.21. Major Trials of IIb/IIIa Antagonists as Adjuncts to Lytics for Acute MI

Study	Antagonist	Setting	Composite Events	Results (Drug vs. Placebo)
TAMI-8[183] (n = 70)	Abciximab	Acute MI (with t-PA)	Rest angina, ECG changes, reinfarction, urgent revascularization, and death at 30 days	13% vs 20%; no excess bleeding in patients receiving t-PA and abciximab
TIMI 14[185] (n = 681)	Abciximab	Acute MI (with SK or t-PA)	TIMI-3 flow at 90 minutes	t-PA + abciximab: 72% Lytic therapy alone: 43%
SPEED[186] (n=305)	Abciximab	Acute MI (with r-PA)	TIMI-3 flow at 60-90 minutes	Abciximab alone: 28% r-PA + abciximab: 63%
GUSTO-IV MI	Abciximab	Acute MI	—	Pending
STOP-AMI[188] (n = 140)	Abciximab	Acute MI (stent + abciximab vs. t-PA	Death, MI, stroke at 6 months; infarct size	8.5% vs. 23.2% (p = 0.02); smaller infarct size with stent/abciximab (14.3% vs. 19.4% of LV)
Intro-AMI[187] (n=342)	Eptifibatide	Acute MI (with t-PA)	TIMI-3 flow at 60 minutes	Better results when eptifibatide given after t-PA; more complete lysis with 50 mg t-PA
IMPACT-AMI[184] (n = 180)	Eptifibatide	Acute MI (with t-PA)	TIMI-3 flow at 90 minutes	66% vs 39% (p = 0.006)
PARADIGM[165] (n = 353)	Lamifiban	Acute MI (with t-PA)	Reperfusion (by continuous ECG at 90 minutes)	80.1% vs 62.5% (p = 0.005)

Acronyms: See Table 34.31, p. 803

Table 34.22. Effects of Abciximab

Effect	Mechanism
Antiplatelet activity	Inhibits platelet cross-linking by fibrinogen
Anticoagulant activity	Inhibits clot retraction; prolongs ACT
Thrombolytic activity	Inhibits factor XIII and PAI-1; displaces fibrinogen
Antiproliferative activity	Nonselective binding to vitronectin receptor
Anti-inflammatory activity	Nonselective binding to Mac-1 receptor on white blood cells

Abbreviations: ACT = activated clotting time; PAI = plasminogen activator inhibitor; Mac-1 = CR3 integrin

Table 34.23. Bleeding Complications in Trials of GPIIb/IIIa Inhibitors

Trial	Agent	Bleeding		Transfusion
		Major	**Minor**	**Transfusion**
EPIC[131]	Abciximab (bolus + infusion)	14.0	16.9	15.0
(n = 2099)	Abciximab (bolus)	11.1	15.4	13.0
	Placebo	6.6	9.8	7.0
	p-value	*< 0.001*	*< 0.001*	*< 0.01*
IMPACT-II[156]	Eptifibatide (135/0.5)*	5.1	11.7	5.6
(n = 4010)	Eptifibatide (135/0.75)*	5.2	14.2	5.9
	Placebo	4.8	9.3	5.2
	p-value	*NS*	*NS*	*NS*
CAPTURE[134]	Abciximab	3.8	4.8	7.1
(n = 1265)	Placebo	1.9	2.0	3.4
	p-value	*0.04*	*< 0.01*	*< 0.01*
RESTORE[159]	Tirofiban	2.4	-	-
(n = 2139)	Placebo	2.1	-	-
	p-value	*NS*		
EPILOG[133]	Abciximab (std. dose heparin)	3.5	7.4	3.3
(n = 2792)	Abciximab (low-dose heparin)	2.0	4.0	1.9
	Placebo	3.1	3.7	3.9
	p-value	*NS*	*< 0.001*	*NS*
EPISTENT[135]	Stent (placebo)	2.2	1.7	2.2
(n = 2399)	Stent (abciximab)	1.5	2.9	2.8
	PTCA (abciximab)	1.4	2.9	3.1
	p-value	*NS*	*NS*	*NS*

Acronyms: See Table 34.31, p. 803

Table 34.24. Safety Issues Related to IIb/IIIa Inhibitors

Issue	Recommendations
Bleeding	**Reduce Preprocedural Risk Factors:** • Identify clinical risk factors (acute MI, low body weight, advanced age). • Identify contraindications (stroke within 2 years, neurosurgery within 6 months, clinically significant GI or GU bleeding with 6 weeks, active internal bleeding, bleeding diathesis, intracranial neoplasm, AV malformation, or aneurysm, severe uncontrolled hypertension, major surgery or trauma within 6 weeks) • For warfarin patients, INR should be < 1.5 **Enhance Procedural Safety:** • Use weight-adjusted heparin (70 U/kg) and abciximab to keep ACT 200-250 seconds; for other IIb/IIIa inhibitors, see Figure 34.1 • Single-wall arterial puncture • Avoid venous sheaths if possible • Use different arterial access site if recent arterial access was achieved (< 2 weeks) • Avoid lytic therapy if possible **Postprocedure Care:** • Avoid post-procedural heparin • Sheaths may be removed during infusion of the IIb/IIIa inhibitor when aPTT ≤ 50 seconds or ACT ≤ 175 seconds. Apply pressure to access site for at least 30 minutes; check site and distal pulses every 15 minutes for 1 hour, then hourly for 6 hours. Keep patient at complete bed rest with head elevated < 30° for 6-8 hours after discontinuation of IIb/IIIa infusion • Nursing care: Avoid IM injections, Foley catheters, NG tubes, and non-compressible sites (e.g., subclavian or jugular vein) for venous access if possible; consider heparin locks for blood drawing
Emergency CABG	• Discontinue infusion of drug and heparin • Obtain ACT in operating room; adjust heparin dose to target ACT (400 sec). Heparin bolus based on ACT: ACT < 200 sec (heparin 4000 U); ACT 200-250 sec (heparin 3500 U); ACT 250-300 sec (heparin 2500 U); ACT 300-350 sec (heparin 1500 U); ACT 350-400 sec (heparin 1000 U); ACT > 400 sec (no additional heparin) • Prophylactic platelet transfusion (6-10 units) • Liberal platelet transfusions after separation from cardiopulmonary bypass
Major hemorrhage	• Discontinue drug and heparin • Platelet transfusions (6-10 units) for abciximab patients • Blood transfusions as necessary • Identify and correct cause
Thrombo-cytopenia	**Platelets > 20,000/mm³ and no Bleeding (Figure 25.1, Table 25.19):** • Stop drug and other agents • Repeat platelet count every 6 hours • If platelet count is not normal within 2-3 days, evaluate other causes **Platelets < 20,000/mm³:** • Stop drug and other agents • Consider prophylactic platelet transfusion (6-10 units) • Repeat platelet counts every 6 hours

Table 34.25. Thrombocytopenia Due to Abciximab or Heparin

	Abciximab (First Exposure)	Abciximab (Re-exposure)	Heparin
Onset	Acute; onset within hours of exposure	Immediate onset within hours of exposure	Subacute; onset within days of exposure
Platelet count	Frequently 20,000-50,000/mm^3; sometimes < 20,000/mm^3	Frequently < 20,000/mm^3	Usually > 50,000/mm^3 (except HIT-2)
Clinical sequelae	Bleeding, particularly when platelet count < 20,000/mm^3	Bleeding is common if not identified early	Thrombosis with HIT-2; bleeding is less common
Recovery	Immediate increase in platelet count 20,000/mm^3 per day after drug discontinuation	Initial increase may be followed by subsequent decrease in platelet count after drug discontinuation	Slow recovery is common after drug discontinuation
Treatment	Stop abciximab; platelet transfusions are indicated for bleeding or platelet count < 20,000/mm^3; IgG does not enhance recovery of platelet count	May not be immediately responsive to initial platelet transfusion; repeat transfusions may be needed; the role of IgG has not been evaluated	Stop heparin; platelet transfusions are not useful.
Laboratory evaluation	Serial platelet counts; identification of abciximab antibodies can be arranged through manufacturer; HACA antibodies may identify patients at risk for thrombocytopenia during readministration	Serial platelet counts; identification of abciximab antibodies can be arranged through manufacturer	Serial platelet counts (Chapter 25)

Abbreviations: HACA = human anti-chimeric antibodies; HIT = heparin-induced thrombocytopenia

Table 34.26. Drug Interactions with Abciximab

Drug	Clinical Impact	Recommendations
Aspirin	No increase in risk of bleeding	Routinely administered with abciximab; no dose adjustment required
Warfarin	About 40% of patients with intracranial hemorrhage while on abciximab occurred in patients on warfarin with INR $\geq$ 1.5	Avoid abciximab in warfarin-treated patients with INR $\geq$ 1.5. If abciximab is mandatory, use FFP (2 units) before abciximab administration
Heparin	Potentiates bleeding, particularly at vascular access sites	Use low-dose weight-adjusted heparin (70 U/kg) and prophylactic (rather than "rescue") abciximab; maintain ACT 200-250 seconds. Avoid post-procedural heparin
Thrombolytics	Potentiates bleeding	Avoid intraprocedural thrombolytic agents, if possible. For lytic patients with acute MI or rescue-PTCA patients after failed lytics, follow heparin recommendations above
Ticlopidine	Weak experimental synergy, but bleeding is not increased	No dose adjustment
Clopidogrel	Clopidogrel monotherapy probably does not increase risk of bleeding. When clopidogrel is given with aspirin, the risk of bleeding is somewhat increased with abciximab	No dose adjustment. Routinely administered with aspirin and abciximab in stent patient

Abbreviations: ACT = activated clotting time; FFP = fresh frozen plasma; INR = international normalized ratio

Table 34.27. Major Trials of Oral GP IIb/IIIa Antagonists

Study	Drug	Setting	Endpoints	Results
Kereiakes[192] (n = 17)	Xemilofiban up to 4 weeks (procedural heparin, aspirin, abciximab)	PCI	Platelet inhibition; safety	Magnitude and extent of platelet inhibition enhanced with combination therapy; no increase in major bleeding
Simpendorfer[193] (n = 30)	Xemilofiban up to 30 days (procedural heparin and aspirin)	PCI for unstable angina	Platelet inhibition; safety	Mucocutaneous bleeding. Severe bleeding in 4 patients (1 death after emergency CABG)
Muller[194] (n = 104)	Fradafiban or lefradafiban up to 7 days (no aspirin)	Healthy volunteers	Platelet inhibition	Continued profound platelet inhibition with oral drug administration
TIMI-12[195] (n = 329)	Sibrafiban up to 28 days (no aspirin)	ACS	Platelet inhibition; safety	Dose-related increase in platelet inhibition; high incidence of minor bleeding
ORBIT[196] (n = 549)	Xemilofiban up to 4 weeks (with aspirin)	After PCI	Platelet inhibition; safety	Dose-related increase in platelet inhibition; no intracranial hemorrhage; low incidence of major bleeding
SOAR[197,198] (n = 259)	Orbofiban up to 3 months (with aspirin)	ACS	Platelet inhibition; safety	Dose-related increase in platelet inhibition; no increase in major bleeding; frequent insignificant/minor bleeding
TIMI-15[199] (n = 192)	Klerval (IV for 24-96 hrs, oral up to 4 weeks)	ACS	Platelet inhibition; safety	Relatively high incidence of thrombocytopenia (13%); limited dose response. Less inhibition with oral drug despite similar receptor occupancy
EXCITE[166] (n = 7232)	Xemilofiban up to 6 months (procedural heparin and aspirin)	PCI	Death, MI, urgent intervention	Placebo vs. xemilofiban 10 mg vs. xemilofiban 20 mg: 30 days (8.1% vs. 8.1% vs. 7.3%, p = NS); 6 months (13.6% vs. 14.1% vs. 12.6%, p = NS). Trend towards higher mortality in low-dose xemilofiban group
OPUS-TIMI 16[167] (n = 10,302)	Orbofiban up to 7 months (with aspirin)	ACS	Death, MI, ischemia-driven or urgent TVR, stroke	Placebo vs. orofiban 50/30 vs. orofiban 50/50: 30 days (10.7% vs. 9.7% vs. 9.3%, p = NS); 7 months (20.5% vs. 20.2% vs. 19.5%, p = NS). Trial halted because of significant excess mortality in low-dose group (1.4% vs. 2.3% vs. 1.6%)

Table 34.27. Major Trials of Oral GP IIb/IIIa Antagonists

Study	Drug	Setting	Endpoints	Results
FROST[200] (n = 531)	Lefradafiban up to 1 month (with heparin, aspirin)	ACS	Bleeding, death, MI, ischemia-driven TVR	High dose (45 mg TID) stopped because of excess major bleeding; no significant difference in composite events; trend toward fewer recurrent ischemic events with 30 mg TID dose
SYMPHONY[168] (n = 9233)	Sibrafiban up to 3 months (without aspirin)	ACS	Death, MI, revascularization	Aspirin: 9.8% Low-dose sibrafiban: 10.1% High-dose sibrafiban: 10%
2nd SYMPHONY[169] (n = 6671)	Aspirin vs. aspirin plus low-dose sibrafiban vs. high-dose sibrafiban alone	ACS	Death, MI, severe recurrent ischemia	[Trial discontinued after SYMPHONY results available] Aspirin: 9.2 % Aspirin + sibrafiban: 9.3% Sibrafiban alone: 10.5%
BRAVO[170] (n = 9200)	Lotrifiban vs. placebo (with aspirin)	Recent ACS; recent neurologic event	Death, MI, stroke, recurrent ischemic TVR	Trial discontinued because of excess mortality (2.7% vs. 2.0%, p = 0.022)

Abbreviations: ACS = acute coronary syndromes; CABG = coronary artery bypass surgery; MI = myocardial infarction; PCI = percutaneous coronary intervention; TVR = target vessel revascularization
Acronyms: See Table 34.31, p. 803

Table 34.28. Results of Rescue IIb/IIIa Inhibitors and Hirulog for Thrombus

Series	N	Adjunctive Therapy	Results
ESPIRT[223] (2001)	77	Rescue eptifibatide for thrombotic complications (42%)	Bailout therapy was associated with more MI (30% vs. 7%, p = 0.01) and urgent PCI at 48 hours (14% vs. 0%, p = 0.03) compared to "no bailout"
Fuchs[228] (2000)	298	Rescue abciximab for thrombus, dissection Type ≥ C, no-reflow, suboptimal result, or distal embolization	Stents in 73%. In-hospital results: death (1.3%); Q-MI (0.7%); non-Q-MI (31%); TLR (4.6%). Late events: death (1.7%); MI (2.7%); TVR (15.1%); EFS at 1-yr (83%)
Velianou[224] (2000)	186	Abciximab (planned 45%; rescue for threatened or acute closure 55%)	In-hospital results (planned vs. rescue): death (1.2% vs. 1.0%); Q-MI (2.4% vs. 2.0%); non-Q-MI (7% vs. 12.9%); TLR (1.2% vs. 0%). 6-month results (planned vs. rescue): death (2.3% vs. 4.0%); MI (9.4% vs. 14.9%); TVR (4.7% vs. 20.8%, p = 0.001)
de Lemos[225] (2000)	92	Rescue abciximab (n = 29) vs. no abciximab (n = 63); TIMI 14 substudy	Abciximab group had greater ST-segment resolution 90-180 minutes after PCI
Piamsomboon[226] (1999)	73	Abciximab (planned 74%; rescue 26%) in acute coronary syndromes with thrombus-containing lesions	Death (1.4%); Q-wave MI (1.4%); non-Q-wave MI (18%). No subacute thrombosis, emergency CABG, or repeat PTCA
Ahmed (1999)	45	Rescue abciximab in degenerated SVG	No benefit on procedural success or major ischemic complications compared to "no-abciximab"; more non-Q-MI in rescue group (40.5% vs. 17.7%)
Fuchs[206] (1999)	186	Rescue abciximab for thrombus and suboptimal PTCA	Procedural success (95.3%); in-hospital MACE (4.7%); non-Q-MI (24.7%); 1-year TLR (24.9%) and EFS (71%)
Haase[208] (1999)	63	Rescue abciximab for thrombus and threatened or acute closure	Repeat PTCA 2 minutes after abciximab. Marked improvement in thrombus score and TIMI flow; MACE (2%); late TVR (15%)
Sullebarger[207] (1999)	17	Planned abciximab and TEC in SVG	Abciximab was associated with higher procedural success (100% vs. 50%) and less distal embolization/no-reflow (0% vs. 30%) compared to "no abciximab"
Barsness (1998)	58	Local delivery of abciximab in thrombotic SVG	Significant improvement in thrombus score and stenosis severity, but not TIMI flow. Adjunctive stent (88%)
Garbarz[214] (1998)	138	Rescue abciximab for thrombus and suboptimal PTCA	Angiographic success in 84% (100% success for stent thrombosis); adjunctive PTCA or stent (100%); MACE (17%); bleeding and vascular complications (27%); transfusion (5%)
Grantham[227] (1998)	185	Planned and unplanned (rescue) abciximab in thrombotic SVG	Procedural success higher with planned abciximab; no impact of abciximab on angiographic (distal embolization, no-reflow) or clinical complications
Henry[213] (1998)	16	Rescue abciximab for acute stent thrombosis	Recurrent thrombosis after PTCA for stent thrombosis may respond to abciximab
Muhlestein[212] (1997)	29	Rescue abciximab for thrombus after PCI	Procedural success (97%), clinical success (93%). Significant improvement in thrombus score and TIMI flow, without distal embolization or no-reflow
Shah[215] (1997)	567	Hirulog vs. heparin for thrombus-containing lesions (Hirulog Angioplasty Study)	Thrombus-containing lesions were associated with more MI (5.1% vs. 3.2%) and abrupt closure (13.6% vs. 8.3%); no difference between hirulog and heparin in acute or late outcomes

Abbreviations: SVG = saphenous vein graft; Q-MI = Q-wave myocardial infarction; MACE = major adverse cardiac events; TLR= target lesion revascularization; EFS = event-free survival; PCI = percutaneous coronary intervention; TIMI = Thrombolysis in Myocardial Infarction

Table 34.29. Recommendations for Platelet Glycoprotein II/IIIa Antagonists

Clinical Setting	Recommendations
Acute MI (lytic therapy)	Abciximab (TIMI-3 flow, ischemic events at 30-days), eptifibatide (TIMI-3 flow, ischemic events at 30-days), and lamifiban (clinical reperfusion but not TIMI flow) all show modest benefit as adjuncts to lytic therapy for ST-elevation acute MI. Further study is needed before GP IIb/IIIa antagonists are routinely used as adjuncts to lytic therapy for acute MI. GUSTO-IV MI results pending.
Acute MI (primary PTCA/Stent)	Trials of abciximab as an adjunct to primary PTCA (RAPPORT, CADILLAC) and stenting (ADMIRAL, CADILLAC) demonstrated variable benefit. In stent patients, data from ADMIRAL are favorable, while data from CADILLAC are not. In PTCA patients, data from CADILLAC are favorable, while data from RAPPORT are not. IIb/IIIa inhibitors reduce acute thrombotic events, but routine use in acute MI is controversial.
Acute MI (rescue PTCA after failed lytic therapy)	Available anecdotal data in small numbers of patients suggest potential benefit for abciximab; further study is needed.
Unstable angina, non-Q-wave MI	There are compelling data to support the routine use of abciximab, eptifibatide, and tirofiban in patients with acute coronary syndromes without ST-elevation referred for PCI. As adjuncts to heparin, aspirin, and β-blockers, these agents decrease early (30-day) cardiac event rates. Benefits are established for tirofiban and eptifibatide in patients not undergoing PCI, but GUSTO-IV ACS failed to show benefit for abciximab.
Percutaneous coronary intervention	There are compelling data to support the routine use of abciximab, eptifibatide, or tirofiban as an adjunct to heparin and aspirin in patients undergoing PCI. Only abciximab has shown long-term (≥ 1 year) mortality benefit in stent patients. Eptifibatide was effective in ESPRIT in reducing short- and mid-term (48-hour, 30-day, 6-month) events. Tirofiban was inferior to abciximab in TARGET.
Rescue use after failed or suboptimal intervention	The value of GP IIb/IIIa antagonists as pretreatment before percutaneous intervention is irrefutable; post-hoc use has not been prospectively studied. Several reports in small numbers of patients suggest potential benefit for "rescue" use in thrombus-containing lesions, stent thrombosis, and abrupt closure, but less benefit in degenerated vein grafts. Disadvantage of "rescue" or post-hoc use is that antecedent high-dose heparin may increase bleeding complications.
Readministration	Readministration is not a concern with tirofiban or eptifibatide. Modest experience with abciximab suggests readministration is feasible, but the risk of severe thrombocytopenia may be higher than after initial exposure. Readministration within 2 weeks of initial exposure is probably safe (before development of HACA). For later re-exposure, H_2-blockers and steroids are not necessary, but close monitoring of platelet counts is recommended to identify thrombocytopenia. Anaphylactic reactions have not been reported.

Acronyms: See Table 34.31, p. 803

PREVENTING ISCHEMIA DURING INTERVENTION

Several agents are commonly used to prevent or attenuate myocardial ischemia during percutaneous intervention (Table 34.30).

A. NITROGLYCERIN is commonly used to treat ischemic chest pain (IV infusion 10-100 mcg/min) and coronary spasm (intracoronary bolus 100-200 mcg; 10-40 mcg per minute IV), but does not prevent or delay the onset of ischemia during balloon inflation. IV nitrates should be used judiciously in patients with hypotension, volume depletion, or right ventricular infarction; preload reduction may exacerbate hypotension and predispose to abrupt closure.[171] Some data suggest that nitrates may induce a heparin-resistant state.[172]

B. BETA-BLOCKERS have been used by some operators to delay the onset and severity of chest pain and ST segment changes, but clear clinical benefit has not been demonstrated. In contrast, beta-blockers are very useful for hypertension and tachycardia not related to hypovolemia; useful agents include propranolol (1 mg IV bolus repeated q 1-2 minutes up to 3-5 mg), metoprolol (5 mg IV bolus repeated every 5 minutes up to 15 mg), or the ultra-short-acting beta-blocker esmolol.[173]

C. CALCIUM ANTAGONISTS. Oral calcium antagonists may be useful for treatment of ischemia associated with hypertension, tachycardia, or coronary vasospasm.[174-178] Intracoronary calcium antagonists are also highly effective in reversing no-reflow (Chapter 21). Caution must be used when parenteral nondihydropyridine calcium antagonists (verapamil or diltiazem) and beta-blockers are administered together, as bradycardia and hypotension may develop in 50% of patients.[179]

TREATMENT OF PERIPROCEDURAL HYPOTENSION

Severe hypotension after intervention can increase the risk of abrupt closure. If blood pressure does not respond immediately to a rapid infusion of saline and discontinuation of nitrates, the systemic circulation must be supported pharmacologically or mechanically (IABP) while the cause is identified and corrected. A variety of pressors have been used for this purpose, including neosynephrine, norepinephrine, dopamine, metaraminol, and dobutamine (Table 34.30).

Table 34.30. Pharmacotherapy for Ischemia and Hypotension During Coronary Intervention

Drug	Indication	Dose
Nitrates	Coronary artery spasm or ischemia unrelated to balloon inflation	Nitroglycerin 100-200 mcg IC bolus; maintenance IV infusion of 10-20 mcg/min, increasing at 10-40 mcg/min increments every 3-5 min until clinical effect or BP < 100 mmHg
β-blockers	Ischemia associated with hypertension and tachycardia	Propranolol 1-2 mg IV; metoprolol 5 mg IV; esmolol 500 mcg/kg IV over 1 min followed by infusion of 25-100 mcg/kg/min; may need to repeat bolus
Calcium antagonists	Ischemia associated with hypertension or tachycardia	Nifedipine 10 mg SL; diltiazem 10-30 mg IV bolus plus infusion of 15 mg over 30-60 min; nicardipine 0.2 mg IC
	Coronary spasm	Nifedipine 10 mg SL; verapamil 100-200 mcg IC; diltiazem 0.5-1.0 mg IC
	No-reflow	Verapamil 100-200 mcg IC up to 2 mg; diltiazem 0.5-2.5 mg slow IC up to 5-10 mg
Vasopressors	Hypotension	Norepinephrine: Initial dose 8-12 mcg/min; titrate to desired blood pressure. Usual maintenance: 2-4 mcg/min. Phenylephrine: Initial dose 0.1-0.18 mg/min; as blood pressure stabilizes, decrease rate to 0.04-0.06 mg/min

Table 34.31. Acronyms of Adjunctive Pharmocotherapy Trials

ACUTE	Antithrombotic Combination Using Tirofiban and Enoxaparin
ADMIRAL	Abciximab Before Direct Stenting in Myocardial Infarction Regarding Acute and Longterm Follow-Up
ATLAST	Antiplatelet Therapy vs. Lovenox Plus Antiplatelet Therapy for Patients with an Increased Risk for Stent Thrombosis
BRAVO	Blockade of the GP IIb/IIIa Receptor to Avoid Vascular Occlusion
CACHET	Comparison of Abciximab Complications with Hirulog Events Trial
CADILLAC	Controlled Abciximab and Device Investigation to Lower Late Angioplasty Complications
CAPTURE	Chimeric c7E3 AntiPlatelet Therapy in Unstable Refractory Angina
ENTICES	Enoxaparin and Ticlopidine after Elective Stenting
EPIC	Evaluation of c7E3 for the Prevention of Ischemic Complications
EPILOG	Evaluation in PTCA to Improve Long Term Outcome with Abciximab GP IIb/IIIa Blockade Study Group
EPISTENT	Evaluation in PTCA to Improve Long Term Outcome with Abciximab GP IIb/IIIa Blockade Study Group - Stent
ERA	Enoxaparin Restenosis after Angioplasty
ERASER	The Evaluation of ReoPro And Stenting to Eliminate Restenosis
ESPRIT	Enhanced Suppression of the Platelet IIb/IIIa Receptor with Integrelin Therapy
ESSENCE	Efficacy and Safety of Subcutaneous Enoxaparin in Non-Q-Wave Coronary Events
EXCITE	Evaluation of Oral Xemilofiban in Controlling Thrombotic Events
FANTASTIC	Full Anticoagulation Versus Aspirin and Ticlopidine
FRAXIS	Fraxiparin in Ischemic Syndromes
FRIC	Fragmin in Unstable Coronary Artery Disease Study
FRISC	Fragmin Fast Revascularization During Instability in Coronary Artery Disease
FROST	French Randomized Optimal Stenting Trial
GRAPE	Glycoprotein Receptor Antagonist Patency Evaluation
GUSTO	Global Utilization of Streptokinase and Tissue Plasminogen Activator for Occluded Coronary Arteries Trial
HELVETICA	Hirudin in a European Trial Versus Heparin in the Prevention of Restenosis after PTCA
IMPACT	Integrelin to Minimize Platelet Aggregation and Prevent Coronary Thrombosis
INTRO-AMI	Integrelin and Reduced dose of Thrombolytics in Acute Myocardial Infarction
ISAR	Intracoronary Stenting and Antithrombotic Regimen Trial
MATTIS	Multicenter Aspirin and Ticlopidine Trial after Intracoronary Stenting
NICE	National Investigators Collaborating on Enoxaparin
OPUS	Oral Glycoprotein IIb/IIIa Inhibition with Orofiban in Patients with Unstable Coronary Syndromes
ORBIT	Oral Glycoprotein IIb/IIIa Receptor Blockade to Inhibit Thrombosis
PARADIGM	Platelet Aggregation Receptor Antagonist Dose Investigation and Reperfusion Gain in Myocardial Infarction
PARAGON	Platelet IIb/IIIa Antagonism for Reduction of Acute Coronary Syndrome in a Global Organization Network
POLONIA	Polish-American Local Lovenox NIR Assessment Study
PRISM	Platelet Receptor Inhibition in Ischemic Syndrome
PURSUIT	The Platelet Glycoprotein IIb/IIIa in Unstable Angina: Receptor Suppression Using Integrilin Therapy
RAPPORT	ReoPro for Acute Myocardial Infarction and Primary PTCA Organization and Randomized Trial Low Molecular Weight Heparin
REDUCE	Reviparin in the Prevention of Restenosis after PTCA
RESTORE	Reviparin in Percutaneous Transluminal Coronary Angioplasty, Randomized Efficacy and Safety of Tirofiban for Outcomes and Restenosis
SOAR	Safety of Orbofiban in Acute Coronary Research
SPEED	Strategies for Patency Enhancement in the Emergency Department
STARS	Stent Anti-thrombotic Regimen Study
STOP-AMI	Stent vs. Thrombolysis for Occluded Coronary Stenosis in Patients with Acute MI
SYMPHONY	Sibrafiban vs. Aspirin to Yield Maximum Protection From Ischemic Heart Events Post-Acute Coronary Syndromes
TACTICS	Treat Angina with Aggrastat (Tirofiban) and Determine Cost of Therapy with an Invasive or Conservative Strategy
TIMI	Thrombolysis In Myocardial Infarction Substudy

REFERENCES

1. Davidson JAH, Boom SJ. Warming lignocaine to reduce pain associated with injection. BMJ 1992;305:617-8.

2. Mader TJ, Playe SJ, Garb JL. Reducing the pain of local anesthetic infiltration: warming and buffering have a synergistic effect. Annals of Emergency Medicine 1994;23:550-4.

3. Lasser EC, et al. Pre-Treatment with Corticosteroids to alleviate reactions to intravenous contrast material. N Engl J Med 1987;317:845-849.

4. Lang DM, Alpern MB, Visintainer PF, et al. Increased risk for anaphylactoid reaction from contrast media in patients on β-adrenergic blockers or with asthma. Ann Intern Med 1991;115:270-276.

5. Mabin TA, Holmes DR Jr., Smith HC, et al. Intracoronary thrombus: Role in coronary occlusion complicating percutaneous transluminal coronary angioplasty. J Am Coll Cardiol 1985; 3:198.

6. Ischinger T, Gruentzig AR, Meier B, Galan K. Coronary dissection and total coronary occlusion associated with percutaneous transluminal coronary angioplasty: Significance of initial angiographic morphology or coronary stenoses. Circulation 1986; 74:1371.

7. Laskey MAL, Deutsch E, Hirshfeld JW, Kussmaul WG, Barnathan E, Laskey WK. Influence of heparin therapy on percutaneous transluminal coronary angioplasty outcome in patients with coronary arterial thrombus. Am J Cardiol 1990; 65:179.

8. Sugrue DD, Holmes DR Jr., Smith HC, et al. Coronary artery thrombus as a risk factor for acute vessel occlusion during percutaneous transluminal coronary angioplasty: Improving results. Br Heart J 1986; 56:62.

9. Deligonul U, Gabliani GI, Caralis DG, Kern MJ, Vandormael MG. Percutaneous transluminal coronary angioplasty in patients with intracoronary thrombus. Am J Cardiol 1988; 62:474.

10. Lincoff A, Popma J, Ellis S, Hacker J, Topol E. Abrupt vessel closure complicating coronary angioplasty: Clinical, angiographic and therapeutic profile. J Am Coll Cardiol 1992; 19:926.

11. De Feyter PJ, van den Brand M, Jaarman G, van Domburg R, Serruys PW, Suryapranata H. Acute coronary artery occlusion during and after percutaneous transluminal coronary angioplasty: Frequency, prediction, clinical course, management, and follow-up. Circulation 1991; 83:927.

12. Ellis SG, Roubin GS, King SB III, Douglas JSJ, Weintraub WS, Thomas RG, et al. Angiographic and clinical predictors of acute closure after native vessel angioplasty. Circulation 1988; 77:372.

13. Reeder GS, Bryant SC, Suman VJ, Holmes DR Jr. Intracoronary thrombus: Still a risk factor for PTCA failure? Cathet Cardiovasc Diagn 1995; 34:191.

14. Tan K, Sulke N, Taub N, Sowton E. Clinical and lesion morphlogic determinants of coronary angioplasty success and complications: current experience. J Am Coll Cardiol 1995; 25:855.

15. Hillegass WB, Ohman EM, O'Hanesian MA, Harrington RA, Faxon DP, Fortin DF, Ellis SG, Stack RS, Holmes DR, Califf RM. The effect of preprocedural intracoronary thrombus on patient outcome after percutaneous coronary intervention. J Am Coll Cardiol 1995; 25:94A.

16. Ferguson JJ, Barasch E, Wilson JM, Strony J, Wolfe MW, Schweiger MJ, Leya F, Bonan R, Isner JM, Roubin GS, Cannon AD, Cleman M, Cabin HS, Adelman B, Bittl JA, and the Heparin Registry Investigators. The relation of clinical outcome to dissection and thrombus formation during coronary angioplasty. J Invas Cardiol 1995; 7:2.

17. Violaris AG, Melkert R, Hermann JR, Serruys PW. Role of angiographically identifiable thrombus on long term luminal renarrowing after coronary angioplasty. Circulation 1996; 93:889.

18. Hattersley PG. Activated coagulation time of whole blood. JAMA 1966; 196:436.

19. Ferguson JJ. All ACTs are not created equal. Tex Heart Inst J 1992; 19:1.

20. Avendano A, Ferguson JJ. Comparison of Hemochron and HemoTec activated coagulation time target values during percutaneous transluminal angioplasty. J Am Coll Cardiol 1994; 23:907.

21. Popma JJ, Weitz J, Bittl JA, Ohman EM, Kuntz RE, Lansky AJ, King SB III. Antithrombotic therapy in patinets undergoing coronary angioplasty. Chest 1998; 114:728S-741S.

22. Hill JD, Dontigny L, de Leval M, Mielke CH Jr. A simple method of heparin management during prolonged extracorporeal circulation. Ann Thorac Surg 1974; 17:129.

23. Bull BS, Korpman RA, Huse WM, Briggs BD. Heparin therapy during extracorporeal circulation: I. Problems inherent in existing heparin protocols. J Thorac Cardiovasc Surg 1975; 69:674.

24. Bull BS, Huse WM, Brauer FS, Korpman RA. Heparin therapy during extracorporeal circulation: II. The use of a dose-response curve to individualize heparin and protamine dosage. J Thorac Cardiovasc Surg 1975; 69:685.

25. Babka R, Colby C, El-Etr A, Pifarre R. Monitoring of intraoperative heparinization and blood loss following cardiopulmonary bypass surgery. J Thorac Cardiovasc Surg 1977; 73:780.

26. Roth JA, Cukingnan RA, Scott CR. Use of activated coagulation time to monitor heparin during cardiac surgery. Ann Thorac Surg 1979; 28:69.

27. Scott JA, Berenstein A, Blumenthal D. Use of the activated coagulation time as a measure of anticoagulation during interventional procedures. Radiology 1986; 158:849.

28. Kopelman HA, Klein LW, Agarwal JB. Adequate heparinization during PTCA: Assessment using activated clotting time. J Am Coll Cardiol 1988; 11:237A.

29. Ogilby JD, Kopelman HA, Klein LW, Agarwal JB. Adequate heparinization during PTCA: Assessment using activated clotting times. Cathet Cardiovasc Diagn 1989; 18:206.

30. Rath B, Bennett DH. Monitoring the effect of heparin by measurement of activated clotting time during and after percutaneous transluminal angioplasty. Br Heart J 1990; 63:18.

31. Dougherty KG, Gaos CM, Bush HS, Leachman DR, Ferguson JJ. Activated clotting times and activated partial

thromboplastin times in patients undergoing coronary angioplasty who receive bolus doses of heparin. Cathet Cardiovasc Diagn 1992; 26:260.

32. Ferguson JJ, Dougherty KG, Gaos CM, Bush HS, Marsh KC, Leachman DR. The relationship between procedural activated clotting times and in-hospital post-PTCA outcome. J Am Coll Cardiol 1994; 23:1061.

33. McGarry TF Jr., Gottlieb RS, Morganroth J, Zelenkofske SL, Kasparian H, Duca PR, Lester RM, Kreulen TH. The relationship of anticoagulation level and complications after successful percutaneous transluminal angioplasty. Am Heart J 1992; 123:1445.

34. Frierson JH, Dimas AP, Simpfendorfer CC, Pearce G, Miller M, Franco I. Is aggressive heparinization necessary for elective PTCA? Cathet Cardiovasc Diagn 1993; 28:279.

35. Narins CR, Hillegass WB Jr., Nelson CL, Tcheng JE, Harrington RA, Phillips HR, Stack RS, Califf RM. Relation between activated clotting time during angioplasty and abrupt closure. Circulation 1996; 93:667.

36. Blumenthal RS, Carter AJ, Resar JR, Coombs V, Gloth ST, Dalal J, Brinker JA. Comparison of bedside and hospital laboratory coagulation during and after coronary intervention. Cathet Cardiovasc Diagn 1995; 35:9.

37. Neuenschwander C, Attenhofer C, Kiowski W, et al. Activated clotting times and heparin need during coronary angioplasty in acute myocardial infarction and angina pectoris. Circulation 1993;88:I-1107.

38. Bittl JA, Ahmed WH. Relation between abrupt vessel closure and the anticoagulant response to heparin or bivalirudin during coronary angioplasty. Am J Cardiol 1998; 82:50P-56P.

39. Snitzer R, Miremath YJ, Lee J, Lasala JM, Eisenberg PR, Winters KJ. Suppression of intracoronary thrombin activity by weight-adjusted heparin administration during coronary interventions. Circulation 1995; 92(Suppl. I):1609.

40. Ferguson JJ, Waly HMF, Le D, Tomakov N, Wilson JM. The effect of body weight and body surface area correction of the distribution of the ACT response to bolus dosese of heparin for PTCA. J Invas Cardiol 1998;10:318-322.

41. Koch KT, Piek JJ, Mulder K, Peters RJG, David GK. Safety of low-dose heparin in elective percutaneous transluminal coronary angioplasty. Eur Heart J 1995; 16(Suppl.):85.

42. Boccara A, Benamer H, Juliard JM, Aubry P, Goy P, Himbert D, Karnillon GJ, Steg PG. A randomized trial of a fixed high dose versus a weight-adjusted low dose of intravenous heparin during coronary angioplasty. Circulation, in press.

43. Aguirre FV, Ferguson JJ, Blankenship JC, Pieper KS, Taylor M, Harrington RA, Rund M, Caracciolo EA, Donohue TJ, Califf RM, Lincoff AM, Tcheng JE, Topol EJ, for the IMPACT-II Investigators. Association of pre-intervention activated clotting times (ACT) and clinical outcomes following percutaneous coronary revascularization: Results from the IMPACT-II trial. J Am Coll Cardiol 1996; 27(Suppl. A):83A.

45. Oltrona L, Eisenberg PR, Lasala JM, Sewall DJ, Shelton ME, Winters KJ. Association of heparin-resistant thrombin activity with acute ischemic complications of coronary interventions. Circulation 1996; 94:2064-2071.

46. Walford CD, Midei MM, Aversano TR, Gottlieb SO, Chew PH, Siu CO, Brin KP, Brinker JA. Heparin after PTCA: Increased early complications and no clinical benefit.

Circulation 1991; 84:II592.

47. Tanjura L, Pinto I, Centemero M, Chaves A, Mattos L, Feres F, Maldonado G, Cano H, Sousa A, Sousa JE. Use of heparin in coronary angioplasty: Randomized trial for prevention of abrupt closure. Eur Heart J 1993; 14:179.

48. Friedman HZ, Cragg DR, Glazier SM, Gangadharan V, Marsalese DL, Schreiber TL, O'Neill WW. Randomized prospective evaluation of prolonged versus abbreviated intravenous heparin therapy after coronary. J Am Coll Cardiol 1994; 24:1214.

49. Pizzuli L, Zirbes M, Fehske W, Pfeiffer D. Omission of intravneous heparin and nitroglycerin following uncomplicated coronary angioplasty: A prospective. Circulation 1995; 92:I74.

50. Rabah M, Mason D, Muller DWM, et al. Heparin after percutaneous intervention (HAPI): A prospective multiventer randomized trial of three heparin regimens after successful coronary intervention. J Am Coll Cardiol 1999;34:461-467.

51. Granger CB, Miller JM, Bovill EG, GA, et al. Rebound increase in thrombin generation and activity after cessation of intravenous heparin in patients with acute coronary syndromes. Circulation 1995;91:1929-1935.

52. Gabliani G, Deligonul U, Kern MJ, et al. Acute closure occlusion occurring after successful percutaneous transluminal coronary angioplasty: Temporal relationship to discontinuation of anticoagulation. Am Heart J 1988;116:696.

53. Chesebro JH, Badimon L, Fuster V. Importance of antithrombin therapy during coronary angioplasty. J Am Coll Cardiol 1991;17:96B-100B.

54. Mabin TA, Holmes DR Jr., Smith HC et al. Intracoronary thrombus: Role in coronary occlusion complicating PTCA. J Am Coll Cardiol 1985;3:198-202.

55. Matthai WH Jr., Kurnik PB, Groh WC, Untereker WJ, Siegel JE. Antithrombin activity during the period of percutaneous coronary revascularization. J Am Coll Cardiol 1999; 33:1248-56.

56. Schachinger V, Allert M, Kasper W et al. Adjuvant intracoronary infusion of antithrombin III during PTCA: Results of a prospective, randomized trial. Circulation 1994;90:2258-2266.

57. Becker PS, Miller VT. Heparin-induced thrombocytopenia. Stroke 1989;20:1449-1459.

58. Kappa J, Fisher C, Todd B, Stenach N, Bell P, Campbell F, Ellison N, Addonizio VP. Intraoperative management of patients with heparin-induced thrombocytopenia. Ann Thorac Surg 1990;49:714-23.

59. Warkentin TE, Levine MN, Hirsh J, Horsewood P, et al. Heparin-induced thrombocytopenia in patients treated with low-molecular-weight heparin or unfractionated heparin. N Engl J Med 1995;332:1330-5.

60. Aster RH. Heparin-induced thrombocytopenia and thrombosis. New Engl J Med 332:1374.

61. Eichinger S, Kyrle PA, Brenner B, et al. Thrombocytopenia associated with low-molecular-weight heparin. Lancet 1991;1:1425-6.

62. Fareed J, Hoppensteadt DA, Walenger JM. Current perspectives on low molecular weight heparins. Seminars in Thromb Heamostasis 1993;19:I-11.

63. Cohen M, Demers C, Gurfinkel EP et al. A comparion of low-molecular-weight-heparin with unfractionated heparin for

unstable coronary artery disease. N Engl J Med 1997;337:447-452.

64. Antman EM, TIMI IIb Investigators. TIMI IIb. Enoxaparin versus unfractionated heparin for unstable angina of non-Q-wave myocardial infarction. A double-blind, placebo-controlled parallel group multicenter trial. Rationale, study design and methods. Am Heart J 1998;135:5353-5360.

65. Zidar JP. Low-molecular-weight heparins in coronary stenting (The ENTICES Trial). Am J Cardiol 1998;82:29L-32L.

66. Karsch KR, Preisack MB, Baildon R, et al. Low molecular weight heparin (reviparin) in percutaneous transluminal coronary angioplasty. Results of a randomized, double blind, unfractionated heparin and placebo-controlled, multicenter trial (REDUCE trial). J Am Coll Cardiol 1996;28:1437-43.

67. Faxon DP, Spiro TE, Minor S, Coté G, Douglas J, Gottlieb R, Califf R, et al. Low molecular weight heparin in prevention of restenosis after angioplasty. Circulation 1994;90:908-914.

68. Zidar JP. ATLAST - Oral presentation. TCT 1999.

69. Rabah MM, Premmereur J, Graham M, Fareed J, Hoppensteadt DA, Khurana S, Grines C. Comparison of an intravneous bolus of enoxaparin versus unfractionated heparin in elective coronary angioplasty. J Am Coll Cardiol 1999; 33:14A (abstract).

70. Kiesz RS, Buszman P, Martin JL, Deutsch E, Rozek MM, Rewicki M, Seweryniak P, Kosmider M, Gaszewska E, Tendera M. Polish-American local lovenox Nir stent assessment study (POLONIA): Final results. JACC 1999; 14A.

71. Kereiakes DJ, Fry E, Barr L, et al. Enoxaparin-abciximab combination for percutaneous coronary intervention: final results of the NICE 4 trial. Am J Cardiol 2000; 86:141.

72. Kereiakes DJ, Grines C, Fry E, et al. Abciximab-enoxaparin interaction during percutaneous coronary intervention: Results of the NICE 1 and 4 trials. J Am Coll Cardiol 2000; 35:92A.

73. Diez JG, Lievano MJ, Croitoru M, Olaya CA, Ferguson JJ. Enoxaparin anticoagulation for percutaneous coronary interventions: A pilot safety study. Circulation 1999; 100:I-188 (Abstract).

74. Ferguson JJ. NICE 3 - Oral presentation. ESC 2000.

75. Cohen M. ACUTE 2 - Oral presentation. AHA 2000.

76. Lefkovits J, Topol E. Direct thrombin inhibitors in cardiovascular medicine. Circulation 1994;90:1522-1536.

77. Topol EJ, Bonan R, Jewitt D, Sigwart U, Kakkar VV, et al. Use of a direct antithrombin, Hirulog, in place of heparin during coronary angioplasty. Circulation 1993;87:1622-1629.

78. Bittl JA, Strony J, Brinker JA, Ahmed WH, et al. Treatment with bivalirudin (Hirulog) as compared with heparin during coronary angioplasty for unstable or post-infarction angina. N Engl J Med 1995;333:764-9.

79. Serruys PW, Herrman JPR, Simon R, Rutsch W, Bode C, et al. A Comparison of Hirudin with heparin in the prevention of restenosis after coronary angioplasty. N Engl J Med 1995;333:757-63.

80. The Global Use of Strategies to Open Occluded Coronary Arteries (GUSTO) IIa Investigators. Randomized trial of intravenous heparin versus recominant hirudin for acute coronary syndromes. Circulation 1994;90:1631-1637.

81. Antman EM, for the TIMI 9A Investigators. Hirudin in acute myocardial infarction, Safety report from the thrombolysis and thrombin inhibition in myocardial infarction (TIMI) 9A trial. Circulation 1994;90:1624-1630.

82. Neuhaus KL, Essen R.v, Tebbe U, Jessel A, Heinrichs H, Mäurer W, et al. Safety Observations from the pilot phase of the randomized r-Hirudin for improvement of thrombolysis (HIT-III) study. Circulation 1994;90:1638-1642.

83. Santos MT, Valles J, Aznar J et al. Prothrombotic effects of Erythrocytes on platelets reactivity. Reduction by aspirin. Circulation 1997; 95:63-68.

84. Rocca B, Fitzgerald GA et al. simply read: Erythrocytes modulate platelet function. Should we rethink the way we give aspirin. Circulation; 1997; 95:11-13

85. Schwartz L, Bourassa MG, Lespérance J, et al. Aspirin and Dipyridamole in the prevention of restenosis after percutaneous transluminal coronary angioplasty. N Engl J Med 1988;318:1714-1719.

86. Mufson L, Black A, Roubin G, et al. A randomized trial of aspirin in PTCA: Effect of high vs. low dose aspirin on major complications and restenosis. J Am Coll Cardiol 1988;11:236A.

87. Ridker PM, Manson JE, Gaziano JM, Buring JE, et al. Low-dose aspirin therapy for chronic stable angina: A randomized, placebo-controlled clinical trial. Ann Intern Med 1991;114:835-839.

88. Chesebro JH, Webster MWI, Smith HC, Frye RI, Holmes DR, et al. Antiplatelet therapy in coronary disease progression: Reduced infarction and new lesion formation. Circulation 1989;80:II-266.

89. Lewis HD Jr, Davis JW, Archibald DG, Steinke WE, Smitherman TC, et al. Protective effects of aspirin against acute myocardial infarction and death in men with unstable angina: Results of a Veterans Administration Cooperative Study. N Engl J Med 1983;309:396-403.

90. Cairns JA, Gent M, Singer J, Finnie KJ, Froggatt GM, Holder DA, Jablonsky G,et al. Aspirin, sulfinpyrazone, or both in unstable angina. N Engl J Med 1985:313:1369-1375.

91. Theroux P, Quimet H, McCans J, Latour JG, Joly P, et al. Aspirin, heparin, or both to treat acute unstable angina. N Engl J Med 1988;319:1105-1111.

92. ISIS-2 Collaborative Group: Randomized trial of intravenous streptokinase, oral aspirin, both or neither among 17,187 cases of suspected acute myocardial infarction: ISIS-2. Lancet 1988;318:349-360.

93. Henderson W, Goldman S, Copeland J, Moritz TE, Harker L. Antiplatelet or anticoagulant therapy after coronary artery bypass surgery: A meta-analysis of clinical trials. Ann Intern Med 1989;743-750.

94. Levin MN, Hirsh L, LandefeldS, raskob G. Hemorrhagic complications of long-term anticoagulant therapy. Chest 1992;102:352S-363S.

95. Alexander JH, Harrington RA, Tuttle RH, Berdan LG, Lincoff AM, Deckers JW, Simoons ML, Guerci A, Hochman JS, Wilcox RG, Kitt MM, Eisenberg PR, Califf RM, Topol EJ, Karsh K, Ruzyllo W, Stepinska J, Widimsky P, Boland JB, and Armstrong PW, on behalf of the PURSUIT Investigators. Prior aspirin use predicts worse outcomes in patients with non-ST-elevation acute coronary syndromes. Am J Cardiol 1999; 83:1147-1151.

96. White CW, Chaitman B, Knudtson ML, et al. Antiplatelet

agents are effective in reducing the acute ischemic complications of angioplasty but do not prevent restenosis: results from the ticlopidine trial. Coronary Artery Dis 1991;2:757.

97. Chronos NA, Patel D, Sigwart U, et al. Intracoronary activation of human platelets following balloon angioplasty despite aspirin and heparin: a flow cytometric study. Circulation 1994;90:I-181.

98. Grotemeyer KH, Scharafinski HW, Husstedt IW. Two-year follow-up of aspirin responder and aspirin non responder. A pilot-study including 180 post-stroke patients. Thromb Tes 1993; 71:397-403.

99. Poggio ED, Kottke-Marchant K, Welsh PA, Brooks LM, Dela Rosa LR, Topol EJ. The prevalence of aspirin resistance in cardiac patients as measured by platelet aggregation and the PFA-100®. J Am Coll Cardiol 1999; 33:254A (abstract).

100. Stiegler H, Fischer Y, Niederau C, Schoebel FC, Borries M, Strauer BE, Leschke M, Reinauer H. Evidence for variable platelet response to low-dose ASA in patients with coronary artery disease. J Am Coll Cardiol 1999; 33:254A (abstract).

101. Di Minno G, Cerbone AM, Mattioli PL. Turco S, et al. Functionally thrombasthenic state in normal platelets following the administration of ticlopidine. J Clin Intest 1985;75:328-338.

102. Maffrand JP, Herbert JM. Effect of clopidogrel and ticlopidine on the binding of [^{3}H]-2 Methyl-Thio-ADP to RAT platelets. Thromb Haemost 1993;69:637.

103. Cattaneo M, Lombardi R, Bettega D et al. Shear-induced platelet aggregation is potentiated by desmopressin and inhibited by Ticlopidine. Arteriosclerosis and Thrombosis 1993;13:393-397.

104. Dembinska-Kiec A, Virgolini I, Rauscha F, et al. Ticlopidine and platelet function in healthy volunteer, Thrombosis Research 1992;65:559-570.

105. Cattaneo M, Akkawat B, Kinlough-Rathbone RL, et al. Ticlopidine facilitates the deaggregation of human platelets aggravated by thrombin. Thrombosis and Hemostasis 1994,71:91-94.

106. Heptinstall S, May JA, Glenn JR, Sanderson HM, et al. Effects of Ticlopidine administered to healthy volunteers on platelet function in whole blood. Thrombosis and Haemostasis 1995;74:1310-5.

107. Leon MB, Baim DS, Popma JJ, Gordon PC, Cutlip DE, Ho KKL, Giambartolomei A, Diver DJ, Lasorda DM, Williams DO, Pocock SJ, Kuntz RE, for the Stent Anticoagulation Restenosis Study Investigators. A clinical trial comparing three antithrombotic-drug regimens after coronary-artery stenting. N Engl J Med 1998; 339:1665-71.

108. Kastrati A, Schühlen H, Hausleiter J, Walter H, Zitzmann-Roth E, Hadamitzky M, Elezi S, Ulm K, Dirschinger J, Neumann F-J, Schömig A. Restenosis after coronary stent placement and randomization to a 4-week combined antiplatelet or anticoagulant therapy. Six month angiographic follow-up of the Intracoronary Stenting and Antithrombotic Regimen (ISAR) trial. Circulation 1997; 96:462-467.

109. Schühlen H, Hadamitzky M, Walter H, Ulm K, Schömig A. Major benefit from antiplatelet therapy for patients at high risk for adverse cardiac events after coronary Palmaz-Schatz stent placement. Analysis of a prospective risk stratification protocol in the Intracoronary Stenting and Antithrombotic Regimen (ISAR) trial. Circulation 1997; 95:2015-2021.

110. Bertrand ME, Legrand V, Boland J, Fleck E, Bonnier J, Emmanuelson H, Vrolix M, Missault L, Chierchia S, Casaccia M, Niccoli L, Oto A, White C, Webb-Peploe M, Van Belle E, McFadden EP. Randomized multicenter comparison of conventional anticoagulation versus antiplatelet therapy in unplanned and elective coronary stenting. The Full Anticoagulation Versus Aspirin and Ticlopidine (FANTASTIC) Study. Circulation 1998; 98:1597-1603.

111. Urban P, Macaya C, Rupprecht H-J, Kiemeneij F, Emanuelsson H, Fontanelli A, Pieper M, Wesseling T, Sagnard L, for the MATTIS Investigators. Randomized evaluation of anticoagulation versus antiplatelet therapy after coronary stent implantation in high-risk patients. The Multicenter Aspirin and Ticlopidine Trial after Intracoronary Stenting (MATTIS). Circulation 1998; 98:2126-2132.

112. Balsano F, Rizzon P, Violi F, et al. Antiplatelet treatment with ticlopidine in unstable angina: A controlled multicenter clinical trial. Circulation 1990;82:17.

113. Hass WK, Easton JD, Adams HP et al. A randomized trial comparing ticlopidine hydrochloride with aspirin for the prevention of stroke in high-risk patients. Ticlopidine Aspirin Stroke Study Group. N Engl J Med 1989;321:501.

114. de Caterina R, Sicari R, Bornane W et al. Benefit/risk profile of combined antiplatelet therapy with Ticlopidine and Aspirin Thrombosis and Haemostasis 1991;65:504-510.

115. Hurana S, Westley S, Mattson J, Safian RD. Is it possible to expedite the antiplatelet effect of Ticlopidine? 1996 Transcatheter Therapeutics (TCT-VIII) meeting Washington Hospital, Washington D.C. J Inv. Card. 1996;8:65.

116. Berger PB, Malcolm RB, David H et al. Safety and efficacy of Ticlopidine for only 2 weeks after successful Intracoronary stent placement. Circulation 1999, 99:248-253.

117. Russo RJ, Stevens KM, Normal SL, et al. Ticlopidine administration after stent placement: frequency of adverse reactions. J Am Coll Cardiol 1997; 29(Suppl. A): 353A.

118. Szto G, Lewis S, Punamiya K, et al. Incidence of neutropenia/fatal thrombocytopenia associated with one month of ticlopidine therapy post coronary stenting. J Am Coll Cardiol 1997;29(Suppl. A):353A.

119. Schrör K. The basic pharmacology of ticlopidine and clopidogrel. Platelets 193; 4:252-61.

120. Savi P, Heilmann E, Nurden P, et al. Clopidogrel: an antithrombotic drug acting on the ADP-dependent activation pathway of human platelets. Clin Appl Thromb/Hemost 1996; 2:35-42.

121. Boneu B, Destelle G. Platelet anti-aggregating activity and tolerance of clopidogrel in atherosclerotic patients. Thromb Haemost 1996; 76:939-43.

122. CAPRIE steering committee. A randomized blinded trial of Clopidogrel versus Aspirin in patients at risk of Ischemic events. Lancet 1996;348:1329-39.

123. Bertrand ME, Rupprecht H-J, Urban P, Gershlick AH, for the CLASSICS Investigators. Double-blind study of the safety of clopidogrel with and without a loading dose in combination with aspirin compared with ticlopidine in combination with aspirin after coronary stenting. The Clopidogrel Aspirin Stent International Cooperative Study (CLASSICS). Circulation 2000; 102:624-629.

124. Bachmann F, Savcic M, Hauert J, Geudelin B, Kieffer G, Cariou R. Rapid onset of inhibition of ADP-induced platelet aggregation by a loading dose of clopidogrel. Eur Heart J 1996; 17(Suppl):263.

125. Bennett CL, Connors JM, Carwile JM, Moake JL, Bell WR, Tarantolo SR, McCarthy LJ, Sarode R, Hatfield AJ, Feldman MD, Davidson CJ, Tsai HM. Thrombotic thrombocytopenia purpura associated with clopidogrel. N Engl J Med 2000; 342(24):1773-7.

126. Bennet CL, Weinberg PD, Rozenberg-Ben-Dror K, Yarnold PR, Kwaan HC, Green D. Thrombotic thrombocytopenia purpura associated with ticlopidine: a review of 60 cases. Ann Intern Med 1998; 128:541-4.

127. Diener HC, Cunha L, Forbes C, et al. European Stroke Prevention Study 2. Dipyridamole and acetylsalicylic acid in the secondary prevention of stroke. J Neurol Sci 1996; 143:1-3.

128. Danchin N, Juilliere Y, Kettani C, Buffet P, et al. Effect of early acute occlusion rate of adjunctive antithrombotic treatment with intravenously administered dipyridamole during percutaneous transluminal coronary angioplasty. American Heart Journal 1994;127:494-8.

129. Heiland UE, Heintzen MP, Klimek WJ, et al. Prevention of abrupt vessel closure following PTCA by intracoronary dipyridamole. A prospectively randomised trial in 1094 consecutive interventions. J Am Coll Cardiol 1997;29(Suppl. A):395A.

130. Lembo NJ, Black AJR, Roubin GS et al. Effect of pretreatment with aspirin versus aspirin plus dipyridamole on frequency and type of acute complications of percutaneous transluminal coronary angioplasty. Am J Cardiol 1990;65:422-426.

131. The EPIC Investigators. Use of a monoclonal antibody directed against the platelet glycoprotein IIb/IIIa receptor in high-risk coronary angioplasty. N Engl J Med 1994; 330:956-961.

132. Topol EJ, Califf RM, Weisman HF, et al. Randomized trial of coronary intervention with antibody against platelet IIb/IIIa integrin for reduction of clinical restenosis: results at six months. Lancet 1994; 343:881-86.

133. The EPILOG Investigators. Platelet glycoprotein IIb/IIIa receptor blockade and low-dose heparin during percutaneous coronary revascularization. N Engl J Med 1997;336:1689-1696.

134. The CAPTURE Investigators. Randomised placebo-controlled trial of abciximab before and during coronary intervention in refractory unstable angina: the CAPTURE study. Lancet 1997; 349:2429-35.

135. The EPISTENT Investigators. Randomized placebo-controlled and balloon-angioplasty-controlled trial to assess safety of coronary stenting with use of platelet glycoprotein-IIb/IIIa blockade. Lancet 1998; 352:87-92.

136. Brener SL, Barr LA, Burchenal JE, et al. Randomized, placebo-controlled trial of platelet glycoprotein IIb/IIIa blockade with primary angioplasty for acute myocardial infarction. ReoPro and Primary PTCA Organization and Randomized Trial (RAPPORT) Investigators. Circulation 1998; 98:734-741.

137. Lincoff AM, Tcheng JE, Califf RM, et al. Sustained suppression of ischemic complications of coronary intervention by GP IIb/IIIa blockade with abciximab: One year outcome in the EPILOG Trial. Circulation 1999; 99:1951-1958.

138. Topol EJ, Ferguson JJ, Weisman HF, et al. Long-term protection from myocardial ischemic events in a randomized trial of brief integrin beta3 blockade with percutaneous coronary intervention. EPIC Investigator Group. Evaluation of Platelet IIb/IIIa Inhibition for Prevention of Ischemic Complications. JAMA 1997; 278:479-84.

139. The Eraser Investigators. Acute platelet inhibition with abciximab does not reduce in-stent restneosis (ERASER Study). Circulation 1999;100:799-806.

140. Topol EJ, Mark DB, Lincoff AM, Cohen E, Burton J, Kleiman N, Talley D, Sapp S, Booth J, Cabot CF, Anderson KM, Califf RM. Outcomes at 1 year and economic implications of platelet glycoprotein IIb/IIIa blockade in patients undergoing coronary stenting: results from a multicentre randomised trial. EPISTENT Investigators. Evaluation of platelet IIb/IIIa inhibitor for stenting. Lancet 1999; 354(9195):2019-24.

141. Marso SP, Lincoff AM, Ellis SG, Bhatt DL, Tanguay JF, Kleiman NS, Hammoud T, Booth JE, Sapp SK, Topol EJ. Optimizing the percutaneous interventional outcomes for patients with diabetes mellitus: results of the EPISTENT (Evaluation of platelet IIb/IIIa inhibitor for stenting trial) diabetic substudy. Circulation 1999; 100(25):2477-84.

142. Barragan P, Beauregard C. Montalescot G, Wittenberg O, Ecollan P, Elhadad S, Villain P, Boulenc JM, Maillard L, Pinton P. Abciximab associated with primary angioplasty and stenting in acute myocardial infarction: The Admiral Study, 6-month results. Circulation 2000; 102(18):II-663 (Abstract).

143. Stone GW. CADILLAC - Oral presentation. TCT 2000.

144. Simoons ML. GUSTO IV ACS - Oral presentation. ESC 2000.

145. Topol EJ. TARGET - Oral presentation. AHA 2000.

146. Berkowitz SD, Sane DC, Sigmon KN, et al. Occurrence and clinical significance of thrombocytopenia in a population undergoing high-risk percutaneous coronary revascularization. J Am Coll Cardiol 1998; 32:311-9.

147. Madan M, Kereiakes DJ, Hermiller JB, Rund MM, Tudor G, Anderson L, McDonald MB, Berkowitz SD, Sketch MH Jr., Phillips HR III, Tcheng JE. Efficacy of *abciximab* readministration in coronary intervention. Am J Cardiol 2000; 85:435-440.

148. Ferguson JJ, Kereiakes DJ, Adgey AA, et al. Safe use of platelet GP IIb/IIIa inhibitors. Am Heart J 1998; 135:S77-89.

147. Tcheng JE, Kereiakes DJ, Braden GA, et al. Safety of abciximab retreatment: final clinical report of the ReoPro readministration registry (R³). Circulation 1998; 19(Suppl.):I-17 (abstract).

149. Gammie JS, Zenati M, Kormos RL, et al. Abciximab and excessive bleeding in patients undergoing emergency cardiac operations. Ann Thorac Surg 1998; 65:465-9.

150. Alvarez JM. Emergency coronary bypass grafting for failed percutaneous coronary artery stenting: increased costs and platelet transfusion requirements after the use of abciximab. J Thorac Cardiovasc Surg 1998; 115:472-3.

153. Boehrer JD, Kereiakes DJ, Navetta FI, et al. Effects of profound platelet inhibition with c7E3 before coronary angioplasty on complications of coronary bypass surgery. Am

J Cardiol 1994; 74:1166-70.

154. Booth JE, Patel VB, Balog C, et al. Is bleeding risk increased in patients undergoing urgent coronary bypass surgery following abciximab? Circulation 1998 (Suppl. 1):I-845 (abstract).

151. Faulds D, Sorkin EM. Abciximab (c7E3 Fab). A review of its pharmacology and therapeutic potential in ischaemic heart disease. Drugs 1994; 48:583-98.

152. Mascelli M, Lance ET, Damaraju L, et al. Pharmacodynamic profile of short-term abciximab treatment demonstrates prolonged platelet inhibition with gradual recovery from GP IIb/IIIa receptor blockade. Circulation 1998; 97:1680-8.

155. Harrington RA, Kleiman NS, Kottke-Marchant K, et al. Immediate and reversible platelet inhibition after intravenous administration of a peptide glycoprotein IIb/IIIa inhibitor during percutaneous coronary intervention. Am J Cardiol 1995; 76:1222-27.

156. The IMPACT-II Investigators. Randomized placebo-controlled trial of effect of eptifibatide on complications of percutaneous coronary intervention: IMPACT-II. Lancet 1997; 349:1422-28.

157. The PURSUIT Trial Investigators. Inhibition of platelet glycoprotein IIb/IIIa with eptifibatide in-patients with acutec coronary syndromes. N Eng J Med 1998; 339:436-43.

158. The ESPRIT Investigators. Novel dosing regimen of eptifibatide in planned coronary stent implantation (ESPRIT): a randomised, placebo-controlled trial. Lancet 2000; 356:2037-44.

159. The RESTORE Investigators. Effects of platelet glycoprotein IIb/IIIa blockade with tirofiban on adverse cardiac event in-patients with unstable angina or acute myocardial infarction undergoing coronary angioplasty. Circulation 1997; 96:1445-53.

160. Gibson CM, Goel M, Cohen DJ, et al. Six-month angiographic and clinical follow-up of patients prospectively randomized to receive either tirofiban or placebo during angioplasty in the RESTORE trial. J Am Coll Cardiol 1998; 32:28-34.

161. PRISM-PLUS study Investigators. Inhibition of the platelet glycoprotein IIb/IIIa receptor with Tirofiban in unstable angina and Non-Q wave myocardial infarction. N Engl J Med 1998; 338:1488-97.

162. Cannon CP. TACTICS/TIMI 18 - Oral presentation. TCT 2000

163. Theroux P, Kouz S, Roy L, et al. Platelet membrane receptor glycoprotein IIb/IIIa antagonism in unstable angina: The Canadian lamifiban study. Circulation 1996;94:899-905.

164. The PARAGON Investigators. International, randomized, controlled trial of lamifiban (a platelet glycoprotein Iib/IIIa inhibitor), heparin, or both in unstable angina. Circulation 1998; 97:2386-95.

165. The PARADIGM Investigators. Combining thrombolytics with the platelet glycoprotein IIb/IIIa inhibitor lamifiban: results of the Platelet Aggregation Receptor Antagonist Dose Investigation and Reperfusion Gain in Myocardial Infarction (PARADIGM) trial. J Am Coll Cardiol 1998; 32:2003-10.

166. O'Neill WW, Serruys P, Knudtson M, van Es GA, Timmis GC, van der Zwaan C, Kleiman J, Gong J, Roecker EB, Dreiling R, Alexander J, Anders R. Long-term treatment with a platelet glycoprotein-receptor antagonist after percutaneous

coronary revascularization. EXCITE Trial Investigators. Evaluation of oral xemilofiban in controlled thrombotic events.

167. Cannon CP, McCabe CH, Wilcox RG, Langer A, Caspi A, Berink P, Lopez-Sendon J, Toman J, Charlesworth A, Anders RJ, Alexander JC, Skene A, Braunwald E, for the OPUS-TIMI 16 Investigators. Oral glycoprotein IIb/IIIa inhibition with orbofiban in patients with unstable coronary syndrome (OPUS-TIMI 16) trial. Circulation 2000; 102:149-156.

168. The SYMPHONY Investigators. Comparison of sibrafiban with aspirin for prevention of cardiovascular events after acute coronary syndromes: a randomised trial. The SYMPHONY Investigators. Sibrafiban versus aspirin to yield maximum protection from ischemic heart events post-acute coronary syndromes. Lancet 2000; 355(9201):337-45.

169. Newby KL. 2nd SYMPHONY - Oral presentation. ACC 2000.

170. Topol EJ, Easton JD, Amarenco P, Califf R, Harrington R, Graffagnino C, Davis S, Diener HC, Ferguson J, Fitzgerald D, Shuaib A, Koudstaal PJ, Theroux P, Van de Werf F, Willerson JT, Chan R, Samuels R, Ilson B, Granett J. Design of the blockade of the glycoprotein IIb/IIIa receptor to avoid vascular occlusion (BRAVO) trial. Am Heart J 2000; 139:927-33.

171. Brown KJ, Prcela L, Kerrick et al. Analysis of hypotension in percutaneous coronary intervention patients. Circulation 1994;90(Part 2)I-205.

172. Chirkov YY, Holmes AS, Chirkova LP, Horowitz JD. Nitrate resistance in platelets from patients with stable angina pectoris. Circulation 1999; 100:129-134.

173. Johansson SR, Lamm C, Bondjers G, et al. Role of beta-adrenergic blockers after percutaneous transluminal coronary angioplasty. Am J Cardiol 1990;66:915-920.

174. Kern MJ, Walsh RA, Barr WK, et al. Improved myocardial oxygen utilization by diltiazem in patients. Am Heart J 1985;110:986-990.

175. Kern MJ, Deligonul U, Labovitz A, et al. Effects of nitroglycerin and nifedipine on coronary and systemic hemodynamics during transient coronary artery occlusion. Am Heart J 1988;115:1164.

176. Serruys PW, van den Brand M, Brower RW. Hugenholtz PG. Regional cardioplegia and cardioprotection during transluminal angioplasty. Which role for nifedipine? Eur Heart J 1984;4:115.

177. Kern MJ, Pearson A, Woodruff R, et al. Hemodynamic and echocardiographic assessment of the effects of diltiazem during transient occlusion of the left anterior descending coronary artery during percutaneous transluminal coronary angioplasty. Am J Cardiol 1989;64:849-855.

178. Hanet C, Rousseau MF, Vincent MF, et al. Myocardial protection by intracoronary nicardipine administration during percutaneous transluminal coronary angioplasty. Am J Cardiol 1987;59:1035-1040.

179. Mager A, Strasberg B, Rechavia E, et al. Clinical significance and predisposing factors to symptomatic bradycardia and hypotension after PTCA. Am J Cardiol 1994;74:1085-1088.

180. Neumann F-J, Kastrati A, Schmitt C, Blasini R, Hadamitzky M, Mehilli J, Gawaz M, Schleef M, Seyfarth M, Dirschinger J, Schömig A. Effect of glycoprotein IIb/IIIa receptor blockade with abciximab on clinical and angiographic restenosis rate after the placement of coronary stents

following acute myocardial infarction. J Am Coll Cardiol 2000; 35:915-21.

181. Lefkovits J, Ivanhoe RJ, Califf RM, Bergelson BA, Anderson KM, Stoner GL, et al for the EPIC Investigators. Effects of platelet glycoprotein IIb/IIIa receptor blockade by a chimeric monoclonal antibody (abciximab) on acute and 6-month outcomes after percutaneous transluminal coronary angioplasty for acute myocardial infarction. Am J Cardiol 1996; 77:1045-51.

182. Van den Merkhof LFM, Zijlstra F, Olsson H, et al. Abciximab in the treatment of acute myocardial infarction eligible for primary percutaneous transluminal coronary angioplasty. J Am Coll Cardiol 1999;33:1538-1532.

183. Kleiman NS, Ohman EM, Califf RM, et al. Profound hibition of platelet aggregation with monoclonal antibody 7E3 Fab after thrombolytic therapy. Results of the thrombolysis and angioplasty in myocardial infarction (TAMI) 8 pilot study. J Am Coll Cardiol 1993;22:81-9.

184. Ohman EM, Kleiman NS, Gacioch G, et al. Combined accelerated tissue-plasminogen activator and platelet glycoprotein IIb/IIIa integrin receptor blockade with Integrillin in acute myocardial infarction. Results of a randomized, placebo-controlled, dose-ranging trial. IMPACT-AMI Investigators. Circulation 1997;95:846-854.

185. Antman EM, Giugliano RP, Gibson CM, et al. Abciximab facilitates the rate and extent of thrombolysis. Results of the thrombolysis in myocardial infarction (TIMI) 14 trial. Circulation 1999;99:2720-2732.

186. Strategies for Patency Enhancement in the Emergency Department (SPEED) Group. Trial of abciximab with and without low-dose reteplase for acute myocardial infarction. Circulation 2000; 101:2788-2794.

187. Zeymer U. INTRO-AMI - Oral presentation. ESC 1999.

188. Schomig A, Kastrati A, Kirschinger J, Mehilli J, Schricke U, Pache J, Martinoff S, Neumann FJ, Schwaiger M. Coronary stenting plus platelet glycoprotein IIb/IIIa blockade compared with tissue plasminogen activator in acute myocardial infarction. Stent versus thrombolysis for occluded coronary arteries in patients with acute myocardial infarction study investigators. N Engl J Med 2000; 343(6):385-91.

189. Moliterno DJ, Harrington RA, Newby KL, et al. Late diverging event curves for surgical following IIb/IIIa antagonism in patients with unstable angina. PARAGON study 1-year follow-up (abstract). J Am Coll Cardiol 1998;31:208A-209A.

190. Harrington RA. PARAGON B - Oral presentation. ACC 2000.

191. The PRISM Sutdy Investigators. A comparison of aspirin plus tirofiban with aspirin plus heparin for unstable angina. The Platelet Receptor Inhibition in Ischemic Syncdrome Management (PRISM) Study Investigators. N Engl J Med 1998;338:1498-1505.

192. Kereiakes DJ, Runyon JP, Kleiman NS, et al. Differential dose-response to oral xemilofiban after antecedent intravenous abciximab: Administration after complex coronary intervention. Circulation 1996;94:906-910.

193. Simpfendorfer C, Kottke-Marchant K, Lowrie M, et al. First chronic platelet glycoprotein IIb/IIIa integrin blockade: A randomized, placebo-controlled pilot study of xemilofiban in unstable angina with percutaneous coronary interventions.

Circulation 1997;96:76-81.

194. Mullter TH, Weisenberger H, Brichl R, et al. Profound and sustained inhibition of platelet aggregation by fradofiban, a nonpeptide platelet glycoprotein IIb/IIIa antagonist, and its orally active prodrug, lefradafiban, in men. Circulation 1997;96:1130-1138.

195. Cannon CP, McCabge CH, Borzak S, et al. Randomized trial of an oral platelet glycoprotein IIb/IIIa antagonist, sibrafiban in patients after an acute coronary syndrome. Results of the TIMI 12 trial. Circulation 1998;97:340-349.

196. Kereiakes DJ, Kleiman, Ferguson JJ, et al. Pharmacodynamic efficacy, clinical safety, and outcomes after prolonged platelet glycoprotein IIb/IIIa receptor blockade with oral xemilofiban: Results of a multicenter, placebo-controlled, randomized trial. Circulation 1998;98:1268-1278.

197. Ferguson JJ, Deedwania PC, Kereiakes DJ, et al. Sustained platelet GP IIb/IIIa blockade with oral orbofiban: Interim pharmacodynamic results of the SOAR study. J Am Coll Cardiol 1998;185A.

198. Deedwania PC, Ferguson JJ, Kereiakes DJ, et al. Sustained platelet GP IIb/IIIa blockade with oral orbofiban: Interim safety and tolerability results of the SOAR study. J Am Coll Cardiol 1998;94A.

199. Giugliana RP, McCabe CH, Sequeira RF, Frey MJ, Henry TD, Piana RN, Tamby JF, Jensen BK, Nicolas SB, Jennings LK, Wise RJ, Braunwald E. First report of an intravenous and oral glycoprotein IIb/IIIa inhibitor (RPR 109891) in patients with recent acute coronary syndromes: results of the TIMI 15A and 15B trials.

200. Akkerhuis KM, Neuhaus KL, Wilcox RG, Vahanian A, Boland JL, Hoffmann J, Baardman T, Nehmiz G, Roth U, Klootwijk AP, Deckers JW, Simoons ML. Safety and preliminary efficacy of one month glycoprotein IIb/IIIa inhibition with lefradafiban in patients with acute coronary syndromes without ST-elevation A phase II study. Eur Heart J 2000; 21(24):2042-2055.

201. Shomig A, Neumann FJ, Kastrati A, et al. A randomized comparison of antiplatelet and anticoagulant therapy after the placement of coronary artery stents. N Engl J Med 1996;334:1084.

202. Albiero R, Hall P, Itoh A, Blengino S, Nakamura S, Martini G, Ferraro M, Colombo A. Results of a consecutive series of patients receiving only antiplatelet therapy after optimized stent implantation. Comparison of aspirin alone versus combined ticlopidine and aspirin therapy. Circulation 1997; 95:1145-1156.

203. Moussa I, Oetgen M, Roubin G, Colombo A, Wang X, Iyer S, Maida R, Collins M, Kreps E, Moses JW. Effectiveness of clopidogrel and aspirin versus ticlopidine and aspirin in preventing stent thrombosis after coronary stent implantation. Circulation 1999; 99:2364-2366.

205. Kleiman NS, Lincoff AM, Sapp SK, Maresh KJ, Topol EJ. Pharmacodynamics of a direct thrombin inhibitor combined with a GP IIb-IIIa antagonist: first experience in humans. Circulation 1999; 100(18):I-328 (Abstract).

206. Fuchs S, Kornowski R, Mehran R, Gruberg L, Satler LF, Pichard AD, Kent KM, Stone GW, Leon MB. Clinical outcomes following "rescue" administration of abciximab in patients undergoing percutaneous coronary angioplasty. J Invas Cardiol 2000; 12:497-501.

207. Sullebarger JT, Dalton RD, Nasser A, Matar FA. Adjunctive abciximab improves outcomes during recanalization of totally occluded saphenous vein grafts using transluminal extraction atherectomy. Cathet Cardiovasc Diagn. 1999;46:107-110.

208. Haase KK, Mahrholdt H, Schroder S, Baumbach A, Oberhoff M, Herdeg C, Karsch KR. Frequency and efficacy of glycoprotein IIb/IIIa therapy for treatmne tof threatened or acute vessel clsoore in 1332 patients undergoing percutaneous transluminal coronary angioplasty. Am Heart J 1999;137:234-240.

209. Albiero R, Hall P, Itoh A, Blengino S, Nakamura S, Martini G, Ferraro M, Colombo A. Results of a consecutive series of patients receiving only antiplatelet therapy after optimized stent implantation. Comparison of aspirin alone versus combined ticlopidine and aspirin therapy. Circulation 1997; 95:1145-1156.

210. Mathew V, Grill DE, Scott CG, Grantham JA, Ting HH, Garratt KN, Holmes DR Jr. The influence of abciximab use on clinical outcome after aortocoronary vein graft interventions. J Am Coll Cardiol 1999; 34(4):1163-9.

211. Faulds D, Sorkin EM. Abciximab (c7E3 Fab). A review of its pharmacology and therapeutic potential in ischaemic heart disease. Drugs 1994; 48:583-98.

212. Muhlestein JB, Karagounis LA, Treehan S, Anderson JL. "Rescue" utilization of abciximab for the dissolution of coronary thrombus developing as a complication of coronary angioplasty. J Am Coll Cardiol 1997;30:1729-1734.

213. Henry P, Boughalem K, Rinaldi JP, Makowski S, Khalife K, Guermonprez JL, Blanchard D. Use of anti-BP IIb/IIIa in acute thrombosis after intracoronary stent implantation. Cathet Cardiovasc Diagn. 1998;43:105-107.

214. Garbarz E, Farah B, Vuillemenot A, Andre F, Angioi M, Machecourt J, Bassand JP, Wolf JE, Danchin N, Prendergast B, Lung B, Vahanian A. "Rescue" abxicimab for complicated percutaneous transluminal coronary angioplasty. Am J Cardiol 1998;82:800-802.

215. Shah PB, Ahmed WH, Ganz P, Bittl JA. Bivalirudin compared with heparin during coronary angioplasty for thrombus-containing lesions. J Am Coll Cardiol 1997;30:1264-1269.

216. FRISC Study Group: Low molecular weight heparin during instability in coronary artery disease. Lancet 1996;347:561-568.

217. Klein W, Buchwalld A, Millis SE, et al. Comparison of low-molecular weight heparin in unfractionated heparin acutely and with placebo for 6-weeks in the management of unstable coronary artery disease: FRIC Study. Circulation 1997;96:61-68.

218. Lindahl B, Venge P, Wallentin L. FRISC Study Group. Relation between Troparin-T and the risk fo subsequent cardiac events in unstable coronary artery disease. Circulation 1996;93:1651-1657.

219. Fragmin and Fast Revascularisation during Instability in Coronary artery disease (FRISC II) Investigators. Long-term low-molecular-mass heparin in unstable coronary-artery disease: FRISC II prospective randomised multicentre study. Lancet 1999; 354:701-9.

220. Gurfinkel EP, Manos EJ, Mejail RI, et al. Low-molecular weight heparin verus regular heparin or aspirin in the treatment of unstable angina and silent ischemia. J Am Coll Cardiol 1995;26:313-318.

221. The FRAXIS Study Group. Comparison of two treatment durations (6 days and 14 days) of a low molecular weight heparin with a 6-day treatment of unfractionated heparin in the initial management of unstable angina or non-Q wave myocardial infarction: FRAX.IS (FRAxiparine in Ischaemic Syndrome). Eur Heart J 1999; 20:1553-1562.

222. Neumann FJ, Blasini R, Schmitt C, et al. Effect of glycoprotein IIb/IIIa receptor blockade on recovery of coronary flow and left ventricular function after the placement of coronary-artery stents in acute myocardial infarction. Circulation 1998;98:2695-701.

223. Cantor W, Hellkamp A, O'Shea J, et al. Bailout platelet GP II/IIIa inhibition in coronary stent implantation: Observations from the ESPRIT trial. J Am Coll Cardiol 2001;37(2):84A

224. Velianou JL, Strauss BH, Kreatsoulas C, et al. Evaluation of the role of abciximab (Reopro) as a rescue agent during percutaneous coronary interventions: In-hospital and six-month outcomes. Cathet Cardiovasc Intervent 2000;51:138-144.

225. deLemos J, Gibson M, Autman EM, et al. Abciximab improves microvascular function after rescue PCI: A TIMI 14 substudy. J Am Coll Cardiol 2000;35:40A.

226. Piamsomboon C, Wong PMT, Mathur A, et al. Does platelet glycoprotein IIb/IIIa receptor antibody improve in-hospital outcome of coronary stenting in high-risk thrombus containing lesions? Cathet Cardiovasc Intervent 1999;46:415-420.

227. Grantham JA, Mathew V, Holmes DR. Antiplatelet therapy with abciximab in percuaneous intervention of thrombus-containing bypass grafts. Circulation 1998;98:17.

228. Fuchs S, Kornowski R, Mehran R, et al. Clinical outcomes following "rescue" administration of abciximab in patient undergoing percutaneous coronary angioplasty. J Invas Cardiol 2000;12:497-501.

229. Yusef, S. Oral presentation. American College of Cardiology meeting, Orlando, Florida, March, 2001

35 CATHETER-BASED TECHNIQUES OF LOCAL DRUG DELIVERY

Raymond G. McKay, M.D.
Robert D. Safian, M.D.

A. RATIONALE FOR LOCAL DRUG DELIVERY. Local delivery of therapeutic agents directly to the site of coronary intervention is currently under active investigation as a new technique to modulate the arterial response to mechanical injury.[1,2] All forms of percutaneous intervention result in a complex sequence of cellular responses resulting from mechanical trauma and subsequent exposure of intramural components to circulating blood. In some cases, these cellular responses may result in adverse clinical outcomes, including abrupt closure from increased platelet deposition and intracoronary thrombus formation, and late restenosis from transformation of normally-quiescent, medial smooth muscle cell into a phenotype that proliferates, migrates to the neointima, and secretes extracellular matrix.

One theory why systemic pharmacologic therapy has been unsuccessful in limiting the biological consequences of vascular injury is that patients are unable to tolerate the high systemic drug concentrations needed to achieve a therapeutic effect. Strategies have been developed to achieve a local therapeutic effect at the site of intervention without the risk of systemic side effects, including local drug delivery catheters, drug-coated metallic stents, endovascular and extravascular drug-eluting polymers, periadventitial drug pumps, cell-targeting techniques designed to locally activate intravenously-administered agents, and gene therapy. The goals of local drug delivery extend beyond the obvious control of thrombosis and restenosis. There may also be a role for angiogenic growth factors to promote neovascularization and for agents to alter endothelial function and vasomotor tone.

B. MECHANISMS OF INTRAMURAL DRUG DEPOSITION. Locally administered drugs exert their therapeutic effect by acting intraluminally during catheter deployment or by persisting in the arterial wall. Three different mechanisms of intramural deposition are possible: passive diffusion, active bulk transfer, and facilitated diffusion (Table 35.1). In *passive diffusion techniques*, drugs are infused via catheters into a closed intraluminal space and allowed to bathe the arterial wall, with intramural deposition occurring by simple diffusion down a concentration or electrochemical gradient. This method is fairly atraumatic and involves little pressure, but drug may be easily lost into sidebranches. With *active bulk transfer*, agents are introduced directly into the wall by hydrostatic pressure or other physical means. Drug delivery is determined by pressure, pore size, and the extent of contact with the arterial wall. Other methods of physical delivery besides hydrostatic pressure can also be used for local delivery, and these techniques may be useful for avoiding barotrauma associated with other devices. With facilitated diffusion, agents are intramurally distributed by means of a substrate-carrier complex that may undergo translational or rotational diffusion.

Table 35.1. Devices for Local Drug Delivery[60]

Passive Diffusion Systems

Double-balloon[4-9]

Hydrogel-coated balloon[30-36,62]

Multichamber balloon

Dispatch catheter[37-43,64,67]

Border catheter

Coated stents[75] (Chapter 26)

Bulk-Transfer Devices

Pressure-driven devices

Porous balloon[65,68,72]

Microporous balloon[26-28,58]

Perforated balloon[10-25]

Transport catheter[29]

Channel balloon[44-48,61,63]

Infusasleeve[49-52]

Non-pressure physical delivery

Iontophoretic balloon[53-55,69,73]

Needle-injection catheter

Infiltrator[59,66,71]

Radioactive stent

Laser balloon

Facilitated Diffusion[70-]

C. **PHARMACOKINETIC CONSIDERATIONS.** Based on *in vitro* and animal studies, the list of possible agents which might have a local therapeutic effect is enormous and includes antiplatelet, antithrombin, thrombolytic, calcium blocking agents, steroids, alcohol, antiproliferative agents, specific growth factor inhibitors, antisense oligonucleotides, and many others. The specific dose, time of administration, and intramural residence time have not been established for any given agent. Moreover, the efficiency of delivery, depth of intramural penetration, and wash-out from the arterial wall is different for each agent depending upon its molecular weight, charge, lipophilicity, receptor binding, affinity for macrophage ingestion, and by differences in catheter designs. All systems vary with respect to efficiency and homogeneity of drug deposition, vascular injury, ability to simultaneously deliver drug and dilate vascular stenoses, and ability to maintain coronary perfusion during drug delivery.

One of the most important aspects of the pharmacokinetics of locally delivered drugs is their *intramural residence time.* Some agents may exert a therapeutic effect despite a short intramural residence time, while other agents may require an intramural residence time of days to weeks in order to achieve a beneficial effect on intimal proliferation and restenosis. The agent may washout from the arterial wall because of diffusion and convection into surrounding tissues, vasa vasorum, lymphatics, and the arterial lumen.[3] Although fluid flux through the arterial wall is relatively slow in a normal artery, it may be accelerated by endothelial denudation. The presence of neovascularization in an atherosclerotic vessel may also impact the dynamics of drug wash-out. A number of catheter-based techniques are currently under investigation to increase drug persistence at the angioplasty site.[1-3] These strategies include the use of drugs contained within non-diffusible biodegradable microparticles, liposomes, gold microparticles, endoluminal polymer "paving" techniques, stents, and thermally-mediated drug delivery.

D. CATHETER-BASED LOCAL DRUG DELIVERY TECHNIQUES (Table 35.1)
1. Passive Diffusion Systems
    a. Double-Balloon Catheter (Figure 35.1). The earliest approach to local drug delivery was the use of the double-balloon catheter.[4-9] The double-balloon catheter (USCI, Billerica, MA) consists of a standard angioplasty shaft with two latex balloons mounted on its distal end and separated by 2 cm. The catheter has four lumens, one for a central guidewire, two for inflating/deflating the balloons, and a fourth for drug infusion. When the catheter is deployed in an artery over a guidewire and the two balloons are inflated, drug may be infused into the closed space between the inflated balloons. The arterial wall is thus bathed in a local intraluminal reservoir of drug, and intramural penetration occurs by passive diffusion or as a result of applied hydrostatic pressure.

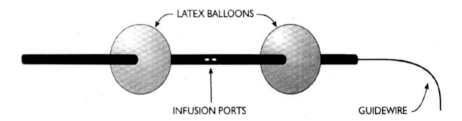

Figure 35.1. The Double-Balloon Catheter

Drugs are infused into the closed space between two inflated balloons.

The double-balloon catheter has been used in several animal models for the delivery of horseradish peroxidase[4] and therapeutically active compounds including heparin,[5] r-hirudin,[6] and t-PA.[7] In addition, at least three groups have also reported successful in-vivo gene transfer with the double-balloon catheter.[8,9] Intramural penetration of agents with this device has been documented with low infusion pressures. In one study, the depth of penetration of horseradish peroxidase was shown to be related to infusion pressure, with complete penetration of the arterial media at 300 mmHg.[4] In a second study, infusion pressures of 150 mmHg were both atraumatic and sufficient for uptake of deoxyribose nucleic acid plasmids into the arterial wall; significant injury was noted at pressures greater than 500 mmHg.[9] Local delivery of heparin to porcine carotid vessels reduced intimal hyperplasia 28 days following balloon angioplasty,[5] and local r-hirudin delivery reduced early platelet deposition and mural thrombus formation compared to systemic therapy.[6] The advantages of the double-balloon catheter include its ability to atraumatically and homogeneously deliver agents at low pressure, and minimize systemic exposure. Disadvantages include the need for prolonged dwell times with total arterial occlusion, loss of drug from sidebranches, and inability to dilate stenoses.

b. **Hydrogel-Coated Balloon (Figure 35.3).** The hydrogel-coated balloon (Boston Scientific Scimed) consists of a standard polyethylene balloon coated with a hydrogel polymer (Hydroplus™). The hydrogel coating consists of an interlacing network of polyacrylic acid chains which adhere to the balloon surface. When the hydrogel comes in contact with an aqueous environment, water is absorbed by the hydrogel and the lattice begins to swell and

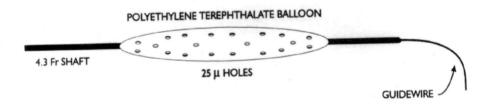

Figure 35.2. The Wolinsky™ Perforated Balloon

Drugs are infused via 28 laser-drilled holes in the balloon surface which are 25 microns in diameter and arranged in longitudinal rows.

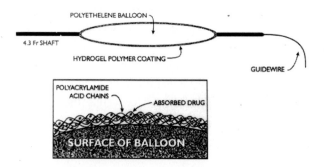

Figure 35.3. The Hydrogel-Coated Balloon

Drugs are absorbed by a hydrogel coating adhered to the balloon surface.

forms a stable matrix of polymer and water. Any agents dissolved in the water will be incorporated into this matrix. The thickness of the coating ranges from 5 microns when dry to 25 microns when fully saturated with water. Intramural drug delivery is achieved during balloon inflation when the hydrogel polymer comes in contact with the intimal surface. Hydrogel compression during balloon inflation results in pressurized diffusion from the polymer into the vessel wall.

The hydrogel balloon has been used for *in vivo* delivery of horseradish peroxidase,[30] heparin,[31] urokinase,[32] PPACK,[33] antisense oligonucleotides [34] and other genes.[35] In all cases, homogeneous intramural penetration of drug has been demonstrated without disruption of the vessel architecture. The *in vivo* delivery of heparin[31] and urokinase[32] in the porcine model significantly decreased platelet deposition following balloon injury. Similarly, hydrogel delivery of heparin[31] and antisense oligomers to c-myb[34] decreased smooth muscle cell proliferation. Pharmacokinetic studies demonstrated that 2-33% of the drug on the balloon surface is intramurally deposited during balloon inflation,[31,32,34] and the depth of drug delivery into the arterial wall is proportional to the inflation pressure and duration.[30] Following local delivery, heparin persists in the arterial wall for as long as 48 hours and antisense oligomers have been detected for at least 24 hours.[31,34] Preliminary studies in patients with urokinase-coated hydrogel balloons demonstrated lysis of intracoronary thrombus and/or reversal of abrupt thrombotic closure without distal embolization or no reflow.[36] The major advantage of the hydrogel system is that it results in homogenous, atraumatic drug delivery while an arterial lesion is dilated. Deficiencies include rapid washoff from the balloon surface, the relatively small amount of drug that can be loaded into the hydrogel coating, and the need for complete vessel occlusion during drug delivery.

c. **Dispatch™ Catheter (Figure 35.4).** The Dispatch catheter (Boston Scientific Scimed) consists of a 4.4F catheter shaft with a 20-mm polyolefin copolymer spiral inflation coil wrapped around a non-porous urethane sheath on its distal tip. When the spiral coil is inflated, it forms both an internal lumen that allows distal coronary perfusion through the inner sheath, and a series of isolated spaces between the catheter's coils, urethane sheath, and arterial wall. Drug is administered through a separate infusion port and is delivered through slits in the shaft of the catheter between the coils of the device. Thus, the arterial wall is bathed in drug that is isolated from blood flowing through the inner urethane sheath.

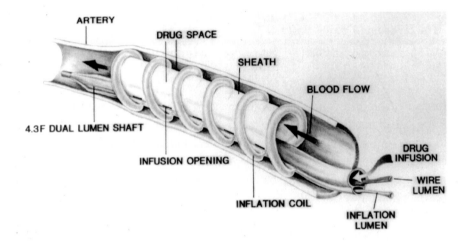

Figure 35.4. The Dispatch™ Catheter

Inflation of the catheter's spiral coil creates an internal lumen for distal coronary perfusion and a series of isolated spaces for drug delivery.

Successful *in vivo* delivery of methylene blue, horseradish peroxidase, heparin, hirudin, urokinase, t-PA, and several genes has been accomplished with the Dispatch catheter in animal models.[37,38] The amount of intramurally deposited heparin is proportional to the infusion time and concentration, with intramural persistence for at least one week.[37] Successful intracoronary deposition of urokinase persists for over 5 hours.[38] In comparison to systemic and intra-arterial infusion, local urokinase delivery with the Dispatch catheter resulted in 10-100-fold greater intramural deposition. The Dispatch catheter was approved for drug delivery by the Food and Drug Administration in December 1993. Since that time, the catheter has been used for as long as 24 hours without significant alteration in coronary blood flow or ventricular function.[39] Preliminary studies demonstrated efficacy for treating thrombus during percutaneous revascularization.[40-43] Unlike other local drug delivery systems, the Dispatch catheter allows prolonged drug delivery and simultaneous perfusion. Limitations include significant ischemia from sidebranch occlusion, inability to dilate a stenosis, and the long duration required for passive drug infusion.

2. **Pressure Driven Systems**
   a. **Wolinsky Perforated Balloon™ Catheter (Figure 35.2).** The Wolinsky perforated balloon catheter (USCI, Billerica, MA) consists of a triple lumen shaft with a distal balloon made of polyethylene terephthalate.[10,11] The balloon has 28 laser-drilled holes which are 25 microns in diameter and arranged in longitudinal rows. During balloon inflation, drug is infused into the balloon and is intramurally deposited by bulk transfer through the balloon's pores. The perforated balloon catheter has been utilized to deliver horseradish peroxidase,[11] heparin,[12] t-PA,[13] methotrexate,[14] doxorubicin,[15] colchicine,[16] thiol protease inhibitor,[17] angiopeptin,[18] antisense oligonucleotides to c-myc,[19] and other gene products.[20,21] The depth of penetration is dependent upon infusion pressure and duration.[11] Intramural persistence has been reported up to 48 hours for heparin, 12-72 hours for c-myc oligomers,[19] and up to two weeks for methotrexate.[14] Studies with local delivery of c-myc oligonucleotides in porcine coronary arteries demonstrated significant inhibition of neointimal hyperplasia following balloon injury.[19] In spite of successful intramural deposition, studies of heparin, methotrexate, doxorubicin, colchicine, TPI, angiopeptin, t-PA, and aurin tricarboxylic acid have not demonstrated a beneficial therapeutic effect.

   The disappointing results with the perforated balloon catheter may be due to trauma from high-pressure jets.[13-15,22-25] Tissue trauma ranges from disruption of the internal elastic lamina, to medial dissection with medial necrosis, to frank arterial perforation. Efforts to limit trauma from the perforated balloon catheter have involved varying the quantity and concentration of drug and changing the design of the catheter.[25] The "jet streaming" effect at any infusion pressure is diminished by increasing the number of pores in the balloon surface.

b. **Microporous Balloon Catheter.** The microporous balloon catheter (Cordis Corporation, Miami Lakes, FL) is a variant of the perforated balloon catheter in which therapeutic agents are locally delivered using a membrane balloon containing thousands of pores less than 1 micron in diameter. This catheter theoretically allows drug delivery via bulk transfer at low pressure, without significant jet effects. A study with horseradish peroxidase demonstrated successful drug delivery to the inner layers of the arterial wall with catheter-induced injury confined to the endothelium.[26] Additional studies demonstrated successful delivery of heparin and low molecular weight heparin.[27,28,58]

c. **Transport™ Catheter.** The Transport catheter (Boston Scientific Scimed, Maple Grove, MN) is a triple lumen catheter with a 3.2F shaft and dual balloons located within one another on its distal tip. One lumen is utilized for inflation of an inner conventional balloon for lesion dilation, a second lumen is for drug infusion through an outer porous balloon, and the third lumen is for a coronary guidewire. The catheter is available in 2.5-4.0 mm balloons. The outer porous balloon contains 36-48 infusion holes depending upon the balloon size. All infusion holes are 250 microns in diameter and are placed circumferentially and centrally within a 10-mm mid-section of the outer balloon. Following dilation with the inner dilating balloon, drug may be infused at 1-3 atm through the outer porous balloon. Preliminary studies demonstrated successful local delivery of t-PA for thrombus-containing lesions.[29] In the United States, the Transport catheter is currently under investigation to treat intracoronary thrombus and acute myocardial infarction.

d. **Channel™ Balloon (Figure 35.5).** The Channel balloon (Boston Scientific Scimed) consists of a standard polyethylene terephthalate balloon mounted on a triple lumen shaft. Surrounding the dilation portion of the balloon are 18 channels which run longitudinally along the surface of the balloon and serve as conduits for delivering agents. Each channel contains one 75 micron pore which connects to a drug infusion port that is independent of the balloon inflation port. When the balloon is inflated to 8 atm through the inflation port, drug can be infused at 2-4 atm through the drug infusion port. The infused drug exits the balloon through the pores in the channels and bathes the arterial wall at low pressure. Successful *in vivo* delivery of horseradish peroxidase,[44] heparin,[44] low molecular weight heparin,[45] urokinase,[46] and several genes[47] has been accomplished.

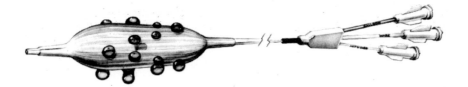

Figure 35.5. The Channel™ Balloon

Drugs are infused into 18 channels which run longitudinally along the surface of the balloon.

Intramural drug deposition correlates with infusion pressure and balloon/artery ratio.[46] Local delivery of heparin with the Channel balloon significantly reduced platelet deposition and mural thrombus formation.[48] The major advantage of the Channel balloon is that successful drug delivery can be achieved with low pressure, with minimal vascular trauma. Disadvantages include a non-homogenous distribution of drug related to the location of the channels on the balloon surface, and the need for arterial occlusion during drug administration.

e. **Infusasleeve™ (Figure 35.6).** The Kaplan-Simpson Infusasleeve (LocalMed, Sunnyvale, CA) is a multi-lumen catheter that is designed to track over a standard PTCA catheter and serve as an adjunctive device for the local delivery. The Infusasleeve has a proximal infusion port, a main catheter or body, and a distal infusion region with multiple sideholes. The central lumen of the Infusasleeve accommodates a standard PTCA catheter and angioplasty guidewire. Following positioning of the standard balloon within the coronary artery, the drug infusion region of the Infusasleeve is positioned along the angioplasty catheter shaft. Drug can then be infused either proximal to, or directly over the balloon during low pressure balloon inflation (i.e., up to 2 atm) to approximate the Infusasleeve directly adjacent to the arterial wall. Previous animal studies with the Infusasleeve demonstrated successful intramural delivery of horseradish peroxidase,[49] heparin,[50] and urokinase,[51] with intramural deposition related to balloon inflation and infusion pressure. Local delivery of heparin in the porcine model successfully inhibited platelet deposition following balloon injury.[50] The device was approved by the FDA in 1994.[52]

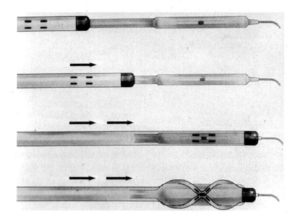

Figure 35.6. The Infusasleeve™

The delivery sleeve is positioned along the shaft of a standard angioplasty catheter for local drug infusion.

3. **Physical Delivery (Non-pressure) Systems**

    a. **Iontophoresis Catheter (Figure 35.7).** Local drug delivery by iontophoresis is based on the concept that an electrical field can be used as a driving force to intramurally deliver charged agents at an angioplasty site.[53] The iontophoresis system (CorTrak Medical, Roseville, MN) consists of a standard angioplasty catheter with a microporous membrane balloon mounted on its distal end. The middle of the membrane balloon, which is contact with the arterial wall during balloon inflation, contains millions of submicron pores for drug delivery. The proximal and distal ends of the membrane balloon are devoid of pores, minimizing drug loss into the bloodstream during iontophoresis. Located under the microporous membrane balloon is an electrode, which is connected to a power source. When the membrane balloon is inflated to 1 atm and an electric current is applied by the power source, charged drug molecules inside the balloon flow through the pores into the arterial wall. Successful in-vivo delivery of hirudin[54] and heparin[55,56] has been accomplished in animals, resulting in tissue concentrations 80 times greater than passive delivery for hirudin, and 13 times greater for heparin. Local iontophoretic delivery of heparin in the porcine model decreased platelet deposition following balloon injury.[55]

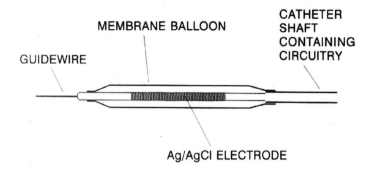

GUIDEWIRE   MEMBRANE BALLOON   CATHETER SHAFT CONTAINING CIRCUITRY

Ag/AgCl ELECTRODE

Figure 35.7. The Iontophoresis Catheter

Drugs are delivered through a membrane balloon in response to a voltage differential between the Ag/AgCl catheter electrode and a return electrode.

    b.   **The Infiltrator™ (Figure 35.8).** The Infiltrator (Interventional Technologies Inc.) consists of a triple lumen balloon catheter (one each for balloon inflation, drug delivery, and guidewire) fitted with 21 metallic InjectorPorts™ mounted on 3 separate InjectorStrips™ on the balloon surface at 120 degrees. During balloon inflation, the InjectorPorts penetrate into the vessel wall, allowing intramural drug delivery. Preliminary studies showed no benefit of intramural delivery of steroids for reducing restenosis.[59] Additional studies using intramural delivery of alcohol and paclitaxel for treatment of stent restenosis are in progress.

E. DRUG DELIVERY CATHETERS APPROVED FOR CURRENT CLINICAL USE

    1.   **Medical-Legal Implications.** Currently, the United States Food and Drug Administration has approved the Dispatch catheter and the Infusasleeve for local drug infusion. Approval for these devices is for *intraluminal* delivery of therapeutic agents, without specific certification for intramural delivery. The hydrogel-coated balloon has also been approved for use, although the hydrogel coating has been specified as a lubricious surface rather than a drug delivery vehicle. The Transport catheter, microporous balloon, Channel balloon, and iontophoresis catheter are investigational.

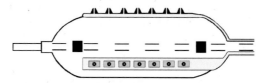

Figure 35.8. The Infiltrator™

Drugs are delivered through InjectorPorts in the drug delivery lumen of the triple lumen balloon catheter during balloon inflation.

2. **The Hydrogel-Coated Balloon.** The hydrogel-coated balloon is available in 0.5 mm sizes from 2.0 to 4.0 mm in diameter. Drugs may be loaded onto the hydrogel balloon by immersion of the inflated balloon into a concentrated drug solution or by "painting" the balloon surface with drug. The amount of fluid (and drug) absorbed by the hydrogel coating is proportional to the balloon surface area and amount of hydrogel available for binding. Relatively larger quantities of drug on the balloon surface can be achieved with "painting."

    In some institutions, urokinase-coated hydrogel balloons are used for treatment of thrombus-containing lesions. Balloons are loaded with urokinase by inflating the balloon to 2 atm pressure, immersing the inflated balloon for 60 seconds in a solution of Abbokinase (Abbott Laboratories, North Chicago, IL) (50,000 units/ml), and deflating the balloon while still in solution. The amount of urokinase absorbed on the balloon surface is approximately 240 units for a 2 mm balloon, 320 units for a 2.5 mm balloon, 420 units for a 3.0 mm balloon, 550 units for a 3.5 mm balloon, and 700 units for a 4.0 mm balloon. The balloon is subsequently positioned over an 0.014-inch angioplasty guidewire through a standard 8F guiding catheter and inflated at the site of thrombus. Balloon sizing is chosen to achieve a balloon/artery ratio of 1:1. Ideally, balloon inflation should be maintained for 2-4 minutes, depending upon the clinical response to coronary occlusion. Following single use, subsequent inflations of the balloon require "reloading" of the hydrogel with urokinase. All hydrogel studies have demonstrated significant wash-off from the balloon surface when the drug-coated balloon is exposed to the intact circulation. For this reason, rapid deployment of the balloon to the site of drug delivery is recommended. Use of a protective sleeve to prevent drug washoff is under investigation.

3. **The Dispatch™ Catheter.** The Dispatch catheter is manufactured with 3.0, 3.5, and 4.0 mm coil sizes, and is deployed within a coronary artery with a 1:1 coil/artery ratio. The catheter is advanced over an 0.014" angioplasty guidewire through a standard 8F guiding catheter and positioned at the drug infusion site, usually after successful predilatation. The coils are inflated with a 50:50 mixture of saline and contrast with a standard indeflator. Inflation of the coils is nominal at 6 atm, with quarter-sizing at 12 atm. In its inflated state, the coils exert 2 atm of radial force on the arterial wall. Contrast injection through the guiding catheter can be used to assess distal coronary perfusion and possible sidebranch occlusion. Following deployment of the catheter and inflation of the device's coils, drug is infused via the drug infusion port using an IMED pump at an infusion rate of 0.5 cc/min. Pressure within the drug infusion port can be measured by connecting a three-way stopcock in series between the IMED infusion pump and the Dispatch catheter, and connecting the side arm of the stopcock to a pressure transducer. This infusion pressure should not exceed 300-400 mmHg at the specified volumetric flow rate. In the event that the fit of the Dispatch catheter within the artery is too "tight" to allow an infusion rate of 0.5 cc/minute without exceeding the pressure limit of 300-400 mmHg, the catheter's coils should be deflated from 6 atm to the highest pressure which allows a flow rate of 0.5 cc/minute with a pressure < 300-400 mmHg. In the event the patient is unable to tolerate initial deployment of the Dispatch catheter because of inadequate distal perfusion or sidebranch occlusion, it may be repositioned or removed.

4. **The Infusasleeve™.** The Infusasleeve is intended for use in conjunction with standard angioplasty catheters. The standard angioplasty catheter is then inserted with its balloon in the deflated state through the proximal end of the Infusasleeve and advanced until the balloon exits the end of the Infusasleeve. The drug infusion region is positioned proximal to the angioplasty balloon. The combined angioplasty catheter-Infusasleeve™ device is then positioned over a 0.014" angioplasty guidewire through a standard 9F guiding catheter to the target lesion. Following dilation with the angioplasty balloon, the Infusasleeve may be positioned along the angioplasty catheter shaft to the target lesion. Drug may be infused through the sleeve proximal, distal, or at the site of the angioplasty balloon. The flow rate for drug infusion is directly related to infusion pressure: 5 ml/min for 10 psi, 15 ml/min for 30 psi, and 25 ml/min for 50 psi. Infusion pressures above 50 psi are undergoing clinical evaluation. In our laboratory, drug infusion is accomplished with the use of a Monarch™ inflation syringe (Merit Medical, Salt Lake City, Utah).

F. **CONCLUSIONS.** The field of catheter-based drug delivery is currently in its earliest stages of development. Multiple drug delivery catheters are being designed and tested,[57] and will probably be available for clinical use in the next several years. Trials in progress include the CORAMI study (local urokinase for acute MI via the Hydrogel balloon), Euro-Dispatch study (heparin after PTCA via the Dispatch catheter), DISTRESS trial (heparin via the Dispatch catheter + PTCA/stenting), DUET trial (urokinase followed by PTCA via the Dispatch catheter), HIPS study (heparin via the Infusasleeve™ + stenting), LHIPS trial (heparin via the Infusasleeve™ + stenting), ITALICS trial (antisense oligonucleotides via the Transport catheter + PTCA/stenting), the local-PAMI trial (heparin via the Infusasleeve™ + PTCA for acute MI), and BARS trial (30% alcohol via the Infiltrator for in-stent restenosis). Comparative studies are needed to assess the relative merits of the different systems with respect to efficiency of drug delivery, effect on vessel architecture, homogeneity of drug deposition, ability to simultaneously dilate vascular stenoses, and limit ischemia from vessel and sidebranch occlusion. Beneficial therapeutic effects on platelet deposition and smooth muscle cell proliferation have been documented with several drugs in animal models, and preliminary human studies have demonstrated successful treatment of intracoronary thrombus. However, additional information is needed on the pharmacokinetics and therapeutic benefit of individual drugs. Moreover, the eventual success of this field may depend upon the success of strategies to prolong intramural drug residence time. Although promising, the ultimate impact of local drug delivery on thrombotic closure and restenosis remains uncertain.

* * * * *

REFERENCES

1. Riessen R, Isner JM. Prospects for site-specific delivery of pharmacologic and molecular therapies. J Am Coll Cardiol 1994;23:1234-44.

2. Lincoff AM, Topol EJ, Ellis SG. Local drug delivery for the prevention of restenosis: Fact, fancy and future. Circulation 1994;90:2070-2083.

3. Wilensky RL, March KL, Gradus-Pizlo I, et al. Methods and devices for local drug delivery in coronary and peripheral arteries. Trends Cardiovasc Med 1993;3:163-170.

4. Goldman B, Blanke H, Wolinsky H. Influence of pressure on permeability of normal and diseased muscular arteries to horseradish peroxidase. Atherosclerosis 1987;65:215-225.

5. Lopez-Sendon J, Sobrino N, Gamallo C, Lorenzo A, et al. Locally delivered heparin reduces intimal hyperplasia and lumen stenosis following arterial balloon injury in swine. European Heart Journal 1993;14(supplement):191 (abstract).

6. Meyer BJ, Fernandez-Ortiz A, Mailhac A, Falk E, et al. Local delivery of r-hirudin by a double-balloon perfusion catheter prevents mural thrombosis and minimizes platelet deposition after angioplasty. Circulation 1994;90:2474-2480.

7. Jorgensen B, Tonnesen KH, Bulow L, et al. Femoral artery recanalization with percutaneous angioplasty and segmentally enclosed plasminogen activator. Lancet 1989;1:1106-8.

8. Nabel EG, Plautz G, Nabel GJ. Site-specific gene expression in vivo by direct gene transfer into the arterial wall. Science 1990;249:1285-8.

9. Nabel EG, Yang Z, Liptay S, et al. Recombinant platelet-derived growth factor B gene expression in porcine arteries reduces intimal hyperplasia in vivo. J Clin Invest 1993;91:1822-9.

10. Wolinsky H, Thung SN. Use of a perforated catheter to deliver concentrated heparin into the wall of the normal canine artery. J Am Coll Cardiol 1990;15:475-81.

11. Wolinsky H, Lin CS. Use of the perforated balloon catheter to infuse marker substances into diseased coronary artery walls after experimental postmortem angioplasty. J Am Coll Cardiol 1991;17:174B-178B.

12. Gimple LW, Gertz SD, Haber HL, Ragosta M, et al. Effect of chronic subcutaneous or intramural administration of heparin on femoral artery restenosis after balloon angioplasty in hypercholesterolemic rabbits. A quantitative angiographic and histopathological study. Circulation 1992;86:1536-46.

13. Gellman J, Enger CD, Sigal SL, True LD, et al. The successful application of a local infusion angioplasty catheter in a rabbit model of focal femoral atherosclerosis. J Am Coll Cardiol 1990;15:164A (abstract).

14. Muller DWM, Topol EJ, Abrams GD, Gallagher K, Ellis SG. Intramural methotrexate therapy for prevention of neointimal thickening after balloon angioplasty. J Am Coll Cardiol 1992;20:460-466.

15. Franklin SM, Kalan JM, Currier JW, Mejias Y, Cody C, Haudenschild CC, Faxon DP. Effects of local delivery of doxorubicin or saline on restenosis following angioplasty in atherosclerotic rabbits. Circulation 1992;86:I-52 (abstract).

16. Wilensky RL, Gradus-Pizlo I, Marck KL, Sandusky GE, Hathaway DR. Efficacy of local intramural injection of colchicine in reducing restenosis following angioplasty in the atherosclerotic rabbitt model. Circulation 1992;86:I-52 (abstract).

17. Wilensky RL, March KL, Hathaway DR. Restenosis in an atherosclerotic rabbit model is reduced by thiol protease inhibitor. J Am Coll Cardiol 1991;17:286A (abstract).

18. Hong MK, Bhatti T, Mathews BJ, Stark KS, et al. Locally delivered angiopeptin reduces intimal hyperplasia following balloon injury in rabbits. Circulation 1991;84:II-72 (abstract).

19. Shi Y, Fard A, Galeo A, Hutchinson HG, et al. Transcatheter delivery of c-myc antisense oligomers reduces neointimal formation in a porcine model of coronary artery balloon injury. Circulation 1994;90:944-951.

20. Flugelman MY, Jaklitsch MT, Newman KD, Casscell W, et al. Low level in vivo gene transfer into the arterial wall through a perforated balloon catheter. Circulation 1992;85:1110-7.

21. Chapman GD, Lim CS, Gammon RS, et al. Gene transfer into coronary arteries of intact animals with a percutaneous balloon catheter. Circ Res 1992;71:27-33.

22. Stadius ML, Collins C, Kernoff R. Local infusion balloon angioplasty to obviate restenosis compared with conventional balloon angioplasty in an experimental model of atherosclerosis. Am Heart J 1993;126:47-56.

23. Lambert CR, Leone JE, Rowland SM. Local drug delivery catheters: functional comparison of porous and microporous designs. Cor Art Dis 1993;4:469-475.

24. Herdeg C, Oberhoff M, Baumbach A, Kamenz J, et al. Application of porous balloon catheter with two different injection pressures: differences in outcome. European Heat Journal 1994:15 (Supplement):561 (abstract).

25. French BA, Mazur W, Finnigan JP, Carter Grinstead W, et al. Gene transfer into intact porcine coronary arteries via infusion balloon catheter: influences of delivery volume and pressure. Circulation 1992;86:I-799 (abstract).

26. Lambert CR, Leone J, Rowland S. The microporous balloon: A minimal trauma local drug delivery catheter. Circulation 1992;86:I-381 (abstract).

27. Thomas CN, Robinson KA, Cipolla GD, Jones M, King SB. In-vivo local delivery of heparin to coronary arteries with a microporous infusion balloon. J Am Coll Cardiol 1994;23:187A (abstract).

28. Lincoff AM, Furst JG, Penn MS, Lee P, MacIssac AI, Chisolm GM, Topol EJ, Ellis SG. Efficiency of solute transfer by a microporous balloon catheter in the porcine coronary model of arterial injury. J Am Coll Cardiol 1994;23:18A (abstract).

29. Cumberland DC, Gunn J, Tsikaderis D, Arafa S, Ahsan A. Initial clinical experience of local drug delivery via a porous balloon during percutaneous coronary angioplasty. J Am Coll Cardiol 1994;23:186A (abstract).

30. Fram DB, Aretz TA, Azrin MA, Mitchel JF, et al. Localized intramural drug delivery during balloon angioplasty using hydrogel-coated balloons and pressure-augmented diffusion. J Am Coll Cardiol 1994;23:1570-7.

31. Azrin MA, Mitchel JF, Fram DB, Pedersen CA, et al. Decreased platelet deposition and smooth muscle cell proliferation following intramural heparin delivery with hydrogel-coated balloons. Circulation 1994:90:433-441.

32. Mitchel JF, Azrin MA, Fram DB, Hong MK, et al. Inhibition of platelet deposition and lysis of intracoronary thrombus during balloon angioplasty with urokinase-coated hydrogel balloons. Circulation 1994:90:1979-88.

33. Nunes GL, Hanson SR, King SB, Sahatjian RA, Scott NE. Local delivery of a synthetic antithrombin with a hydrogel-coated angioplasty balloon inhibits platelet-dependent thrombosis. J Am Coll Cardiol 1994;23:1578-83.

34. Azrin MA, Mitchel JF, Pedersen C, Curley TM, et al. Inhibition of smooth muscle cell proliferation in-vivo following local delivery of antisense oligonucleotides to c-myb during angioplasty. J Am Coll Cardiol 1994;23:396A (abstract).

35. Riessen R, Rahimizadeh H, Blessing E, Takeshita S, et al. Arterial gene transfer using pure DNA applied directly to a hydrogel-coated angioplasty balloon. Hum Gene Ther 1993;4:749-58.

36. Mitchel JF, Hirst JA, Kiernan FJ, Fram DB, et al. Local, intracoronary thrombolysis using urokinase-coated hydrogel balloons. Circulation 1994;90(4):I-493 (abstract).

37. Fram DB, Mitchel JF, Azrin MA, Schwedick MW, et al. Local heparin delivery in porcine coronary arteries with the Dispatch catheter: delivery, washout and effect on platelet deposition following balloon angioplasty. Circulation 1994;90(4):I-493 (abstract).

38. Mitchel JF, Fram DB, Palme DF, Foster R, et al. Enhanced local thrombolysis with urokinase using the Dispatch catheter. Circulation 1995;91:785-793.

39. Camenzind E, di Mario C, de Jaegere P, de Feyter P, et al. Left ventricular and coronary hemodynamics during local drug delivery with a new infusion catheter: First experience in humans. European Heat Journal 1994;15 (Supplement):561 (abstract).

40. McKay RG, Fram DB, Kiernan FJ, Hirst JA, et al. Localized thrombolysis of intracoronary thrombus using a new drug delivery system - the Dispatch catheter. Cathet Cardiovasc Diagn 1994;33:181-188.

41. Mitchel JF, McKay RG. Treatment of acute stent thrombosis with local drug delivery systems. Cathet Cardiovasc Diagn 1995;34:149-154.

42. Mitchel JF, Fram DB, Palme DF, Foster R, et al. Enhanced intracoronary thrombolysis using the Dispatch catheter. Circulation 1994;90(4):I-493 (abstract).

43. Mitchel JF, Fram DB, Hirst JA, Kiernan FJ, et al. Local dissolution of intracoronary thrombus with urokinase using the Dispatch catheter: clinical studies. J Am Coll Cardiol 1995;25:347A (abstract).

44. Hong MK, Wong SC, Farb A, Mehlman MD, et al. Feasibility and drug delivery efficiency of a new balloon angioplasty catheter capable of performing simultaneous local drug delivery. Cor Art Dis 1993;4:1023-1027.

45. Hong MK, Wong SC, Haudenschild CC, Mehlman MD, et al. Local delivery with low molecular weight heparin by the Channel balloon during simultaneous angioplasty in atherosclerotic rabbit iliac arteries. Circulation 1994;90(4):I-157 (abstract).

46. Mitchel JF, Fram DB, Azrin MA, Bow L, et al. Localized intracoronary delivery of urokinase with the Channel balloon: pharmacokinetics of drug delivery and washout. J Am Coll Cardiol 1995;25:347A (abstract).

47. Feldman LJ, Steg PG, Zheng LP, Barry JJ, et al. Efficient percutaneous adenovirus-mediated arterial gene transfer using a channelled angioplasty balloon. Circulation 1994;90(4):I-20 (abstract).

48. Thomas CN, Barry JJ, King SB, Scott NA. Local delivery with heparin with a PTCA infusion balloon inhibits platelet-dependent thrombosis. J Am Coll Cardiol 1994;23:4A (abstract).

49. Kaplan AV, Kermode J, Grant G, Klein E, et al. Intramural delivery of marker agent in ex vivo and in vivo models using a novel drug delivery sleeve. J Am Coll Cardiol 1994;23:187A (abstract).

50. Moura A, Lam JYT, Hebert D, Letchacovski G, et al. Local heparin delivery decreases the thrombogenicity of the balloon-injured artery. Circulation 1994;90(4):I-449 (abstract).

51. Azrin MA, Mitchel JF, Bow LM, Alberghini TV, et al. Local delivery of urokinase to porcine coronary arteries using the Localmed infusion sleeve. J Am Coll Cardiol 1995;25:347A (abstract).

52. Kaplan AV, Vandormael M, Bartorelli A, Hofman M, et al. Local delivery at the site of angioplasty with a novel drug delivery sleeve: Initial clinical series. J Am Coll Cardiol 1995;25:286A (abstract).

53. Chien YW, Banga AK: Iontophoretic delivery of drugs: Overview of historical development. J Pharm Sci 1989;78:353-354.

54. Fernandez-Ortiz A, Meyer BJ, Mailhac A, Falk E, et al. A new approach for local intravascular drug delivery. The iontophoretic balloon. Circulation 1994;89:1518-1522.

55. Mitchel JF, Azrin MA, Schwedick MW, Bow LM, et al. Local delivery of heparin with a novel iontophoretic catheter - quantitative heparin delivery and effect on platelet deposition following balloon angioplasty. Circulation 1994;90(4):I-492 (abstract).

56. Mitchel JF, Azrin MA, Fram DB, Feroze H, et al. Localized intracoronary delivery of heparin with iontophoresis. J Am Coll Cardiol 1995;25:285A (abstract).

57. Local Drug Delivery. Cathet & Cardiovasc Diagn 1997;41(3): Special issue.

58. Oberhoff M, Baumbach A, Hermann T, et al. Local and systemic delivery of low-molecular-weight heparin following PTCA: Acute results and 6-month follow-up of the initial clinical experience with the porous balloon (PILOT-Study). Cathet Cardiovasc Diagn 1998;44:267-274.

59. Reimers B, Moussa I, Akiyama T, et al. Persistent high restenosis after local intrawall delivery of long-acting steroids before coronary stent implantation. J Invas Cardiol 1998;10:323-331.

60. Gonschior P. Local drug delivery for restenosis and thrombosis-progress? J Invasc Cardiol 1998;10:528-532.

61. Hong MK, Wong SC, Barry JJ, et al. Feasibility and efficacy of locally delivered enoxaprarin via the channeled balloon catheter on smooth muscle cell proliferation following balloon injury in rabbits. Cathet Cardiovasc Diagn 1997;41:241-245.

62. Glazier JJ, Hirst JA, Kiernan FJ, et al. Site-specific intracoronary thrombolysis with urokinase-coated hydrogel balloons: Acute and follow-up studies in 95 patients. Cathet Cardiovasc Diagn 1997;41:246-253.

63. Mitchel JF, Barry JJ, Bow L, et al. Local urokinase delivery with the Channel balloon: Device safety, pharmcokinetics of intracoronary drug delivery, and efficacy of thrombolysis. Cathet Cardiovasc Diagn 1997;41:254-260.

64. Glazier JJ, Kiernan FJ, Bauer HH, et al. Treatment of thrombotic saphenous vein bypass grafts using local urokinase infusion therapy with the dispatch catheter. Cathet Cardiovasc Diagn 1997;41:261-267.

65. Oberhoff M, Herdeg C, Baumbach A, et al. Time course of smooth muscle cell proliferation after local drug delivery of low-molecular-weight heparin using a porous balloon catheter. Cathet Cardiovasc Diagn 1997;41:268-274.Pavlides GS, Barath P, Maginas A, et al. Intramural drug delivery by direction injection within the arterial wall: First clinical experience with a novel intracoronary delivery-infiltrator system. Cathet Cardiovasc Diagn 1997;41:287-292.

66. Baumbach A, Oberhoff M, Bohnet A, et al. Efficacy of low-molecular-weight heparin delivery with the dispatch catheter following balloon angioplasty in the rabbit iliac artery. Cathet Cardiovasc Diagn 1997;41:303-307.

67. Herdeg C, Oberhoff M, Baumbach A, et al. Local drug delivery with porous balloons in the rabbit: Assessment of vascular injury for an improvement of application parameters. Cathet Cardiovasc Diagn 1997;41:308-314.

68. Mitchell JF, Azrin MA, Fram DB, et al. Localized delivery of heparin to angioplasty sites with iontophoresis. Cathet Cardiovasc Diagn 1997;41:315-232.

69. Dev V, Eigler N, Fishbein MC, et al. Sustained local drug delivery to the arterial wall via biodegradable microspheres. Cathet Cardiovasc Diagn 1997;41:324-332.

70. Barath P, Popov A, Dillehay GL, et al. Infiltrator angioplasty balloon catheter: A device for combined angioplasty and intramural site-specific treatment. Cathet Cardiovasc Diagn 1997;41:333-341.

71. Robinson KA, Chronos NAF, Schieffer E, et al. Endoluminal local delivery of PCNA/cdc2 antisense oligonucleotides by porous balloon catheter does not affect neointimal formation or vessel size in the pig

coronary artery model of postangioplasty restenosis. Cathet Cardiovasc Diagn 1997;41:348-353.

72. Robinson KA, Chronos NAF, Schieffer E, et al. Pharacokinetics and tissue localization of antisense oligonucleotides in balloon-injury pig coronary arteries after local delivery with an iontophoretic balloon catheter. Cathet Cardiovasc Diagn 1997;41:354.

73. Glazier JJ, Jiang AJ, Crilly RJ, Spears JR. Laser balloon angioplasty combined with local intracoronary heparin therapy: Immediate and short-term follow-up results. Am Heart J 1997;134:266-273.

74. Stack R. Local drug delivery: The development of a drug delivery stent. J Invas Cardiol 8:396-397.

PERIPHERAL VASCULAR INTERVENTION

36

Christopher J. White, MD
Stephen R. Ramee, MD
Phillip J. Bendick, Ph.D.
Robert D. Safian, MD

There are compelling reasons for cardiologists to participate in the global approach to the patient with vascular disease. First, atherosclerosis is a "systemic" disease resulting in the frequent association of coronary and peripheral vascular disease (Table 36.1). Second, coronary artery disease is the most common cause of morbidity and mortality in patients with vascular disease.[1,2] Finally, experienced interventional cardiologists have the technical skills to perform peripheral vascular intervention.[133] Nevertheless, the American College of Cardiology, the American Heart Association, the American Society of Cardiovascular Interventionists, the Society of Cardiovascular Interventional Radiologists, and the Society of Cardiac Angiography and Intervention have published disparate guidelines for peripheral angioplasty.[134-140] Recently the Society of Cardiac Angiography and Interventions published revised guidelines for peripheral angioplasty and defined two types of certification:[141] Limited certification (for iliac and renal artery angioplasty), and unrestricted certification (for the broad scope of peripheral vascular intervention).

PATHOPHYSIOLOGY OF PERIPHERAL VASCULAR DISEASE

Patients with coronary artery disease frequently have symptomatic peripheral vascular disease.[131,132] Historically, patients with severe ischemia have been treated by surgical revascularization,[3,4] but endovascular interventional techniques have broadened the indications and utilization of percutaneous revascularization.[5-7] The purpose of the diagnostic evaluation of peripheral vascular disease is to identify the sites of obstruction and to determine if patients are suitable candidates for percutaneous and/or surgical revascularization. The pathophysiology of lower extremity atherosclerotic disease is similar to coronary artery disease, since the disease progresses slowly, and ischemic symptoms develop when diameter stenosis exceeds 60%.[8] As the stenosis increases, there is gradual progression of claudication; when multiple arterial segments are involved, chronic ischemia may cause progressive rest pain, ulceration, gangrene, and limb loss. (In contrast, cerebral ischemia is usually associated with plaque ulceration and thromboembolism, rather than progressive stenosis to occlusion.) It is helpful to consider lower extremity vascular obstruction in three anatomic zones (Figure 36.1):[131]

1. **Inflow Tract.** The infrarenal aorta and iliac arteries make up the inflow tract to the lower extremities and are often affected by diffuse atherosclerosis. The most severe lesions are typically found at the aortic bifurcation involving the origin of the common iliac arteries, or at the iliac bifurcation involving the origin of the external and internal iliac arteries. Aorto-iliac disease usually causes claudication in the hips and buttocks, but may extend into the thighs and calves upon further exertion. Femoral artery

pulses may or may not be diminished, depending on the degree of proximal disease.[132]

2. **Outflow Tract.** The outflow tract extends from the inguinal ligament to just below the knee, and consists of the common femoral, superficial femoral, and popliteal arteries (the femoropopliteal system). The common femoral artery and the mid-segment of the popliteal artery are often spared from significant atherosclerosis. The superficial femoral artery may be involved throughout its length, and the most critical lesions are often observed near the adductor hiatus.[3]

3. **Runoff Bed.** The runoff bed consists of the tibioperoneal trunk, anterior tibial artery, posterior tibial artery, and peroneal artery (the trifurcation vessel system) in the lower leg. The proximal segments of these vessels are frequently diseased, limiting distal runoff to the foot. Diabetic patients comprise a unique population with regard to distribution of atherosclerosis in the lower extremities. One-third of diabetics with peripheral atherosclerosis have disease limited to the lower leg trifurcation vessels, one-third have disease limited to the aortoiliac or femoropopliteal vessels, and one-third have multiple segmental disease involving the inflow, outflow, and runoff systems.[9,10] (By contrast, atherosclerotic disease in nondiabetics is equally divided between isolated lesions of the inflow/outflow tract and multiple segmental lesions involving the runoff vessels.) Trifurcation lesions in diabetics are often not amenable to surgical bypass, but sometimes can be treated percutaneously.

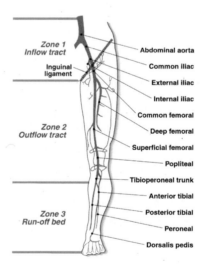

Figure 36.1. Arterial Circulation of the Lower Extremity

Zone 1: In-flow tract (abdominal aorta, common iliac artery, and external iliac artery)
Zone 2: Outflow tract; extends from the inguinal ligament to the knee (common femoral artery, superficial femoral artery, and popliteal artery)
Zone 3: Run-off bed (anterior tibial artery, posterior tibial artery, and peroneal artery)

Table 36.1. Arterial Occlusive Disease: Pathophysiology and Outcome

Distribution	Organ	Symptoms	Pathophysiology	Morbidity
Coronary	Heart	Angina	Progressive stenosis, thrombosis	MI, CHF, death
Carotid/vertebral	Brain	TIA	Ulceration, embolization	Stroke, death
Iliofemoral	Legs	Claudication	Progressive stenosis, occlusion	Tissue loss
Renal	Kidney	None*	Progressive stenosis, occlusion	CRF, death

Abbreviations: CHF = congestive heart failure; CRF = chronic renal failure; MI = myocardial infarction; TIA = transient ischemic attack

* Symptoms are secondary to other end-organ injury, such as the heart (angina, pulmonary edema), the brain (intracranial hemorrhage, stroke), or the kidney (end-stage ischemic nephropathy leading to uremia)

DIAGNOSIS AND EVALUATION OF PERIPHERAL VASCULAR DISEASE

A. **LOWER EXTREMITY VASCULATURE.** The clinical history helps determine the likelihood of ischemia and the degree of functional impairment. The quality of pulses can help localize the site(s) of obstruction, but is unreliable for estimating disease severity.[11]

1.   **Ankle-Brachial Index.** Objective data are provided by the ankle-brachial index (ABI), defined as the ratio of systolic blood pressure in the ankle to systolic blood pressure in the upper arm (Table 36.2).[12-14] Brachial systolic pressure should be measured in both arms and the higher value used to calculate the right and left ABI. Ankle systolic pressures are measured with a standard adult blood pressure cuff (12 x 23 cm bladder) wrapped snugly around the ankle, with the lower edge of the cuff just above the malleoli. Using a Doppler pencil probe to monitor the signal from the posterior or anterior tibial artery, the cuff is inflated to 30 mmHg above systolic pressure to temporarily occlude flow; as the cuff is slowly deflated (2-4 mmHg per second), the pressure at which a Doppler flow signal is heard is recorded as the ankle systolic pressure.

2.   **Duplex Ultrasound.** Further noninvasive evaluation is provided by duplex ultrasound, which allows direct real-time ultrasound imaging of obstructive lesions and simultaneous assessment of hemodynamic significance by Doppler. The entire peripheral arterial tree from the abdominal aorta to the tibial arteries can be surveyed if necessary (Figures 36.1, 36.2). Stenosis severity can be estimated from Doppler flow signals or Doppler velocity spectra (Table 36.3).[15-18]

B. **CAROTID CIRCULATION.** Duplex ultrasound can be used to evaluate atherosclerotic disease in the cerebrovascular circulation (Table 36.4, Figure 36.3), but it is important to emphasize that widely accepted objective criteria for significant carotid disease have not been firmly established. At present, the most sensitive criterion is the absolute peak velocity (APV) at end-diastole at the site of stenosis; velocity recordings > 100 cm/sec suggest a high likelihood of severe stenosis and the need for further evaluation.

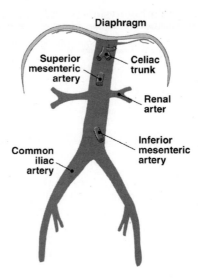

Figure 36.2. The Abdominal Aorta and Branches

C. **RENAL AND MESENTERIC ARTERIES.** The renal arteries, celiac axis, and superior mesenteric artery (SMA) may all be evaluated at their origin from the abdominal aorta (Table 36.5).[19] The renal-to-aortic peak systolic velocity ratio (RAR) is used to evaluate the renal arteries—the Doppler flow signal from the suprarenal aorta is used as a reference signal—while absolute velocities are used to evaluate the celiac trunk and superior mesenteric artery (SMA). Patients should be fasting for at least 8 hours prior to the examination. Normal resting flow waveforms in the renal arteries and celiac axis consist of low distal vascular resistance with good antegrade flow throughout diastole. In contrast, distal vascular resistance in the SMA is relatively high in the fasting state, resulting in a Doppler waveform that has a very sharp systolic peak and minimal antegrade flow in late diastole. Following a caloric challenge, vascular resistance in the gut decreases sharply, with an attendant increase in end-diastolic flow velocity. In the normal mesenteric circulation, the SMA end-diastolic velocity should double (compared to fasting) within 30 minutes of a caloric challenge.

D. **SUBCLAVIAN ARTERY.** A systolic pressure difference ≥ 20 mmHg between the two arms suggests significant subclavian artery obstruction; reversal of flow in the ipsilateral vertebral artery by Doppler is diagnostic of hemodynamically-significant subclavian stenosis. Direct evaluation of the subclavian artery by duplex ultrasound may reveal post-stenotic turbulence for subtotal stenoses, or damped waveforms consistent with total occlusion and collateral reconstitution (Table 36.3).

Table 36.2. Correlation of Ankle-Brachial Index with Clinical Presentation and Lesion Severity

ABI	Symptoms	Disease Severity
> 1.30	Indeterminate	Medial wall calcification; nondiagnostic.
0.90 - 1.25	Asymptomatic	No hemodynamically-significant lesions
0.60 - 0.90	Claudication	Single segment stenosis or well-collateralized occlusion
0.30 - 0.60	Claudication	Multiple segment disease
0.15 - 0.30	Rest pain	Multiple segment total occlusions
< 0.15	Impending tissue loss	Multiple segment total occlusions

Abbreviations: ABI = ankle-brachial index

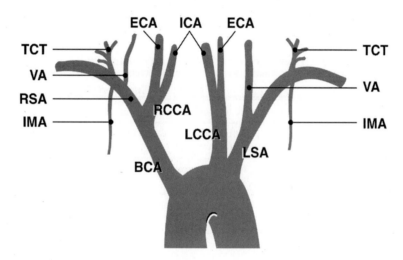

Figure 36.3. Arch of the Aorta and Great Vessels

BCA = brachiocephalic (innominate) artery; LCCA = left common carotid artery; LSA = left subclavian artery; RSA = right subclavian artery; RCCA = right common carotid artery; ICA = internal carotid artery; ECA = external carotid artery; VA = vertebral artery; IMA = internal mammary artery; TCT = thyrocervical trunk.

Table 36.3. Qualitative Assessment of Doppler Flow Signals (Lower and Upper Extremity)

Flow Pattern	Characteristics	Significance
Normal	Multiphasic flow signal with a brisk, well-defined, high-pitched systolic peak; low-pitched signals during diastole; transient reversal of flow during early diastole	No significant obstruction
Damped	Slow systolic upstroke with a poorly-defined systolic peak; slowly diminishing flow from systole through diastole, with antegrade flow during the entire cardiac cycle	Significant proximal obstruction
Absent	No flow signal	Total occlusion; absent collateral reconstitution
Hyperemia	Sustained hyperemic flow throughout diastole	Markedly diminished peripheral vascular resistance; characteristic of an arteriovenous fistula or arterial conduit supplying a distal runoff bed with significant inflammatory reaction (e.g., cellulitis)

Table 36.4. Doppler Velocity Criteria for Grading Severity of Internal Carotid Artery Stenosis

Diameter Stenosis (%)	Spectrum Characteristics
< 20	No increase in V_p relative to proximal arterial segment; minimal spectral broadening
20 - 49	> 30% increase in V_p relative to proximal artery segment; V_p < 125 cm/sec; spectral broadening throughout pulse cycle
50 - 75	> 100% increase in V_p relative to proximal arterial segment; V_p < 125 cm/sec; spectral broadening throughout pulse cycle
> 75	Spectrum similar to 50-75% diameter stenosis, with absolute end-diastolic velocity > 100 cm/sec

Abbreviations: V_p = peak systolic velocity

Table 36.5. Duplex Ultrasound Criteria for the Renal and Mesenteric Arterial Systems[19]

Arterial System	Duplex Criteria for Significant Stenosis*
Renal artery	Renal/Aortic Ratio (RAR) > 3.5 and peak systolic velocity > 180 cm/sec
Celiac trunk	Peak systolic velocity > 200 cm/sec
Superior mesenteric artery (SMA)	Peak systolic velocity > 275 cm/sec; failure to increase postprandial end-diastolic velocity by at least 2-fold compared to fasting velocity (within 30 minutes)

* Significant stenosis is defined as renal artery stenosis > 60%; iliac or SMA stenosis > 70%

CONSIDERATIONS FOR PERCUTANEOUS REVASCULARIZATION

Percutaneous transluminal angioplasty (PTA), stents, atherectomy, laser, and peripheral intra-arterial thrombolysis (PIAT) are complementary techniques used to improve symptoms of claudication, reverse critical limb ischemia, and avert or limit the extent of vascular bypass surgery and limb loss (Table 36.6). Clinical indications for percutaneous and surgical revascularization are similar, and optimal treatment depends on clinical and angiographic data and target lesion location (Table 36.7).[20-36] Regardless of which technique is employed, all patients should undergo aggressive risk factor modification to limit atherosclerosis and improve cardiovascular prognosis. Aspirin is essential for all patients, and lipid-lowering therapy is recommended to meet NCEP guidelines and achieve LDL-cholesterol levels < 100 mg/dL. Other risk reduction measures are described in Chapter 41. Pentoxifylline (Trental) is frequently prescribed to improve claudication and exercise capacity, but most contemporary studies show no benefit compared to placebo. In contrast, cilostazol (Pletal) resulted in significant improvement in walking distance compared to pentoxifylline or placebo, but is contraindicated in patients with heart failure. Other medications which show promise include naftidrofuryl, propionyl-L-carnitine, and prostaglandin E1, but none are yet available (Table 36.8). Patients with critical limb ischemia should generally be evaluated by angiography to identify targets for surgical and percutaneous revascularization. Amputation is sometimes the only therapeutic option, but full mobility is achieved in < 50% of patients and 2-year mortality is almost 40%. Investigational therapies showing promise for critical limb ischemia include intravenous prostanoids and gene therapy[308] (Table 36.1).

A. **ADJUNCTIVE MEDICATION.** Aspirin should be given at least 24 hours before PTA and indefinitely after PTA. Nifedipine (10 mg SL) or nitroglycerin (100-200 mcg intra-arterial) is often recommended before crossing target lesions in the renal artery and infrapopliteal vessels to minimize spasm. Heparin (5000 units IV) should be administered before the lesion is crossed with a guidewire, but ideal ACT guidelines have not been clearly defined. After intervention, sheath removal should be performed when the ACT is < 175 seconds. Post-procedure heparin (to maintain the PTT at 60-80 seconds for 12-24 hours) is sometimes recommended for infrapopliteal PTA, severe dissection, and in slow-flow states, but proof of efficacy is lacking. Clopidogrel (75 mg daily) is commonly employed for 2-4 weeks after stenting, but data to support its use in this setting are lacking.

B. **VASCULAR ACCESS.** Safe and secure vascular access is critical, and thoughtful planning is essential. Arterial access should be achieved as close as possible to the target lesion (Table 36.9). Retrograde (Figure 36.4) and antegrade (Figure 36.5) techniques are commonly performed using a single wall puncture; a Potts-Cournand needle or micropuncture set is typically used for axillary and brachial artery punctures to minimize arterial spasm (Figure 36.6). Placement of an appropriate arterial sheath facilitates exchange of catheters and guidewires.

1. **Contralateral Femoral Artery Approach ("Crossover" Technique).** This route often provides a better angle for reaching stenoses in the distal external iliac, common femoral, and proximal

superficial or profunda femoral arteries; for thrombolytic therapy of occluded femoropopliteal grafts; and for gaining access to the superficial femoral artery when the ipsilateral antegrade approach is difficult (as in obese patients). A contralateral approach is also useful in the presence of a high common femoral artery bifurcation,[143,144] and for bilateral lower extremity percutaneous revascularization, angioplasty of the internal iliac arteries, or renal transplant artery intervention. Access is achieved by retrograde puncture of the contralateral femoral artery, followed by advancement of a guidewire to the aortoiliac bifurcation. A Cobra catheter, Simmons Sidewinder, or internal mammary artery catheter is then used to direct the wire down the opposite iliac artery (Figure 36.7). A stiff Teflon-coated guidewire (Amplatz or Rosen guidewire) may be used to further advance the catheter around the bifurcation.

2. **Antegrade Common Femoral Artery Approach.** Target lesions in the mid-superficial femoral artery or the tibial vessels are generally approached by ipsilateral antegrade common femoral artery access. The most important landmark is the mid-portion of the femoral head, which virtually always identifies the common femoral artery. Access at the level of the inguinal crease will frequently result in puncture of the superficial or profunda femoral artery, which will increase the risk of bleeding and vascular complications; puncture of the profunda femoral artery precludes further endovascular intervention on the superficial femoral or tibioperoneal arteries.

3. **Left Axillary Artery Approach (Figure 36.8).** This approach was used in the past when access could not be obtained via the femoral artery, but has been replaced in most centers by the percutaneous brachial approach. To obtain axillary artery access:
   1. Abduct the left arm and place hand under the patient's head.
   2. Obtain baseline axillary, brachial, radial, and ulnar pulses.
   3. Locate the puncture site of the axillary artery along the lateral axillary fold over the proximal humerus; this will allow the underlying bone to provide support during compression.
   4. Administer local anesthesia carefully and avoid deep penetration; an axillary hematoma may compress the brachial plexus.
   5. Fix the artery firmly at the intended puncture site with left index and middle fingers on either side of the pulse to avoid displacement of the axillary artery.
   6. Enter the axillary artery at a 45° angle and insert an appropriate guidewire. Use of a micropuncture kit, vascular sheath (5-7F), and vasodilators will minimize spasm.

4. **Brachial or Radial Access.** See Chapter 2.

5. **Popliteal Artery Access.** The popliteal approach is potentially useful for several situations, including failed antegrade approaches, flush occlusion of the superficial femoral artery, occlusion of the superficial femoral artery associated with extensive collaterals, ostial superficial femoral artery lesions, common femoral artery lesions, and acute angulation of the aortic bifurcation precluding femoral crossover.[145,146] Absolute contraindications to popliteal artery puncture include known aneurysms of the popliteal artery and presence of a Baker's cyst. The popliteal artery

courses anteriorly and medially to the popliteal vein, increasing the risk of puncture of the popliteal vein.[147] However, there is minimal overlap of the artery and vein cephalad to the joint space; the most reliable landmark is 6.5 cm cephalad to the femorotibial joint space, the needle directed from medial to lateral.

C. DIAGNOSTIC ANGIOGRAPHY

1. **Imaging Suite.** Imaging equipment is largely based on physician preference, although a C-arm capable of oblique views with cranial and caudal angulation for "head-to-toe" digital acquisition is essential. Interventional cardiologists may consider a multipurpose biplane cineangiographic suite, with an AP plane for cardiac imaging (equipped with a 5/7/9-inch image intensifier) and a lateral plane for peripheral diagnostic and interventional procedures (equipped with a 9/12/16-inch image intensifier). Angulation of the image intensifier is necessary to resolve bifurcation lesions (aorta, iliac, femoral, tibioperoneal) and to optimally visualize aorto-ostial lesions (renal, mesenteric). Cineangiographic imaging is ideal to assess blood flow and is preferred by most cardiologists over standard cut-film; cineangiographic images of interest may be selected and printed in place of cut-film. Images may be obtained with digital subtraction techniques, which requires less contrast and removes nonvascular structures from the image. "Panning" the table must be avoided to prevent motion artifact.

2. **Radiographic Contrast.** Low osmolar ionic (Hexabrix) or non-ionic (Visipaque, Omnipaque) radiographic contrast is preferred for peripheral angiography to avoid patient discomfort. In patients at substantial risk for contrast-induced renal failure, visceral and lower extremity arteriography may be performed with gadolinium or CO_2, provided digital subtraction techniques are available.[272]

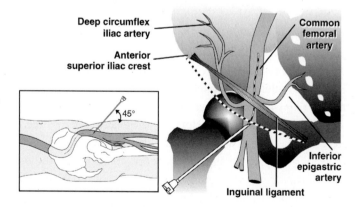

Figure 36.4. Common Femoral Artery: Retrograde Puncture

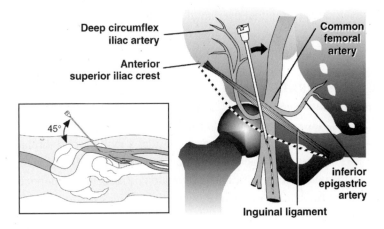

Figure 36.5. Common Femoral Artery: Antegrade Puncture

3. **Imaging Technique.** It is essential to demonstrate the vascular segment preceding the target lesion ("inflow") and the vascular segment distal to the target vessel ("outflow").

4. **Outcome Assessment.** The Society of Vascular Surgery has adopted guidelines for classification of acute (Table 36.10) and chronic (Table 36.11) limb ischemia and criteria for outcome assessment (Table 36.12).[148] Quantitative angiography, the current standard for coronary intervention, should be strongly considered for assessment of angiographic results.

D. **CROSSING THE LESION.** Diagnostic angiography should be performed using appropriate catheters (Figure 36.9) and radiographic views (Table 36.13) to delineate the lesion and major branch vessels.[37] After baseline angiography, the lesion should be crossed with a wire based on operator preference, such as a soft-tip floppy straight wire (Wholey wire, Magic-torque wire), a hi-torque floppy wire, an angled Glidewire, or a TAD (tapered attenuated diameter) wire. For subtotal stenoses, it may be useful to advance a transfer catheter (e.g., 4F Glide catheter) just proximal to the lesion and cross the lesion with the guidewire. If necessary, the transfer catheter can be advanced across the lesion and the initial guidewire exchanged for a heavy-duty wire; PTA can then be performed as indicated. In difficult chronic occlusions or lesions with severe angulation, access to the lesion and distal vascular bed can often be achieved with coronary angioplasty guidewires, such as the 0.018-inch gold Glidewire, 0.018-inch Roadrunner wire, 0.014-inch Choice PT wire, or 0.014-inch Crossit-wire.

E. **BALLOON CATHETER SELECTION.** Balloon size is estimated by measuring the diameter of the reference artery distal to the target lesion from cut-film or DSA images. If estimates are based on cut-film, the balloon will be oversized by 10-15% due to geometric magnification. Once the balloon is positioned using anatomic landmarks, DSA road-mapping, or external markers (such as a hemostat), it is inflated using 50% contrast for 30-60 seconds. If a "waist" persists despite 2-3 inflations, a larger balloon or higher inflation pressures are considered. Repeat angiography and transluminal pressure gradients are useful to assess the final result.[38] Typical balloon sizes are described in Table 36.14.

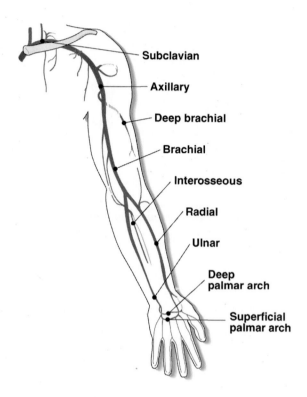

Figure 36.6. Arterial Circulation of the Upper Extremity

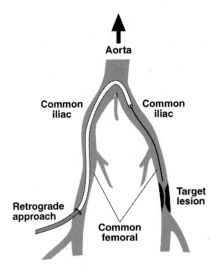

Figure 36.7. Peripheral Angioplasty: Contralateral Femoral Artery Approach

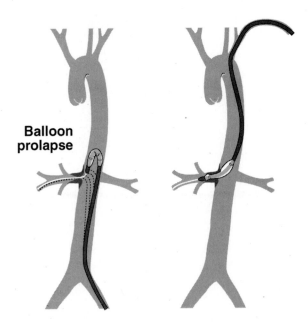

Figure 36.8. Peripheral Angioplasty: Brachial Artery Approach

Application	Name	Tip shape
Aortography Venacavography Pulmonary arteriography *(with tip deflector wire)*	Pigtail	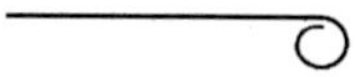
Pulmonary arteriography	Grollman	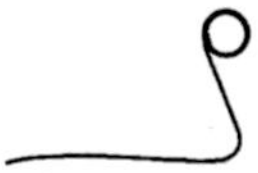
Iliac and antegrade femoral angiography	Straight-flush	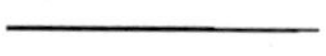
	Multipurpose (curve)	
Inferior mesenteric artery; hooking contralateral iliac	IMA (single hook)	
Left gastric arteriography	LGA	
Visceral and extremity	Cobra C1-C3 C2 and C3 have wide primary curves, for adults	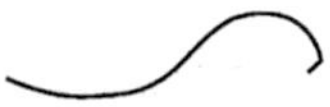
Selective renal arteriography	Renal Curve Right Judkins Coronary Simmons Sidewinder	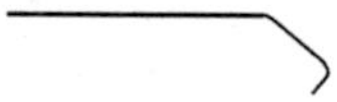
Aortic arch and subclavian	Modified Headhunter Simmons Sidewinder	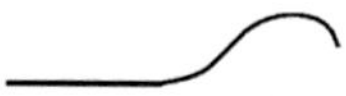
Visceral and cerebral selective arteriography *(shape must be reformed in the artery)*	Simmons Sidewinder 1: narrow aorta 2: normal aorta 3: wide aorta 4: elongated aorta (numbered by increasing radius of primary curve)	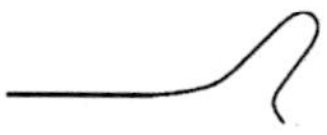

Figure 36.9. Peripheral Angioplasty: Catheter Selection

Table 36.6. Goals of Therapy for Lower Extremity Vascular Disease

Goal	Therapy
Prevent limb loss and adverse cardiovascular events	Vigorous risk factor modification to limit atherosclerosis, including aspirin (or clopidogrel), smoking cessation, control of diabetes and hypertension, lipid-lowering therapy, aerobic exercise, weight control, and possibly ACE inhibitors
Treat critical limb ischemia	Vigorous evaluation for possible surgical and/or percutaneous revascularization; amputation may be needed in patients who are unsuitable for revascularization. New strategies include intravenous prostanoids (PGI_2, PGE_1) and gene therapy
Improve pain-free walking distance	Regular exercise program (30 minutes 3 times per week for 6 months) and medical therapy (Table 36.8); revascularization for refractory claudication

Table 36.7. Indications and Contraindications for Peripheral Vascular Intervention

Target Vessel	Indications	Relative Contraindications	Absolute Contraindications
Aorta[20,21]	• Short stenosis of infrarenal aorta without other aortic disease • Buttock or lower extremity claudication or impotence	• Stenosis > 4 cm in infrarenal aorta • Stenosis resulting in blue-toe syndrome • Stenosis 2-4 cm associated with diffuse infrarenal atherosclerosis • Total occlusion of aorta	• Stenosis associated with abdominal aortic aneurysm
Peripheral artery[20,21]	• Intermittent claudication • Critical limb ischemia (rest pain, ulceration, gangrene, poor wound healing) • Improve inflow or outflow, before or after vascular bypass surgery • Bypass graft stenosis or anastomotic lesion • Impending amputation (to improve the level)	• Ulcerated plaque with atheroemboli • Long total occlusions (iliac > 4 cm, SFA > 10 cm), unless converted to shorter occlusion by thrombolysis • Long segment of infrapopliteal disease • Heavy, eccentric calcification • Lesion in or adjacent to an essential collateral	• Mild or moderate stenosis with no significant pressure gradient • Stenosis immediately adjacent to an aneurysm • Embolic occlusion
Renal artery[22-34]	• Renal artery stenosis > 50% and ≥ 1 factor in Table 36.31 • Renal transplant arterial stenosis or bypass stenosis producing hypertension, azotemia, or both	• Long occlusion • Stenosis associated with renal artery aneurysm	• Irreversible renal dysfunction • Hemodynamically-insignificant stenosis • Medically-unstable patient • Renal size < 6 cm
Visceral/ mesenteric[35,36]	• Chronic mesenteric ischemia (unexplained weight loss with postprandial pain and chronic nausea, vomiting, diarrhea) with significant stenoses or occlusion of ≥ 2 visceral vessels or acute symptoms in a patient who is not a surgical candidate. At this time surgery remains the first line of treatment	• Stenosis > 3 cm or ostial lesion of superior mesenteric or celiac artery • Occlusion of visceral vessels • Acute mesenteric ischemia	

Abbreviations: SFA = superficial femoral artery

Table 36.8. Medical Therapy for Claudication

Medication	Mechanism	Comments
Pentoxifylline (Trental)	Poorly understood; decreases fibrinogen, platelet adhesiveness, whole blood viscosity	FDA-approved for claudication; randomized trials show inconsistent benefit compared to placebo (dose: 400 mg TID)
Cilostazol (Pletal)	Phosphodiesterase-III inhibitor; vasodilator; inhibits platelet aggregation	FDA-approved for claudication; significant improvement in walking distance compared to placebo or pentoxifylline; may require 12 weeks to achieve a clinical response; contraindicated in heart failure (dose: 50-100 mg BID)
Naftidrofuryl	5-hydroxytryptamine-2 receptor antagonist	Available in Europe; increase in walking distance compared to placebo
Propionyl-L-carnitine	Improves energy metabolism in ischemic muscle	Available in Europe; significant improvement in walking distance, especially in patients with severe functional impairment
Beraprost sodium	PGI_2 analog with antiplatelet and vasodilating properties	Available in Europe; significant improvement in walking distance; may decrease adverse cardiac events

Table 36.9. Site of Vascular Access for Peripheral Vascular Intervention

Arterial Approach	Target Lesion Location
Retrograde femoral	Aorta; common iliac; proximal external iliac; renal; visceral
Antegrade femoral	Superficial femoral; profunda femoral; popliteal; infrapopliteal
Contralateral femoral (retrograde)[+]	Internal iliac and branches; distal external iliac; common femoral; can be used for femoral and popliteal vessels if antegrade approach is not feasible
Left brachial	Indicated if femoral access is not feasible
Left axillary	Indicated if no other routes are available

+ Internal mammary, Simmons Sidewinder, or Cobra catheter may be used to access the contralateral iliac artery

Table 36.10. Clinical Assessment of Acute Limb Ischemia[148]

Category	Description	Capillary Fill	Muscle Weakness	Sensory Loss	Doppler Signals Arterial	Venous
Viable	No risk	Intact	None	None	Audible	Audible
Threatened	Salvageable	Slow	Mild	Mild	Inaudible	Audible
Irreversible	Amputation	Absent	Profound	Profound	Inaudible	Inaudible

Table 36.11. Assessment of Chronic Limb Ischemia[148]

Grade	Category	Description	Criteria
0	0	No symptoms	Normal GXT
I	1	Mild claudication	Completes GXT; symptoms at > 500 yards; post-exercise ASP > 50 mmHg
	2	Moderate claudication	May complete GXT; symptoms at 50-500 yards
	3	Severe claudication	Fails GXT; symptoms at < 50 yards; post-exercise ASP < 50 mmHg
II	4	Rest pain	Resting ASP < 40 mmHg
	5	Minor tissue loss	Resting TSP < 40 mmHg
III	6	Major tissue loss	Resting TSP < 40 mmHg

Abbreviations:ASP = ankle systolic pressure; GXT = graded exercise test; TSP = toe systolic pressure

Table 36.12. Clinical Assessment After Revascularization: Limb Status Grade [148]

+3 = Markedly improved; normalized; no symptoms; ABI ≥ 9

+2 = Moderately improved; one category improved; ABI improved by > 0.10 but not normalized

+1 = Minimally improved; no category change but ABI < 0.1 improved

 0 = No change

-1 = Minimally worse; no category change; ABI > 0.1 decreased

-2 = Moderately worse; one category worse or unexpected minor amputation

-3 = Markedly worse; more than one category worse or unexpected major amputation

Table 36.13. Radiographic Views for Peripheral Angiography and Intervention[37]

Target Vessel	Projection
Carotid bifurcation	AP and oblique or lateral
Aortic arch (to open arch)	AP and LAO
Aortic arch (for brachiocephalic vessels)	45° LAO
Origin of mesenteric vessels	Lateral
Origin of renal arteries	Right: 15° RAO* Left: 15° LAO*
Common iliac bifurcation	Right: 15-30° LAO* Left: 15-30° RAO*
Common femoral bifurcation	Right: 15-30° RAO* Left: 15-30° LAO*

Abbreviations: AP = anteroposterior; LAO = left anterior oblique; RAO = right anterior oblique
* Varying degrees of cranial and caudal angulation may be necessary

Table 36.14. PTA and Balloon Size

Target Vessel	Balloon Diameter (mm)*
Common iliac artery	8 - 10
External iliac artery	6 - 8
Common femoral or superficial femoral artery	4 - 6
Popliteal artery	3 - 5
Tibial or peroneal artery (below trifurcation)	< 4**
Renal artery	4 - 8

*   Balloon length varies from 2-10 cm; use the shortest balloon to straddle the lesion, and kissing balloons for bifurcation lesions.
** Coronary balloons may be useful.

INDICATIONS AND RESULTS OF ENDOVASCULAR INTERVENTION

PTA success may be defined angiographically (residual stenosis < 15-20%), hemodynamically (no residual pressure gradient at rest, < 10 mmHg after nitroglycerin), or clinically (increase in ABI > 0.15, limb salvage, relief of claudication, or improvement in hypertension or renal function).[39] The lack of a single definition for PTA success and inconsistencies in the inclusion of technical failures when reporting long-term patency has made it difficult to compare different studies.[40] The selection of patients for lower extremity endovascular intervention should be guided by, but not limited to, accepted indications for surgical revascularization of peripheral vascular disease. For lower extremity revascularization, success, complications, and restenosis rates improve as intervention moves caudad from the inflow circulation (aortoiliac), to the outflow circulation (femoropopliteal), to the runoff bed (tibioperoneal).

AORTOILIAC INTERVENTION (Table 36.15)

A. **INDICATIONS.** Accepted indications for aortoiliac angioplasty (PTA) include lifestyle-limiting claudication, ischemic rest pain, non-healing ischemic ulcerations, gangrene, and the need to preserve vascular access. Focal, nontotal occlusions are ideal for PTA or stenting, whereas total occlusions are better suited for surgery (Table 36.13). AHA guidelines for iliac artery angioplasty are shown in Table 36.16.

B. **BALLOON ANGIOPLASTY (Table 36.15).** The procedural success rate of PTA for "optimal" aortoiliac stenoses is > 90% and 5-year patency is 80-85%. Immediate success (33-85%) and 2-4-year patency (75-100%) are lower for total occlusions.[149-151]

C. **STENTS.** Stents have dramatically improved the results of PTA.[152-162] Balloon-expandable stents have greater radial force and allow greater precision for placement in ostial lesions, whereas self-expanding stents are more flexible, can be easily delivered from a contralateral femoral approach, allow for normal vessel tapering, and are well-suited for long lesions (Table 36.17). Because iliac vessels are usually > 7 mm in diameter, the risk of thrombosis and restenosis after stenting is quite low.

   1. **Planned Stenting.** PTA vs. Palmaz stents have been evaluated in two randomized trials in patients with iliac stenoses, followed for up to 4 years.[163] Using life-table analysis, clinical benefit was achieved in 91% of stent patients at 1 year, 84% at 2 years, and 69% at 4 years; angiographic patency was 92-94% for stents and 69% for PTA[163,164] (Table 36.18).

   2. **Provisional Stenting.** Procedural success was 91% and 6-month patency was 99% for Palmaz stents after failed or suboptimal iliac angioplasty.[165] At 4 years, primary and secondary patency

were 86% and 95%, respectively. Excellent results have also been achieved with Wallstents after failed iliac angioplasty,[166] with 1-year patency in 95%, 2 year patency in 88%, and 4-year patency in 82%.[167] In a randomized trial of iliac PTA and provisional stenting compared to planned stenting in iliac arteries, final translesional pressure gradients and overall procedural success (89% vs. 81%) and quality of life at 2 years were similar.[168,305] Although stents were avoided in 63% of lesions, longer follow-up is necessary to evaluate the efficacy of this approach.

3. **Adjunctive Stent Placement.** Iliac stent placement may be also be used as an adjunct to surgical revascularization in selected patients. When iliac stenosis and superficial femoral arterial occlusion coexist in the same patient, iliac PTA and stenting can be used to secure inflow, followed by infrainguinal bypass to revascularize the outflow circulation. Using this strategy in patients with rest pain or tissue loss, limb salvage and patency rates at 5 years were 93% and 72%, respectively,[169] comparable to surgical reports.[171,171] A similar strategy can be employed to preserve inflow for femorofemoral bypass:[172] Outcomes at 7 years after femorofemoral bypass were similar for patients who did and did not require angioplasty or stenting of the inflow iliac artery.

Table 36.15. Classification of Aortoiliac Lesions for Percutaneous Intervention

Favorable	Unfavorable
Stenoses (nontotal occlusion)	Total occlusions
Noncalcified	Calcified
Discrete (≤ 3 cm)	Length ≥ 5 cm
Patent run-off vessels	Disease in run-off vessels
No diabetes	Diffuse diabetic arteriopathy
Aortoiliac occlusive disease	Aortoiliac aneurysmal disease
In-situ stenoses	Atheroembolic disease

Table 36.16. AHA Guidelines for Iliac Artery Angioplasty

Category	Lesion Description	Treatment Recommendations
1	Noncalcified, concentric lesion < 3 cm	PTA is procedure of choice
2	Noncalcified stenosis 3-5 cm Calcified or eccentric stenosis < 3 cm	Well-suited for PTA
3	Stenosis length 5-10 cm Chronic occlusion < 5 cm	Amenable to PTA; surgery may have longer patency
4	Stenosis length > 10 cm Chronic occlusion > 5 cm Associated abdominal aortic aneurysm	Surgery is superior to PTA

Abbreviations: PTA = percutaneous transluminal angioplasty

Table 36.17. Stents for Peripheral Vascular Disease

Self-Expanding Stents
   Thermal Memory (nitinol)
      SMART stent (Cordis)
      Memotherm (Bard)
      Symphony (Boston Scientific)
      IntraCoil (IntraTherapeutics)
      Dynalink, Acculink (Guidant)
   Spring-Loaded (stainless-steel)
      Wallstent (Boston Scientific)

Balloon-Expandable Stents
   Palmaz, Corinthian (Cordis)
   MegaLink (Guidant)
   Flexible Biliary, Extra Support Biliary Plus, Bridge X3 Biliary (Medtronic)
   Double strut, XS (IntraTherapeutics)

Covered Stents
   Wallgraft (Boston Scientific Scimed)
   Others: Corvita, World Medical, Hemobahn

Table 36.18. Results of Aortoiliac Angioplasty and Stenting[54-56,306,307]

| Target Vessel | Success (%) | Long-Term Patency (%) | | |
		1-year	2-year	3-year
Aorta	83 - 100	83 - 100	83 - 96	70 - 92
Iliac artery	73 - 100	63 - 100	58 - 95	32 - 92
Aortoiliac bifurcation	100	-	87	-

Abbreviations: FMD = fibromuscular dysplasia; ARAS = atherosclerotic renal artery stenosis; - = not reported

FEMORAL-POPLITEAL ARTERY INTERVENTION (Table 36.19)

A. **INDICATIONS.** The indications for femoral-popliteal artery intervention are similar to those for aortoiliac intervention and include lifestyle-limiting claudication, rest pain, and threatened limb loss with non-healing ulcers or gangrene. However, the benefit of percutaneous revascularization for superficial femoral artery (SFA) disease is not as well-established as aortoiliac intervention. In general, better immediate and long-term outcomes are achieved in nondiabetics with claudication and focal (< 5 cm) stenoses compared to diabetics with critical limb ischemia and long (> 7 cm) occlusions.

B. **BALLOON ANGIOPLASTY.** Procedural success for femoropopliteal PTA is 70-97%; success is higher for stenoses than for total occlusions,[173-175] and patency at 3-5 years is 50%-70%. [150,151] A randomized trial of PTA vs. femoropopliteal bypass surgery in selected patients with severe stenoses demonstrated similar event-free survival and ankle-brachial indices at 3 years. The long-term patency of femoropopliteal PTA depends on several clinical and angiographic characteristics (Table 36.20).[177-181] Factors favorably influencing late outcome include proximal, noncalcified, focal stenoses in patients with claudication; adverse factors include distal disease, total occlusion, critical limb ischemia, and poor run-off.[166,169,184,185]

C. **STENTS.** In general, it is difficult to interpret the results of stenting in the femoropopliteal circulation for several reasons. First, older studies employed large vessel stents with high metal surface areas, which led to high recurrence rates. Second, warfarin was commonly prescribed rather than current antiplatelet therapy, which may have contributed to stent thrombosis and reocclusion. Third, newer nitinol stents may be easier to precisely cover the lesion (no shortening) and may have less restenosis than stainless steel stents. Finally, "restenosis" may be less important than "patency"; secondary 2-year patency rates of 70-80% are not substantially different than 2-year patency after bypass surgery.[302] Possible indications for provisional stenting in the femoropopliteal circulation are described in Table 36.21. Using these criteria, technical success was achieved in 99% of patients,[182] and 6-month restenosis rates were 4.4% for the proximal SFA, 9.8% for the mid-SFA, 18% for the distal SFA, and 20% for the popliteal artery. Risk factors for stent restenosis are shown in Table 36.22. Although primary patency for Palmaz stents decreased from 81% at 1 year to 65% at 4 years, secondary patency was > 95%.[182] Among 15 cases in which self-expanding Wallstents were utilized after failed PTA, 20-month primary patency was 20% and secondary patency was 54%.[166] While these results were less favorable than for Palmaz stents, the patient populations were not comparable. One advantage of self-expanding stents (such as the Wallstent, IntraCoil, or SMART stent) in the femoropopliteal circulation is that there is no risk of external compression or deformation of the stent, as with balloon-expandable stents.

Table 36.19. Impact of Target Vessel Location and Morphology on PTA Success[21,22,57-65]

Characteristic	Location	Immediate Success (%)	3-Year Patency (%)
All lesions	Iliofemoral	90	75
	Femoropopliteal	85	60
Ideal lesion*	Iliofemoral	95	90
	Femoropopliteal	90	75
Poor lesion**	Iliofemoral		-
	Femoropopliteal	70	20

Abbreviations: PTA = percutaneous transluminal angioplasty; - = not reported
* Focal stenosis; good runoff; claudication
** Occlusion length > 9 cm; poor runoff; limb salvage

Table 36.20. Determinants of Vessel Patency After Femoropopliteal Angioplasty[52]

Variable	2-Year Patency (%)	p-Value
Claudication	64	0.06
Critical limb ischemia	50	
2-3 vessel run-off	68	0.02
0-1 vessel run-off	49	
Single stenosis	74	0.06
Multiple stenoses	63	
Occlusion length < 10 cm	59	0.06
Occlusion length ≥ 10 cm	47	
Diabetes	68	0.05
No diabetes	54	
Male	68	0.06
Female	56	

Table 36.21. Potential Indications for Stenting After Femoropopliteal PTA[182]

Residual diameter stenosis > 30%

Flow-limiting dissection

Restenosis after PTA

Abbreviations: PTA = percutaneous transluminal angioplasty

Table 36.22. Risk Factors for Restenosis After Femoropopliteal Stenting[182]

Lesion length > 3 cm

Vessel diameter < 7 mm

Multiple stents

INFRAPOPLITEAL INTERVENTION (Table 36.23)

A. **INDICATIONS.** Infrapopliteal PTA is generally reserved for patients with severe ischemia, such as rest pain, tissue necrosis, or threatened limb loss. These patients usually have limited options for surgical revascularization, and unsuccessful PTA is sometimes followed by amputation.[195-198]

B. **BALLOON ANGIOPLASTY.** Procedural success for infrapopliteal PTA is 85% and 2-year patency varies from 40-85%.[192-197] The small size of these arteries often mandates the use of coronary angioplasty wires and balloons.[200,201] Although restenosis rates are high, PTA frequently enhances blood flow to heal ischemic ulcers, even if restenosis occurs.

C. **STENTS.** In our practice, stents are reserved for bail-out indications, not for planned interventions. Given the small size of these arteries, coronary stents are frequently employed.

Table 36.23. Results of Infrapopliteal Angioplasty[67-69]

Series	N	Success (%)			Complications (%)	
		Technical	Early	Late	Major	Minor
Bull[69] (1992)	168	83	77	67	11	8
Brown[67] (1988)	12	75	66	50	17	-
Schwarten[68] (1988)	98	97	88	86	2	1

RENAL ARTERY INTERVENTION

A. **INCIDENCE OF RENAL ARTERY STENOSIS.** The two most common causes of renal artery stenosis are fibromuscular dysplasia (FMD) and atherosclerotic renal artery stenosis (ARAS). FMD is rare, occurs most often in women < 50 years of age, and affects the distal half of the renal arterial circulation. In contrast, ARAS is highly prevalent among elderly patients with other manifestations of atherosclerosis, and typically affects the renal artery ostium and proximal vessel (Table 36.24). The prevalence of ARAS increases from < 5% of patients under age 50 to 60% of patients > 50 years with hypertension, other manifestations of coronary or peripheral vascular disease, and unexplained chronic renal insufficiency (Table 36.25). ARAS is also progressive; nearly 60% of patients with renal artery stenosis < 50% will develop progressive stenosis or occlusion within 2-4 years (Table 36.26).

B. **CLINICAL MANIFESTATIONS.** Since renal artery stenosis is not associated with symptoms until there is end-organ injury, the diagnosis relies on a high index of suspicion and confirmation by noninvasive or imaging modalities. Clinical features which increase suspicion for renal artery stenosis are shown in Table 36.27. In general, there are two distinct clinical syndromes associated with renal artery stenosis: hypertension and ischemic nephropathy (Table 36.28). In patients with FMD, hypertension is usually renin-dependent (renovascular hypertension) and relief of obstruction usually improves or cures hypertension. In contrast, the vast majority of patients with ARAS have essential hypertension, which usually persists despite successful renal artery revascularization. Patients with ARAS and malignant or accelerated hypertension often have a component of renin-dependent hypertension superimposed on a background of essential hypertension. Renal revascularization often corrects the malignant phase and improves blood pressure control. Ischemic nephropathy, defined as renal ischemia leading to excretory dysfunction, is a common manifestation of ARAS but virtually never occurs with FMD.

C. **DIAGNOSIS.** Functional studies and vascular imaging studies are used to confirm the diagnosis of renal artery stenosis (Table 36.29), but none are suitable as mass-screening tools. Imaging studies are most important to establish the diagnosis when used in patients with high clinical suspicion for renal artery stenosis. The best imaging method is dependent on local skills and preference, but usually involves magnetic resonance angiography (MRA) or renal duplex ultrasound (RDU) (Table 36.30). Patients who require coronary angiography may be considered for abdominal aortography and renal angiography if risk factors for renal artery stenosis are present (Table 36.31). Functional studies (e.g., captopril-stimulated renin, renal vein renin) which assess activation of the renin-angiotensin system are not useful in patients with suspected ARAS due to the high prevalence of essential (not renovascular) hypertension.

D. **INDICATIONS.** Indications for renal artery revascularization are controversial and have not been established by any randomized trial (Table 36.32). Stenting is the preferred method of percutaneous revascularization for aorto-ostial lesions, restenosis lesions, and following suboptimal PTA (residual stenosis ≥ 30% or dissection).

1. **Hypertension.** Patients with refractory hypertension and FMD should be treated with PTA; cure of hypertension is expected in > 75% of such patients (Table 36.33). In contrast, patients with refractory hypertension and ARAS are rarely cured by any form of surgical or percutaneous revascularization (Table 36.34), although blood pressure may be easier to manage and medication requirements may decrease.[241]

2. **Renal Insufficiency.** Patients with moderate renal insufficiency (serum creatinine > 2 mg/dL) and ARAS may benefit from percutaneous revascularization by stabilizing or reversing renal dysfunction, although this has not been confirmed in any randomized study (Table 36.35). Renal revascularization for unilateral ARAS in the setting of advanced renal dysfunction (serum creatinine > 3 mg/dL) does not impact overall renal function since severe bilateral parenchymal disease is present. In contrast, patients with bilateral renal artery stenosis may benefit from bilateral renal revascularization, although it is often difficult to distinguish advanced parenchymal disease from ischemic nephropathy. Several factors have been proposed to help make this distinction, but the value of any single factor in a given patient has uncertain predictive value. In our experience, thinning of the renal cortex and poor cortical blood flow are often associated with irreversible nephropathy. Several studies identified baseline creatinine > 1.5 mg/dL as the strongest independent predictor of late morbidity and mortality after surgical or percutaneous revascularization (Table 36.36), suggesting that renal revascularization should not be delayed until there is marked elevation of creatinine.

3. **Renal Preservation.** Revascularization of isolated renal artery stenosis (without uncontrolled hypertension or elevated creatinine) to preserve renal function is controversial. Nuclear split renal function studies may be useful to identify asymmetry in renal perfusion and serve as a baseline for late follow-up. Our preference is to revascularize unilateral renal artery stenosis if ipsilateral blood flow is ≤ 40% of total renal blood flow. A randomized trial is currently in progress to address this issue.

4. **Unstable Angina or Heart Failure.** Renal artery stent placement in patients with refractory hypertension, unstable angina or heart failure, and unilateral or bilateral renal artery stenosis resulted in improved blood pressure control in 74% of patients at 6 months.[220,221]

E. **CONTRAINDICATIONS.** Patients with bulky, ulcerative atherosclerosis in the abdominal aorta ("shaggy" aorta) are at increased risk for cholesterol emboli during catheter manipulation in the infrarenal aorta using the femoral approach. In such patients, brachial access should be considered. Patients with renal artery aneurysms may be at higher risk of rupture or perforation during renal intervention. Diffuse intrarenal atherosclerosis and poor cortical blood flow usually indicate advanced nephrosclerosis. In general, renal revascularization should not be considered to preserve renal function in these patients.

F. BALLOON ANGIOPLASTY (Table 36.37). PTA is the accepted treatment for FMD associated with renovascular hypertension refractory to medical therapy.[223-227] In contrast, PTA for ARAS is associated with poor procedural success[228-234] and 6-month restenosis rates > 50%.[235] Aorto-ostial renal artery lesions are unsuitable for PTA because of elastic recoil and dissection.[236-239] A randomized trial of PTA vs. stenting for ARAS has progressed slowly because of operator unwillingness to use PTA alone.

G. STENTS (Table 36.37). Renal artery stenting is more effective than PTA for improving residual stenosis and abolishing translesional pressure gradients.[239] Techniques for renal stenting include the "bare-wire" technique (which is now obsolete), catheter-exchange techniques, direct guide technique, and the "no-touch" technique (Table 36.38).[271] There are no FDA-approved renal stents, although several balloon-expandable stents have been employed and many companies are developing low-profile balloon expandable stents for renal revascularization. Contemporary procedural success rates are 90-100% and restenosis rates at 1 year are 10-25%.[240,241] Precision of stent placement and the need for radial support (especially for aorto-ostial lesions) favor use of balloon-expandable stents over self-expanding stents.

H. COMPLICATIONS. Complications of renal artery stenting are described in Table 36.39.

I. CONTEMPORARY APPROACH TO PATIENTS WITH RENOVASCULAR DISEASE. There is now a simplified approach to the diagnosis of renal artery stenosis, which relies on a high-index of suspicion (based on clinical markers associated with renal artery stenosis) and confirmation by vascular imaging studies (Figure 36.10). Patients with confirmed renal artery stenosis undergo baseline evaluation to determine the extent of renal impairment based on serum creatinine, urinalysis, and nuclear assessment of GFR (total and single-kidney GFR). Patients are then stratified into treatment groups based on the extent of renal artery stenosis (unilateral vs. bilateral) and the presence of end-organ injury (Figure 36.11). Revascularization is generally recommended for patients with unilateral or bilateral disease and end-organ injury, and for patients with unilateral disease and hypoperfusion to the involved kidney. Patients with chronic renal failure rarely benefit from unilateral renal artery revascularization since advanced parenchymal disease is invariably present.

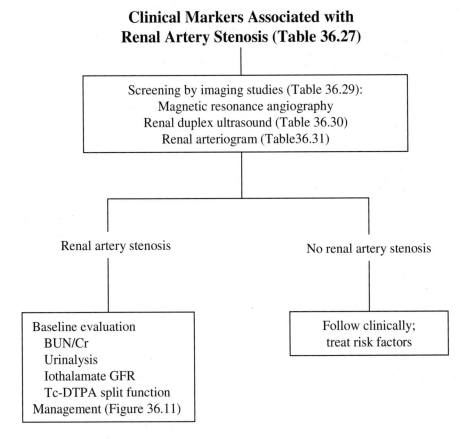

Figure 36.10. Approach to Suspected Renovascular Disease

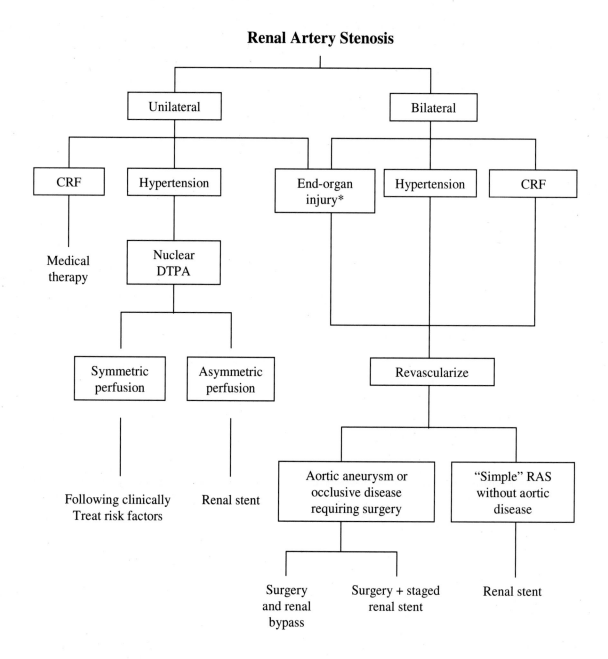

Figure 36.11. Management of Renal Artery Stenosis

CRF = chronic renal failure; RAS = renal artery stenosis
* Hypertensive emergency with TIA, stroke, intracranial hemorrhage, unstable angina, MI, pulmonary edema, or severe retinopathy

Table 36.24. Renal Artery Stenosis: Comparison of Fibromuscular Dysplasia and Atherosclerotic Renal Artery Stenosis (ARAS)

	Fibromuscular Dysplasia	ARAS
Natural history	Progressive dissection, thrombosis	Progressive stenosis, occlusion
Etiology	Unknown	Atherosclerosis
Incidence	Rare	Common
Age	< 50	> 50
Gender	Female >> Male	Female = Male
Location	Mid, distal 1/3	Ostial, proximal 1/3
Hypertension syndrome	Renovascular hypertension	Essential hypertension
Excretory dysfunction	None	Common
Comorbidities	Few	Coronary artery disease, peripheral vascular disease, diabetes mellitus
Primary treatment	Antihypertensive therapy with angiotensin converting enzyme inhibitor	Control atherosclerosis (aspirin, smoking cessation, risk factor modification)
Revascularization	PTA for refractory hypertension	Stent for refractory hypertension and possibly ischemic nephropathy; surgery may be reasonable for severe renal and aortic disease

Abbreviations: ARAS = atherosclerotic renal artery stneosis; PTA = percutaneous transluminal angioplasty

Table 36.25. Estimated Prevalence of Renal Artery Stenosis

Patient Population	Prevalence (%)
General population	0.1
Age < 50 with hypertension	4-5*
Age > 50 with:	
Hypertension	15[+]
Hypertension + CAD	20-30[+]
Malignant hypertension	30[+]
Hypertension + CAD + PVD	40-60[+]
Hypertension + CAD + CRF	40-60[+]

Abbreviations: CAD = coronary artery disease; CRF = chronic renal failure PVD = peripheral vascular disease
*   Fibromuscular dysplasia
\+   Atherosclerotic renal artery stenosis

Table 36.26. Natural History of Atherosclerotic Renal Artery Stenosis

Study	N	Follow-up (mos)	Progression (%)	Occlusion (%)
Caps[208] (1998)	170	33	51	9
Zierler[215] (1994)	80	-	42	11
Tollefson[183] (1991)	48	54	53	9
Schreiber[213] (1984)	85	52	44	16

Table 36.27. Clinical Markers Associated with Renal Artery Stenosis

Hypertension	Renal Function	Other
Abrupt onset, age < 50* Abrupt onset, age > 50** Accelerated hypertension Malignant hypertension	Unexplained acute or chronic azotemia ACEI-induced azotemia	Unilateral small kidney Unexplained hypokalemia Abdominal bruit Flank bruit Severe retinopathy "Flash" pulmonary edema CHF with normal LV function

Abbreviations: ACEI = angiotensin converting enzyme inhibitor; CHF = congestive heart failure; LV = left ventricular
* Fibromuscular dysplasia
**Atherosclerotic renal artery stenosis

Table 36.28. Renovascular Syndromes

	Renin-dependent Hypertension	Hypertension and RAS	Ischemic Nephropathy
Patient Characteristics			
Age	< 50	> 50	> 50
Gender	Female > Male	Female = Male	Female = Male
Comorbidities	Few	PVD, CAD, DM	PVD, CAD, DM
Etiology	FMD > ARAS	ARAS >> FMD	ARAS
Treatment			
Primary	ACEI	Risk factor modification	Risk factor modification
Secondary*	PTA	Stent	Stent, surgery

Abbreviations: ACEI = angiotensin converting enzyme inhibitor; ARAS = atherosclerotic renal artery stenosis; CAD = coronary artery disease; DM = diabetes mellitus; FMD = fibromuscular dysplasia; PTA = percutaneous transluminal angioplasty; PVD = peripheral vascular disease
* If primary treatment fails

Table 36.29 Renal Artery Stenosis: Noninvasive Assessment

Study	Rationale	Advantages	Disadvantages
— PHYSIOLOGIC STUDIES TO ASSESS RENIN-ANGIOTENSIN ACTIVATION —			
Peripheral renin activity (PRA)	Measure PRA relative to sodium excretion	Assess activation of RAS	Not useful as a screening test for ARAS; low predictive accuracy for RVH; influenced by medications and other conditions
Captopril-stimulated renin	Captopril induces a decrease in perfusion pressure distal to a stenosis	Enhances renin release from stenotic kidney	Not useful as a screening test for ARAS; low predictive accuracy for RVH; influenced by medications and other conditions
Renal vein renin	Relative comparison of renin release from each kidney	Lateralization predicts improvement in BP after revascularization	Failure to lateralize does NOT predict failure to improve BP; not useful as a screening test; influenced by medications and other conditions
— FUNCTIONAL STUDIES TO ASSESS OVERALL RENAL FUNCTION —			
Serum Cr	Measures overall renal function	Easy to measure; inexpensive blood test	Poor screening test for renovascular disease; not sensitive to early changes in renal mass or single-kidney function
Urinalysis	Assess urinary sediment and degree of proteinuria	Easy to measure; inexpensive urine test	Nonspecific; poor screening test for renovascular disease; influenced by many other conditions
Nuclear GFR	Measures overall GFR	Accurate in patients with normal and impaired renal function	Expensive; time consuming (3-6 hrs); not suitable as a screening test for renovascular disease
— PERFUSION STUDIES TO ASSESS DIFFERENTIAL RENAL BLOOD FLOW —			
Captopril renography (Tc-MAG3)	Captopril-induced fall in filtration pressure amplifies differences in renal perfusion	Normal study excludes RVH when renal function is normal	Not useful as a screening test for ARAS; unreliable when serum Cr > 2 mg/dL
Nuclear split function (Tc-DTPA or Tc-MAG3)	Estimates fractional flow to each kidney	Allows calculation of single-kidney GFR; asymmetry in renal blood flow suggests renovascular disease	Less reliable with advanced renal dysfunction or with obstructive uropathy
— VASCULAR IMAGING TECHNIQUES —			
Intravenous DSA	Images the renal arteries	Intravenous injection	Low sensitivity; contrast load may be deleterious in patients with renal dysfunction; not a useful screening test
Renal duplex ultrasound (RDU) (Table 36.30)	Images the renal arteries and measures flow velocity to assess stenosis severity	Inexpensive; widely available; noninvasive	Heavily dependent on operator technique; less useful in obese patients or those with FMD or accessory renal arteries

Table 36.29 Renal Artery Stenosis: Noninvasive Assessment

Study	Rationale	Advantages	Disadvantages
— VASCULAR IMAGING TECHNIQUES (cont.) —			
Magnetic resonance angiography (MRA)	Images the renal arteries and perirenal aorta	Excellent images; useful in patients with renal dysfunction; noninvasive	Expensive; less useful for FMD; imaging artifacts with stents
Computed tomography angiography (CTA)	Images the renal arteries and perirenal aorta	Excellent images; no artifacts with stents; noninvasive	Not widely available; contrast load may be deleterious in patients with renal dysfunction
Digital subtraction arteriography (DSA)	Images the renal arteries, aorta, and intrarenal circulation	Excellent images; allows physiologic assessment (pressure gradients)	Invasive; contrast load may be deleterious in patients with renal dysfunction

Abbreviations: ARAS = atherosclerotic renal artery stenosis; BP = blood pressure; Cr = serum creatinine; FMD = fibromuscular dysplasia; GFR = glomerular filtration rate; RAS = renin-angiotensin system

Table 36.30. Renal Duplex Ultrasound Criteria for Renal Artery Stenosis[79]

	Peak Systolic Velocity	Renal-to-Aorta Ratio
Normal	< 180 cm/sec	< 3.5
Diameter stenosis < 60%	≥ 180 cm/sec	< 3.5
Diameter stenosis 60-95%	≥ 180 cm/sec	> 3.5
Total occlusion	No renal signal	No renal signal

Table 36.31. Possible Indications for Renal Arteriography During Cardiac Catheterization*

Malignant hypertension

Persistent hypertension despite 3 or more medications

Unexplained heart failure or flash pulmonary edema

Known asymmetry in renal dimensions

Unexplained serum Cr > 1.5 mg/dL

ACEI-induced renal failure

Abbreviations: ACEI = angiotensin converting enzyme inhibitor; Cr = serum creatinine
*   Renal angiography is reasonable in patients with refractory hypertension or signs/symptoms of end-organ injury to brain, heart, or kidneys

Table 36.32. Therapeutic Options for Patients with Renal Artery Stenosis

Treatment	Impact on Hypertension	Impact on Nephropathy	Comments
Medical therapy	Effective for control of hypertension	No confirmed benefit for reversing or stabilizing renal function	Mandatory for risk-factor modification (ASA, lipid-lowering therapy, smoking cessation). Good randomized trials are needed to assess impact of medical therapy
PTA	Effective for refractory hypertension in patients with FMD; not superior to medical therapy in patients with ARAS	Uncertain role; complex relationship between revascularization vs. complications (distal embolization, contrast nephropathy)	Not useful for ostial ARAS because of suboptimal results
Stents	Not evaluated in patients with FMD; effective for achieving "statistical" improvement in blood pressure; not clearly superior to medical therapy	Same as for PTA. Anecdotal experience suggests benefit if patient does not have advanced nephropathy or parenchymal disease	Treatment of choice in most patients with ARAS if revascularization is needed
Bypass surgery	Not employed for FMD; not clearly useful in patients with ARAS	Anecdotal experience suggests possible benefit in the absence of advanced renal dysfunction	Used infrequently in patients with extensive aortic aneurysmal or occlusive disease; perioperative mortality 2-6%

Abbreviations: ARAS = atherosclerotic renal artery stenosis; FMD = fibromuscular dysplasia; PTA = percutaneous transluminal angioplasty

Table 36.33. Long-term Outcome After Angioplasty for Hypertension and Renal Artery Stenosis

Series	Follow-up (mos)	Etiology	Hypertension (%)		
			Cured	Improved	No Response
Lossino[48] (1994)	60	FMD	57	21	21
		ARAS	12	51	37
Tegtmeyer[24,46,47] (1992)	39	FMD	37	63	0
		ARAS	25	55	20
Miller[27] (1985)	6	FMD	85	15	0
		ARAS	25	58	17
Sos[25,33] (1983)	16	FMD	59	33	8
		ARAS	27	60	13

Abbreviations: FMD = fibromuscular dysplasia; ARAS = atherosclerotic renal artery stenosis

Table 36.34. Impact of Renal Artery Revascularization on Hypertension

Study	N	Technique	Cure (%)
Burket[274] (2000)	127	Stent	8
DRASTIC[268] (2000)	78	PTA	7
Rocha-Singh[273] (1999)	150	Stent	6
Rodriguez-Lopez[270] (1999)	108	Stent	11
Dorros[317] (1998)	163	Stent	1
Henry[326] (1996)	151	Stent	20
Iannone[318] (1996)	63	Stent	7
Hansen[319] (1992)	200	Surgery	21
Weibull[235] (1991)	61	Surgery	15
Canzanello[231] (1989)	100	PTA	11

Abbreviations: PTA = percutaneous transluminal angioplasty

Table 36.35. Impact of Renal Artery Revascularization on Renal Function

Study	N	Technique	Stable/Improved (%)	Worse (%)
Watson[269] (2000)	33	Stent	72	28
Rodriguez-Lopez[270] (1999)	105	Stent	96	4
ven de Ven[267] (1999)	24	Stent	92	8
Rocha-Singh[273] (1999)	150	Stent	92	8
Steinbach[324] (1997)	222	Surgery	71	29
Taylor[320] (1997)	29	Stent	62	38
Harden[321] (1997)	32	Stent	69	31
Iannone[318] (1996)	63	Stent	82	18
Dorros[240] (1995)	70	Stent	78	22
Pattynama[325] (1994)	40	PTA	60	40
Libertino[322] (1992)	91	Surgery	84	16
Hansen[319] (1992)	70	Surgery	85	15
Brendenberg[323] (1992)	40	Surgery	80	20
Weibull[235] (1991)	61	Surgery	85	15
Rees[80] (1991)	28	Stent	86	14

Abbreviations: PTA = percutaneous transluminal angioplasty

Table 36.36. Predictors of Outcome After Renal Artery Revascularization

Outcome Predictors	Risk Ratio
Predictors of Mortality[317]	
Baseline Cr ≥ 1.5 mg/dL	5.0
Diabetes	2.5
Age ≥ 70	1.9
Predictors of Improvement in Blood Pressure[273]	
Baseline MAP > 110 mmHg	2.9
Bilateral renal artery stenosis	4.6

Abbreviations: Cr = serum creatinine; MAP = mean arterial pressure

Table 36.37. Results of Percutaneous Renal Artery Revascularization

Series	Technique	N	Initial Success (%)	Long-term Patency (%)	Follow-up (months)
Burket[274] (2000)	Stent	127	100	-	-
van de Ven[267] (1999)	PTA (ostial)	42	57	29	6
	Stent (ostial)	42	88	75	
Rodriguez-Lopez[270] (1999)	Stent	108	98	-	-
Rocha-Singh[273] (1999)	Stent	150	97	88	13
White[84] (1995)	Stent	98	99	72	-
Tegtmeyer[41] (1984)	PTA	149	94	93*	72
Sos[25] (1983)	PTA	101	79	-	-
Colapinto[42] (1982)	PTA	68	85	81	36
Puijlaert[44] (1981)	PTA	54	96	70	-
Schwarten[45] (1981)	PTA	70	93	71	6
Katzen[43] (1979)	PTA	17	94	75	12

Abbreviations: PTA = percutaneous transluminal angioplasty; - = not reported
* Includes successful redilatations

Table 36.38. Renal Artery Stenting Techniques

Technique	Description	Comments
Bare-wire technique	Selective engagement of renal artery with 4-6F diagnostic catheter. Wire is advanced to distal vessel, exchanged for a support wire, and catheter is removed. PTA/stenting is performed, relying on landmarks	Only advantage is to minimize sheath size. Lack of support and inability to inject contrast are strong arguments against this technique
Catheter-exchange technique	Selective engagement of renal artery with 4-6F diagnostic catheter. Wire is advanced to distal vessel and exchanged for a support wire; catheter is removed and replaced by a guiding catheter or long sheath. PTA/stenting is performed	Safe technique to minimize contact between guide and infrarenal aorta; requires multiple exchanges; useful for aorto-ostial stenoses
Direct guide technique	Direct selective engagement with a guiding catheter	Guiding catheter manipulation in the aorta may scrape the aorta or injure the renal artery ostium. Acceptable technique for non-ostial renal artery stenosis and when the perirenal aorta does not have significant plaque
No-touch technique[271]	Modification of the direct guide technique. The guide catheter is advanced to the peri-renal aorta, leaving a 0.035-inch guidewire extending beyond the catheter tip. After crossing the lesion with a suitable guidewire, the 0.035-inch wire is removed and the guide positioned at the ostium. PTA/stenting is performed	Useful technique to minimize contact between the guide and aorta for those who prefer a direct guide technique. Sometimes may be difficult to cross the lesion, since guide alignment may not be coaxial.

Table 36.39. Complications of Renal Artery Stent Placement

Study	N	Technique	Success	Complications (%)					
				Death	Bleeding	VSR	Emb or occl	CE	RS
van de Ven[267] (1999)	42	PTA	57	-	19	5	5	10	71
	42	Stent	88	-	19	7	7	10	25
Rocha-Singh[273] (1999)	150	Stent	97	1.5	-	-	5.9	-	
White[241] (1997)	-	Stent	-	-	7	1	2	-	-

Abbreviations: CE = cholesterol embolization; Emb or occl = renal embolism or occlusion; RS = restenosis; VSR = vascular repair

DIALYSIS ACCESS INTERVENTION

A. **INDICATIONS.** The most common types of dialysis access are the endogenous arteriovenous fistula (using the radial or ulnar artery in a side-to-side anastomosis with its adjacent vein) and the polytetrafluoroethylene (PTFE) graft (between the brachial artery and the brachial or cephalic vein). Both types of access are subject to failure, with patency rates of 60-70% at 1 year and 50% at 4 years.[242] Failure is most frequently due to intimal hyperplasia, thrombosis, and stenosis at the anastomosis or in the draining veins (Table 36.40). Subclavian vein stenoses due to trauma from temporary dialysis catheters can also occur. Failed access is a frequent cause of hospitalization, and PTA has been shown to decrease the rate of PTFE graft failure,[243] avoid repeat surgical revisions, and prolong the functional life of the dialysis access site (Table 36.41).[244-246]

B. **BALLOON ANGIOPLASTY.** In one study, PTA success was 96% and restenosis occurred in 20%. Repeat PTA is feasible.[247,248]

C. **STENTS.** Stents may overcome some of the problems of PTA.[249-251] In our experience, Palmaz stents and Wallstents allow resumption of hemodialysis within 24 hours in 97% and continued use of the access site in 90% at 5 months.

D. **THROMBOLYSIS.** In the past, thrombosed dialysis access sites were managed with surgical thrombectomy and revision. However, successful recanalization with catheter-directed thrombolytic agents, thrombectomy with the AngioJet, and PTA can be achieved in up to 90% of patients, which may be a reasonable alternative to surgical thrombectomy.

Table 36.40. Frequency and Location of PTFE Graft Failure for Dialysis Access

Location	Graft Failure (%)
Venous anastomosis	58-77
Arterial anastomosis	7-19
Central/distal vein	< 10
Unknown	4-35

Table 36.41. Advantages of PTA for Dialysis Fistula Stenoses

Additional vein is not needed

Patency rates are equivalent to surgical revision

No need for temporary dialysis access

Outpatient procedure

SUBCLAVIAN AND INNOMINATE INTERVENTION

A. **INDICATIONS.** Patients with subclavian or innominate artery occlusive disease may have vertebrobasilar symptoms (subclavian "steal" syndrome, due to flow reversal in the vertebral artery), upper extremity claudication, limb-threatening ischemia, or myocardial ischemia (when antegrade flow to the internal mammary artery bypass graft is compromised) (Table 36.42). The conventional treatment in the past was carotid-to-subclavian artery bypass,[252] which was associated with substantial morbidity (15-33%) and mortality (5-8%).[253,254]

B. **PTA AND STENTS (Table 36.43).** Percutaneous intervention may be preferable to surgery in patients with symptomatic subclavian or innominate artery stenosis, although total occlusions may increase the risk of embolic complications.[254,255] Stents have facilitated treatment, with success rates approaching 100% in published studies.[256,257]

Table 36.42. Indications for Subclavian and Innominate Artery Revascularization

Subclavian Steal Syndrome

Upper extremity claudication

Myocardial ischemia due to compromised flow to internal mammary artery graft

Compromised flow to axillary-femoral bypass graft

Preservation of flow to internal mammary artery in patients requiring coronary artery bypass surgery

Preservation of flow to subclavian artery in patients requiring subclavian-carotid bypass surgery

Table 36.43. Stenting of the Innominate or Subclavian Artery

Study	N	Success	Comments
Hadjipetrou[295] (1999)	108	97	Death/CVA (0%); minor complications (6%); recurrence at 20-months (3%)
Al-Mubarak[296] (1999)	38	92	No complications; restenosis at 20-months (6%); recurrent symptoms (9%)
Al-Mubarak[296] (1999)	136	100	Metanalysis
Sullivan[86] (1995)	33	94	Distal embolization (6%); vertebral artery occlusion (3%); vascular injury (12%)
Registry	258	97	No major complications; minor complications (3.2%). Outcome at 9-months: restenosis (11%); primary patency (89%); secondary patency (98.5%)

EXTRACRANIAL CAROTID ARTERY INTERVENTION

A. **BACKGROUND.** The treatment of extracranial carotid artery disease requires an in-depth understanding of the anatomy of the extra- and intracranial circulations (Figure 36.12) and the natural history, pathophysiology, and treatment of cerebrovascular disease (Table 36.44). The risk of stroke due to extracranial carotid disease is dependent on stenosis severity, plaque characteristics (ulcerated, soft, fibrotic), collateral circulation, and symptomatic status of the patient. Symptomatic patients have a much higher risk of cerebrovascular events than asymptomatic patients, and patients with more severe (> 90%) stenoses have a worse prognosis. In stark contrast to myocardial ischemia and infarction, cerebrovascular symptoms are more often due to thromboembolism (80%) than in-situ occlusion of the carotid artery (20%) (Table 36.1). The clinical impact of occlusive carotid artery disease is very dependent on intracranial collateral circulation (Circle of Willis), formed by the posterior circulation (vertebral and basilar arteries) and the contralateral internal carotid artery. To appropriately assess the potential significance of a carotid occlusion, the intracranial circulation should be defined by selective angiography.

B. **NON-INVASIVE DIAGNOSIS.** Baseline evaluation begins with a careful history (for neurologic and other symptoms of atherosclerosis) and physical examination (to establish baseline neurological status, auscultate for cervical and clavicular bruits, and measure bilateral brachial artery pressure). Non-invasive assessment should include duplex ultrasound to estimate disease severity and characterize the plaque (Table 36.4). Magnetic resonance angiography (MRA) can be performed to image the carotid and intracranial circulations, and a CT scan (with and without contrast) is useful to identify prior cerebral infarction.

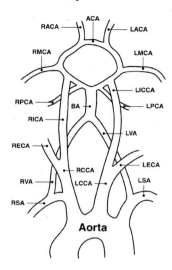

Figure 36.12. Extracranial and Intracranial Circulation

ACA = anterior communicating artery; BA = basilar artery; R/L ACA = right/left anterior cerebral artery; R/L CCA = right/left common carotid artery; R/L ECA = right/left external carotid artery; R/L ICA = right/left internal carotid artery; R/L MCA = right/left middle cerebral artery; R/L PCA = right/left posterior cerebral artery; R/L SA = right/left subclavian artery; R/L VA = right/left verterbral artery

C. ANGIOGRAPHY. We recommend diagnostic angiography using nonionic contrast and 5 or 6F diagnostic catheters, beginning with a pigtail catheter for arch aortography and then selective extracranial and intracranial carotid and vertebral angiography. It is important to record delayed images to identify collateral vessels, and to be aware of the potential risks of catheter manipulation (in the Asymptomatic Carotid Artery Study [ACAS], stroke due to diagnostic angiography occurred in 1.2%).

D. CAROTID ENDARTERECTOMY TRIALS. Large-scale randomized trials in symptomatic (NASCET, ECST) and asymptomatic (ACAS) patients with carotid stenosis consistently demonstrated 20-50% reductions in the 30-day risk of death and stroke in patients treated with carotid endarterectomy (CEA) compared to medical therapy (Table 36.45).[264-266] Relative risk reduction for ipsilateral stroke was greatest in symptomatic patients with severe (> 70%) carotid stenosis, less pronounced in symptomatic patients with moderate carotid stenosis (50-69%), and statistically insignificant in symptomatic patients with mild carotid stenosis (< 50%) (Table 36.47). Based on these data, the AHA Stroke Council issued guidelines for CEA and set benchmarks for perioperative death and stroke; centers (or surgeons) which fail to meet these benchmarks will not achieve significant benefits compared to medically treated patients (Table 36.46). In summary, data from randomized trials suggest that medical therapy may be appropriate for symptomatic patients with carotid stenosis < 50% and for asymptomatic patients with carotid stenosis < 60%, and that CEA should be considered for symptomatic patients with carotid stenosis > 70% and asymptomatic patients with carotid stenosis ≥ 60% (Tables 36.48, 36.49). It is important to appreciate that in asymptomatic patients with carotid stenosis > 60%, up to 55% of subsequent strokes are caused by lacunar infarction or cardiac embolism (as opposed to carotid stenosis),[275] suggesting that without analysis of the cause of stroke, the relative benefit of endarterectomy may be overestimated.

E. INDICATIONS FOR PTA AND STENTING. No stents are currently approved for carotid revascularization. At this time we recommend that all patients considered for carotid stenting be enrolled in investigational protocols approved by the hospital's Institutional Review Board. Patients not participating in an FDA-approved trial of carotid stenting and who meet criteria for carotid revascularization should be considered for endarterectomy. Carotid stenting may be considered in poor surgical candidates (by vascular surgical criteria) or those who refuse surgery and understand their treatment options and associated risks (Table 36.50). Contraindications to carotid stenting are described in Table 36.51. Dispassionate oversight by an independent neurologist is strongly encouraged for patients undergoing CEA or carotid stenting. In a metanalysis of 16,000 patients undergoing CEA, the overall risk of perioperative death was 1.6% and death or stroke was 5.6%. However, the incidence of stroke was 3-4-fold higher if an independent neurologist was involved rather than a single surgeon (Table 36.52).

F. STENTS. The technique of carotid stenting is undergoing continued evolution (Table 36.53). The world's largest experience was recently reported,[291] including early and late results of 5210 carotid stent procedures in 4757 patients (Table 36.54). More than half of the physicians contributing to this registry are cardiologists.[291] Based on data from 36 centers worldwide, overall procedural success was 98.4%. Complications within 30 days included TIA in 2.8%, minor stroke in 2.7%, major stroke in 1.5%, and death in 0.8%. The combined incidence of all strokes and death at 30 days was 5%. Outcomes at 12 months included restenosis in 3.5% and neurologic events in 1.4%. There appeared to be an important learning curve, with the rate of major complications decreasing by 2-fold after performance of 50 procedures. Other single-centers reported similar results [135-138] (Table 36.54). In general, 75% of patients treated by carotid stenting would have been ineligible for CEA based on NASCET and ACAS exclusion criteria. Since these patients are at higher risk than those in published randomized CEA trials, direct comparison of results may not be appropriate. Current stents were developed for use in iliac arteries and are not ideal. Cerebral protection devices to prevent distal embolization and the use of platelet IIb/IIIa receptor antagonists are under investigation.

G. COMPLICATIONS. In-hospital complications after carotid stenting include hemodynamic disturbances (hypotension, bradycardia), distal embolization, stroke, MI, and death (Table 36.55). The risk of distal embolization and stroke are higher in patients with more advanced symptoms and greater stenosis severity (Table 36.56). Persistent limitations of carotid stenting may soon be overcome (Table 36.57).

H. LATE OUTCOMES. Late outcomes after carotid stenting include mechanical problems (stent crush or deformation), restenosis (defined by duplex ultrasound criteria or angiography), stroke, and death (Table 36.58). Strong independent predictors of stent restenosis included female gender (odds ratio 3.5) and multiple stents (odds ratio 2.4); weaker predictors included age > 75 and final stenosis diameter.[278] Late clinical outcome was similar for men and women.[279] Treatment of carotid stent restenosis is problematic, but repeat angioplasty, stent removal and endarterectomy, vein graft interposition, and temporal-to-middle cerebral artery bypass have been employed in some cases.[290]

I. **DISTAL EMBOLIC PROTECTION DEVICES.** Because of concerns about distal embolization, a number of devices have been developed to trap and remove embolic debris during carotid intervention. In general, there are 3 classes of embolic protection devices: balloon occlusion devices, filters, and catheter occlusion devices (Tables 36.59, 36.60). The largest published experience is with the PercuSurge GuardWire, which is currently being evaluated in two large registries in Europe (CAFÉ-Europe) and the United States (CAFÉ-USA). Preliminary experience suggests that the average duration of balloon occlusion using the GuardWire system (7 minutes) is poorly tolerated in approximately 8% of patients.[276,277,280] The risk of intolerance to balloon occlusion is difficult to predict, but seems greater in patients with baseline diameter stenosis < 75%.[276] Using transcranial Doppler techniques, distal protection is associated with a marked reduction of microembolic signals during all aspects of the carotid stent procedure, although the clinical impact has yet to be defined.[281,282,284] The CAFÉ (Carotid Artery Free of Emboli) trials will be supplanted by SHELTER (Stenting of High-Risk Extracranial Lesions Trial with Emboli Removal), which will utilize the PercuSurge GuardWire and the new rapid-exchange Wallstent (to reduce occlusion duration).

J. **GLYCOPROTEIN PLATELET RECEPTOR ANTAGONISTS.** The role of abciximab and other platelet receptor antagonists has not yet been defined. Anecdotal experience in small numbers of patients suggests safety, but the impact of adjunctive antiplatelet therapy requires further study. The risk of intracranial hemorrhage appears to be < 1%.[288,289,294]

K. **VERTEBRAL ARTERY STENTING.** Surgical and percutaneous approaches to vertebral artery revascularization are relatively uncommon and success rates are variable. Important limitations of vertebral artery angioplasty include elastic recoil and dissection, which are readily resolved with stents. Preliminary experience with balloon-expandable stents suggest high procedural success rates (98%), few complications, and infrequent (< 6%) restenosis at 1 year.[286]

L. **SUMMARY.** Based on available data, the AHA issued an advisory about carotid stenting, which is summarized in Table 36.61.

Table 36.44. Cause and Risk of Stroke in Asymptomatic Internal Carotid Artery Disease[275*]

Etiology of Stroke	5-Year Risk of Stroke	Risk Factors
Large-vessel stroke	10%	Diabetes Severe carotid stenosis Silent brain infarction
Cardioembolic stroke	2%	Prior myocardial infarction Angina Hypertension
Lacunar stroke	6%	Age ≥ 75 Hypertension Diabetes Severe carotid stenosis

* 60-99% stenosis

Table 36.45. Randomized Trials of Carotid Endarterectomy vs. Medical Therapy

Trial	N	Symptoms	Stenosis (%)	Death/Stroke (%) (at 30 days)	Benefit	RRR
ACAS[258] (1995)	1662	No	≥ 60	2.3	Yes	20
VA Study[328] (1993)	444	No	≥ 50	4.4	No	9.9
MACE (1992)	71	No	≥ 50	8.3	No	-
CASANOVA (1991)	233	No	≤ 90	3.0	No	22
VA Study[329] (1991)	189	Yes	≥ 50	6.6	No	-7.8
ECST[261] (1991)	778	Yes	≥ 82	7.5	Yes	36.3
NASCET[259] (1991)	659	Yes	70-99	5.8	Yes	52.5
Shaw (1984)	41	Yes	-	35	No	-14.3
Fields (1970)	372	Yes	-	10.2	No	1.5

Abbreviations: ACAS = Asymptomatic Carotid Atherosclerosis Study; ECST = European Carotid Surgery Trial; NASCET = North American Symptomatic Carotid Endarterectomy Trial; RRR = relative risk reduction for carotid endarterectomy compared to medical therapy

Table 36.46. AHA Stroke Council Guidelines for Carotid Endarterectomy

Clinical Profile	Target: Perioperative Stroke/Death*
Asymptomatic	< 3%
Transient ischemic attack	< 5%
Stroke	< 7%
Repeat carotid endarterectomy	< 10%

* Carotid endarterectomy does not reduce the risk of stroke/death if the actual rate of perioperative stroke/death is higher than the "target" outcome

Table 36.47. Long-term Outcome After Carotid Endarterectomy

Study	Diameter Stenosis (%)	Follow-up (yrs)	Treatment	Ipsilateral Stroke (%)	Major Stroke (%)	All Stroke/Death (%)
NASCET[259]	70	2	CEA (n = 328)	9.0*	3.7	15.8
			MED (n = 331)	26.0	13.1	32.3
			RRR (%)	*65*	*72*	*51*
NASCET[259]	50-69	5	CEA (n = 430)	15.7**	2.8	18.3
			MED (n = 428)	22.2	7.2	25.2
			RRR (%)	*29*	*61*	*27*
NASCET[259]	< 50	5	CEA (n = 678)	19.9	36.2	-
			MED (n = 690)	18.7	37	-
			RRR (%)	*6*	*2*	
ECST[261]	> 80	3	CEA (n = 356)	6.8*	9.7	14.9
			MED (n = 220)	20.6	25.8	26.5
			RRR (%)	*67*	*62*	*44*
ACAS[258]	> 60	5	CEA (n = 825)	5.1***	6.4	25.6
			MED (n = 834)	11.0	9.1	31.9
			RRR (%)	*54*	*29*	*20*

Abbreviations: CEA = carotid endarterectomy; MED = medical therapy; RRR = relative risk reduction
* $p < 0.001$
** $p < 0.05$
*** $p < 0.01$

Table 36.48. Recommendations for Carotid Endarterectomy

Symptom Status	Carotid Stenosis (%)	Recommendation	Trials
Symptomatic	0-29	Medical therapy	ECST
	30-49	Medical therapy	ECST, NASCET
	50-69	Variable	ECST, NASCET
	70-99	Carotid endarterectomy	ECST, NASCET
Asymptomatic	< 60	Medical therapy	
	≥ 60	Carotid endarterectomy	ACAS

Abbreviations: ACAS = Asymptomatic Carotid Atherosclerosis Study; ECST = European Carotid Surgery Trial; NASCET = North American Symptomatic Carotid Endarterectomy Trial

Table 36.49. Summary of Carotid Endarterectomy for Symptomatic Carotid Stenosis

At 2 years, the relative risk of ipsilateral stroke after carotid endarterectomy vs. medical therapy is:

65% less if diameter stenosis > 70% (p < 0.001)

29% less if diameter stenosis = 50-69% (p < 0.05)

3.8% less if diameter stenosis < 50% (p = NS)

Benefit of carotid endarterectomy is lost if perioperative death/stroke rate exceeds 5%

Table 36.50. Limitations of Carotid Endarterectomy

Anatomic Factors

　　Cervical scarring (radiation therapy, radical neck dissection)

　　Intracranial lesion

　　Extracranial submandibular or intrathoracic lesion

　　Severe cervical spine disease or fixation preventing neck extension

Clinical Factors

　　High-risk coronary disease (unstable angina, MI < 1 month, left main disease)

　　Severe COPD ($FEV_1 < 1.0$)

　　Carotid endarterectomy restenosis

　　Contralateral carotid occlusion

　　Less benefit in asymptomatic women

　　Heart failure, class III-IV

　　Bleeding diathesis

Table 36.51. Contraindications to Carotid Stenting

Absolute Contraindication

　　Intracranial aneurysm

　　Intraluminal thrombus

　　Unable to give informed consent

Relative Contraindication

　　Tortuous, calcified arch vessels

　　No femoral vascular access

Table 36.52. Symptomatic Carotid Stenosis: Metanalysis of Carotid Endarterectomy*[326]

Study Characteristic	Death (%)	Stroke/Death (%)
Prospective	1.9 (1.3-2.6)	5.5 (3.9-7.3)
Retrospective	1.5 (1.2-1.8)	5.1 (4.3-5.8)
Independent neurologist	1.4 (0.2-2.7)	7.7 (5.0-10.2)
Neurologist author	1.8 (1.2-2.5)	6.4 (4.6-8.1)
Multiple surgeons	1.7 (1.4-1.9)	5.5 (4.8-6.1)
Single surgeon	0.7 (0.4-1.0)	2.3 (1.8-2.7)
Overall (n = 15,956 patients)	1.6%	5.6%

* In multiple published studies including nearly 16,000 patients, the reported risk of adverse outcomes was lowest for single surgeon authors and highest for independent neurologists

Table 36.53. Carotid Artery Stenting: Transfemoral Technique

Perform arch aortography with 5F pigtail catheter (LAO 50-60°).

Selective catheterization of either innominate artery or left common carotid artery with a 5F catheter (JB1 or 2, Vitek, Simmons) and a flexible 0.035-inch guidewire (Glidewire, Magic-torque, Wholey, Storq). Position the catheter proximal to the carotid bifurcation and ensure an ACT of 300 seconds.

Inject sufficient contrast to define the carotid bifurcation, and advance the 0.035-inch guidewire into the external carotid artery.

Exchange the 5F catheter for a 7-8F sheath (Shuttle Flexor sheath, Arrow sheath) or a 9F Multipurpose guiding catheter, and position the tip proximal to the carotid bifurcation. Remove the 0.035-inch guidewire.

Perform selective carotid arteriography in the AP, lateral, and/or oblique projections to define the anatomic landmarks and stenosis. Cross the target lesion with a 0.018-inch flexible guidewire (Roadrunner). The platinum tip of the wire should not be intracranial.

Predilate the stenosis with a 4.0 x 30-40 mm balloon, and then deploy a self-expanding stent (e.g., Wallstent, Smart stent) in the lesion. A residual stenosis < 20% is acceptable, and pursuit of better lumen enlargement is not recommended because of the risk of embolization and vessel injury.

Table 36.54. Carotid Artery Stenting: Success and Complications

Study	Setting	N	Success (%)	30-day (%)		Restenosis (%)
				Stroke/TIA	Death	
Shawl[292] (2000)	High-risk	170	99	2.9	0	2
Wholey[291] (2000)	Multiple	4757	98.4	7.0	0.8	3.5
Gupta[293] (2000)	Inoperable	100	100	6	0	2
Tan[283] (2000)	CEA restenosis	70	97	1.4	0	-
Shawl[285] (2000)	Age < 80 Age > 80	194 76	99 100	3.5 1.3	0 0	- -
Henry[287] (2000)	High-risk	290	99	4.5	0.3	4
Bergeron (1999)	-	99	-	1	0	-
Al-Mubarak[266] (1999)	High-risk	44	100	2.2	4.5	0
Waigand[265] (1998)	Severe CAD	50	-	2.0	4*	6
Wholey[262] (1998)	Multiple	2048	99	1.3	2.7	4.8
Henry (1998)	-	174	-	2.8	0	-
Criado (1997)	-	33	100	0	0	3
Yadav[263] (1997)	High-risk	112	-	8.0	0.9	4.9
Roubin (1996)	-	146	99	6.2	0.7	< 5
Yadav[264] (1996)	CEA restenosis	25	100	4	0	0

Abbreviations: CAD = coronary artery disease; CEA = carotid endarterectomy; TIA = transient ischemic attack
* All deaths occurred after CABG

Table 36.55. Complications of Carotid Stenting

Complication	Incidence	Comments
Hemodynamic changes	30-60%	Hypotension and bradycardia may occur in up to 60% of patients, particularly during right carotid stenting. Most episodes are transient, but sometimes hypotension persists for 6-10 hrs. Pressors are required in 30%; temporary pacemakers are rarely needed.
Distal embolization	< 3%	Most common cause of stroke after stenting. Transcranial Doppler studies show frequent embolization (for stents and CEA), but clinical events are less frequent. May be reduced or eliminated by distal embolic protection devices. The impact of GP IIb/IIIa inhibitors is under evaluation.
Stroke	0-10%	Overall, the risk of any ipsilateral stroke was 5.5%, but persistent neurologic defects > 30 days after stenting occurred in 1-3% of patients. Cerebral hemorrhage is usually fatal.
Myocardial infarction	~ 0.2%	Nonfatal MI is rare.
Death	~ 0.6%	Most deaths are due to cardiovascular causes.
Hyperperfusion syndrome	NR	More common in patients with bilateral carotid stenosis and hypertension who undergo bilateral stenting at the same time. Patients may develop transient focal deficits which resolve quickly. Findings by angiography, MRI, and CT are usually negative.
Spasm	10-15%	Usually transient and readily responsive to nitroglycerin.
Dissection	NR	Edge dissections are sometimes seen in tortuous vessels, and can be avoided in most cases by using low-pressure inflations and by resisting the temptation to enlarge a mild residual lesion.
External carotid artery (ECA) occlusion	NR	Generally no sequelae. In patients without collaterals, may cause jaw claudication. If the ECA supplies collaterals via the ophthalmic artery, patency should be re-established, if possible.

NR = not reported

Table 36.56. Risk Factors for Complications After Carotid Stenting

Clinical Factors	Anatomic Factors
Age > 80	Tortuous arch vessels
Prior stroke	Calcified arch vessels
Large neurologic deficit	Subtotal occlusion/high-grade stenosis
Cerebral atrophy	Target lesion calcification
Unstable neurologic symptoms	Target lesion thrombus
Diffuse severe vascular disease	Long lesion ("string" sign)
	Tortuous internal carotid artery
	Coexistent proximal common carotid stenosis

Table 36.57. Limitations of Carotid Stenting

Lack of ideal hardware

Lack of experience

Management of intracranial complications is not defined

Treatment for restenosis

Stent compression (balloon-expandable stents)

Table 36.58. Late Outcomes After Carotid Stenting

Outcome	Incidence	Comments
Stent deformation	~ 2%	More frequent with balloon-expandable stents than self-expanding stents; due to loss of apposition of the stent to the vessel wall.
Restenosis	5-10%	Most definitions rely on duplex ultrasound or quantitative angiography. Presumably due to intimal proliferation, which may be associated with progressive stenosis rather than embolization.
Stroke/death	< 10%	Stroke-free survival at 1-year is generally > 93%.

Table 36.59. Devices for Distal Protection*

Balloon-Occlusion Devices
 PercuSurge GuardWire[+]

Filter Devices
 Cordis Angioguard
 Guidant Accunet
 EPI Filter
 Medtronic device
 Bard device
 Mednova filter
 Microvena TRAP
 Intratherapeutics Intraguard
 Boston Scientific Sentinel Wire

Catheter-Occlusion Devices
 Parodi Guiding KJ
 Coppi Invatec Guiding KT
 Kachel catheter

+ SAFER trial demonstrated a marked reduction in ischemic complications in vein grafts (Chapter 17); CAFÉ trials in progress in US and Europe; SHELTER trial pending
* Courtesy of Dr. Max Amor and Dr. Michel Henry

Table 36.60. Comparison of Designs of Distal Embolic Protection Devices*

Type	Advantages	Disadvantages
Balloon-occlusion devices	• Easy to use • Compatible with devices • Aspirates large and small particles • Reliably traps debris	• No antegrade flow • 5-8% intolerant • Balloon-induced injury • Not as steerable as PTCA wires • Difficult to image during the procedure
Filter devices	• Preserves antegrade flow • Contrast imaging is possible throughout the procedure	• May not capture all debris • Difficult to evaluate retrieval of debris during the procedure • Filters may "clog" • Delivery catheters may cause embolization before filter deployment
Catheter-occlusion devices	• Transient reversal of flow in internal carotid artery	• More cumbersome to use than other devices

* Courtesy of Dr. Max Amor and Dr. Michel Henry

Table 36.61. Summary of AHA Advisory on Carotid Stenting

Observations

Benefit/risk of CEA is well-defined

Benefit/risk of stenting is not well-defined

Training criteria are absent

Surgical revascularization for acute occlusion is not available

Surgical alternative (CEA) is relatively safe and inexpensive

Recommendations

Carotid stenting should be limited to well-designed randomized studies with dispassionate oversight

Ad hoc stenting is not recommended

A registry approach to gather initial experience and training is reasonable, using a multispecialty team

*Abbreviation*s: CEA = carotid endarterectomy

OTHER TECHNIQUES IN PERCUTANEOUS VASCULAR INTERVENTIONS

Thrombolytic therapy is an important adjunct to PTA and stents. Atherectomy and laser have been evaluated, while the role of endoluminal grafting awaits further definition.

A.   **PERIPHERAL INTRA-ARTERIAL THROMBOLYSIS (PIAT).** PIAT consists of direct intra-arterial infusion of fibrinolytic agents to restore blood flow to an ischemic limb caused by thrombotic or embolic occlusion (Figure 36.13, Table 36.62). Such therapy can often convert a long occlusion into a short occlusion or discrete stenosis, limiting the extent of surgical revascularization or making the lesion more amenable to percutaneous intervention. Although no thrombolytic agent has received FDA-approval for peripheral vascular use, urokinase was the most commonly used agent for PIAT, due to its advantages over streptokinase (shorter infusion time, fewer complications)[92,93] and tPA (lower cost, fewer hemorrhagic complications);[94,95] however, urokinase is no longer available in the United States (Table 36.63). Patients undergoing PIAT must be monitored closely for signs of bleeding, particularly access site bleeding, retroperitoneal hemorrhage, and intracranial hemorrhage. Routine laboratory studies should be obtained every 6-8 hours during the infusion including complete blood and platelet counts, aPTT, and fibrinogen levels. If the fibrinogen level falls to < 150 mg/dL, it should be remeasured in 2-4 hours. A fibrinogen level < 100 mg/dL identifies a patient with a systemic fibrinolytic condition, which we believe is an indication for termination of the infusion due to the risk of hemorrhage.

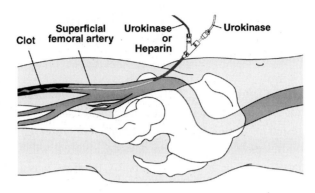

Figure 36.13. Peripheral Intra-Arterial Thrombolysis (PIAT)

1. **Indications.** Indications for PIAT include acute limb-threatening ischemia from thrombotic or embolic occlusion,[96-99] and claudication associated with chronic total occlusion (Tables 36.62, 36.64). Usual contraindications include recent stroke, internal bleeding, recent cardiopulmonary resuscitation, uncontrolled hypertension, severe coagulopathy, and the presence of a non-viable limb. Several clinical and angiographic variables can be used to predict successful thrombolysis (Table 36.65).

2. **Technique.** The goal of PIAT is to deliver the lytic directly into the target lesion, so the puncture site should be carefully chosen to allow the most direct access (Table 36.9). Unlike embolectomy, lysis is not traumatic to the endothelium and can potentially dissolve distal thrombi in run-off vessels (Table 36.66).[198] After baseline angiography, the thrombus is probed with a guidewire. Acute thrombus usually allows easy passage of a guidewire, but organized (chronic) thrombus may be resistant. After entering the lesion, a multi-sidehole catheter is passed over the guidewire, and a transthrombus bolus of lytic agent is administered using a pulsed-spray technique.[99] Typically, a bolus of urokinase (150-250,000 IU) was given over a 20-minute period, followed by a slow intra-arterial infusion (4000 IU/min for 2 hours, then 2000 IU/min for 2 hours, and then 1000 IU/min for 24-72 hours). For patients without sensorimotor deficits, the transthrombus bolus was often followed by low-dose infusion of 1000 IU/hr.[100] Since urokinase is no longer available in the United States, tPA is often used at a dose of 0.5-2.0 mg/hr for 12-24 hours (usually without a bolus), although some prefer weight-adjusted tPA at 0.05-0.10 mg/kg/hr. Intravenous heparin is started as soon as the thrombus is crossed with a wire, using a bolus of 70 U/kg followed by an infusion of 600-1000 U/hr to maintain the aPTT at 2.0-2.5 times control. Angiography is repeated at 4 and 12 hours, and every 12 hours thereafter. Lysis is terminated for successful recanalization, bleeding complication, or failure. Underlying stenotic or occlusive lesions are treated promptly

with PTA, atherectomy, or surgical revascularization.[98,100] Another approach to PIAT is to deliver a continuous infusion of the thrombolytic agent at multiple levels to increase the surface area of treatment. Multiple catheters or infusion wires arranged in a coaxial configuration are used for this purpose. Angiography is repeated every 4-8 hours and the catheters are advanced as needed to maintain contact with the thrombus.

3. **Lytics Used for PIAT (Tables 36.67, 36.68).** The standard agent for PIAT was urokinase.[70-74] In the United States, urokinase is no longer available and has been replaced by rt-PA and r-PA. For rt-PA the suggested infusion is 0.05-0.10 mg/kg/hr; we prefer adjunctive heparin to keep the aPTT at 60-80 seconds, although some centers do not use heparin with rt-PA. A single randomized trial reported similar efficacy for urokinase and rt-PA, but there was a trend toward less bleeding with urokinase.[75]

4. **Results of PIAT.** Procedural success rates with PIAT are 60-95%.[99,101] Long-term patency is 80% at 2 years and correlates with correction of the underlying stenosis.[91,97,98,102,103] Grafts with no identifiable stenosis have long-term patency of only 10%.[104] Several prospective randomized comparisons of PIAT vs. surgical revascularization for patients with acute lower limb ischemia showed better outcomes for PIAT (Table 36.69).

5. **Complications of PIAT (Table 36.70).**[105-109] The most common complication of PIAT is bleeding at the puncture site, which occurs in 3-20%. Other complications include intracranial hemorrhage (0.5-2.0%), acute MI (8%), distal embolization (12%), acute limb ischemia (2%; more common in patients with popliteal aneurysms), compartment syndrome (2%), pericatheter thrombus (5%),[91] and oliguria and increased creatinine (< 3%).

6. **Adjunctive Therapy.** Mechanical thrombectomy catheters may be useful as adjuncts to or substitutes for prolonged lytic infusions (Table 36.71).

B. **ATHERECTOMY (Table 36.72).** Mechanical atherectomy for peripheral arterial disease has undergone extensive evaluation.[110-115] Directional atherectomy, TEC, the Kensey catheter, and Rotablator have received FDA-approval for peripheral revascularization. With the exception of the Kensey catheter, all depend on the ability to pass a guidewire through the lesion. Initial success after directional atherectomy is 87-100%. Results are better in the iliac than femoropopliteal circulation,[185-191] but restenosis rates are still 14-52%. For popliteal stenoses in patients with claudication, 2-year patency was 45% and major complications occurred in 5%. Directional atherectomy is not useful for distal vessels < 6 mm in diameter, long total occlusions, calcified lesions, or for limb salvage. Despite early enthusiasm for directional atherectomy, several large series suggest worse results compared to PTA,[39,116-118] although it has been successfully applied to ulcerated atheromas causing "blue-toe syndrome" and stenoses in vein grafts.[119,120] Directional atherectomy is rarely used in contemporary practice because of the superiority of stent implantation. The rotational atherectomy devices achieved initial success rates of 80%, with 6-month patency in 40% and 2-year patency in only 15%. Similar to all other angioplasty techniques, the worst results were observed in long occlusions in the femoro-popliteal system and in limb salvage cases.

C. **LASER ABLATION.** The status of laser angioplasty is under re-evaluation. In a prospective study of 78 total occlusions, procedural success was 97%,[55] but in-hospital thrombosis occurred in 8%. Arterial patency was 47% at 1 year and 40% at 2 years; lesion length > 10 cm, poor run-off, and calcified lesions had unacceptable reocclusion rates.[121-128] There is renewed interest in laser revascularization of long chronic occlusions of the SFA (Chapter 30).

D. **ENDOLUMINAL STENT GRAFTS.** Numerous stent grafts have been developed for nonsurgical repair of abdominal aortic aneurysms and thoracic aortic dissection (Table 36.73). In the United States, the AneuRx and Ancure devices are approved by the FDA, and other devices are in various stages of evaluation. Suitability for endovascular aneurysm repair is dependent on several anatomic features, which include the diameter and length of the proximal neck (between the renal arteries and proximal aneurysm), the diameter and length of the distal neck (between the distal aneurysm and the iliac bifurcation), and the presence of an iliac artery aneurysm (Table 36.74). Potential complications including conversion to open repair and the presence of endoleaks are important limitations of currently available devices (Table 36.75). In one study comparing endovascular repair to open surgical reconstruction, survival at 6 years was similar, but endovascular repair was associated with less resource utilization and lower cost.[301]

E. **COARCTATION OF THE AORTA.** Occasionally, adults with native or recurrent coarctation of the aorta are considered for percutaneous revascularization (Table 36.76). Results of PTA and stenting have generally been favorable in terms of gradient reduction and improvement in blood pressure. Long-term results and the relative merits compared to surgical repair have not yet been defined.

Table 36.62. General Goals of PIAT

Acute Limb Ischemia	Chronic Limb Ischemia
Restore antegrade flow by thrombolysis	Recanalize a chronic total occlusion
Lyse thrombus in distal runoff circulation	Restore proximal vessel patency to facilitate distal bypass
Convert urgent to elective surgical revascularization	
Limit the extent of surgical revascularization	
Alter the level of amputation when limb salvage fails	
Restore patency of distal branches not suitable for thrombectomy	

Abbreviations: PIAT = peripheral intra-arterial thrombolysis

Table 36.63. Thrombolytic Agents for PIAT

	Streptokinase	Urokinase*	r-PA	rt-PA
Pharmacology				
Fibrin affinity	Low	Low	Low	High
Fibrin specificity	Low	Low	Moderate	High
Half-life	23 min+	15 min	13-16 min	< 5 min
Clot penetration	Unknown	Unknown	Yes	No
Immunogenic	Yes	Yes	No	No
Platelet activation	Yes	No	No	No
Clinical Utility				
Rate of lysis	Slow	Slow	Very rapid	Rapid
Hemorrhage	19%	6-12%	10-12%	Not defined
Clinical success	60-70%	75-90%	80-90%	Not defined
Need for heparin	Yes	Yes	Unknown	Possible
Dose: bolus	-	250,000 U	≤ 2.0 mg	-
infusion	-	50,000-100,000 U/hr	0.5-1.0 mg/hr**	0.5-2.0 mg/hr

Abbreviations: PIAT = peripheral intra-arterial thrombolysis; r-PA = recombinant plasminogen activator (Reteplase); rt-PA = recombinant tissue-type plasminogen activator (Alteplase)
*   Distribution halted by the FDA over concerns of Reovirus contamination
**   Some prefer weight-adjusted tPA (0.05-0.10 mg/kg/hr)
+   Half-life of streptokinase-plasminogen activator complex

Table 36.64. Signs of Acute Limb Ischemia

Rest pain

Limb pallor

Absent pulses

Cold extremity

Paralysis or paresthesia

Table 36.65. PIAT: Predictors of Successful Thrombolysis

Factor	Favorable	Unfavorable
Guidewire	Penetrates occlusion	Proximal to occlusion
Occlusion duration	Hours to days	Months to years
Occlusion length	< 5 cm	> 10 cm
Distal runoff	Present	Absent
Distal Doppler signals	Audible	Absent

Abbreviations: PIAT = peripheral intra-arterial thrombolysis

Table 36.66. Advantages of PIAT vs. Surgical Embolectomy

Not traumatic to vascular endothelium

Visualization of culprit lesion

Improves distal run-off

Easily combined with adjunctive PTA

Abbreviations: PIAT = peripheral intra-arterial thrombolysis; PTA = percutaneous transluminal angioplasty

Table 36.67. Comparison of Lytic Agents for Lower Extremity Acute Ischemia[203]

	Streptokinase (n = 200)	Urokinase (n = 200)	t-PA (n = 65)
Bypass Graft (%)			
Success*	72	97	94
Failure	28	3	6
Native Artery (%)			
Success*	34	74	87
Failure	66	21	13

Abbreviations: tPA = tissue plasminogen activator
* $p < 0.001$ for bypass graft vs. native artery; UK and tPA were similar (p = ns) and superior to SK ($p < 0.001$)

Table 36.68. Complications of PIAT for Acute Lower Extremity Ischemia[203]

Complication (%)	Streptokinase (n = 200)	Urokinase (n = 200)	t-PA (n = 65)
Fever	51	2	0
Nausea	18	17	6
Major bleed	28	6*	12
Stroke	2	0	2
Death	4	0**	2

Abbreviations: t-PA = tissue plasminogen activator; PIAT = peripheral intra-arterial thrombolysis
*   UK vs. SK, p < 0.01; UK vs. tPA, p = 0.09
** UK vs. SK, p < 0.001; UK vs. tPA, p = 0.25

Table 36.69. Randomized Trials of Thrombolytic Therapy vs. Surgery for Acute Lower Extremity Ischemia

Trial	Lytic Agent	Comments
TOPAS[309] (1998)	r-UK	UK with less need for surgical revascularization at 6 and 12 months, but more bleeding complications (12.5% vs. 5.5%, p < 0.01). Similar need for amputation in both groups
Comerota[311] (1996)	UK	In patients with occluded bypass grafts < 14 days, UK was associated with less amputation (20% vs. 48%, p < 0.05). If the duration of ischemia was > 14 days, patients treated with UK had more adverse events (81% vs. 46%, p < 0.001) and recurrent ischemia
Ouriel[105] (1994)	UK	UK with better 1-yr EFS (84% vs. 58%, p < 0.001) and fewer major complications (16% vs. 49%, p < 0.001), but more bleeding complications (11% vs. 2%, p = 0.06). Similar degrees of limb salvage at 1 and 12 months
STILE[310] (1994)	tPA, UK	Lytic infusion with less death, amputation, secondary revascularization, and shorter hospital stay. No difference between tPA and UK

Abbreviations: EFS = event-free survival; PIAT = peripheral intra-arterial thrombolysis; r = recombinant; STILE = Surgery vs. Thrombolysis for Ischemia of the Lower Extremity; tPA = tissue plasminogen activator; TOPAS = Thrombolysis or Peripheral Arterial Surgery; UK = urokinase

Table 36.70. Complications of PIAT

Complication	Comments
Allergic reactions (fever, rigors)	Common with streptokinase; rare with other agents; treated with acetaminophen

Hemorrhage
  Access site bleeding (3-20%)
  Intracranial hemorrhage (0.5-2%)
  Graft extravasation
	
	Lowest risk with urokinase
	Lowest risk with urokinase
	The fibrin seal in knitted Dacron grafts may leak; such patients should not receive lytic therapy. Woven Dacron and PTFE grafts are not prone to extravasation

Distal embolization (5-12%)	May be due to partial thrombolysis and secondary embolization, or to inadvertent mechanical disruption by guidewires or infusion catheters. Seems to be more common during treatment of acute arterial emboli or thrombosed PTFE grafts, rather than occluded native vessels or vein grafts
Catheter-induced thrombosis	Can be reduced by delivering lytic agent or heparin through the infusion catheter and vascular sheath (proximal to the target lesion)

Abbreviations: PIAT = peripheral intra-arterial thrombolysis; PTFE = Teflon

Table 36.71. Mechanical Thrombectomy Devices*

Motor-driven Devices (clot fragmentation)
  Amplatz Clot Buster
  Terotola Device
  Rotarex

Ultrasound Devices (clot dissolution)
  Angiosonics device

Hydrodynamic Thrombectomy (Venturi effect)
  AngioJet (Possis)
  Hydrolyser (Cordis)
  Oasis (Boston Scientific Scimed)
  Thrombektomat

* Courtesy of Dr. Max Amor and Dr. Michel Henry

Table 36.72. Comparison of PTA and Atherectomy for Peripheral Vascular Disease

Technique	Success (%)	Complications (%)	Patency* (%)
Balloon	90	8-12	70
Atherectomy	90	20-30	15-45

* Patency at 2-3 years

Table 36.73. Aortic Stent Grafts

Product	Manufacturer	Description
AneuRx	Medtronic AVE	Modular system; Dacron graft externally supported by nitinol stent rings over entire length. FDA-approved
Talent	Medtronic AVE/World Medical	Fully-supported modular system with nitinol stent and polyester graft. Bare cephalad stent may allow suprarenal deployment
Ancure	Guidant-EVT	Unibody woven polyester graft with balloon-expandable stents at each end; FDA-approved
Endo Stent Graft	Endotex	Modular stent graft with etched sheet of nitinol lined with Dacron
Hemobahn	Prograft-Gore	Self-expanding nitinol stent with ultra-thin PTFE
Vanguard	Boston Scientific Scimed	Modular system with outer Dacron cover and inner nitinol self-expanding stent

Table 36.74. Classification of Abdominal Aortic Aneurysm

Classification	Proximal Neck (cm)	Distal Cuff (cm)	Iliac Aneurysm	Suitability for ELG
I	> 1.5	> 2	Absent	Yes
IIA	> 1.5	< 2	Absent	Yes
IIB	> 1.5	< 2	Proximal	Possible
IIC	> 1.5	< 2	Diffuse	Possible
III	< 1.5	< 2	Absent	No

Abbreviations: ELG = endoluminal graft

Table 36.75. Potential Complications of Aortic Stent Grafts

Complication	Comments
Conversion to open repair	Incidence 5%; perioperative mortality 11%
Endoleaks	Incidence 10-15%; due to persistent blood flow outside the vascular graft but inside the aneurysm. Most seal spontaneously, but may lead to further aneurysm expansion/rupture
Post-implantation syndrome	Common. Presents as low-grade fever, malaise, diaphoresis, thrombocytopenia; some patients experience DIC
Renal artery obstruction	Covered stents may partially or completely occlude the main or accessory renal arteries
Cholesterol embolization	Similar to cholesterol embolization associated with other catheter-based interventions

Table 36.76. PTA or Stenting for Coarctation of the Aorta in Adults

Series	N	Age	Type	Device	Success	Comments
Koerselman[297] (2000)	18	14-67	Native	PTA	100	Improvement in hypertension and translesional pressure gradient; no late aneurysms at 1 year
Marshall[298] (2000)	33	5-60	Native, recurrent	Stent	97	Improvement in hypertension, translesional pressure gradient, and LVEDP; no late aneurysms at 27 months

Abbreviations: LVEDP = left ventricular end-diastolic pressure; PTA = percutaneous transluminal angioplasty

* * * * *

REFERENCES

1. Criqui MH: Peripheral arterial disease and subsequent cardiovascular mortality: a strong and consistent association. Circulation 1990;82:2246-7.

2. Hertzer NR: The natural history of peripheral vascular disease: Implications for its management. Circulation 1991;83:I-12-19.

3. Rutherford RB. Evaluation and selection of patients for vascular surgery. In Rutherford RB (ed). Vascular Surgery, Third Edition. WB Saunders, Philadelphia 1989;10-16.

4. Smith RB, Fulenwider JT. Reversed autogenous vein graft for lower extremity occlusive disease. In Ernst CB, Stanley JC (eds). Current Therapy in Vascular Surgery. BC Decker, Toronto, 1987;206-210.

5. Veith FJ. The impact of nonoperative therapy on the clinical management of peripheral arterial disease. In Yao JST, Pearce WH (eds). Technologies in Vascular Surgery. WB Saunders, Philadelphia, 1991;402-411.

6. Graor RA, Gray BH. Interventional treatment of peripheral vascular disease. In Young JR, Graor RA, Olin JW, et al (eds). Peripheral Vascular Diseases. Mosby, St Louis, 1991;111-133.

7. Salles-Cunha Sx, Andros G. Preoperative duplex scanning prior to infrainguinal revascularization. Surg Clin of NA 1990;70:41-59.

8. Strandness DE Jr, Sumner DS. Hemodynamics for Surgeons. Grune & Stratton, New York, 1975.

9. Bendick PJ, Glover JL, Kuebler TJ, et al. Progression of atherosclerosis in diabetics. Surgery 1983;93:834-838.

10. Krajewski LP, Olin JW. Atherosclerosis of the aorta and lower extremity arteries, In Young JR, Graor RA, Olin JW, et al. Peripheral Vascular Diseases. Mosby, St Louis, 1991;179-200.

11. Strandness DE Jr. Noninvasive vascular laboratory and vascular imaging. In Young JR, Graor RA, Olin JW, et al. Peripheral Vascular Diseases. Mosby, St Louis, 1991;39-69.

12. Yao JST. Hemodynamic studies in peripheral arterial disease. Br J Surg 1970;57:761-770.

13. Bridges RA, Barnes RW. Segmental limb pressures. In Kempczinski RF, Yao JST (eds). Practical noninvasive vascular diagnosis, second edition. Year Book Medical Publishers, Chicago, 1987;112-126.

14. Binnington HB. Segmental limb pressures, doppler waveforms, and stress testing. In Hershey FB, Barnes RW, Sumner DS (eds). Noninvasive diagnosis of vascular disease. Appleton Davies, Pasadena, California, 1984;16-23.

15. Jager KA, Ricketts HJ, Strandness DE Jr. Duplex scanning for the evaluation of lower limb disease. In Bernstein EF (ed). Noninvasive diagnostic techniques in vascular disease. Mosby, St Louis, 1985;619-631.

16. Kohler TR, Nance DR, Cramer M, et al. Duplex scanning for diagnosis of aortoiliac and femoropopliteal disease: a prospective study. Circulation 1987;76:1074-1080.

17. Strandness DE Jr. Duplex Scanning in Vascular Disorders. Raven Press, New York,1990;121-145.

18. Bandyk DF. Postoperative surveillance of infrainguinal bypass. Surg Clin NA 1990;70:71-85.

19. Vascular Technology, Vol II of Vascular Registry Review and Vascular Educational Program, 1995. Society of Vascular Technology, Lanham, MD.

20. Standards of Practice Committee of the Society of Cardiovascular and Interventional Radiology. Guidelines for percutaneous transluminal angioplasty. Radiology 1990;177: 619-626.

21. Schwarten DE, Tadavarthy SM, Castaneda-Zuniga WR. Aortic, iliac, and peripheral arterial angioplasty. In Castaneda-Zuniga WR. Tadavarthy SM (eds). Interventional Radiology. 2ed. Williams & Wilkins, Baltimore, 1992;378-421.

22. Becker GJ, Katzen BT, Dake, MD. Noncoronary angioplasty. Radiology, 1989;170:921-940.

23. Pickering TG. Diagnosis and evaluation of renovascular hypertension: indications for therapy. Circulation 1991;83:I-147-I-154.

24. Tegtmeyer CJ, Kellum CD, Ayers A. Percutaneous transluminal renal angioplasty of renal arteries: Results and long term follow-up. Radiol 1984;153:77-84

25. Sos TA, Pickering TG, Sniderman K, et al. Percutaneous transluminal renal angioplasty for renovascular hypertension due to atherosclerosis and fibromuscular dysplasia. N Engl J Med 1983;309:274-279.

26. Gerlock AJ, MacDonnell RC Jr, Smith CW, et al. Renal transplant arterial stenosis: percutaneous transluminal angioplasty. Am J Roentgen 1983;140:325-331.

27. Miller GA, Ford KK, Braun SD, et al. Percutaneous transluminal angioplasty vs. surgery for renovascular hypertension. Am J Roentgen 1985;144:447-450.

28. Kuhlman U, Greninger P, Gruntzig A, et al. Long term experience in percutaneous transluminal dilation of renal artery stenosis. Am J Med 1985;79:692-698.

29. Martin LG, Casarella WJ, Gaylord GM. Azotemia caused by renal artery stenosis: treatment by percutaneous angioplasty. Am J Roentgen 1988;150:839-844.

30. Pickering TG, Sos TA, Saddekni S, et al. Renal angioplasty in patients with azotemia and renovascular hypertension. J Hypertension 1986;4:s667-s669.

31. Pickering TG, Sos Ta, Vaughan ED, et al. Predictive value and changes of renin secretion in hypertensive patients with unilateral renovascular disease undergoing successful renal angioplasty. Am J Med 1984;76:398-404.

32. Martin EC, Mattern RF, Baer L, et al. Renal angioplasty for hypertension: predictive factors for long term success. Am J Roentgen 1981;137:921-924.

33. Sos TA. Angioplasty for the treatment of azotemia and renovascular hypertension in atherosclerotic renal artery disease. Circulation 1991;83:I-162--I-166.

34. Pickering TG, Devereux RB, James GD, et al. Recurrent pulmonary edema in hypertension due to bilateral renal artery stenosis: treatment by angioplasty or surgical revascularization. Lancet 1988;9:551-552.

35. Sniderman, KW. Transluminal angioplasty in the management of chronic intestinal ischemia. In Strandness and Van Breda D (eds), Vascular Diseases: Surgical and Interventional Therapy. New York: Churchill Livingstone, 1994. pp. 803-809.

36. Roberts L, Wertman DA, Mills SR, et al: Transluminal angioplasty of the superior mesenteric artery: an alternative to surgical revascularization. Am J Roentgen 141;1039:1983.

37. Kandarpa, K. Handbook of cardiovascular and interventional radiologic procedures, 1st ed. Little, Brown and Company,

Boston, 1989.

38. Kaufman SL, Barth KH, Kadir S. et al. Hemodynamics measurements in the evaluation and follow-up of transluminal angioplasty of the iliac and femoral arteries. Radiol 1982;142:329-336.

39. Becker GJ. Femoropopliteal angioplasty, atherectomy, stents. Second International Symposium on Cardiovascular and Interventional Radiology. Harvard Medical School/Brigham and Women's Hospital, Vol. 1, 1994:53-65.

40. Johnston KW. Femoral and popliteal arteries: reanalysis of results of balloon angioplasty. Radiol 1992;183:767-771.

41. Tegtmeyer CJ, Kellum CD, Ayers C. Percutaneous transluminal angioplasty of the renal artery: results and long-term follow-up. Radiol 1984;153:77-84.

42. Colapinto RF, Stronell RD, Harries-Jones EP, et al. Percutaneous transluminal dilatation of the renal artery: follow-up studies on renovascular hypertension. Am J Roentgen 1982;139:727-732.

43. Katzen BT, Chang J, Knox WG. Percutaneous transluminal angioplasty with the Gruntzig balloon catheter: a review of 70 cases. Arch Surg 1979;114:1389-1399.

44. Puijlaert CBAJ, Boomsma JHB, Ruijs JHJ, et al. Transluminal renal artery dilatation in hypertension: technique, results and complications in 60 cases. Urol Radiol 1981;2:201-210.

45. Schwarten DE. Percutaneous transluminal renal angioplasty. Urol Radiol 1981;2:193-200.

46. Tegtmeyer CJ, Sos TA. Techniques of renal angioplasty. Radiol 1986;161:577-586.

47. Tegtmeyer CJ, Selby JB. Percutaneous transluminal angioplasty of the renal arteries. In WR Castaneda-Zuniga and SM Tadavarthy (eds), Interventional Radiology (2nd ed). Baltimore: Williams & Wilkins, 1992, pp 364-377.

48. Lossino F, Zuccala A, Busato F. Renal artery angioplasty for renovascular hypertension and preservation of renal function: long-term angiographic and clinical follow-up. Am J Roentgen 1994;16.2:853-7.

49. Gardiner GA, Meyerovitz MF, Stokes KR, Clouse ME, Harrington DP, Bettmann MA. Complications of transluminal angioplasty. Radiol 1986;159:201-208.

50. Weibull H, et al. Complications after percutaneous transluminal angioplasty in the iliac, femoral and popliteal arteries. J Vasc Surg, 5: 681-686, 1987.

51. Plecha FR, et al. The early results of vascular surgery in patients 75 years of age and older: an analysis of 3259 cases. J Vasc Surg, 2: 767-774, 1985.

52. Thomson, KR. Longterm results of renal artery stenting: the Australian experience. Harvard Medical School/Brigham and Women's Hospital Second International Symposium on Cardiovascular and Interventional Radiology. 1994, Vol I, 892-6.

53. Sos TA. Renal angioplasty: optimal techniques, long-term results. Harvard Medical School/Brigham and Women's Hospital Second International Symposium on Cardiovascular and Interventional Radiology. 1994, Vol. I, 75-75N.

54. Capek P, Mclean GK, Berkowitz HD. Femoropopliteal angioplasty: Factors influencing long-term success. Circulation 1991;83:I-70-I-80.

55. Rholl KS and von Breda A, percutaneous intervention for aortoiliac disease. In: Vascular Diseases: Surgical and Interventional Therapy. 1994, Churchill Livingston, New York.

56. Gallino A, Mahler F, Probst P, Nachbur B. Percutaneous transluminal angioplasty of the arteries of the lower limbs: a 5-year follow-up. Circulation 1984;70:619-623.

57. van Andel GJ, van Erp WF, Krepel VM et al. Percutaneous transluminal dilatation of the iliac artery: long-term results. Radiol 1985;156:321-323.

58. Johnston KW, Rae M, Hogg S, et al. 5-year results of a prospective study of percutaneous transluminal angioplasty. Ann Surg 1987;206:403-413.

59. Wilson SE, Wolf GL, Cross AP. Percutaneous transluminal angioplasty versus operation for peripheral arteriosclerosis: report of a prospective randomized trial in a selected group of patients. J Vasc Surg 1989;9:1-9.

60. Rutherford RB, Durham J. Percutaneous balloon angioplasty for arteriosclerosis obliterans: long-term results. In Yao JST, Pearce WH (eds). Technologies in Vascular Surgery. W.B. Saunders, Philadelphia, 1992;329-345.

61. Colapinto RF, Stronell RD, Johnston KW. Transluminal angioplasty of complete iliac obstructions. Am J Roentgen 1986;146:859-862.

62. Schwarten DE. Clinical anatomical considerations for non-operative therapy in tibial disease and the results of angioplasty. First international symposium on cardiovascular and interventional radiology. Harvard Medical School/Brigham and Women's Hospital, 1992: pp 196-205.

63. Berkowitz HD, Spence RK, Frieman DB, et al. Long-term results of transluminal angioplasty of the femoral arteries. In Dotter CT, Gruntzig A, Schoop W, et al. (eds). Percutaneous transluminal angioplasty. Springer-Verlag, Berlin 1983;207-214.

64. Jeans WD, Armstrong S, Cole SE, et al. Fate of patients undergoing transluminal angioplasty for lower limb ischemia. Radiol 1990;177;559-564.

65. Rutherford RB, Patt A, Kumpe DA. The current role of percutaneous transluminal angioplasty. In Greenhalgh KM, Jamieson CW, Nicolaides AN (eds). Vascular Surgery: Issues in Current Practice. Grune & Stratton, London, 1986;229-244.

66. Adar R, Critchfield GC, edsdy DM. A confidence profile analysis of the results of femoro-popliteal percutaneous transluminal angioplasty in the treatment of lower-extremity ischemia. J Vasc Surg 1989;10:57-67.

67. Brown KT, Schoenberg NY, Moore, ED, Saddekni S. Percutaneous transluminal angioplasty of infrapopliteal vessels: preliminary results and technical considerations. Radiol 1988;169:78-78.

68. Schwarten DE Cutcliff WB. Arterial occlusive disease below the knee: treatment with percutaneous transluminal angioplasty performed with low profile catheters and steerable guide wires. Radiol 1988;169:71-74.

69. Bull PG, Mendel H, Hold M, et al. Distal popliteal and tibioperoneal tibioperoneal transluminal angioplasty: long-term follow-up. J Vasc Interv Radiol 1992;3:15-53.

70. Schwarten DE. Clinical and anatomical considerations for nonoperative therapy in tibial disease and the results of angioplasty. Circulation 1991;83:86-90.

71. Horvath W, Oertl M, Haidinger D. Percutaneous transluminal angioplasty of crural arteries. Radiol 1990;177:565-569.

72. Tamura S, Sniderman KW, Beinart C, et al. Percutaneous

transluminal angioplasty of the popliteal artery and its branches. Radiol 1982;143:645-648.

73. The North American Cerebral Percutaneous Transluminal Angioplasty Register (NACPTAR) Investigators. Update of the immediate angiographic results and in-hospital central nervous system complications of cerebral percutaneous transluminal angioplasty. Circulation 1995;92:I-382.

74. Rutherford RB, Becker GJ. Standards for evaluating and reporting the results of surgical and percutaneous therapy for peripheral arterial disease. Radiol 1991;181:277-281.

75. Saeed M. Aortoiliac and renal artery stenting. In: Kandarpa K and Aruny J, (eds). Handbook of Interventional Radiologic Procedures, 2nd edition. Boston: Little Brown, 1996. pp. 103-114.

76. Richter GM, Roeren T, Brado M, Noeldge G. Renal artery stents: Long-term results of a European trial. Society of Cardiovascular and Interventional Radiology Meeting Abstracts, J. Vasc Interv Radiol, 4: 47, 1993.

77. Becker GJ, Palmaz JC, Rees CR, et al. Angioplasty-induced dissections in human iliac arteries: management with Palmaz balloon-expandable intraluminal stents. Radiol 1990;176:31-38.

78. Rees CT, Palmaz JC, Garcia O, et al. Angioplasty and stenting of completely occluded iliac arteries. Radiol 1989;172:953-959.

79. Williams JB, Watts PW, Nguyen VA, Peterson CL. Balloon angioplasty with intraluminal stenting vs the initial treatment modality in aortoiliac occlusive disease. Am J Surg 1994;168:202-204.

80. Rees CR, Palmaz JC, Becker GJ, et al. Palmaz stent in atherosclerotic stenoses involving the ostia of the renal arteries. Preliminary report of a multi-center study. Radiol 1991;181:507-514.

81. Richter GM, Noeldge G, Roeren T, et al. Further analysis of the randomized trial: Primary iliac stenting vs. PTA. Harvard Medical School (BWH 2nd Intl'l Symposium of CVIR). 1994, vol 1, 52-52 L.

82. Palmaz JC, Laborde JC, Rivera FJ, et al. Stenting of the iliac arteries with the Palmaz stent: experience from a multicenter trial. Cardiovasc Interven Radiol 1992;15:291-297.

83. Henry M, Amor M, Henry I, Ethevenot G, et al. Placement of Palmaz-Schatz in femoropopliteal arteries: A 6-year experience. Factors influencing restenosis and longterm results. Circulation 1995;92:I-58.

84. White CJ, Ramee SR, Collins TJ, Jenkins JS, et al. Stent placement for unfavorable renal artery stenosis. Circulation 1995;92:I-129.

85. Bacharach JM, Olin JW, Sullivan TM, et al. Renal artery stents: early patency and clinical followup. Circulation 1995;92:I-128.

86. Sullivan TM, Bacharach JM, Childs MB. PTA and primary stenting of the subclavian and innominate arteries. Circulation 1995;92:I-383.

87. Iyer SS, Yadav S, Vitek J, Wadlington V, et al. Technical approaches to angioplasty and stenting of the extracranial carotid arteries. Circulation 1995;92:I-383.

88. Diethrich EB, Lopez JR, Galarza L. Stents for vascular reconstruction in the carotid arteries. Circulation 1995;92:I-383.

89. Diethrich EB, Papazoglou CO, Lopez JR, Lopez-Galarza L. Endoluminal grafts for aneurysm exclusion and intraluminal bypass in the superficial femoral arteries. Circulation 1995;92:I-377.

90. Gomes AS, Moore WS, Quinones-Baldrich WJ, et al. Treatment of abdominal aortic aneurysm with the EVT-EGS endograft. Circulation 1995;92:I-127.

91. Slonim SM, Dake MD, Semba CP, Razavi MK, et al. True lumen obliteration in complicated aortic dissection: endovascular management. Circulation 1995;92:I-127.

92. Belkin M, Belkin B, Buckman CA, et al. Intra-arterial fibrinolytic therapy: efficacy of streptokinase vs urokinase. Arch Surg 1986;121:769-773.

93. Van Breda A, Groar RA, Katzen BT, et al. Relative cost-effectiveness of urokinase versus streptokinase in the treatment of peripheral vascular disease. J Vasc Interv Radiol 1991;2:77-87.

94. Graor RA, Olin J, Bartholomew JR, et al. Efficacy and safety of intraarterial local infusion of streptokinase, urokinase and tissue plasminogen activator for peripheral arterial occlusion: a retrospective review. J Vasc Med Biol;1990:310-5.

95. Meyerovitz MF, Goldhaber SZ, Reagan K, et al. Recombinant tissue-type plasminogen activator versus urokinase in peripheral arterial and graft occlusions: a randomized trial. Radiol 1990;175:75-78.

96. McNamara TO. Thrombolysis as an alternative initial therapy for the acutely ischemic limb. Sem Vasc Surg 1992;5:89-98.

97. Gardiner GA, Koltun W, Kandarpa K, et al: Thrombolysis of occluded femoropopliteal grafts. Am J Roentgen 1986;147:621-626.

98. Sullivan KL, Gardiner GA, Kandarpa K, et al. Efficacy of thrombolysis in infrainguinal bypass grafts. Circulation 1991;83:I-99 - I-105.

99. Valji K, Roberts AC, Davis GB, Pulsed spray thrombolysis of arterial and bypass graft occlusions. Am J Roentgen 1991;156:617-21.

100. McNamara TO. Thrombolysis treatment for acute lower limb ischemia. In Strandness D and Van Breda A (eds). Vascular Diseases: Surgical and Interventional Therapy. New York: Churchill-Livingstone, 1994. pp 355-378.

101. McNamara TO, Bomberger RA: Factors affecting initial and six month patency rates after intra-arterial thrombolysis with high dose urokinase. Am J Surg 1986;152:709-712.

102. Hoch JR, Tullis MJ, Acher CW et al. Thrombolysis vs. surgery as the initial management for native artery occlusion: efficacy, safety and cost. Surgery, 1994;116:649-56.

103. Durham JD, Rutherford RB. Assessment of long-term efficacy of fibrinolytic therapy in the ischemic extremity. Sem Intervent Radiol 1992;9:166-173.

104. Belkin M, Donaldson MG, Whittemore AD, et al. Observation of the use of thrombolytic agents for thrombotic occlusion of infrainguinal vein grafts. J Vasc Surg 1990;11:289-96.

105. Ouriel K, Shortell CK, DeWesse JA, et al. A comparison of thrombolytic therapy with operative revascularization in the initial treatment of acute peripheral arterial ischemia. J Vasc Surg 1994;19:1021-30.

106. McNamara TO, Goodwin SC, Kandarpa K. Complications of thrombolysis. Semin in Intervent Radiol. 1994;II:134-144.

107. Smith CM, Yellin AE, Weaver FA, et al. Thrombolytic therapy

for arterial occlusion: a mixed blessing. Am J Surg 1994;116: 649-56;discussion 656-7.

108. Galland RB, Earnshaw JJ, Baird RN et al. Acute limb deterioration during intra-arterial thrombolysis. Br J Surg 1993;80: 1118-20.

109. Kandarpa K. Regional intraarterial thrombolysis. In: Kandarpa K and Aruny J.(eds), Handbook of Interventional Radiological Procedures. Boston: Little Brown, 1996;59-68.

110. Queral LA, Criado FJ, Patten P et al. Long-term results of Simpson atherectomy. In Yao JST, Pearce WH (eds). Technologies in Vascular Surgery. W.B. Saunders, Philadelphia, 1992;366-372.

111. Simpson JB, Selmon MR, Robertson GC et al. Transluminal atherectomy for occlusive peripheral vascular disease. Am J Cardiol 1988;61:96G-101G.

112. Ahn SS, Eton D, Mehigan JT. Preliminary clinical results of rotary atherectomy. In Yao JST, Pearce WH (eds). Technologies in Vascular Surgery. W.B. Saunders, Philadelphia, 1992;388-401.

113. Snyder SO, Wheeler JR, Gregory RT et al. Kensey catheter: early results with a transluminal endarterectomy tool. J Vasc Surg 1988;8:541-543.

114. Wholey MH, Smith JAM, Godlewski BS, et al. Recanalization of total arterial occlusions with the Kensey dynamic angioplasty catheter. Radiol 1989;172:95-98.

115. Ahn SS, Auth D, Marcus D, et al. Removal of focal atheromatous lesions by angioscopically guided high-speed rotary atherectomy: preliminary experimental observations. J Vasc Surg 1988;7:292-300.

116. Dorros G, Lewin RF, Sachdev N, et al: Percutaneous atherectomy of occlusive peripheral vascular disease: stenoses and/or occlusions. Cathet Cardiovasc Diagn 1989;18:1-6.

117. McLean GK. Percutaneous peripheral atherectomy. J Vasc Interv Radiol 1993;4:465-480.

118. Johnson DE, Hinohara T, Selmon MR, et al: Primary peripheral arterial stenoses and restenoses excised by transluminal atherectomy: a histopathological study. J Am Coll Cardiol 1990 15:410-425.

119. Dolmatch BL, Rholl KS, Moskowitz LB, et al. Blue toe syndrome: treatment with percutaneous atherectomy. Radiol 1989;172:799-804.

120. Katzen BT, Becker GJ, Benenati JF, et al. Long-term follow-up of directional atherectomy in the femoral and popliteal arteries. (abstr). J Vasc Interv Radiol 1992;3:38-39.

121. Rosenthal D. Hot-tip laser angioplasty: a three year follow-up study. In Yao JST, Pearce WH (eds). Technologies in Vascular Surgery. W.B. Saunders, Philadelphia, 1992;357-365.

122. Rosenthal D, Pesa FA, Gottsegen WL, et al. Thermal laser balloon angioplasty of the superficial femoral artery: a multicenter review of 602 cases. J Vasc Surg 1989;14:152-159.

123. White RA, Grundfest WS. Lasers in Cardiovascular Disease. Year Book Medical Publishers, Chicago, 1987.

124. Choy DSJ. History of lasers in medicine. Thorac Cardiovasc Surg 1988;36:114-117.

125. Litvack F, Grundfest WS, Adler L, et al. Percutaneous excimer-laser and excimer-laser-assisted angioplasty of the lower extremities: results of initial clinical trial. Radiol 1989;172:231-235.

126. McCarthy WJ, Vogelzang RL, Nemcek AA Jr, et al. Excimer laser-assisted femoral angioplasty: early results. J Vasc Surg 1991;13:607-614.

127. McCarthy WJ, Vogelzang RL, Pearce WH et al. Excimer laser treatment of femoral artery atherosclerosis. In Yao JST, Pearce WH (eds). Technologies in Vascular Surgery. W.B. Saunders, Philadelphia, 1992;346-356.

128. Perler BA, Osterman FA, White RI et al. Percutaneous laser probe femoropopliteal angioplasty: a preliminary experience. J Vasc Surg 1989;10:352-357.

129. Yadav S, Roubin G, Iyver S, et al. Immediate and late outcome after carotid angioplasty (PTA) and stenting. J Am Coll Cardiol 1996;27:277A.

130. Isner JM, Rosenfeld K: Redefining the treatment of peripheral artery disease. Role of percutaneous revasculariation. Circulation 1993;88:534-1557.

131. Graor RA, Whitlow P. Coronary artery disease associated with peripheral vascular disease. In Young JR, Graor RA, Olin JW, et al (eds). Peripheral Vascular Diseases. Mosby, St Louis, 1991;201-213.

132. Glover JL, Bendick PJ, Dilley RS, et al. Efficacy of balloon catheter dilatation for lower extremity atherosclerosis. Surgery 1982;91:560-565.

133. White CJ, Ramee SR, Collins TJ, et al. Initial results of peripheral vascular angioplasty performed by experienced interventional cardiologists. Am J Cardiol 1992;69:1249-1250.

134. Levin DC, Becker GJ, Dorros G, et al. Training standards for physicians performing peripheral angioplasty and other percutaneous peripheral vascular interventions. Circulation 1992;86:1348-1350.

135. Spies JB, Bakal CW, Burke DR, et al. Guidelines for percutaneous transluminal angioplasty. Radiology 1990;177:619-626.

136. Wexler L, Levin D, Dorros G, et al. Training standards for physicians performing peripheral angioplasty: new developments. Radiology 1991;178:19-21.

137. Cowley JM, King SB III, Baim D, et al. Guidelines for performance of peripheral percutaneous transluminal angioplasty. Cathet Cardiovasc Diagn 1988;21:128-129.

138. Ryan TH, Klocke FJ, Reynolds WA, et al. Clinical competence in percutaneous transluminal coronary angioplasty: a statement for physicians from the ACP/ACC/AHA Task Force on Clinical Privileges in Cardiology. J Am Coll Cardiol 1990;15:1469-1474.

139. Pentecost MJ, Criqui MH, Dorros G, et al. Guidelines for peripheral percutaneous transluminal angioplasty of the abdominal aorta and lower extremity vessels. A statement for health professionals from a special writing group of the Councils on Cardiovascular Radiology, Arteriosclerosis, Cardio-Thoracic and Vascular Surgery, Clinical Cardiology, Epidemiology and Prevention of the American Heart Association. Circulation 1994;89: 511-531.

140. Spittell JA, Nanda NC, Creager MA, et al. Recommendations for peripheral transluminal angioplasty: training and facilities. American College of Cardiology Perpheral Vascular Disease Committee. J Am Coll Cardiol 1993;21:546-8.

141. Babb JD, Collins TJ, Cowley MJ, et al. Revised guidelines for

the performance of peripheral vascular intervention. Cathet Cardiovasc Intervent 1999;46:21-23.

142. Spijkerboer AM, Scholten FG, Mali WPT, VanSchaik JP. Anterograde puncture of the femoral artery: morphologic study. Cardiovascular Radiology 1990;176:57-60.

143. Kaufman SL. Angioplasty from the contralateral approach: Use of a guiding catheter and coaxial angioplasty balloons. Radiology 1990;177:577-578.

144. White CJ, Nguyen M, Ramee SR. Use of a guiding catheter for contralateral femoral artery angioplasty. Cathet and Cardiovasc Diagn 1990;21:15-17.

145. Tonnesen KH, Sager P, Karle A, et al. Percutaneous transluminal angioplasty of the superficial femoral artery by retrograde catheterization via the popliteal artery. Cardiovasc. Intervent Radiol 1988;11:127-131.

146. Zaitoun R, Iyer SS, Lewin RF, Dorros G. Percutaneous popliteal approach for angioplasty of superficial femoral artery occlusions. Cathet and Cardiovasc Diagn 1990;21:154-158.

147. Trigauz JP, VanBeers B, DeWispelaere, JF. Anatomic relationship between the popliteal artery and vein: a guide to accurate angiographic puncture. Am J Roentgen 1991;157:1259-1262.

148. Rutherford RB, Flanigan P, Gupta, S., et al. Suggested standards for reports dealing with lower extremity ichemia. J Vasc Surg 1986;4:80-94.

149. Johnston, KW. Balloon angioplasty: predictive factors for long-term success. Semin Vasc Surg 1989;3:117-122.

150. Gallino A, Mahler F, Probst P, Nachbur B. Percutaneous transluminal angioplasty of the arteries of the lower limbs: a 5 year follow-up. Circulation 1984;70:619-623.

151. Cassarella WJ. Noncoronary angioplasty. Curr Prob Cardiol 1986;11:141-174.

152. Becker GJ, Palmaz JC, Rees CR, et al. Angioplasty-induced dissections in human iliac arteries: management with Palmaz balloon-expandable intraluminal stents. Radiology 1990;176:31-38.

153. Katzen, BT, Becker GJ. Intravascular stents: status of development and clinical application. Surg Clin North Am 1992;72:941-957.

154. Palmaz JC, Richter GM, Noeldge G, et al. Intraluminal stents in atherosclerotic iliac artery stenosis: preliminary report of a multicenter study. Radiology 1988;168:727-731.

155. Palmaz JC, Carcia OJ, Schatz RA, et al. Placement of balloon-expandable intraluminal stents in iliac arteries: first 171 procedures. Radiology 1990;174:969-975.

156. Sullivan TM, Childs MB, Bacharach JM, et al. Percutaneous transluminal angioplasty and primary stenting of the iliac arteries in 288 patients. J Vasc Surg 1997;25:829-39.

157. Murphy KD, Encarnacion CE, Le VA, Palmaz JC. Iliac artery stent placement with the Palmaz stent: follow-up study. J Vasc Intervent Radiol 1995;6:321-329.

158. Sapoval MR, Chatellier G, Long AL, et al. Self-expandable stents for treatment of iliac artery obstructive lesions: long-term success and prognostic factors. Am J Radiol 196;166:1173-1179.

159. Laborde JC, Palmaz JC, Rivera FJ, et al. Influence of anatomic distribution of atherosclorosis on the outcome of revascularization with iliac stent placement. J Vasc Intervent Radiol 1995;6-513-521.

160. Kichikawa K, Uchida H, Yoshioka T, et al. Iliac artery stenosis and occlusion: Preliminary results of treatment with Gianturco expandable metallic stents. Radiology 1990;177:799-802.

161. Rees CR, Palmaz JC, Garcia O, et al. Angioplasty and stenting of completely occluded iliac arteries. Radiology 1989;172:953-959.

162. Ballard JL, Taylor FC, Starks SR, Killen JD. Stenting without thrombolysis for aortoiliac occlusive disease: experience in 14 high-risk patients. Ann Vasc Surg 1995;9:453-58.

163. Palmaz JC, Laborde JC, Rivera FJ, et al. Stenting of the iliac arteries with the Palmaz stent: experience from a multicenter trial. Cardiovasc Intervent Radiol 1992;15:291-297.

164. Richter GM, Noeldge G, Roeren T, et al. First long-term results of a randomized multicenter trial: iliac balloon-expandable stent placement versus regular percutaneous transluminal angioplasty. In Lierman D (ed). State of the Art and Future Developments, Morin Heights, Canada, Polyscience, 1995 pp 30-35.

165. Henry M, Amor M, Thevenot G, et al. Palmaz stent placenent in iliac and femoropopliteal arteries: primary and secondary patency in 310 patients with 2 -4 year follow up. Radiology 1995;197:167-174.

166. Zollikofer C, Antonucci F, Pfyffer M et al. Arterial stent placement with use of the Wallstent: midterm results of clinical experience. Radiology 1991;179:449-456.

167. Varwerk D, Gunther RW, Schurmann K, Wendt G. Aortic and iliac stenosis: follow-up results of stent placement after insufficient balloon angioplasty in 118 cases. Radiology 1996;198:45-48.

168. Tetteroo E, Haaring C, van der Fraff Y, et al. Intraarterial pressure gradients after randomized angioplasty or stenting of iliac artery lesions. Dutch Iliac Stent Trial Study Group. Cardiovasc Intervent Radiol 1996;19:411-417.

169. Peterkin GA, Belkin M, Cantelmo NL, et al. Combined transluminal angioplasty and infrainguinal reconstruction in multilevel atherosclerotic disease. Am J Surg 1990;`60:277-279.

170. Kalman PG, Hosang M, Johnston KW, Walker PM. The currrent role for femorofemoral bypass. J Vasc Surg 1987;6:71-76.

171. Rafferty TD, Avellone JC, Farrell CJ, et al. A metropolitan experience with infrainguinal revascularization: operative risk and late results in Northeastern Ohio. J Vasc Surg 1987;6:365-371.

172. Perler BA and Williams GM. Does donor iliac artery percutaneous transluminal or stent placement influence the results of femorofemoral bypass? Analysis of 70 consecutive cases with long-term follow-up. J Vasc Surg 1996;24:363-370.

173. Capek P, McLean Gk, Berkowitz HD. Femoropopliteal angioplasty: Factors influencing long-term success. Circulation 1991;83 (Supp I):70-80.

174. Morgenstern B, Getrajdman GI, Laffey KJ, et al. Total occlusions of the femoropopliteal artery: high technical success rate of conventional balloon angioplasty. Radiology 1989;172:937-940.

175. Becquemin J. Effect of ticlopidine of the long-term patency of saphenous vein grafts in the legs. N Engl J Med 1997;337:1726-1731.

176. Wilson SE, Wolf, GL, Cross AP. Percutaneous transluminal angioplasty versus operation for peripheral arteriosclerosis: Report of a prospective randomized trial in a selected group of patients. J Vasc Surg 1989;9:1-9.

177. Jens WD, Armstrong S, Cole SEA, et al. Fate of patients undergoing transluminal angioplasty for lower-limb ischemia. Radiology 1990;177:559-564.

178. Stokes KR, Strunk HM, Campbell DR, et al. Five-year results of iliac and femoropopliteal angioplasty in diabetic patients. Radiology 1990;174:977-982.

179. Hewes RC, White RI Jr, Murray RR, et al. Long-term results of superficial femoral artery angioplasty. Am J Radiol 1986;146:1025-1029.

180. Murray RR, Hewes RC, White RI Jr., et al. Long-segment femoropopliteal stenoses: is angioplasty a boon or a bust? Radiology 1987;162:473-476.

181. Miner E, Ahmadi A, Koppensteiner R, et al. Comparison of effects of high-dose and low-dose aspirin on restenosis after femoropopliteal percutaneous transluminal angioplasty. Circulation 1995;91:2167-2173.

182. Henry M, Amor M, Thevenot G, et al. Palmaz stent placement in iliac and femoropopliteal arteries: Primary and secondary patency in 310 patients with 2 - 4 year follow up. Radiology 1995;197:167-174.

183. Tollefson DF, Ernst CB. Natural history of atherosclerotic renal artery stenosis associated with aortic disease. J Vasc Surg 1993;14:327-331.

184. Visona A Perissinotto C, Lusiani L et al. Percutaneous excimer laser angioplasty of lower-limb vessels: results of a prospective 24-month follow-up. Angiology 1998;49:91-98.

185. Von Polnitz A, Nerlich A, Berger H, Hofling B. Percutaneous peripheral atherectomy: angiographic and clinical follow-up of 60 patients. J Am Coll Cardiol 1990;15:682-688.

186. Kim D, Gianturco LE, Porter DH, et al. Peripheral directional atherectomy: 4 year experience. Radiology 1992;183:773-778.

187. Dorros G, Lewin R, Sachdev N, Mathiak L. Percutaneous atherectomy of occlusive peripheral vascular disease: stenoses and/or occlusions. Cathet Cardiovasc Diagn 1989;18:1-6.

188. Graor RA, Whitlow Pl. Transluminal atherectomy for occlusive peripheral vascular disease. J Am Coll Cardiol 1990;15:1551-1558.

189. Bates ER, O'Neill WW, Topol EJ. Percutaneous atherectomy catheters. Cardiol Clin 1988;6:373.

190. Simpson JB, Selmon MMR, Robertson GC, et al. Transluminal atherectomy for occlusive peripheral vascular disease. Am J Cardiol 1988;61:91G-101G.

191. Schwarten DE, Katzen BT, Simpson JB, Cutcliff WB. Simpson catheter for percutaneous transluminal removal of atheroma. Am J Radiol 1988;150:799-801.

192. Ratner SE, Reilly CH, Gudas CJ. Percutaneous transluminal angioplasty in the treatment of ischemic disease of the lower extremity. J Foot Surg 1983;22:86-91.

193. Schwarten DE, Cutliff WB. Arterial occlusive disease below the knee: treatment with percutaneous transluminal angioplasty performed with low-profile catheters and steerable guide wires. Radiology 1988;169:71-74.

194. Casarella WJ. Percutaneous transluminal angioplasty below the knee: new techniques, excellent results. Radiology 1988;169:271-272.

195. Widlus DM, Osterman FA Jr. Evaluation and percutaneous management of atherosclerotic peripheral vascular disease. J Am Coll Cardiol 2989;21:3148-3154.

196. Matsi PJ, Manninen HI, Suhonen MT, et al.. Critical lower-limb ischemia: prospective trial of angioplasty with 1-36 months of follow-up. Radiology 1993;188:381-387.

197. Dorros G, Lewin RF, Jamnadas P, Mathiak LM. Below-the-knee angioplasty: tibioperoneal vessels, the acute outcome. Cathet Cardiovasc Diagn 1990;19:170-178.

198. Graor RA, Risius B, Young JR, et al. Thrombolysis of peripheral arterial bypass grafts. Surgical thrombectomy compared with thrombolysis. J Vasc Surg 1988;Feb;7(2)347-355.

199. Kandarpa K, Chopra PS, Aruny JE, et al. Intraarterial thrombolysis of lower extremity occlusions: prospective, randomized comparison of forced periodic infusion and conventional slow continuous infusion. Radiology 1993;188:861-867.

200. McNamara TO, Bomberger RA, Merchant RF. Intra-arterial urokinase as the initial therapy for acutely ischemic lower limbs. Circulation 1991;83 (suppl I):I-106--I-119.

201. Scott DJ, Wyatt MG, Murphy YG, et al. Intra-arterial streptokinase infusion in acute lower limb ischemia. Br J Surg 1991;78:732-734.

202. Lonsdale RG, Berridge DC, Earnshaw JJ, et al. Recombinant tissue-type plaminogen activator is superior to streptokinase for local intra-arterial thrombolysis. Br J Surg 1992;79:272-275.

203. Graor RA, Olin J, Bartholomew JR, et al. Efficacy and safety of intraarterial local infusion of streptokinase, urokinase or tissue plasminogen activator for peripheral arterial occlusion: a retrospective review. J Vasc Med Biol 1990;2:310-315.

204. Meyerovitz MF, Goldhaber SZ, Reagen K, et al. Recombinant tissue-type plasminogen activator versus urokinase in peripheral arterial and bypass graft occlusions: A randomized study. Radiology 1990;175:75-78.

205. Meyrier A, Buchet P, Simon P, et al. Atheromatous renal disease. Am J Med 1988;85:139-146.

206. Choudhri AH, Cleland JGF, Rowlands PC, et al. Unsuspected renal artery stenosis in peripheral vascular disease. Br Med J 1990;301:1197-1198.

207. Jean WJ, Al-Bittar I, Xwicke DL, et al. High incidence of renal artery stenosis in patients with coronary artery disease. Cathet Cardiovasc Diagn 1994;32:8-10.

208. Caps MT, Perissinotto C, Zieler RE, et al. Prospective study of atherosclerotic disease progression in the renal artery. Circulation 1998;98:2866-72.

209. Novick AC, Pohl MA, Schreiber M, et al. Revascularization for preservation of renal function in patients with atherosclerotic renovascular disease. J Urol 1983;129:9007-912.

210. Kaylor WM, Novick AC, Ziegelbaum M, Vidt DG. Reversal of end stage renal failure with surgical revascularization in patients with atherosclerotic renal artery occlusion. J Urol 1989;141:486-488.

211. Meany TF, Dustan HP, Novick AC. Natural history of renal arterial disease. Radiology 1968;9:877-887.

212. Greco BA and Breyer JA. The natural history of renal artery stenosis: who should by evaluated for suspected ischemic nephropathy? Semin Neph 1996;16:2-11.

213. Schreiber MJ, Pohl MA, Novick AC. The natural history of theroslerotic and fibrous renal artery disease. Urol Clin N Am 1984;11:383-392.

214. Wollenweber J, Sheps SG, Davis GD. Clinical course of atherosclerotic renovascular disease. Am J Cardiol 1968;21:60-71.

215. Zieler RE, Bergelin RO, Isaacson JA, et al. Natural history of atherosclerotic renal artery stenosis: a prospective study with duplex ultrasonography. J Vasc Surg 1994;19:250-258.

216. Novick AC, Pohl MA, Schreiber M, et al. Revascularization for preservation of renal function in pateints with atherosclerotic renovascular disease. J Urol 1983;129:907-912.

217. Kaylor WM, Novick AC, Ziegelbaum M, et al. Reversal of end stage renal failure with surgical revascularization in patients with atherosclerotic renal artery occlusion. J Urol 1989;141:486-488.

218. Pickering TG, Devereux RB, James GD, et al. Recurrent pulmonary edema in hypertension due to bilateral renal artery stenosis: treatment by angioplasty or surgical revacularisation. Lancet 1988;Sept:551-552.

219. Messina LM, Zelenock GB, Yao KA, et al. Renal revascularization for recurrent pulmonary edema in patients with poorly controlled hypertension and renal insufficiency: a distinct subgroup of patients with arteriosclerotic renal artery occlusive disease. J Vasc Surg 1992;15:73-82.

220. Tami LF, McElderry MW, Al-Adli, et al. Renal artery stenosis presenting as crescendo angina pectoris. Cath Cardiovasc Diag 1995;35:252-256.

221. Khosia S, White CJ, Collins TJ, et al. Effects of renal artery stent implantation in patients with renovascular hypertension presenting with unstable angina or congestive heart failure. Am J Cardiol 1997;80:363-366.

222.. Scoble JE. Is the 'wait-and-see' approach justified in atherosclerotic renal artery stenosis? Nephrol Dial Trans 1995;4:588-589.

223. Tegtmeyer CJ, Brown J, Ayers CA, et al. Percutaneous transluminal angioplasty for the treatment of renovascular hypertension. J Am Med Assoc 1981;246:2068-70.

224. Archibald GR, Beckmann CF, Libertino JA. Focal renal artery stenosis caused by fibromuscular dysplasia: treatment by percutaneous transluminal angioplasty. Am J Radiol 1988;151:593-6.

225. Cluzel P, Raynaud A, Beyssen B, et al. Stenosis of renal branch arteries in fibromuscular dysplasia: results of percutaneous transluminal angioplasty. Radiology 1994;193:227-32.

226. Soulen MC. Renal angioplasty: underutilized or overvalued? Radiology 1994;193:19-21.

227. Ramsay LE, Waller PC. Blood pressure response to percutaneous transluminal angioplasty for renovascular hypertension: an overview of published series. Br Med J 1990;300:569-572.

228. Greminger P, Steiner A, Schneider E, et al. Cure and improvement of renovascular hypertension after percutaneous transluminal angioplasty of renal artery stenosis. Nephrol 1989;51:362-6.

229. Sos TA, Pickering TG, Sniderman K, et al. Percutaneous transluminal renal angioplasty in renovascular hypertension due to atheroma or fibromuscular dysplasia. N Engl J Med 1983;309:274-9.

230. Libertino JA and Beckman CF. Surgery and percutaneous angioplasty in the management of renovascular hypertension. Urologic Clin North Am 1994;21:235-43.

231. Canzanello VJ, Millan VG, Stiegel JE, et al. Percutaneous transluminal renal angioplasty in management of atherosclerotic renovascular hypertension: results in 100 patients. Hypertension 1989;13:163-72.

232. Klings J, Mali WP, Puijlaert CB et al. Percutaneous transluminal renal angioplasty initial and long-term results. Radiology 1989;13:163-172.

233. Plouin PF, Darne B, Chattelier G, et al. Restenosis after a first transluminal percutaneous renal angioplasty. Hypertension 1993;21:89-96.

234. Martin LG, Cork RD, Kaufman SL. Long-term results of angioplasty on 110 patients with renal artery stenosis. J Vasc Interv Radiol 1992;3:619-26.

235. Weibull H, Bergqvist D, Jonsson K et al. Long term results after percutaneous transluminal angioplasty of atherosclerotic renal artery stenosis: the importance of intensive follow up. Eur J Vasc Surg 1991;5:291-301.

236. Sos TA, Pickering TG, Phil D, et al. Percutaneous transluminal renal angioplasty in revascular hypertension due to atheroma or fibromuscular dysplasia. N Engl J Med 1983;309:274-279.

237. Brawn LA, Ramsey LE. Is improvement real with percutaneous transluminal angioplasty in the management of renovascular hypertension? Lancet 1987;2:1313-1316.

238. Cicuto KP, McLean G, Oleaga J. Renal artery stenosis: anatomic classification for percutaneous angioplasty. Am J Roentgenol 1981;137:599-601.

239. Dorros G, Prince C, Mathiak L. Stenting of a renal artery stenosis achieves better relief of the obstructive lesion than balloon angioplasty. Cathet Cardiovasc Diagn 1993;29:191-8.

240. Dorros G, Jaff M, Jain A, et al. Follow-up of primary Palmaz-Schatz stent placement for atherosclerotic renal artery stenosis. Am J Card 1995;75:1051-5.

241. White CJ, Ramee SR, Collins TJ, et al. Renal artery stent placement: utility in difficult lesions for balloon angioplasty. J Am Coll Cardiol 1997;30:1445-50.

242. Kumpe DA, Cohen MAH, Druham JD. Treatment of failing and failed hemodialysis access sites: comparison of surgical treatment with thrombolysis/angioplasty. Sem Vasc Surg 1992;5:118-127.

243. Schwab SJ, Raymond JR, Saeed M, et al. Prevention of hemodialysis fistula thrombosis. Early detection of venous stenosis. Kidney Int 1989;36:707-711.

244. Saeed M, Newman GE, McCann RL, et al. Stenoses in dialysis fistulas: treatment with percutaneous angioplasty. Radiology 1987;164:693-697.

245. Martin EC, Diamond NG, Casarella WJ. Percutaneous transluminal angioplasty in non-atherosclerotic disease. Radiology 1980;135:27-33.

246. Gordon DH, Glanz S, Butt KM, et al. Treatment of stenotic lesions in dialysis access fistulas and shunts by transluminal angioplasty. Radiology 1982;143:53-58.

247. Ramee ST, Rees AF, Jusseri FE, et al. Percutaneous angioplasty for preservation of dialysis access: immediate

results and follow-up. (Abstract) Circulation 1991;84(Suppl II):II-292.

248. Dapaunt O, Feurstein M, Rendl KH, et al. Transluminal angioplasty versus conventional operation in the treatment of hemodialysis fistula stenosis: results from a 5-year study. Br J Surg 1987;74:1004-1005.

249. Vorwerk D, Grnther RW, Bohndorf K, et al. Follow-up results after stent placement in failing arteriovenous shunts: a three year experience. Cardiovasc Intervent Radiol 1991;14:285-289.

250. Quinn SF, Schuman ES, Hall L, et al. Venous stenoses in patients who undergo hemodialysis: treatment with self-expandable endovascular stents. Radiology 1992;183:499-504.

251. Beathard GA. Gianturco self-expanding stent in the treatment of stenosis in dialysis access grafts. Kidney Int 1993;43:872-887.

252. Lee NS, Jones HR Jr. Extracranial cerebrovascular disease. Cardiol Clin 1991;9:523-534.

253. Beebe HG, Stard R, Johnson ML, et al. Choices of operation for subclavian vertebral arterial disease. Am J Surg 1980;139:616-623.

254. Dorros G, Lwein RF, Jamnadas P, et al. Peripheral transluminal angioplasty of the subclavian and innominate arteries utilizing the brachial approach: acute outcome and follow-up. Cathet Cardiovasc Diagn 1990;19:71-76.

255. Gershony G, Basta L, Hagan AD. Correction of subclavian artery stenosis by percutaneous angioplasty. Cathet Cardiovasc Diagn 1990;21:165-169.

256. Hadjipetrou P, Cox S, Piemonte T, et al. Percutaneous revascularization of atherosclerotic obstruction of aortic arch vessels. J Am Coll Cardiol 1999;33:1238-35.

257. Jain SP, Zhang SY, Khosla S, et al. Subclavian and innominate artery stenting: acute and long-term results. J Am Coll Cardiol 1998;31:63A.

258. ACAS Investigators. Endarterectomy for asymptomatic carotid artery stenosis. JAMA 1995;273:1421-28.

259. NASCET Investigators. Beneficial effect of carotid endarterectomy in symptomatic patients with high grade carotid stenosis. N Engl J Med 1991;325:445-53.

260. Barnett HJM, Taylor DW, Eliasziw M, et al. Benefit of carotid endarterectomy in patients with symptomatic moderate or severe stenosis. N Engl J Med 1998;339:1415-25.

261. ECST Investigators. Randomized trial of endarterectomy for recently symptomatic carotid stenosis: final results of the MRC Euoropean Carotid Surgery Trial (ECST). Lancet 1998;351:1379-87.

262. Wholey MH, Wholey M, Bergeron P, et al. Current global status of carotid artery stent placement. Cath and Cardiovasc Diagn 1998;44:1-6.

263. Yadav JS, Roubin GS, Iyer S, et al. Elective stenting of the extracranial carotid arteries. Circulation 1997;95:376-381.

264. Yadav JS, Roubin GS, King P, et al. Angioplasty and stenting for restenosis after carotid endarterectomy: initial experience. Stroke 1996;27:2075-2079.

265. Waigand J, Gross CM, Uhlich F, et al. Elective stenting of carotid artery stenosis in patients with severe coronary artery disease. Eur Heart J 1998;19:1365-1370.

266. Al-Mubarak N, Roubin GS, Gomez CR, et al. Carotid artery stenting in patients with high neurologic risks. Am J Cardiol 1999;83:1141-13.

267. van de Ven PJG, Kaatee R, Beutler JJ, et al. Arterial stenting and balloon angioplasty in ostial atherosclerotic renovascular disease: a randomized trial. Lancet 1999;353:82-86.

268. van Jaarsveld BC, Krijnen P, Pieterman H, et al. The effect of balloon angioplasty on hypertension in atherosclerotic renal-artery stenosis. N Engl J Med 2000;342:1007-14.

269. Watson PS, Hadjipetrou P, Cox SV, et al. Effect of renal artery stenting on renal function and size in patients with atherosclerotic renovascular disease. Circulation 2000;102:1671-1677.

270. Rodriguez-Lopez JA, Werner A, Ray LI, et al. Renal artery stenosis treated with stent deployment: indications, technique, and outcome for 108 patients. J Vasc Surg 1999;29:617-24.

271. Feldman RL, Wargovich TJ, Bittl JA. No-touch technique for reducing aortic wall trauma during renal artery stenting. Cathet Cardiovasc Intervent 1999;46:245-248.

272. Spinosa DJ, Matsumoto AH, Angle JF, et al. Renal insufficiency: Usefulness of gadolinium-enhanced renal angiography to supplement CO_2-enhanced renal angiography for diagnosis and percutaneous treatment. Radiology 1999;210:663-672.

273. Rocha-Singh KJ, Mishkel GJ, Katholi RE, et al. Clinical predictors of improved long-term blood pressure control after successful stenting of hypertensive patients with obstructive renal artery atherosclerosis. Cathet Cardiovasc Intervent 1999;47:167-172.

274. Burket MW, Cooper CJ, Kennedy DJ, et al. Renal artery angioplasty and stent placement: predictors of a favorable outcome. Am Heart J 2000;139:64-71.

275. Inzitari D, Eliasziw M, Gates P, et al. The causes and risk of stroke in patients with asymptomatic internal-carotid artery stenosis. N Engl J Med 2000;342:1693-700.

276. Tuebler T, Schlueter M, Sievert H, et al. Protected carotid artery stenting: increased risk of balloon intolerance in patients with a baseline diameter stenosis $\leq 75\%$. Circulation 2000;102:II-476.

277. Henry M, Klonaris C, Amor M, et al. Stent supported carotid artery angioplasty: the beneficial effect of cerebral protection. Circulation 2000;102:II-476.

278. Khan MA, Liu MW, Chio FL, et al. Predictors of restenosis after successful carotid stenting. Circulation 2000;102:II-476.

279. New GS, Roubin GS, Iyer SS, et al. Is there a gender difference in outcomes following carotid artery stenting? Circulation 2000;102:II-476.

280. Roubin GS, Mehran R, Iyer SS, et al. Carotid stent-supported angioplasty with distal neuro-protection using the Guardwire™; Initial results from the carotid angioplasty free of emboli (CAFE-USA) trial. Circulation 2000;102:II-825.

281. Al-Mubarak N, Roubin GS, New GS, et al. Does distal balloon occlusion during carotid artery stenting reduce microembolization? Circulation 2000;102:II-825.

282. Whitlow PL, Katzan IL, Dagirmanjian A, et al. Embolization during protected versus unprotected carotid stenting. Circulation 2000;02:II-175.

283. Tan WA, Jarmolowski CR, Eles G, et al. Long-term outcomes of percutaneous carotid artery revascularization (PCA) for post-endarterectomy (CEA) restenosis. J Am Coll

Cardiol2000;ACCIS:85A.

284. Whitlow PL, Lylyk P, Londero H, et al. Protected carotid stenting with the PercuSurge guardwire: results from a multi specialty study group. J Am Coll Cardiol 2000;ACCIS:85A.

285. Shawl FA, Kadro WY, Lapetina F, et al. Outcome of carotid stenting in symptomatic octogenarians and non-octogenarians. J Am Coll Cardiol 2000;ACCIS:85A.

286. Jain SP, Ramee SR, White CJ, et al. Treatment of atherosclerotic vertebral artery disease by endoluminal stenting: results from a US multicenter registry. J Am Coll Cardiol 2000;ACCIS:86A.

287. Henry M, Amor M, Klonaris HC, et al. Angioplasty and stenting of extracranial carotid arteries in high-risk patients. J Am Coll Cardiol 2000;ASSIS:22A.

288. Cecena FA, Hoelzinger DH, Miller JA, Abu-Sharka S. The platelet IIb/IIIa inhibitor abciximab as adjunctive therapy in carotid stenting of potential thrombotic lesions. J Interven Cardiol 1999;12:355-362.

289. Kapadia SR, Bajzer CT, Ziada KM, et al. Initial experience of glycoprotein IIb/IIIa inhibition with abciximab during carotid stenting: a safe adjunctive therapy. J Am Coll Cardiol 2000;ACCIS:86A.

290. Schievink WI, Thompson RC, Lavine SD, Yu JS. Superficial temporal artery to middle cerebral artery bypass and external carotid reconstruction for carotid restenosis after angioplasty and stent placement. Mayo Clin Proc 2000;75:1087-1090.

291. Wholey MH, Wholey M, Mathias K, et al. Global experience in cervical carotid artery stent placement. Cathet Cardiovasc Intervent 2000;50:160-167.

292. Shawl F, Kadro W, Domanski MJ, et al. Safety and efficacy of elective carotid artery stenting in high-risk patients. J Am Coll Cardiol 2000;35:1721-8.

293. Gupta A, Bhatia A, Ahuja A, et al. Carotid stenting in patients older than 65 years with inoperable carotid artery disease: A single-center experience. Cathet Cardiovasc Intervent 2000;50:1-8.

294. Winkley JM, Adams HP. Potential role of abciximab in ischemic cerebrovascular disease. Am J Cardiol 2000;85:47C-51C.

295. Hadjipetrou P, Cox S, Piemonte T, Eisenhauer A. Percutaneous revascularization of atherosclerotic obstruction of aortic arch vessels. J Am Coll Cardiol 1999;33:1328-45.

296. Al-Mubarak N, Liu MW, Dean LS, et al. Immediate and late outcomes of subclavian artery stenting. Cathet Cardiovasc Intervent 1999;46:169-172.

297. Koerselman J, de Vries H, Jaarsma W, et al. Balloon angioplasty of coarctation of the aorta: A safe alternative for surgery in adults: immediate and mid-term results. Cathet Cardiovasc Intervent 2000;50:28-33.

298. Marshall AC, Perry SB, Keane JF, Lock JE. Early results and medium-term follow-up of stent implantation for mild residual or recurrent aortic coarctation. Am Heart J 2000;139:1054-60.

299. Neinaber CA, Fattori R, Lund G, et al. Nonsurgical reconstruction of thoracic aortic dissection by stent-graft placement. N Engl J Med 1999;340:1539-45.

300. Dake MD, Kato N, Mitchell S, et al. Endovascular stent-graft placement for the treatment of acute aortic dissection. N Engl J Med 1999;340:1546-52.

301. Moore WS, Kashyap VS, Vescera CL, et al. Abdominal aortic aneurysm. A 6-year comparison of endovascular versus transabdominal repair. Ann Surg 1999;230:298-308.

302. Ansel GM. Endovascular treatment of superficial femoral and popliteal arterial occlusive disease. J Invas Cardiol 2000;12:382-388.

303. Brevetti G, Hiehm C, Lambert D. European multicenter study on propionyl-L-carnitine in intermittent claudication. J Am Coll Cardiol 1999;34:1618-24.

304. Lievre M, Morand S, Besse B, et al. Oral beraprost sodium, a prostaglandin I_2 analogue, for intermittent claudication. A double-blind, randomized, multicenter controlled trial. Circulation 2000;102:426-431.

305. Bosch JL, van der Graaf Y, Hunink MGM. Health-related quality of life after angioplasty and stent placement in patients with iliac artery occlusive disease. Results of a randomized controlled clinical trial. Circulation 1999;99:3155-3160.

306. Scheinert D, Schroder M, Balzer JO, et al. Stent-supported reconstruction of the aortoiliac bifurcation with the kissing balloon technique. Circulation 1999;100[suppl II]:II295-II300.

307. Al Mubarak N, Liu MW, Dean LS, et al. Primary stenting of infrarenal abdominal aortic stenosis: A report of seven cases and review of the literature. J Interv Cardiol 2000;13:107-111.

308. Lazarous DF, Unger EF, Epstein SE. Basic fibroblast growth factor in patients with intermittent claudication: results of a phase I trial. J Am Coll Cardiol 2000;36:1239-44.

309. Ouriel K Veith FJ, Seashore AA, et al. A comparison of recombinant urokinase with vascular surgery as initial treatment for acute arterial occlusion of the legs. N Engl J Med 1998;338:1105-1111.

310. The STILE Investigators. Results of a prospective randomized trial evaluating surgery versus thrombolysis for ischemia of the lower extremity. Ann Surg 1994;220:251-268.

311. Comerota AJ, Weaver FA, Haskias JD, et al. Results of a prospective randomized trial of surgery vs. thrombolysis for occluded lower extremity bypass grafts. Am J Surg 1996;172:105

312. Safian RD, Textor SC. Renal artery stenosis: Hypertension and ischemic nephropathy. N Engl J Med 2001 (In press).

313. Caps MT, Perissinotto C, Zierler E, et al. Prospective study of atherosclerotic disease progression in the renal artery. Circulation 1998;98:2866-2872.

314. Zierler RE, Bergelin RO, Isaacson JA, et al. Natural history of renal artery stenosis: a prospective study with duplex ultrasound. J Vasc Surg 1994;19:250-258.

315. Schreiber MJ, Pohl MA, Novick ACL The natural history of atherosclerotic and fibrous renal artery disease. Urol Clin North Am 1984;11:383-392.

316. Tollefson DE, Ernst CB. Natural history of atherosclerotic renal artery stenosis associated with aortic disease. J Vasc Surg 1991;14:327-331.

317. Dorros G, Jaff M, Mathiak L, et al. Four-year follow-up of Palmaz-Schatz stent revascularization as treatment for atherosclerotic renal artery stenosis. Circulation 1998;98:642-647.

318. Iannone LA, Underwood PL, Nath A, et al. Effect of primary balloon expandable renal artery stents on long-term patency,

renal function, and blood pressure in hypertensive and renal insufficiency patients with renal artery stenosis. Cathet Cardiovasc Diagn 1996;37:243-250.

319. Hansen KH, Starr MS, Sands E, et al. Contemporary surgical management of renovascular disease. J Vasc Surg 1992;15:319-331.

320. Taylor A, Sheppard D, Macleod MJ, et al. Renal artery stent placement in renal artery stenosis: technical and early clinical results. Clinical Radiology 1997;52:451-457.

321. Harden PN, Macleod MJ, Rodger RSC, et al. Effect of renal-artery stenting on progression of renovascular renal failure. Lancet 1997;349:1133-1136.

322. Libertino JA, Bosco PJ, Ying CY, et al. Renal revascularization to preserve and restore renal function. J Urol 1992;147:1485-1487.

323. Brehdenberg CE, Sampson LN, Ray FS, et al. Changing patterns in surgery for chronic renal artery occlusive disease. J Vasc Surg 1992;15:1018-1024.

324. Steinbach F, Novick AC, Campbell S, et al. Long-term survival after surgical revascularization for atherosclerotic renal artery disease. J Urol 1997;158:38-41.

325. Pattynama PM, Becker GJ, Brown J, et al. Percutaneous angioplasty for atherosclerotic renal artery disease: effect on renal function in azotemic patients. Cardiovasc Intervent Radiol 1994;17:143-6.

326. Henry M, Amor M, Henry I, et al. Stent placement in the renal artery; three year experience with the Palmaz stent. J Vasc Interv Radiol 1996;7:343-50.

327. Rothwell PM, Slattery J, Warlow CP. A systematic review of the risks of stroke and death due to endarterectomy for symptomatic carotid stenosis. Stroke 1996;27(2):260-50

328. VA Asymptomatic Carotid Artery Stenosis Trial New Engl J Med 1993;328:221.

329. Mayberg MR, Wilson SE, Yatsu F, et al. Carotid endarterectomy and prevention of cerebral ischemia in symptomatic carotid stenosis. Veterans affaris Cooperative Studies Program 309 Trialist Group. JAMA 1991;266(23):3289-94.

37 BALLOON VALVULOPLASTY

Simon Dixon, M.D.
Robert D. Safian, M.D.

PERCUTANEOUS BALLOON MITRAL VALVULOPLASTY

Patients with mild-to-moderate mitral stenosis (i.e., valve area > 2.0 cm^2) are usually asymptomatic or have only mild dyspnea; treatment consists of prophylaxis for rheumatic fever and infectious endocarditis, warfarin for atrial fibrillation or embolism, and beta-blockers for exercise-induced dyspnea. In contrast, patients with "critical" mitral stenosis (i.e., valve area < 1.0 cm^2) usually present with incapacitating dyspnea; when pulmonary hypertension and right heart failure supervene, peripheral edema, orthopnea and paroxysmal nocturnal dyspnea dominate the clinical picture. Atrial fibrillation eventually develops in 80% of these patients and may be complicated by systemic thromboembolism in 20%. Percutaneous balloon mitral valvuloplasty (PBMV), first introduced by Inoue in 1984 and later used by others,[1-6] is now considered the treatment of choice for selected patients with critical mitral stenosis.[165-167] Randomized trials suggest that the results of PBMV are similar to those of open commissurotomy and better than closed commissurotomy.[158] Antegrade transseptal [7-15]and retrograde transarterial left atrial catheterization techniques have been described.[16-18]

A. **MECHANISM OF MITRAL VALVULOPLASTY.** Closed surgical commissurotomy and PBMV increase orifice diameter and leaflet mobility by separating fused commissures and fracturing calcified nodules.[26-29] In contrast to open surgical commissurotomy (performed under direct vision using circulatory arrest and cardiopulmonary bypass), PBMV and closed commissurotomy have little or no impact on subvalvular thickening or chordal involvement. In bioprosthetic mitral stenosis, where the mechanism of stenosis is calcification and fibrosis of the cusps rather than commissural fusion, balloon dilatation may result in severe mitral regurgitation; surgery is preferred in these patients.[30-33]

B. **PREPROCEDURAL EVALUATION.** Once the diagnosis of mitral stenosis is established, 2-D and transesophageal echocardiography (TEE) are recommended to assess the extent of mitral valve thickening, calcification, leaflet mobility, subchordal disease, and mitral regurgitation. Findings by 2-D echocardiography can be used to generate an "echo score," which has important prognostic impact on the immediate and long-term results after PBMV (Table 37.1).[8] TEE is particularly useful in evaluating left atrial thrombus, especially in patients with atrial fibrillation. Patients with cavitary thrombus should be treated with anticoagulants for 2-3 months prior to valvuloplasty.[157] Persistent thrombus is a contraindication to PBMV, although small numbers of patients with thrombus limited to the left atrial appendage have undergone PBMV with TEE guidance.[19-22] A prior history of embolism in the absence of thrombus on TEE is not a contraindication to PBMV.[23-25]

Table 37.1. Mitral Valve Echo Score Based on Morphologic Features*

Feature	Grade	Definition
Leaflet mobility	1	Highly mobile valve; only leaflet tips restricted
	2	Normal mobility (mid portion and base of leaflet)
	3	Valve moves forward in diastole, mainly from the base
	4	No forward movement of leaflets in diastole
Leaflet thickening	1	Leaflets normal in thickness (4-5mm)
	2	Mid portion of leaflets normal; thickening of margins (5-8mm)
	3	Moderate thickening of entire leaflet (5-8mm)
	4	Marked thickening of leaflet (>8 mm)
Subvalvular disease	1	Minimal thickening just below mitral leaflets
	2	Thickening of chordal structures extending up to one-third of the chordal length
	3	Thickening extends to distal third of the chords
	4	Extensive thickening and shortening of all chordal structures to papillary muscles
Calcification	1	Single area of increased echo brightness
	2	Scattered areas of brightness confined to leaflet margins
	3	Brightness extends into mid portion of leaflets
	4	Extensive brightness throughout the leaflets

* Echo score is determined by adding the individual scores for leaflet mobility, leaflet thickening, subvalvular disease, and calcification. Three-year freedom from death, mitral valve replacement, or repeat PBMV is approximately 86%, 82%, 68%, and 40% for echo scores of < 4, 5-8, 9-12, and 13-16, respectively.

C. **TECHNIQUE.** Diagnostic right and left heart catheterization and left ventriculography should be performed prior to PBMV, to assess the severity of mitral stenosis and mitral regurgitation. The two general approaches to PBMV are the antegrade transvenous approach and the retrograde transarterial approach.

     1. **Antegrade Transvenous Approach (Inoue Technique; Single or Double-Balloon Technique).** This approach requires transseptal left heart catheterization:

         a. **Technique of Transseptal Left Heart Catheterization.** An 8F sheath is introduced into the right femoral vein and exchanged for a modified 8F Mullins sheath and dilator, which is advanced over a 0.032-inch J-guidewire into the superior vena cava. The guidewire is removed, a Brockenbrough needle is advanced to within a few millimeters of the tip of the dilator, and the needle is then flushed and connected to a transducer for continuous pressure

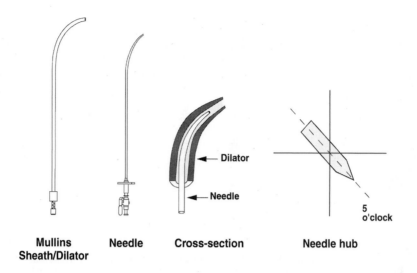

Figure 37.1. Catheters Used for Transseptal Catheterization

A.   Mullins sheath and dilator
B.   Brockenbrough needle and stylet
C.   Correct position of needle inside the dilator
D.   Orientation of arrow on needle hub. When hub marker is approximately 5 o'clock, the tip of the needle is in correct position

monitoring (Figure 37.1). There are several techniques for crossing the interatrial septum; the easiest is to orient the arrow on the Brockenbrough handle to 5 o'clock while monitoring the position of the needle in the AP projection. In this position, as the sheath, dilator, and needle are withdrawn along the shadow of the spine, the needle tip will descend over the top of the aortic knob, and then drop into the fossa ovalis. Further slight pullback and then gentle re-advancement of the Mullins sheath and dilator will usually produce a "catching" sensation, indicating that the tip is in the fossa ovalis. This position can be confirmed by further imaging in a standard 30° RAO projection, which should demonstrate that the needle is directed toward the atrial side of the AV groove. Similarly, fluoroscopy can be employed in the lateral projection (Figure 37.2), confirming a posterior orientation of the needle toward the left atrium. In some cases, a high left atrial pressure may result in flattening and posterior displacement of the fossa ovalis. If the fossa cannot be easily identified as described above, the needle can be oriented more posteriorly by turning the arrow to 6 o'clock. In some cases, it may be necessary to repeat the entire approach after adding an extra bend to the tip of the Brockenbrough needle. In difficult cases, transesophageal echo may be especially useful for identifying the fossa ovalis. Once proper position is achieved, the Mullins sheath and dilator are gently advanced into the fossa (which may result in transient pressure damping),and the Brockenbrough needle

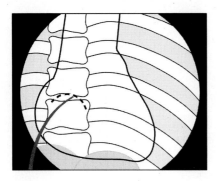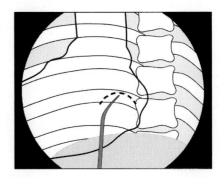

Figure 37.2. Transseptal Puncture

Orientation of needle in antero-posterior (A) and left lateral (B) views. The dotted line represents the limbus of the fossa ovalis.

is advanced across the atrial septum to the left atrium, which is usually associated with a slight "popping" sensation. In general, the AP and RAO projections result in mild foreshortening of the atrial septum and left atrium; it is therefore preferable to advance the needle into the left atrium in a 60°-90° LAO projection. Transseptal catheterization described above is safe: Perforation leading to tamponade has been reported in 1.3%, and mortality in < 0.1%.[34]

b. Inoue Technique. The Inoue balloon catheter is a 12F, 70-cm long polyvinyl chloride catheter with two central coaxial lumens. The inner lumen allows pressure measurement and passage of a guidewire, and the outer lumen is for balloon inflation. Balloon size is based on patient height: balloon size in mm = height (cm; rounded to the nearest 0) divided by 10, and added to 10. The stainless steel guidewire is inserted into the left atrium through the Mullins sheath until the coiled tip touches the superior wall of the left atrium. After dilating the groin and atrial septum, the Inoue balloon is carefully advanced over the guidewire into the left atrium and across the mitral valve. The distal balloon is partially inflated and then pulled back and anchored in the mitral valve; full balloon inflation is completed to dilate the mitral valve. After deflating the balloon, left atrial pressure is remeasured. If an inadequate result is obtained, the balloon can be advanced and inflated to larger size (the Inoue balloon diameter is adjustable within 4 mm). When the dilation process is complete, the balloon catheter is removed and final measurements obtained. A lower cost, double-lumen reusable Accura balloon may be comparable to the Inoue balloon.[154]

c. **Single or Double-Balloon Technique.** Following transseptal catheterization, heparin is administered, and a balloon-tipped flotation catheter is advanced through the Mullins sheath into the left atrium, left ventricle, and the ascending aorta. One (single-balloon technique) or two (double-balloon technique) 0.035" J wires are then advanced through the balloon-tipped catheter into the aorta, after which the interatrial septum is dilated with an 8-mm balloon. After septostomy, one (25 mm) or two (18, 20 mm) balloons are advanced across the mitral valve and inflated using a hand-held syringe (Figure 37.3). The final balloon size depends on the patient's size; for patients with a small body habitus (< 60 kg), it is reasonable to start with a single 25-mm balloon, with further increases depending on hemodynamics. A single 25-mm balloon has an inflated area of 4.9 cm^2; combined 15-mm and 20-mm balloons inflate to 5.51 cm^2; and two 18-mm balloons inflate to 5.78 cm^2. PBMV is most effective using inflated balloons > 4.9 cm^2. Following dilation, the balloons are removed and the flotation catheter is advanced to the left atrium for repeat pressure measurements.

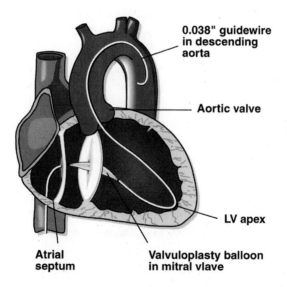

0.038" guidewire in descending aorta

Aortic valve

LV apex

Atrial septum

Valvuloplasty balloon in mitral vlave

Figure 37.3. Percutaneous Balloon Mitral Valvuloplasty (PBMV)

d. Metallic Valvulotome. Recently, a reusable metallic valvotomy device was developed to increase the cost-effectiveness of percutaneous mitral valvuloplasty.[151] The device can be expanded from 30-40 mm in diameter, and is inserted using standard transseptal technique.

e. Multi-Track System. Two separate balloons are positioned on a single guidewire. The first catheter, with only a distal guidewire lumen, is introduced into the vein and then advanced into the mitral orifice. A rapid exchange balloon catheter is then advanced over the same guidewire. Once both balloons are side-by-side, simultaneous inflations are performed.[168]

2. Retrograde Transarterial Approach. The left ventricle is entered retrograde with a pigtail catheter via the femoral artery and exchanged for a special steerable left atrial catheter. The steering wire is retracted and a "J" is formed in the left ventricular apex. To enter the left atrium, the 45° LAO and 45° RAO projections are used. Ventriculography in these views can define the mitral valve plane and facilitate cannulation of the left atrium. After the guidewire enters the left atrium, the left atrial catheter is exchanged for a pigtail catheter to obtain pressure measurements and calculation of mitral valve area. The pigtail catheter is exchanged for a standard valvuloplasty balloon catheter using a single or double balloon technique.

D. RESULTS

1. Hemodynamics Results (Tables 37.2, 37.3). PBMV produces immediate improvement in hemodynamic and clinical status in most patients.[9-12,14,15,17,25,35-44,169-172] In general, there is a 50-70% decrease in transmitral gradient and a 50-100% increase in mitral valve area (Figure 37.4). Approximately 10% of patients have persistent mitral valve areas < 1.0 cm^2. Valve areas are smaller after PBMV with single balloons than double balloons, and results with the Inoue balloon are similar to the double balloon technique (Table 37.3).[10,42-44] Several reports confirm the effectiveness of PBMV after previous percutaneous valvuloplasty[173] or surgical commissurotomy[45-48,174-176] (although symptom recurrence is more frequent at 6 months),[45-47] and for pregnant women with mitral stenosis.[25,49-53,177,178] PBMV may also be effective in selected patients with significant calcific mitral stenosis[179] or moderate mitral regurgitation,[180] and in elderly patients considered unsuitable for surgery.[181] Immediate results of the metallic valvulotome appear to be similar to those of balloon valvuloplasty.[151]

2. Complications (Table 37.4). Serious complications include death (0-1.6%), thromboembolic events (0-6.5%), and severe mitral regurgitation requiring valve replacement (0.9%-3%). Transient heart block and pericardial tamponade occur infrequently ($< 5\%$) with transseptal techniques.[34,182] An echocardiographic score based on valve morphology has been established to identify patients at risk of developing severe mitral regurgitation after percutaneous mitral valvulotomy.[183,184] While a left-to-right shunt is detected in 20% of patients immediately after transseptal PBMV, the shunt ratio is usually < 1.5 and decreases over the next 6 months in the majority of cases.[55-58]

3. Long-term Results (Tables 37.5, 37.6). In general, improvements in hemodynamic and clinical status persist in the majority of patients.[11,15,17,35,39,40,42,59-61,152] However, restenosis (loss of $\geq 50\%$

of the original gain in mitral valve area) develops in 7-24% of patients within 5 years. Factors adversely affecting long-term outcome include high echo score, elevated left ventricular end-diastolic pressure, and higher NYHA functional class; predicted 5-year event-free survival is 60-84% and 13-41% in patients with ≤ 1 risk factor and ≥ 2 risk factors, respectively.[8] Total survival and event-free survival at 2 years were 98% and 79% for patients with an echo score ≤ 8, and 72% and 39% for patients with echo score > 8. The strongest independent predictors of event-free survival at 2-4 years were mitral valve morphology reflected by the echo score, baseline and post-procedure mitral valve area, and post-procedure mean pulmonary capillary wedge pressure.[62,152,153,163,164] The relative risk of an adverse cardiac event after PBMV is 3.6 times higher in patients with preexisting mitral regurgitation, despite excellent initial results.[156]

Table 37.2. Immediate Results of PBMV

Series	Technique	N (pts)	MVA (cm^2)		MVG (mm Hg)	
			Pre	Post	Pre	Post
Iung[169] (1999)	1, 2, I	1024	1.1	1.9	10	5
Leon[170] (1999)	I, D	734	0.9 AF 0.9 SR	1.7 2.0	13 AF 16 SR	5 5
Hernandez[171] (1999)	I	561	1.0	1.8	-	-
Cribier[151] (1999)	MV	153	1.0	2.2	20	4
Shephanadis[153] (1998)	R	441	1.0	2.1	18	6
Lau[155] (1998)	I	68	0.8	1.7	13	5
Orrange[152] (1997)	2, I	132	1.0	1.9	14	6
Fawzy[150] (1996)	I	220	0.7	1.7	15	6
Chen[15] (1995)	I	4832	1.1	2.1	18	5
Arora[35] (1994)	2, I	600	0.8	2.2	27	4
Block[36] (1994)	1, 2	570	0.9	2.0	16	6
Vahanian[25] (1994)	2, I	790	1.1	2.1	15	6
Stephanadis[37] (1994)	R	154	1.0	2.2	16	6

Abbreviations: MVA = mitral valve area; MVG = transmitral valve gradient; I = Inoue technique; 1 = single balloon technique; 2 = double balloon technique; R = retrograde (transarterial) technique; MV = metallic valvulotome; AF = atrial fibrillation; SR = sinus rhythm; PBMV = percutaneous balloon mitral valvuloplasty

Table 37.3. Immediate Results and Technique of PBMV

Series	N (pts)	Technique	MVA (cm^2) Pre	Post	MVG (mmHg) Pre	Post
Kang[172]	152	I	0.9	1.8	16	7
(1999)	150	D	0.9	1.9	17	6
Nanjappa[154]	400	A	0.8	1.9	15	5
(1998)	512	I	0.9	2.0	16	5
Park[42]	59	I	0.9	1.9	-	-
(1993)	61	2	0.9	2.0	-	-
Ribeiro[43]	9	I	0.8	1.8	-	-
(1993)	9	2	0.8	1.9	-	-
NHLBI[10]	114	1	0.9	1.7	14	7
(1992)	591	2	1.0	2.0	14	6
Bassand[44]	161	2	1.0	2.0	13	5
(1991)	60	I	1.1	2.0	12	5

Abbreviations: MVA = mitral valve area; MVG = transmitral valve gradient; I = Inoue technique; 1 = single balloon technique; 2 = double balloon technique; R = retrograde (transarterial) technique; - = not reported; A = Accura balloon

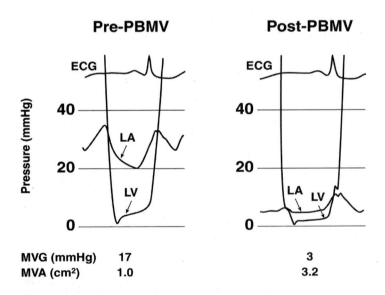

	Pre-PBMV	Post-PBMV
MVG (mmHg)	17	3
MVA (cm²)	1.0	3.2

Figure 37.4. PBMV: Immediate Hemodynamic Results

PBMV results in a decrease in mitral valve gradient (MVG) and an increase in mitral valve area (MVA). Pressure in the left atrium (LA) decreases, and there is no change in the left ventricular (LV) diastolic pressure.
PBMV = percutaneous balloon mitral valvuloplasty

Table 37.4. Complications of PBMV

Series	N (pts)	Death (%)	Emb/CVA (%)	Perf/Tamp (%)	MR (%)
Kang[172] (1999)	302	0.3	-	-	6.0
Iung[169] (1999)	1024	0.4	0.3	0	3.4
Leon[170] (1999)	734	3.1 AF 0.5 SR	2.0 AF 0.8 SR	1.1 AF 0.5 SR	2.6 AF 4.0 SR
Hernandez[171] (1999)	561	-	-	-	4.5
Cribier[151] (1999)	153	0	0.6	0.6	1.2
Shephanadis[153] (1998)	441	0.2	-	-	3.4
Nanjappa[154] (1998)	912	0.2	0	1.0	0.5
Orrange[152] (1997)	132	4.5	-	1.5	6
Fawzy[150] (1996)	220	0	0	0.9	1.4
Chen[15] (1995)	4832	0.1	0.5	0.8	0.4
Arora[35] (1994)	600	1.0	0.5	1.3	1.0
Block[36] (1994)	570	0.5	1.0	1.0	1.4
Vahanian[25] (1994)	810	0.5	3.6	0.9	3.5
Stephanadis[37] (1994)	155	0.6	0	0	1.3
Feldman[38] (1993)	260	1.1	0.7	0.7	2.7
NHLBI[10] (1992)	737	1.6	1.7	0.4	-
Cohen[11] (1992)	146	1.0	2.0	4.0	2.7
Stephanadis[17] (1992)	86	0	0	0	1.2

Abbreviations: Emb/CVA = embolic event or stroke; Perf/Tamp = cardiac perforation or tamponade; MR = severe mitral regurgitation; AF = atrial fibrillation; PBMV = percutaneous balloon mitral valvuloplasty; SR = sinus rhythm; - = not reported

Table 37.5. Clinical Follow-up After PBMV

Series	N (pts)	Follow-up (months)	Restenosis (%)	RePBMV (%)	MVR (%)	Death (%)
Kang[172] (1999)	302	51	17 I 13 D	3.3 I 2.0 D	4.6 I 6.6 D	1.3 I 1.3 D
Iung[169] (1999)	1024	49	-	-	17.9	6.1
Leon[170] (1999)	672	66	-	6.1 AF 6.1 SR	24.0 AF 23.6 SR	15.5 AF 7.6 SR
Hernandez[171] (1999)	561	39	10	0.9	9.8	5.0
Stephanadis[153] (1998)	385	42	9.1	0.5	4.9	0.3
Orrange[152] (1997)	126	29	20	4.5	15	5
Iung[163] (1996)	528	32	7.6	0.9	6.7	1.5
Chen[15] (1995)	4832	32	5.2	0.4	-	-
Arora[35] (1994)	600	37	1.7	0.3	0.2	-
Chan[59] (1994)	253	20	23.5	3.6	10.3	3.9
Pan[39] (1993)	350	38	11.7	0.6	5.1	1.7
Chen[60] (1992)	85	60	6.8	1.1	4.7	-
Cohen[11] (1992)	146	36	18	4.1	12.4	22.1
Stephanadis[17] (1992)	84	24	15.4	-	3.6	-

Abbreviations: AF = atrial fibrillation; MVR = mitral valve replacement; PBMV = percutaneous balloon mitral valvuloplasty; RePBMV = repeat PBMV; SR = sinus rhythm; - = not reported

Table 37.6. Hemodynamic Follow-up After PBMV

Series	N (pts)	Follow-up (years)	Technique	MVA (cm²)		
				Pre	Post	F/U
Hernandez[171] (1999)	561	39	I	1.0	1.8	1.7
Chen[159] (1998)	202	8.1	I	1.0	2.1	1.7
Chen[15] (1995)	-	2.6	I	1.1	2.1	1.8
Park[42] (1993)	-	1	I, 2	0.9	1.9	1.7
Chen[60] (1992)	85	5	I	1.1	2.0	1.8
Block[61] (1992)	41	2	1, 2	1.1	1.8	1.6
Stephanadis[17] (1992)	26	2	R	0.9	2.0	1.9

Abbreviations: I = Inoue technique; 1 = single balloon technique; 2 = double balloon technique; R = retrograde (transarterial) technique; MVA = mitral valve area; PBMV = percutaneous balloon mitral valvuloplasty; - = not reported

Table 37.7. Randomized Trials of PBMV and Surgery

Study	Technique	N	Months	MVA (cm²)			RS (%)
				Baseline	Post	F/U	
Farhat[158] (1998)	PBMV	30	6	0.9	-	2.2	6.6
	OMC	30		0.9	-	2.2	6.6
	CMC	30		0.9	-	1.6	37
Reyes[162] (1994)	PBMV	30	36	0.9	2.1	2.4	10
	CMC	30		0.9	2.0	1.8	13
Arora[161] (1993)	PBMV	100	24	0.8	2.4	2.0	5
	CMC	100		0.8	2.2	1.9	4
Turi[160] (1991)	PBMV	20	8	0.8	1.6	1.6	-
	CMC	20		0.9	1.6	1.8	-

Abbreviations: PBMV = percutaneous balloon mitral valvuloplasty; OMC = open mitral commissurotomy; CMC = closed mitral commissurotomy; MVA = mitral valve area; RS = restenosis; F/U = follow-up; MVA = mitral valve area

4. **Predictors of Early Outcome.** Clinical, echocardiographic, hemodynamic, and procedural factors associated with a less successful immediate outcome after PBMV include:[8,10-12,39,63-69] advanced age (only 50% of patients > 65 years achieve a final valve area > 1.5 cm^2);[77,78] rhythm other than sinus; high echo score (although some patients with high scores have good results); mitral valve calcification (mitral valve area after PBMV was smaller in calcified than noncalcified valves, 1.8 vs. 2.1 cm^2); and treatment with smaller balloons. Factors not affecting the early results of PMBV include severity of mitral stenosis[71] and mild-to-moderate mitral or aortic regurgitation.[72,73,156] Elevated pulmonary artery pressure has been variably associated with an adverse outcome.[74-76]

5. **Comparison of Different Techniques and Surgical Commissurotomy.** Selection of the technique for mitral valvuloplasty is based primarily on personal experience and available equipment. In appropriate hands, all techniques are effective and safe.[10,42-44,79-83] In studies comparing double balloons to the Inoue technique, final valve area was slightly larger after double balloons (2.0-2.2 vs. 1.7-2.0 cm^2), but the degree of mitral regurgitation and intracardiac shunting were similar. No studies have directly compared transarterial and transseptal techniques. PBMV and surgical techniques (closed and open commissurotomy[84-86]) have been shown to achieve similar early results, although in one report, mitral valve area at 3 years was greater in patients treated with PBMV (2.4 vs. 1.8 cm^2) (Table 37.7).[86]

PERCUTANEOUS BALLOON AORTIC VALVULOPLASTY

Aortic stenosis (AS) in adults is most commonly caused by degenerative calcification of a congenital bicuspid valve. Characterized by a long latent period during which progressive stenosis and left ventricular (LV) hypertrophy occur, patients with severe AS may remain asymptomatic for many years. However, once symptoms develop, prognosis is poor: Life-expectancy for those with angina, syncope, and heart failure is 5 years, 3 years, and 2 years, respectively.

Percutaneous balloon aortic valvuloplasty (PBAV) was first performed in children with aortic stenosis,[87] and later applied to adults with degenerative calcific aortic stenosis.[88,91] Although PBMV has become a viable alternative to surgical commissurotomy for select patients with mitral stenosis, PBAV has not become a viable alternative to aortic valve replacement (AVR) in adults. AVR is the standard treatment for adults with symptomatic aortic stenosis and is typically associated with marked hemodynamic improvement, regression of LV hypertrophy, enhanced LV performance, and increased survival;[94,96] perioperative mortality rates are 1.5-5% but may be as high as 15-40% for emergency operations or in patients with severe LV dysfunction and shock.[97] The impact of advanced age per se is somewhat controversial: some studies of AVR in patients > 70 years reported perioperative mortality rates of 12-33%,[98,99] but contemporary studies report perioperative mortality rates < 10%.[100,101] Actuarial 1- and 5-year survival rates are 83% and 67% for octogenarians treated with isolated AVR for aortic stenosis, which is similar to the actuarial survival of octogenarians without aortic stenosis.[100]

A. **MECHANISM OF AORTIC VALVULOPLASTY.** Post-mortem and intraoperative studies indicate that the mechanisms of PBAV include fracture of calcified nodules, separation of fused commissures (rheumatic aortic stenosis), and simple stretching of valve leaflets. Although leaflet mobility and orifice dimensions improve, valve leaflets remain severely deformed, calcified, and stenotic.[102]

B. **PREPROCEDURAL EVALUATION.** Adults with clinical evidence of aortic stenosis should undergo 2-D echocardiography to evaluate valve function and morphology, and left ventricular performance. Right and left heart catheterization, coronary angiography, and aortography are recommended to assess the extent of coronary artery disease and aortic insufficiency.

C. **TECHNIQUE.** The two potential approaches for PBAV are the retrograde arterial approach and the antegrade transvenous approach:

1. **Retrograde Arterial Approach (Figure 37.5).** The most common approach to PBAV is the retrograde femoral arterial approach. (A retrograde brachial approach may also be used if femoral arterial access cannot be achieved.) To perform PBAV using the retrograde femoral approach:

   - Place an 8F sheath in the left femoral vein for right heart catheterization, cardiac output determination, and central access in the event a temporary pacemaker is needed.
   - Place an arterial monitoring line in the left femoral or radial artery.
   - Perform left heart catheterization via the right femoral artery (or brachial artery) using a 7F angled pigtail catheter and a long (30-cm) 8F introducing sheath; heparin (3000-5000 units) should be administered intravenously after arterial access is obtained. Simultaneous LV and systemic pressures may be obtained via the pigtail catheter and arterial sidearm, or by using an 8F double-lumen pigtail catheter, which permits pressure measurements in close proximity to the aortic valve. Special care must be taken to adequately flush the proximal lumen, since a damped pressure will falsely overestimate the transaortic valve gradient and degree of aortic stenosis.
   - Cross the aortic valve with the pigtail catheter using a 0.038-inch straight guidewire. After baseline hemodynamic measurements are obtained, a 280-cm 0.038-inch J-guidewire should be placed in the left ventricle; a large curve should be fashioned on the distal end of the guidewire to conform to the shape of the apex.
   - Exchange the 8F arterial sheath and pigtail for a 12F introducing sheath and a 20 mm x 50 mm valvuloplasty balloon (or alternatively an Inoue balloon).[186] Position the balloon across the aortic valve, and inflate the balloon with dilute contrast using a hand-held syringe. If blood pressure allows, balloon inflations of 30-60 seconds are desirable.
   - After 2-4 inflations, the valvuloplasty balloon is exchanged for the pigtail catheter for repeat hemodynamic assessment. Once the desired result is achieved (generally a 50% reduction in gradient), the procedure is terminated. Vascular sheaths may be removed when the ACT is less than 150 seconds.

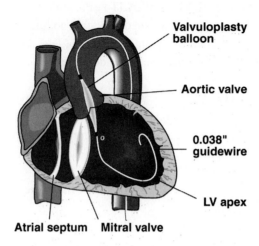

Figure 37.5. Percutaneous Balloon Aortic Valvuloplasty (PBAV)

2. **Antegrade Transvenous Approach.** The antegrade transvenous approach requires transseptal left heart catheterization, as described for balloon mitral valvuloplasty. This techniques should be reserved for operators experienced in transseptal techniques and in circumstances where retrograde crossing of the aortic valve is impossible.

3. **Single vs. Multiple Balloon Techniques.** PBAV may be performed using single or multiple balloons; multiple balloon techniques seem to achieve slightly larger valve areas, but no difference in late outcome. In most patients, the simplest approach is the single balloon technique using a 20 mm balloon; if necessary, larger or multiple balloons may be used.[103]

D. RESULTS
1. **Hemodynamic Results (Table 37.8).** PBAV results in a 50-70% decrease in aortic valve gradient and a 40-60% increase in aortic valve area (Figure 37.6). Despite these results, all patients still have severe AS. The hemodynamic results are similar for retrograde or antegrade approaches, and for single or multiple balloons.[103-110]

Table 37.8. Immediate Hemodynamic Results of PBAV

Series	N (pts)	Approach	AVA (cm²)		AVG (mm Hg)	
			Pre	Post	Pre	Post
Lieberman[185] (1995)	165	R	0.5	0.7	68	38
Block[104] (1994)	375	All	0.5	0.9	61	27
Letac[105] (1993)	406	S, R	0.6	1.0	72	29
Safian[103] (1991)	225	S, R	0.6	0.9	67	33
NHLBI[106] (1991)	674	All	0.5	0.8	65	31
McKay[107] (1991)	492	All	0.5	0.8	60	30

Abbreviations: PBAV = percutaneous balloon aortic valvuloplasty; S = single balloon; R = retrograde approach; AVA = aortic valve area; AVG = transaortic valve gradient

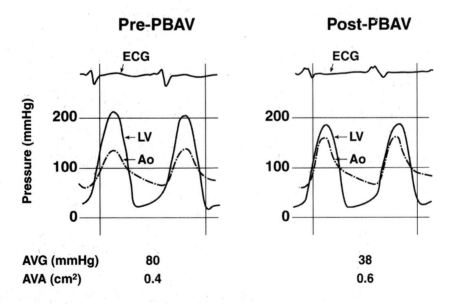

Figure 37.6. PBAV: Immediate Hemodynamic Results

PBAV results in a decrease in aortic valve gradient (AVG) and an increase in aortic valve area (AVA). Left ventricular (LV) pressure decreases, and aortic (AO) pressure increases.

Table 37.9. Complications of PBAV

Series	N (pts)	Death (%)	CVA (%)	Perf (%)	MI (%)	AI (%)	Vasc (%)
Block[104] (1994)	308	5.0	2.0	0.3	0.5	0.00	9.0
Safian[103] (1991)	225	3.1	0.4	1.2	0.5	0.8	7.5
Isner[112] (1991)	492	2.6	-	1.8	-	0.8	-
NHLBI[106] (1991)	672	3.0	4.6	1.0	1.0	1.0	27
McKay[107] (1991)	492	7.5	2.2	1.8	0.2	1.0	11
Cribier[111] (1990)	334	4.5	1.4	0.6	0.3	0.00	13.1
Lewin[108] (1989)	125	10.4	3.2	0.00	1.6	1.6	9.6

Abbreviations: PBAV = percutaneous balloon aortic valvuloplasty; CVA = stroke; Perf = cardiac perforation; MI = myocardial infarction; AI = severe aortic insufficiency; Vasc = vascular injury requiring surgical repair or blood transfusion; - = not reported

2. **Complications (Table 37.9).** Major clinical complications are not infrequent and include death (2.6-10.4%), cerebrovascular events (0.4-4.6%), cardiac perforation (0-1.8%), myocardial infarction (0.3-1.6%), severe aortic insufficiency (0-1.6%), and vascular injury requiring blood transfusion and/or vascular repair (7.5-27%).[103,104,106-108,111,112] Procedure-related mortality is more common in acutely decompensated patients with severe LV dysfunction. Cardiac perforation may be caused by the guidewire or balloon catheter. Sudden hemodynamic collapse during the procedure is usually due to cardiac tamponade or aortic valve disruption,[113-116] while worsening congestive heart failure immediately after PBAV is usually due to aortic insufficiency.[117,118] Other reported complications include transient complete heart block,[119] mitral valve rupture,[120,121] and bacterial endocarditis.[122]

3. **Long-term Results (Table 37.10).** In contrast to balloon mitral valvuloplasty, the long-term results of PBAV are poor. Available studies of 1-3-year follow-up report a high incidence of late cardiac events, including death in 30-60%, aortic valve replacement in 7-27%, and repeat balloon valvuloplasty in 4-22%.[103,106,108,111,185] Acute and long-term results of repeat PBAV are similar to initial PBAV.[123-125]

4. **Predictors of Late Outcome.** The poor long-term results of PBAV are secondary to several factors, including persistent severe aortic stenosis despite successful dilation, a high incidence (30-60%) of early restenosis, the presence of concomitant severe coronary artery disease, and associated noncardiac comorbid diseases. The most important determinants of event-free survival are those associated with baseline LV performance,[126-131,185] not improvement in valve area. In a study of 205 valvuloplasty patients, event-free survival correlated with baseline LV ejection fraction, LV systolic pressure, aortic systolic pressure, and percent reduction in valve gradient; baseline pulmonary wedge pressure was inversely related to outcome.[126] Although overall event-free survival at 2-years was 25%, it was only 4% in patients with all 3 baseline adverse predictors. Patients with severe LV dysfunction who underwent PBAV had long-term results similar to those of untreated aortic stenosis.[126]

5. **Comparison of Balloon Valvuloplasty and Aortic Valve Replacement (Table 37.11).** There are no prospective randomized studies of PBAV and AVR. However, a single center observational study reported the superiority of AVR in octogenarians with symptomatic aortic stenosis: in-hospital mortality rates were similar, but event-free survival at 22 months was 78% in AVR patients but only 6.5% in PBAV patients.[132]

E. **RECOMMENDATIONS.** Available data are compelling: Aortic valve replacement is the preferred treatment for virtually all adults with symptomatic aortic stenosis. Octogenarians with aortic stenosis should not be denied the opportunity for valve replacement based on age alone. Nevertheless, there may be selected patients for whom PBAV may be considered:

1. **Severe LV Dysfunction.** Some adult patients with aortic stenosis have severely depressed ejection fractions (EF < 25%), which may be explained by factors such as critical aortic stenosis and afterload mismatch, previous myocardial infarction, coexisting hypertensive heart disease, advanced mitral regurgitation, or cardiomyopathy. Although patients with LV dysfunction due to critical aortic stenosis and afterload mismatch will improve after aortic valve replacement, it is difficult to identify these patients using standard clinical criteria. In contrast, patients with aortic stenosis and LV dysfunction secondary to causes other than afterload mismatch may not have improvement in LV performance after aortic valve replacement. Thus, PBAV may be used to identify a subgroup of patients who are likely to improve after AVR. In such patients, significant improvement in LV ejection fraction is observed in 40-50% of patients 3 months after PBAV;[133] these patients should be considered for AVR to improve survival, since late outcome after PBAV alone is poor.[134,135] The role of PBAV in improving mitral regurgitation associated with aortic stenosis is controversial: some studies suggest benefit,[136] but others do not.[137]

Table 37.10. Clinical Follow-up After PBAV

Series	N (pts)	F/U (months)	Death (%)	AVR (%)	rePBAV (%)
Lieberman[185] (1995)	165	47	60	25	19
Safian[103] (1991)	225	24	40	27	22
NHLBI[106] (1991)	648	36	60	13	4
Cribier[111] (1990)	300	16	30	19	17
Lewin[108] (1989)	125	12	42	7	8

Abbreviations: AVR = aortic valve replacement; F/U = follow-up interval (months); PBAV = percutaneous balloon aortic valvuloplasty; rePBAV = repeat PBAV

Table 37.11. Comparison of PBAV and AVR[132]

	PBAV (n = 46)	MVA (n = 23)
Age (yrs)	80	78
Preop AVG (mmHg)*	105	107
In-hospital death (%)	6.5	8.7
Follow-up at 22 mos. (%)		
Death	52	13
AVR	35	0.00
EFS	6.5	78
Total survival		
1-yr	75	83
2-yr	47	83
3-yr	33	75

Abbreviations: AVR = aortic valve replacement; AVG = transaortic valve gradient; EFS = event-free survival; PBAV = percutaneous balloon aortic valvuloplasty
* Doppler gradient

2. **Low-Gradient, Low-Output State.** Symptomatic patients with aortic stenosis, a low cardiac output, and a low transaortic valve gradient are at high risk for perioperative death after AVR and have a poor long-term prognosis. In these patients, PBAV may identify a subgroup of patients with hemodynamic and clinical improvement, who might then be considered for AVR.[138]

3. **Cardiogenic Shock.** PBAV may be a life-saving procedure in select patients with aortic stenosis and cardiogenic shock. However, because in-hospital mortality is high and long-term prognosis is poor, patients who survive hospitalization should be strongly considered for AVR.[139-145]

4. **Preoperative Palliation Before Noncardiac Surgery.** PBAV may be considered in some patients with aortic stenosis who require urgent noncardiac surgery.[146-148] In these patients, PBAV results in significant hemodynamic improvement, similar to that observed in other patients treated with PBAV. In spite of this hemodynamic improvement, there are no data to suggest that routine PBAV will improve the perioperative risks of noncardiac surgery. In fact, in one study of 48 patients with severe aortic stenosis, careful monitoring during anesthesia resulted in no major complications, despite the need for vascular, orthopedic, abdominal, and other forms of surgery without preoperative PBAV.[149] We empirically proceed with valvuloplasty in patients with overt heart failure or systolic blood pressures < 100 mmHg who require urgent noncardiac surgery. In other patients without heart failure or hypotension, we recommend noncardiac surgery without preoperative PBAV; monitoring of systemic and pulmonary artery pressure is useful to avoid hypovolemia and vasodilation, which could have adverse consequences for patients with significant aortic stenosis.

* * * * *

REFERENCES

1. Inoue K, Owaki T, Nakamura T, et al. Clinical application of transvenous mitral commissurotomy by a new balloon catheter. J Thorac Cardiovas Surg. 1984;87:394-402.
2. Lock JE, Khalilulah M, Shrivastava S, et al. Percutaneous catheter commissurotomy in rheumatic mitral stenosis. N Engl J Med 1985;313:1515-1518.
3. Al Zaibag MA, Kasab SA, Ribeiro PA, et al. Percutaneous double-balloon mitral valvuloplasty for rheumatic mitral valve stenosis. Lancet 1986;1:757-761.
4. McKay RG, Lock JE, Keane JF, et al. Percutaneous mitral valvuloplasty in an adult patient with calcific rheumatic mitral stenosis. J Am Coll Cardiol 1986;7:1410-1415.
5. Palacios IF, Lock JE, Keane JF, et al. Percutaneous transvenous balloon valvuloplasty in a patient with severe calcific mitral stenosis. J Am Coll Cardiol 1986;7:1416-1419.
6. Babic UU, Pejac P, Djurisic Z, et al. Percutaneous transarterial balloon valvuloplasty for mitral valve stenosis. Am J Cardiol 1986;57:1101-1104.
7. Brockenbrough EC, Braunwald E. A new technique for left ventricular angiocardiography and transseptal left heart catheterization. Am J Cardiol 1960;6:1062.
8. Palacios IF, Block PC, Wilkins GT, et al. Follow-up of patients undergoing percutaneous mitral balloon valvotomy. Analysis of factors determining restenosis. Circulation 1989;79:573-579.
9. Vahanian A, Michel PL, Cormier B, et al. Results of percutaneous mitral commissurotomy in 200 patients. Am J Cardiol 1989;63:847-852.
10. The National Heart, Lung, and Blood Institute Balloon Valvuloplasty Registry Participants Multicenter Experience with Balloon Mitral Commissurotomy: NHLBI Balloon Valvuloplasty Registry report on immediate and 30-day follow-up results. Circulation 1992;85:448-461.
11. Cohen DT, Kuntz RE Gorday SP, et al. Predictors of longterm

outcome after percutaneous balloon mitral valvuloplasty. N Engl J Med 1992;327:1329-1335.

12. Abascal VM, Wilkins GT, O'Shea JP, et al. Prediction of successful outcome in 130 patients undergoing percutaneous mitral valvotomy. Circulation 1990;82:448-456.

13. Palacios IF, Tuzcu ME, Weyman AF, et al. Clinical follow-up of patients undergoing percutaneous mitral balloon valvotomy. Circulation 1995;91:671-676.

14. Nobuyoshi M, Hameishi N, Dimura T, et al. Indications, complications, and short-term clinical outcome of percutaneous transvenous mitral commissurotomy. Circulation 1989;80:782-792.

15. Chen CR, Cheng TO. Percutaneous balloon mitral valvuloplasty by the Inoue technique. A multicenter study of 4832 patients in China. Am Heart J 1995;129:1197-1203.

16. Orme EC, Wray RB, Mason JW. Balloon mitral valvuloplasty via retrograde left atrial catheterization. Am Heart J 1989;117:680-683.

17. Stefanadis C, Stratos C, Pitsaves C, et al. Retrograde nontransseptal balloon mitral valvuloplasty immediate results and Longterm follow-up. Circulation 1992;85:1760-1767.

18. Bahl VK, Juneya R, Thatar D, et al. Retrograde nontransseptal balloon mitral valvuloplasty for rheumatic mitral stenosis. Cathet Cardiovasc Diagn 1994;33:331-334.

19. Yeh K-H, Hung J-S, Wu C-J, Fu M. Safety of inoue balloon mitral commissurotomy in patients with left atrial appendage thrombi. Am J Cardiol 1995;75:302-304.

20. Hung J. Mitral stenosis with left atrial thrombi: Inoue balloon catheter technique. New York: Igakushoin Medical, 1992:280-293.

21. Fu M, Hung J-S, Lee C-B, Cherng W-J. Coronary neovascularization as a specific sign for left atrial appendage thrombus in mitral stenosis. Am J Cardiol 1991;67:1158-1160.

22. Chen WJ, Chen MF, Liau CS, Chung C. Safety of percutaneous transvenous balloon mitral commissurotomy in patients with mitral stenosis and thrombus in the left atrial appendage. Am J Cardiol 1992;70:117-119.

23. Chow WH, Chow TS, Yip A, Cheung KL. Percutaneous balloon mitral valvotomy in patients with history of embolism. Am J Cardiol 1993;71:1243-1244.

24. Kamalesh M, Burger AJ, Shubrooks SJ. The use of transesophageal echocardiography to avoid left atrial thrombus during percutaneous mitral valvuloplasty. Cathet Cardiovasc Diagn 1993;28:320-322.

25. Vahanian A, Acar J. Mitral valvuloplasty: The French Experience. In: Topol EJ, Editor. Textbook of Interventional Cardiology; Philadelphia, WB Saunders, 1994.

26. McKay RG, Lock JE, Safian RD, et al. Balloon dilation of mitral stenosis in adult patients: post morterm and percutaneous mitral valvuloplasty studies. J Am Coll Cardiol 1987;9:723-731.

27. Block PC, Palaeios IF, Jacobs ML, et al. Mechanism of percutaneous mitral valvotomy. Am J Cardiol 1987;59:178-179.

28. Kaplan JD, Isner JM, Karas RH, et al. In vitro analysis of mechanisms of balloon valvuloplasty of stenotic mitral valves. Am J Cardiol 1987;59:318-323.

29. Hogan K, Ramaswamy K, Losordo DW, et al. Pathology at mitral commissurotomy performed with the Inoue catheter: implication for mechanisms and complications. Cathet Cardiovasc Diagn 1994;32(Suppl 2):42-51.

30. Lin PJ, Chang J-P, Chu J-J, Chang C-H. Balloon valvuloplasty is contraindicated in stenotic mitral bioprostheses. Am Heart J 1994;127:724-726.

31. Calvo OL, obrino N, Gamallo C, Oliver J. Balloon percutaneous valvuloplasty for stenotic bioprosthetic valves in the mitral position. Am J Cardiol 1987;60:736-737.

32. Cox D, Friedman P, Selwyn A, Lee R, JA B. Improved quality of life after successful balloon valvuloplasty of a stenosed mitral bioprosthesis. Am Heart J 1989;118:839-41.

33. Babic U, Gruijicic S, Vucinic M. Balloon valvuloplasty of bioprosthesis. Int J Cardiol 1991;30:230-2.

34. Roelke M, Smith AJ, Palacios IF. The technique and safety of transseptal left heart catheterization: the Massachusetts General Hospital experience with 1279 procedures. Cathet Cardiovasc Diagn 1994;32:332-339.

35. Arora R, Kalra G, Murty G, et al. Percutaneous transatrial mitral commissurotomy: Immediate and intermediate results. J Am Coll Cardiol 1994;23:1327-32.

36. Block PC, Palacios IF. Aortic and mitral balloon valvuloplasty. The US Experience. In: Topol EJ, Editor. Textbook of Interventional Cardiology; Philadelphia, WB Saunders, 1994.

37. Stephanadis, Toutouzas P. Retrograde nontransseptal mitral alvuloplasty. In: Topol EJ, Editor. Textbook of Interventional Cardiology; Philadelphia, WB Saunders, 1994.

38. Feldman T, Carroll JD, Herrmann HC, Holmes DR. Effect of balloon size and stepwise inflation technique on the acute results of Inoue mitral commissurotomy. Cathet Cardiovasc Diagn 1993;28:199-205.

39. Pan M, Medina A, deLexo JS, Hernandez E. Factors determining late success after mitral balloon valvulotomy. Am J Cardiol 1993;71:1181-1185.

40. Hung J, Chern M, Wu J, Fu M. Short and longterm results of catheter balloon percutaneous transvenous mitral commissurotomy. Am J Cardiol 1991;67:854-862.

41. Ruiz CE, Allen J, Lau F. Percutaneous double balloon valvotomy for severe rheumatic mitral stenosis. Am J Cardiol 1990;65:473-477.

42. Park SJ, Kim JJ, Park SW, et al. Immediate and one-year results of PBMV using Inoue and double-balloon techniques. Am J Cardiol 1993;71:938-943.

43. Ribeiro PA, Fawzy ME, Arafat MA, Dunn B. Comparison of mitral valve area results of balloon mitral valvotomy using the Inoue and double balloon techniques. Am J Cardiol 1991;68:687-688.

44. Bassand J, Schiele F, Bernard Y, Anguenot T. The double-balloon and Inoue techniques in percutaneous mitral valvuloplasty: comparative results in a series of 232 cases. J

Am Coll Cardiol 1991;18:982-989.

45. Davidson CT, Bashore TM, Mickel M, et al. Balloon mitral commissurotomy after previous surgical commissurotomy. The NHLBI balloon valvuloplasty registry participants. Circulation 1992;86:91-99.

46. Jang I-K, Block P, Newell J, Tuzcu M, Palacios I. Percutaneous mitral balloon valvotomy for recurrent mitral stenosis after surgical commissurotomy. Am J Cardiol 1995;75:601-605.

47. Serra A, Bonan R, Lefevre T, Barraud P. Balloon mitral commissurotomy for mitral restenosis after surgical commissurotomy. Am J Cardiol 1993;71:1311-1315.

48. Rediker D, Block P, Abascal V. Mitral balloon valvuloplasty for mitral restenosis after surgical commissurotomy. J Am Coll Cardiol 1988;11:252-256.

49. Glantz JC, Pomerantz RM, Cunningham MJ, et al. Percutaneous balloon valvuloplasty for severe mitral stenosis during pregnancy: a review of therapeutic options. Obstet Gyn Surg 1993;48:503-508.

50. Kalra G, Arora R, Kahn J, Nigam M. Percutaneous mitral commissurotomy for severe mitral stenosis during pregnancy. Cathet Cardiovasc Diagn 1994;33:28-30.

51. Iung B, Cormier B, Elias J, Michel P. Usefulness of percutaneous balloon commissurotomy for mitral stenosis during pregnancy. Am J Cardiol 1994;73:398-400.

52. Safian R, Berman A, Sachs B, et al. Percutaneous balloon mitral valvuloplasty in a pregnant woman with mitral stenosis. Cathet Cardiovasc Diagn 1988;15:103-108.

53. Esteves CA, Ramos AIO. Effectiveness of percutaneous balloon mitral valvotomy during pregnancy. Am J Cardiol 1991;68:930-934.

54. Herrmann HC, Lima JA, Feldman T, et al. Mechanisms and outcome of severe mitral regurgitation after Inoue balloon valvuloplasty. J Am Coll Cardiol 1993;22:783-9.

55. Thomas MR, Monaghan MJ, Metealfe JM, et al. Residual atrial septal defects following balloon mitral valvuloplasty using different techniques. A transthoracic and transesophageal study demonstrating an advantage of the Inoue balloon. Eur Heart J 1992;13:496-502.

56. Arora R, Jolly N, Kalra GS, et al. Atrial septal defect after balloon mitral valvuloplasty: a transesophageal echocardiographic study. Angiology 1993;44:217-221.

57. Cequier A, Bonan R, Serra A, et al. Left to right shunting after percutaneous mitral valvuloplasty. Incidence and longterm hemodynamic follow-up. Circulation 1990;81:1190-1197.

58. Casale P, Block PC, O'Shea JP, et al. Atrial septal defect after percutaneous mitral balloon valvuloplasty: Immediate results and follow-up. J Am Coll Cardiol 1990;15:1300-1304.

59. Chan C, Berland J, Cribier A, Rocha P. Results of percutaneous transseptal mitral commissurotomy in patients 40 years and above with those under 40 years of age: Immediate and 5-year follow-up results. Cathet Cardiovasc Diagn 1994;32:223-230.

60. Chen CR, Cheng To, Chen JY, et al. Longterm results of percutaneous mitral valvuloplasty with the Inoue balloon catheter. Am J Cardiol 1992;70:1445-8.

61. Block PC, Palacios IF, Block EH, et al. Late (two-year) follow-up after percutaneous mitral balloon valvotomy. Am J Cardiol 1992;69:537-554.

62. Pavlides GS, Nahhas GT, London J, et al. Predictors of long-term event-free survival after percutaneous balloon mitral valvuloplasty. Am J Cardiol 1997;79:1370-1374.

63. Wilkins GT, Weyman AE, Abascal VM, et al. Percutaneous mitral valvotomy: An analysis of echocardiographic variables related to outcome and the mechanism of dilation. Br Heart J 1988;60:299-308.

64. Herrmann HE, Wilkins GT, Abascal VM, et al. Percutaneous balloon mitral valvotomy for patients with mitral stenosis. Analysis of factors influencing early results. J Thorac Cardiovasc Surg 1988;96:33-38.

65. Abascal VM, Wilkins GT, Choong CY, et al. Mitral regurgitation after percutaneous balloon mitral valvuloplasty in adults: Evaluation by pulsed Doppler echocardiography. J Am Coll Cardiol 1988;11:257-263.

66. Come PC, Riley MF, Diver DJ, et al. Noninvasive assessment of mitral stenosis before and after percutaneous balloon mitral valvuloplasty. Am J Coll Cardiol 1988;61:817-825.

67. Reid CL, Chandraratna AN, Kawamishi DT, et al. Influence of mitral valve morphology on double-balloon catheter balloon valvuloplasty in patients with mitral stenosis. Analysis of factors predicting immediate and 3-month results. Circulation 1989;80:515-524.

68. Reid CL, Otto CM, Davis KB, et al. Influence of mitral valve morphology on mitral balloon commissurotomy: Immediate and six-month results from the NHLBI Balloon Valvuloplasty Registry. Am Heart J 1992;124:657-665.

69. Complications and mortality of percutaneous balloon mitral commissurotomy. A report from the National Heart, Lung, and Blood Institute Balloon Valvuloplasty Registry. Circulation 1992;85:2014-2024.

70. Tuzcu Em, Block PC, Griffin B, et al. Percutaneous mitral balloon valvotomy in patients calcific mitral stenosis: Immediate and longterm outcome. J Am Coll Cardiol 1994;23:1604-1609.

71. Herrmann HE, Feldman T, Isner JM, et al. Comparison of results of percutaneous balloon valvuloplasty in patients with mild and moderate mitral stenosis. Am J Cardiol 1993;71:1300-1303.

72. Alfonso F, Macaya C, Hernandex R, et al. Early and late results of PBMV for mitral stenosis associated with mild mitral regurgitation. Am J Cardiol 1993;71:1304-1310.

73. Chen CR, Cheng TO, Chen JY, et al. Percutaneous balloon mitral valvuloplasty for mitral stenosis with and without associated aortic regurgitation. Am Heart J 1993;125:128-137.

74. Alfonso F, Macaya C, Hernandez R, et al. Percutaneous mitral valvuloplasty with severe pulmonary artery hypertension. Am J Cardiol 1993;72:325-330.

75. Wisenbaugh T, Essop R, Middlemost S, Skoularigis J. Effects

of severe pulmonary hypertension on outcome of balloon mitral valvotomy. Am J Cardiol 1992;70:823-825.

76. Dev V, Shrivastrava S. Time course of changes in pulmonary vascular resistance and the mechanism of regression of pulmonary arterial hypertension after balloon mitral valvuloplasty. Am J Cardiol 1991;67:439-442.

77. Tuzcu EM, Block PC, Griffin BP, et al. Immediate and lLongterm outcome of percutaneous mitral valvotomy in patients 65 years and older. Circulation 1992;85:963-971.

78. Shapiro LM, Hassanein H, Crowley JJ. Mitral balloon valvuloplasty in patients > 70 years of age with severe mitral stenosis. Am J Cardiol 1995;75:633-636.

79. Kasper W, Wollschlager H, Gerbel A, et al. Percutaneous mitral balloon valvuloplasty: a comparative evaluation of two transatrial techniques. Am Heart J 1992;124:1562-6.

80. Abdullah M, Halim M, Rajedran V. Comparison between single (Inoue) and double balloon mitral valvuloplasty. Immediate and short-term results. Am Heart J 1992;123:1581-1588.

81. Rihal CS, Nishimura RA, Reeder GS, et al. Percutaneous balloon mitral valvuloplasty: Comparison of double and single (Inoue) techniques. Cathet Cardiovasc Diagn 1993;29:183-190.

82. Manga P, Landless P, Gebka M. Comparative results of PBMV using the Trefoil/Biofoil and Inoue balloon techniques. Int J Cardiol 1994;43:21-25.

83. Zhang HP, Gamra H, Allen J, Lau F, Ruiz C. Comparison of late outcome between inoue balloon and double-balloon techniques for percutaneous mitral valvotomy in a matched study. Am Heart J 1995;130:340-4.

84. Shrivastava S, Mathur A, Der V, et al. Comparison of immediate hemodynamic response to closed mitral commissurotomy, single balloon and double balloon mitral valvuloplasty in rheumatic mitral stenosis. J Thorac Cardiovasc Surg 1992;104:1262-7.

85. Turi ZG, Reyes VP, Raju BS, et al. Percutaneous balloon versus surgical closed commissurotomy for mitral stenosis: a prospective randomized trial. Circulation 1991;83:1179-1185.

86. Reyes VP, Raju BS, Wynne J, et al. Percutaneous balloon valvuloplasty compared with open surgical commissurotomy for mitral stenosis. N Engl J Med 1994;331:961-967.

87. Lababidi Z, Wu JR, Walls JT. Percutaneous balloon aortic valvuloplasty. Results in 23 patients. Am J Cardiol 1984;53:194-197.

88. Cribier A, Saoudi N, Berland J, et al. Percutaneous transluminal valvuloplasty of acquired aortic stenosis in elderly patients: An alternative to valve replacement? Lancet 1986;1:63-67.

89. McKay R, Safian RD, Lock J, Mandell V. Balloon dilatation of calcific aortic stenosis in elderly patients: postmortem, intraoperative, and percutaneous valvuloplasty studies. Circulation 1986;74:119-125.

90. Frank S, Johnson A, Ross J. Natural history of valvular aortic stenosis. British Heart J. 1973;35:41-46.

91. Lombard JT, Selzer A. Valvular aortic stenosis. A clinical and hemodynamic profile of patients. Ann Int Med 1987;106:292-298.

92. Turina J, Hess O, Sepulcri F, Kravenbuehl HP. Spontaneous course of aortic valve disease. Eur Heart J 1987;8:471-483.

93. O'Keefe JH, Vlietstra RE, Bailey KR, Holmes DR. Natural history of candidates for balloon aortic valvuloplasty. Mayo Clin Proc 1987;62:986-991.

94. Smith N, McAnulty J, Rahimtoola S. Severe aortic stenosis with impaired left ventricular function and clinical heart failure: Results of valve replacement. Circulation 1978;58:255-264.

95. Kennedy W, Doces J, Stewart D. Left ventricular function before and following aortic valve replacement. Circulation 1977;56(6):944-950.

96. Pantely G, Morton M, Rahimtoola S. Effects of successful, uncomplicated valve replacement on ventricular hypertrophy, volume and performance in aortic stenosis and in aortic incompetence. J Thorac Surg 1978;75:383-391.

97. Magovern J, Pennock J, Campbell D, Pae W. Aortic valve replacement and combined aortic valve replacement and coronary artery bypass grafting: Predicting high risk groups. J Am Coll Cardiol 1987;9:38-43.

98. Copeland J, Griepp R, Stinson E, Shumway N. Isolated aortic valve replacement in patients older than 65 years. JAMA 1977;237:1578-1581.

99. Edmunds H, Stephenson L, Edie R, Ratcliffe M. Open-heart surgery in octogenarians. N Engl J Med 1988;319:131-136.

100. Levinson JR, Akins CW, Buckley MJ, et al. Octogenarians with aortic stenosis: outcome after aortic valve replacement. Circulation 1989;80:I-49-I-56.

101. Fremes S, Goldman B, Ivanov J, Weisel R. Valvular surgery in the elderly. Circulation 1989;80:I77-90.

102. Safian RD, Mandell VS, Thurer RE, et al. Postmortem and intraoperative balloon valvuloplasty of calcific aortic stenosis in elderly patients: Mechanisms of successful dilatation. J Am Coll Cardiol 1987;9:655-660.

103. Safian RD, Kuntz RE, Berman AD. Aortic valvuloplasty. Cardiol Clin 1991;9:289-299.

104. Block P, IF P. Aortic and mitral balloon valvuloplasty: The United States experience. In: Topol EJ, Editor. Textbook of Interventional Cardiology; Philadelphia, WB Saunders, 1994.

105. Letac B, Cribier A. Aortic balloon dilatation as a treatment of aortic stenosis: what are the indications? J Interven Cardiol 1993;6:1-6.

106. NHLBI Balloon Valvuloplasty Registry Participants. Percutaneous balloon aortic valvuloplasty. Acute and 30-day follow-up results in 674 patients from the NHLBI Balloon Valvuloplasty Registry. Circulation 1991;84:2383-2397.

107. McKay RG for the Mansfield Scientific Aortic Valvuloplasty Registry Investigators. Overview of acute hemodynamic results and procedural complications. J Am Coll Cardiol

1991;17:485-491.

108. Lewin R, Dorros G, King J, Mathiak L. Percutaneous transluminal aortic valvuloplasty: acute outcome and follow-up of 125 patients. J Am Coll Cardiol 1989;14:1210-1217.

109. Isner JM, Salem DN, Desnoyers MR, Fields CD. Dual balloon technique for valvuloplasty of aortic stenosis in adults. Am J Cardiol 1988;61:583-589.

110. Block PC, Palacios IF. Comparison of hemodynamic results of anterograde versus retrograde percutaneous balloon aortic valvuloplasty. Am J Cardiol 1987;60:659-662.

111. Cribier A, Gerber L, Letac B. Percutaneous Balloon Aortic Valvuloplasty: The French Experience,. Philadelphia: WB Saunders, 1990. (Eds) Topol,E. Textbook of Interventional Cardiology; vol p.849.

112. Isner JM. Acute catastrophic complications of balloon aortic valvuloplasty. J Am Coll Cardiol 1991;17:1436-1444.

113. Lewin RF, Dorros G, King JF, Seifert PE. Aortic annular tear after valvuloplasty: The role of aortic annulus echocardiographic measurement. Cathet Cardiovasc Diagn 1989;16:123-129.

114. Seifert PE, Auer JE. Surgical repair of annular disruption following percutaneous balloon aortic valvuloplasty. Ann Thorac Surg 1988;46:242-243.

115. Vrolix M, Piessens J, Moerman P, et al. Fatal aortic rupture: An unusual complication of percutaneous balloon valvuloplasty for acquired valvular aortic stenosis. Cathet Cardiovasc Diagn 1989;16:119-122.

116. Lembo NJ, King SB, Roubin GS, Hammami A. Fatal aortic rupture during percutaneous balloon valvuloplasty for valvular aortic stenosis. Am J Cardiol 1987;60:733-736.

117. Dean LS, Chandler JW, Saenz CB, Baxley WA. Severe aortic regurgitation complicating percutaneous aortic valve valvuloplasty. Cathet Cardiovasc Diagn 1989;16:130-132.

118. Sadaniantz A, Malhotra R, Korr KS. Transient acute severe aortic regurgitation complicating balloon aortic valvuloplasty. Cathet Cardiovasc Diagn 1989;17:186-189.

119. Plack RH, Porterfield JK, Brinker JA. Complete heart block developing during aortic valvuloplasty. Chest 1989;96:1201-1203.

120. deUbago J, dePrada JAV, Moujir F, Olalla JJ. Mitral valve rupture during percutaneous dilation of aortic valve stenosis. Cathet Cardiovasc Diagn 1989;16:115-118.

121. Farb A, Galloway J, Davis R, et al. Mitral valve laceration and papillary muscle rupture secondary to percutaneous balloon aortic valvuloplasty. Am J Cardiol 1992;69:829-830.

122. Cujec B, McMeekin J, Lopez J. Bacterial endocarditis after percutaneous aortic valvuloplasty. Am Heart J 1988;115:178-179.

123. Ferguson J, Garza R. Efficacy of multiple balloon aortic valvuloplasty procedures. J Am Coll Cardiol 1991;17:1430-1435.

124. Kuntz R, Tosteson, Anna, Maitland L, Gordon P. Immediate results and longterm follow-up after repeat balloon aortic valvuloplasty. Cathet Cardiovasc Diagn 1992;25:4-9.

125. Koning R, Cribier A, Asselin C, et al. Repeat balloon aortic valvuloplasty. Cathet Cardiovasc Diagn 1992;26:249-254.

126. Kuntz RE, Tosteson AN, Berman AD, et al. Predictors of event-free survival after balloon aortic valvuloplasty. N Engl J Med 1991;325:17-23.

127. Otto C, Mickel M, Kennedy W, et al. Three-year outcome after balloon aortic valvuloplasty: Insights into prognosis of valvular aortic stenosis. Circulation 1994;89:642-650.

128. O'Neill WW. Predictors of longterm survival after percutaneous aortic valvuloplasty: report of the Mansfield Scientific Balloon Aortic Valvuloplasty Registry. J Am Coll Cardiol 1991;17:193-198.

129. Holmes D, Nichimura R, Reeder G. In-hospital mortality after balloon aortic valvuloplasty: frequency and associated factors. J Am Coll Cardiol 1991;17:189-192.

130. Legrand V, Beckers J, Fastrez M, et al. Longterm follow-up of elderly patients with severe aortic stenosis treated by balloon aortic valvuloplasty. Importance of hemodynamic parameters before and after dilatation. Eur Heart J 1991;12:451-457.

131. Davidson C, Harrison K, Pieper K, Harding M. Determinants of one-year outcome from balloon aortic valvuloplasty. Am J Cardiol 1991;68:75-80.

132. Bernard Y, Etievent J, Mourand J, et al. Longterm results of percutaneous aortic valvuloplasty compared with aortic valve replacement in patients more than 75 years old. J Am Coll Cardiol 1992;20:796-801.

133. Safian R, Warren S, Berman A, et al. Improvement in symptoms and left ventricular performance after balloon aortic valvuloplasty in patients with aortic stenosis and depressed left ventricular ejection fraction. Circulation 1988;78:1181-1191.

134. Berland J, Cribier A, Savin T, et al. Percutaneous balloon valvuloplasty in patients with severe aortic stenosis and low ejection fraction: Immediate results and 1-year follow-up. Circulation 1989;79:1189-1196.

135. Davidson CJ, Harrison K, Leithe M, Kisslo K. Failure of balloon aortic valvuloplasty to result in sustained clinical improvement in patients with depressed left ventricular function. Am J Cardiol 1990;65:72-77.

136. Come P, Riley M, Berman A, et al. Serial assessment of mitral regurgitation by pulsed doppler echocardiography in patients undergoing balloon aortic valvuloplasty. J Am Coll Cardiol 1989;14:677-682.

137. Adams P, Otto C. Lack of improvement in coexisting mitral regurgitation after relief of valvular aortic stenosis. Am J Cardiol 1990;66:105-107.

138. Nishimura R, Holmes D, Michela M. Follow-up of patients with low output, low gradient hemodynamics after percutaneous balloon aortic valvuloplasty: the Mansfield Scientific Aortic Valvuloplasty Registry. J Am Coll Cardiol 1991;17:828-833.

139. Moreno P, Jank I-K, Newell J. The role of percutaneous aortic balloon valvuloplasty in patients with cardiogenic shock and

critical aortic stenosis. J Am Coll Cardiol 1994;23:1071-1075.

140. Smedira NG, Ports TA Merrick SH, et al. Balloon aortic valvuloplasty as a bridge to aortic valve replacement in critically ill patients. Ann Thorac Surg 1993;55:914-916.

141. Friedman H, Cragg D, O'Neill W. Cardiac resuscitation using emergency aortic balloon valvuloplasty. Am J Cardiol 1989;63:387-8.

142. Desnoyers M, Salem D, Rosenfield K, et al. Treatment of cardiogenic shock by emergency aortic balloon valvuloplasty. Ann Int Med 1988;108:833-5.

143. Losordo D, Ramaswamy K, Rosenfield K, Isner J. Use of emergency balloon dilation to reverse acute hemodynamic decompensation developing during diagnostic cardiac catheterization for aortic stenosis (bailout valvuloplasty). Am J Cardiol 1989;63:388-9.

144. Brady S, Davis C, Kussmaul W, Laskey W. Percutaneous aortic balloon valvuloplasty in octogenarians: Morbidity and mortality. Ann Int Med. 1989;110:761-766.

145. Cribier A, Remadi F, Koning R, et al. Emergency balloon valvuloplasty as initial treatment of patients with aortic stenosis and cardiogenic shock. N Engl J Med 1992;326:646.

146. Levine MJ, Berman AD, Safian RD, Diver DJ. Palliation of valvular aortic stenosis by balloon valvuloplasty as preoperative preparation for noncardiac surgery. Am J Cardiol 1988;62:1309-1310.

147. Roth R, Palacios I, Block P. Percutaneous aortic balloon valvuloplasty: Its role in the management of patients with aortic stenosis requiring major noncardiac surgery. J Am Coll Cardiol 1989;13:1039-1041.

148. Hayes SN, Holmes DR, Nishimura RA, Reeder GS. Palliative percutaneous aortic balloon valvuloplasty before noncardiac operations and invasive diagnostic procedures. Mayo Clin Proc 1989;64:753-757.

149. O'Keefe JH, Shub C, Rettke SR. Risk of noncardiac surgical procedures in-patients with aortic stenosis. Mayo Clin Proc 1989;64:400-405.

150. Fawzy ME, Mimish L, Sivanandam V, et al. Advantage of Inoue balloon catheter in mitral balloon valvotomy: Experience with 220 consecutive patients. Cathet Cardiovasc Diagn 1996;38:9-14.

151. Cribier A, Eltchaninoff H, Koning R, et al. Percutaneous mechanical mitral commissurotomy with a newly designed metallic valvulotome. Immediate results of the initial experience in 153 patients. Circulation 1999;99:793-799.

152. Orrange SE, Kawanishi DT, Lopex BM, et al. Actuarial outcome after catheter balloon commissurotomy in patients with mitral stenosis. Circulation 1997;95:382-389.

153. Stefanadis CI, Stratos CG, Lambrou SG, et al. Retrograde nonttransseptal balloon mitral valvuloplasty: Immediate results and intermediate long-term outcome in 441 cases—A multicenter experience. J Am Coll Cardiol 1998;32:1009-1016.

154. Nanjappa MC, Dorros G, Kikkeri S, et al. The Indian experience of percutaneous transvenous mitral commissurotomy: Comparison of the triple lumen (Inoue) double lumen (Accura) variable sized single balloon with regard to procedural outcome and cost savings. J Interven Cardiol 1998;11:107-112.

155. Lau KW, Ding ZP, Quek, et al. Long-term (36-63 month) clinical and echocardiographic follow-up after Inoue balloon mitral commissurotomy. Cathet Cardiovasc Diagn. 1998;43:33-38.Zhang HP, Yen GS, Allen JW, et al. Comparison of late results of balloon valvotomy in mitral stenosis with versus without mitral regurgitation. Am J Cardiol 1998;81:51-55.

156. Kang DH, Song JK, Chae JK, et al. Comparison of outcomes of percutaneous mitral valvuloplasty versus mitral valve replacement after resolution of left atrial appendage thrombi by warfarin therapy. Am J Cardiol 1998;81:97-100.

157. Farhat MB, Ayari M, Maatouk F, et al. Percutaneous balloon versus surgical closed and open mitral commissurotomy. Seven-year follow-up results of a randomized trial. Circulation 1998;97:245-250.

158. Chen CR, Cheng TO, Chen JY, et al. Long-term results of percutaneous balloon mitral valvuloplasty for mitral stenosis: A follow-study to 11 years in 202 patients. Cathet Cardiovasc Diagn. 1998:43:132-139.

159. Turi ZG, Reyes VP, Raju S, et al. Percutaneous balloon versus surgical closed commissurotomy for mitral stenosis. A prospective, randomized trial. Circulation 1991;83:1179-1185.

160. Arora R, Nair M, Kalra GS, et al. Immediate and long-term results of balloon and surgical closed mitral valvulotomy: A randomized comparative study. Am Heart J 1993;125:1091-1094.

161. Reyes VP, Raju BS, Wynne J, et al. Percutaneous balloon valvuloplasty compared with open surgical commissurotomy for mitral stenosis. N Engl J Med 1994;331:961-967.

162. Iung B, Cormier B, Ducimetiere P, et al. Functional results 5 years after successful percutaneous mitral commissurotomy in a series of 528 patients and analysis of predictive factors. J Am Coll Cardiol 1996;27:407-414.

163. Dean LS, Mickel M, Bonan R, et al. Four-year follow-up of patients undergoing percutaneous balloon mitral commissurotomy. A report from the National Heart, Lung, and Blood Institute Balloon Valvuloplasty Registry. J Am Coll Cardiol 1996;28:1452-1457.

164. Palacios IF. Farewell to surgical mitral commissurotomy for many patients. Circulation 1998;97:223-226.

165. Cheng TO, Holmes DR. Percutaneous balloon mitral valvuloplasty by the Inoue balloon technique: the procedure of choice for treatment of mitral stenosis. Am J Cardiol 1998;81:624-628.

166. Bonow RO, Carabello B, de Leon AC, et al. ACC/AHA guidelines for the management of patients with valvular heart disease. Executive summary. A report of the American College of Cardiology/American Heart Association Task

Force on Practice Guidelines (Committee on management of patients with valvular heart disease). J Am Coll Cardiol 1998;32:1486-1582.

167. Bonhoeffer P, Esteves C, Casal U, et al. Percutaneous mitral valve dilatation with the Multi-Track system. Cathet Cardiovasc Intervent 1999;48:178-183.

168. Iung B, Garbarz E, Michaud P, et al. Late results of percutaneous mitral commissurotomy in a series of 1024 patients. Analysis of late clinical deterioration: frequency, anatomic findings and predictive factors. Circulation 1999;99:3272-3278.

169. Leon MN, Harrell LC, Simosa HF, et al. Mitral balloon valvotomy for patients with mitral stenosis in atrial fibrillation. J Am Coll Cardiol 1999;34:1145-52.

170. Hernandez R, Banuelos C, Alfonso F, et al. Long-term clinical and echocardiographic follow-up after percutaneous mitral valvuloplasty with the Inoue balloon. Circulation 1999;99:1580-1586.

171. Kang DH, Park SW, Song JK, et al. Long-term clinical and echocardiographic outcome of percutaneous mitral valvuloplasty. Randomized comparison of Inoue and double-balloon techniques. J Am Coll Cardiol 1999;35:169-75.

172. Pathan AZ, Mahdi NA, Leon MN, et al. Is redo percutaneous mitral balloon valvuloplasty (PMV) indicated in patients with post-PMV mitral restenosis. J Am Coll Cardiol 1999; 34: 49-54.

173. Iung B, Garbarz, Michaud P, et al. Percutaneous mitral commissurotomy for restenosis after surgical commissurotomy. Late efficacy and implications for patient selection. J Am Coll Cardiol 2000; 35: 1295-1302.

174. Gupta S, Vora A, Lokhandwalla Y, et al. Percutaneous balloon mitral valvotomy in mitral restenosis. Eur Heart J 1996; 17: 1560-1564.

175. Jang IK, Block PC, Newell JB, et al. Percutaneous mitral balloon valvuloplasty for recurrent mitral stenosis after surgical commissurotomy. Am J Cardiol 1995; 75: 601-605.

176. Mangione JA, Lourenco RM, dos Santos ES, et al. Long-term follow-up of pregnant women after percutaneous mitral valvuloplasty. Cathet Cardiovasc Intervent 2000; 50: 413-417.

177. Cheng TO. Percutaneous Inoue balloon valvuloplasty is the procedure of choice for symptomatic mitral stenosis in pregnant women. Cathet Cardiovasc Intervent 2000; 50: 418.

178. Abraham KA, Chandrasekar B, Rajagopal S, et al. Percutaneous transvenous mitral commissurotomy for significant calcific mitral stenosis: utility of the stepwise balloon dilatation technique and follow-up results. J Invasive Cardiol 1999; 11: 345-350.

179. Lau K-W, Ding Z-P, Hung J-S. Percutaneous Inoue balloon valvuloplasty in patients with mitral stenosis and associated moderate mitral regurgitation. Cathet Cardiovasc Diagn 1996; 38: 1-7.

180. Sutaria N, Elder AT, Shaw TR. Longterm outcome of percutaneous mitral balloon valvotomy in patients aged 70 and over. Heart 2000; 83: 433-8.

181. Hung JS, Lau KW, Lo PH, et al. Complications of Inoue balloon mitral commissurotomy: impact of operator experience and evolving technique. Am Heart J 1999; 138: 114-21.

182. Padial LR, Freitas N, Sagie A, et al. Echocardiography can predict which patients will develop severe mitral regurgitation after percutaneous mitral valvulotomy. J Am Coll Cardiol 1996; 27: 1225-31.

183. Padial LR, Abascal VM, Moreno PR, et al. Echocardiography can predict the development of severe mitral regurgitation after percutaneous mitral valvuloplasty by the Inoue technique. Am J Cardiol 1999; 83: 1210-3.

184. Lieberman EB, Bashmore TM, Hermiler JB, et al. Balloon aortic valvuloplasty in adults: failure of procedure to improve long-term survival. J Am Coll Cardiol 1995; 26: 1522-8.

185. Eisenhauer AC, Hadjipetrou P, Piemonte TC. Balloon aortic valvuloplasty revisited: the role of the Inoue balloon and transseptal antegrade approach. Cathet Cardiovasc Intervent 2000; 50: 484-491.

SPECIAL CONSIDERATIONS FOR CATH LAB PERSONNEL

38

Harold Z. Friedman, M.D.
Alan Bennett, R.C.I.S.
Kevin L. Kelco, M.A., R.C.I.S.

Patients well-suited for percutaneous revascularization include those with lifestyle-limiting angina pectoris despite medical therapy, patients at high-risk for myocardial infarction or sudden cardiac death due to high-grade stenoses which supply large amounts of viable myocardium, and individuals considered poor operative candidates due to severe co-existing medical illness or absence of suitable bypass conduits. Patients previously considered unsuitable for PTCA are now routinely considered for percutaneous coronary intervention (PCI) due to advances in PTCA hardware, improved operator experience, and availability of potent antiplatelet agents and other interventional technologies, particularly stents and atherectomy. Through technological advances, cath lab personnel duties have become substantially more complex. Patient care involves allaying fears and monitoring vital signs, identifying conditions which may result in case postponement, anticipating and reacting to procedural complications, participating in the actual performance of the case, and expertly troubleshooting equipment malfunctions. This chapter has been written specifically for cath lab technicians and nurses with the intention of providing an overview of the organizational framework of the interventional laboratory, defining specific responsibilities, and detailing patient management strategies and technical considerations involved in the performance of complex coronary interventional procedures. In this regard, an overview of patient evaluation, equipment selection, troubleshooting, and identification and management of procedure-related complications is presented.

PREPROCEDURAL CONSIDERATIONS

A. **STAFF RESPONSIBILITIES.** The cardiac catheterization lab must function as a critical care unit. More than 95% of cases performed in the interventional suite are successful but 5% may result in myocardial infarction, emergency CABG, or death. Although the risk of major ischemic complications has been associated with specific angiographic and clinical findings, serious complications such as anaphylaxis, ventricular tachycardia or fibrillation, pulmonary edema, and shock can occur without warning. All cath lab personnel must be able to handle any deterioration in patient status, from delivering advanced cardiac life support to troubleshooting equipment failure. The catheterization lab can be a cold and intimidating environment for patients. Staff can alleviate anxiety by attending to the patient's needs, keeping them covered, and communicating with the family. Awareness of patient comfort often reveals early warning signals of impending complications, including restlessness (hypoxia); somnolence (hypoventilation); nausea, hives, itching, and rhinorrhea (precursors to anaphylax); bladder discomfort (need for Foley catheterization); and lower quadrant abdominal pain and distention (retroperitoneal hemorrhage).

Our experience suggests that a minimum of two nurses/technologists with overlapping responsibilities should be routinely assigned to an interventional lab:

1. **Scrub Nurse/Technologist (duties often performed by circulating nurse/technologist):**
   a. Sterile preparation of catheterization site(s).
   b. Placement of sterile covers on image intensifier and lead shield.
   c. Preparation of all necessary sterile materials and pack.
   d. Assist physician during procedure by passing or exchanging guidewires, injecting contrast material, or panning the x-ray table.
   e. Perform CPR.

2. **Circulating Nurse/Technologist:**
   a. Confirm type of interventional procedure and needed equipment before case.
   b. Place ECG patches.
   c. Insert peripheral IV.
   d. Administer sedation and other medications, and reassure the patient throughout the procedure.
   e. Inspect for hemostasis and stability of vascular sheaths.
   f. Data collection (image intensifier angulation, equipment use).
   g. Obtain accessory equipment and supplies during procedure.
   h. Monitor pressures.
   i. Monitor oxygen saturation by pulse oximetry.
   j. Monitor activated clotting times (ACT).
   k. Assure quality assurance in compliance with Joint Commission on Accreditation of Hospital Organization (JCAHO) guidelines before each case.
   l. In the event of CPR, place metal support under head of table and remind physician to place table over the main pedestal. (Otherwise, CPR is not effective)
   m. Assist ventilation with Ambu bag in the event of respiratory failure or CPR.

3. **Monitoring Nurse/Technologist:**
   a. Confirm the patient's signature for consent.
   b. Acquire pertinent preprocedural laboratory information and baseline demographic data.
   c. Continuously monitor hemodynamic pressures, waveforms, heart rate, rhythm and ST segments, and relay data to the physician. Alert physician if CPR is not effective (generated pressure ≤ 60 mmHg).
   d. Document resuscitative efforts and maintain procedural log.
   e. Record drugs, duration of radiation exposure, and contrast volume.
   f. Inspect equipment before each procedure and troubleshoot when necessary (see below).
   g. Arrange bed transfers.
   h. Register implantable devices (stents, IVC filters, etc) with manufacturer.

B. **PATIENT CARE.** Amidst an endless stream of new equipment designs (high-pressure balloons, cutting balloons, low-profile balloons, autoperfusion balloons), new devices (atherectomy, lasers, stents), and new imaging modalities (intravascular ultrasound, angioscopy, Doppler wire) lies the commitment to patient care. Attention to the patient's needs is of primary importance. Successful coordination of responsibilities requires organization. A preprocedural checklist is one of the keys to a safe procedure; if complications develop, a checklist ensures that important details are not overlooked.

Preprocedural Check List:
- Is there signed consent?
- Does the patient have a functioning IV?
- Are the patient's vital signs stable (temp < 37.5°, systolic BP > 90 mmHg or < 200 mmHg)? If not, notify the physician immediately.
- Does the patient have abnormal laboratory values which may indicate a severe medical illness and necessitate postponement of the procedure (hemoglobin <10 or >17gm/dL; WBC >15,000 or platelets <100,000/mm^3; Na$^+$ >155 or <120 meq/L; K$^+$ <3.3 or >6.0 meq/L; creatinine >1.8 mg/dL; PT >1.2 x control)?
- Has a type and cross-match request been received by the blood bank?
- Is there a recent ECG on the chart?
- Is there a history of dye or latex allergy and was the patient premedicated? If not, notify the physician. Note any adverse reaction during previous intervention. Use latex-free supplies if indicated.
- Has the patient been taking at least one aspirin a day for 24 hours prior to the procedure? If not, notify physician. This is extremely important, since patients not taking aspirin have a higher risk of ischemic complications.
- If the patient has an elevated (>2.0 gm/dL) creatinine, has he/she been well-hydrated?
- Record amplitude of peripheral pulses and locate with Doppler and mark if needed.
- Consider Foley catheter for complex procedures.
- Apply defibrillation pads in acute MI patients.
- Assure O$_2$ delivery, suction, and defibrillation are functional.
- Place the patient on pulse oximetry and continuous blood pressure monitoring.

C. **CONSCIOUS SEDATION (Chapter 34).** Drugs used for sedation vary greatly between institutions. Opiates, barbiturates, and benzodiazepines are used commonly. The dose should be titrated according to the patient's clinical status. Intravenous drugs should be given slowly over several minutes and not as a bolus. Naloxone (0.4-2 mg IV up to 10 mg in 10 minutes) and flumazenil (0.2 mg IV over 15 seconds repeated as needed every 60 seconds up to 1 mg) must be immediately available to reverse excessive sedation from opiates and benzodiazepines, respectively. One common regimen includes the use of intravenous dilaudid plus versed or diazepam. Medications used for conscious sedation may need to be reduced or withheld in the setting of:
- Advanced age
- Chronic renal failure

- Respiratory insufficiency or hypoxia
- Liver disease
- Hypotension
- Mental status depression

D. ASSESSMENT OF PROCEDURAL RISK AND CASE PREPARATION (Chapter 4). Patient and lesion characteristics have been identified that increase the risk of percutaneous intervention. An estimate of procedural risk should be ascertained prior to each case. High-risk lesion characteristics are associated with an increased likelihood of acute closure (e.g., complex coronary artery dissection, degenerated saphenous vein graft, diffuse disease, thrombus-containing lesion, angulated lesion). High-risk patient characteristics are associated with an increased risk of death should acute closure develop (e.g., left main coronary artery disease, left ventricular dysfunction, multivessel disease, age > 70 years old). High-risk patient characteristics are more important determinants of overall procedural risk:

Patient Risk	+	Lesion Risk	=	Procedural Risk
High		High		Highest
High		Low		High
Low		High		Intermediate
Low		Low		Low

High-risk patients typically require modifications of patient preparation, drug therapy, and angioplasty technique. All potential complications must be anticipated by the cath lab team; additional safety measures are highlighted in Table 38.1.

INTRAPROCEDURAL CONSIDERATIONS

A. STAFF RESPONSIBILITIES. During an interventional case, the cardiologist is focused on the angiographic image, the performance of the balloon or device, and the patient. The cath lab staff must focus on three things:

Table 38.1. Safety Measures for High-Risk Procedures

Measure	Rationale
Bilateral inguinal prep	Need for IABP, CPS
Baseline and continuous 12-lead ECG monitor	Useful for comparison
Decrease sedation	Marginal cardiovascular and respiratory reserve
R-2 pads	Immediate cardioversion capabilities
Low-osmolar contrast	Minimize hypotension/LV dysfunction/arrhythmias
Pulmonary artery catheter	Monitor intravascular volume; avoid heart failure
Arterial blood gases	Maintain optimal oxygenation
CCU monitoring post-procedure	Quick recognition and treatment of catastrophic complications

1. **Patient Clinical Status.** This includes but is not limited to ECG, blood pressure, respiration, arterial oxygen saturation (by pulse oximetry), level of consciousness, and comfort. IV patency should be checked periodically to ensure that medications are not extravasating subcutaneously Fluid totals should be tracked and drips should not be allowed to run dry (something that can easily happen in long cases in a darkened lab). **The staff must monitor the contrast bottle at all times: Arterial air emboli can be fatal!** This also applies to contrast used in the power injector. Air ventriculograms have occurred.

2. **Equipment Operation.** This involves safe and optimal functioning of all devices and equipment. The moving C-arm is a powerful motorized device capable of inflicting damage to equipment, patient, and staff. The staff must observe and prevent collisions with IVAC's, monitors, ventilators, etc. and pay special attention to heat unit alarms, error messages, circuit breaker problems, and collision alarms.

3. **Completeness of Data.** In any interventional case, meticulous recording of procedure details is essential, especially if data are used for research. Obtaining and documenting ACT values every 20 minutes, monitoring contrast, and notifying the physician if contrast volume exceeds 300 ml are vital details which have implications for patient care. Balloon inflation time and pressure, number of atherectomy or laser passes, and patient complaints should be entered into the database.

B. **EQUIPMENT SELECTION (Chapter 1)**
1. **Sheaths.** The majority of PTCA procedures employ 6F to 8F arterial sheaths, whereas most atherectomy devices mandate use of 8F to 10F sheaths. Extra-long sheaths can be used to span tortuous femoral and iliac vessels and improve guide catheter movement and torque-control. Floppy-tipped or hydrophilic guidewires are used to traverse highly diseased or tortuous arterial

segments. Venous access is established in high-risk cases with 5F to 8F sheaths, permitting fluid resuscitation, administration of medications, and insertion of a temporary pacemaker or pulmonary artery catheter as necessary.

2. **Guide Catheters.** Right and left Judkins 4.0 angioplasty guide catheters are selected most often. Sidehole catheters are often used when vessels appear small or catheter pressure damping occurs. An early left main trunk bifurcation might favor a standard catheter with a short-tip or a 3.5 Judkins curve if the LAD is the target vessel. Left Amplatz and geometric catheters provide better support compared to Judkins curves. In addition, an enlarged aortic root favors a larger Judkins (4.5-6.0), Amplatz, or geometric curve. The physician's goal in all cases is to optimize coaxial alignment between the catheter tip and long axis of the proximal target vessel.

3. **Guidewires.** Several guidewire designs are available, each with different degrees of flexibility and steerability. Soft, flexible wires are preferred in the vast majority of cases; however, stiffer wires may be necessary in some complex cases.

4. **Balloons.** Balloon catheters come in one of two basic designs: Balloon over-the-wire and balloon on-the-wire systems. With balloon over-the-wire systems, both wire and balloon move independently. The principal advantage of this system is the ability to maintain lesion access (i.e., the wire remains across lesion throughout the procedure) if acute closure occurs or if balloon upsizing is required. Balloon on-the-wire systems are "fixed systems"; both guidewire and balloon are bonded together and cannot move independently. The principal advantage of this system is its extremely low profile, which may be of particular value when over-the-wire systems fail due to proximal tortuosity, diffuse disease, or high-grade stenosis. In addition, single operators may favor a fixed-wire or monorail (rapid-exchange) system due to its simplicity of use. Long balloons (30-40mm) may be used to treat diffuse coronary disease or lesions located on highly angulated segments. Autoperfusion catheters have sideholes proximal and distal to its balloon and allow passive delivery of arterial blood to the ischemic myocardial bed during balloon inflation, when patients develop severe angina or hypotension.

C. **SUBOPTIMAL RESULTS.** Major ischemic complications develop in 2-4% of elective cases and may result in acute myocardial infarction, emergency surgery, or death. For the technician or nurse, the key is to plan ahead, anticipate complications, and meet physician needs. Attention should be directed to new ECG changes, hypotension, and chest pain that might otherwise escape early detection. One should anticipate the need for intra-aortic balloon pump support, temporary transvenous pacing, a pulmonary artery catheter, new medications, or a different balloon or device. In all such cases, therapy is directed toward restoring normal antegrade blood flow and treating spasm (Chapter 19), thrombus (Chapter 9), perforation (Chapter 22), and dissection (Chapter 20). In particular, knowledge and awareness of all types of stents in the hospital inventory is crucial to procedural success and safety, since stents are the most important mechanical tool for treating dissection, reversing abrupt closure, and preventing ischemic complications (Chapter 26).

D. MAJOR INTRAPROCEDURAL COMPLICATIONS. Acute complications during angioplasty most frequently include bradycardia/asystole, ventricular tachycardia/fibrillation, hypotension/shock, and allergic reactions. In many cases, the technician or nurse may be the first person to recognize the diagnosis, observe the change in patient condition, and initiate treatment. The causes and treatments for commonly encountered complications are listed in Table 38.2.

E. SPECIAL PROCEDURES

    1. Stents (Chapter 26). These devices reduce restenosis, are the treatment of choice for dissection abrupt closure, and are implanted in 50-80% of all patients referred for percutaneous intervention. If intravascular ultrasound is desirable, the technologist should be proficient in image processing. Absolute familiarity with all stents designs (balloon-expandable and self-expanding stents) and adjunctive equipment (high-pressure balloons, intravascular ultrasound, extra-support guidewires) is essential.

    2. Rotablator Atherectomy (Chapter 27). Technologist responsibilities in these cases include equipment setup and operation, safety concerns particular to this device, and documentation and preservation of device components in the event of malfunction. Equipment assembly requires a cylinder of compressed nitrogen to drive the burr. If pressure falls below 400 psi the tank should be changed to avoid malfunction during the procedure. There should be easy access to a burr

Table 38.2. Common Intraprocedural Management Problems

Complication	Cause	Treatment
Bradycardia or asystole	Ionic contrast Hypoxia Vagal response AV node ischemia Bezold-Jarish reaction	Cough Oxygen IV atropine, fluids Treatment of ischemia Temporary pacer
Ventricular tachycardia or fibrillation	Catheter-induced Guidewire-induced Contrast Ischemia	Remove catheter; immediate cardioversion/defibrillation; switch to low osmolar contrast; replete K^+, Mg^{++}; consider IV amiodarone or lidocaine
Hypotension	Artifact Dehydration Medications Ischemia/infarction Pericardial tamponade VT/VF Dye reaction	Recalibrate transducer; tighten O-ring on Y-adapter Saline bolus Stop nitrates Dopamine/dobutamine Pericardiocentesis Cardioversion/defibrillation Epinephrine; consider IABP or CPS
Hives or bronchospasm	Dye allergy	Diphenhydramine; hydrocortisone; epinephrine; ABGs/pulse oximetry (see Table 34.1)

compatibility chart to ensure selection of a guiding catheter with adequate inner lumen diameter to accept the appropriate burr. A liter bag of saline or lactated Ringers should be purged of air and pressurized to at least 200 mmHg. Depending on physician preference, a "cocktail" of heparin, nitroglycerin, and calcium antagonist may be added. Sterile contrast tubing without an air chamber or Y-branches should be selected to avoid air emboli, and air bubbles should be flushed out. Vigilance on the part of the technologist can prevent a catastrophic air embolus. It is up to the technologist to frequently check the pressurized flush solution and to alert the physician to air in the system. Other possible complications include no-reflow, bradycardia, or asystole during rotablation. For no-reflow (Chapter 21), be prepared to administer large doses of intracoronary verapamil and anticipate the need for a pacing electrode, connector cables, and an external pulse generator. The generator should be checked just before the case for battery function. Nothing should be left to chance. Drops in RPM more than 5000 indicate resistance against the lesion and are associated with increased risk for dissection and large particle formation. The physician should "peck" at the lesion to avoid drops in RPM and excessive heat generation. The technologist should <u>not</u> increase the RPM in that situation (it will generate more heat), but rather advise the physician of excessive deceleration. As with any other medical device, if a malfunction occurs (with or without injury to the patient), care must be taken to comply with all requirements of the federal government's Safe Medical Devices Act. It is the technologist's responsibility to immediately document the details of any incident and save all components of the system for further investigation by the hospital's Biomedical Engineering Department.

3.   **Directional Coronary Atherectomy (Chapter 28).** Directional coronary atherectomy (DCA) is indicated for a small subset of complex angioplasty patients, particularly those with ostial LAD or bifurcation stenoses. Contraindications to DCA include vessel diameter < 2.5mm, marked proximal vessel angulation or tortuosity, heavy lesion calcification, and degenerated saphenous vein grafts. Catheter design and function are presented in Chapter 28. Some degree of ischemia commonly occurs during directional atherectomy due to mechanical obstruction by the device or guiding catheter. Coronary artery dissection, thrombosis, perforation, and intimal disruption secondary to nosecone trauma have been described. The technologist should have 10% formalin or other preservative available if atherectomy tissue is sent for histologic examination. Availability of these resources must be assured by the technologist before the case begins.

4.   **Excimer Laser Coronary Angioplasty (ELCA) (Chapter 30).** ELCA may be used for long lesions, diffusely diseased coronary segments, and ostial narrowings. It can also be used for stenoses resistant to high pressure and calcified lesions that cannot be crossed or dilated with a balloon, but these cases are generally treated by Rotablator. ELCA systems are considered "cold" lasers; their mode of action is to break apart chemical bonds in the atheroma. They differ from thermal-laser balloons which rely on heating and welding effects. Safety precautions require that all personnel and patients undergoing laser procedures wear protective eye glasses. The laser system may require specialized maintenance with special attention to power elements, lenses and power output, based on catheter size and energy density. Flushing with saline is considered

essential with ELCA to reduce the risk of dissection. Adjunctive balloon angioplasty or stenting is performed after lasing in more than 90% of cases. Contraindications to ELCA include severe lesion eccentricity, marked angulation or proximal vessel tortuosity, and true bifurcation lesions.

5. **Cardiopulmonary Support (CPS) (Chapter 6).** CPS (femoral vein to femoral artery bypass) is specifically designed for hemodynamic support of patients with severe LV dysfunction or circulatory collapse. Portable CPS requires 20 minutes of preparation and the assistance of a hemoperfusionist thoroughly familiar with the system. Arterial cannulas are 18-20F and are based on body size. Considerable physician experience is also required to avoid complications. In order to avoid consumption of coagulation factors, a bolus of 30,000 units of heparin is typically given and the ACT level maintained at >400 seconds. Frequent monitoring of the ACT and arterial blood gases is required to avoid anemia, metabolic acidosis, and hypoxemia. Following case completion, the patient is transferred to a specially-designed stretcher with extra thick padding to increase patient comfort during prolonged immobilization (12-24 hours); necessary features include the ability to be lowered closer to the floor than conventional stretchers, and a siderail configuration that does not interfere with the CPS lines. Distal pulses should be checked frequently. The patient may remain on the stretcher, minimizing bed-to-bed transfers and accidental dislodgement of cannulae.

6. **Prolonged Thrombolytic Infusion (Chapter 9).** This form of adjunctive pharmacotherapy is sometimes used to recanalize occluded saphenous vein grafts and native coronary arteries. A standard 7 or 8F guiding catheter is seated in the target vessel. The guidewire is advanced into the artery as far as possible and a hollow core wire or multiple hole perfusion catheter is advanced until it abuts or enters the occlusion. The angioplasty guidewire is then removed, leaving a conduit through which a thrombolytic is selectively infused. The entire system must be sutured and secured to the patient's leg (Chapter 9). Tape and dressings can be applied to further secure the system since any movement jeopardizes equipment position and procedural success. **Since this is an intracoronary infusion it is essential that absolutely no bubbles are present in the infusion line.** Sterile stopcocks are attached to the infusion system to permit exit of bubbles and contrast injection during follow-up angiography. Forceful flushing is contraindicated because of ongoing clot dissolution and possible embolization. The thrombolytic infusion typically lasts 12-24 hours and the patient must remain supine with vascular sheaths in-situ. A secure vascular sheath, bladder catheterization, and continuous sedation are important patient care considerations. Successful infusion results in partial clot lysis and improved antegrade blood flow, and is typically followed by further intervention on any residual stenosis.

F. **TROUBLESHOOTING.** Technical problems commonly encountered during the interventional procedure include abnormal pressure on monitor, temporary venous pacemaker malfunction, power injector failure, x-ray equipment malfunction, and intra-aortic balloon pump malfunction. A systematic step-by-step approach will often identify and solve most simple problems (Tables 38.3-38.6).

Table 38.3. Pressure Monitoring Problems

Waveform	Assessment	Options
Absent	Reversed or broken transducers Disconnected cable Pressure tubing disconnected Hemostatic valve open Incorrect zero Incorrect scale	Notify physician Secure and clean cable connection Flush pressure lines Check for back-bleeding Recalibrate system Replace transducer
Low amplitude	Incorrect scale Valve/stopcock open to air Twisted catheter or tip obstructed	Reset scale Recalibrate system Flush pressure lines Observe catheter tip placement and shaft on fluoroscopy
Overshoot	Air	Flush system Change electronic filter setting
Drift	Transducer setup	Refill strain gauge membrane with fluid

POSTPROCEDURAL CONSIDERATIONS

This is a critical period when control of patient care is transferred to the technician or nurse, who must confirm the security of vascular sheaths, oxygen supply, and infusion of medication. The patient should be pain-free and prepared for transfer. Concurrently, patient needs must be assessed. Patient anxiety and complaints often reveal warning signs of impending complications, including chest pain (vessel reocclusion), shortness of breath (hypoxia, heart failure), palpitations (arrhythmia), nausea, hives, itching (precursor to anaphylaxis), lower quadrant abdominal pain and distention (retroperitoneal bleeding), leg swelling (expanding hematoma), and leg pain (possible development of limb-threatening ischemia within hours). Therefore, it is critical that the technician understand the assessment and management of chest pain, rhythm disorders, bleeding, and limb pain.

Chest pain is the most important post-procedural complication since it may herald abrupt vessel closure. Multiple factors must also be considered and ruled out before the patient returns to the interventional lab. Bleeding is relatively uncommon after coronary intervention despite the use of systemic anticoagulation, platelet glycoprotein IIb/IIIa receptor antagonists, and large arterial sheaths. If difficulties with vascular sheaths are observed, hematoma formation should be monitored closely. Bleeding may be encountered within the GI tract or the pericardium (as a result of an occult perforation). Rhythm disturbances, extremity pain, and confusion are additional problems. Early recognition, accurate diagnosis, and prompt treatment will have a major impact on patient outcome (Table 38.8).

Table 38.4. Assessment of Temporary Ventricular Pacemaker (TVP) Malfunction

No Pacing Spike

Check and clean cable connections

Confirm appropriate generator lead connection (atrial vs ventricular)

Check pacing mode (demand/asynchronous)

Check pacing rate set (generator > patient)

Increase output to maximum

Recheck battery indicator.

Replace cable and/or generator

Confirm generator switch on

Spike without Capture

Confirm that catheter position is level with apex of right ventricle or right ventricular outflow tract

Increase pacemaker generator output to maximum; determine threshold and set output 2-3 times above this

Observe for signs of perforation: hypotension, chest pain, ST-segment elevation on ECG, hiccoughs, friction rub on auscultation

Intermittent Capture

Confirm catheter position

Check generator settings; reset to increased heart rate

Recheck threshold

Failure to Capture

Check generator sensing threshold and set 2-3 below this

Check catheter position

Table 38.5. Simple Causes of Power Injector Failure

Improperly loaded injection syringe

Syringe compartment latch not secure

Trigger cable short circuit

Insufficient contrast for programmed injection

Always purge air from injector syringe and extension tubing before connecting to catheters.

Table 38.6. Simple Causes of X-Ray Equipment Malfunction

No Image

Inappropriate monitor brightness and contrast

Accidental activation of reset or "panic" buttons

Auto dose exposure mode not on (KV freeze mode is on)

Generator error (check message and reset)

No film magazine on camera*

Magazine sensor malfunction*

No Cine

Cine mode not selected on control board*

Film magazine misaligned, misloaded, or film torn*

No film*

"Overspeed" trip activated on camera*

Loose cable from cine camera to image intensifier*

Incorrect use of foot pedals for digital cine mode*

C-arm Failure

Proximity or safety switch bent, broken, or triggered (check image intensifier, collimator, table base position)

Biplane lateral arm out of "park" position

Collision of X-ray tube or image intensifier requiring manual override

* These are relevant to institutions which utilize cine-film

Table 38.7. Common Intraprocedural Equipment and Drug Delivery Problems

Problem	Recommendations
IVUS and Doppler FloWire Recording over videotape of previous cases No blank tape for recording No logbook record for retrieval of cases in the future Lost tapes and photos of past cases	• Put a small team of IVUS and Doppler specialists in charge of maintaining tapes and data • Immediately following case place archival tape and records in an image library as would be done with cine films or CD's of digital images
Intra-aortic balloon pump (IABP) IABP console not plugged in, batteries not charged Helium tank empty Wrench for opening tank missing Missing or broken EKG, pressure or slave cables Incompatibility between catheter helium tubing connector and safety disk port of console Excess noise from catheter whip on waveform	• Daily quality assurance checklist to ensure readiness of pump in emergency • Spare cables and adapters nearby • In-line oscillation filter available
Transvenous Pacemaker Generator batteries dead No cables	• Quality assurance checklist before each case to ensure readiness in emergency

Table 38.7. Common Intraprocedural Equipment and Drug Delivery Problems

Problem	Recommendations
Defibrillator Unit not plugged in and charging Dried gel left on paddles from previous use No defibrillator gel available Wrong mode (synchronous or asynchronous) selected Shorter staff persons unable to reach over patient with paddles	• Quality assurance checklist before each case to ensure readiness in emergency • Step stool for added height in achieving proper paddle pressure
Airway management Oral airway missing No stethoscope Oxygen extension tubing for connecting Ambu bag missing Laryngoscope battery not working Suction canister liners still dirty from previous case Tubing to wall suction and to patient reversed	• Quality assurance checklist before each case to ensure readiness in emergency • Have spare parts (including spare stethoscope) located nearby
Drugs Errors in drug calculations	• Quick reference sheets for drug calculations available in lab • Drug manual with "recipes" for drugs updated frequently • Computer drug database accessible to hemodynamic monitoring staff person
Pulmonary artery catheter Catheter clotted Catheter contaminated, unable to reposition from right ventricle or to "wedge" position	• Attach to pressurized flush bag as soon as possible when case is completed • Insert sterile sleeve on catheter when prepping before insertion • Dress catheter as soon as possible when case is completed, including double male adapter for monitoring right atrial pressure
Pericardiocentesis No phlebotomy tubing or liter vacutainer bottles No wedge for positioning patient at 45 degree angle No fenestrated drape sheet for prepping subxiphoid area	• Quality assurance checklist before each case to ensure readiness in emergency

Table 38.8. Common Postprocedural Management Problems

Problem	Cause	Assessment
Chest pain	• Ischemia • Pericardial perforation • Reflux esophagitis • Musculoskeletal	• Compare pre, intra, and postprocedural ECGs • Pain similar to pain on balloon inflation? • Response to nitrates and antacids • Check vital signs and pulsus paradoxicus
Arrhythmia	• Nausea/vagal effect • AV node (RCA) ischemia • Drug effect • Hypoxia	• Check ECGs for acute change as above • Check medications and dosage • Check oxygen saturation or ABG
Tachycardia/hypotension	• Ischemia • Hypovolemia • Drug Effect • Congestive failure	• Check blood pressure in both arms • Ischemia evaluation as above • Response to saline fluid bolus and Trendelenburg. • Check lower quadrant for retroperitoneal bleed • Check breath sounds for pulmonary edema
Bleeding	• Local • Retroperitoneal • Gastrointestinal • Pericardial	• Local compression • Check vascular sheath • Check ACT, CBC; consider protamine • Pericardiocentesis • Surgical evaluation
Limb pain	• Ischemia • Emboli • Retroperitoneal hematoma (femoral nerve compression)	• Check for loss of pulse (use Doppler) • Look for livedo reticularis • Examine for quadriceps weakness? • Check for IABP or possible sheath movement
Mental status change	• Stroke • Oversedation • Hypoxia • Hypoglycemia • Lidocaine	• Look for focal motor deficits • Give naloxone or flumazenil as needed • Check ABG, oxygen saturation • Give glucose • Stop lidocaine

LABORATORY LOGISTICS AND SAFETY

A. MATERIAL MANAGEMENT

1. **Room Supplies.** It is advisable to stock each lab to minimize confusion. Basic items should always be in similar arrangements, including IV lines, solutions, needles, sutures, standard diagnostic and PTCA catheters, drug cassettes, and emergency medications. Expensive devices and custom catheters should be centralized and dispensed individually. Several computerized systems are available to track and control inventory; a bar code system is extremely effective.

2. **Sterile Packs.** Contents are tailored to the specific needs of a particular cath lab and are often dictated by physician preference. The cost of the packaging should be offset by improved efficiency. Different packs for brachial cutdown and femoral and radial approaches are available.

3. **Specialty Carts.** These carts are dedicated to a single interventional procedure and contain all equipment needed to complete that case. Carts are ideal for specialized techniques such as valvuloplasty, laser, atherectomy, and stenting. The carts are portable, easy to use, and consolidate inventory storage.

4. **ACLS Equipment.** Standard equipment for ACLS should be present in each catheterization suite. A cassette of commonly used drugs facilitates storage and access. The entire cassette should be rotated periodically for complete restocking by the pharmacy. In addition, a "crash cart" containing a defibrillator, intubation supplies, and ACLS medications must be present in every room. The contents of the cart are usually sealed as a quality assurance measure. In addition to the cassette and crash cart system, certain medications should be immediately available at all times, such as lidocaine, nitroglycerin, and dopamine.

5. **Quality Assurance.** The quality assurance process is an integral part of cath lab function and should begin before the patient enters the interventional laboratory. It is mandatory that the monitoring technician complete a checklist ensuring that all appropriate equipment, medications, and ACLS support devices are ready. The basic list should apply to all cardiac procedures. It is best to physically check each device: squeeze the Ambu bag; turn on suction; pull defibrillator paddles out of holder; turn pacemaker generator on and off. This checklist must be completed, signed, and should accompany the patient chart. The key to every emergency situation is being prepared ahead of time.

B. **RADIATION PROTECTION.** Radiation exposure is a concern to all members of the interventional team (Chapter 39). Table 38.9 includes tips to minimize individual exposure. The importance of lead shielding, maintaining proper distance from the tray source, and rotating responsibilities in the lab deserve emphasis. Exposure is similar in biplane and monoplane systems provided that total fluoroscopy and cine time is the same. The average radiation dose for diagnostic angiography is roughly equal to that for simple PTCA. During angioplasty, fluoroscopy time is longer than during diagnostic angiography, whereas cine time, which causes the highest radiation exposure, is shorter. Film badge monitoring is intended to provide important information about radiation exposure.

Table 38.9. Methods to Reduce Radiation Exposure

Keep distance from the patient (inverse square law)

Select the minimum collimation possible

Set image intensifier as close as possible to the patient

Do not reach into the radiation beam with hands

Use unit components for "shadowing" as designed

Wear radiation protection clothing at all times (apron, glasses, thyroid shield)

Use pulsed fluoroscopy whenever available

Where possible, use cine operation with 15 or 30 f/s

Utilize leaded glass shields between staff and X-ray tube.

* * * * *

39 RADIATION PRINCIPLES AND SAFETY

Cheryl Culver Schultz, M.S.
Vincent McCormick, M.S.
Janice Campbell, M.S.

The volume of interventional cardiology procedures is increasing rapidly. Since x-rays have biological effects which pose a risk to human health, the challenge is to optimize image quality while minimizing radiation exposure to the patient and staff.[1-5] This chapter provides a brief overview of the characteristics of ionizing radiation, production of x-rays, basic operational features of the x-ray equipment, biological effects of radiation, and radiation protection principles which are the keys to the safe delivery of radiation.

TYPES OF RADIATION

A. **DEFINITIONS.** Radiation refers to energy in transit, and can be categorized by physical properties such as *particulate* and *electromagnetic* emission. Particulate radiation consists of atomic or subatomic particles that have kinetic energy, including beta particles (electrons with a negative charge), positrons (electrons with a positive charge), protons (positive charge), and neutrons (neutral charge). In contrast, electromagnetic radiation is generated by oscillating electrical and magnetic fields traveling at the speed of light, and exhibit characteristic wavelength and frequency. The electromagnetic spectrum consists of a wide range of energies, including radiowaves, microwaves, visible light, x-rays, and gamma rays. X-rays and gamma rays have the shortest wavelength, highest energy, and most penetrating power.

When x-ray and gamma ray photons interact with matter, energy is transferred to an orbital electron in an atom of the absorbing medium, resulting in *excitation* (the electron is moved from its orbit to a more distant orbit) or *ionization* (the electron is completely ejected from the atom). X-rays are a form of ionizing radiation, whereas lower energy electromagnetic radiation such as microwaves are nonionizing forms of radiation. Ionizing radiation is important clinically because it produces *free radicals*, which can cause tissue damage.

B. **RADIATION DOSE.** The amount of energy transferred from ionizing radiation to living tissue is often referred to as the "radiation dose," but factors such as age, gender, tissue sensitivity, volume of tissue irradiated, and rate of delivery all influence the tissue response to radiation. Three units of radiation are routinely used to describe the "radiation dose": the Roentgen, the gray (or rad), and the sievert (or rem).

  1. **Exposure and Exposure Rate.** Exposure refers to the amount of ionizing radiation the patient is exposed to, and is expressed as Roentgen (R). The exposure rate can be directly measured with a survey instrument or ionization detector, expressed as R/minute or milli-R/hour.

2. **Absorbed Dose**. The absorbed dose refers to the amount of radiation needed to transfer a certain amount of energy (1 joule/kg), and is expressed as gray (Gy) or rad (1 gray = 100 rad). The absorbed dose varies with different types of tissue: 0.95 rad/R for soft tissue and 5.0 rad/R for bone.

3. **Dose Equivalent.** To account for different biological effects of radiation, dose equivalent was defined as the absorbed dose multiplied by the quality factor, expressed as sievert (Sv) or rem (1 sievert = 100 rem). For x-rays, the quality factor is 1, so the gray and sievert are equal. For practical purposes, the rad, rem, and Roentgen have approximate numerical equivalence in the x-ray energy range used in the cardiac cath lab.

PRODUCTION OF X-RAYS

A. **OPERATION OF THE X-RAY TUBE.** The X-ray tube assembly consists of a filament, a rotating tungsten target (anode), and an evacuated glass tube (Figure 39.1). When a current is applied to the filament, electrons are released and accelerated towards the target by a high-voltage electric potential. X-rays are produced when electrons collide and are completely stopped by the target (called *characteristic* x-rays), and when electrons are rapidly decelerated after striking the target (called *Bremsstralung or "braking" radiaton"*).

B. **TUBE SETTINGS.** The x-ray tube produces x-rays with different energies, and the maximum energy is dependent on the voltage across the x-ray tube (kVp, kilovolt potential), as displayed on the control console during the exposure. Electrons that are accelerated across a potential of 100 kV produce x-rays with a maximum energy of 100 kiloelectron volts. Increasing the kVp produces higher energy x-rays, which have greater penetrating power for larger patients, increases the intensity of the x-rays, and decreases image contrast. The optimum setting for iodinated contrast in the coronary arteries is usually 70-80 kVp for adults and 60 kVp for children. Some low-energy x-rays are inadequate for imaging purposes and result in needless radiation exposure to the patient. Copper or aluminum filters are placed between the x-ray tube and the patient to absorb low energy x-rays. The intensity of x-rays and image brightness is directly related to the current (mA) passing through the filament.

C. **X-RAY INTERACTIONS.** When x-rays are generated by the x-ray tube, there are three outcomes as they interact with the patient: absorption, scatter, and transmission. Higher density materials absorb more x-rays. Iodinated radiographic contrast increases the density of blood, thus enhancing image contrast between vascular structures and adjacent soft tissue. Although higher kVp can increase x-ray energy and transmission, these potential benefits are offset by increases in scattered radiation and decreased image contrast. Other factors which increase scattered radiation include larger patients and lower magnification (larger field of view).

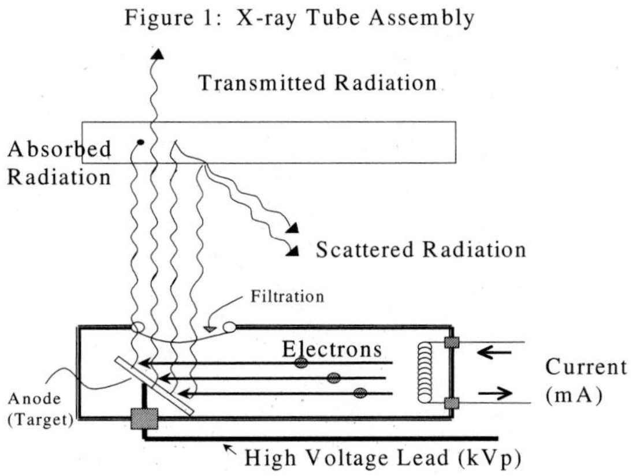

Figure 1: X-ray Tube Assembly

Figure 39.1. X-ray Tube Assembly

X-RAY IMAGE ACQUISITION

A. **FLUOROSCOPY.** Fluoroscopy is a routine type of x-ray examination used for dynamic imaging; when used for visualization of blood vessels, it is called angiography. To enhance the visibility of small guidewires, high sensitivity image intensifiers are used to amplify the brightness of the image. X-rays transmitted through the patient enter the input phosphor, which emits light that is then converted to electrical energy. The electrical energy is amplified and converted back into light at the output phosphor. The output phosphor of the image intensifier is coupled to a television pickup tube which converts the light pattern into an electrical signal, which forms the image on the monitor (Figure 39.2).

B. **CINE ANGIOGRAPHY AND DIGITAL ANGIOGRAPHY.** In conventional cine angiography, light exiting the output phosphor is divided by a beam-splitting mirror, which diverts part of the light beam to the TV monitor (for fluoroscopic imaging), and the rest of the beam to the cine camera lens (which refocuses the light onto cine film). Standard cine cameras use 35 mm film at frame rates of 15-60 frames/sec (15-30 fps for coronary angiography; 60 fps for ventriculography); higher frame rates have higher radiation doses. In many labs, cine has been replaced by digital angiography, which utilizes computerized digital processing techniques to acquire and display images.[6] Once the image is captured by the image intensifier and optically coupled to a television camera, the video signal is digitized and stored in computer memory for subsequent display and manipulation. Digital image acquisition will soon replace cine film due to lower radiation doses and opportunities for image processing.

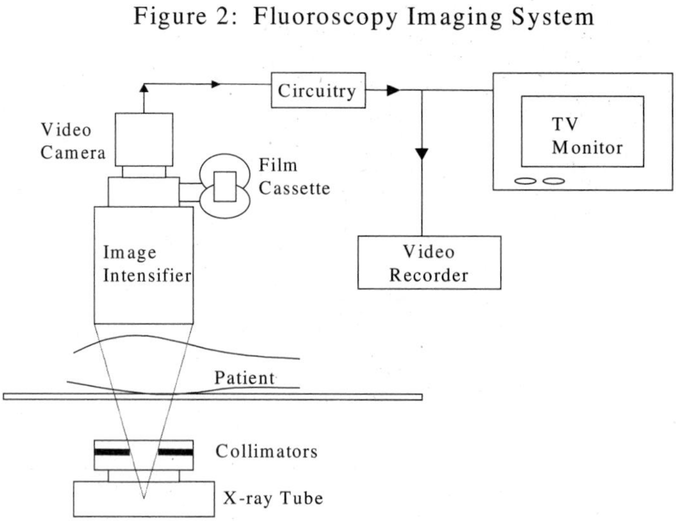

Figure 2: Fluoroscopy Imaging System

Figure 39.2. Fluoroscopy Imaging System

IMAGE QUALITY

A. **AUTOMATIC BRIGHTNESS CONTROL.** Modern fluoroscopy equipment automatically adjusts the kVp and mA to optimize image quality. This automatic brightness control (ABC) or automatic exposure control (AEC) uses an electronic sensor to measure light at the output phosphor, and adjusts the x-ray tube mA and/or kVp to maintain brightness. Increases in kVp enhance brightness but decrease contrast, while increases in mA enhance brightness. Manually-operated controls have been replaced by automatic systems, which determine kVp and mA for optimal image quality and prevent flaring. Properly functioning ABC and AEC produce images of constant average brightness.

B. **COLLIMATION.** Modern fluoroscopic equipment is designed so that the x-ray tube cannot produce x-rays unless the image intensifier is in position to intercept the entire beam. To prevent unnecessary irradiation, collimators are used to restrict the size of the x-ray field (Figure 39.2). These are motor driven metal or lead shutters located just outside the x-ray tube that confine the x-ray beam to the maximum area recorded on the cine film or displayed on the TV monitor. The collimators are used to manually adjust the field size to the area of interest.

C. **FIELD SIZE AND MAGNIFICATION.** Most cardiac catheterization laboratories utilize image intensifiers with 3 field sizes and modes of magnification to optically adjust the field size and magnification (Figure 39.3): low magnification mode (9-11 inch field size), intermediate magnification mode (6-7 inch field size), and high magnification mode (4-5 inch field size). Usually, exposure factors automatically increase during magnification to compensate for the decreased brightness that results from spreading the smaller field over the full viewing area. As the field size decreases with magnification, the local patient dose rate must increase to compensate for the loss of brightness from the image intensifier. Since scatter decreases, image quality improves. With digital software, the operator can enlarge an image without an increase in dose to the patient. Optical magnification can also be enhanced by lowering the table height and/or raising the image intensifier; both increase patient dose and scattered radiation.

D. **PATIENT RADIATION DOSE (Table 39.1)**

The FDA limits the dose rate for standard fluoroscopy with AEC to 10 R/minute, but "high dose," "high-contrast," "high output, or "boosted," exposure modes can be used by applying additional pressure to the foot pedal or changing settings on the control panel. A continuous audible signal is required in the "boosted mode." The FDA limits the dose to 20 R/minute in the boosted mode, although units capable of much higher exposure rates exist.[6,7] Pulsed fluoroscopy may reduce exposure by 30-50%. There is no exposure limit if film or digital images are produced. Patient radiation dose is dependent on several factors, including x-ray tube factors (kVp, filtration, exposure mode, and collimation), image intensifier factors (field size, magnification mode), distance factors (table height, intensifier height, oblique projections), and patient factors (size).

1. **X-ray Tube Factors.** Tube factors such as kVp and filtration are largely independent of the operator, whereas collimation and exposure mode (fluoroscopy, "boosted" fluoroscopy, cine) are operator-dependent.

2. **Image Intensifier Factors.** The patient dose from fluoroscopy also depends on field size and magnification. For fluoroscopy, the entrance or skin radiation exposure rate typically ranges from 1-2 R/minute in the 9-inch mode and 2-5 R/minute in the smaller magnification modes. Since most radiation is absorbed by the patient, the exposure exiting the patient is less than 1% of the entrance exposure rate. For 10 minutes of fluoroscopy, the patient's skin exposure is 10-50 R, equivalent to 10 to 50 rads.

3. **Distance.** If the x-ray tube is too close to the patient, harmful skin radiation may result; the intensity of x-rays decreases as the table height increases (inverse square law). The standard practice is to maintain a minimum distance of 18 inches between the x-ray tube and the patient. The height of the operator may influence the table position, since a taller operator will usually raise the table, decreasing the patient dose. The image intensifier should be positioned as close to the patient as possible, and care should be used in oblique and lateral orientations to maintain a safe distance between the tube and patient.

4. **Exposure Factors.** Patient exposure also depends on several exposure factors. Typically the input phosphor of the image intensifier requires an exposure rate of 1.0 microR/frame for cine. If the frame rate increases from 15 to 30 frames per second, then twice the number of x-rays are needed, doubling the patient's radiation dose. Cine image sharpness is usually not noticeably different with 15 frames/second unless the patient is tachycardic; digital images are routinely acquired at 15 frames/second, reducing patient exposure.

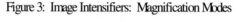

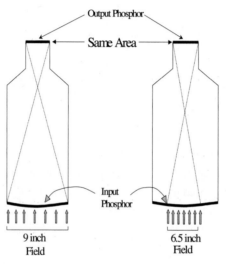

Figure 39.3. Image Intensifiers: Magnification Modes

Table 39.1. Factors That Increase Patient Radiation Dose[8-10]

X-ray Tube Factors
    Hi kVp techniques*
    Inadequate filtration*
    "Boosted" exposure mode**
    Collimation**

Image Intensifier Factors
    High magnification modes (small field size)**

Distance
    Lower table height**
    Higher image intensifier height**
    Lateral and oblique projectors**

Exposure Factors
    Prolonged or repeated cine runs**
    Longer fluoroscopy times**
    Higher frame rates**

Patient Factors
    Small body size*

*   Factors that are preset or automatic
**   Factors that are at the discretion of the physician

RADIATION BIOLOGY

A. **ENVIRONMENTAL RADIATION EXPOSURE.** All living things are exposed to background ionizing radiation: People in rocky areas receive more terrestrial radiation, whereas others living at high altitudes receive more cosmic radiation. Most natural radiation is from radon, a gas product from the decay of natural uranium. Ionizing radiation also comes from man-made sources, such as medical and dental x-rays, fallout from nuclear weapons, nuclear power industries, and occupational exposures (Table 39.2). Medical exposures including diagnostic radiology, nuclear medicine, and radiation therapy represent the largest source of man-made radiation. Radiation doses to the US population from natural and man-made sources are approximately 1 mRem/day; 15% of the radiation dose is from medical sources.

B. **RADIATION INJURY**
    1. **General Considerations.** Radiobiological research has amassed more information about the effects of ionizing radiation on living systems than nearly any other physical or chemical agent. The biological effects of radiation on humans are classified as *stochastic* or *deterministic*. Stochastic effects are considered non-threshold; risk is proportional to dose, but there is no safe threshold below which the risk is zero (e.g., radiation-induced leukemia). These stochastic effects are the principal health risk from medical radiation exposure, and form the basis for radiation protection programs.

Deterministic effects are those where the severity of injury increases with dose, but there is a threshold dose below which the effect is not seen. Examples of deterministic effects are cataracts, erythema, fibrosis, and necrosis.[11]

2. **Damage and Repair.** Radiation-induced injury begins with chemical changes at the atomic and molecular level, similar to those produced by other physical or chemic agents. Cellular injury is mostly induced by generation of ions and free radicals, rather than heat, and DNA is the most critical target. If DNA damage cannot be repaired, permanent DNA and/or chromosome breaks may occur, leading to somatic effects in the exposed individual and/or genetic effects in their offspring.

3. **Somatic Effects.** Somatic effects may be observed early (within days to weeks of exposure) or late (within month to years of exposure). Early effects develop in proliferating cell systems, particularly those that are the most radiosensitive (skin, ocular lens, testes, intestines, esophagus). Delayed effects occur many months after exposure, and are often seen in nerves, muscles, and other radioresistant cell types. Damage is usually expressed as fibrosis or scar. Carcinogenesis is the most important delayed somatic effect. The data on radiation exposure to humans comes from atomic bomb survivors, medical exposures, occupational exposures, and high background radiation areas. Although the dose-response relationship for the development of cancer at high doses is well established, there are insufficient data to assess the risk of cancer after exposure to low doses, due to the natural incidence of cancer. At the present time, there is no conclusive evidence that doses from diagnostic angiography pose any hazard to adult patients, but the potential should not be disregarded in young adults, pediatric patients, or in radiosensitive tissues such as the breast. Acute reactions usually involve the skin and adjacent tissues, since cells at the base of the epidermis are the most sensitive to radiation. Injury is dependent on the exposure rate, total dose, age, health of the patient, and skin site. The onset of the reaction may take up to two weeks.

Many cardiac catheterization labs have modes of operation where dose rates are higher than 0.2 Gy/min (20 rad/min); potential skin injury can be observed during prolonged procedures (Table 39.3). To prevent skin injury during long procedures, the operator should be familiar with FDA recommendations: 1) Change the tube angle to change the irradiated area and minimize skin injury; 2) Use replay features instead of repeated exposures; 3) Limit lateral and oblique projections, which yield high skin doses because the x-ray tube is closer to the patient; 4) For prolonged exposures, increase the table height and lower the image intensifier; 5) Use the "boosted mode" only when necessary. The FDA also suggests that facilities develop clinical protocols for the safe use of interventional fluoroscopy, and that the absorbed radiation dose should be recorded on the patient record after prolonged interventional procedures.[13] Methods for directly monitoring the patient's radiation doses are currently being developed.

4. **Effects on the Developing Embryo and Fetus.** Occasionally, genes and DNA spontaneously change, leading to spontaneous mutations; the prevalence of these mutations is termed the mutation frequency. The mutation frequency can be altered by viruses, chemicals, pollutants, and radiation.

Table 39.2. Average Radiation Dose to the U.S. General Public (mrem/year)[12]

Natural Background	
Cosmic rays	30-70
External terrestrial	10-100
Internal	10-20
Radon	200
Subtotal	300
Medical Sources	
X-rays	39
Radiopharmaceuticals	14
Subtotal	53
Man-made Sources	
Fallout (weapons testing)	3
Nuclear poser industry	<1
Consumer products	3-4
Airline travel	0.6
Subtotal	7-9
TOTAL	360

The embryo and fetus are most sensitive to ionizing radiation during the first 6 weeks of gestation, when a woman is usually unaware of the pregnancy. As a result, the National Commission on Radiation Protection recommends that pregnancy be ruled out in all females of child-bearing age prior to exposure to diagnostic x-rays or fluoroscopy.[14] The outcome of radiation exposure to the embryo and fetus depends on the stage of development: Exposure during pre-implantation (0 - 10 days after conception) results in a high incidence of prenatal death, doses as low as 0.1 Gy (10 rad) may be fatal during this time. (Surviving embryos usually exhibit no visible abnormality.) Exposure during organogenesis (2nd - 8th week) may result in severe abnormalities of the central nervous and skeletal systems. Irradiation on different gestational days will result in different abnormalities; the greatest variety of congenital abnormalities is produced when exposure occurs during the 23rd to 37th day of gestation. The most common abnormalities include microcephaly, hydrocephaly, abnormal appendages, spina bifida, and blindness. As the dose of radiation increases above 0.5 Gy (50 rad), the likelihood of malformations increases. The fetus becomes more radioresistant during the third trimester, and higher doses are necessary to produce damage. The fetal growth stage in humans begins at day 45 and continues to term. Exposure during this period may produce anomalies of the nervous system and sense organs. Much of the damage induced during this period may not manifest until later in life.

Table 39.3. Radiation-Induced Injuries[13,15]

Effect	Threshold Dose (rad)	Hours of Fluoroscopy Time		Onset of Effect
		@ 2 rad/min	@ 20 rad/min	
Erythema	200-600	1.7-5.0	0.17-0.5	Hours to 10 days
Epilation	300-700	2.5-5.8	0.25-0.58	3 weeks
Pericarditis	800	6.7	0.33	>10 weeks
Dermal necrosis	1800	15.0	1.5	>10 weeks

RADIATION SAFETY AND PROTECTION

As understanding of the biological effects of radiation has evolved, so have the standards for radiation protection. To properly protect the patient, physician, and others from the potentially harmful effects of radiation, the interventionalist should consistently practice basic principles of radiation protection.

A. **RECOMMENDED DOSE LIMITS FOR IONIZING RADIATION.** The maximum permissible dose of ionizing radiation to workers, the general public, and the embryo-fetus from occupational exposure is regulated by strict state and federal standards (Table 39.4).[16] The mean annual whole body dose equivalent for all medical workers in the United States is 70 millirem/year, which is well below the maximum permitted radiation dose for occupational workers (5,000 mrem/year).[17] Unquestionably, the highest occupational exposure to radiation occurs during x-ray procedures.

B. **RADIATION PROTECTION FOR THE INTERVENTIONALIST.**[18-20] Cardiac catheterization laboratories are constructed with 1.5 mm of lead or equivalent shielding to protect individuals in the control room and adjacent areas from exposure to ionizing radiation. Only personnel whose presence is required should remain in the cath lab during x-ray procedures. The primary source of radiation to the interventionalist is scatter radiation from the patient during fluoroscopy and cine acquisition; the dose rate close to the patient can be as high as 0.3 rem per hour. The three common principles for protecting the operator against radiation exposure are *time, distance, and shielding*. Radiation dose is proportional to exposure duration and inversely proportional to the square-root of distance from the patient (Figure 39.4). Lead is the most common material used for shielding, and critical organs (lung, GI tract, gonads, breast, and bone marrow) should be properly shielded during all procedures. A lead apron with an equivalent of 0.5 mm of lead in the front panel is mandatory, and lead in the back panel (0.25 mm lead equivalence) provides additional protection. Custom fit lead aprons may optimize comfort and reduce cervical and back strain without compromising radiation protection. It is important to verify that lighter non-lead aprons meet the standard of 0.5 mm of lead equivalence throughout the range of kVp used in the cath lab. A thyroid shield (0.5 mm of lead equivalence) is recommended to shield the sternum, upper breast, and thyroid gland. Leaded eyeglasses with side shields reduce the exposure to the eyes, and depending on the composition of the eyeglasses, can also improve visual acuity. Leaded eyeglasses are recommended for staff with collar-badge doses approaching 15 rem per year, and for interventionalists in training. The hands are relatively insensitive to radiation, but receive the highest radiation dose. Commercially available leaded surgical gloves provide only a small reduction in hand exposure, and are no substitute for keeping hands out of the radiation field. Each cardiac cath lab should also be equipped with supplemental lead shielding to reduce scatter, including table-mounted lead drapes, ceiling-mounted lead acrylic shields, and specially designed rolling lead acrylic shields with optional lead drapes. Supplemental shielding should always be used when the operator remains in the room.

C. **PERSONNEL DOSIMETRY.** Interventionalists who work in the cath lab are commonly assigned two radiation badges, one on the collar outside the lead apron to estimate the doses to the eyes and the unshielded shoulders, and the second underneath the lead apron.[21] The lead apron reduces the radiation dose at the waist to 10% of the collar dose, at 75 kVp. The effective dose equivalent is best estimated by averaging the two dosimeters. Compliance with the radiation badge monitoring program is critical for radiation safety. Based on 15,000 cardiac procedures from 1984-1988, the mean dose equivalent per procedure was 4 ± 2 millirem.[22] The highest doses were delivered to physicians-in-training (5 rem per year). These radiation doses are consistent with other medical facilities that have busy cardiac catheterization services.

Table 39.4. Recommended Dose Limits For Occupational Exposure to Ionizing Radiation[16]

Effective Dose Limits - Occupational Exposure	
Annual	5000 millirem
Cumulative	1000 millirem x age
Annual Dose Limits for Tissues - Occupational	
Lens of eye	15,000 millirem
Skin, hands, and feet	50,000 millirem
Embryo fetus, total	500 millirem
Embryo fetus, monthly	50 millirem
Annual Public Exposure - Nonoccupational	
Annual effective dose	100-500 millirem
Lens of the eye	1500 millirem
Skin, hands, and feet	5000 millirem
Negligible Individual Annual Dose	1 millirem

Figure 4: Scatter Radiation Doses in mR/h

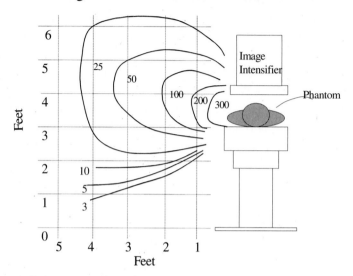

Figure 39.4. Scatter Radiation Doses (mR/h)

E. **RADIATION PROTECTION FOR WOMEN OF CHILD-BEARING AGE.** Protecting the unborn fetus from radiation exposure is of paramount importance. Current regulations restrict the radiation dose to the embryo and fetus to 500 millirem for the entire gestation and a monthly dose < 50 millirem, for women who declare their pregnancy in writing to their employer. Pregnancy does not preclude working in the cardiac catheterization lab. The individual's radiation history should be reviewed to determine if these dose limits are likely to be reached and if any special precautions are appropriate. Maternity lead aprons provide an extra 1 mm of lead equivalence and use of a properly fitting wrap-around lead apron provides the same radiation protection for the fetus (1 mm lead equivalent apron provides protection from 99% of radiation exposure at 75 kVp). Fetal radiation badges should be worn on the abdomen underneath the lead apron, and provide a monthly record of fetal exposure. When pregnancy is reported, it is important to review the cardinal principles of radiation protection: minimize exposure time, maximize distance from the x-ray source, and use available shielding.

F. **QUALITY ASSURANCE.** The x-ray equipment should be tested to assure optimal function, compliance with state and federal regulations, and radiation protection for the patients and staff.[23,24] X-ray output and exposure rates should be measured annually in all modes. The entrance exposure dose is a measure of the exposure rate at the skin surface and varies from unit to unit and patient to patient. Resolution is the ability of an imaging system to reproduce fine detail and is commonly evaluated using line pair testing. Contrast refers to the ability to distinguish tissue density, and low contrast resolution the ability to differentiate objects of similar density. Both high and low contrast test tools should be used regularly according to established operating parameters, and should be compared to baseline performance for that equipment and adjusted accordingly.

The x-ray beam is composed of photons of varying energies (the maximum energy is the kVp) and filtration of lower energy photons results in beam "hardening." Regulations require a minimum filter thickness (e.g., an aluminum equivalent of 2.5 mm to 3.5 mm depending on kVp), and compliance is verified annually by measuring the Half Value Layer (HVL) of the beam, defined as the thickness of aluminum that is required to reduce the intensity of the beam to half its original intensity. Other annual tests evaluate beam-limiting devices, collimators, beam alignment (to verify that the image intensifier intercepts the entire beam and that the beam is perpendicular to its face), automatic brightness control, accuracy of kVp, focal spot size, and video equipment (i.e., automatic gain control). An imaging system is only as good as the video equipment on which it is viewed. Resolution problems or distortions introduced by the video system can seriously impair the ability to evaluate small vessels and structures. The tests discussed above are commonly performed by a medical physicist, biomedical engineer, or trained technical staff. However, the interventionalist may be the first to notice a change in image quality.

CORONARY BRACHYTHERAPY

Radiation therapy that involves placement of radioactive materials in close proximity to the treatment site is referred to as brachytherapy, which means "short distance" therapy. Brachytherapy to prevent restenosis following coronary intervention involves placement of a sealed radioactive source into the target vessel. The dose ranges from 15 to 30 gray (1500-3000 rad) with dwell times of 2-45 minutes. Two classes of radionuclides are currently under investigation for preventing restenosis: *gamma emitters*, which give off photons similar to an x-ray, and *beta emitters*, which give off subatomic particles. Cath labs are designed for low energy x-rays, and structural shielding may not be adequate for higher energy gamma sources such as Ir-192. Beta emitters such as Sr-90 and P-32 are non-penetrating forms of radiation; adequate shielding against beta emitters is found in most cath labs. Brachytherapy is discussed in Chapter 24.

*****

REFERENCES

1. Pepine CJ, Allen HD, Bashore TM and the members of the American College of Cardiology and American Heart Association Ad Hoc Task Force on Cardiac Catheterization. ACC-AHA guidelines for cardiac catheterization and cardiac catheterization laboratories. Journal of the American College of Cardiology 1991;18:1149-1182.

2. Moore RJ. *Imaging Principles of Cardiac Angiography.* Carle Place, NY: Nuclear Associates, 1993.

3. Curry TS, Dowdey JE, Murry RC. *Christensen's Introduction to the Physics of Diagnostic Radiology.* 4th ed. Philadelphia, Lea & Febiger, 1990.

4. Bushong SC. *Radiologic Science for Technologists: Physics, Biology, and Protection.* 4th ed. St. Louis, CV Mosby Co., 1988.

5. Sprawls, P. *Physical Principles of Medical Imaging.* 2nd ed, Aspen Publishers, Inc., 1993.

6. Cagnon CH, Benedict SH, et. al. Exposure Rates in High-Level-Control Fluorsocopy for Image Enhancement. Radiology 1991;178:643-646.

7. Gray JE, Holmes DR., Schueler BA. High dose and interventional radiological examinations including efficacy issues. In: *Radiation Protection in Medicine.* Proceedings of the Twenty-Eighth Annual Meeting of the National Council on Radiation Protection and Measurements, Washington DC, NCRP, 1993.

8. Faulkner K. The potential for reducing exposure in x-ray imaging. In: *Frey DC, Sprawls P, eds. The Expanding Role of Medical Physics in Diagnostic Imaging.* Madison, WI, Advanced Medical Publishing, 1997.

9. Wagner LK, Archer BR. *Radiation Management for Fluoroscopy for Physicians.* Partners in Radiation Management, 1995.

10. Shope TB. Radiation-induced skin injuries from fluoroscopy. Radiographics 1996;16:1195-1199.

11. Hall EJ. *Radiobiology for the Radiologist,* 4th ed. Philadelphia, PA, J.B. Lippincott Co., 1994.

12. National Council on Radiation Protection and Measurements. Ionizing Radiation Exposure of the Population of the United States. NCRP Report No. 93. Bethseda, Maryland, NCRP Publications, 1987.

13. Food and Drug Administration. Public health advisory: avoidance of serious x-ray induced skin injuries to patients during fluoroscopically-guided procedures. Rockville, MD, Center for Devices and Radiological Health. FDA, September 9, 1994.

14. National Council on Radiation Protection and Measurements. Medical Radiation Exposure of Pregnant and Potentially Pregnant Women. NCRP Report No. 54. Bethesda, MD, NCRP, 1977.

15. American Association of Physicists in Medicine. *Managing the Use of Fluoroscopy in Medical Institutions,* AAPM Report No. 58. Madison, WI, Medical Physics Publishing, 1998.

16. National Council on Radiation Protection and Measurements. Limitation of Exposure to Ionizing Radiation. NCRP Report No. 116. Bethesda, Maryland, NCRP Publications, 1993.

17. National Council on Radiation Protection and Measurements. Implementation of the Principle of as Low as Reasonably Achievable (Alara) for Medical and Ental Personnel. NCRP Report No. 107. Bethesda, Maryland, NCRP Publications, 1990.

18. Marx VM. Interventional Procedures: Risks to Patients and Personnel. In: *Radiation Risk: A Primer.* American College of Radiology. Reston, VA: American College of Radiology, 1996.

19. Bateman LF. Perspective: safety matters in fluoroscopy. Advance for Radiology & Radiation Oncology 1998; July: 46-49.

20. Balter S. Teaching radiation safety to invasive fluoroscopists. In: Frey DC, Sprawls P, eds. *The Expanding Role of Medical Physics in Diagnostic Imaging.* Madison, WI, Advanced Medical Publishing, 1997.

21. Rosenstein M. Personnel Dosimetry Issues in Interventional Radiology. In: *Radiation Protection in Medicine,* Proceedings of the Twenty-Eighth Annual Meeting of the National Council on Radiation Protection and Measurements, Washington DC, NCRP, 1993.

22. Renaud L. A 5-y follow-up of the radiation exposure to in-room personnel during cardiac catheterization. Health Physics 1992; 62(1): 10-15.

23. Martin MC. Fluoroscopy System Evaluation. In: Frey DC, Sprawls P, eds. *The Expanding Role of Medical Physics in Diagnostic Imaging.* Madison, WI, Advanced Medical Publishing, 1997.

24. National Council on Radiation Protection and Measurements. *Quality Assurance for Diagnostic Imaging Equipment,* Report No. 99. Washington, DC, NCRP, 1988.

40 ATHEROSCLEROSIS AND THROMBOSIS

Michael Peterson, M.D.
George Dangas, M.D., Ph.D.
Valentin Fuster, M.D., Ph.D.

Atherosclerotic coronary artery disease is the leading cause of death in the United States. Medical therapy is aimed at halting the progression of atherosclerosis and limiting the propensity for plaque rupture and thrombosis. Optimal treatment requires an understanding of the various mechanisms involved in atherogenesis, thrombosis, and fibrinolysis. Earlier theories suggested that atherosclerosis was either a primary disorder of the endothelial cell with secondary lipid accumulation (encrustation theory); a primary lipid disorder with secondary effects promoting intimal proliferation (lipid theory); or a disorder due to endothelial injury, making it more susceptible to lipid accumulation (response-to-injury theory). Fuster expanded the response-to-injury hypothesis by suggesting a broader scheme for vascular injury (Table 40.1), beginning with functional changes in endothelial permeability.

STAGES OF ATHEROSCLEROSIS

Atherosclerosis is characterized by repetitive injury, inflammation, and repair within the vascular wall. Endothelial injury is though to be the initial event, resulting in an early lesion that progresses through advanced stages (Table 40.2), affecting all components of the arterial wall (Table 40.3).

Table 40.1. Classification of Vascular Injury

Vascular Injury	Description	Implications
Type I	Functional changes in endothelium with minimal structural change; characterized by increased lipoprotein permeability and leucocyte adhesion	Earliest identifiable form of vascular injury; initiates atherosclerosis
Type II	Endothelial denudation and minor thrombosis	More advanced injury promotes further atherosclerosis; slowly progressive
Type III	Deeper injury to media which may precipitate severe thrombosis	Leads to rapid progression of chronic atheroma by ulceration and thrombosis; cause of acute coronary syndromes

Table 40.2. The Stary Classification of Atherosclerotic Lesions

Type	Lesion	Histology	Decade of Onset
I	Initial lesion	Macrophages, isolated foam cells	≥1st
II	Fatty streak	Intracellular lipids, smooth muscle cells	
III	Preatheroma	Extracellular lipid	≥3rd
IV	Atheroma	Core of extracellular lipid	
V	Fibrous plaque	Increased smooth muscle and collagen	≥4th
VI	Ruptured plaque	Mural thrombus	
VII, VIII	Fibrocalcific lesions	Mineralization with minimal lipids	≥5th

From Stary HC. Composition and classification of human atherosclerotic lesions.
[Vi rch Arch Pathol Anat 1992;421:277-290].

A. **ENDOTHELIAL INJURY: THE INITIAL EVENT OF ATHEROSCLEROSIS.** The initial injury to the endothelium is a localized inflammation in response to hyperlipidemia, tobacco, diabetes mellitus, hypertension, homocystinemia, and other factors. (Figure 40.1). The precise mechanisms for endothelial cell injury are unknown. Recent hypotheses suggest an early, subtle injury, leading to functional changes (including alterations in permeability, cell turnover and synthesis) which precede subsequent histologic changes (Type I vascular injury, Table 40.1). Early endothelial dysfunction is manifest as impaired fibrinolysis (↑ PAI-1, ↓ t-PA) and abnormal vasoreactivity (↓ nitric oxide). Numerous factors are known to be associated with early endothelial dysfunction (Figure 40.1), and hyperlipidemia appears to be the most important. Most atherosclerotic lipid is derived from LDL-cholesterol, which enters cells by active and passive mechanisms. Active mechanisms play a minor role in atherosclerosis. In contrast, passive LDL uptake, particularly by endothelial cells and macrophages

Table 40.3. Histopathology of Atherosclerosis

Component	Normal Vessel	Atherosclerotic Vessel
Endothelium	Cellular monolayer; fibrinolysis, nitric oxide synthesis	Thickened; impaired fibrinolysis; platelet adhesion and activation
Intima	Thin layer	Thickened; inflammatory cell and smooth muscle cell migration and proliferation
Media	Smooth muscle cells	Abnormal vasomotion (endothelium/ nitric oxide dependent)
Adventitia	Connective tissue, fibroblasts	(?) Arterial remodeling; (?) role of vasa vasorum; other unknown effects

(so-called "scavenger" pathway), permits massive lipid accumulation and plays an important role in atherosclerosis. Oxidation of LDL by endothelial cells and leucocytes initiates a critical series of events resulting in expression of endothelial surface adhesion molecules (E-selection, P-selection, VCAM, ICAM), and further recruitment of leucocytes (Figure 40.2). Expression of endothelial surface adhesion molecules leads to further changes in cellular function and interactions, including increased adherence of leucocytes to endothelial cells, enhanced oxidation and uptake of LDL by macrophages and leucocytes (via the "scavenger" pathway), and accumulation of large pools of intracellular lipid (foam cells). Interactions between leucocytes and endothelial cells lead to further endothelial dysfunction. Other factors such as diabetes, smoking, hypertension, infection, homocysteine, and high blood shear rate may be independently atherogenic, and may amplify endothelial injury and plaque progression. Several infectious agents have also been shown to cause damage to vessel endothelium and smooth muscle cells, both directly and indirectly (via activation of macrophages and T-cells or by immune-mediated cross-reactivity to endothelial-derived heat-shock proteins). Evidence of *Chlamydia pneumoniae, Helicobacter pylori,* cytomegalovirus, and other herpes viruses have been reported in atherosclerotic plaques.

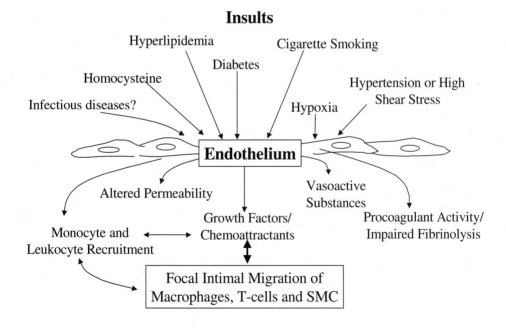

Figure 40.1. Endothelial Injury and Atherosclerosis

Atherosclerosis is due to endothelial injury leading to a localized inflammatory response. The various causes of injury and pathways leading to local inflammation offer potential targets for prevention and treatment of atherosclerosis. SMC = smooth muscle cells.

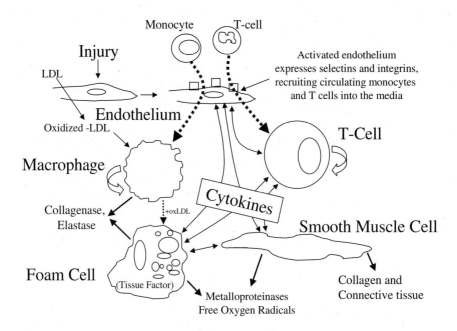

Figure 40.2. Cellular Interactions in Atherosclerosis

Various cell types activate each other and themselves, amplifying the atherosclerotic process to produce intimal thickening and extracellular matrix formation. Note the importance of LDL cholesterol: it is both a primary insult leading to endothelial dysfunction, and in its oxidized form it converts intimal macrophages into foam cells teaming with tissue factor. The cellular products collagenase, elastase, metalloproteinases and free oxygen radicals increase the propensity for plaque rupture and thrombosis by digesting the fibrous cap and inactivating important anti-atherothrombotic molecules such as nitric oxide.

B. **THE SLOW PHASE OF PROGRESSIVE ATHEROSCLEROSIS.** The Stary classification is recognized as a convenient framework for understanding the progression of atherosclerosis, plaque interaction, and vascular thrombosis (Figure 40.3). Early endothelial cell injury and dysfunction ultimately progress to microscopic accumulation of leucocytes with small intracellular lipid deposits (Stary I lesion) and microscopic fatty streaks (Stary II lesion). Intracellular lipid pools become so large that they disrupt normal cellular function, ultimately leading to pools of extracellular lipid. Further disruption of the internal elastic lamina by foam cells and extracellular lipid leads to the mature fatty streak, or preatheroma (Stary III lesion). The process thus far is considered to be slow, clinically silent, and may be reversible with appropriate risk factor modification.

C. **RUPTURE-PRONE PLAQUES: STARY IV-VA LESIONS**. Atheroma is formed as extracellular lipid pools coalesce into a lipid core (Stary IV lesion) with intact media and adventitia (Figure 40.3). The early fibrous cap (Stary Va lesion) develops as a result of smooth muscle cell proliferation and collagen synthesis. Lesions with greater collagen synthesis, less inflammation, and smaller lipid cores (Stary Vb and Vc lesions) characterize the classic fibroatheroma and typically manifest slow plaque progression. In contrast, greater lipid accumulation and inflammation in the Stary Va lesion may make the boundary between the fibrous cap and lipid core more susceptible to high shear stress and rupture. In addition, inflammatory cell production of matrix metalloproteinases, collagenases, gelatinases, and stromelysins further weaken vulnerable plaques and increase their propensity to rupture.

D. PLAQUE RUPTURE AND THROMBOSIS. Rupture of Stary IV or Va lesions leads to formation of the complicated fibroatheroma (Stary VI lesion), characterized by plaque hemorrhage, necrosis, ulceration, and thrombosis (Figure 40.3).   The lipid core is the most thrombogenic substrate of all atherosclerotic plaque contents due to its high concentration of tissue factor. Other local and systemic factors also contribute to increased thrombogenicity after plaque rupture (Table 40.5). Vasospasm and plaque erosion may also expose the lipid core and induce thrombosis. Complete thrombotic occlusion manifests clinically as ST-elevation (Q-wave) MI, while nonocclusive mural thrombus typically presents as unstable angina or non-Q-wave MI. The amount of angiographic thrombus has been correlated with the severity of clinical presentation of acute coronary syndromes.   If the intrinsic fibrinolytic system prevails, residual mural thrombus may regress, organize, and transform the lesion to a stable Stary Vb/c lesion. In cases of repetitive injury, rupture, and healing, the lesion may progress to chronic total occlusion (see below).

E. INTERMEDIATE PROGRESSION OF ATHEROSCLEROSIS. If "vulnerable" Stary Type Va lesions do not rupture, smooth muscle cell proliferation and fibrosis may transform the plaque to the more "stable" Stary Vb/c lesions. Calcification (Stary VII lesion) and severe fibrosis (Stary VIII lesion) characterize advanced forms of chronic atherosclerosis, associated with severe stenosis and total occlusion.

Table 40.4. Characteristics of Vulnerable Plaques

Characteristic	Causes
Mechanical propensity to rupture	Increased wall stress High shear rate Soft lipid-rich core Stiff, thin fibrous cap
Digestion of fibrous cap	Local inflammation Increased matrix metalloproteinases Mechanical erosion of shoulders
Limited elasticity	Decreased smooth muscle cells Degraded collagen and elastin
Other	Increased temperature (?) Positive adaptive remodeling (?) Lipoprotein (a) (?)

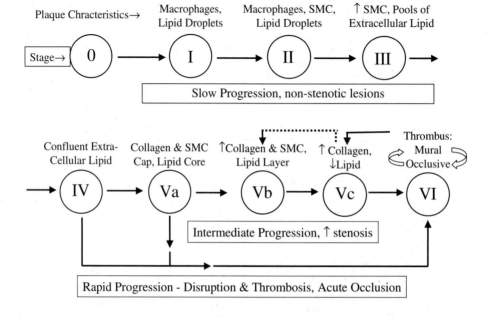

Figure 40.3. Atherosclerosis Progression in Humans: The Stary Classification

Initially plaques evolve slowly, but may acutely rupture or gradually stenose over time. SMC = smooth muscle cells.

Table 40.5. Factors Contributing to Increased Thrombogenicity Following Plaque Rupture

Factor	Mechanism
Local Thrombogenic Factors	
Apoptosis of macrophages	Macrophages serve as a defense mechanism against the accumulation of lipoproteins in the vessel wall. When they undergo programmed cell death (apoptosis), multiple enzymes and tissue factor are released leading to potent procoagulant activity
Oxidized LDL in plaques	Direct activation of platelets
Lipoprotein (a)	Thrombogenic substrate; detected in higher concentrations in unstable and macrophage-rich plaques
Systemic Procoagulant Factors	
Circulating monocytes and neutrophils	May be involved in local tissue factor expression
Acute and chronic inflammation	Caused by infection or autoimmune reaction; may augment the local thrombotic process
Other factors	Increased blood thrombogenicity due to cigarette smoking, catecholamine release, hyperlipidemia, hyperfibrinogenemia, and elevated serum lipoprotein(a) and homocysteine may augment the local thrombotic response. Statins have antithrombotic properties, highlighting the importance of risk factor modification

F. TARGETED THERAPY FOR CORONARY ARTERY DISEASE. Therapy of CAD is aimed at plaque stabilization and preventing thrombosis (Table 40.6), by aggressive cholesterol reduction with "statins" (to decrease LDL cholesterol and maintain plaque integrity), risk factor modification, and antithrombotic therapy (Chapter 41).

THROMBOSIS AND FIBRINOLYSIS

Thrombosis is central to the pathogenesis of coronary artery disease, and occurs by activation of two complementary systems: platelets and the coagulation cascade. A multitude of phospholipids, glycoproteins, enzymes, and other factors are involved in platelet plug formation (primary hemostasis) and fibrin formation (secondary hemostasis), as summarized in Tables 40.8 and 40.9.

Table 40.6. Targeted Therapy of Atherosclerotic Disease (see Chapter 41)

TARGET: Decrease Vessel Injury and Stabilize Plaque (Long-term Goal)

Aggressive Risk Factor Modification
- Smoking cessation
- Control hypertension, diabetes
- Treat dyslipidemia ($\downarrow$LDL, $\downarrow$Lp(a), $\uparrow$HDL, $\downarrow$triglyceride) with statins and others
- Possible vitamin B_{12} and folate supplements for elevated homocysteine

Decrease Blood Shear Rate
- Vasodilators
- Mechanical revascularization

Unknown Effects
- Antioxidant supplements
- Antibiotics
- Anti-COX_2 therapy, fish oil/omega-3 fatty acid supplements

TARGET: Treat Endovascular Thrombosis (Short and Long-term Goals)

Antiplatelet Therapy
- COX_1 inhibition (aspirin)
- ADP receptor inhibitors (ticlopidine, clopidogrel)
- GP IIb/IIIa receptor inhibitors (abciximab, eptifibatide, tirofiban)
- Thrombin receptor inhibitors (?)

Antithrombin Therapy
- Heparin
- Low-molecular-weight heparins
- Direct antithrombins (e.g., hirudin)

Tissue Factor Pathway Inhibitor

Fibrinolytic Therapy

PLATELETS AND THROMBUS FORMATION

A. **OVERVIEW.** The injured vessel wall exposes von Willebrand factor, collagen, vitronectin, fibronectin, and other adhesive molecules, which induce platelet adhesion, activation, and aggregation.

B. **PLATELET ADHESION.** Platelet adhesion is initiated by von Willebrand factor (vWF) binding to the platelet glycoprotein (GP) Ib receptor. This pathway is activated in stenoses with high shear stress.

C. **PLATELET ACTIVATION.** The local thrombogenic environment exposes platelets to multiple activators (Figure 40.4); these factors trigger events within the platelet, including release of granules and conformational changes in the GP IIb/IIIa receptor complex. The constitutive form of cyclo-oxygenase (COX_1) metabolizes arachidonic acid to thromboxane, which further increases expression and conformational change of GP IIb/IIIa receptors. Platelet activation is dependent upon local signals from other activated cells, local concentration of coagulation factors and fibrinogen, and the degree of flow impairment.

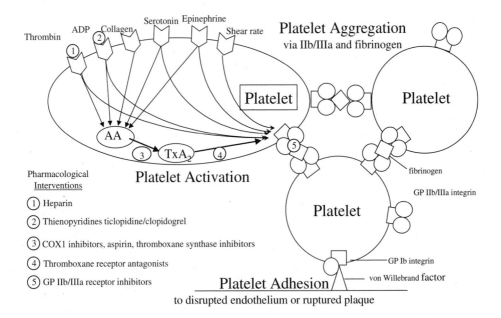

Figure 40.4. Platelet Activation

Platelet activators can be the specific targets of pharmacological intervention. However, the final common pathway for platelet aggregation is dependant on GP IIb/IIIa receptor activation. AA = arachidonic acid; COX = cyclo-oxygenase; Tx = thromboxane.

D. PLATELET AGGREGATION. Activation of the GP IIb/IIIa receptor complex constitutes the final common pathway for platelet aggregation and is a critical event in thrombosis. The GP IIb/IIIa receptors are the most abundant integrin on the platelet membrane. They bind fibronectin, vWF, and vitronectin for *adhesion* to the vessel surface, and bind fibrinogen and vWF for *aggregation* to other platelets. Fibrinogen is the most important ligand of the GP IIb/IIIa receptor. It can bind to two receptors simultaneously, providing a molecular platelet-to-platelet bridge. Ultimately, platelet aggregates and cross-linked fibrin form fresh thrombus, which matures and organizes over time with the recruitment of monocytes, erythrocytes, and smooth muscle cells.

COAGULATION CASCADE

A. OVERVIEW. Primary hemostasis results in the formation of loosely adherent platelet aggregates at the site of vessel injury or plaque rupture. Secondary hemostasis involves activation of the coagulation cascade and formation of cross-linked fibrin, which reinforces the primary hemostatic plug and results in fresh clot. Exposure of tissue factor from the vessel wall initiates the extrinsic pathway of coagulation and is the principal mechanism for thrombin generation and fibrin deposition following plaque rupture (Figure 40.5).

B. TISSUE FACTOR. Tissue factor is a highly thrombogenic low molecular weight glycoprotein concentrated in vessel wall macrophages and vulnerable plaque. Following plaque rupture, tissue factor is exposed to circulating blood and initiates the extrinsic coagulation pathway by forming a high affinity complex with factors VII/VIIa. The tissue factor/VIIa complex in turn activates factors IX and X, leading to thrombin generation. Although alternative pathways for thrombin generation exist, tissue factor achieves a rapid and dramatic activation of the entire cascade, thus occupying a pivotal role in thrombosis following plaque rupture. Tissue factor pathway inhibitor (TFPI), a recombinant peptide, is a potentially novel agent for antithrombotic therapy.

C. THROMBIN. Thrombin (factor IIa) has a critical role in clot formation, by converting fibrinogen to fibrin, activating clotting factors V and VIII, and serving as a potent stimulus for platelet activation and aggregation. The formation and polymerization of fibrin is crucial to clot stabilization and propagation, converting the unstable primary platelet plug into an adherent "red" thrombus. In addition, thrombin induces smooth muscle cell proliferation, contributing to atherogenesis; both platelet activation and thrombin-induced smooth muscle cell proliferation are mediated via a specific thrombin receptor on the cell membrane. Indirect thrombin inhibitors (unfractionated and low-molecular-weight heparin) and direct thrombin inhibitors (hirudin) have important anticoagulant effects in a variety of disorders characterized by clot formation and propagation.

D. FIBRINOLYTIC SYSTEM. The intrinsic fibrinolytic system degrades thrombus via breakdown of fibrin by plasminogen (Figure 40.6), which is activated by tissue-type plasminogen activator (t-PA) or urokinase-type plasminogen activator (u-PA). These activators are counteracted by PAI-1 and plasminogen activator (PAR) in endothelial cells. The process of fibrin breakdown releases D-dimers and other D-polymers.

ANTITHROMBOTIC THERAPY (Chapter 34)

A. OVERVIEW. Antithrombotic therapies target different elements of the two keys to thrombus formation: platelets and thrombin (Figures 40.4. 40.5, Table 40.6).

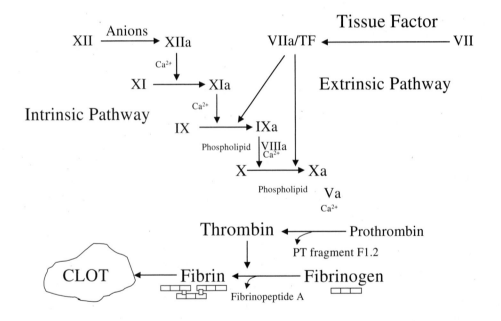

Figure 40.5. The Coagulation Cascade

Two pathways leading to thrombin generation and fibrin deposition. After plaque rupture, exposed tissue factor initiates the extrinsic pathway of coagulation by directly activating factor VII. Thrombin (factor IIA) is responsible for the conversion of fibrinogen to fibrin, further activation of coagulation factors, and stimulation of platelet aggregation. Various antithrombins are used in clinical practice: Hirudin is a direct thrombin inhibitor; unfractionated heparin works via antithrombin to antagonize thrombin and factor Xa; low-molecular-weight heparin also binds with antithrombin, but much more selectively inhibits factor Xa than thrombin.

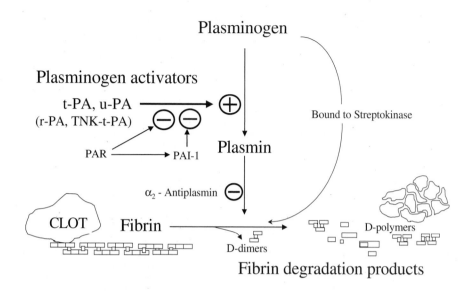

Figure 40.6. The Intrinsic Fibrinolytic System

Intravascular fibrinolysis is primarily initiated by t-PA. Produced by the endothelium, its major stimulus is fibrin and its major inhibitor is PAI-1 (from endothelium and platelets). Reteplase is a truncated form of t-PA that is less fibrin specific. A mutant of t-PA, TNK-t-PA, has a longer half-life, allowing for bolus administration. Streptokinase binds plasminogen and makes it plasmin-like, but is not inhibited by α_2-antiplasmin. PAR = plasminogen activator receptor, PAI-1 = plasminogen activator inhibitor.

B. **ANTIPLATELET THERAPY.** Antiplatelet agents used in clinical practice work by blocking the production of platelet agonists (aspirin), by inhibiting the binding of platelet agonists to their receptors (ticlopidine, clopidogrel), or by antagonizing GP IIb/IIIa receptors directly (abciximab, eptifibatide, tirofiban):

- Aspirin irreversibly binds platelet cyclo-oxygenase (COX_1), thereby preventing platelet thromboxane production.
- Ticlopidine and clopidogrel inhibit the binding of adenosine diphosphate (ADP) to its platelet receptor. However, platelet activation is still possible even with inhibition of ADP and COX_1 pathways.
- GP IIb/IIIa inhibitors (abciximab, eptifibatide, tirofiban) block the final pathway of platelet aggregation.

Table 40.7. Mediators of Atherosclerosis

Factor	Description
LDL cholesterol	Primary cause of endothelial dysfunction; increases lipid content in plaque and propensity for plaque rupture
Oxidized LDL	Primary cause of endothelial dysfunction; increases lipid content in plaque and propensity for plaque rupture; induces transformation of macrophages into foam cells. Oxidized LDL facilitates further lipid accumulation and inflammation
HDL cholesterol	Involved in reverse transport of LDL cholesterol from lipid-rich plaque
Lipoprotein (a)	LDL-like particle with unique plasminogen-like molecule (apo [a]); atherothrombogenic; accumulates in macrophages
Tobacco, diabetes, hypertension	Atherothrombogenic; cause of abnormal vasomotion, endothelial dysfunction, and impaired lipoprotein metabolism
Homocysteine	By-product of protein metabolism; cause of endothelial dysfunction; linked to increased thrombogenicity
ICAM, VCAM	Adhesion molecules; upregulated during atherogenesis; facilitates adhesion of circulating cells to vessel wall; proinflammatory
Circulating monocytes and neutrophils	Inflammatory cells localize at injury site; enter vessel wall and release proinflammatory cell products
Circulating T-cells	Inflammation (? direct atherogenic role)
Subendothelial macrophages	Proinflammatory; associated with antibody production; ingest oxidized LDL cholesterol; contain high concentrations of tissue factor, which activates the extrinsic pathway of coagulation
Smooth muscle cells	Involved in capsid digestion, inflammation, plaque rupture, increased plaque volume, restenosis
Oxygen free radicals	Responsible for oxidation of LDL; induces neointimal inflammation; cause of endothelial dysfunction
Endothelial dysfunction	Thrombogenic, abnormal vasomotion
Nitric oxide	Normal vasomotion, anti-thrombogenic

C. **ANTITHROMBIN THERAPY.** The effect of heparins (including unfractionated and low-molecular-weight analogs) and direct antithrombins (r-hirudin, PEG-hirudin, hirulog) are directed at the thrombin pathway. Unfractionated heparin binds to antithrombin to potentiate inhibition of factors Xa and IIa (thrombin). Low-molecular-weight heparins (LMWH) exert their activity by non-selective inhibition of factor Xa (and to a lesser extent factor IIa). LMWH produces predictable levels of anticoagulation which is not accurately measured by the activated partial thromboplastin time (aPTT). Neither unfractionated nor LMWH bind clot- or matrix-bound thrombin, in contrast to direct antithrombins. Tissue factor pathway inhibitor (TFPI) is a protein that blocks multiple elements of the coagulation cascade, particularly factors VIII and IX. TFPI may become a useful agent to inhibit the thrombin pathway. Warfarin antagonizes the vitamin K dependent factors of the coagulation system (factors II, VII, IX, X), inhibiting

Table 40.8. Mediators of Primary Hemostasis (Platelet Plug Formation at Site of Injury)

Factor	Description
Glycoprotein Ia/IIa	Specific platelet collagen receptor responsible for initial platelet adhesion to collagen fibrils in vascular subendothelium
von Willibrand factor (vWf)	Adhesive glycoprotein that allows platelets to remain attached to vessel wall despite high shear forces
Epinephrine, collagen, thrombin	Platelet agonists that bind to platelet surface receptors
Phospholipase C and phospholipase A	Platelet membrane enzymes activated by binding of platelet agonists to cell surface receptors
Phosphatidylinositol and phosphatidylcholine	Major membrane phospholipids acted upon by phospholipase C and phospholipase A to release arachidonic acid
Arachidonic acid	Fatty acid precursor of thromboxane A_2
Cyclooxygenase	Enzyme responsible for metabolism of arachidonic acid to thromboxane A_2; inhibited by aspirin
Thromboxane A_2	By-product of platelet arachidonic acid metabolism; potent platelet aggregator
Inositol triphosphate (IP$_3$)	By-product of membrane phospholipid metabolism; responsible for increasing platelet cytosolic calcium; induces phosphorylation of myosin-like chains, which interact with platelet actin to induce changes in platelet shape
Diacylglycerol	By-product of platelet phospholipid metabolism; activates protein kinase C, which phosphorylates cell proteins to regulate platelet granule secretion
Prostacyclin	Endothelial cell product of arachidonic acid metabolism; increases intraplatelet cyclic AMP to inhibit platelet aggregation
Calcium, serotonin, ADP	Released from dense platelet granules into plasma following platelet activation
von Willibrand factor, fibronectin, thrombospondin, platelet-derived growth factor (PDGF), heparin-neutralizing protein (platelet factor 4)	Released from alpha granules into plasma following platelet activation
ADP	Induces conformational change in GP IIb/IIIa receptor so it can bind fibrinogen; inhibited by clopidogrel
Fibrinogen	Most important ligand for GP IIb/IIIa receptor; binds two receptors simultaneously, providing platelet-to-platelet bridge; contains hexapeptide domain specific for gamma-chain fibrinogen binding; can bind RGD tripeptide-containing domain
Glycoprotein IIb/IIIa receptor	Vital common pathway for platelet aggregation; binds fibronectin, von Willibrand factor, vitronectin for adhesion to vessel surface; binds fibrinogen and von Willibrand factor for aggregation to other platelets
Platelet-derived growth factor	Stimulates growth and migration of smooth muscle cells in vessel wall

Table 40.9. Mediators of Secondary Hemostasis (Plasma Reactions Leading to Fibrin Formation)

Factor	Description
Hageman factor (factor XII), high-molecular-weight kininogen (HMWK), prekallikrein (PK)	Plasma proteins that form a complex on vascular subendothelial collagen to initiate the contact (intrinsic) phase of coagulation
Tissue factor	Cell membrane phospholipid that is exposed after injury; combines with calcium and factor VII to initiate extrinsic phase of coagulation
Factor X activation	Point in coagulation cascade in which the contact (intrinsic) system and the tissue factor-dependant (extrinsic) system merge; results in conversion of prothrombin to thrombin
Factors II (prothrombin), VII, IX, X	Requires calcium and vitamin K for activity; site of warfarin effect
Thrombin	Responsible for conversion of fibrinogen to fibrin; activates factors V, VIII, XIII; stimulates platelet aggregation
Fibrinopeptides A and B	Released from alpha and beta chains of fibrinogen during thrombin-mediated metabolism
Fibrin polymer	Insoluble gel product of fibrin monomers
Factor XIIIa	Cross-links and stabilizes fibrin polymer
Tissue factor pathway inhibitor (TFPI)	Protein that blocks multiple elements of the intrinsic pathway, particularly factors VIII and IX; becomes the dominant regulator of thrombin generation

both extrinsic and common pathways and indirectly decreasing thrombin production. Since thrombin itself is a potent platelet activator, antithrombin drugs may also decrease platelet activation. Likewise, since thrombin generation occurs on the platelet membrane, potent antiplatelet drugs (i.e., GP IIb/IIIa inhibitors) may act as anticoagulants.

D. **FIBRINOLYTIC THERAPY.** Streptokinase activates plasminogen to plasmin indirectly, whereas urokinase and recombinant t-PA act directly. Fibrin greatly increases the affinity of t-PA for plasminogen, specifically on the thrombus site, resulting in less systemic activation. Genetic recombinant technology has developed new thrombolytic agents such as reteplase (r-PA) and the Thr103 mutant (rt-PA-TNK), allowing for specific, direct thrombolysis, with long clearance times after bolus administration. Since the fibrinolytic process activates platelets directly, residual mural thrombus and the underlying thrombogenic plaque can promote further thrombus formation. Hence, fibrinolytic therapies require adjunctive antithrombotic therapies targeted to platelets and thrombin.

E. **SUMMARY.** Atherosclerosis is a dynamic, repetitive process of injury, inflammation and repair. The resulting atherosclerotic plaque progresses through phases leading to or progressive stenosis or acute plaque rupture and thrombosis. Platelet aggregation and thrombin-driven fibrin formation are the main targets of antithrombotic therapies.

Table 40.10. Mediators of the Fibrinolytic System

Factor	Description
t-PA and urokinase	Endothelial cell products; principal activators of fibrinolytic system; inhibited by PAI-I
Plasminogen	Absorbed onto fibrin clot; acted upon by t-PA and u-PA
Plasmin	Degrades fibrin polymer to small fragments which are cleared by macrophage-monocyte system
Plasminogen activator inhibitor (PAI-1)	Released from endothelial cells; directly inhibits t-PA and u-PA
Antithrombin, Protein C, Protein S, tissue factor pathway inhibitor (TFPI)	Inhibitors of coagulation cascade; limit propagation of thrombus from beyond site of injury

* * * * *

CARDIOVASCULAR RISK REDUCTION

James H. O'Keefe, Jr. M.D.
Christie M. Ballantyne, M.D.
Norman M. Kaplan, M.D.
Mark Freed, M.D.

41

Atherosclerotic vascular disease is the leading cause of morbidity and mortality in the United States: 12 million Americans have coronary artery disease (CAD), 4 million have had strokes, and millions have peripheral vascular disease. Treatment of hypertension and dyslipidemia reduces the risk of myocardial infarction and stroke by 25-80%. This chapter provides a step-by-step guide to the diagnosis, evaluation, and management of dyslipidemia and hypertension. Adjunctive preventive measures aimed at halting atherosclerosis, stabilizing plaques, preventing thrombosis, and improving prognosis are also described.

TREATMENT OF DYSLIPIDEMIA

A. **DEFINITION.** Dyslipidemia is defined as an undesirable or abnormal plasma lipid status. Common lipid abnormalities include low high-density lipoprotein (HDL) cholesterol, and elevated total cholesterol, low-density lipoprotein (LDL) cholesterol, lipoprotein(a), triglycerides, and small, dense LDL particles (Tables 41.1, 41.2). These abnormalities can be found alone or in combination.

B. **PREVALENCE.** Approximately 50% of adults in the United States have elevated total cholesterol levels. Even though 40% of patients with coronary artery disease have "normal" total cholesterol (< 200 mg/dL), most have some other form of dyslipidemia. Despite marked benefits of lipid therapy, dyslipidemias are grossly undertreated: 70% of high-risk patients without coronary disease and 80% of patients with coronary disease do not meet the National Cholesterol Education Program (NCEP) guidelines.

C. **RISK FACTORS.** Elevated total and LDL cholesterol, and low HDL cholesterol are important treatable risk factors for atherosclerosis. For each 1% decrease in LDL cholesterol and 1% increase in HDL cholesterol, the risk of cardiovascular events decreases by 2% and 3%, respectively. Other important modifiable risk factors include elevated levels of triglycerides, lipoprotein (a), small, dense LDL particles, homocysteine, C-reactive protein, and fibrinogen.

D. **SCREENING.** Routine screening for dyslipidemia is recommended by the NCEP for all Americans over age 20, since early recognition and treatment improves event-free survival.

Table 41.1. Common Dyslipidemias

Dyslipidemia	Comments
Elevated LDL cholesterol	For every 1% reduction in LDL cholesterol, the risk of cardiovascular events is decreased by 2%. Statins are the drug class of choice; bile acid sequestrants and niacin are useful adjuncts
Low HDL cholesterol	HDL cholesterol < 40 mg/dL in men and < 45 mg/dL in women are more powerful predictors of CAD risk than elevated total or LDL cholesterol. Weight loss, exercise, smoking cessation, monounsaturated and omega-3 fatty acids, niacin, statins, fibrates, and estrogens raise HDL levels. Progestins, androgens, beta-blockers, probucol, nicotine, and possibly thiazide diuretics lower HDL levels
Elevated triglycerides	Independent risk factor for CAD. Target level $\leq$ 150 mg/dL. Weight loss, exercise, and a Mediterranean diet lower triglyceride levels. Drug therapy includes niacin, fibrates, or fish oil; statins can be used for mixed dyslipidemia (increased triglyceride, increased LDL cholesterol)
Atherogenic dyslipidemia	Common in patients with CAD. Characterized by increased triglycerides, decreased HDL cholesterol, and normal LDL cholesterol; associated with insulin resistance. Rapid progression of atherosclerosis is common. Treatment consists of lifestyle changes (exercise, weight loss, smoking cessation) and drug therapy (niacin, fibrates, statins; combination therapy is often needed)
Elevated lipoprotein (a)	LDL-like particle with unique glycoprotein apo(a) moiety. Proatherogenic and prothrombotic. Niacin and estrogen reduce Lp (a) levels; statins and lifestyle modifications have little or no effect. Optimal treatment is unknown

Table 41.2. Fredrickson Classification of Hyperlipidemias

Phenotype	ICD-9 codes	Lipoprotein(s) Elevated	Plasma TC	Plasma TG	Atherogenicity	Relative Frequency*
I	272.3	Chylomicrons	Normal to +	++++	Not routinely seen	<1%
IIa	272.0	LDL	++	Normal	Marked	10%
IIb	272.2	LDL and VLDL	++	++	Marked	40%
III	272.2	IDL, β-VLDL	++	+++	Marked	<1%
IV	272.1	VLDL	Normal to +	++	Yes	45%
V	272.4	VLDL and chylomicrons	+ to ++	++++	Yes	5%

Abbreviations: TC = total cholesterol; TG = triglyceride; LDL = low density lipoprotein; IDL = intermediate density lipoprotein; VLDL = very low density lipoprotein
* Approximate percentages of US patients with hyperlipidemia
+ to ++++ = increasing degrees of plasma elevation

E. **BENEFITS OF LIPID THERAPY.** Acute coronary syndromes are caused by vulnerable plaques (with extensive inflammation, lipidrich cores, and thin fibrous caps) which ulcerate and rupture, leading to thrombotic occlusion. The beneficial effects of lipid therapy are due more to plaque stabilization than to reduction in stenosis severity, as plaque regression is modest and does not account for the 25-80% reduction in major cardiovascular events. Plaque stabilization occurs quickly (within weeks to months with aggressive treatment) and is related to resorption of lipid deposits, decrease in inflammation, and enhancement of fibrous cap integrity. In addition, lipid-lowering therapy improves endothelial function, resulting in beneficial vasodilatory, antithrombotic, and anti-inflammatory effects. For most patients, treatment of dyslipidemia and other risk factors is the best way to improve long-term prognosis. Several large randomized trials have shown reduction in morbidity and mortality with statin therapy for primary and secondary prevention. A metanalysis has shown that for every 1% reduction in total cholesterol there is a 1% reduction in total mortality and a 1.5% reduction in cardiovascular mortality.

F. **DIAGNOSIS AND TREATMENT OF DYSLIPIDEMIA.** The diagnosis, evaluation, and treatment of dyslipidemia in patients with and without coronary artery disease are summarized in Figures 41.1 and 41.2. The absolute risk for coronary disease can be estimated from the Framingham equation (Table 41.3). Once a dyslipidemia is identified, it is important to screen for secondary and genetic causes of dyslipidemia (Tables 41.4, 41.5). Blood glucose, thyroid and liver function tests, urinalysis, and review of medications and use of alcohol will identify most secondary causes. If severe hypercholesterolemia is present (total cholesterol > 300 mg/dL) or a genetic disorder is discovered, a family history and measurement of cholesterol are needed in other family members. Diet modification and other hygienic measures (exercise, weight control, smoking cessation) are considered first-line therapy for all patients with dyslipidemia (Table 41.6). In most patients this will improve lipid levels only modestly (total cholesterol lowering < 10%). Drug therapy should be initiated *concurrently* with nonpharmacologic measures in: (1) Patients with diabetes or established coronary artery, peripheral vascular, or cerebrovascular disease with LDL cholesterol ≥130 mg/dL; (2) Patients with very high LDL cholesterol levels (> 220 mg/dL); and (3) Patients at markedly increased risk for coronary disease (e.g., multiple clustered risk factors) with LDL cholesterol ≥160 mg/dL. The choice of drug therapy depends on the patient's lipid profile and other characteristics (Tables 41.7, 41.8). Major uses and prescribing information for the various cholesterol-lowering drugs are described in Tables 41.9 and 41.10, and administration guidelines for combined use of statins and fibrates are listed in Table 41.11. It is important to repeat total cholesterol, assess dietary compliance, and reinforce lifestyle changes at 4-6 weeks and 3 months after beginning therapy. If LDL cholesterol is not adequately reduced at 4-6 weeks, drug dosage should be increased. If drug monotherapy does not reduce LDL cholesterol to target, combination therapy should be considered. Once LDL cholesterol is at an acceptable level, total cholesterol should be monitored every 2-3 months during the first year of therapy and every 4-6 months thereafter, and a lipid profile should be repeated yearly. Patients who fail therapy may benefit from fish oil, referral to a lipid specialist, LDL apheresis, or ileal bypass surgery. Common management pitfalls are listed in Table 41.12.

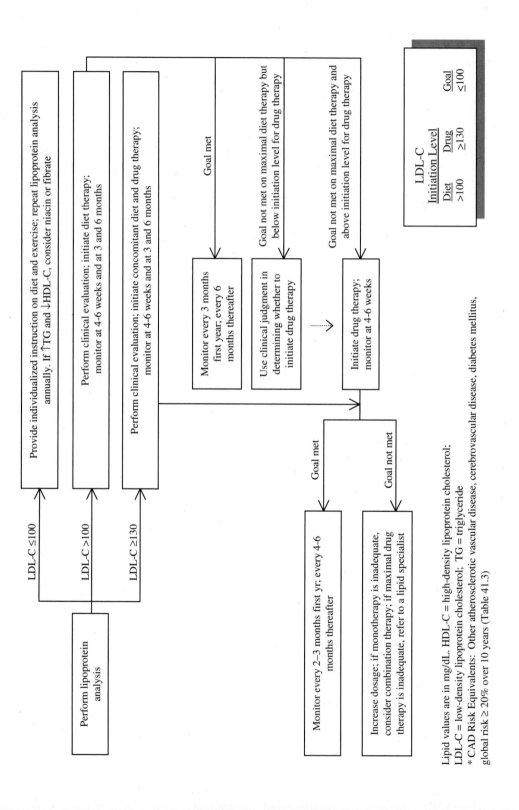

Figure 41.1. Assessment and Treatment of Dyslipidemia in Adults WITH Coronary Artery Disease

Lipid values are in mg/dL. HDL-C = high-density lipoprotein cholesterol;
LDL-C = low-density lipoprotein cholesterol; TG = triglyceride
* CAD Risk Equivalents: Other atherosclerotic vascular disease, cerebrovascular disease, diabetes mellitus, global risk ≥ 20% over 10 years (Table 41.3)

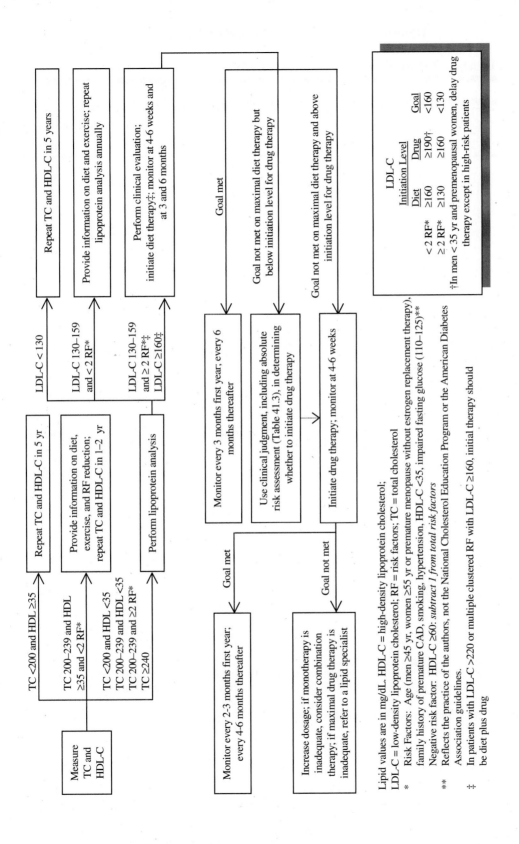

Lipid values are in mg/dL. HDL-C = high-density lipoprotein cholesterol;
LDL-C = low-density lipoprotein cholesterol; RF = risk factors; TC = total cholesterol

*   Risk Factors: Age (men ≥45 yr, women ≥55 yr or premature menopause without estrogen replacement therapy),
family history of premature CAD, smoking, hypertension, HDL-C <35, impaired fasting glucose (110–125)**
Negative risk factor: HDL-C ≥60: *subtract 1 from total risk factors*

** Reflects the practice of the authors, not the National Cholesterol Education Program or the American Diabetes
Association guidelines.

‡   In patients with LDL-C >220 or multiple clustered RF with LDL-C ≥160, initial therapy should
be diet plus drug

Figure 41.2. Assessment and Treatment of Dyslipidemia in Adults WITHOUT Coronary Artery Disease

Table 41.3. Global Absolute Risk Score: Estimating Risk of Coronary Artery Disease*

STEP 1: Determine Total Risk Points

Risk Factor	Risk Points Men	Risk Points Women
Age, years		
<35	−1	−9
35–39	0	−4
40–44	1	0
45–49	2	3
50–54	3	6
55–59	4	7
60–64	5	8
65–69	6	8
70–74	7	8
Total cholesterol (mg/dL)		
<160	−3	−2
160–199	0	0
200–239	1	1
240–279	2	2
≥280	3	3
HDL cholesterol (mg/dL)		
<35	2	5
35–44	1	2
45–49	0	1
50–59	0	0
≥60	−2	−3
Systolic BP (mmHg)		
<120	0	−3
120–129	0	0
130–139	1	1
140–159	2	2
≥160	3	3
Diabetes mellitus		
No	0	0
Yes	2	4
Smoking		
No	0	0
Yes	2	2
TOTAL RISK POINTS	____	____

STEP 2: Assess Risk of Coronary Disease

Total Risk Points	10-Year Absolute Risk Men	10-Year Absolute Risk Women
≤ −2		1%
−1	2%	2%
0	3%	2%
1	3%	2%
2	4%	3%
3	5%	3%
4	7%	4%
5	8%	4%
6	10%	5%
7	13%	6%
8	16%	7%
9	20%	8%
10	25%	10%
11	31%	11%
12	37%	13%
13	45%	15%
14	≥53%	18%
15	≥53%	20%
16	≥53%	24%
≥ 17	≥53%	≥27%

* In general, a 10-year absolute risk ≥ 20% would be considered high, 10-20% risk would generally be considered moderate, and < 10% risk would be considered low. By comparison, patients with stable angina have mortality rates of approximately 2% per year.

Sources: Circulation 1998;97:1837-1847, Circulation 1999;100:1481-1492

Table 41.4. Common Causes of Secondary Dyslipidemias

Cause	Effects on Plasma Lipids			Comments
	Total-C	**TG**	**HDL-C**	
Diabetes mellitus *Type 1*	None or ↓	None or ↑	None or ↑	Lipid values vary greatly and are dependent on glycemic control, ranging from ↑TG and ↓HDL-C with poor control to ↓TG and ↑HDL-C with very tight control
Type 2	None or ↑	↑	↓	Although poor glycemic control leads to ↑TG and ↓HDL-C, even optimal glycemic control will usually not normalize dyslipidemia
Hypothyroidism	↑	↑	None or ↑	Receptor-mediated clearance of LDL is partly dependent on thyroid hormone activity. Effects on HDL are inconsistent
Obesity		↑	↓	High waist/hip girth associated with poor prognosis and insulin resistance
Primary biliary cirrhosis	↑	↑	↑ early ↓ late	Increased fraction of free cholesterol. Abnormal lipoprotein (lipoprotein X) is present, an immature form of HDL
Obstructive liver disease	↑↑	None	↑	Mildly ↑ LFTs, particularly GGT, may be secondary to hyperlipidemia and not causative
Cushing's syndrome	↑	↑↑	-	
Cigarette smoking	-	-	↓	Lowers HDL cholesterol by an average of 5-10 mg/dL
Nephrotic syndrome	↑↑	↑ to ↑↑	None or ↓	Low or normal cholesterol levels suggest a poor prognosis
Uremia	Usually none	↑	None or ↓	Improved HDL cholesterol and triglyceride levels are often noted after renal transplantation
Drugs *Thiazides*	None or ↑	None or ↑	None	Dose-dependent effects
β-blockers	None	↑	↓	β-blockers with ISA may ↑ HDL levels. Cardioselective agents affect lipid levels less
Estrogens	↓	↑	↑	Transcutaneous preparations have minimal effect on lipids
Progestins	↑	↓	↓	Effects are generally opposite those of estrogen
Androgens	↑	↓	↓	Effects are more prominent if taken orally
Glucocorticoids	↑	↑	↑	Direct relation between total cholesterol level and prednisone dose
Cyclosporine	↑↑	None or ↑	None	Also may increase risk of myositis with statin therapy
Alcohol	None	↑↑	↑	May dramatically increase triglycerides, particularly during binges
Protease inhibitors	↑	↑↑	None or ↓	May dramatically increase triglycerides

Abbreviations: Total-C = total cholesterol; TG = triglycerides; HDL-C = HDL cholesterol; VLDL = very low density lipoprotein; LPL = lipoprotein lipase; LCAT = lecithin-cholesterol acyltransferase; LFT = liver function test; ISA = intrinsic sympathomimetic activity

Table 41.5. Primary (Genetic) Dyslipidemias

Dyslipidemia	Description	Treatment
Familial hyper-cholesterolemia (FH)	Markedly elevated total cholesterol and LDL cholesterol levels: total cholesterol in homozygotes 600-1200 mg/dL, in heterozygotes 350-500 mg/dL. Triglycerides generally $\leq$ 200 mg/dL, HDL cholesterol may be reduced. Xanthelasma, tendon xanthomas, corneal arcus, premature atherosclerosis	High-dose statin therapy. The more potent statins, such as high-dose atorvastatin or simvastatin, are usually necessary. May require additional therapy with bile acid sequestrants or nicotinic acid. Rarely, LDL apheresis may be required
Defective apo B-100	Similar phenotype to FH, with severely elevated LDL cholesterol and clinical findings that can include tendinous xanthomas and corneal arcus	High-dose statin therapy, combined as necessary with bile acid sequestrants or nicotinic acid.
Polygenic hypercholesterolemia	Cholesterol elevation generally less than in heterozygous FH. Xanthomas very rare. High prevalence: approximately 1/20	Appropriate treatment depends on sex, age, LDL cholesterol, and CAD risk. Severe cases should be treated as in heterozygous FH, although combination drug therapy may not be necessary
Familial combined hyperlipidemia	Elevated cholesterol (250-350 mg/dL), triglyceride (250-500 mg/dL), or both. No unique clinical features	Treat with appropriate agent(s)—statins, fibrates, niacin—to normalize lipid elevation(s)
Type III hyperlipidemia (familial dysbeta-lipoproteinemia)	Elevated cholesterol (300-600) mg/dL and triglycerides (400-800 mg/dL, but may be higher). Xanthomas (tuberous, tuberoeruptive, palmar, tendinous), xanthelasmas, corneal arcus, premature atherosclerosis. Expression of disorder may result from hypothyroidism, obesity, estrogen deficiency, or glucose intolerance	Low saturated fat diet and weight control, supplemented as needed with statins/fibrates to decrease remnant particles. Niacin may be helpful but should be used only with careful monitoring in patients with impaired glucose metabolism
Familial hypertriglyceridemia	Triglyceride typically 200-500 mg/dL in type IV phenotype; >1000 mg/dL in type V phenotype. Total cholesterol only moderately elevated; LDL cholesterol and HDL cholesterol reduced. Abdominal pain, pancreatitis, eruptive xanthomas, hepatosplenomegaly, abnormal glucose tolerance, hyperuricemia, CAD	Treat as described for elevated triglycerides
Familial chylomicronemia	Rare; autosomal recessive inheritance (consanguinity common). Recurrent acute pancreatitis, eruptive xanthomas, retinal lipemia, hepatosplenomegaly, psychoneurologic manifestations (paresthesias of the hands, memory loss). In heterozygotes, triglyceride may be normal or mildly elevated. In homozygotes, fasting triglyceride level may be >1000 mg/dL	Diet low in simple carbohydrates and <10% fat; medium-chain triglyceride intake helpful. Avoid alcohol; control body weight. Drugs usually do not improve triglycerides in these patients.
Familial low HDL cholesterol (hypoalpha-lipoproteinemia)	Very rare. HDL cholesterol varies with the genetic defect but may be <10 mg/dL. Clinical manifestations may include corneal opacities, xanthomatosis, tonsil anomalies, neuropathy, hepatosplenomegaly, and amyloidosis	Patients should be referred to a lipid specialist for treatment

Table 41.6. Hygienic Measures to Reduce Cardiovascular Risk

Measure	Comments
Diet	Mediterranean diet (increased consumption of alpha-linolenic acid and omega-3 fatty acids) is a reasonable alternative to Step I/II AHA diets (Tables 41.19, 41.20)
Physical activity	Lifestyle-based exercise program is effective in reducing cardiovascular risk. Exercise does not need to be done all at once; goal is to accumulate 30 minutes of adequate physical activity on most days of the week
Weight control	Caloric intake and energy expenditure should be adjusted to maintain body-mass index (BMI) of 21-25 kg/m^2 and waist circumference < 102 cm in men and < 88 cm in women. Drug therapy (sibutramine, orlistat) is useful for BMI > 30 kg/m^2 (or > 27 kg/m^2 if multiple risk factors are present). Behavior modification techniques (self-monitoring, stress management, social support) improve compliance
Smoking cessation	Identify all tobacco users at *every* visit and strongly urge them to quit. Help with a quit plan (Table 41.23), provide practical counseling, and recommend approved pharmacotherapy and a local quit-smoking program to all patients (Table 41.22)
Alcohol	Small amounts ($\leq$ 1 ounce/day) of alcohol may be cardioprotective, but benefit is offset by increased risk of cancer, strokes, accidents with $\geq$ 3 drinks/day

Table 41.7. Drug Therapy Based on Lipid Profile

Dyslipidemia	Lipid Profile (mg/dL)	Recommended Agent(s)[1]	Comments
High LDL-C, normal TG	LDL-C ≥ 190 TG < 150	*Monotherapy*: statin *Combination*: BAS + statin; BAS + niacin; statin + niacin[2]	Homozygous FH requires the attention of a lipid specialist. BAS is preferred as monotherapy if liver disease is present
	LDL-C 160-190 TG < 150	*Monotherapy*: statin; alternative: BAS, niacin	Statins, niacin and BAS have proven long-term safety profiles. The Lipid Research Clinics Trial showed a 19% reduction in nonfatal MI with cholestyramine
Mixed hyperlipidemia	LDL-C 160-190 TG 150-400	*Monotherapy*: statin; alternative: niacin, FIB *Combination*: statin + niacin[2]; statin + FIB[3]; FIB + BAS	The Coronary Drug Project, a secondary-prevention trial, showed a 27% reduction in nonfatal MI with niacin. The Helsinki Heart Study showed a decrease in the incidence of CHD with gemfibrozil. FIB is preferred if diabetes or peptic ulcers are present
Elevated triglycerides	LDL-C < 130 TG > 400	*Monotherapy*: niacin, FIB, fish oils *Combination*: FIB + fish oils, niacin + fish oils, FIB + niacin	Fish oils may be used as adjunctive therapy. Treat to decrease the risk of pancreatitis. Niacin worsens diabetes control and may activate peptic ulcer disease. Avoid FIB in patients with gallbladder disease
Isolated low HDL-C	LDL-C < 130 TG < 150 HDL-C < 35	*Monotherapy*: niacin, FIB, statin *Combination*: niacin + FIB, niacin + statin, FIB + niacin	Low HDL-C greatly increases CHD risk even in the absence of elevated LDL-C. In VA-HIT, gemfibrozil raised HDL-C by 6% and reduced relative risk for nonfatal MI or coronary death by 22%

Abbreviations: BAS = bile-acid sequestrant (colesevelam, cholestyramine, colestipol); FIB = fibric-acid derivative (fenofibrate, gemfibrozil); statin = HMG-CoA reductase inhibitor (atorvastatin, cerivastatin, fluvastatin, lovastatin, pravastatin, simvastatin); niacin = nicotinic acid

* The following guidelines are based on the general activity of the drugs. However, drug selection is a highly individualized process and should take into account factors such as tolerance, compliance, and the unique medical condition of the patient

1. In patients with low HDL-C, consider an agent that will increase HDL-C as well as lower LDL-C and/or triglyceride. Severe elevations of LDL-C and/or triglyceride may require combination therapy. Avoid all drugs during pregnancy

2. Increased risk for myopathy and hepatitis

3. Increased risk for myopathy

Table 41.8. Effective Cholesterol-Lowering Drugs: Indications and Major Effects on Lipids

Class	Agent	Effect on LDL-C	Effect on HDL-C	Effect on TG	Major Use	Contraindications
HMG-CoA reductase inhibitors (statins)	Atorvastatin Cerivastatin Fluvastatin Lovastatin Pravastatin Simvastatin	↓20-60%	↑5-15%	↓10-30%	Hypercholesterolemia (elevated LDL-C levels) and primary and secondary prevention. Overwhelmingly the drug class of choice for elevated LDL-C levels. Highly effective for lowering LDL-C and preventing cardiovascular and cerebrovascular events	Absolute: active or chronic liver disease Relative: previous intolerance to statins due to myalgias, elevated liver function tests, other side effects
Nicotinic acid (niacin)	Immediate-release (crystalline) form Sustained-release forms (e.g., Niaspan)	↓10-25%	↑15-35%	↓20-50%	Useful in nearly all dyslipidemias. Uniquely effective in atherogenic dyslipidemia (elevated triglycerides, depressed HDL-C, mild to moderately elevated LDL-C levels). Also used for patients with elevated Lp(a) levels. Also useful as adjunctive therapy for mixed dyslipidemia	Absolute: active or chronic liver disease Relative: severe gout, uncontrolled type 2 diabetes, active peptic ulcer disease
Bile acid sequestrants	Colesevelam Cholestyramine Colestipol	↓10-20%	↑3-5%	usually not affected; may ↑	Moderate hypercholesterolemia in premenopausal females and other patients in whom systemic drug therapy is felt to be undesirable (sequestrants are not absorbed out of the GI tract). Also useful as adjunctive therapy	Absolute: markedly elevated triglyceride levels (>500 mg/dL) Relative: triglyceride levels between 200-500 mg/dL (bile acid sequestrants can elevate triglyceride levels further)
Fibric acid derivatives	Gemfibrozil Clofibrate Fenofibrate	↓10-15%*	↑10-15%	↓20-50%	Severe hypertriglyceridemia, atherogenic dyslipidemia, especially in patients with type 2 diabetes. Not indicated for patients with isolated LDL-C elevation	Absolute: hepatic or severe renal dysfunction, primary biliary cirrhosis, gallbladder disease, patients on existing therapy with cyclosporine and statin Relative: combined therapy with statins (occasional occurrence of severe myopathy or rhabdomyolysis)

↑ = increases; ↓ = decreases; LDL-C = LDL cholesterol; HDL-C = HDL cholesterol; TG = triglycerides

* ↓ 10-15% with ↑ baseline LDL-C; may ↑ LDL-C with ↑ baseline TG

Table 41.9. Effective Cholesterol-Lowering Drugs: Dosage and Side Effects

Class	Dosage and Administration	Side Effects and Precautions
HMG-CoA reductase inhibitors	Atorvastatin: 10-80 mg/d Cerivastatin: 0.4-0.8 mg/d Fluvastatin: 20-80 mg/d Lovastatin: 20-80 mg/d Pravastatin: 20-40 mg/d Simvastatin: 10-80 mg/d Generally more effective when taken at night; atorvastatin can be taken anytime. Maximum lipid effects in 2-4 weeks	If elevations in liver transaminases $\geq$ 3 times normal persist, therapy should be discontinued until levels normalize, then reinitiated at a reduced dosage or with a different statin. Rare cases of rhabdomyolysis and acute renal failure or death have occurred, usually in association with fibrates, antifungals (azole derivatives), cyclosporine, or erythromycin. Follow administration guidelines when statins and fibrates are used in combination (Table 41.10); discontinue if myopathy is diagnosed
Niacin	Immediate-release form: 250 mg QD-BID; gradual titration over 1-3 weeks to 1 gm BID-TID (with meals) Sustained-release form (Niaspan): 500 mg at bedtime after a low-fat snack; titrated over 4-6 weeks to 1-2 gm at bedtime	Cutaneous flushing and GI upset are common side effects. A once-daily formulation (Niaspan) and premedication with aspirin (81-325 mg 30 minutes to 6 hours before niacin) may reduce flushing. Increased risk for myopathy and hepatitis when combined with a statin; avoid combination in patients with hepatic or renal disease, and in those receiving cyclosporine, erythromycin, or itraconazole. Other side effects include increased serum glucose (up to 25% in Type II diabetics), elevated hepatic enzymes in 1-2% (rare chronic liver disease, hepatic failure), atrial fibrillation, orthostatic hypotension, and acanthosis nigricans
Bile acid sequestrants	Colesevelam: 3750-4375 mg/d in 1 or 2 divided doses Cholestyramine: 4-8 gm/d; gradually titrated up to 12-24 gm/d in 2 or 3 divided doses Colestipol: 5-10 gm/d; gradually titrated up to 15-30 gm/d in 2 or 3 divided doses	Constipation is a common (fluid and fiber intake often help); mild increase in hepatic enzymes; impaired intestinal absorption of many drugs (warfarin, digoxin, thiazides, beta-blockers) requires administration 1 hour before or 4 hours after bile acid sequestrants
Fibrates	Gemfibrozil: 1200 mg/d in 2 divided doses 30 minutes before morning and evening meals Fenofibrate: 200 mg/d; 67 mg/d in renal insufficiency or when combined with statins	Use with extreme caution, if at all, in patients severe hepatic or renal insufficiency. Myositis or myopathy may occur, especially in patients with pre-existing renal insufficiency or those taking statins (follow administration guidelines in Table 41.10 when fibrates and statins are used in combination; discontinue if myopathy is diagnosed). Fibrates potentiate the effect of oral anticoagulants and increase the risk for bleeding (may need to decrease warfarin dose by up to 30%)

Table 41.10. Administration Guidelines for Combination Therapy with Statins and Fibrates

DO:
- Document the need for combination therapy such as failure to respond to monotherapy in a high-risk patient (CAD or CAD equivalent)
- Instruct patients to stop both drugs if they ever develop severe muscle soreness, pain, or weakness
- Instruct patients to stop the medication (at least one) if they ever become acutely ill, dehydrated, require antibiotics, or are admitted to the hospital for any cause
- Check baseline renal function, liver function, and creatine kinase
- In patients on full-dose fibrate, begin with a low dose of statin
- In patients on moderate statin dose, begin with a low dose of fibrate (fenofibrate 67 mg/d, gemfibrozil 300 mg BID)

DO NOT:
- Do not use in patients with impaired liver function
- Do not use in patients with impaired renal function (creatinine ≥2.0 mg/dL)
- Do not use in patients receiving cyclosporine or tacrolimus
- Do not use in patients on chronic erythromycin or antifungal (itraconazole, ketoconazole) therapy
- Do not use in patients >70 years of age
- Do not use high dose of statins (80 mg of atorvastatin, simvastatin, or lovastatin) in combination with fibrates
- Do not use cerivastatin (listed as contraindication in package insert)

Abbreviations: CAD = coronary artery disease

Table 41.11. Treatment of Special Patient Populations with Dyslipidemia

Group	Treatment
Young adult males and premenopausal females	Emphasis on diet and lifestyle; consider drug therapy for extreme elevation of LDL (> 220 mg/dL), multiple risk factors, of strong family history
Postmenopausal females	Topical estrogen preferred to oral estrogen, which may exacerbate hypertriglyceridemia. When indicated, oral estrogens should be used in low-dose
Elderly patients	Drug therapy should not be withheld; statins reduce coronary events and stroke
Diabetics	Aggressive therapy is required with diet and drugs, even in the absence of coronary disease. Target LDL ≤ 100 mg/dL. Treatment of dyslipidemia and hypertension are more important for improving cardiovascular prognosis than intensive glycemic control

Table 41.12.　Common Pitfalls in Dyslipidemia Management

Pitfall	Description	Recommendation
Failure to screen and initiate therapy in patients with CAD	A minority (25-35%) of CAD patients with dyslipidemia receive statins	Obtain a lipid profile in all patients with CAD and begin statin therapy for LDL cholesterol > 100-130 mg/dL. If lipid levels are not measured during the first 24 hours of hospitalization for acute coronary syndromes, discharge the patient on a statin. If LDL cholesterol is excessively depressed (< 50-70 mg/dL) during outpatient follow-up, statins can be reduced or discontinued
Inadequate dosing of antidyslipidemic medications	Most physicians fail to titrate statins to a range needed to achieve LDL levels recommended by the NCEP guidelines	Patients with CAD should be started on high-dose therapy (atorvastatin 10 mg/d, cerivastatin 0.4 mg/d, fluvastatin 80 mg/d, lovastatin 40 mg/d, pravastatin 40 mg/d, simvastatin 20 mg/d). Once in the target range, lipid levels should be rechecked every 6-12 months
Failure to measure and treat HDL cholesterol	Many CAD patients with average or only mildly elevated total and LDL cholesterol levels have very low HDL levels	All adult patients should be screened for total and HDL cholesterol. In CAD patients with low HDL cholesterol, NCEP guidelines recommend niacin even if LDL cholesterol is <100 mg/dL
Failure to treat markedly elevated triglycerides	Severe hypertriglyceridemia is an independent risk factor for CAD	Weight loss and exercise are beneficial. Effective drug therapy includes fibrates, nicotinic acid, and fish oil (not statins). Triple therapy may be required. Metformin and PPAR-γ agonists are beneficial in diabetics
Cessation of therapy because of minor elevations of CPK or hepatic transaminases	Minor elevations in CPK or hepatic enzymes are common and generally benign	Rhabdomyolysis or severe hepatic disease is rarely seen with lipid-lowering monotherapy. Since CPK elevations occur frequently even in patients on placebo (~30%), statins should not be stopped for mild increases in CPK (< 3 times normal) or hepatic transaminases (< 2 times normal)
Lack of patient follow-up	50% of patients discontinue lipid therapy during the first year without consulting a physician	Patients who are started on lipid therapy should be given a definite plan with periodic follow-up visits and face-to-face feedback, either with a physician or nurse

TREATMENT OF HYPERTENSION

A. **BLOOD PRESSURE GOALS (Figure 41.3).** Blood pressure should be reduced to < 140/90 mmHg for the general population. Lower targets have been established for patients who are post-MI or have renal insufficiency or heart failure ($\leq$ 130/85 mmHg), for patients with diabetes mellitus ($\leq$ 130/80 mmHg), and for patients with renal insufficiency and proteinuria > 1 gram per day ($\leq$ 125/75 mmHg). To achieve maximum cardiovascular and renovascular protection, *systolic and diastolic* blood pressure should be reduced to established targets.

B. **RECOGNITION OF SPECIAL FORMS OF HYPERTENSION.** It is important to recognize "white-coat" and pseudohypertension, which often lead to overdiagnosis and overtreatment, and curable (secondary) forms of hypertension.

1. **"White-Coat" Hypertension.** Defined as hypertension that occurs only during doctors office visits, white-coat hypertension is responsible for $\geq$ 20% of apparent hypertension. The diagnosis should be suspected in patients with persistent elevations in blood pressure but without target organ damage, and is confirmed by ambulatory and home blood pressure levels consistently $\leq$ 135/85 mmHg. Over 10 years, white-coat hypertension is associated with little if any increased risk for end-organ damage. Treatment consists of lifestyle modifications and close follow-up. Drug therapy is reserved for persistent elevations in blood pressure.

2. **Pseudohypertension.** When the cuff pressure needed to compress calcified, rigid brachial arteries exceeds intraarterial pressure, an artificial elevation in blood pressure may occur. Pseudohypertension should be suspected in elderly patients with evidence of generalized atherosclerosis, in patients whose radial artery can still be palpated when blood pressure exceeds auscultatory systolic blood pressure (Osler's sign), and in patients with persistently elevated blood pressures who develop hypotensive symptoms during drug therapy. For a true blood pressure reading, intra-arterial recording should be considered.

3. **Secondary Hypertension.** Secondary hypertension is hypertension that can be ascribed to an identifiable cause, and affects 5-10% of the total hypertensive population. Indications for work-up include history, physical exam, and labs suggesting a secondary cause (Table 41.13), resistance to triple drug therapy, blood pressure worsening after a period of good control, accelerated or malignant hypertension, or a negative family history with diastolic BP > 110 mmHg. In elderly patients with multiple risk factors for atherosclerosis and poorly controlled hypertension, renal artery stenosis should be considered (Chapter 36).

C. **DRUG THERAPY.** The choice of initial drug therapy should be individualized and based on patient characteristics and the presence of associated conditions (Table 41.14). In general, most patients should be started on a low dose of a long-acting once-daily drug that can be titrated slowly based on the patient's age and response. About 50% of patients respond to monotherapy. In high-risk patients (BP ≥ 180/110 mmHg, clinical cardiovascular disease, target organ damage), intervals between adding new drugs and changing existing regimens can be reduced. Persons with BP ≥ 200/120 mmHg and symptomatic target organ damage should be considered for hospitalization. If the initial drug has no effect on blood pressure or causes bothersome side effects, another drug from a different drug class should be substituted. If a partial response is obtained and the drug is well tolerated, a second agent from a different drug class is added. If a diuretic is not initially chosen it should probably be added next since it will enhance the effect of most antihypertensives. If target blood pressure is still not attained, additional drugs from other classes are added. Before proceeding to each successive treatment step, it is important to examine potential reasons for lack of responsiveness (Table 41.17), including pseudoresistance, nonadherence to therapy, volume overload, drug-related causes, associated conditions, and secondary causes of hypertension (Table 41.13). Elevated BP alone in asymptomatic patients without new or worsening target organ damage rarely requires emergency control. Indications and effects of common antihypertensive drug classes are described in Table 41.15.

D. **COMBINATION DRUG THERAPY.** Once-daily, low-dose combination therapy can also be used for the initial treatment of hypertension, in which a full dose of one drug is replaced by smaller doses of two or more drugs. The different mechanisms of action may result in fewer side effects and better blood pressure control, especially in the resistant hypertensive. Additionally, for the 50% of patients (and 75% of diabetics) who require more than one antihypertensive drug, once-daily low-dose combination therapy may improve compliance. Useful combinations for initial therapy include a diuretic with a beta-blocker, calcium antagonist, ACE inhibitor, or angiotensin II receptor blocker. For subsequent therapy, various combinations may be used, including an ACE inhibitor plus calcium antagonist, a diuretic plus adrenergic blocker plus vasodilator, or a beta-blocker plus calcium antagonist. Drug combinations that should be avoided include two drugs from the same class (e.g., two beta-blockers), a centrally-acting agent and a beta-blocker, and a beta-blocker with diltiazem or verapamil.

E. **STEPDOWN THERAPY.** Monotherapy ultimately provides adequate blood pressure control for more than 50% of patients. If blood pressure has been well-controlled on two drugs for ≥ 6 months, gradual withdrawal of the first drug may be attempted. Close monitoring is advised since hypertension may return after a delayed period of months to years. Attempts to completely discontinue antihypertensive therapy are not recommended without sustained and substantial improvements in lifestyle.

G. **OPTIMIZING PATIENT COMPLIANCE (Table 41.16).** Since 50% or more of hypertensive patients adjust or discontinue antihypertensive therapy on their own, education about dietary, lifestyle, and pharmacologic measures is essential. Patients should be encouraged to record and report their BP prior to their morning drug dose (to ensure protection against the surge in BP upon awakening) and in the early evening (to ensure coverage throughout the day).

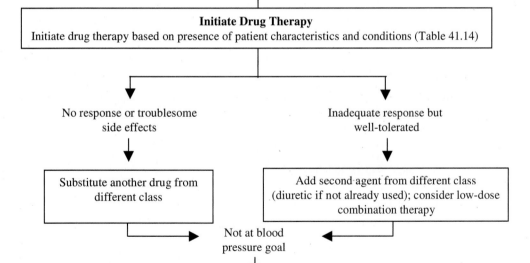

Begin or Continue Lifestyle Modifications

- Lose weight if overweight
- Limit alcohol to no more than 1 oz (30 mL) of ethanol per day (eg, 24 oz [720 mL] of beer, 10 oz [300 mL] of wine or 2 oz [60 mL] of 100-proof whiskey). Limit to 5 oz [15 mL] per day for women and lighter-weight people
- Increase aerobic physical activity (30-45 min most days of the week)
- Reduce sodium intake to no more than 100 mmol/d (2.4 g of sodium or 6 g of sodium chloride)
- Maintain adequate intake of dietary potassium (approximately 90 mmol/d)
- Maintain adequate intake of dietary calcium and magnesium for general health
- Stop smoking for overall cardiovascular health
- Increase dietary intake of fruits, vegetables and grains; reduce intake of dietary saturated fat and cholesterol

Not at Blood Pressure Goal
General population: < 140/90 mmHg
Post-MI, heart failure, or renal insufficiency: ≤ 130/85 mmHg
Diabetes mellitus: ≤ 130/80 mmHg
Renal insufficiency with proteinuria ≥ 1 gm/d: ≤ 125/75 mmHg

Initiate Drug Therapy
Initiate drug therapy based on presence of patient characteristics and conditions (Table 41.14)

No response or troublesome
side effects

Inadequate response but
well-tolerated

Substitute another drug from
different class

Add second agent from different class
(diuretic if not already used); consider low-dose
combination therapy

Not at blood
pressure goal

Continue adding agents from other classes (diuretic if not already used)
Exclude causes of resistant hypertension (Table 41.17)
Consider referral to a hypertension specialist

Figure 41.3. Treatment of Hypertension

Table 41.13. Causes of Secondary Hypertension

Cause	Features
Renovascular hypertension	Age < 30 years, diastolic pressure ≥ 120 mmHg, recent onset or exacerbation of hypertension (<2 years), malignant hypertension, systolic-diastolic bruit in epigastrium or upper quadrants of abdomen, refractory hypertension, acquired resistance to antihypertensive therapy especially in elderly patients, deterioration in renal function after ACE inhibitors or angiotensin II receptor blockers.
Pheochromocytoma	Spells of headache, palpitations, tachycardia, inappropriate perspiration, tremor and pallor, unusually labile blood pressure, recent weight loss, recent onset or discovery of diabetes, malignant hypertension, pressor response to antihypertensive drugs or during induction of anesthesia, refractory hypertension. (Symptoms are usually but not necessarily paroxysmal.)
Hyperthyroidism	Palpitations, tremor, weight loss, sweating, increased appetite.
Primary aldosteronism	Unprovoked hypokalemia with inappropriate kaliuresis (24-hour urinary potassium ≥ 40 mEq and serum potassium ≤ 3.5 mEq/L), refractory hypertension.
Cushing's syndrome	Characteristic body habitus, skin changes, muscle weakness, osteoporosis.
Coarctation of the aorta	Absent, delayed, or diminished pulses in lower extremities, especially in patients age < 30 years.
Medications	Birth control pills, amphetamines (diet pills, cold capsules, nasal spray), MAO inhibitors (e.g., phenelzine [Nardil], tranylcypromine [Parnate], isocarboxazid [Marplan]), tricyclic antidepressants (e.g., amitriptyline [Elavil], desipramine [Norpramin], nortriptyline [Aventyl], imipramine [Tofranil], doxepin [Sinequan]), cocaine abuse, adrenal steroids, exogenous thyroid hormone, cyclosporine, erythropoietin
Others	Renal parenchymal disease, alcohol > 2 oz. per day, acromegaly, hypothyroidism, hypercalcemia (hyperparathyroidism), congenital adrenal hyperplasia, pregnancy-induced, neurological disorders (increased intracranial pressure, sleep apnea, quadriplegia, acute porphyria, familial dysautonomia, lead poisoning, Guillain-Barre syndrome), acute stress (surgery, psychogenic hyperventilation, hypoglycemia, burns, alcohol withdrawal, sickle cell crisis, after resuscitation, perioperative), and systolic hypertension (aortic valvular insufficiency, arteriovenous fistula, patent ductus arteriosus, thyrotoxicosis, Paget's disease of bone, beriberi, rigidity of aorta)

Table 41.14. Treatment of Essential Hypertension Based on Patient Characteristics

Subset	Drug Therapy	Comments
Angina	ACE inhibitor, β-blocker, or 2nd generation calcium antagonist (amlodipine, felodipine)	Reduce BP gradually to prevent hypotensive episodes and myocardial ischemia. Thiazide diuretics should be used in low doses, due to unfavorable effects of higher doses on insulin resistance, lipids, and electrolytes
Blacks	Diuretic, calcium antagonist, or α-β-blocker. β-blockers and ACE inhibitors are less effective as monotherapy, but may be indicated for diabetic nephropathy, LVH, systolic dysfunction, CAD, or post-MI. More than one drug is often required; consider low-dose combination therapy	Lifestyle modification is extremely important, due to the high prevalence of cigarette smoking, obesity, and type 2 diabetes. Blacks are also very responsive to reductions in salt intake
COPD with bronchospasm or asthma	Calcium antagonist, ACE inhibitor, or ARB	β-blockers and α-β-blockers increase airway resistance and may provoke bronchospasm. ACE inhibitor-induced cough may complicate bronchospastic disease; ARBs can be used if a cough develops. In patients with severe COPD ("blue bloaters") who utilize hypoxic pulmonary vasoconstriction to minimize V/Q mismatch, calcium blockers may worsen gas exchange
Diabetes	ACE inhibitor/ARB* + thiazide diuretic. If BP remains elevated, follow with a calcium antagonist and then a low-dose beta-blocker. More than one drug is normally required. ACE inhibitor + dihydropyridine calcium antagonist combination may have additive antiproteinuric effects. If orthostatic BP changes are present, use standing BP to guide therapy	Treat to BP $\leq$ 130/80 mmHg (or $\leq$ 125/75 mmHg if renal insufficiency or proteinuria > 1 gm/d). The HOT study demonstrated a 51% reduction in cardiovascular events for diabetics treated to a diastolic BP target of 80 mmHg vs. 90 mmHg. ACE inhibitors slow the progression of nephropathy and provided better cardioprotection than calcium antagonists in ABCD and FACET trials despite similar degrees of blood pressure lowering
Elderly (age > 65)	Diuretic, calcium antagonist, ACE inhibitor or ARB, started at low dose to avoid postural hypotension. β-blockers are effective, but have not been shown to be cardioprotective and cause more side effects. If orthostatic hypotension is present, use standing BP to guide therapy	Exclude pseudohypertension and white-coat hypertension prior to initiating therapy. Dementia was reduced by 50% in elderly patients treated with a dihydropyridine calcium antagonist in the Syst-Eur trial. Sudden onset of hypertension in the elderly suggests renal artery stenosis
Heart failure, systolic dysfunction	ACE inhibitor, ARB*, diuretic, α-β-blocker (carvedilol), or a cardioselective β-blocker (bisoprolol, metoprolol)	A second-generation calcium antagonist (amlodipine, felodipine) can be added for angina or resistant hypertension

Table 41.14. Treatment of Essential Hypertension Based on Patient Characteristics

Subset	Drug Therapy	Comments
High cholesterol	ACE inhibitor, ARB, calcium antagonist, or low-dose diuretic	Non-pharmacologic therapy may lower BP, improve lipid profile, and reduce cardiovascular risk. Calcium antagonists, ACE inhibitors, and ARBs have no effect on plasma lipids. β-blockers increase triglycerides (10-15%) and decrease HDL (10%), but have no effect on total cholesterol; β-blockers with ISA may increase HDL. High-dose thiazide diuretics increase total cholesterol (5%) and triglycerides (20-25%), but have no effect on HDL. Low-dose diuretics have few if any effects on lipids
Left ventricular hypertrophy (LVH)	ACE inhibitor, ARB*, calcium antagonist, or β-blocker. Preload reducing agents (nitrates, diuretics) may cause hypotension in patients with LVH and severe diastolic dysfunction	Weight loss, low sodium diet, and all drugs except direct vasodilators have been shown to decrease LV mass and wall thickness. ACE inhibitors appear to cause the most regression
Myocardial infarction, post	β-blocker (without ISA), ACE inhibitor, ARB*	β-blockers and ACE inhibitors prevent recurrent MI and reduce long-term mortality. Diltiazem or verapamil can be used if β-blockers prove ineffective following non-Q-wave MI with preserved LV function
Peripheral vascular disease	ACE inhibitor, ARB*, vasodilator or calcium antagonist	Avoid non-selective β-blockers, which may cause peripheral vasoconstriction and increase symptoms. Claudication may worsen as BP is lowered
Renal insufficiency (creatinine > 2 mg/dL)	Diuretic (loop diuretics require multiple daily high doses; metolazone is effective once daily), calcium antagonist, or labetalol. Combination therapy is often required and minoxidil may be needed for refractory cases. Avoid potassium-sparing diuretics and potassium supplements. Patients with proteinuric nephropathy should be treated with an ACE inhibitor or ARB*. Many BP medications are excreted by the kidneys and require dose adjustment	Treat to BP $\leq$ 130/85 mmHg (or $\leq$ 125/75 mmHg if proteinuria > 1 gm/d). Control of BP slows the progression of renal failure. Since volume excess contributes significantly to hypertension, diuretics are often used alone or in combination with other agents. Thiazide diuretics (except metolazone) are ineffective in patients with glomerular filtration rates < 30 cc/min. ACE inhibitors decrease proteinuria and slow functional deterioration in diabetic and other proteinuric nephropathies. If creatinine rises $\geq$ 1 mg/dL after starting an ACE inhibitor or ARB, suspect renal artery stenosis
Systolic hypertension (isolated) in the elderly	Thiazide diuretic or dihydropyridine calcium antagonist, starting at low dose and adjusting in small increments. Lower BP slowly to reduce the risk of cerebral ischemia. If heart failure or diabetic nephropathy is present, an ACE inhibitor or ARB* should be considered	Exclude white-coat hypertension and pseudohypertension, and obtain multiple BP measurements before starting therapy. Low-dose diuretics and long-acting dihydropyridine calcium antagonists (nitrendipine and nifedipine) decreased the risk of stroke, MI, and heart failure by 25-45% over 2 years

Abbreviations: ACE = angiotensin converting enzyme; ARB = angiotensin receptor blocker; ARB* = ARB for patients who develop an intolerant cough to ACE inhibitors

Table 41.15. Indications and Effects of Outpatient Antihypertensives

Drug Class	1° Indications	METABOLIC + PHYSIOLOGIC EFFECTS								
		Chol	TG	HDL	K⁺	Mg⁺	Uric acid	Insulin resistance	LVH regression	2° cardio-protection
ACE inhibitors	Proteinuric nephropathy; post-MI; CHF; vascular disease; diabetes	0	0	0	↑	0	0	↓	↓↓	2
Angiotensin II receptor blockers	Intolerance to ACE inhibitor (e.g., cough); indications evolving	0	0	0	↑	0	0	0, ↓	probably ↓	0
β-blockers without ISA	Post-MI, migraine, tremor, tachycardia	0/↑	↑↑	↓	↑	0	0	↑↑	↓	0
β-blockers with ISA	Post-MI, migraine, tremor, tachycardia	0	↑	0	0	0	0	↑	↓	0
Calcium antagonists	Elderly, blacks, CAD, renal insufficiency	0	0	0	0	0	0	0	↓↓	Perhaps with verapamil or diltiazem
Diuretics**	Elderly, blacks, renal insufficiency, CHF	↑	0	0	↓	↓	↑	↑	↓	0
Central α-blockers	Sedative effect desired	0	0	0	0	0	0	?	↓	?
Peripheral α-blockers	Diabetes, dyslipidemia, BPH	↓	↓	↑	0	0	0	↓	↓	?
Vasodilators	Peripheral vascular disease, vasculitis	↓	0	0	0	?	0	?	0	0

0 = no significant effect; ↑ (↓) = increased (decreased) effect; ? = unknown or no consistent group effect; CAD = coronary artery disease; CHF = congestive heart failure; ISA = intrinsic sympathomimetic activity; BPH = benign prostatic hypertrophy
* Similar to ACE inhibitors for systolic heart failure in ELITE II trial
** Lower doses cause fewer adverse effects

Table 41.16. General Guidelines to Improve Patient Adherence to Antihypertensive Therapy

Be aware of the problem and be alert to signs of patient nonadherence

Establish the goal of therapy: to reduce blood pressure to near normotensive levels with minimal or no side effects

Educate the patient about the disease and its treatment
    Discuss the silent nature of the disease
    Discuss the need for lifelong treatment
    Discuss common rationalizations given to justify discontinuing medications on own
    Encourage visits and calls to allied health personnel
    Allow the pharmacist to monitor therapy
    Give feedback to the patient via home BP readings
    Make contact with patients who do not return

Keep care inexpensive and simple
    Do the least workup needed to rule out secondary causes
    Obtain follow-up laboratory data only yearly unless indicated more often
    Use home blood pressure readings
    Use nondrug, low-cost therapies
    Use once-daily doses of long-acting drugs
    Use generic drugs and break larger doses of tablets in half
    If appropriate, use combination tablets
    Tailor medication to daily routines

Prescribe according to pharmacologic principles
    Add one drug at a time
    Start with small doses, aiming for 5- to 10-mmHg reductions at each step
    Prevent volume overload with adequate diuretic and sodium restriction

Be willing to stop unsuccessful therapy and try a different approach

Anticipate side effects

Adjust therapy to reduce side effects that do not spontaneously disappear

Continue to add effective and tolerated drugs, stepwise, in sufficient doses to achieve the goal of therapy

Table 41.17. Causes of Resistant Hypertension

Category	Causes
Pseudoresistance	"White-coat hypertension" or office evaluations, pseudohypertension in older patients, use of regular cuff on very obese arm
Nonadherence to therapy	Most common cause of resistance. Results from lack of awareness about silent nature of disease and use of medications that are too expensive, inconvenient, confusing or cause side effects
Volume overload	Inadequate diuretic therapy (most common cause after non-adherence to therapy), excess salt intake, progressive renal damage (nephrosclerosis), fluid retention from reduction in blood pressure
Drug-related causes	Doses too low, wrong type of diuretic, inappropriate combinations, rapid inactivation (e.g., hydralazine). May also be caused by drug actions and interactions with sympathomimetics, nasal decongestants, appetite suppressants, cocaine and other illicit drugs, caffeine, oral contraceptives, adrenal steroids, licorice (as may be found in chewing tobacco), cyclosporine, tacrolimus, erthyropoeitin, antidepressants, nonsteroidal anti-inflammatory drugs. Review all medications to detect negative drug interactions. Be sure to give drugs an appropriate time to work (i.e., weeks) before declaring them ineffective
Associated conditions	Smoking, increasing obesity, sleep apnea, insulin resistance/hyperinsulinemia, ethanol intake more than 1 oz (30 ml) per day, anxiety-induced hyperventilation or panic attacks, chronic pain, intense vasoconstriction (arteritis), organic brain syndrome (e.g., memory deficit), identifiable (secondary) cause of hypertension, especially renovascular hypertension (responsible for 20% of resistant hypertension in non-blacks; less common in blacks)

Adapted from JNC VI (JAMA 1997;278:1065)

ADJUNCTIVE THERAPY TO PREVENT ATHEROTHROMBOSIS

In addition to control of dyslipidemia, the risk for atherothrombotic events may also be reduced by therapies that control hypertension and target mechanisms such as thrombosis and oxidation.

EVIDENCE-BASED THERAPY

A. **ANTIPLATELETS**
   1. **Aspirin.** Aspirin has been consistently shown to prevent MI and stroke in patients at risk for atherosclerotic vascular disease. Although aspirin does not prevent atherosclerosis, it does inhibit platelet function and decreases the likelihood that an occlusive thrombus will form at the site of an

inflamed and ulcerated atherosclerotic plaque. The optimal aspirin dose is between 81 and 325 mg daily. Doses in excess of 325 mg per day are associated with increased risk of gastrointestinal bleeding in a dose-dependent fashion. Enteric-coated or buffered forms of aspirin are no less likely to cause gastrointestinal bleeding than soluble aspirin. Low-dose aspirin (81-162 mg) should be considered for patients on an ACE inhibitor or with a history of serious bleeding, especially from the gastrointestinal tract. All patients with coronary artery disease should be on aspirin therapy unless a very strong contraindication exists (e.g., anaphylaxis). Aspirin should also be used in high-risk primary prevention (2 or more risk factors) and in middle-aged or older patients with elevated LDL cholesterol, increased high-sensitivity C-reactive protein, or hypertension.

2. **Clopidogrel (Plavix).** Clopidogrel interferes with ADP-mediated platelet activation and is somewhat more effective at platelet inhibition than aspirin. These two agents have additive effects when used in combination. Clopidogrel has been shown to be improve event-free survival in CAD patients compared to aspirin in the Clopidogrel versus Aspirin in Patients at Risk of Ischemic Events (CAPRIE) secondary prevention study involving 19,185 patients, particularly in patients with peripheral vascular disease. Results of the CURE trial (aspirin plus clopidogrel vs. aspirin alone for acute coronary syndromes) have recently been reported (Table 34.32, p. 779). The safety profile of clopidogrel is similar to low-dose aspirin, with a rare incidence of thrombotic thrombocytopenic purpura. Clopidogrel is indicated for use in aspirin-intolerant patients or those at high risk for cardiovascular or cerebrovascular events.

3. **Ticlopidine (Ticlid).** Ticlopidine is an antiplatelet agent with a structure and mechanism of action similar to clopidogrel. This agent has been found to be more effective than aspirin following coronary stenting and in preventing recurrent ischemic stroke in high-risk patients. However, occasional life-threatening neutropenia and thrombotic thrombocytopenic purpura (TTP) have limited its use. Clopidogrel, with similar efficacy but a lower incidence of serious adverse effects, is generally used instead of ticlopidine when these agents are indicated.

B. **LOW-DOSE FISH OIL.** In the GISSI Prevention Study, 1 g/d (850 mg of DHA and EPA) of fish oil, a dose too low to affect lipid levels, significantly reduced total mortality by 20%, due in large part to a 45% reduction in sudden cardiac death.

C. **ACE INHIBITORS**
1. **Overview.** Angiotensin converting enzyme (ACE) inhibitors block the conversion of angiotensin I to angiotensin II and inhibit the breakdown of bradykinin, resulting in physiologic benefits that confer unique cardioprotective and renoprotective properties to this class of drugs. ACE inhibitors have been shown to improve prognosis in a wide variety of cardiovascular disorders, including hypertension, heart failure, asymptomatic LV dysfunction, MI, post-coronary revascularization procedures, and proteinuric nephropathy. Potential mechanisms for improved cardiovascular prognosis include lowering of blood pressure, improved endothelial function, and reduction in LVH and arterial wall mass.

2. **Heart Outcomes Prevention Evaluation (HOPE) Trial.** Compelling data from the HOPE trial demonstrated an important role for ACE inhibitors in the primary and secondary prevention of atherosclerotic vascular disease and in the development of new-onset diabetes mellitus (NEJM 2000;342:145). In this large randomized trial, involving 9,297 patients with atherosclerotic arterial disease (prior MI, prior stroke, or peripheral arterial disease) or diabetes plus one additional risk factor (hypertension, elevated total cholesterol, depressed HDL cholesterol, smoking, or microalbuminuria), patients receiving ramipril (10 mg/d) had a 22% reduction in a composite endpoint of MI, stroke, or death from cardiovascular disease. Additionally, significant risk reduction was noted for most individual endpoints, including all-cause mortality (16%), MI (20%), stroke (32%), cardiac arrest (38%), and revascularization procedures (15%). Also noted was a reduction in the development of new-onset diabetes mellitus by 34% (p < 0.001). The beneficial effects of ramipril in HOPE were observed consistently among all subgroups—with and without diabetes, hypertension, or cardiovascular disease; older or younger than age 65—and were independent of the effects of concomitant cardiovascular medications (such as aspirin, β-blockers, lipid-lowering agents, or other blood pressure drugs). Ramipril has recently been approved to reduce the risk of MI, stroke, and death from cardiovascular causes in patients 55 years or older at high risk of developing a major cardiovascular event because of a history of coronary artery disease, stroke, peripheral arterial disease, or diabetes that is accompanied by at least one other cardiovascular risk factor (hypertension, elevated total cholesterol levels, low HDL levels, cigarette smoking, or documented microalbuminuria). Ramipril can be used in addition to other needed treatment, including antihypertensive, antiplatelet, and lipid-lowering therapy. The recommended starting dose is 2.5 mg once daily for 1 week, increased to 5 mg once daily for the next 3 weeks, then increased as tolerated to a maintenance dose of 10 mg once a day (which may be given in 2 divided doses for patients who have hypertension or who are post-MI).

3. **Recommendations.** ACE inhibitors are generally safe, well-tolerated, and affordable. Patients with atherosclerotic vascular disease, diabetes, or insulin resistance should therefore be considered for ACE inhibitor therapy unless they have an intolerable cough, systolic blood pressure consistently below 100-110 mmHg, or renal failure (creatinine > 2.5 mg/dL). Angiotensin receptor blockers are not equivalent to ACE inhibitors, but nevertheless may be a reasonable alternative for patients who are intolerant to ACE inhibitor therapy.

D. **DIET THERAPY AND LIFESTYLE MODIFICATION.** Dietary modification, weight control, smoking cessation, and increased physical activity are important for all patients with coronary artery disease (Table 41.16). In patients who also require drug therapy for dyslipidemia or hypertension, drugs should be added to, not substituted for, diet and lifestyle modification.

1. **Mediterranean-Style Diet.** Increasing evidence suggests that a Mediterranean-style diet (Tables 41.18, 41.19) may play an important role in the prevention of clinical cardiovascular disease. In contrast to the standard American Heart Association Step I and Step II Diets (Table 41.20), which emphasize restriction of total fat, saturated fat, and cholesterol, the Mediterranean diet includes up to 30% of calories from fat, predominantly in the form of monounsaturated and omega-3 fatty acids.

The Lyon Diet Heart Study was a randomized trial of 605 post-MI patients comparing a Mediterranean diet providing increased levels of alpha-linolenic acid (from olive oil and canola oil) to usual dietary instruction. Patients in the Mediterranean diet group were instructed to consume more fish, bread, and root and green vegetables; eat less meat; have fruit at least once daily; and use canola-based margarine and olive oil as a fat source. After 4 years, patients on the Mediterranean diet showed a 70% reduction in all-cause mortality (p = 0.03). The rate of cardiovascular death and nonfatal MI was 1.32 per 100 patient years in the treated group compared to 5.55 per 100 patient years in the control group (p = 0.001). The GISSI Prevention study randomized 11,324 Italian men and women (who presumably were eating a Mediterranean diet) with MI within the preceding 3 months to omega-3 fatty acids (850-882 mg/d), vitamin E (300 mg/d), both, or neither. After 3.5 years, the omega-3 group had a significant 20% reduction in all-cause mortality and 45% reduction in sudden cardiac death. In DART (Diet and Reinfarction Trial), 2033 men with prior MI were randomized to receive different types of dietary advice to prevent another MI. After 2 years, the group told to increase their omega-3 intake by eating oily fish (e.g., salmon, herring, mackerel) at least twice weekly had a 29% reduction in overall mortality (p < 0.05). These studies suggest that the type of fat, not only the amount, determines cardiovascular health. It is reasonable to recommend a Mediterranean diet as an alternative to the standard AHA low-fat diet as part of a comprehensive program to reduce cardiovascular risk.

2. **Smoking Cessation.** Compared to age-matched nonsmokers, persons who smoke one pack of cigarettes per day are twice as likely to suffer an MI or stroke, and twice as likely to die from heart disease. By 12-18 months after quitting, most of the increased risk for CAD has disappeared; by 3-5 years, the risk for cardiovascular events is no different than for a nonsmoker. A patient's chance of quitting is doubled if a physician makes a strong statement about the medical necessity of smoking cessation. Bupropion hydrochloride and nicotine replacement therapy also increase the likelihood of successful quitting (Table 41.21). The U. S. Public Health Service has recently issued practice guidelines for treating tobacco use and dependence (Table 41.22).

POSSIBLE BENEFIT FOR PREVENTION OF ATHEROTHROMBOSIS

A. **FOLIC ACID.** Folic acid lowers elevated levels of homocysteine, an amino acid by-product of protein metabolism associated with adverse cardiovascular prognosis (particularly in patients with CAD). All adults should be encouraged to take at least 400 mcg of folic acid daily by diet and/or supplementation. Foods rich in folate include broccoli, spinach, and other green leafy vegetables, citrus fruits, asparagus, and beans. Because of the lack of outcome trials, currently there are no consensus panel recommendations on criteria for measurement of homocysteine. In our practices, we measure homocysteine in patients with premature or severe atherosclerosis. Folic acid supplementation as well as supplementation with vitamins B_6 and B_{12} have been shown to decrease homocysteine levels by approximately 15-30%. If elevated homocysteine levels are present, folic acid (800-1600 mcg per day) in conjunction with vitamin B_{12} (250 mcg per day) and vitamin B_6 (20-25 mg per day) should be considered.

B. **ANTIOXIDANTS.** Oxidation of LDL cholesterol is required for LDL to accumulate into evolving atherosclerotic plaque. However, there is no clear evidence that antioxidants (vitamin E, vitamin C, beta-carotene) reduce cardiovascular events.

C. **ESTROGEN REPLACEMENT THERAPY.** Observational studies of hormone replacement therapy suggested decreased risk for MI and cardiovascular death in women with established CAD or multiple risk factors. However, no benefit on nonfatal MI or cardiovascular death was demonstrated in the randomized Hormone Estrogen Replacement Study (HERS), and estrogen provided no angiographic benefit in the ERA trial. Definitive evidence to support routine use of hormone replacement therapy in women for the prevention of cardiovascular disease is lacking. The ongoing Women's Health Initiative trial involving more than 63,000 women will provide information on the use of estrogen for primary prevention.

Table 41.18. Basic Components of a Mediterranean Diet

Component	Benefits
Omega-3–rich[1] fish 1-2 times per week or omega-3 supplements[2]	Reduces all-cause mortality and sudden cardiac death post-MI; lowers triglycerides (high doses) and blood pressure; improves insulin resistance; boosts the immune system; may help prevent cancer, arthritis, depression, Alzheimer's disease.
Monounsaturated cooking oils (olive, flaxseed, or canola)	Does not increase LDL cholesterol or decrease HDL cholesterol (unlike high saturated fat or highly refined carbohydrate intake). "Metabolically neutral" calorie source for people with insulin resistance.
Fresh fruit and vegetables (5-10 servings per day); aim for a wide variety	High concentrations of vitamins, minerals, fiber, and phytochemicals[3] help prevent heart disease, stroke, and many types of cancer (colon, stomach, prostate).
Vegetable protein from nuts and beans 1-2 times per week	Lowers LDL cholesterol; improves digestion; may reduce CHD and certain cancers. Nuts are an excellent source of protein, monounsaturated fat, fiber, and minerals. Beans contain high-quality protein, fiber, potassium, and folic acid.[4]
Limit saturated fats to < 10-20 grams per day	Saturated fats increase LDL cholesterol, which promotes atherosclerosis and increases the risk of CHD and stroke. Saturated fats are also linked to certain cancers.
Avoid trans fats	Trans fats are manufactured from vegetable oils and are used to enhance the taste and extend the shelf-life of fast foods, French fries, packaged snacks, commercial baked goods, and most margarines. Trans fats may be more atherogenic than saturated fats. Food manufacturers are not required to list trans fats on food labels; instruct patients to avoid foods with "hydrogenated" or "partially hydrogenated" vegetable oil as first or second ingredient—these contain trans fats.
Increase dietary to fiber to 20-30 grams per day	Lowers LDL cholesterol; improves insulin resistance; reduces the risk of heart disease and diabetes; protects against colon cancer, and possibly breast cancer, irritable bowel syndrome, diverticulitis and hemorrhoids; prevents constipation.
At least one source of high-quality protein with every meal	Produces satiety that lasts longer than high carbohydrate meals (reduces hunger and cravings); maintains muscle mass and bone strength. Lack of protein increases the risk of breast cancer, diabetes, and osteoporosis.

Adapted from The Omega Diet, by A. Simopoulos, MD

1. The typical American diet consists of an unhealthy ratio (>15:1) of omega-6:omega-3 essential fatty acids, favoring excessive production of proinflammatory, prothrombotic, and vasoconstrictive mediators of the arachidonic acid cascade (e.g., leukotrienes, thromboxane). Increasing consumption of omega-3 essential fatty acids helps regulate inflammation, thrombogenicity, arrhythmogenicity, and vascular tone.
2. Omega-3 supplements should be considered for patients with documented CHD, especially if risk factors for sudden death are present (LV dysfunction, LVH, ventricular dysrhythmias).
3. Phytochemicals are naturally occurring chemicals found in plants—many of them plant pigments—that act as free radical scavengers and protease inhibitors, among others. Examples include lycophene, beta-carotene, indoles, thiocyanates, lutein, resveratrol, ellagic acid, genistein, and allium.
4. Folic acid lowers homocysteine levels, a by-product of methionine metabolism associated with atherosclerosis.

Table 41.19. How to Incorporate a Mediterranean Diet into Daily Living

Step	Choose	Go Easy On	Avoid
Eat omega-3 rich food 1-2 times per week	Salmon, trout, herring, water-packed tuna, sardines, mackerel, flaxseed, spinach, purslane, fish oil supplements	Raw shellfish (due to danger of infection risk, including hepatitis A and B)	Deep-fried fish, fish sticks, fish from seriously contaminated water
Switch vegetable oils	Flaxseed oil, extra virgin cold pressed olive oil or canola oil (check the label), mayonnaise from olive or canola oil	High-oleic safflower, sunflower, or soybean oil	Corn oil, safflower oil, sunflower oil, palm oil, peanut oil, any other kind of oil, mayonnaise
Load up on fresh fruit and vegetables	Fresh fruit: 3 to 5 daily. Fresh vegetables: 4 to 6 daily. Aim for a wide variety	Fruit juice (no more than 1-2 cups per day), dried fruit, canned fruit	Vegetables or fruit prepared in heavy cream sauces or butter
Add nuts and beans 1-2 times per week	Soybeans, kidney beans, lentils, navy beans, split peas, all other kinds of beans, most nuts	Heavily salted nuts	Stale or rancid nuts
Limit saturated fats to 10-20 grams per day; eat at least one source of high-quality protein with every meal	Fish, lean cuts of fresh meat with fat trimmed off, chicken and turkey without skin, nonfat or lowfat dairy products (skim milk, yogurt, low-fat cottage cheese), dark chocolate, egg whites or egg substitute, omega-3–enriched eggs	Processed lowfat meats (bologna, salami, other luncheon meats), 2% milk, "lite" cream cheese, part-skim mozzarella cheese, milk chocolate, egg yolks (3-4 per week)	Prime-grade fatty cuts of meat, goose, duck, organ meats (liver, kidneys), sausages, bacon, full-fat processed meats, hot dogs, whole milk, cream, full-fat cheeses, cream cheese, sour cream, ice cream
Say "no" to trans fats	Stanol-enriched margarine (Benecol, Take Control)	Commercial peanut butter, water crackers and other crackers that contain no fat, bagels	Fast food, French fries and other deep-fried food, chips and other packaged snacks, most commercial baked goods and margarines
Add more fiber; aim for 20-30 grams per day	Whole-grain breads and cereals, oats, brown rice, whole grain pasta, potatoes with skin (baked, boiled, or steamed), whole-grain bagels	Pasta, white rice, mashed instant potatoes, plain bagels, dinner rolls, egg noodles	Sweetened cereals, white bread, crackers, table sugar, honey, syrup, candy, and all highly processed foods
Drink at least 64 ounces of water per day	Each day, drink 8 glasses of pure, non-chlorinated water. Additional drinks: skim milk (up to 4 glasses); pure fruit juice (up to 2 glasses); tea, especially green tea (up to 4 cups); smoothie made with nonfat yogurt and fresh fruit	Coffee (regular or decaf), 1% or 2% milk, artificially sweetened fruit juice (with "corn syrup" in the label), sports drinks, artificially flavored soft drinks, alcohol	Sugared soft drinks, milkshakes, excess alcohol

Table 41.20. Guidelines for Dietary Therapy: NCEP Step I and Step II Diets*

Food Composition	Step I Diet	Step II Diet
Total fat	≤ 30% of total calories	Same
Saturated fat	8-10% of total calories	< 7% of total calories
Polyunsaturated fat	Up to 10% of total calories	Same
Monounsaturated fat	Up to 15% of total calories	Same
Carbohydrates	≥55% of total calories (more than half as complex carbohydrates from whole grains, fruits, and vegetables)	Same
Protein	~15% of total calories	Same
Cholesterol	< 300 mg/d	< 200 mg/d
Total calories	Sufficient to achieve and maintain desirable body weight.	

* The Step I Diet also serves as the dietary recommendations of the NCEP for the general public. The more intensive Step II Diet is designed for patients with established CHD or atherosclerotic disease, or for whom the Step I Diet has proven insufficient. The assistance of a registered dietician is often useful in maintaining compliance.

Table 41.21. Drug Therapy for Smoking Cessation*

Pharmacotherapy	Precautions/ Contraindications	Adverse Effects	Dosage and Duration
First-line Bupropion HCl (Zyban®)	History of seizures or eating disorder	Insomnia; dry mouth	150 mg every morning for 3 days then 150 mg twice daily (begin treatment 1-2 weeks prior to quit). Treat for 7-12 weeks; maintenance up to 6 months
Nicotine gum	Concurrent cigarette smoking is contraindicated due to the risk of nicotine overdose	Mouth soreness; dyspepsia	*1-24 cigarettes/d:* 2 mg gum (up to 24 pieces/d) ≥ *25 cigarettes/d:* 4 mg gum (up to 24 pieces/d). Treat up to 12 weeks
Nicotine inhaler	Concurrent cigarette smoking is contraindicated due to the risk of nicotine overdose	Local irritation of mouth and throat	6-16 cartridges/d for up to 6 months
Nicotine nasal spray	Concurrent cigarette smoking is contraindicated due to the risk of nicotine overdose	Nasal irritation	8-40 doses/d for 3-6 months
Nicotine patch	Concurrent cigarette smoking is contraindicated due to the risk of nicotine overdose	Local skin reaction; insomnia	21 mg/24 h (4 weeks), then 14 mg/24 h (2 weeks), then 7 mg/24 h (2 weeks). Alternative: 15 mg/16 h (8 weeks)
Second-line Clonidine	Rebound hypertension	Dry mouth; drowsiness; dizziness; sedation	0.15-0.75 mg/d for 3-10 weeks
Nortriptyline	Risk of arrhythmias	Sedation; dry mouth	75-100 mg/d for 12 weeks

* The information contained in this table is not comprehensive. First-line pharmacotherapies have been approved for smoking cessation by the Food and Drug Administration; second-line agents have not. From: The U.S. Public Health Service Clinical Practice Guidelines for Treating Tobacco Use and Dependence (JAMA 2000;283:3224).

Table 41.22. Strategies to Assist Patients Willing to Quit Smoking

Step	Strategies for Implementation
Help the patient with a quit plan	• Set a quit date • Tell family, friends, and coworkers about quitting; request understanding and support • Anticipate withdrawal symptoms and how to resist urges and cravings (clean the house; take a 5-minute walk; do stretching exercises; call a nonsmoking friend and talk) • Throw out ashtrays; clean clothes and car • Learn as much about how to quit smoking as possible. Useful sources for reading materials include the American Heart Association (7272 Greenville Avenue, Dallas, TX 75231, 800-242-8721), American Cancer Society (1599 Clifton Road, NE, Atlanta, GA 30329, 800-227-2345), American Lung Association (1740 Broadway, 14th floor, New York, NY 10019, 800-586-4872)
Provide practical counseling	• Total abstinence is essential: "Not even a single puff after the quit date" • Identify what helped and what hurt in previous quit attempts • Discuss challenges/triggers and how to overcome them successfully • Since alcohol can cause relapse, the patient should abstain from alcohol while quitting • Patients should encourage housemates to quit with them or not to smoke in their presence • Provide a supportive clinical environment while encouraging the patient during the quit attempt: "My office staff and I are available to assist you"
Recommend the use of approved pharmacotherapy (Table 41.22)	• Bupropion may be more effective than NRT for achieving permanent cessation of tobacco use, but there are insufficient data to rank-order first-line therapies. Some synergy between the two approaches may exist. Sustained-release bupropion and nortriptyline are well-suited for patients with a history of depression • Combining the nicotine patch with either nicotine gum or nicotine nasal spray may increase long-term abstinence rates compared to single-NRT treatment • The nicotine patch in particular is safe in patients with cardiovascular disease and has been shown not to cause adverse cardiovascular effects. However, the safety of these products has not been established for the immediate post-MI period or in patients with unstable angina. • Long-term therapy may be helpful for smokers who report persistent withdrawal symptoms

Abbreviations: MI = myocardial infarction; NRT = nicotine replacement therapy
Adapted from: The U.S. Public Health Service Clinical Practice Guidelines for Treating Tobacco Use and Dependence (JAMA 2000;283:3224)

* * * * *

VI

Summary of Tables, Figures, and Index

SUMMARY OF TABLES AND FIGURES

Chapter 26. CORONARY STENTS

Chapter 41. CARDIOVASCULAR RISK REDUCTION

INDEX

Interventional Cardiology Publications

Visit the Physicians' Press Bookstore
at www.physicianspress.com

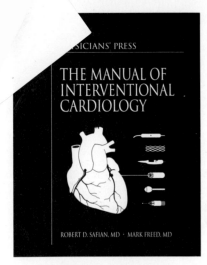
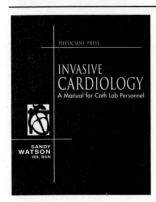
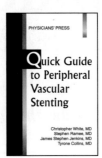
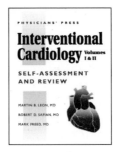

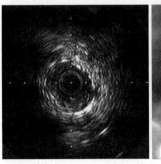
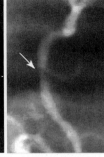
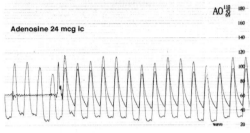
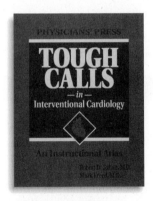
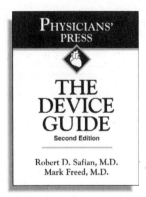
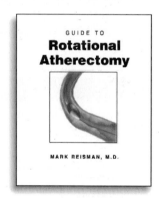

LIST OF TIT

1	Manual of Interventional Cardiology - 3rd Edition Hard cover & Pocket Companion	$129.95
2	Invasive Cardiology: A Manual for Cath Lab Personnel	$54.95
3	Quick Guide to Peripheral Vascular Stenting	$39.95
4	Interventional Cardiology: Self-Assessment & Review Volumes I & II: 750 Questions & Answers	$69.95
5	Interactive IVUS and Pressure-Flow CD-ROMs **5a. IVUS:** CD-ROM: $395; **5b.** Workbook: $39; **5c.** Both: $425 **5d. Pressure-Flow:** CD-ROM: $195; **5e.** Workbook: $39; **5f.** Both: $225 **5g.** IVUS & Pressure-Flow **CD-ROMs:** $450 **5h.** IVUS & Pressure-Flow CD-ROMs & Workbooks: $500	
6	The Device Guide – 2nd Edition	$39.95
7	Tough Calls in Interventional Cardiology	$69.95
8	Guide to Rotational Atherectomy *(with CD-ROM: $69.95)*	$59.95

SHIPPING CHARGES

TOTAL PURCHASE	USA UPS Ground; arrives 3–7 days	OUTSIDE USA* US Postal Surface Arrives 6–8 weeks	US Postal Air Arrives 10-14 Days	Express Air UPS, FEDEX, DHL arrives 2-5 Days
$1–35	Add $4	Add $10	Add $20	Add $30
$36–90	Add $7	Add $15	Add $30	Add $60
$91–150	Add $12	Add $20	Add $50	Add $75
$151–400	Add $14	Add $25	Add $60	Add $90
$401–750	Add $16	Add $30	Add $70	Add $120
$751–1000	Add $20	Add $35	Add $80	Add $150
$1000 +	Add $30	Add $50	Add $100	Add $180

30-day Money Back Guarantee

You will be notified if shipping charges exceed those posted

4 Ways to Order:

By Phone:
USA: (800) 642-5494
Outside USA:
(248) 616-3023

By Fax:
(248) 616-3003

By Internet:
www.physicianspress.com

By Mail:
**Physicians' Press
620 Cherry Street
Royal Oak, Michigan
USA 48073**

FAX/MAIL ORDER FORM *(please print)*

ITEM	QUANTITY	TOTAL
_____	_____	_____
_____	_____	_____
_____	_____	_____
_____	_____	_____
_____	_____	_____

Sales Tax *(MI residents add 6%*
Canadian residents add 7% GST) _____

Shipping Charge _____

Total U.S. Dollars _____

For shipping outside USA, check one:
☐ Express Air
☐ US Postal Air
☐ US Postal Surface

☐ Check Enclosed
(US Dollars from US Bank)
☐ Bill Me
☐ Credit Card: ☐ Visa ☐ MasterCard ☐ AMEX

Credit Card No.: _____

Exp. Date:_____ Signature: _____

Name _____

Address _____

_____

_____

_____

Phone (important): _____

Fax: _____

e-mail: _____

*Your phone number is important —
please be sure to include it.*